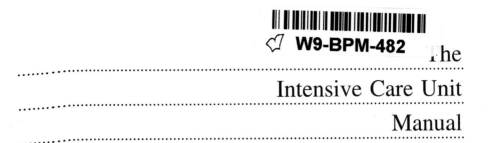

W9-BPM-482

The
Intensive Care Unit
Manual

The
Intensive Care Unit
Manual

Edited by
Paul N. Lanken, MD

Professor of Medicine
Chief, Critical Care Section
Pulmonary, Allergy, and Critical Care Division
University of Pennsylvania School of Medicine

Medical Director (1987–1999), Medical Intensive Care Unit
Hospital of the University of Pennsylvania, Philadelphia, Pennsylvania

Associated Editors
C. William Hanson III, MD

Associate Professor of Anesthesia, Surgery, and Internal Medicine
University of Pennsylvania School of Medicine
Section Chief, Critical Care Medicine
Department of Anesthesia
Medical Director, Surgical Intensive Care Unit
Hospital of the University of Pennsylvania, Philadelphia, Pennsylvania

Scott Manaker, MD, PhD

Associate Professor of Medicine and Pharmacology
Pulmonary, Allergy, and Critical Care Division
University of Pennsylvania School of Medicine
Director of Clinical Documentation, Department of Medicine
Hospital of the University of Pennsylvania, Philadelphia, Pennsylvania

W.B. SAUNDERS COMPANY
A Harcourt Health Sciences Company
Philadelphia   London   New York   St. Louis   Sydney   Toronto

W.B. SAUNDERS COMPANY
A Harcourt Health Sciences Company

The Curtis Center
Independence Square West
Philadelphia, Pennsylvania 19106

Library of Congress Cataloging-in-Publication Data

The intensive care unit manual / [edited by] Paul N. Lanken, C. William Hanson III, Scott Manaker.—1st ed.

p.   cm.

ISBN 0–7216–2197–X

1. Critical care medicine—Handbooks, manuals, etc.   I. Lanken, Paul N.
   II. Hanson, C. William (Clarence William), 1955–   .   III. Manaker, Scott.
[DNLM: 1. Intensive Care—methods.   WX 218 I608 2001]

RC86.8.I585 2001   616'.028—dc21

DNLM/DLC   98-40583

Acquisitions Editor: Richard Zorab
Project Manager: Agnes Hunt Byrne
Production Manager: Frank Polizzano
Illustration Specialist: Walt Verbitski

THE INTENSIVE CARE UNIT MANUAL   ISBN 0–7216–2197–X

Printed in the United States of America.

Last digit is the print number: 9   8   7   6   5   4   3   2   1

To our teachers, colleagues, and students
Most importantly, to our families

CONTRIBUTORS

Michael Acker, MD
Associate Professor of Surgery, University of Pennsylvania School of Medicine; Surgical Director, Heart Transplantation and Mechanical Assist Programs, Hospital of the University of Pennsylvania, Philadelphia, Pennsylvania
Cardiac Surgery

Jennifer Aldrich, MD
Adjunct Assistant Professor of Medicine, University of Pennsylvania School of Medicine; Director of HIV Clinical Services, Philadelphia Department of Health, Philadelphia, Pennsylvania
Rational Use of Antibiotics

Harry L. Anderson III, MD
Clinical Associate Professor of Surgery, University of Pennsylvania School of Medicine, Division of Trauma and Surgical Critical Care, Philadelphia; Attending Surgeon, St. Luke's Hospital, Bethlehem, Pennsylvania
Hemorrhagic Shock and Other Low Preload States

Paul Atkins, MD
Professor of Medicine, University of Pennsylvania School of Medicine; Director, Allergy Programs, Hospital of the University of Pennsylvania, Philadelphia, Pennsylvania
Allergies to Antibiotics

Victor M. Aviles, MD
Assistant Professor of Medicine, Pennsylvania State University College of Medicine, Hershey; Associate Director, Morgan Cancer Center, Lehigh Valley Hospital, Allentown, Pennsylvania
Care of the Cancer Patient with Neutropenia or Thrombocytopenia

Elizabeth Cordes Behringer, MD
Associate Clinical Professor of Anesthesiology and Surgery, University of California, Irvine, College of Medicine, Irvine; Director, Fellowship in Critical Care Medicine, Department of Anesthesia, University of California, Irvine, Medical Center, Irvine, California
Airways and Emergency Airway Management

Shawn J. Bird, MD
Associate Professor of Neurology, University of Pennsylvania School of Medicine; Director, Electromyography Laboratory, Hospital of the University of Pennsylvania, Philadelphia, Pennsylvania
Acute Neuromuscular Weakness

Kathleen A. Brady, MD
Instructor of Medicine, University of Pennsylvania School of Medicine,
Philadelphia, Pennsylvania
Rational Use of Antibiotics

Patrick J. Brennan, MD
Associate Professor of Medicine, Division of Infectious Diseases, University of
Pennsylvania School of Medicine; Hospital Epidemiologist and Director of
Infection Control, University of Pennsylvania Health System, Philadelphia,
Pennsylvania
Community Acquired Pneumonia

Paul S. Brown, Jr, MD
Assistant Professor of Surgery, Division of Cardiovascular and Thoracic Surgery,
University of Texas Medical School at Galveston, Galveston, Texas
Approach to the Trauma Patient; Thoracic Trauma

David J. Callans, MD
Associate Professor of Medicine, Cardiovascular Division, University of
Pennsylvania School of Medicine, Philadelphia, Pennsylvania
Arrhythmias (Bradycardias)

Jeffrey P. Carpenter, MD
Associate Professor of Surgery, University of Pennsylvania School of Medicine,
Philadelphia, Pennsylvania
Major Vascular Procedures

Melissa D. Cohen, MD
Attending Pulmonologist, Winthrop University Hospital, Mineola; North Shore
University Hospital, Manhasset, New York
*Acute Respiratory Failure Due to Asthma and Chronic Obstructive Pulmonary
Disease*

Malcolm Cox, MD
Professor of Medicine and Associate Dean, Network and Primary Care
Education, University of Pennsylvania School of Medicine, Philadelphia,
Pennsylvania
Disorders of the Serum Sodium Concentration

Kelly D. Davis, MD
Adjunct Faculty, University of Pennsylvania School of Medicine, Philadelphia;
Senior Director, Clinical Research and Development, Wyeth-Ayerst Laboratories,
Radnor, Pennsylvania
Thyroid and Adrenal Disorders

Frederick DeClement, MD, FACS
Clinical Professor of Surgery, Temple University School of Medicine; Co-
Director, Burn Unit, Temple University Hospital, Philadelphia, Pennsylvania
Burns

Horace M. DeLisser, MD

Assistant Professor of Medicine, Pulmonary, Allergy, and Critical Care Division, University of Pennsylvania School of Medicine, Philadelphia, Pennsylvania
End-of-Life Care; The Challenge to Wean Patient

David DeNofrio, MD

Assistant Professor of Medicine, Tufts University School of Medicine; Medical Director, Lifespan Cardiac Transplantation Program, New England Medical Center, Boston, Massachusetts
Cardiogenic Pulmonary Edema

Clifford S. Deutschmann, MD, FCCM

Professor of Anesthesia and Surgery, University of Pennsylvania School of Medicine; Director of Fellowship/Critical Care Medicine, Department of Anesthesia, Hospital of the University of Pennsylvania, Philadelphia, Pennsylvania
Perioperative Approach to the High-Risk Surgical Patient

Jeffrey D. Edelman, MD

Assistant Professor of Medicine, Pulmonary and Critical Care Division, Oregon Health Sciences University School of Medicine, Portland, Oregon
Nosocomial Infections

Ashraf A. Elshami, MD

Pulmonologist, Central Plains Clinic, Sioux Falls, South Dakota
Falling Urine Output and Rising Creatinine Levels; Fever, Hypothermia, or a Rising White Blood Cell Count

Nancy Evans-Stoner, RN, MSN, CNSN

Clinical Nurse Specialist, Clinical Nutrition Support Services, Hospital of the University of Pennsylvania, Philadelphia, Pennsylvania
Nutritional Therapy

Douglas O. Faigel, MD

Assistant Professor of Medicine, Oregon Health Sciences University School of Medicine; Director, Gastrointestinal Endoscopy, Portland Veterans Affairs Medical Center, Portland, Oregon
Acute Pancreatitis

George M. Feldman, MD

Professor of Internal Medicine and Physiology, Virginia Commonwealth University, Medical College of Virginia; Chief, Renal Section, Hunter Holmes McGuire Veterans Affairs Medical Center, Richmond, Virginia
Metabolic Acidoses and Alkaloses

F. Michael Ferrante, MD
Professor of Anesthesia, University of Pennsylvania School of Medicine; Director, Pain Management Center, University of Pennsylvania Health System, Philadelphia, Pennsylvania
Management of Postoperative Pain

Victor A. Ferrari, MD
Assistant Professor of Medicine and Radiology, University of Pennsylvania School of Medicine; Associate Director, Cardiac Noninvasive Imaging Laboratory, Hospital of the University of Pennsylvania, Philadelphia, Pennsylvania
Pericardial Tamponade

David Fish, MD
Associate Professor, Department of Anesthesia, Temple University School of Medicine; Chairman, Anesthesia and Director of Critical Care, Fox Chase Cancer Center, Philadelphia, Pennsylvania
How to Read and Understand the Anesthesia Record

Neil Fishman, MD
Assistant Professor of Medicine, University of Pennsylvania School of Medicine; Director, Antimicrobial Management Program, University of Pennsylvania Health System, Philadelphia, Pennsylvania
Rational Use of Antibiotics

Kevin R. Fox, MD
Associate Professor of Medicine, Hematology/Oncology Division, University of Pennsylvania School of Medicine, Philadelphia, Pennsylvania
Care of the Cancer Patient with Neutropenia or Thrombocytopenia

Ian Frank, MD
Associate Professor of Medicine, University of Pennsylvania School of Medicine; Director, Antiretroviral Clinical Research, Hospital of the University of Pennsylvania, Philadelphia, Pennsylvania
Care of the Patient Infected with the Human Immunodeficiency Virus

Neil Freedman, MD
Pulmonologist, Lake Forest, Illinois
Sleep Disturbances in the Intensive Care Unit

Andrew Freese, MD
Associate Professor of Neurosurgery, Jefferson Medical College of Thomas Jefferson University; Vice Chairman, Deptartment of Neurosurgery, Thomas Jefferson University Hospital, Philadelphia, Pennsylvania
Spinal Injury

Linda Fried, MD
Assistant Professor of Medicine, University of Pittsburgh School of Medicine;
Chief, Peritoneal Dialysis, Veterans Affairs Pittsburgh Healthcare System,
Pittsburgh, Pennsylvania
Acute Renal Failure and Rhabdomyolysis

Barry Fuchs, MD
Assistant Professor of Medicine, University of Pennsylvania School of Medicine;
Medical Director, Medical and Intermediate Intensive Care Units, Hospital of the
University of Pennsylvania, Philadelphia, Pennsylvania
Acute Arterial Desaturation

Yevgeniy Gincherman, MD
Emergency Medicine Resident, Hospital of the University of Pennsylvania,
Philadelphia, Pennsylvania
Major Pulmonary Embolism

Gregory G. Ginsberg, MD
Associate Professor of Medicine, Gastroenterology Division, University of
Pennsylvania School of Medicine; Director of Endoscopic Services, Hospital of
the University of Pennsylvania, Philadelphia, Pennsylvania
Upper Gastrointestinal Bleeding

Stephen Gluckman, MD
Associate Professor of Medicine, University of Pennsylvania School of Medicine;
Director, Infectious Disease Clinical Service, Hospital of the University of
Pennsylvania, Philadelphia, Pennsylvania
Acute Central Nervous System Infections

Andrew N. Goldberg, MD
Associate Professor, University of California-San Francisco, San Francisco, CA
Swallowing and Communication Disorders

Joseph H. Gorman III, MD
Instructor of Surgery, University of Pennsylvania School of Medicine,
Philadelphia, Pennsylvania
Necrotizing Fasciitis and Related Soft Tissue Infections

Robert C. Gorman, MD
Assistant Professor of Surgery, University of Pennsylvania School of Medicine,
Philadelphia, Pennsylvania
Necrotizing Fasciitis and Related Soft Tissue Infections

Jonathan Gottlieb, MD
Professor of Medicine, Jefferson Medical College of Thomas Jefferson
University; Senior Vice President for Clinical Affairs, Thomas Jefferson
University Hospital, Philadelphia, Pennsylvania
Approach to Supportive Care and Noninvasive Bedside Monitoring

Michael D. Grossman, MD
Assistant Professor of Surgery, Division of Traumatology and Surgical Critical
Care, University of Pennsylvania School of Medicine, Philadelphia; Chief,
Trauma and Surgical Critical Care, St. Lukes Hospital, Bethlehem, Pennsylvania
Major Abdominal Surgery: Postoperative Considerations

Indira Gurubhagavatula, MD, MPH
Instructor of Medicine, University of Pennsylvania School of Medicine,
Philadelphia, Pennsylvania
Limb Swelling

John Hansen-Flaschen, MD
Professor of Medicine, Chief, Pulmonary, Allergy, and Critical Care Division,
University of Pennsylvania School of Medicine, Philadelphia, Pennsylvania
*Sedation and Paralysis During Mechanical Ventilation: Treating Distress and
Agitation*

C. William Hanson III, MD, FCCM
Associate Professor of Anesthesia, Surgery, and Internal Medicine, University of
Pennsylvania School of Medicine; Section Chief, Critical Care Medicine,
Department of Anesthesia, Medical Director, Surgical Intensive Care Unit,
Hospital of the University of Pennsylvania, Philadelphia, Pennsylvania
*Sedation and Paralysis During Mechanical Ventilation: Use of Neuromuscular
Blocking Agents; Assessment and Monitoring of Hemodynamic Function;
Vascular Access Issues and Procedures; Approach to the Trauma Patient*

Fred Henretig, MD
Professor of Pediatrics and Emergency Medicine, University of Pennsylvania
School of Medicine; Medical Director, Poison Control Center, Director, Clinical
Toxicology, Children's Hospital of Philadelphia, Philadelphia, Pennsylvania
Drug Overdoses and Toxic Ingestions

Daniel O. Hensell, MD, FACS, FCCM
Instructor in Surgery, Temple University School of Medicine; Co-Director, Burn
Unit, Temple University Hospital, Philadelphia, Pennsylvania
Burns

Irving M. Herling, MD
Associate Professor of Medicine, University of Pennsylvania School of Medicine;
Director, Consultative Cardiology, Hospital of the University of Pennsylvania,
Philadelphia, Pennsylvania
Cardiogenic Shock and Other Pump Failure States

William S. Hoff, MD
Assistant Professor of Surgery, University of Pennsylvania School of Medicine,
Philadelphia; Chairman, Department of Traumatology, Brandywine Hospital,
Coatesville, Pennsylvania
Extremity and Major Vascular Trauma

Roberta J. Hunter, MD
Gastroenterologist, Lewis-Gale Clinic, Salem, Virginia
Lower Gastrointestinal Bleeding and Colitis

Leigh Jefferies, MD
Associate Professor of Pathology and Laboratory Medicine, University of
Pennsylvania School of Medicine; Associate Director, Transfusion Service,
Hospital of the University of Pennsylvania, Philadelphia, Pennsylvania
Transfusion Reactions

Kevin D. Judy, MD
Assistant Professor, Department of Neurosurgery, University of Pennsylvania
School of Medicine, Philadelphia, Pennsylvania
Craniotomy

Marc J. Kahn, MD
Associate Professor of Medicine, Internal Medicine Residency Program Director,
Associate Director for Student Programs, Tulane University School of Medicine,
New Orleans, Louisiana
*Thrombocytopenia; Hemolytic Anemia; Idiopathic and Thrombotic
Thrombocytopenias*

Donald R. Kauder, MD
Associate Professor of Surgery, Division of Trauma and Surgical Critical Care,
University of Pennsylvania School of Medicine, Philadelphia, Pennsylvania
Rational Use of Blood Products

Bruce D. Klugherz, MD
Assistant Professor of Medicine, University of Pennsylvania School of Medicine;
Director, Cardiac Catheterization Laboratory, Philadelphia Veterans Affairs
Medical Center, Philadelphia, Pennsylvania
Chest Pain and Myocardial Ischemia

Sidney M. Kobrin, MD
Associate Professor of Medicine, Renal Electrolyte and Hypertension Division,
University of Pennsylvania School of Medicine, Philadelphia, Pennsylvania
Renal Replacement Therapy

Michael L. Kochman, MD, FACP
Associate Professor of Medicine, Gastroenterology Division, University of
Pennsylvania School of Medicine, Philadelphia, Pennsylvania
Lower Gastrointestinal Bleeding and Colitis

Daniel M. Kolansky, MD
Assistant Professor of Medicine, University of Pennsylvania School of Medicine;
Attending Staff, Hospital of the University of Pennsylvania, Philadelphia,
Pennsylvania
Chest Pain and Myocardial Ischemia

Mark J. Kotapka, MD
Chairman, Neurosurgery, Albert Einstein Medical Center, Philadelphia, Pennsylvania
Head Trauma

Paul N. Lanken, MD
Professor of Medicine, Chef, Critical Care Section, Pulmonary, Allergy, and Critical Care Division, University of Pennsylvania School of Medicine; Medical Director (1987–1999), Medical Intensive Care Unit, Hospital of the University of Pennsylvania, Philadelphia, Pennsylvania
Approach to Acute Respiratory Failure; Mechanical Ventilation; Weaning and Extubation; Vascular Access Issues and Procedures; Nosocomial Infections; End-of-Life Care; Ventilator Alarm Situations; Brain Death and Management of Potential Organ Donors; Prognosis After Cardiopulmonary Arrest; Acute Respiratory Distress Syndrome

Todd M. Lasner, MD
Neurosurgeon, Miami, Florida
Increased Intracranial Pressure

Ebbing Lautenbach, MD, MPH
Fellow, Division of Infectious Diseases, University of Pennsylvania School of Medicine, Philadelphia, Pennsylvania
Community Acquired Pneumonia

Jin-Moo Lee, MD, PhD
Instructor of Neurology, Washington University School of Medicine; Attending Physician, Barnes-Jewish Hospital, St. Louis, Missouri
Stroke

Gary R. Lichtenstein, MD
Associate Professor of Medicine, Gastroenterology Division, University of Pennsylvania School of Medicine; Director, Inflammatory Bowel Diseases Center, Hospital of the University of Pennsylvania, Philadelphia, Pennsylvania
Diarrhea Developing in the Intensive Care Patient; Ileus

Evan Loh, MD
Associate Professor of Medicine, University of Pennsylvania School of Medicine; Medical Director, Heart Failure/Cardiac Transplant Program, Director, Coronary Care Unit, Hospital of the University of Pennsylvania, Philadelphia, Pennsylvania
Cardiogenic Pulmonary Edema

David W. Low, MD
Associate Professor of Surgery, Division of Plastic Surgery, University of Pennsylvania School of Medicine; Attending Surgeon, Hospital of the University of Pennsylvania and Children's Hospital of Philadelphia, Philadelphia, Pennsylvania
Major Tissue Flaps

Michael R. Lucey, MD, FRCPI
Associate Professor of Medicine, University of Pennsylvania School of Medicine; Director of Hepatology and Medical Director, Liver Transplant Program, Hospital of the University of Pennsylvania, Philadelphia, Pennsylvania
Acute Liver Failure

Steven A. Malosky, MD
Cardiologist, Eisenhower Medical Center, Desert Regional Medical Center, Rancho Mirage, California
Pericardial Tamponade

Scott Manaker, MD, PhD
Associate Professor of Medicine and Pharmacology, Pulmonary, Allergy, and Critical Care Division, University of Pennsylvania School of Medicine; Director of Clinical Documentation, Department of Medicine, Hospital of the University of Pennsylvania, Philadelphia, Pennsylvania
Septic Shock and Other Low Afterload States; Falling Urine Output and Rising Creatinine Levels; Fever, Hypothermia, or a Rising White Blood Cell Count; Hypertensive Episodes; Hypotensive Episodes or Falling Hemoglobin; Smoke and Carbon Monoxide Inhalation

Francis E. Marchlinski, MD
Professor of Medicine, University of Pennsylvania School of Medicine; Director, Cardiac Electrophysiology, Hospital of the University of Pennsylvania, Philadelphia, Pennsylvania
Arrhythmias (Tachycardias)

Paul Marcotte, MD, FRCS(C), FACS
Assistant Professor of Neurosurgery, University of Pennsylvania School of Medicine, Philadelphia, Pennsylvania
Spinal Injury

David J. Margolis, MD, MSCE
Associate Professor of Dermatology and Epidemiology, University of Pennsylvania School of Medicine, Philadelphia, Pennsylvania
Skin Rashes and Pressure Ulcers

Addison K. May, MD
Assistant Professor of Surgery and Anesthesiology, University of Alabama School of Medicine; Director, Surgical Intensive Care Unit, University of Alabama Hospital, Birmingham, Alabama
Rational Use of Blood Products

Joseph R. McClellan, MD
Chairman, Department of Cardiovascular Medicine and Surgery, Hamot Medical Center, Erie; Formerly Medical Director, Cardiac Care Unit, Hospital of the University of Pennsylvania, Philadelphia, Pennsylvania
Acute Coronary Syndromes: Acute Myocardial Infarction and Unstable Angina

C. Crawford Mechem, MS, MD
Assistant Professor, Emergency Medicine, University of Pennsylvania School of Medicine; EMS Medical Director, Philadelphia Fire Department, Philadelphia, Pennsylvania
Hypothermia and Hyperthermia

David C. Metz, MD
Associate Professor of Medicine, Division of Gastroenterology, University of Pennsylvania School of Medicine; Co-Director, Gastrointestinal Physiology Laboratory, Director, Acid-Peptic Disease Program, Hospital of the University of Pennsylvania, Philadelphia, Pennsylvania
Acute Pancreatitis

Bonnie L. Milas, MD
Assistant Professor of Anesthesiology, University of Pennsylvania School of Medicine, Philadelphia, Pennsylvania
Thoracic Aortic Aneurysms and Dissections

Marc E. Mitchell, MD
Assistant Professor of Surgery, University of Pennsylvania School of Medicine, Philadelphia, Pennsylvania
Major Vascular Procedures

Lori J. Morgan, MD
Assistant Professor of Surgery, University of Iowa College of Medicine; Department of Surgery, University of Iowa Hospitals and Clinics, Iowa City, Iowa
Barotrauma and Chest Tubes

Mark A. Morgan, MD
Deceased; Former Associate Professor of Obstetrics and Gynecology, University of Pennsylvania School of Medicine, Philadelphia, Pennsylvania
Care of the Maternal-Fetal Unit; Obstetric and Postobstetric Complications

Jon B. Morris, MD
Associate Professor of Surgery, Associate Dean for Clinical Education, University of Pennsylvania School of Medicine; Attending Surgeon, Hospital of the University of Pennsylvania, Philadelphia, Pennsylvania
Necrotizing Fasciitis and Related Soft Tissue Infections

David G. Morrison, MD, PhD
Hematologist/Oncologist, Montgomery Cancer Center, Montgomery, Alabama
Idiopathic and Thrombotic Thrombocytopenias

Christen M. Mowad, MD
Assistant Professor of Dermatology, Pennsylvania State University College of Medicine, Hershey; Director of Contact Dermatitis, Geisinger Medical Center, Danville, Pennsylvania
Skin Rashes and Pressure Ulcers

James L. Mullen, MD
Professor of Surgery, University of Pennsylvania School of Medicine; Associate Executive Director, Hospital of the University of Pennsylvania, Philadelphia, Pennsylvania
Nutritional Therapy

Michael L. Nance, MD
Assistant Professor of Surgery, University of Pennsylvania School of Medicine; Attending Surgeon, Pediatric General and Thoracic Surgery, Children's Hospital of Philadelphia, Philadelphia, Pennsylvania
Abdominal Trauma

R. John Naranja, Jr., MD
Clinical Instructor, Department of Orthopedics, University of North Dakota School of Medicine, Grand Forks; Major, USAF, Minot Air Force Base Hospital, Minot, North Dakota
Major Orthopedic Procedures

Frederick A. Nunes, MD
Assistant Professor of Medicine, Gastroenterology Division, University of Pennsylvania School of Medicine, Philadelphia, Pennsylvania
Care of the Patient with End-Stage Liver Disease

Christopher D. O'Brien, MD
Instructor of Medicine, University of Pennsylvania School of Medicine, Philadelphia, Pennsylvania
Smoke and Carbon Monoxide Inhalation

Liza C. O'Dowd, MD
Pulmonary, Allergy, and Critical Care Division, Instructor of Medicine, University of Pennsylvania School of Medicine, Philadelphia, Pennsylvania
Allergies to Antibiotics

Harold I. Palevsky, MD
Associate Professor of Medicine, University of Pennsylvania School of Medicine; Chief, Pulmonary and Critical Care Section, Presbyterian Medical Center; Director, Pulmonary Vascular Disease Program, University of Pennsylvania Health System, Philadelphia, Pennsylvania
Major Pulmonary Embolism

Paul M. Palevsky, MD
Associate Professor of Medicine, University of Pittsburgh School of Medicine; Chief, Renal Section, Veterans Affairs Pittsburgh Healthcare System, Pittsburgh, Pennsylvania
Acute Renal Failure and Rhabdomyolysis

Reynold A. Panettieri, Jr., MD

Associate Professor of Medicine, University of Pennsylvania School of Medicine; Adjunct Associate Professor, Wistar Institute; Director, Comprehensive Asthma Program, University of Pennsylvania Health System, Philadelphia, Pennsylvania
Acute Respiratory Failure Due to Asthma and Chronic Obstructive Pulmonary Disease

Samuel Parry, MD

Assistant Professor, Division of Maternal-Fetal Medicine, Department of Obstetrics and Gynecology, University of Pennsylvania School of Medicine, Philadelphia, Pennsylvania
Care of the Maternal-Fetal Unit; Obstetric and Postobstetric Complications

Jeanmarie Perrone, MD

Assistant Professor, Department of Emergency Medicine, University of Pennsylvania School of Medicine; Attending Physician and Toxicologist, Department of Emergency Medicine, Hospital of the University of Pennsylvania, Philadelphia, Pennsylvania
Drug Overdoses and Toxic Ingestions

Matthew F. Philips, MD

Chief Resident, Department of Neurosurgery, Hospital of the University of Pennsylvania, Philadelphia, Pennsylvania
Head Trauma

Alberto Pochettino, MD

Assistant Professor of Surgery, University of Pennsylvania School of Medicine; Attending Surgeon, Division of Cardiothoracic Surgery, Hospital of the University of Pennsylvania, Philadelphia, Pennsylvania
Thoracic Aortic Aneurysms and Dissections; Cardiac Surgery

Eric C. Raps, MD

Deceased; Former Associate Professor of Neurology, University of Pennsylvania School of Medicine, Philadelphia, Pennsylvania
Change in Mental Status or New-Onset Seizures; Stroke

James F. Reilly, MD

Clinical Assistant Professor of Surgery, University of Pennsylvania School of Medicine, Philadelphia; Associate Trauma Program Director, St. Luke's Hospital, Bethlehem, Pennsylvania
Extremity and Major Vascular Trauma

Patrick M. Reilly, MD

Assistant Professor of Surgery, Division of Trauma/Surgical Critical Care, University of Pennsylvania School of Medicine, Philadelphia, Pennsylvania
Major Abdominal Surgery: Postoperative Considerations

Daniel J. Reily, BS, RRT
Administrative Director of Respiratory Care Services and Pulmonary Diagnostic
Services, Hospital of the University of Pennsylvania, Philadelphia, Pennsylvania
Ventilator Alarm Situations

John R. Roberts, MD
Associate Professor of Surgery, Vanderbilt University School of Medicine; Chief,
General Thoracic Surgery, Vanderbilt Medical Center, Nashville, Tennessee
Thoracic Surgical Patient

Cynthia B. Robinson, MD
Assistant Adjunct Professor, Pulmonary, Allergy, and Critical Care Division,
University of Pennsylvania School of Medicine, Philadelphia; Director, Clinical
Research, Pulmonary, SmithKline Beecham Pharmaceuticals, Collegeville,
Pennsylvania
Acute Hypercapnic Episodes

Keith M. Robinson, MD, MSc
Associate Professor of Rehabilitation Medicine, University of Pennsylvania
School of Medicine; Chief of Service, Rehabilitation Medicine, Pennsylvania
Hospital, Philadelphia, Pennsylvania
Rehabilitation Interventions

Charles H. Rodenberger, MD
Staff Physician, Lancaster General Hospital, Lancaster, Pennsylvania
Electrolyte Disorders

Bruce R. Rosengard, MD
Assistant Professor of Surgery, University of Pennsylvania School of Medicine;
Director, Heart-Lung Transplantation, Hospital of the University of Pennsylvania,
Philadelphia, Pennsylvania
Thoracic Surgical Patient

Michael F. Rotondo, MD
Professor of Surgery, East Carolina University School of Medicine; Chief of
Trauma and Surgical Critical Care, Pitt County Memorial Hospital, Greenville,
North Carolina
Abdominal Trauma

Michael W. Russell, MD
Assistant Professor of Anesthesia, University of Pennsylvania School of
Medicine, Philadelphia, Pennsylvania
Perioperative Approach to the High-Risk Surgical Patient

Brian H. Sarter, MD
Clinical Assistant Professor, Jefferson Medical College of Thomas Jefferson
University, Philadelphia, Pennsylvania; Attending Cardiologist/
Electrophysiologist, Christiana Care Hospital, Christiana, Delaware
Arrhythmias (Bradycardias)

Joseph B. Schellenberg, MD
Adjunct Clinical Professor, Pennsylvania State University College of Medicine, Hershey; Pulmonologist, Lehigh Valley Hospital Center, Allentown, Pennsylvania
Brain Death and Management of Potential Organ Donors

Henry J. Schiller, MD
Assistant Professor of Surgery, State University of New York, College of Medicine; Director, The Clark Burn Center, State University of New York, Health Science Center, Syracuse, New York
Hemorrhagic Shock and Other Low Preload States

Richard J. Schwab, MD
Assistant Professor of Medicine, University of Pennsylvania School of Medicine; Medical Director, Penn Center for Sleep Disorders, Hospital of the University of Pennsylvania, Philadelphia, Pennsylvania
Sleep Disturbances in the Intensive Care Unit; Obesity Hypoventilation Syndrome

Michael B. Shapiro, MD, FACS, FCCP
Assistant Professor of Surgery, Division of Trauma and Surgical Critical Care, University of Pennsylvania School of Medicine; Co-Medical Director, Surgical Intensive Care Unit, Hospital of the University of Pennsylvania, Philadelphia, Pennsylvania
Barotrauma and Chest Tubes

Andrew Siderowf, MD
Assistant Professor of Neurology, University of Pennsylvania School of Medicine, Philadelphia, Pennsylvania
Status Epilepticus

Frank E. Silvestry, MD
Assistant Professor of Medicine, Cardiovascular Division, University of Pennsylvania School of Medicine, Philadelphia, Pennsylvania
Cardiogenic Shock and Other Pump Failure States

Melissa A. Simonian, MEd, CCC-SLP
Clinical Instructor, Department of Otorhinolaryngology, University of Pennsylvania School of Medicine; Supervisor, Division of Speech-Language Pathology, Hospital of the University of Pennsylvania, Philadelphia, Pennsylvania
Swallowing and Communication Disorders

Steven R. Sloan, MD, PhD
Instructor, Harvard Medical School; Associate Blood Bank Director, Children's Hospital, Boston, Massachusetts
Transfusion Reactions

Mark M. Stecker, MD, PhD
Assistant Professor of Neurology, Department of Neurology, University of Pennsylvania School of Medicine, Philadelphia, Pennsylvania
Status Epilepticus

Daniel H. Sternman, MD
Assistant Professor of Medicine, University of Pennsylvania School of Medicine; Director of Interventional Pulmonology, Hospital of the University of Pennsylvania, Philadelphia, Pennsylvania
Hypertensive Episodes

Brian R. Stotland, MD
Assistant Professor of Medicine, Gastroenterology Division, Boston University School of Medicine, Boston, Massachusetts
Upper Gastrointestinal Bleeding

Harold M. Szerlip, MD, MS(Ed)
Professor and Associate Chairman, Department of Medicine, Tulane University School of Medicine; Chief, Tulane Medical Service, Medical Center of Louisiana at New Orleans, New Orleans, Louisiana
Diabetic Ketoacidosis, Nonketotic Hypertonic Hyperglycemia, and Alcoholic Ketoacidosis

Darren B. Taichman, MD, PhD
Instructor in Medicine, Pulmonary and Critical Care Division, University of Pennsylvania School of Medicine; Attending Physician, Hospital of the University of Pennsylvania, Philadelphia, Pennsylvania
Prognosis After Cardiopulmonary Arrest

James W. Teener, MD
Clinical Assistant Professor, University of Minnesota—Duluth School of Medicine; Stroke Center Director, SMDC Health System, Duluth, Minnesota
Change in Mental Status or New-Onset Seizures; Acute Neuromuscular Weakness

Erica R. Thaler, MD
Assistant Professor of Otorhinolaryngology, University of Pennsylvania School of Medicine, Philadelphia, Pennsylvania
Airways and Emergency Airway Management

Karen J. Tietze, PharmD
Professor of Clinical Pharmacy, Philadelphia College of Pharmacy, University of the Sciences in Philadelphia, Philadelphia, Pennsylvania
Pharmacokinetics and Drug Interactions

Gregory Tino, MD
Assistant Professor of Medicine, Pulmonary, Allergy, and Critical Care Division, University of Pennsylvania School of Medicine; Director, Pulmonary Outpatient Practices, Hospital of the University of Pennsylvania, Philadelphia, Pennsylvania
Limb Swelling

Mitchell D. Tobias, MD

Assistant Professor of Anesthesia, University of Pennsylvania School of Medicine; Director of the Inpatient Pain Service, Hospital of the University of Pennsylvania, Philadelphia, Pennsylvania
Management of Postoperative Pain

Raymond Townsend, MD

Associate Professor of Medicine, Renal-Electrolyte and Hypertension Division, University of Pennsylvania School of Medicine; Director, Hypertension Program, Hospital of the University of Pennsylvania, Philadelphia, Pennsylvania
Hypertensive Crisis

Frank Trudo, MD

Staff Physician, Pulmonary and Critical Care, Virtua Memorial Hospital of Burlington County, Mt. Holly, New Jersey
Obesity Hypoventilation Syndrome

Edward J. Vresilovic, Jr., MD, PhD

Assistant Professor, University of Pennsylvania School of Medicine; Chief, Orthopedic Spine Service, Hospital of the University of Pennsylvania, Philadelphia, Pennsylvania
Major Orthopedic Procedures

Alan G. Wasserstein, MD

Associate Professor of Medicine, Renal-Electrolyte and Hypertension Division, University of Pennsylvania School of Medicine; Director, Renal Outpatient Programs, Hospital of the University of Pennsylvania, Philadelphia, Pennsylvania
Care of the Patient With End-Stage Renal Disease

Gerald L. Weinhouse, MD

Assistant Professor of Medicine, Mount Sinai School of Medicine of the City University of New York, New York, New York
Massive Hemoptysis and Diffuse Pulmonary Hemorrhage

Stuart J. Weiss, MD, PhD

Assistant Professor of Anesthesia, University of Pennsylvania School of Medicine, Philadelphia, Pennsylvania
How to Read and Understand the Anesthesia Record

Kathy M. Witta, RN, MSN, CRNP

Nursing Clinical Preceptor, University of Pennsylvania Graduate School of Nursing; Gerontological Nurse Practitioner, Hospital of the University of Pennsylvania, Philadelphia, Pennsylvania
The Challenge to Wean Patient

Eric T. Wittbrodt, PharmD, BCPS
Assistant Professor of Clinical Pharmacy, University of the Sciences in Philadelphia; Clinical Assistant Professor of Medicine, Medical College of Pennsylvania–Hahnemann University School of Medicine, Philadelphia, Pennsylvania
Pharmacokinetics and Drug Interactions

Dina R. Yazmajian, MD
Cardiologist, Abington Memorial Hospital, Abington, Pennsylvania
Arrhythmias (Tachycardias)

Eric L. Zager, MD
Associate Professor of Neurosurgery, University of Pennsylvania School of Medicine; Attending Surgeon, Department of Neurosurgery, Hospital of the University of Pennsylvania, Philadelphia, Pennsylvania
Increased Intracranial Pressure

Fuad N. Ziyadeh, MD
Professor of Medicine, Renal-Electrolyte and Hypertension Division, University of Pennsylvania School of Medicine; Attending Nephrologist, Hospital of the University of Pennsylvania, Philadelphia, Pennsylvania
Electrolyte Disorders

Jonathan Zuckerman, MD
Assistant Professor of Medicine, University of Vermont College of Medicine, Burlington, Vermont; Director, Adult Cystic Fibrosis Program, Maine Medical Center, Portland, Maine
Hypotensive Episodes or Falling Hemoglobin

PREFACE

"Why does the world need another ICU textbook?" asked one prospective contributor shortly after this project began. It was not exactly what I had expected to hear at the time. It turned out, however, to be an excellent question, whose answer, like a landmark on the horizon, has guided this book along its journey to completion. The answer lies in my original vision for this book: to create a manual of critical care medicine that would be especially useful for housestaff in medical, cardiac, and surgical intensive care units (ICUs). As such, it would have to be *comprehensive, concise,* and *practical.*

The book needed to be *comprehensive* to help ICU housestaff perform many jobs successfully—no matter what kind of ICU they were in. If the book had a motto, it would be "It's all here!" The 98 chapters of *The Intensive Care Unit Manual* encompass the scope and complexity of critical care medicine that ICU housestaff encounter. Included are not only descriptions of common, important disorders that result in ICU admission, but also instructions about how to evaluate and manage problems that arise *after* ICU admission. The book covers the practices of many specialists, and its content reflects both the medical literature and literally hundreds of "author-years" of critical care experience.

The book had to be *concise* to make it readable for ICU housestaff who are often on-call. But making it concise mandated that contributors and editors drastically condense many chapters without disrespecting the importance of their topics. One contributor not so subtly commented to me that entire books had been written about his assigned topic—as he handed me his 8 pages of galley proofs.

If the book were not *practical,* it would have missed its mark entirely. For housestaff on call in ICUs, critical care medicine is first and foremost a practical endeavor. They need practical resources to help them deal with the practical problems that arise in the ICU setting.

Do not read *The Intensive Care Unit Manual* as if it were a novel. Instead, read the parts you need to take care of your patients. The first three sections of the book contain basic ICU principles and practices, and care of "generic" and "special" patients. Next come the *problem-based* chapters that focus on evaluation and management of problems arising *after* ICU admission. The final section contains a traditional menu of common *ICU admitting diagnoses* followed by chapters pertaining to *postoperative ICU care* after major surgery and trauma.

As you use this manual "in the trenches," you may discover important topics that were omitted or need more emphasis. How can this manual be more useful for you? We welcome your opinions and feedback, preferably by email (lanken@mail.med.upenn.edu).

This book is the product of many people. I greatly appreciate all their contributions and encouragement. I especially want to thank Richard Zorab, Editor-in-Chief, Medicine of W.B. Saunders Company. Not only did he share my vision for this book from its start but, more importantly, he also has been absolutely essential in the challenging process of transforming that vision into this final product.

PAUL N. LANKEN, MD

CONTENTS

Section III
CARE OF SPECIAL INTENSIVE CARE UNIT PATIENTS

Section V
PRESENTING PROBLEMS FOR INTENSIVE CARE UNIT ADMISSION

Cardiovascular

Infectious

Neurologic

Obstetric

Pulmonary

1 Approach to Acute Respiratory Failure

Paul N. Lanken

The nearly ubiquitous presence of mechanical ventilators in the intensive care unit (ICU) reflects how commonly patients in the ICU suffer from acute respiratory failure. In caring for these patients, ICU clinicians must decide when to start, change, or stop assisted ventilation. Knowing the mechanism that caused a patient's acute respiratory failure helps in making these decisions and in determining what needs to improve so that the patient can breath spontaneously again.

Despite having many causes, acute respiratory failure results from only a few basic pathophysiologic mechanisms. Thus, a mechanism-based approach to evaluation and management can be applied to a wide spectrum of patients with acute respiratory failure of different causes. Knowing the mechanism of respiratory failure involved in specific clinical disorders allows the ICU clinician to direct treatment effectively and efficiently.

DEFINITIONS

Acute respiratory failure is the final common pathway for diverse clinical disorders. *Acute* refers to an onset usually measured in terms of minutes or hours. *Respiratory failure* indicates a severe impairment of pulmonary gas exchange; it is categorized into two types. *Hypercapnic respiratory failure* occurs when a patient's $PaCO_2$ rises to greater than normal, that is, greater than 45 mm Hg. *Hypoxemic respiratory failure* occurs when a patient's PaO_2 falls so low that it is life-threatening or has serious adverse physiologic effects. For example, in cases of hypoxemic respiratory failure, PaO_2 is often less than 55 mm Hg despite administration of high, potentially toxic concentrations of oxygen. A PaO_2 of 55 mm Hg corresponds to a modestly reduced arterial hemoglobin saturation of about 88%. This is near the "top" of the steep part of the oxyhemoglobin dissociation curve and further decrements result in steep, linear falls in arterial O_2 content (see Appendix A for oxyhemoglobin dissociation curves).

FOUR COMPONENTS OF THE RESPIRATORY SYSTEM

The *respiratory system* can be regarded as having four functional and structural components: (1) the central nervous system (CNS) component (chemoreceptors, the controller [respiratory center in the medulla], and CNS efferents), (2) the chest bellows component (composed of the peripheral nervous system, respiratory muscles, and the chest wall and soft tissues surrounding the lung), (3) the airway component, and (4) the alveolar component. Together they form the *effector arm* of the respiratory system's feedback and control loop (Fig. 1–1).

When all four components function correctly, their sequential actions result in normal pulmonary gas exchange.

1

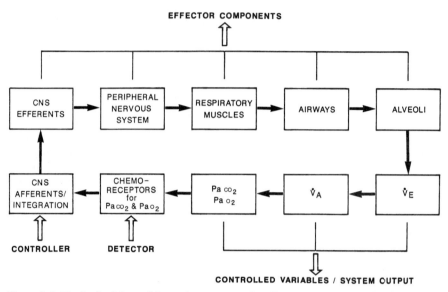

Figure 1–1. The feedback loop of the respiratory system. Its effector components consist of the central nervous system (CNS) drive to ventilate, neural connections to the respiratory muscles, the muscles themselves, conducting airways, and alveoli. The controlled variables (system output) consists of minute ventilation ($\dot{V}_E$), alveolar ventilation ($\dot{V}_A$), Pa_{CO_2}, and Pa_{O_2}. Changes in Pa_{O_2} and Pa_{CO_2} are detected by peripheral and central chemoreceptors (detector), which then send information to the CNS respiratory center (controller). The controller maintains homeostasis by increasing or decreasing activity of the effector components in response to abnormalities in Pa_{O_2} or Pa_{CO_2}. (From Lanken PN: Respiratory failure. In: Carlson RW; Geheb MA [eds]: Principles and Practice of Medical Intensive Care. Philadelphia: WB Saunders, 1993, pp 754–763.)

1. The CNS controller initiates respiratory drive by generating neural output. The rate and intensity of its output are determined by the feedback provided by peripheral chemoreceptors (monitoring Pa_{O_2} and Pa_{CO_2}) and central chemoreceptors (monitoring Pa_{CO_2} or its effects) and by input from other neural sources.
2. The neural impulses from the CNS controller traverse the spinal cord and the phrenic and other motoneurons and reach the diaphragm and other respiratory muscles.
3. In response, these muscles expand the chest cavity, displace adjacent abdominal contents, and produce negative (subatmospheric) pleural pressure within the thorax.
4. This negative pressure is transmitted to the alveoli, creating a gradient between the alveoli and atmospheric pressure at the mouth. In response, air flows through the conducting airways to the alveoli, leading to lung inflation.
5. Finally, alveolar O_2 passively diffuses across the alveolar-capillary membrane so that red blood cells become fully equilibrated with alveolar Po_2 as they pass through alveolar capillaries. The same process, but in the reverse direction, occurs for CO_2.

RESPIRATORY PUMP AND CONTROL OF Paco$_2$

Under normal conditions, the feedback and control loop (see Fig. 1–1) maintains the system's set point for Paco$_2$ at 40 mm Hg. Pathologic conditions, however, can move this set point up or down. Under such circumstances, the CNS controller tries to achieve the "proper" level of Paco$_2$ at this new set point by changing minute ventilation.

Because the actions of the respiratory system's first three components (CNS, chest bellows, and airway) determine a patient's minute ventilation, they have been called the *respiratory pump*. Minute ventilation can be increased or decreased by the respiratory pump by changing tidal volume, respiratory rate, or both (Table 1–1, Equation 1). Since this pump controls Paco$_2$ levels, failure of one or more of its components can result in hypercapnic respiratory failure.

Although the respiratory pump changes minute ventilation (abbreviated as $\dot{V}_E$, since one measures *expired* minute ventilation), how those changes affect Paco$_2$

Table 1–1. Basic Physiologic Equations

....

Equation 1: $\dot{V}_E = V_T \times RR$
where $\dot{V}_E$ is the expired minute ventilation, V_T the tidal volume, and RR the respiratory rate.

Equation 2: $Paco_2 = K \times \dot{V}co_2/\dot{V}_A$
where K is a constant (863 mm Hg), $\dot{V}co_2$ is CO_2 production per minute and $\dot{V}_A$ is alveolar ventilation.

Equation 3: $V_T = V_A + V_D$
where V_A is the part of the tidal volume that contributes to alveolar ventilation and V_D is the dead space, i.e., that part of the tidal volume not contributing to gas exchange.

Equation 4: $\dot{V}_E = \dot{V}_A + \dot{V}_D$
where $\dot{V}_A$ is alveolar ventilation ($\dot{V}_A = V_A \times RR$) and $\dot{V}_D$ is dead space ventilation ($\dot{V}_D = V_D \times RR$).

Equation 5: $\dot{V}_D = V_D \times RR = V_D (\dot{V}_E/V_T) = (V_D/V_T) \times \dot{V}_E$
where RR $= \dot{V}_E/V_T$ by rearranging Equation 1 and V_D/V_T is the dead space to tidal volume ratio.

Equation 6: $\dot{V}_E = [\dot{V}_A + \dot{V}_D] = \dot{V}_A + \dot{V}_E (V_D/V_T)$
where $\dot{V}_D$ in Equation 4 is replaced by $\dot{V}_E (V_D/V_T)$ as derived in Equation 5.

Equation 7: $\dot{V}_E = \dot{V}_A/(1 - V_D/V_T)$
which is derived by solving equation 6 for $\dot{V}_E$.

Equation 8: $\dot{V}_A = \dot{V}_E \times (1 - V_D/V_T)$
which is derived by solving Equation 6 for $\dot{V}_A$.

Equation 9: $Paco_2 = K \times \dot{V}co_2/\{1 - V_D/V_T) \times \dot{V}_E\}$
after right-hand side of Equation 8 is substituted for $\dot{V}_A$ in Equation 2.

Equation 10: $Paco_2 \times \dot{V}_E = K \times \dot{V}co_2/(1 - V_D/V_T)$
which is derived from Equation 9 by rearrangement of the term $\dot{V}_E$.

Equation 11: $\dot{V}_E = K \times \dot{V}co_2/\{Paco_2 \times (1 - V_D/V_T)\}$
which solves Equation 10 for $\dot{V}_E$.

Equation 12 (Alveolar Gas Equation): $PAO_2 = PIO_2 - PACO_2/R$
where PAO_2 is mean ideal alveolar Po_2, PIO_2 the inspired Po_2, $PACO_2$ is alveolar Pco_2 estimated as equal to $Paco_2$, and R is the respiratory ratio, usually assumed to be 0.8 (except when $FIO_2 = 1.0$, $R = 1$). R is the non–steady-state equivalent of the steady-state respiratory quotient, RQ, which is defined as $RQ = \dot{V}co_2/\dot{V}o_2$.

....

depend on associated changes in *alveolar ventilation,* $\dot{V}_A$ (Table 1–1, Equation 2). Unlike $\dot{V}_E$, which is measurable by a spirometer, $\dot{V}_A$ is a theoretical quantity that cannot be measured directly but can be illustrated if the lung is viewed as a *two-compartment model.* In this model, the lung has an alveolar space (for gas exchange) and a dead space (for convective gas flow) (Table 1–1, Equation 3). The latter includes anatomic dead space (the trachea and other conducting airways) and alveolar dead space (alveoli with ventilation/perfusion ratios [V/Q] >1.0). In this model, minute ventilation, $\dot{V}_E$, is the *sum* of alveolar ventilation, $\dot{V}_A$, and dead space ventilation, $\dot{V}_D$ (Table 1–1, Equation 4) or, alternatively, can be expressed as a function of alveolar ventilation and ratio of dead space to tidal volume (V_D/V_T) (Table 1–1, Equation 7).

If V_D/V_T and $\dot{V}CO_2$ (Table 1–1, Equation 10) remain constant, $Paco_2$ has a *hyperbolic* relationship with $\dot{V}_E$ (since the right-hand side of Equation 10 would be a constant). Figure 1–2 illustrates this relationship and how changes in $\dot{V}_E$ affect $Paco_2$ at different values of V_D/V_T.

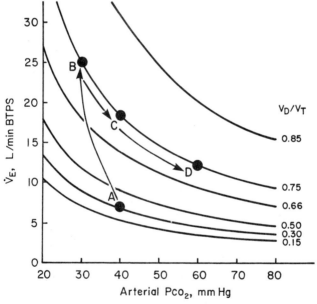

Figure 1–2. Changes in $Paco_2$ and minute ventilation during three phases of status asthmaticus (see text for details). Isopleths of equal V_D/V_T indicate the level of minute ventilation ($\dot{V}_E$) (ordinate) that is needed to achieve a certain level of $Paco_2$ (abscissa) for an individual with an assumed value for O_2 consumption of 200 mL/min. Normally (point A) $V_D/V_T = 0.3$, $Paco_2 = 40$ mm Hg, and $\dot{V}_E = \sim 7$ L/min. If V_D/V_T increases to 0.75 and if a new, lower value of $Paco_2$ is used as the "set point" ($Paco_2$ decreases from 40 mm Hg to 30 mm Hg), the patient needs to achieve $\dot{V}_E$ of ~ 25 L/min (point B). Point C represents the "crossover" point at which the $Paco_2$ is normal despite $\dot{V}_E$ falling to ~ 18 L/min due to onset of respiratory muscle fatigue. Finally, at point D, the patient has acute respiratory failure with elevated $Paco_2$ despite a $\dot{V}_E$ that has decreased further from point B or C but remains greater than at baseline (point A). (Adapted from Selecky P, Wasserman K, Klein M, et al: A graphic approach to assessing interrelationships among minute ventilation; arterial carbon dioxide tension, and ratio of physilogic lead space to tidal volume in patients on respirators. Ann Rev Respir Dis 117:181–184, 1978.)

RESPIRATORY MUSCLE FATIGUE

The respiratory muscles, like any skeletal muscle, may *fatigue*, that is, become unable to produce a contraction of normal strength when stimulated by a certain neural input. Although this condition is reversible if the muscle is allowed to rest, some fatigued skeletal muscles may take up to 24 hours to recover fully to a nonfatigued state.

Acute respiratory muscle fatigue results from an *imbalance* between ventilatory capacity and "demand" for ventilation. Ventilatory capacity is represented by the maximal sustainable ventilation, that is, the maximal ventilation that an individual can maintain indefinitely without respiratory muscle fatigue developing (this is usually equal to 50% of one's maximal voluntary ventilation). The *demand* for ventilation is the spontaneous minute ventilation required to achieve the $PaCO_2$ set by the CNS controller. Increases in spontaneous minute ventilation increase the mechanical load imposed on the respiratory muscles. If this load continues to increase, eventually it results in respiratory muscle fatigue.

At rest a normal person has a great deal of "ventilatory reserve"; for example, their maximal sustainable ventilation often exceeds their resting minute ventilation by tenfold. Pathologic processes can reduce maximal sustainable ventilation while increasing demand for ventilation. As shown in Equation 11 (Table 1–1), increased "ventilatory demand" ($\dot{V}_E$) can result either from an increase in V_D/V_T or $\dot{V}CO_2$, or from a decrease in the $PaCO_2$ set point (see Fig. 1–2). When ventilatory capacity approximates demand for ventilation, patients are breathing on the brink of hypercapnic respiratory failure. Further reductions in maximal sustainable ventilation or increases in demand result in an unsustainable load on the respiratory muscles and lead to *respiratory muscle fatigue*. Hypercapnic respiratory failure soon follows.

FAILURE OF COMPONENTS OF THE RESPIRATORY SYSTEM

As noted earlier, disorders that impair one or more component of the respiratory system can result in acute respiratory failure. In the evaluation of ICU patients with respiratory failure, identifying which of the respiratory system components has failed is essential in directing therapy. Although the effects of failure of a *single* component are described later, many patients in the ICU experience respiratory failure from the simultaneous or sequential failure of *multiple* components, and successful treatment requires taking such complexities into account.

Central Nervous System Component

Acute respiratory failure arising from impaired CNS drive commonly occurs in cases of intentional overdoses of sedatives, opioids, or other drugs that can depress CNS drive, for example, tricyclic antidepressants. Iatrogenic causes arise from the therapeutic use of opioids and sedatives.

The pathophysiologic mechanism of acute respiratory failure is illustrated in Figure 1–3. Arterial blood gases typically show an acute respiratory acidosis (Table

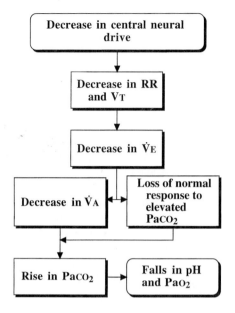

Figure 1–3. Schematic flow diagram of how impaired CNS respiratory drive results in acute hypercapnic respiratory failure. As CNS respiratory drive falls, so do respiratory rate and tidal volume. This decreases minute ventilation ($\dot{V}_E$) (see Table 1–1, Equation 1) and alveolar ventilation ($\dot{V}_A$) (see Table 1–1, Equation 8). The latter, in turn, results in a rise in Pa_{CO_2} (see Table 1–1, Equation 2). In these circumstances, there is a loss of the normal response to the elevated Pa_{CO_2}, which then results in acute respiratory acidosis (see Table 1–2).

1–2). Hypoxemia results from the effect of CO_2 retention on alveolar P_{O_2} (Pa_{O_2}), (Table 1–1, Equation 12). The difference between Pa_{O_2} and Pa_{O_2} ($P(A-a)_{O_2}$) is the "$A-a$ difference" (also called the "$A-a$ gradient"). Although $P(A-a)_{O_2}$ may be normal (≤ 20 mm Hg when breathing ambient air) in patients with impaired CNS drive, it is often increased because of associated atelectasis (see Table 1–2). The latter develops because of small tidal volume breathing and loss of sighs (extra-large spontaneous tidal volumes).

Specific treatment includes reversing the CNS depression by giving a pharmacologic agent, if available–for example, intravenous administration of naloxone for opioid-induced decreased respiratory drive. Many drugs that depress respiration, however, do not have effective antidotes. In these circumstances, one should intubate the patient to provide ventilation and to protect against aspiration of gastric contents (because as a rule the gag reflex is also depressed or absent).

Chest Bellows Component

Respiratory muscle weakness is a common example of failure of the chest bellows component (see Chapter 67). Specific clinical disorders that produce such weakness include Guillain-Barré syndrome (acute demyelinating polyneuropathy), generalized myasthenia gravis, and cervical spinal cord injury involving the phrenic motoneurons (C3–5). Disorders of the thoracic cage and subdiaphragmatic soft tissues may also contribute to acute hypercapnic respiratory failure. Examples include acute thoracic injuries (multiple rib fractures with severe pain during breathing), certain postoperative states (after multiple rib thoracoplasty), and other mechanical limitations to lung expansion (tense ascites).

The pathophysiologic mechanism of acute respiratory failure is illustrated in

Table 1–2. Tyical Changes in Arterial Blood Gases in Acute Respiratory Failure

MECHANISM OF ACUTE RESPIRATORY FAILURE	pH	Pa_{CO_2}	Pa_{O_2}	SERUM HCO_3	$P(A-a)_{O_2}$
Failure of central nervous system component	↓	↑	↓	WNL	WNL or ↑†
Failure of chest bellows component	↓	↑	↓	WNL	↑†
Failure of airway component					
Asthma flare					
Early phase (before respiratory failure)	↑	↓	WNL (or ↓)	WNL	↑
"Crossover point"	WNL	WNL	↓	WNL	↑
Very severe obstruction and respiratory muscle fatigue	↓	↑	↓	WNL	↑
COPD flare					
Nonchronic CO_2 retainer	↓	↑	↓	WNL	↑
Chronic CO_2 retainer					
During base line	WNL	↑	↓	↑	↑
During flare	↓	↑↑	↓	↑	↑
Failure of alveolar component					
Before respiratory muscle fatigue	↑	↓	↓↓	WNL	↑↑
After respiratory muscle fatigue	↓	↑	↓↓	WNL	↑↑

†If atelectasis or pneumonia is present.
↑, increased; ↑↑, very increased; ↓, decreased; ↓↓, very decreased; WNL, within normal limits; COPD, chronic obstructive pulmonary disease; $P(A-a)_{O_2} = Pa_{O_2} - Pa_{O_2}$, where Pa_{O_2} is alveolar P_{O_2}.

Figure 1–4. Neuromuscular disorders lead to acute respiratory failure primarily by limitations in ventilatory capacity (although some increase in ventilatory demand occurs because of a relatively increased V_D/V_T due to decreased V_T in the face of constant V_D). Although adequate CNS respiratory drive exists, transpulmonary pressures are diminished because of disruption of neuronal transmission at any point along the neuromuscular pathway from spinal cord to diaphragms or from intrinsic weakness of the respiratory muscles themselves.

These patients exhibit a pattern of small tidal volume breathing at a rapid rate, so-called rapid shallow breathing. They also cannot take large breaths or sighs. Because sighs are essential for renewing the surface tension–lowering activity of surfactant, virtually all patients who cannot take deep breaths for whatever reason (muscle weakness, pain, tachypnea) or who have their spontaneous sighs suppressed (by opioids and sedatives) experience significant microatelectasis (not visible on chest radiograph) or macroatelectasis (radiographically evident as subsegmental, segmental, or lobar atelectasis), or both. Patients with neuromuscular weakness also often have poor gag reflexes and ineffective coughs and thus may develop an aspiration pneumonia.

Arterial blood gases in patients with acute respiratory failure due to neuromuscular weakness resemble those with impaired central neural drive but usually with more hypoxemia and a greater $P(A-a)_{O_2}$ due to commonly associated atelectasis or aspiration pneumonia, or both (see Table 1–2).

Although specific therapy depends on the particular condition resulting in respiratory failure, the generic approach includes positive-pressure mechanical

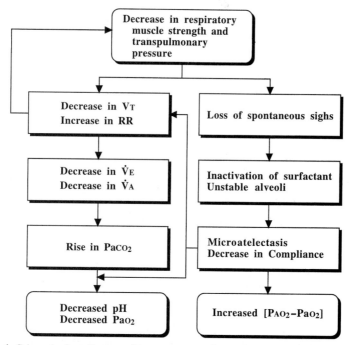

Figure 1–4. Schematic flow diagram of how neuromuscular weakness results in acute hypercapnic respiratory failure. Initially an increased respiratory rate compensates for decreased tidal volumes and maintains normal alveolar ventilation ($\dot{V}_A$) and $Paco_2$ (mediated by the normal response to elevated $Paco_2$). Eventually, however, with progressive weakness, this compensation fails and $Paco_2$ rises with an associated acute respiratory acidosis (see Table 1–2). The increase in $P(A-a)o_2$ ($Pao_2 - Pao_2$) is due to commonly associated atelectasis or aspiration pneumonia, or both.

ventilation via tracheal intubation. Alternatively, if aspiration is not a significant concern, many patients can be effectively managed with noninvasive positive-pressure ventilation delivered via a nasal or facial continuous positive airway pressure (CPAP) mask (see Chapter 77).

Airway Component

Two common examples of impairment of the airway component leading to hypercapnic respiratory failure are status asthmaticus (a severe asthma flare) and acute decompensation of chronic obstructive pulmonary disease (COPD flare) (see Chapter 74).

Pathophysiologic Mechanism of Respiratory Failure

The mechanism of CO_2 retention in both disorders is multifactorial (Fig. 1–5). The capacity for ventilation decreases because of limited expiratory flow and minute ventilation due to airway obstruction. Airway obstruction plus a rapid respiratory rate results in dynamic hyperinflation (the cause of "auto–positive end-expiratory

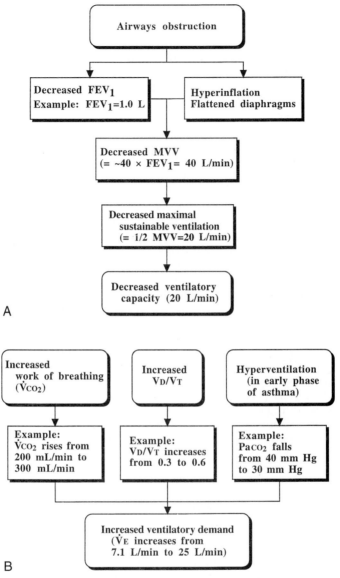

Figure 1–5. *A,* Schematic flow diagram of how airway obstruction leads to decreased ventilatory capacity. The decreased FEV_1 and mechanical disadvantage induced by flattening of the domes of the hemidiaphragms lead to a decreased maximal voluntary ventilation (MVV), which can be approximated as $40 \times FEV_1$. Maximal sustainable ventilation normally equals approximately 50% of MVV (although this may be increased in patients with chronic respiratory disorders) so that a patient with severe airway obstruction as represented by FEV_1 of 1 L would have a maximal sustainable ventilation of only about 20 L/min (compared with a normal range of 100–200 L/min). *B,* While capacity for ventilation is falling, demand for ventilation simultaneously increases. This increased demand occurs because (1) CO_2 production increases (arising from increased O_2 consumption due to greatly increased work of breathing through obstructed airway), (2) V_D/V_T markedly increases (due to V/Q mismatch on a microscopic level with many alveoli having V/Q ratios >1.0), and (3) the set point for $Paco_2$ decreases (due to vagal afferent stimuli to the CNS controller). The overall end result of these changes as calculated by Equation 11 (see Table 1–1) shows a more than threefold increased ventilatory demand. If this demand for 25 L/min persisted in a patient whose capacity was only 20 L/min, respiratory muscle fatigue would result.

pressure [auto-PEEP]", also called intrinsic PEEP) (see Chapter 2). This limits minute ventilation by flattening the domes of the hemidiaphragms and compromising the normal length-force relationship of the diaphragm. These changes decrease ventilatory capacity (see Fig. 1–5A), and other changes (see Fig. 1–5B) increase demand for ventilation. They combine to set the stage for development of respiratory muscle fatigue.

Arterial Blood Gases in Severe Asthma Flares

On their way to acute respiratory failure, patients with severe asthma flares often pass through *three* phases (see Table 1–2). In the *first phase*, patients have mild to moderate degrees of airway obstruction and exhibit *hypocapnia* with $Paco_2$ in the range of 30 to 33 mm Hg. This hyperventilation reflects increased respiratory input to the CNS controller from pulmonary vagal afferent receptors, for example, irritant receptors in airway epithelium, and other neural afferents stimulated by the asthma flare. This is usually accompanied by mild hypoxemia and an increased $P(A-a)o_2$ due to V/Q mismatch.

In the *second phase*, as the airway obstruction becomes more severe, the respiratory muscles begin to fatigue and $Paco_2$ rises to about 40 mm Hg. Known as the *crossover point,* this "normal" $Paco_2$ is actually ominous because it represents a rise from prior *hypocapnic* levels and may indicate that respiratory muscle fatigue and hypercapnic respiratory failure are imminent. In a patient in status asthmaticus, a "normal" $Paco_2$ should definitely be considered *abnormal,* and the patient should be monitored closely for respiratory failure.

In the *third phase*, extreme airway obstruction leads to respiratory muscle fatigue and acute respiratory acidosis with an elevated $Paco_2$ (see Table 1–2). Hypoxemia is universal unless supplemental oxygen is given. Unlike COPD patients with chronic CO_2 retention, an elevated serum bicarbonate level is atypical in patients with an asthma flare because the latter typically do not have chronic CO_2 retention.

Arterial Blood Gas Changes in Chronic Obstructive Pulmonary Disease Flares

Arterial blood gases in COPD patients who are *not* chronic CO_2 retainers are similar to those observed in acute asthma flares (see Table 1–2). COPD patients with chronic CO_2 retention, however, have high serum bicarbonate concentrations at baseline because of renal compensation for the chronic respiratory acidosis. Acting as a buffer, the elevated bicarbonate results in a smaller fall in arterial pH as $Paco_2$ rises during an acute decompensation (see Table 1–2).

Therapy

Initial management of both asthma and COPD flares includes supplemental oxygen, inhaled bronchodilators, intravenous glucocorticosteroids, and antibiotics (if a bacterial respiratory infection is suspected) (see Chapter 74). Although giving oxygen to nonintubated patients with COPD flares can worsen hypercapnia in about two thirds of cases, one should still aim to achieve adequate oxygenation in these patients. If life-threatening gas exchange and acid-base abnormalities develop, one should use positive-pressure mechanical ventilation. Since noninvasive ventilation in patients with COPD flares has been shown to be effective and less expensive than conventional mechanical ventilation in those who tolerate it, this method of ventilation should be attempted in most patients who are still breathing spontaneously and can mobilize their respiratory secretions (see Chapter 77).

Alveolar Component

Disorders that severely impair the function of the alveolar component of the respiratory system result in *hypoxemic* respiratory failure. As a rule, they also result in acute *hyercapnic* respiratory failure. These patients typically present with diffuse alveolar flooding due to cardiogenic or noncardiogenic pulmonary edema, diffuse pulmonary hemorrhage syndrome, or extensive pneumonia.

Hypoxemic respiratory failure occurs as a result of pathophysiologic changes in gas exchange set into motion by the alveolar flooding (Fig. 1–6). Arterial blood gas measurements show severe hypoxemia despite the patient breathing high concentrations of oxygen. This profound resistance to oxygen arises from the presence of a large right-to-left shunt across the lungs. Early in these disorders, *hypo*capnia and acute respiratory alkalosis are common; later, however, *hyper*capnia occurs because of respiratory muscle fatigue (see Table 1–2). The mechanism of hypercapnic respiratory failure is multifactorial (see Chapter 73).

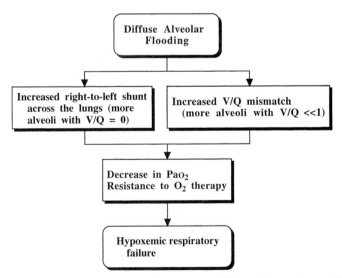

Figure 1–6. Alveolar flooding decreases ventilation to zero (V/Q = 0) or nearly zero (V/Q <<1.0) for many alveoli. The former represents true right-to-left shunts because the P_{O_2} of the mixed venous blood that passes through capillaries of these alveoli remains unchanged. Alveoli with very low V/Q represent so-called physiologic shunts because their low V/Q results in very low alveolar P_{O_2}. Hypoxemia due to right-to-left shunts is resistant to supplemental oxygen therapy because the supplementary oxygen does not decrease the shunt fraction.

Therapy includes specific treatment of the causative agent (such as bacterial pneumonia) and mechanical ventilation to restore safe levels of arterial oxygenation. Large right-to-left shunt fractions should be treated by decreasing the shunt fraction (and not by giving high concentrations of oxygen alone). One does this for patients with intravascular volume overload by lowering pulmonary capillary pressure by diuresis (see Chapter 51). For patients with acute respiratory distress syndrome (ARDS), one should lower pulmonary capillary pressure and add PEEP during mechanical ventilation as well. If ARDS occurs as part of the syndrome of multiple organ system failure, however, one needs to balance the beneficial effects of PEEP and diuresis on improving hypoxemia with their potentially adverse effects on nonpulmonary organ dysfunction (see Chapter 73).

BIBLIOGRAPHY

Kelsen SG, Criner GJ: Pump failure: The pathogenesis of hypercapnic respiratory failure in patients with lung and chest wall disease. In: Fishman AP, Elias JA, Fishman JA, et al (eds): Pulmonary Diseases and Disorders, 3rd ed. New York: McGraw-Hill, 1998, pp 2605–2625.
This chapter describes mechanisms of acute and chronic respiratory failure, with emphasis on respiratory muscle fatigue (77 references).

Lanken PN: Respiratory failure. In: Carlson RW, Geheb MA (eds): Principles and Practice of Medical Intensive Care. Philadelphia: WB Saunders, 1993, pp 754–763.
This chapter reviews the mechanisms of acute respiratory failure and factors reducing ventilatory capacity and increasing ventilatory demand (40 references).

Roussos C, Macklem PT: The respiratory muscles. N Engl J Med 307:786–797, 1982.
This is the classic description of the respiratory pump and its relationship to hypercapnic respiratory failure.

Selecky P, Wasserman K, Klein M, et al: A graphic approach to assessing interrelationships among minute ventilation, arterial carbon dioxide tension and ratio of physiologic dead space to tidal volume in patients on respirators. Am Rev Respir Dis 117:181–184, 1978.
This article provides information and details validating the graph presented in Figure 1–2.

2   Mechanical Ventilation

Paul N. Lanken

Knowing how mechanical ventilators ventilate, their common operating modes, and the complications associated with their use is a basic but essential skill for all intensive care unit (ICU) clinicians. This chapter presents these topics along with the physical and physiologic principles with which ICU clinicians need to be familiar in order to use mechanical ventilation rationally and safely.

Modern ventilators have their origins in respirators that were designed to duplicate the physiology of normal breathing. In the 1920s, Drinker and coworkers developed the so-called "iron lung" to treat patients with paralytic poliomyelitis. This ventilator applied subatmospheric pressure externally to the patient's thorax and abdomen in order to produce airflow and ventilation. Although these early devices were lifesaving for some patients, they had serious limitations: (1) inability to suction respiratory secretions because the trachea was not intubated, (2) inability to generate moderate-to-high intrapulmonary pressures (as a result, patients with stiff lungs or obstructed airways could not be adequately ventilated), and (3) limited access to the patient's body for nursing or emergency medical care (because the ventilator enclosed all of the patient's body except the head).

THE "GENERIC" POSITIVE PRESSURE VENTILATOR

In contrast to the iron lung, which applied *negative pressure* to the thorax, virtually all ventilators used in ICUs today apply *positive pressure* to the airways and lungs. For this reason, current ventilators as a class are referred to as *positive pressure ventilators*.

The superiority of this type of ventilator was originally demonstrated by its use with patients with paralytic poliomyelitis. Bjorn Ibsen, an anesthetist, started the modern era of positive pressure ventilation during the 1952 Copenhagen poliomyelitis epidemic. He used cuffed endotracheal tubes combined with hand-compressed bag ventilation to successfully ventilate hundreds of patients with respiratory failure due to paralytic poliomyelitis. Subsequent milestones include automating delivery of the breaths by machines, adding monitors to ensure safe and effective ventilation, and, finally, adding microprocessors to control the ventilator's electromechanical functioning and to monitor the patient-ventilator interface.

Although modern microprocessor-controlled ventilators have a large array of settings, controls, and displays on their consoles, all positive pressure ventilators operate by the same basic elements and parameters (Fig. 2–1 and Table 2–1). The mode of ventilation selected and the patient's specific clinical circumstances should determine the exact settings.

PRINCIPLES AND PRACTICE OF POSITIVE PRESSURE VENTILATION

The effectiveness and safety of mechanical ventilation depend on numerous elements. First are the *mechanical properties* of the patient's respiratory system.

13

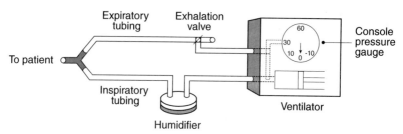

Figure 2–1. Model of basic elements of a volume-cycled ventilator. The ventilator delivers a preset tidal volume (symbolized by the piston and cylinder) via the inspiratory tubing and humidifier to the patient. The exhalation valve is closed by positive pressure during inspiration. At the start of exhalation, the valve opens and the expired gas exits the circuit via the expiratory tubing (normally the exhaled gas re-enters the ventilator to monitor its volume). The pressure gauge on the console reflects pressure proximal to the inspiratory tubing. (Modified from Lanken PN: Mechanical ventilation. In: Fishman AP [ed]: Pulmonary Diseases and Disorders, 2nd ed. New York: McGraw-Hill, 1988.)

Table 2–1. Basic Ventilator Parameters and Typical Initial Settings

PARAMETER	SETTINGS*	RANGE	COMMENTS
Mode	A/C		Use A/C mode for patients not breathing spontaneously and for starting assisted ventilation.
Respiratory rate	7–8 BPM	5–35 BPM	For patients without spontaneous breathing efforts, set rate to achieve a desired $Paco_2$ guided by ABGs.
			For spontaneously breathing patients in A/C or IMV mode, set rate 2–3 BPM below spontaneous rate.
Tidal volume	700 mL	300–1200 mL	Without assisted ventilation, *spontaneous* tidal volumes are normally ~5 mL/kg IBW (or ~350 mL for a 70-kg IBW patient); traditionally, ventilators have used larger tidal volumes (~10 mL/kg) to prevent atelectasis and to counteract the patient's sensation of "air hunger."
Fio_2	1.00	0.21–1.0	Start at 1.0 and taper as guided by Pao_2 or Sao_2.
Inspiratory flow rate	60 L/min	50–100 L/min	Flows are set higher when patient has a high respiratory rate or "air hunger" or to decrease inspiratory time.
Sigh volume	1000 mL	900–1500 mL	Adjust sigh volume in a given patient to produce Pplat of 30 cm H_2O (because transpulmonary pressure of ~35 cm H_2O inflates a normal lung to total lung capacity). Set sigh rate for 5–6/h (the rate of spontaneous sighs).
I:E ratio	1:2	2:1 to 1:4	Usually a derived, not a preset, parameter.

*Initial settings for 70-kg IBW adult with normal lungs (see Chapter 12, Table 12–1 for IBW formulas). Set initial rate higher (12–14 BPM) if lung disease is present, e.g., asthma and COPD.

ABGs, arterial blood gases; A/C, assist/control; BPM, breaths per minute; Fio_2, fractional concentration of inspired oxygen; IBW, ideal body weight; I:E, inspiratory time to expiratory time; Pplat, plateau pressure; Sao_2, arterial O_2 saturation; IMV, intermittent mandatory ventilation; COPD, chronic obstructive pulmonary disease.

Second is the *degree of synchrony* between the patient and the ventilator, that is, the interface between the patient and the ventilator. Finally, complications of positive pressure ventilation generally result from its misuse or from abnormal respiratory mechanics rather than from intrinsically damaging effects of the ventilator.

Ventilating the Respiratory System

The respiratory system resembles a balloon in that it inflates during inspiration, followed by passive deflation during expiration (Fig. 2–2). This model has two mechanical elements: *compliance* and *resistance*. Compliance relates the gas volume in the balloon to the pressure inside the balloon under static conditions. It determines the balloon's internal pressure (static recoil pressure) after inflation to a certain volume. Resistance determines the inspiratory pressure needed to achieve a certain inspiratory airflow as well as how fast the lungs empty during expiration.

As a rule, when adults are being mechanical ventilated via an endotracheal tube or tracheostomy tube, the respiratory system is a "closed" system and has no leaks (Fig. 2–2). Under these circumstances, the following relationship holds during inspiration:

$$Pprox = \Delta P_{AW} + P_{ALV} = [R(airways) \times flow] + P_{ALV}$$

(Equation 1)

where Pprox is the pressure at the proximal end of the artificial airway during inspiration; ΔP_{AW}, the pressure drop across the airways during inspiration; R(air-

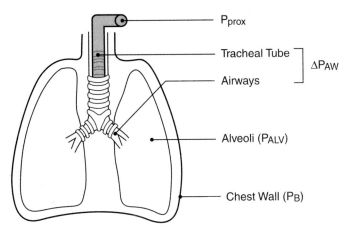

Figure 2–2. The respiratory system (lungs plus chest wall) is a closed system during ventilation with a cuffed endotracheal tube. See Equation 1 for relationships among pressures. Pprox, pressure at proximal end of endotracheal tube; ΔP_{AW}, pressure drop across airways during inspiration as a result of resistance of artificial and natural airways; P_{ALV}, alveolar pressure (equal to the static recoil pressure of the respiratory system); P_B, barometric pressure. (Modified from Lanken PN: Mechanical ventilation. In: Fishman AP [ed]: Pulmonary Diseases and Disorders, 2nd ed. New York: McGraw-Hill, 1988.)

ways), airway resistance; flow, the inspiratory flow rate; and Palv, the alveolar pressure during inspiration.

Equation 1 indicates that the proximal airway pressure during inspiration is the sum of two components: (1) a dynamic component, ΔPaw, representing the pressure drop that occurs as air flows into the lungs (as a result of resistance of artificial and natural airways), and (2) a static component, Palv, the mean pressure in alveoli, which represents the static recoil pressure of the lungs and chest wall. This pressure is determined by the increase in lung volume above functional residual capacity (FRC), the volume in the lungs at end-expiration.

Pressure-Volume Curves of the Respiratory System

Static Pressure-Volume Curve

As noted earlier, changes in lung volume above FRC during inspiration relate to the recoil pressure of the respiratory system (Fig. 2–3A). The *compliance of the respiratory system* incorporates both lung compliance and chest wall compliance and is expressed as follows:

$$Cstat = \Delta V/\Delta P \qquad \text{(Equation 2)}$$

where Cstat is the static compliance of the respiratory system, ΔV is a change in volume, and ΔP is the corresponding change in pressure.

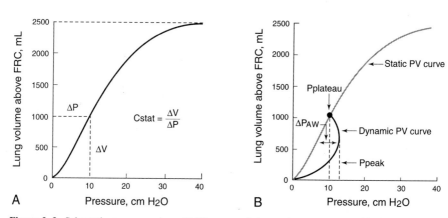

Figure 2–3. Schematic pressure-volume (P-V) curves of the respiratory system, with the static recoil pressure of the respiratory system (Palv in Figure 2–2) as abscissa. *A,* Static P-V curve. A tidal volume of 1000 mL results in recoil pressure of 10 cm H_2O. Because compliance of the respiratory system (Cstat) is equal to the change in volume (ΔV) above functional residual capacity (FRC) divided by the change in pressure (ΔP), Cstat = (1000 mL/10 cm H_2O) = 100 mL/cm H_2O (a normal value). Note that the curve flattens at higher pressures as total lung capacity is approached. *B,* Dynamic P-V curve of 1000 mL tidal volume superimposed on the static P-V curve in *A.* The difference between the two curves (ΔPaw) represents the pressure drop across the airways resulting from airway resistance. Note that peak pressure (Ppeak) exceeds the end-inspiratory static pressure (Pplateau) by ~2 cm H_2O, reflecting normal airway resistance. (Modified from Lanken PN: Mechanical ventilation. In: Fishman AP [ed]: Pulmonary Diseases and Disorders, 2nd ed. New York: McGraw-Hill, 1988.)

In general, ΔP equals the plateau pressure (Pplateau) minus the end-expiratory pressure (which equals zero unless positive end-expiratory pressure [PEEP] is present). One measures Pplateau as the change in airway pressure after a certain tidal volume has been delivered by use of an inspiratory pause (0.5-second pause) at end-inspiration. While monitoring Cstat over time, one should use the same tidal volume for each Pplateau measurement. Normal respiratory system compliance is 50 to 100 mL/cm H_2O, that is, the lungs expand by 50 to 100 mL for every 1 cm H_2O of static distending pressure. *Low* respiratory system compliance is common in ICU patients and, if present, needs special consideration during ventilator management. A low Cstat indicates that the respiratory system is "stiffer" than normal. This may be due to stiff lungs, such as those caused by pulmonary edema, or a stiff chest wall, resulting from edema of the chest wall or taut, dilated loops of bowel encroaching into the chest.

A *high* Cstat usually does not affect ventilator care as much as a low Cstat. A high Cstat may reflect abnormal lungs that have lost their elastic recoil because of emphysema or an abnormal chest wall that has low compliance, such as that caused by neuromuscular blocker–induced paralysis or multiple rib fractures and a "flail chest."

Dynamic Pressure-Volume Curve

The *static* pressure-volume curve of the respiratory system, discussed earlier, applies only when there is no airflow, that is, at end-inspiration or end-expiration. When air is flowing into or out of the lung, resistance to airflow comes into play (see Equation 1 and Fig. 2–3B).

BASIC MODES OF VENTILATION

All ventilators used in the ICU setting can provide three basics modes of ventilation: (1) assist/control (A/C) mode, (2) pressure support (PS) mode, and (3) intermittent mandatory ventilation (IMV) mode. Although this chapter describes only these basic three modes, most microprocessor-controlled ventilators can provide additional modes of assisted ventilation or combine several modes.

Assist/Control Mode

The term *assist/control mode* arises from two traditional methods of ventilation used in early ventilators: (1) assist mode, which allows a patient with spontaneous breathing efforts to initiate the desired machine delivered tidal volume, and (2) control mode, which provides machine breaths without regard to the patient's pattern of breathing. The latter is now obsolete because it "locks out" patients even if they are making spontaneous efforts to breathe. Furthermore, studies have indicated that total lack of use of the respiratory muscles rapidly leads to disuse atrophy. This can be prevented, in part, by providing neural stimuli for muscular contractions (e.g., those provided by the assist mode), even if the ventilator provides most of the work of breathing.

Settings

The *control mode* is straightforward because the operator sets only two primary parameters, respiratory rate and tidal volume (Fig. 2–4*A*). Most ventilators function as *volume-cycled ventilators*, in which inspiration ceases after the preset tidal volume is delivered to the patient. Unless there is a leak in the system, such as around the cuff of a tracheal tube or through a chest tube, or unless peak inspiratory pressure exceeds the "pop-off" pressure (the threshold set for the peak pressure alarm), the patient should receive all of the preset tidal volume. The combination of rate and tidal volume, therefore, defines the minute ventilation that the patient receives. Other ventilator parameters in the control mode include volume and frequency of sigh breaths (see Table 2–1). Sighs are physiologic and occur during normal spontaneous respirations. They are extra large (12 to 15 mL/kg) breaths, occurring at 6 to 10 times per hour. Sighs are normally essential in the renewal of surfactant's surface activity and are used during mechanical ventilation to prevent alveolar instability and development of microatelectasis.

The *assist mode* adds two features of operation to the control mode (Fig. 2–4*B*). First, the ventilator can detect a patient's inspiratory effort (by detecting the negative pressure deflection from baseline in the inspiratory circuit or by detecting the beginning of patient-initiated airflow through the ventilator's demand valve). When that inspiratory effort exceeds a certain threshold, the patient "triggers" the ventilator to begin delivery of the preset inspiratory tidal volume. The timing of the start of the next inspiration is defined by the set respiratory rate or by the patient's spontaneous rate, whichever is higher. For example, if the preset rate is 10 breaths/min, the ventilator provides a tidal volume every 6 seconds unless it detects the patient's spontaneous inspiratory effort earlier. If it does, it resets the start of the next ventilator-initiated breath to be 6 seconds from the start of that patient-initiated breath.

The second additional feature of the assist mode allows the patient to inspire from the ventilator's demand valve (which is similar to the demand valve of SCUBA [self-contained underwater breathing apparatus] gear). This occurs during inspiration if the patient's inspiratory flows exceed those generated by the ventilator or if the patient continues to inspire after the preset tidal volume has been delivered. In this manner, the patient's actual tidal volumes can be larger than the ventilator's set tidal volume (Fig. 2–4*B*). On occasion, patients breathing vigorously can also set off the ventilator's low inspiratory pressure alarm by continually inspiring during machine inspiration (see Chapter 48 for more information about alarms).

Mechanical Considerations

In volume-cycled ventilation, such as in A/C mode, the delivered tidal volume is less than the preset tidal volume if the peak inspiratory pressure (PIP) exceeds the threshold for the peak pressure alarm. For any given tidal volume and inspiratory flow rate, PIP is determined by two factors relating to the patient's mechanics (as expressed by Equations 1 and 2): airway resistance and static compliance of the respiratory system. If the PIP exceeds the threshold for the ventilator's peak pressure alarm, the remaining tidal volume is "dumped" (allowed to escape from the system) and is not delivered to the patient. This may occur if the patient

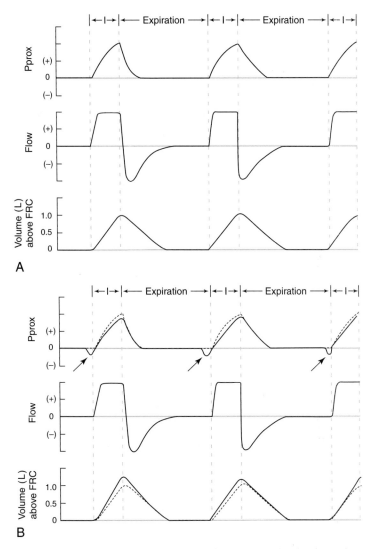

Figure 2–4. Schematic pressure, flow, and volume waveforms in control and assist modes. *A*, Control mode. Flow is delivered as a square wave during inspiration. During this mode, the patient makes no spontaneous efforts to breathe. Note that the tidal volume is 1.0 L. *B*, Assist mode. Each inspiration is triggered by the patient's spontaneous breathing effort *(arrows)*. Note that the pressure waveform is distorted from the control mode *(dashed curves)* because of the patient's continued efforts to breath during inspiration. Also note that the delivered tidal volume is greater than the 1.0 L delivered previously in the control mode *(dashed curves)*. This is because the patient's continued inspiratory efforts took additional volume from the ventilator's demand valve. Pprox, pressure at proximal end of endotracheal tube; FRC, functional residual capacity; I, inspiration; (+), inspiratory flow; (−), expiratory flow.

actively resists the machine delivered inspiration (termed *bucking* or *fighting* the ventilator) or coughs (both of which decrease compliance of the respiratory system). Another common cause of high PIPs is if the patient's airway resistance increases, such as in an airway that is partially blocked by respiratory secretions or by the patient biting the endotracheal tube.

Clinical Considerations

The A/C mode of ventilation is indicated for patients without spontaneous respiratory efforts, such as in paralyzed and apneic patients, or for patients with potential loss of their breathing efforts. The latter include patients with drug overdoses who wax and wane in their depressive effects on central nervous system respiratory drive. It is also the mode of choice to provide therapeutic hyperventilation.

Numerous studies have indicated that spontaneously breathing patients with a high ventilatory drive often continue to have a high work of breathing while on A/C mode. In these conditions, they make strenuous efforts to breathe during machine-delivered inspirations, as reflected by negative esophageal pressure swings during machine inspiration. As a consequence, if such patients were put on A/C mode because of respiratory muscle fatigue, this mode may not effectively "unload" their respiratory muscles, that is, put their respiratory muscles at rest to allow for full recovery from skeletal muscle fatigue.

In the case of patients who have high respiratory rates while on A/C mode, one must first check that the ventilator's triggering sensitivity is not excessive (which could lead to ventilator self-cycling and high respiratory rates). One can address the problem of ventilated patients who continue to make strong inspiratory efforts on A/C mode by increasing inspiratory flow rates and checking for auto-PEEP (auto–positive end-expiratory pressure, described later). If auto-PEEP is present, it should be treated as discussed later. If the tachypnea persists, one may need to suppress the patient's high respiratory drive pharmacologically, such as with more sedation (see Chapter 4), in order to provide a respite for the patient's respiratory muscles. Changing to PS mode of ventilation is another alternative.

Pressure Support Mode

Pressure support differs from A/C mode in how it provides assisted ventilation. Instead of delivering a preset tidal volume, PS delivers a preset pressure. When it detects that the patient is starting to inhale, it provides a certain level of pressure to the inspiratory circuit. The result is a synchronized inspiratory pressure "boost" that assists the patient's own efforts in order to augment the patient's spontaneous tidal volume and to unload the patient's respiratory muscles (Fig. 2–5A). The boost stops when the ventilator detects that inspiratory flow has decreased to a certain degree.

Settings

One should set the level of PS to achieve a certain tidal volume during the patient's spontaneous breathing. Often, a trial-and-error approach is used to arrive

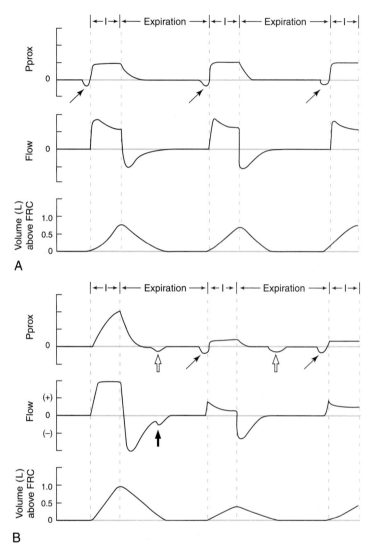

Figure 2–5. Schematic pressure, flow, and volume waveforms in pressure support (PS) and intermittent mandatory ventilation (IMV) modes. *A*, PS mode. Patient triggers each breath *(arrows)*, resulting in a pressure assist during inspiration, which results in a tidal volume of 0.75 L. *B*, IMV mode. The first breath is a machine-delivered tidal volume of 1.0 L, not triggered by the patient. The second breath, 0.5 L, represents the patient's spontaneous breath (enhanced by a low level of PS). The *vertical open arrows* indicate two inspiratory efforts that were not sensed by the ventilator. Note that the first of these *(solid vertical arrow)* distorts the expiratory flow waveform (compare with Figure 2–4*A* or 2–4*B*). FRC, functional residual capacity; Pprox, pressure at proximal end of endotracheal tube; I, inspiration; (+), inspiratory flow; (−), expiratory flow.

at the appropriate level of PS. The respiratory rate is the patient's spontaneous respiratory rate. Backup minute ventilation is available on some modern ventilators as a safety feature if patients stop or slow their breathing or if tidal volumes fall because of fatigue or changes in lung mechanical properties.

Mechanical Considerations

As noted earlier, tidal volumes in PS may fall if the mechanical properties of the patient's respiratory system change or the patient's respiratory muscles become fatigued. Instead of delivering a certain preset tidal volume, as in A/C or IMV mode, PS provides only the desired level of pressure support during a patient-initiated inspiration. What size tidal volume this pressure generates depends on the inspiratory effort, the duration of the inspiratory flow, the airway resistance, and the respiratory system compliance. If any of these factors fluctuate over time, tidal volumes at the same PS also fluctuate. In addition, the respiratory rate on PS is the patient's *spontaneous* respiratory rate. Because this may also change over time, the need for backup ventilation should be self-evident. Certain ventilators can provide a backup ventilation when they detect an exhaled minute ventilation lower than threshold setting.

Clinical Considerations

As noted earlier, ICU clinicians set the level of inspiratory pressure support, not a certain tidal volume or respiratory rate. Because tidal volumes may change at the same selected level of PS as a result of changes in airway resistance and Cstat, PS is less attractive when these mechanical properties are expected to fluctuate, such as in acute asthma flares. Likewise, PS mode is problematic when apneas or hypopneas occur. If the PS mode is used in these conditions, having a backup system of ventilation is necessary.

Intermittent Mandatory Ventilation Mode

The IMV mode consists of two types of ventilation (see Fig. 2–5*B*). The first type of ventilation in synchronized IMV is identical to that in A/C mode, and it provides machine-delivered tidal volumes at a preset respiratory rate. In current ventilators, these IMV breaths are synchronized with the patient's spontaneous breaths so that they do not "stack" on top of the patient's spontaneous breaths. The second type of ventilation allows the patient to breathe spontaneously from the ventilator's demand valve. The volume and the rate of these spontaneous breaths depend on the patient's respiratory drive and the mechanical properties of the patient's respiratory system.

Settings

The primary settings for IMV mode include IMV rate and tidal volume. In addition, in order to compensate for the airway resistance of the artificial airway, a low level of pressure support (5 to 8 cm H_2O) is often added to aid the spontaneous breaths (see Fig. 2–5B).

Mechanical Considerations

As in the A/C mode, the operator sets the IMV tidal volumes. Their corresponding peak inspiratory pressures are also determined by the mechanical properties of resistance and compliance.

Clinical Considerations

Although synchronized IMV was originally developed as a weaning mode from mechanical ventilation, some ICU clinicians use synchronized IMV as their standard mode of mechanical ventilation, weaning or not. This practice probably reflects the style of their institution or clinical training. Because of a lack of studies of comparing outcomes of patients ventilated with A/C mode or IMV under nonweaning conditions, there are no data indicating which mode results in better outcomes. In the absence of compelling results to the contrary, either mode can be used successfully for assisted ventilation, but one mode may be better than the other in some circumstances.

For example, for patients with respiratory muscle fatigue, some clinicians have expressed concern that even though IMV rates provide for adequate CO_2 removal, they may be set too low to provide adequate unloading of the respiratory muscles. In addition, as discussed in Chapter 3, two clinical trials comparing methods of weaning indicated that IMV was the *slowest* weaning method. IMV has a physiologic advantage over A/C mode, however, when there is auto-PEEP (intrinsic PEEP). The patient's spontaneous breaths in IMV provide negative intrathoracic pressures that counterbalance the positive intrathoracic pressure of the auto-PEEP and IMV breaths.

Some ICU clinicians use IMV when they encounter patients with hyperventilation and a severe respiratory alkalosis. These patients breathe at high respiratory rates on A/C mode because of an increased central nervous system respiratory drive. Simply switching the patient from A/C to IMV mode does not solve the problem of alkalosis unless the patient's respiratory muscles become fatigued during IMV. This is clearly not a desirable outcome. Likewise, adding extra dead space or locking out the patient (by setting the triggering threshold high) should not be used, because both methods may also induce respiratory muscle fatigue. Under these conditions, it is more appropriate to decrease the patient's high drive pharmacologically, such as with anxiolytics if the high rates are due to anxiety, opioids, or even paralysis for other states of centrally mediated hyperventilation (see Chapter 4).

Noninvasive Ventilation

Noninvasive ventilation has established itself in recent years as a safe and effective approach for certain patients with acute or chronic respiratory failure. For some, such as those with obesity-hypoventilation syndrome, it is the method of choice for assisted ventilation (see Chapter 77). Noninvasive ventilation generally uses a nasal or "full-face" continuous positive airway pressure (CPAP) mask. How well the mask is sealed on the face is important. Getting a good seal depends on the pliability and the shape of the mask as well as the skill of the ICU staff in selecting and fitting the mask to the patient.

For treatment of patients with acute respiratory failure, noninvasive ventilation employs the same positive pressure volume-cycled ventilators as those used in invasive ventilation. When only partial rather than complete assistance in ventilation is needed, one can utilize less complex, bilevel respiratory assist devices that provide low-to-moderate levels of PS. These levels are called *inspiratory positive airway pressure* (IPAP) and *expiratory positive airway pressure* (EPAP). These devices (some of which are not approved by the United States Food and Drug Administration for use as a ventilator and lack many of the ventilator's monitoring and alarm systems) should be used selectively. Good candidates include patients with the obesity-hypoventilation syndrome (see Chapter 77) and those who have recently been extubated and need transient ventilatory assistance, with the alternative being re-intubation.

Noninvasive ventilation is also an effective therapy for dyspnea. In selected patients with acute respiratory failure who have made the decision not to be intubated, it has been successfully used as part of the palliative care being used to treat severe dyspnea.

Settings

Noninvasive ventilation delivered by conventional ventilators uses the same settings as invasive ventilation except that tidal volume and respiratory rate need to be increased because tidal volume leaks are common. Settings for use of bilevel respiratory assist devices are presented in Chapter 77, Table 77–5.

Mechanical Considerations

One should anticipate that noninvasive ventilation will have an inspiratory air leak from the mouth if a nasal CPAP mask or nasal "pillows" (soft bulbous cannulas that make a good fit into the patient's nares) are used. Leaks are less common around the mask when a full-face CPAP mask is used. Interventions such as use of a chin strap or changing from a nasal mask to a full-face mask may help. In general, once the best-fitting mask is in place, one adjusts the tidal volume such that the measured exhaled tidal volumes are in the desired range. If exhaled volumes are not measurable, one follows $Paco_2$, usually with the help of an arterial catheter.

Clinical Considerations

Indications for noninvasive ventilation are increasing as its usefulness is being explored in different disorders. Controlled studies have shown it to be an effective, safe, and less costly option than invasive ventilation in patients with congestive heart failure and acute cardiogenic pulmonary edema and in certain patients with chronic obstructive pulmonary disease (COPD) flares. However, patients with

COPD who need frequent tracheal suctioning or have a poor cough are not good candidates for noninvasive ventilation. Finally, it is contraindicated in patients who have had recent esophageal or gastrointestinal surgery in whom distending the esophagus or stomach with air would be unsafe.

PATIENT MANAGEMENT DURING MECHANICAL VENTILATION

Monitoring and Alarms

Monitoring patients receiving mechanical ventilation is essential to their safe management. This monitoring takes many forms that anticipate potential problems related to (1) the intrinsic function of the ventilator, (2) the ventilator-patient interface, and (3) the patient's physiologic status. These are discussed more fully in Chapter 48.

Dyssynchrony Between Patient and Ventilator

Lack of synchrony between the patient and the ventilator in terms of breathing patterns is probably the most common complication of mechanical ventilation. Usually, the patient is dyspneic and struggling to breathe so that lack of synchrony between patient and ventilator means continued respiratory distress for the patient and a possibly increased risk of barotrauma. Dealing with interface problems between the patient and the ventilator is more of an art than a science once physiologic causes of the distress, such as hypercapnia and hypoxemia, are ruled out. Experienced respiratory care practitioners and ICU nurses should be sought for guidance in making ventilator adjustments and in calming the distressed patient by reassurance or medications. Because most patients receiving invasive ventilation are receiving sedatives, these can be increased in dosage, if necessary, to improve synchrony between the patient and the ventilator (see Chapter 4).

Complications of Mechanical Ventilation

A host of complications are associated with intubation and mechanical ventilation (Table 2–2). Many of these are discussed in detail in Chapters 11, 24, 26 to 28, 32, and 48. Salt and water retention are believed to occur primarily through the effects of positive pressure ventilation on cardiac output and renal perfusion, but decreases in secretion in atrial natriuretic factor may also play a role.

Patient Dysphoria

Having an endotracheal tube in one's trachea, feeling suffocated from secretions that need suctioning, or enduring painful sensations during suctioning are unpleasant and frightening experiences for awake and alert ICU patients on mechanical ventilation. These are in addition to the pain, fear, and other physical and emotional

Table 2–2. Complications of Mechanical Ventilation

....

Gas Exchange Problems

Acute respiratory alkalosis due to overventilation of patients with chronic CO_2 retention
Hyperventilation, including ventilator "self-cycling" due to sensitivity being set too low
Hypoventilation, especially due to cuff leaks or inappropriate settings or mode
Hypoxemia due to atelectasis (secretions, lack of turning, or tube malposition)

Tube Problems

Intubation of right main branches
Excessive airway resistance due to kinking, clogging, and so on
Self-extubation
Tracheomalacia due to excessive cuff pressures (>25 cm H_2O)

Other Problems

Auto-PEEP with hypotension
Barotrauma, including tension pneumothroax
Dysphoria (due to endotracheal tube and suctioning)
Microatelectasis and macroatelectasis
Nosocomial pneumonia
Sodium and water retention
Ventilator-associated lung injury ("volutrauma") (see Chapter 73)

....

PEEP, positive end-expiratory ventilation.

discomforts caused by their underlying conditions or their other ICU interventions. For these reasons, virtually all noncomatose patients on ventilators should be treated for dysphoric sensations, such as with benzodiazepines for anxiolysis, sedation, and amnesia and opioids for sedation and analgesia (see Chapter 4).

AUTO-PEEP (INTRINSIC PEEP)

Definition and Detection

Auto-PEEP is defined as the presence of positive alveolar pressure at the start of a new inspiration that is not due to applied PEEP (Fig. 2–6). Levels of auto-PEEP can range from trivial (1 to 2 mm Hg) with no adverse effects to substantial (>20 mm Hg), causing severe, life-threatening problems. It has also been called "occult PEEP" because it does not appear on the pressure gauge of the ventilator (Fig. 2–6C). Its presence, however, can be reliably inferred by inspection of the ventilator's display of waveforms for pressure and flow (Fig. 2–7). Some degree of auto-PEEP is present in all patients with significant airway obstruction during mechanical ventilation.

Certain ventilators can measure auto-PEEP in spontaneously breathing patients by using a shutter valve that activates at the end of expiration and then measuring the pressure in the tubing circuit after it equilibrates with alveolar pressure. One can also estimate its magnitude by making a well-timed occlusion of the expiratory port just before the start of inspiration (see Fig. 2–6D).

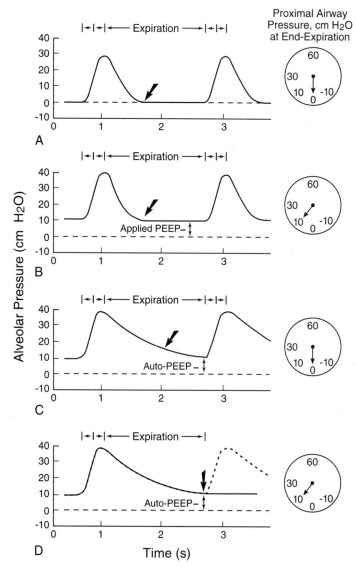

Figure 2–6. Schematic alveolar pressures during ventilation in A/C mode (without triggering by patient). *A*, No applied PEEP and no auto-PEEP. Note that alveolar pressure returns to baseline well before start of next breath *(arrow)*. *B*, 10 cm H_2O of applied PEEP with no auto-PEEP. Again, note return of pressure to baseline *(arrow)*. *C*, No applied PEEP with 10 cm H_2O of auto-PEEP. Note the delay in return of the alveolar pressure to baseline *(arrow)* and that the pressure gauge of the ventilator (representing proximal airway pressure at end-expiration) does not detect the auto-PEEP. *D*, If one stops expiratory flow just prior to start of next breath *(arrow)*, the pressure gauge indicates the presence of auto-PEEP and estimates its magnitude. I, inspiration; PEEP, positive end-expiratory pressure. (Modified from Lanken PN: Mechanical ventilation. In: Fishman AP [ed]: Pulmonary Diseases and Disorders, 2nd ed. New York: McGraw-Hill, 1988.)

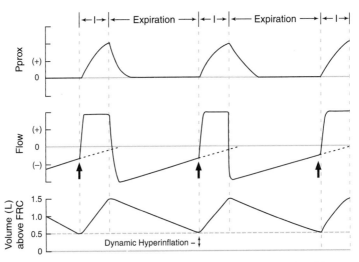

Figure 2–7. Schematic diagram of mechanical ventilation on assist/control mode (with no spontaneous breathing efforts), as in Figure 2–4A, but with airway obstruction and auto-PEEP. Note that the expiratory flow does not reach zero before the onset of the next breath *(arrow)*, resulting in dynamic hyperinflation. Delaying the start of the next breath until expiratory flow *(dashed line)* reaches zero would prevent auto-PEEP. PEEP, positive end-expiratory pressure; FRC, functional residual capacity; Pprox, pressure at proximal end of endotracheal tube; I, inspiration; (+), inspiratory flow; (−), expiratory flow.

Physiology, Adverse Effects, and Management

Auto-PEEP arises when there is insufficient time for full expiration such that the lungs do not return to their baseline FRC by the start of the next breath. This leads to stacking of the new breath before full expiration of the prior breath and results in a new, increased FRC (see Figs. 2–6 and 2–7). This process of stacking continues until the patient's FRC reaches a new equilibrium. This stacking is also referred to as *dynamic hyperinflation*. High levels of auto-PEEP and dynamic hyperinflation can cause several problems. First, in patients intubated for asthma, the increased risk of *barotrauma* at high levels of auto-PEEP correlates best with the degree of dynamic hyperinflation. In addition, auto-PEEP may cause *hypotension* and *falls in cardiac output*, especially in hypovolemic patients. These cardiovascular effects arise because auto-PEEP makes the pleural pressure more positive during the respiratory cycle. This, in turn, decreases venous return to the thorax (the "central tourniquet" effect), with the end result being decreased cardiac preload (see Chapter 7).

In addition to these hemodynamic effects, auto-PEEP can result in patients struggling to breathe during mechanical ventilation and interfere with weaning. In both instances, the problem lies in the need for the patient's spontaneous inspiratory efforts to first overcome the positive alveolar pressure caused by the auto-PEEP before being able to trigger the ventilator. If auto-PEEP reaches 15 to 20 cm H_2O or more, overcoming this extra elastic load can result in respiratory muscle fatigue and prolonged ventilatory support.

One can easily diagnose the presence of auto-PEEP–induced hypotension if the

Table 2–3. Managing Auto-PEEP

....

Address Causes of Auto-PEEP

Treat underlying bronchospasm and airway inflammation (see Chapter 74)
Prolong expiratory time relative to inspiratory time
    Shorten inspiratory time
        Increase inspiratory flow rate
        Decrease tidal volume
    Decrease respiratory rate
Change from A/C mode to IMV mode

Address Effects of Auto-PEEP

Expand intravascular volume
Give vasopressors for blood pressure support (if hypotensive)

....

A/C, assist/control; IMV, intermittent mandatory ventilation; PEEP, positive end-expiratory pressure.

blood pressure quickly (almost instantaneously) returns to normal when patients are removed from the ventilator temporarily, such as for tracheal suctioning. Transient removal from the ventilator allows patients with auto-PEEP enough time to empty their lungs. Management of auto-PEEP and its adverse effects are described in Table 2–3.

PEARLS AND PITFALLS

One can determine how much to change minute ventilation to get the desired change in $Paco_2$ by using a graphic approach (see Appendix B, Fig. 1) or its algebraic equivalent (Equation 3). This can avoid the common problem of overventilation of chronic CO_2-retaining patients.

$$Paco_2(1) \times \dot{V}E(1) = Paco_2(2) \times \dot{V}E(2) \qquad \text{(Equation 3)}$$

where $Paco_2(1)$ is the $Paco_2$ with the baseline minute ventilation, $\dot{V}E(1)$, and $Paco_2(2)$ is the $Paco_2$ predicted to occur after the minute ventilation is changed to another value, $\dot{V}E(2)$. Because this equation assumes that ratio of dead space to tidal volume (V_D/V_T) and $\dot{V}CO_2$ remain constant despite changes in minute ventilation, minute ventilation must be increased or decreased only by *changing respiratory rate*, that is, without changes in tidal volume or ventilatory mode.

BIBLIOGRAPHY

Drinker P, McKhann CF: The use of a new apparatus for the prolonged administration of artificial respiration. I. A fatal case of poliomyelitis. JAMA 92:1658–1660, 1929.
    This is the landmark paper describing the successful first trial of the "iron lung" in which an 8-year-old with polio was ventilated for 122 hours.
Hill NS: Noninvasive mechanical ventilation: Does it work, for whom and how? Am Rev Respir Dis 147:1050–1055, 1993.
    This is a review of the use of noninvasive ventilation.

Hillberg RE, Johnson DC: Noninvasive ventilation. N Engl J Med 337:1746–1752, 1997.
This is a review of noninvasive ventilation, including bilevel ventilatory assist devices, and their use in chronic and acute respiratory failure and congestive heart failure.

Ibsen B: The anaesthetist's viewpoint on the treatment of respiratory complications in poliomyelitis during the epidemic in Copenhagen, 1952. Proc R Soc Med 47:72–74, 1954.
This is the classic description of the first widespread use of positive pressure ventilation resulting in impressive survival rates.

Jubran A, Tobin MJ: Monitoring during mechanical ventilation. Clin Chest Med 17:453–474, 1996.
This is a comprehensive review of monitoring of different types, including arterial blood gases, capnography, and pulmonary mechanics.

MacIntyre NR: New modes of mechanical ventilation. Clin Chest Med 17:411–421, 1996.
This is a review comparing and contrasting new modes and concepts in mechanical ventilation.

MacIntyre NR: Respiratory function during pressure support ventilation. Chest 89:677–683, 1986.
This is an early description of the use of pressure support mode of ventilation.

Marini JJ, Rodriguez RM, Lamb V: The inspiratory workload of patient-initiated mechanical ventilation. Am Rev Respir Dis 134:902–909, 1986.
This study describes the extent of continued inspiratory efforts while on assist mode of ventilation.

Meyer TJ, Hill NS: Noninvasive positive pressure ventilation to treat respiratory failure. Ann Intern Med 120:760–770, 1994.
This is a comprehensive, state-of-the-art review of multiple studies utilizing positive pressure noninvasive ventilation in both acute and chronic respiratory failure, including the indications for and mechanisms of nocturnal ventilation.

Nava S, Ambrosino N, Clini E, et al: Noninvasive mechanical ventilation in the weaning of patients with respiratory failure due to chronic obstructive pulmonary disease. A randomized, controlled trial. Ann Intern Med 128:721–728, 1998.
This recent study of patients intubated for a COPD flare compared switching with noninvasive ventilation for weaning starting at 48 hours after intubation compared with remaining on conventional ventilation. Those switched had faster weaning (with a mean of 10.2 days vs. 16.6 days, higher probability of weaning and 60-day survival, and shorter ICU stay.

Pepe PE, Marini JJ: Occult positive end-expiratory pressure in mechanically ventilated patients with airflow obstruction: The auto-PEEP effect. Am Rev Respir Dis 126:166–170, 1982.
This was the first description of auto-PEEP in the ICU setting and how to measure it.

Tobin MJ: Mechanical ventilation. N Engl J Med 330:1056–1061, 1994.
This is a concise review, including weaning methods, by one of the experts in the field.

3   Weaning and Extubation

Paul N. Lanken

Critical care clinicians routinely "liberate" their patients from mechanical ventilation to allow them to resume breathing on their own. Although the transition from assisted to spontaneous ventilation traditionally has been referred to as "weaning," the process does not have to be gradual or time-consuming. Even though stopping assisted ventilation may be a long ordeal for some patients, it is accomplished over a relatively short period for most.

This chapter discusses two basic questions: (1) When should mechanical ventilation be stopped and the patient extubated? and (2) How should mechanical ventilation be stopped?

The answer to the first question is "as soon as it is safe and reasonably likely that the patient can succeed in breathing spontaneously and protect his or her airway." To determine this point accurately, several critical tasks should be performed. First, obtain a history of the patient's health and respiratory status at baseline, before development of acute respiratory failure. Second, appreciate the mechanism and pathophysiology of the patient's respiratory failure (see Chapter 1) or other reasons why the patient was started on assisted ventilation. Third, clarify how far the patient has come along his or her path to recovery. Fourth, assess the patient's current physiologic capacities to maintain adequate oxygenation, ventilation, and airway protection.

In answer to the second question, mechanical ventilation should be stopped by the safest and fastest available method. To decide this, one needs to understand the pros and cons of the ways used to discontinue mechanical ventilation and their relative efficacy and safety based on experience and results of controlled clinical trials.

WHEN TO STOP ASSISTED VENTILATION?–THE "FIRST FIX WHAT'S BROKEN" APPROACH

In this approach, one starts with the underlying assumption that patients cannot be successfully removed from mechanical ventilation unless the problems causing their respiratory failure in the first place are treated and reversed. To accomplish this, one should begin by identifying how the patient's respiratory failure developed (see Chapter 1). Failure of nonrespiratory organ systems that contributed to or even precipitated the need for mechanical ventilation (e.g., cardiac arrest resulting from a primary cardiac arrhythmia) also need to be addressed appropriately before mechanical ventilation is stopped.

This approach can be especially helpful when diverse disease processes and complications are involved. For example, a patient being mechanically ventilated immediately after undergoing heart surgery may have a depressed central nervous system drive to breathe because of the effects of intraoperative opioids. The function of the patient's chest bellows may be compromised by the operative incision and associated pain, by pleural effusions, or by phrenic nerve dysfunction resulting from exposure to cold cardioplegia. Furthermore, the patient's airway may be obstructed if he or she has chronic obstructive pulmonary disease (COPD), and alveolar gas exchange may be compromised by atelectasis and pulmonary edema. Finally, a shivering patient may be reacting to hypothermia after bypass surgery.

Predictably, the workload on the patient's respiratory pump (also referred to as ventilatory demand) is increased by the presence of an increased ratio of dead space to tidal volume (V_D/V_T), airflow obstruction, pulmonary edema, atelectasis, and increased CO_2 production (from the shivering) (Table 3–1). At the same time, ventilatory pump capacity is limited by the surgical incision and pain, loss of lung volume from multiple causes, and respiratory muscle dysfunction caused by phrenic nerve injury, poor diaphragmatic perfusion, electrolyte disorders, and possibly residual effects of neuromuscular blockers (Table 3–2).

CATEGORIES OF PROBLEMS TO CONSIDER AND FIX

Neurologic Impairment and Central Nervous System Drive Problems

Three categories of neurologic impairment may prevent or delay successful discontinuation of assisted ventilation and extubation:

1. Loss of upper airway protective reflexes
2. Decreased level of consciousness
3. Effects on the central respiratory drive by hypoventilation syndromes or metabolic acid-base disturbances

Loss of Upper Airway Protection

After extubation, some patients may be at risk of clinically significant aspiration or failure to clear their respiratory secretions. Both can prevent patients from being able to maintain spontaneous breathing. Before extubation, patients must be

Table 3–1. Factors and Causes Increasing Ventilatory Demand

FACTORS	CAUSES
Increased V_D/V_T	Acute respiratory distress syndrome, asthma, emphysema, pulmonary emboli
Increased oxygen consumption	Fever, increased work of breathing, morbid obesity, sepsis, shivering, trauma
Increased respiratory quotient (increased CO_2 production relative to O_2 consumption)	Excessive carbohydrate feeding
Decreased set point for Pa_{CO_2}	Anxiety, central neurogenic hyperventilation, hepatic failure, hypoxemia, metabolic acidosis, renal failure, sepsis

From Lanken PN: Respiratory failure: An overview. In: Carlson RW, Geheb MA (eds): Principles and Practice of Medical Intensive Care. Philadelphia: WB Saunders, 1993, pp 754–763.

V_D/V_T, dead space-to-tidal volume ratio.

Table 3–2. Factors and Examples Reducing Ventilatory Capacity

CATEGORIES AND FACTORS	EXAMPLES
Decreased Respiratory Muscle Strength	
Fatigue of respiratory muscle	During recovery period from fatigue, high respiratory rates, increased inspiratory time
Disuse atrophy	Prolonged mechanical ventilation; status-postphrenic nerve injury or transection
Malnutrition	Protein-calorie starvation
Electrolyte abnormalities	Low phosphate, low potassium
Alteration in force-length relationship of the hemidiaphragms	Flattened domes of diaphragms caused by dynamic hyperinflation
Drug-induced weakness	Effects of neuromuscular blocking drugs
Increased Muscular Energetics or Decreased Substrate Supply	
High elastic work of breathing	Low lung or chest wall compliance, high respiratory rates
High resistive work of breathing	Expiratory airways obstruction, high flow rates
Decreased perfusion of diaphragm	Circulatory shock states, anemia
Abnormal Respiratory Mechanics	
Flow limitation	Bronchospasm, upper airway obstruction, airways secretions
Loss of lung volume	Atelectasis, lung resection, pleural effusions
Other restrictive defects	Incisional or other pain-limiting inspiration; tense abdomen caused by ileus, peritoneal dialysis, or ascites

From Lanken PN: Respiratory failure: An overview. In: Carlson RW, Geheb MA (eds): Principles and Practice of Medical Intensive Care. Philadelphia: WB Saunders, 1993, pp 754–763.

assessed for the presence of adequate cough and gag reflexes and the ability to cough well enough to clear their secretions (Table 3–3). If patients lack a good cough or are otherwise unable to clear secretions by themself, weaning patients from assisted ventilation can progress but extubation should be delayed. If the patient cannot adequately protect his or her airway or clear tracheal secretions, in general, it is safest to proceed with an elective tracheostomy. This allows a secure access to the airways for suctioning secretions and is more comfortable than

Table 3–3. Criteria for Adequate Protection of Upper Airway*

1. **Cough reflex:** present and judged at least moderate in strength
2. **Volitional coughing:** patient can cough on command with good strength
3. **Tracheal secretions:** not voluminous, not tenacious, not requiring suctioning at hourly intervals or less, and mobilizable by the patient's efforts
4. **Gag reflex:** present and at least moderate in strength

*Criteria 1 through 3 must be met before extubation. If only criterion 4 is not fulfilled, the patient can be extubated except if there is a high risk of massive aspiration, such as with partial small bowel obstruction. In all cases, swallowing function after extubation must be carefully tested before any oral intake (see Chapter 24).

continuation of an endotracheal tube. A tracheostomy is also useful for monitoring aspiration of oral fluids during assessment of swallowing function.

The presence of swallowing dysfunction should be assessed in all recently extubated patients before oral intake. This is especially important in patients with poor or absent gag reflexes and in patients with tracheostomies who can breathe off the ventilator for sustained periods (see Chapter 24).

Decreased Mental Status

Intensive care unit (ICU) patients commonly have a decreased level of consciousness, sometimes because they are heavily sedated. Level of consciousness influences attempts at weaning and extubation in three major ways. First, a depressed mental status may result in loss of upper airway protection, as discussed earlier. Patients with decreased mental status may also have decreased respiratory drive. As long as respiratory drive is persistently absent or minimal, assisted ventilation is necessary. However, when the lack of respiratory drive is due to the absence of chemical stimuli to breathe, a tapering of assistance in breathing is reasonable and often effective. For example, well-oxygenated patients who are alkalemic because of iatrogenic hyperventilation while on mechanical ventilation may not breathe until their $Paco_2$ levels are allowed to return to normal.

Second, it is important to be aware of patients with a history of central or obstructive apneas or who have a central hypoventilation syndrome, such as obesity hypoventilation syndrome (see Chapter 77), or periodic breathing, such as Cheyne-Stokes breathing. Attempts to wean a patient with sleep apnea and hypoventilation by a ventilator mode that depends on the patient initiating breaths, such as pressure support, will be unsuccessful. Doing so may make it seem that the patient is unweanable when, in fact, the patient may only require ventilatory assistance at night. As another point of caution, because patients with obesity hypoventilation syndrome and other central hypoventilation syndromes usually lack normal responsiveness to elevations in $Paco_2$, they do not exhibit respiratory distress when $Paco_2$ increases. This may give the ICU staff the false impression that they are breathing fine during a trial of spontaneous breathing when, in fact, their $Paco_2$ has doubled.

Third, in contrast to patients who do not breathe enough, some patients breathe too much. For example, patients who have had a brainstem stroke may breathe with a marked tachypnea as a result of central neurogenic hyperventilation. As a rule, adults cannot sustain persistent respiratory rates of more than 36 to 40 breaths per minute; eventually they will develop respiratory muscle fatigue. Suppression of respiratory drive by high-dose opioids may be successful in such patients, allowing them to be weaned.

Metabolic Acid-Base Disorders

Central nervous system drive can be altered by either metabolic acidosis or metabolic alkalosis. On the one hand, patients with a metabolic acidosis (serum HCO_3^- <18–20 mEq/L) must "blow down" their $Paco_2$, that is, hyperventilate, to keep arterial pH in the normal range. This means that elevated alveolar and minute ventilation are required when breathing spontaneously (see figure in Appendix B).

This requirement for extra ventilation may tilt the balance between ventilatory capacity and demand in favor of demand and lead to respiratory muscle fatigue. In this case, one should first treat the metabolic acidosis to elevate serum HCO_3^- to a level that does not tax the patient's capacity to maintain respiratory compensation.

On the other hand, patients with a severe metabolic alkalosis (serum HCO_3^- >45–55 mEq/L) have no pH stimulus to breathe when their $Paco_2$ is 40 mm Hg. Hypercapnia develops as respiratory compensation for the acidosis. Hypercapnia in such a patient may be mistakenly attributed to respiratory muscle fatigue and delay weaning.

Another common problem relating to elevated serum HCO_3^- levels or, more precisely, the lack thereof, is the patient with COPD and chronic CO_2 retention whose serum HCO_3^- is above normal as a result of renal compensation for the chronic respiratory acidosis. If mechanical ventilation reduces $Paco_2$ to normal and if serum HCO_3^- likewise decreases to normal (as should occur in the absence of a stimulus for renal compensation), these patients, as a rule, develop increasing respiratory acidosis, dyspnea, tachypnea, and, eventually, respiratory muscle fatigue when assisted ventilation is discontinued. The preferred approach is to ventilate patients with COPD and chronic CO_2 retention to keep their $Paco_2$ at an elevated level, close to baseline. This also tends to maintain the baseline elevated serum HCO_3^- so that, when the patient's pulmonary function has returned toward its baseline, weaning has a reasonable chance to be successful.

Chest Bellows and Peripheral Nervous System Problems

Respiratory Muscle Weakness

In some patients, respiratory muscle weakness occurs as a primary event, for example, when a neuromuscular disorder directly weakens the muscles; in others, it occurs secondary to effects of critical illness or respiratory failure (see Table 3–2), for example, when fatigued respiratory muscles are not yet recovered fully (which may take up to 1 day). Alternatively, the muscles may atrophy, such as occurs with disuse or protein malnutrition. Other deleterious factors for muscle function include metabolic disorders such as hypophosphatemia and hypokalemia. Severe hyperinflation, such as results from airflow obstruction and auto–positive end-expiratory pressure (auto-PEEP), compromises the efficiency of the length-tension relationship of the normally situated diaphragm and exacerbates the effects of muscle weakness.

Changes in Chest Bellows Function

Various factors can limit lung or chest expansion. One important factor is the effects of incisions in postoperative states and degree of pain control. For example, prior to modern pain management strategies (see Chapter 85), on the first postoperative day, a patient's vital capacity often decreased to only about 25% of preoperative values after thoracotomy or even after open cholecystectomy. Other common factors include flail chest after accidents or closed chest cardiac resuscitation; pleural effusions; major atelectasis; and effects of abdominal distension due to air, ascites, dialysate, or edema.

Airways Problems

Airflow Obstruction

If severe airways obstruction was the reason for respiratory failure, it must be reversed before the patient can be weaned. Standard regimens usually accomplish this after several days, although some patients may recover more slowly than others. For example, injuries to airways from smoke inhalation may be particularly refractory. Consequences of acute airways obstruction include decreased ventilatory capacity as a result of airflow obstruction and a compromise in the force-tension relationship resulting from hyperinflation (flatting the domes of the diaphragms). In addition, as a rule, ventilatory load is increased by a markedly increased V_D/V_T, increased resistive work of breathing, and tachypnea (caused by vagal afferents stimulating the respiratory drive).

Inspiratory Loading due to Auto-PEEP

An additional important inspiratory load arises from effects of auto-PEEP on triggering the ventilator or opening the ventilator's demand valve. To trigger the ventilator, the patient's inspiratory efforts must be detected by the ventilator. This is usually done by setting the ventilator to recognize a certain negative pressure, for example, -1 cm H_2O, in the inspiratory circuit as the triggering threshold. If auto-PEEP is present, however, the patient's inspiratory efforts must overcome *both* the auto-PEEP and the threshold negative pressure in order to trigger the ventilator (see Chapter 2, Fig. 2–7).

For example, if auto-PEEP is high (>12–15 cm H_2O), a substantial extra burden is added to the inspiratory muscles to the point of causing respiratory muscle fatigue. In these circumstances, having 14 cm H_2O auto-PEEP present with the triggering sensitivity set at -1 cm H_2O is like setting the sensitivity at -15 cm H_2O. Although such a high sensitivity setting would be recognized as contraindicated and potentially deleterious for weaning patients, the presence of high auto-PEEP may go unappreciated and untreated. Treatment of auto-PEEP during weaning trials should combine more aggressive treatment of the underlying airway obstruction plus external PEEP that is equal to, or almost equal to, the level of auto-PEEP present. Adding external PEEP to the inspiratory circuit "resets" the sensitivity level. In the example used here, adding 14 cm H_2O external PEEP would restore the sensitivity to -1 cm H_2O for the patient's inspiratory muscles. Some ventilators can measure auto-PEEP as part of their monitoring package. Otherwise, one can estimate its value by occluding the expiratory tubing or port just before start of the next inspiration and reading the pressure in the circuit on the pressure gauge of the ventilator or the digital readout (see Fig. 2–7).

Performing a Tracheostomy to Facilitate Weaning

Traditionally, recommendations for a tracheostomy were commonly made after about 2 weeks of mechanical ventilation (see Chapter 24). The purpose of the tracheostomy was to facilitate weaning and to provide an airway that was more secure and comfortable than the endotracheal tube. Gradually, however, intensivists have become more comfortable with the practice of extending the period of use of endotracheal tubes beyond 2 weeks, depending on when they anticipate the patient can be extubated.

One additional reason why tracheostomy tubes tend to facilitate weaning in patients on mechanical ventilation for several weeks or more has recently become apparent. Such patients have a previously unrecognized source of increased work of breathing and auto-PEEP: their endotracheal tube. Recently, it was reported that replacement of an endotracheal tube with a tracheostomy of the *same* internal diameter resulted in significant *decreases* in work of breathing and in auto-PEEP. The problems with the removed endotracheal tubes were studied in vitro and their added resistance was accounted for by the presence of a microlayer of secretions and other build-up on its inner surface. Previously, this microlayer was identified as a reservoir for microorganisms that are dislodged into the lower respiratory tract with every suctioning. In addition, it appears that it also may delay weaning because of its mechanical properties in patients with borderline pulmonary function and prolonged ventilatory support. This finding adds a new layer of concern to the practice of trying to extend the use of endotracheal tubes and adds another factor in favor of timely tracheostomy in the challenge to wean patient.

Alveolar Flooding Problems

Problems with failure of the alveolar component predominantly are reflected by (1) the persistent need for high FIO_2 (≥ 0.5) and for PEEP (>5 cm H_2O), (2) the high elastic work of breathing (caused by stiff lungs), and (3) an increased drive to breathe, causing tachypnea (resulting from vagal and phrenic afferents). The lung stiffness and the restrictive defect produced by flooding of alveoli with edema fluid also limits ventilatory capacity.

Even though supplementary high-flow oxygen can be supplied to patients after discontinuation of mechanical ventilation, as a rule, a conservative approach is taken with regard to requiring a threshold level of adequate oxygenation before extubation (Table 3–4). If mechanisms to maintain normoxia are borderline before weaning, the risk of hypoxemia increases after weaning.

Table 3–4. Criteria for Adequate Capacity for Oxygenation*

....

1. **Ability** to achieve an arterial oxygen saturation ≥ 92–95% or PaO_2 >60 mm Hg with
   FIO_2 ≤ 0.5 and
   PEEP ≤ 5 cm H_2O and
   PaO_2/FIO_2 >200
2. **Trend** of FIO_2 and PEEP in the right direction:
   FIO_2 (at present) equal to or lower than the FIO_2 used the previous day
   PEEP (at present) equal to or lower than the PEEP used the previous day
3. **Stability** in oxygenation as demonstrated by no episodes of arterial desaturation
   $<88\%$ in the prior 24 h

....

*All three criteria need to be present at the time of assessment.
PEEP, positive end-expiratory pressure; FIO_2, fraction of inspired oxygen.

Problems from Nonrespiratory Organ Systems

Some common problems that interfere with stopping assisted ventilation are cardiovascular. These include left ventricular failure with pulmonary edema (often occult or refractory to therapy), atrial and ventricular arrhythmias, episodic or persistent hypotension with continuing vasopressor therapy, and low cardiac output states with poor perfusion of other organs such as kidneys or liver.

Patients with acute respiratory failure plus end-stage renal disease or acute renal failure may also be problematic to wean. First, they are susceptible to intravascular volume overload with pulmonary edema. In addition, they have the metabolic acidosis associated with their renal failure. Despite intensive intermittent hemodialysis, it is difficult to sufficiently elevate serum HCO_3^- to compensate for chronic CO_2 retention in COPD patients on a ventilator. This alone makes successful weaning unlikely.

Likewise, patients with end-stage liver disease (ESLD) have their own set of difficulties in weaning. If they have active gastrointestinal bleeding from varices or from severe coagulopathy, they need airway protection to prevent aspiration of blood. They also usually have ascites, which, if severe, compromises the chest bellows and full descent of the diaphragms or causes pleural effusions and a restrictive defect or both. Finally, ESLD by itself causes hyperventilation, which increases ventilatory load.

When to Stop Assisted Ventilation?–Testing for Physiologic Capacities

To do well after stopping assisted ventilation and extubation, patients need to have adequate function in three major capacities:

1. Capacity to protect and clear their upper airway.
2. Capacity to oxygenate
3. Capacity to ventilate

Criteria for assessing the adequacy of each capacity are presented in Tables 3–3 to 3–6.

A number of other parameters have traditionally been used to assess whether patients are able to be removed from the ventilator. Some that are used to predict ability to breathe spontaneously are vital capacity greater than 10 mL/kg, maximum inspiratory pressure less than -20 cm H_2O, resting minute ventilation less than 10 L/min, maximum voluntary ventilation greater than 2 times the resting minute ventilation, and V_D/V_T less than 0.6. Prospective trials of these parameters, however, indicated that their predictive value as screening tests was poor and that the single screening test with the most utility was the rapid-shallow breathing index (Table 3–5).

Rather than using single test or a set of physiologic tests to make the determination of adequacy of capacity to ventilate, some intensivists have adopted the use of trials of spontaneous breathing after patients have met certain screening criteria similar to those listed in Tables 3–4 to 3–6. The steps of this

Table 3–5. Assessing Ventilatory Capacity: Screening Criteria

....

Patient Must First Pass All Criteria Listed

Absence of serious cardiac arrhythmias
Absence of hemodynamic instability and off vasopressors (except low-dose dopamine)
Presence of respiratory efforts
Oxygenation criteria met (see Table 3–4)
Respiratory rate-to-tidal volume ratio <105 breaths/min/L*
Adequate capacity to cough and clear secretions (see Table 3–3)

....

*Perform the test only if all the preceding criteria in the table are met. Test: Allow patient to breath spontaneously for 1 min with 5 cm H_2O continuous positive airway pressure, no change in FIO_2, and no mandatory breaths. Use ventilator to measure minute ventilation and respiratory rate and obtain tidal volume by dividing the minute ventilation by the rate.

screening process are often written as unit-based protocols that are managed by ICU respiratory care providers and nurses. Management of these protocols by persons other than physicians permits screening to be performed on a daily basis routinely, before physician rounds. In ICUs that use these protocols in this manner, they have become established as effective tools for timely removal of the ventilator and extubation. Controlled studies indicate that such protocols lead to shorter periods of mechanical ventilation and ICU length of stay without an increase in rate of reintubations compared with decisions that are made without using such protocols.

Table 3–6. Assessing Ventilatory Capacity: Trial of Spontaneous Breathing

....

1. **Screening criteria:** Patient must have passed all criteria listed in Table 3–5 earlier on same day.
2. **Preparatory steps:**
   Place patient as upright as possible in bed.
   Reassure patient about breathing on his or her own.
   Suction airway well, ensure that monitoring is in place, and note baseline vital signs.
   Keep FIO_2 the same as on the ventilator or increase current FIO_2 by 0.1.
   Select one: CPAP with PS = 5 cm H_2O, Flow-Bye mode, or T-piece.
3. **Trial of spontaneous breathing***
   Plan to allow patient to breath spontaneously for up to 2 h.
       Monitor ECG, pulse, respiratory rate, tidal volumes (if on CPAP or Flow-Bye), SaO_2 by pulse oximetry, blood pressure, and signs of dyspnea or other serious problems (e.g., angina).
   Stop the trial earlier for any of the following indications:
   Respiratory rate >35 breaths/min for >5 min
   Arterial O_2 saturation <90%
   Heart rate >140 beats/min or sustained changes >20% over or under baseline rate
   Serious arrhythmias
   Systolic blood pressure >180 mm Hg or <90 mm Hg
   Moderate or severe respiratory distress (increased anxiety or diaphoresis)
4. **Successful trial:** The patient breathes without mechanical ventilation for 2 h.

....

*Modified from Ely EW, Baker AM, Dunagan DP, et al: Effect on the duration of mechanical ventilation of identifying patients capable of breathing spontaneously. N Engl J Med 335:1864–1869, 1996.

CPAP, continuous positive airway pressure; ECG, electrocardiogram; PS, pressure support; SaO_2, oxygen saturation.

Successful Trial of Spontaneous Breathing

Test Characteristics

If a patient passes the screening criteria (see Table 3–5) and the trial of spontaneous breathing (see Table 3–6), and if he demonstrates adequate capacity to protect and clear his or her upper airway (see Table 3–3), then he or she should be considered a good candidate for extubation. To make the final decision regarding stopping ventilation and extubation, however, one should consider the combination of screening criteria and trial as a diagnostic test having a false-positive rate (patient passes test but needs to be reintubated) and false-negative rate (patient fails the test but can ventilate spontaneously successfully). The percent of extubated patients passing the test but needing to be reintubated within 48 hours (i.e., the false-positive rate) ranges from 4 to 18%. These results necessitate a certain period of intense monitoring in the ICU after stopping mechanical ventilation or extubation. How long this degree of monitoring should be continued depends on one's clinical assessment of each patient because specific risk factors for reintubation have not been well defined by prospective studies. If the patient needs ventilatory support after extubation, one should consider applying *noninvasive* ventilation first, before reintubation (see Chapter 77).

Extubation Steps

In general, extubation is carried out through a series of steps: (1) explain to the patient about the extubation, (2) sit the patient erect in bed, (3) suction the airways, (4) suction secretions that may have pooled above the cuff, (5) deflate the cuff and remove the artificial airway, and (6) treat the patient with an appropriate level of supplemental oxygen.

Postextubation Upper Airway Obstruction

Upper airway obstruction and stridor occur in a few percent of patients over the first approximately 60 minutes after extubation. If this occurs, the patient should be monitored closely for respiratory failure. Treatment includes inhaled alpha-adrenergic agents (to vasoconstrict blood vessels), intravenous corticosteroids (e.g., 60 mg methylprednisolone), and noninvasive ventilation. If stridor progresses to respiratory failure, reintubation is needed. Some patients may be known to be at high risk for upper airway obstruction after extubation (e.g., persons intubated for smoke inhalation, stridor, or acute epiglottitis). In these cases, it is prudent to check the patency of the supraglottic space surrounding the endotracheal tube before extubation. Although this can be done by direct inspection using a fiberoptic nasopharyngoscope, a simpler approach is to test for an air leak when the cuff of the endotracheal tube is deflated. If the patient's air leak around the deflated cuff is nil or modest (<100 mL per breath), one can assume that supraglottic obstruction is present and, on that basis, delay extubation until direct inspection of the upper airway confirms adequate space around the tube.

Unsuccessful Trial of Spontaneous Breathing

Failing the Trial

If a patient fails the trial of spontaneous breathing (see Table 3–6), in general, the patient should be considered as "not ready" for stopping assisted ventilation and extubation. In certain cases, however, the patient may be unsuccessful in the trial but still may be able to breathe successfully on his or her own (a false-negative result). It is unclear what fraction of patients who fail the trial are truly able to breathe spontaneously but it is assumed to be small. In borderline cases, the final decision whether to extubate should be based on one's clinical judgment, taking into account more than just the dichotomous results of the breathing trial.

For patients failing the trial who are judged not capable of ventilating adequately on their own, most intensivists would begin a trial of weaning (see Weaning Trials). In addition, one should review the clinical situation to optimize ventilatory capacity and decrease demand on the ventilatory system (see Tables 3–1 and 3–2). The ICU clinician's task is to identify which factors might be contributing to the patient's problem and to address treatable conditions appropriately to facilitate weaning.

Some ICUs that use noninvasive ventilation extensively have reported improved outcomes for patients intubated for COPD flares when they change those patients over to noninvasive ventilation after 48 hours of invasive ventilation. This shift applied only to patients with good mental status and ability to cough and clear secretions. The effectiveness and safety of this method, however, needs confirmation before it is recommended for widespread adoption by other ICUs.

Weaning Trials

All weaning techniques are based on the assumption that many patients on mechanical ventilation with poor ventilatory capacity can benefit from "training" their respiratory muscles, much like athletes do in training to improve their performance. Although this assumption seems reasonable from a physiologic perspective, the optimal clinical tactics to train respiratory muscles in most patients on mechanical ventilators remain undefined. Recent randomized, controlled clinical trials, however, have been helpful in this regard in suggesting that certain approaches work more effectively than others.

Two controlled clinical trials that studied discontinuing mechanical ventilation after 1 to 4 or more weeks of use have been reported. The studies found that weaning by once- or twice-daily T-piece trials or by pressure support were superior to weaning by synchronized intermittent mandatory ventilation (SIMV) in terms of producing shorter lengths of stay on mechanical ventilation. T-piece trials are limited periods of spontaneous ventilation during which the patient is off the ventilator and breathing through a plastic T-shaped accessory (hence the name, T-piece) (Fig. 3–1).

Despite these results, some ICUs still use IMV for weaning based on their personal or institutional experiences. For example, in "Challenge to Wean" patients, that is, patients with prolonged ventilator dependency (>30 days), factors other than the specific weaning method used also seem important in successful

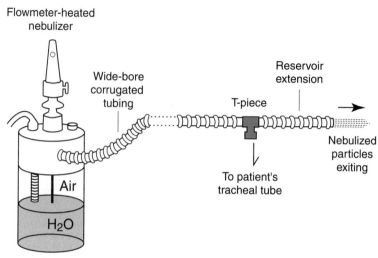

Flowmeter-heated nebulizer

Wide-bore corrugated tubing

Reservoir extension

T-piece

Nebulized particles exiting

To patient's tracheal tube

Air

H_2O

Figure 3–1. Equipment utilized in a T-piece trial. Oxygen is mixed with entrained ambient air in a heated nebulizer chamber to produce a specific FIO_2. This is then delivered to the patient's tracheal tube via wide-bore tubing and the T-piece. The extension tubing is used to prevent inspiration of ambient air. (From Lanken PN: Weaning from mechanical ventilation. In: Fishman AP [ed]: Update: Pulmonary Diseases and Disorders. New York: McGraw-Hill, 1982.)

outcomes. These include providing good nutrition, establishing sleep hygiene, setting goals, and using a multidisciplinary team to provide a program of comprehensive care (see Chapter 23).

T-Piece Trials (CPAP Trials)

This method stops assisted ventilation abruptly when one places the patient on a T-piece or equivalent. Using the continuous positive airway pressure (CPAP) mode of the ventilator with zero PEEP and 5 to 7 cm H_2O of pressure support (to overcome airway resistance of the tube) is considered by many to be nearly equivalent to a T-piece trial but with the added benefit of extensive monitoring. Some ventilators also have a special mode, which can be used as a substitute for a T-piece trial but without losing the ventilator's monitoring capabilities. The patient starts breathing on his or her own, usually for the duration that was tolerated during trial of spontaneous breathing, then that duration is gradually increased. If respiratory distress develops before the target time period is finished and the patient cannot be assisted in his or her efforts with coaching (or mild anxiolysis if anxiety is the main problem), then the patient is returned to the ventilator for a rest period. A repeat T-piece trial is usually attempted later that same day, but, depending on the clinical circumstances, it may be delayed until the morning of the next day in order to further improve the patient's clinical situation.

If the patient breathes well for one full 2-hour period, some clinicians would extubate the patient at that point; others would extubate after several such 2-hour periods of successful breathing, especially if the patient had undergone a prolonged course of mechanical ventilation. Because of their abrupt transition from 100%

Table 3–7. Pressure Support Weaning Protocol*

....

1. Place patient on a level of pressure support (PS) to keep the patient's respiratory rate at 25 breaths/min.
2. After 120 min at this level of PS with no signs of distress (see Table 3–5) and respiratory rate (RR) ≤25 breaths/min, decrease PS by 2–4 cm H_2O. If distress develops or RR >25 breaths/ min, go to step 5.
3. After each time period, as in step 2, decrease PS by 2–4 cm H_2O and observe for distress or RR >25 breaths/min.
4. After 120 min at PS of 5 cm H_2O without distress or RR >25 breaths/min, extubate the patient.
5. If distress develops or RR >25 breaths/min, return to the next higher level. Allow at least 2 h for recovery to baseline before lowering PS again.
6. To promote rest and sleep, return patient to the next higher PS level or to full ventilatory support (PS level used in step 1 or assist-control mode) in the evening and at night.

....

Modified from Esteban A, Frutos F, Tobin MJ, et al: A comparison of four methods of weaning patients from mechanical ventilation. N Engl J Med 332:345–350, 1995.

*Patient is assumed to have met all the airway protection criteria in Table 3–3, the oxygenation criteria in Table 3–4, and the nonpulmonary screening criteria listed in Table 3–5.

assisted breaths to 100% unassisted breaths, T-piece or similar methods of weaning may not work as well as a weaning method that provides a tapering of support in patients with congestive heart failure. For these patients, the complete loss of positive pressure ventilation when they are removed from the ventilator may exacerbate their congestive heart failure, resulting in dyspnea and respiratory distress.

Pressure Support Weaning Protocol

The protocol for pressure support weaning (Table 3–7) allows patients to be weaned over the course of 1 day if they prove themselves capable of unassisted breathing. Finishing the weaning trial by 7 or 8 PM is important because many ICUs traditionally avoid continuing active weaning and extubation after this time in the evening. This restriction is out of concern for lack of availability for close monitoring of the weaning or of the recently extubated patient because fewer staff are generally on duty.

BIBLIOGRAPHY

Brochard L, Rauss A, Benito S, et al: Comparison of three methods of gradual withdrawal from ventilatory support during weaning from mechanical ventilation. Am J Respir Crit Care Med 150:896–903, 1994.
Landmark clinical trial compared weaning methods; it found that pressure support had shorter weaning duration than T-piece trials or IMV (which was the slowest method). Reintubation rate within 48 hours was 7.3%

Chao DC, Scheinhorn DJ: Weaning from mechanical ventilation. Crit Care Clin 14:799–817, 1998.
This is an excellent recent review article with 79 references.

Diehl J, El Atrous S, Touchard D, et al: Effects of tracheotomy on work of breathing. Am J Respir Crit Care Med 159:383–388, 1999.

This study documents decreased work of breathing when endotracheal tubes were replaced by tracheotomy tubes of the same internal diameter.

Ely EW, Baker AM, Dunagan DP, et al: Effect on the duration of mechanical ventilation of identifying patients capable of breathing spontaneously. N Engl J Med 335:1864–1869, 1996.
Clinical trial established the efficacy of respiratory therapist driven protocols for trials of spontaneous ventilation. Reintubation rate within 48 hours was 4%.

Esteban A, Frutos F, Tobin MJ, et al: A comparison of four methods of weaning patients from mechanical ventilation. N Engl J Med 332:345–350, 1995.
This is the second landmark clinical trial comparing weaning methods; it found that once or twice daily T-piece trials were superior to pressure support or IMV (which again was the slowest method). Reintubation rate within 48 hours was 17.7%.

Kollef MH, Shapiro SD, Silver P, et al: A randomized, controlled trial of protocol directed weaning from mechanical ventilation. Crit Care Med 25:567–574, 1997.
This study found that weaning by protocols managed by ICU nurses or respiratory therapists vs. nonprotocol weaning resulted in shorter duration of mechanical ventilation with no adverse effects.

Nava S, Ambrosino N, Clini E, et al: Noninvasive mechanical ventilation in the weaning of patients with respiratory failure due to chronic obstructive pulmonary disease. A randomized, conrolled trial. Ann Intern Med 128:721–728, 1998.
This controlled clinical trial found that noninvasive ventilation during weaning reduced weaning time and ICU length of stay among COPD patients who initially required intubation and ventilation.

Stroetz RW, Hubmayr RD: Tidal volume maintenance during weaning with pressure support. Am J Respir Crit Care Med 152:1034–1040, 1995.
The study found that clinicians could not accurately predict who was ready for weaning based on clinical impressions alone, thus documenting the need for objective measurements.

Yang KL, Tobin M: A prospective study of indexes predicting the outcome of trials of weaning from mechanical ventilation. N Engl J Med 324:1445–1450, 1991.
This is the classic article that systematically compared the value of various parameters to predict weaning success or failure. It found that the rapid shallow breathing index preformed best.

4

Sedation and Paralysis During Mechanical Ventilation

Treating Distress and Agitation

John Hansen-Flaschen

Sedating drugs are almost universally used to treat distress or agitation experienced by patients undergoing mechanical ventilation in the intensive care unit (ICU). Sedating drugs are psychoactive medications that exert a calming effect on thought or behavior. Medications commonly used for this purpose include benzodiazepines, opioids, neuroleptic agents, and intravenous anesthetics such as propofol.

There are four categories of indications for the use of sedating drugs or analgesics during mechanical ventilation: (1) to alleviate patient distress, (2) to control agitation, (3) to provide sedation and amnesia during pharmacologic paralysis, and (4) to provide analgesia, anxiolysis, or amnesia for bedside procedures or special situations. To a large degree, the third and fourth categories represent strategies to *prevent* agitation and distress rather than to *relieve* symptoms that are occurring. Procedures or special situations in this regard include endotracheal intubation, bedside procedures such as cardioversion or percutaneous tracheostomy, diagnostic imaging studies such as computed tomography or magnetic resonance imaging, alcohol or sedative drug withdrawal, and terminal withdrawal of mechanical ventilation (for the latter, see Appendix C).

DISTRESS

Distress is a global term for suffering, strain, or misery affecting the body or mind. The term is particularly apt in the care of mechanically ventilated patients in whom it is often easier to discern that distress is present than to determine the precise nature of that distress. Nevertheless, it is important to identify the type of distress present whenever possible because different types are best treated differently.

Four Types of Distress

Four types of distress are common during the acute phase of respiratory failure: (1) pain, (2) dyspnea, (3) anxiety, and (4) delirium.

Pain. Pain is an unpleasant physical and emotional sensation associated with a potentially harmful stimulus or an actual tissue injury. Pain is probably underappreciated in the ICU and undertreated even when recognized. For example, analgesics may be withheld deliberately for fear of exacerbating hypotension, creating addiction, or masking evolution of clinical problems such as the evaluation of an acute abdomen. More often, perhaps, the pain of a silent patient fails to register

45

as a priority to clinicians in the context of other serious problems that also require attention.

Dyspnea. Contrary to a common misperception, shortness of breath or dyspnea often is not relieved by restoration of adequate arterial blood gases during mechanical ventilation for acute respiratory failure. One reversible cause is a lack of coordination between mechanically assisted respiration and the breathing efforts of the patient. Increasing inspiratory flow rates or changing mode of ventilation, such as from assist-control to pressure support (see Chapter 2), may relieve the dyspnea in some instances. If adjustments to mechanical ventilation and person-to-person reassurance fail to relieve dyspnea, administration of a drug to relieve it is appropriate.

Dyspnea is also commonly experienced during weaning from prolonged mechanical ventilation; indeed, some degree of dyspnea may be unavoidable as patients who have weak respiratory muscles are retrained during weaning trials to sustain spontaneous respiration.

Anxiety. Anxiety is defined as a diffuse and unpleasant emotion of apprehension that is not associated with a specific threat. In the ICU, the overriding apprehension is the fear of death. In addition, helplessness, dependency, and the inability to predict upcoming events contribute to anxiety during mechanical ventilation, as do pain, dyspnea, and the disturbed perceptions associated with delirium.

Delirium. Delirium is defined as an acute, reversible disturbance of consciousness and cognitive function that fluctuates in severity. Its characteristics include defective perception, reduced short-term memory, confusion, disorientation, and hallucinations that are often visual in nature. The cognitive impairment of a delirious patient typically fluctuates and may take on a diurnal pattern that is worse in the evening. In the ICU, delirium is sometimes referred to as "sun downing" or the "ICU syndrome" (see Chapter 44).

The causes of delirium during mechanical ventilation for respiratory failure include neurologic injuries; sleep deprivation; severe cardiovascular, hematologic, and respiratory disorders; endocrine and metabolic disturbances; and a variety of toxins. Drug withdrawal is another common cause of delirium during the first several days after admission. Drugs used in the treatment of critically ill patients, notably benzodiazepines and anticholinergic drugs, can also cause or exacerbate delirium.

Agitation

In the ICU, *agitation* is a manifestation of distress; it refers to excessive or detrimental motor activity associated with internal tension. Repetitive, nonproductive movement is the hallmark of agitated behavior. In contrast to tremors, seizures, and myoclonic movements, agitation is volitional and often, although not invariably, purposeless.

A mildly agitated patient might be described as vaguely uneasy or "fidgety." Intermittent mild agitation does not necessarily require pharmacologic treatment to suppress it but rather the intensivist should evaluate and treat the patient for the causes of the agitation listed previously. At the other extreme, severe agitation threatens placement of vascular catheters and access tubes. It can severely compromise respiratory and cardiovascular life support as well. Unnecessary exertion can promote respiratory and metabolic acidosis by increasing the production of carbon dioxide and lactic acid. Even minor motor activity can cause transient, potentially severe hypoxemia in patients with severe acute respiratory distress syndrome.

ASSESSMENT OF PATIENT WITH DISTRESS OR AGITATION

Assessing for the presence of distress or signs of agitation should be a routine component of the bedside evaluation of patients during mechanical ventilation. One should first observe the patient's spontaneous behavior for agitation. A semiquantitative scale of severity of agitation (Table 4–1) can be used to facilitate communication among ICU nurses and physicians and to document the patient's status on the ICU flow sheet. Alternately, some physicians use the Ramsey scale to document level of consciousness as a reflection of the degree of sedation (Table 4–2).

After assessing for agitation, one should next verify that the patient can see, hear, understand, and respond appropriately to simple questions. Because critically ill patients are often separated from their eyeglasses or hearing aids, a special effort may be needed to communicate with them. Vision, hearing, and the ability to respond can all be confirmed by asking a single question: "Show me that you understand by blinking your eyes this many times (questioner shows two or three fingers)."

Responsive patients should then be asked about their comfort using direct questions that intubated patients can answer yes or no by some unambiguous movement: "Do you have any pain now?" "Are you short of breath now?" One should ask questions in the present tense because many patients experience short-term memory deficits that preclude meaningful answers about their experiences in the recent past. Affirmative responses are followed when appropriate with additional questions that can be answered by movement or gesture, for example, "Is the breathing tube painful?" or "Point to where you feel the pain." If a patient is experiencing pain, anxiety, or dyspnea, the severity of distress should be evaluated

Table 4–1. Bedside Scale for Recording Levels of Agitation

SCORE	LEVEL OF AGITATION	DESCRIPTION
P	None	Neuromuscular blocking agent in effect and patient is paralyzed
0	None	Patient is calm; movements are appropriate, coordinated, and do not interfere with treatment
1	Mild	Movements are occasionally inappropriate or excessive Muscle tone may be increased
2	Moderate	Patient is fidgety or changes body position frequently Vascular access and tubes are not threatened Ventilation is not compromised
3	Severe	Patient poses immediate threat to self or staff Excessive movements repeatedly threaten vascular access and tubes, cause frequent episodes of hypoxemia, or repeatedly trigger peak pressure alarm on ventilator

From Hansen-Flaschen J: Treatment of agitation and distress in mechanically ventilated patients. In: Fishman AP (ed): Fishman's Pulmonary Diseases and Disorders, 3rd ed. New York: McGraw-Hill, 1998.

Table 4–2. Ramsey Scale for Assessment of Sedation

LEVEL	STATE	DESCRIPTION
1	Awake	Anxious, and agitated or restless, or both
2	Awake	Awake, cooperative, oriented and tranquil
3	Awake	Awake, responds to commands only
4	Asleep	Brisk response to light glabellar tap or loud noise
5	Asleep	Sluggish response to light glabellar tap or loud noise
6	Asleep	No response to light glabellar tap or loud noise

From Ramsay M, Savege T, Simpson B, et al: Controlled sedation with alphaxalone-alphadalone. Br Med J 2:656–659, 1974.

on a scale of 1 to 10, for example, using a Visual Analog Pain scale (see Chapter 85, Fig. 85–1). Quantitation of distress determines the urgency of treatment and guides drug dosing.

PHARMACOLOGIC TREATMENT OF DISTRESS AND AGITATION

The optimal treatment of agitation and distress during mechanical ventilation in the ICU has not been determined. The recommendations presented here favor generic, relatively nontoxic drugs and are consistent with current knowledge regarding the pharmacology of intravenous (IV) sedation for critically ill patients.

Routine Treatment of Ventilated Patients with Opioids or Benzodiazepines

Most conscious patients receiving mechanical ventilation for respiratory failure, especially those with endotracheal or nasotracheal tubes, should be routinely treated with an opioid or a benzodiazepine or both (Tables 4–3 and 4–4). The rationale for this recommendation is based on the inherent discomfort of the artificial airway and the distress due to acute respiratory failure. This rule, however, assumes the absence of contraindications, such as the need to follow serial mental status or neurologic examinations without confounding effects of sedating agents. It does not apply to patients with tracheostomy tubes in place because discomfort from this tube is much less than that from endotracheal or nasotracheal tubes.

The choice of initial agent and the use of additional agents depend on the specifics of the clinical situation, as noted further on, as well as on the sedating practices adopted in individual ICUs. One recommended practice is to treat all endotracheally intubated patients receiving mechanical ventilation who are exhibiting mild-to-moderate levels of agitation (score 1 or 2 in Table 4–1) or who communicate that they are having pain, anxiety, or dyspnea. Patients with mild-to-moderate agitation or distress, who have been *previously unexposed* to these types of drugs, one can start with low-dose fentanyl, for example, 50 to 100 μg IV bolus followed by 50 to 100 μg/h infusion (see Table 4–3), or low-dose lorazepam,

Table 4–3. Opioid Dosing During Mechanical Ventilation

DRUG	INITIAL INTRAVENOUS DOSE*	FOLLOW-UP DOSES	CONTINUOUS INTRAVENOUS INFUSION DOSAGE, COST, AND COMMENTS
Fentanyl	50 μg–100 μg given over 2–3 min	Repeat every 5–10 min to therapeutic effect	Start by infusing one quarter to one half the loading dose/h, typically 25–125 μg/h (costing $2–7 for 24-h dose); infusions >1.0 mg/h may be necessary to treat refractory pain or agitation (100 μg/h of fentanyl is approximately equivalent to 2.5 mg/h of morphine)
Morphine sulfate	2–10 mg given over 2–3 min	Repeat every 10–15 min to therapeutic effect	Start by infusing one quarter to one half the loading dose/h, typically 1–4 mg/h (costing $1–3 for 24-h dose); infusion >25–50 mg/h may be necessary to treat refractory pain or agitation
Hydromorphone	See Comments	See Comments	Second-line opioid used when high-dose fentanyl (≥1 mg/h) or morphine (≥25 mg/h) is ineffective (due to a "ceiling effect") or requires a large volume of fluid for delivery; initially use 4–8 mg/h of hydromorphone (costing $8–15 for 24-h dose) as a substitute for 1000 μg/h of fentanyl and then adjust dose to effect; (1.5 mg/h of hydromorphone is approximately equivalent to 40 μg/h of fentanyl)

*These doses are for patients who are *not* tolerant to opioids; dosages for tolerant patients may exceed these by 10- to 30-fold.

Costs reflect approximate hospital acquisition cost of the drug in the year 2000.

for example, 0.5 to 2.0 mg IV bolus followed by 0.5 to 1.0 mg/h infusion (see Table 4–4). Some intensivists use a combination of these two agents at similar starting doses, aiming for synergistic effects and less toxicity from each individual agent. For patients who have been *previously exposed* to sedating drugs or opioids, the same drugs are recommended but their dosages need to be increased and titrated to effect (see Tables 4–3 and 4–4).

For patients with moderate-to-severe distress (scores 2 or 3 in Table 4–1), an individualized approach must be used based on the cause of the distress or agitation, as described earlier, and the clinical urgency of the situation. Therapies to use under these clinical circumstances are described in the sections that follow.

Emergent Treatment of Acute, Severe Agitation

In a ventilator-dependent patient, acute, severe agitation (score 3 in Table 4–1) requires immediate attention. If a quick, directed examination does not reveal a correctable cause for agitation, such as a ruptured endotracheal tube balloon or obstructed endotracheal tube, empirical treatment with a high dose of a sedative,

Table 4–4. Benzodiazepine Dosing During Mechanical Ventilation

DRUG	INITIAL INTRAVENOUS DOSE*	FOLLOW-UP DOSES	CONTINUOUS INTRAVENOUS INFUSION DOSAGE, COST, AND COMMENTS
Lorazepam	0.5–2 mg (maximal rate of 2 mg/min)	Repeat every 5–15 min to effect (as tolerated)	Start with 1 mg/h after IV load (use 50% of loading dose if patient is very agitated); typical infusions of 1–5 mg/h (costing $10–50 for 24-h dose); to adjust dose up, give 1-mg bolus and then increase infusion rate by 1 mg/h; for intermittent therapy, give 1–3 mg every 4–12 h
Midazolam	1–2 mg (maximal rate of 2 mg/min)	Repeat every 2–5 min to effect (as tolerated)	Start with 1 mg/h after IV load (use 50% of loading dose if patient is very agitated); typical infusions of 1–5 mg/h (costing $38–188 for 24-h dose); half-life is too short to use as intermittent IV therapy
Diazepam	See Comments	See Comments	Second-line agent; used when more than 2 wk of mechanical ventilation with heavy sedation is anticipated; to change to diazepam from lorazepam, give 5–10 mg diazepam IV every 1–2 h for every 10 mg/h of lorazepam on first day of conversion (CNS drug levels may fall 15–30 min after bolus because of redistribution during this period); over the next 3 days, the injection interval can be increased to 4–12 h as clinically tolerated

*Start with lower dose in elderly; patients previously exposed to benzodiazepines will need higher doses.
Costs reflect approximate hospital acquisition cost of the drug in the year 2000.
CNS, central nervous system; IV, intravenous.

either an opioid or a benzodiazepine or both (see Tables 4–3 and 4–4), is indicated. In addition, if the episode is severe with the need for immediate control of the agitation, a rapidly acting neuromuscular blocking agent, such as pancuronium or vecuronium, should also be administered (see Table 4–7). Neuromuscular blockade should not be continued beyond the duration of action of an initial bolus, however, unless the patient fails to tolerate return of muscle activity despite deep sedation.

IV infusion of propofol, an intravenous anesthetic also commonly used in the ICU for heavy sedation, is an alternative for control of acute, severe agitation (Table 4–5). This highly lipid soluble drug has an exceptionally rapid onset and offset of action but may cause hypotension when administered rapidly. Its chief advantage is rapid recovery of alertness after the dose is decreased or the drug withdrawn. Its use for sedation is described in more detail later.

Treatment of Moderate, Sustained Agitation

To treat moderately severe agitation, one should start with a single sedating drug given intravenously—an opioid, a benzodiazepine, or a neuroleptic agent, chosen as described further on. One should titrate the dose to effect by giving additional bolus doses followed by increases in the maintenance infusion rate, remembering

Table 4–5. Propofol Dosing During Mechanical Ventilation

INITIAL INTRAVENOUS DOSE	FOLLOW-UP DOSES	CONTINUOUS INTRAVENOUS INFUSION DOSAGE, COST, AND COMMENTS
0.3 mg/kg/h (avoid rapid bolus)	Increase the infusion rate by increments of 0.3–0.6 mg/kg/h at 3- to 5-min intervals to therapeutic effect (as tolerated hemodynamically)	Continue propofol infusion at the final loading infusion rate, typically 0.6–6 mg/kg/h (costing $38–380 for 24-h dose); adjust propofol infusion rate to maintain desired level of sedation. Reduce dose in elderly, debilitated, or hypotensive patients; rapid IV bolus injection can result in hypotension

that it is usually unnecessary to abolish nonproductive movement altogether. For example, under most circumstances, titrating the drug so that the patient appears relatively calm (score 1 in Table 4–1) is appropriate.

There is no absolute upper limit to the infusion dose of sedating drugs for mechanically ventilated patients. Indeed, uncommonly large doses (10 to 30 times usual) are sometimes needed to control agitation in this setting, particularly for patients who have acquired a tolerance to sedating drugs or have chronically used alcohol. The risk of adverse effects, however, increases with higher doses.

The choice of sedating drugs for persistent, moderately severe agitation depends on the form of distress that is thought to cause the agitation. Other important considerations include adverse effects, pharmacokinetics, and cost. Shorter-acting drugs with few or no active metabolites, such as midazolam or lorazepam, are preferred in the acute phase of treatment because their sedating effects are more controllable. Proprofol is another short-acting, sedating agent that should be considered. Inexpensive, longer-acting drugs, such as diazepam, can be used for long-term sedation provided that care is taken to avoid a "sedation hangover" that delays weaning from mechanical ventilation.

Opioids to Treat Dyspnea or Pain

The cause of dyspnea experienced during mechanical ventilation is not well understood; however, limited published experience in other settings suggests that opioids may be more effective in relieving dyspnea than are benzodiazepines. They are also the preferred systemic agents to relieve pain (see Chapter 85). Benzodiazepines, neuroleptic agents, and neuromuscular blocking agents do not provide analgesia by themselves.

Because they are inexpensive and familiar, fentanyl and morphine are the opioids commonly used for continuous IV administration in the ICU (see Table 4–3). Since fentanyl lacks the vasodilatory effects of morphine, it is the preferred opioid to use in patients receiving mechanical ventilation, especially in those with intravascular volume contraction or hypotension. Fentanyl is also preferred for use in patients with renal failure because an active metabolite of morphine (morphine-6-glucuronide) accumulates in renal failure; this prolongs the action of morphine relative to fentanyl.

A continuous infusion of fentanyl (or morphine) should be instituted after an initial loading dose. Subsequent boluses should be repeated at 5- to 10-minute intervals as guided by signs of distress or by the use of a visual analogue or numeric distress scale in appropriate patients until pain or dyspnea is relieved. Occasionally, a patient-controlled infusion pump can be used to dose opioids for mechanically ventilated patients who are sufficiently alert and capable (see Chapter 85).

Benzodiazepines to Treat Anxiety

In patients mechanically ventilated for acute respiratory failure, anxiety that does not respond to nonpharmacologic measures should be treated with an IV benzodiazepine (see Table 4–4). Because the anxiolytic efficacy and adverse effects of the commonly used IV benzodiazepines are similar, selection should be based primarily on pharmacokinetic considerations and cost.

Lorazepam is recommended when the anticipated duration of parenteral sedation is less than 2 weeks. A continuous infusion of midazolam can be used instead of lorazepam, but the total cost of sedation may be greater (see Table 4–4). Midazolam can also be given by patient-controlled infusion. The control offered patients by self-administration of a benzodiazepine may in itself help to limit anxiety under certain circumstances, such as prolonged, difficult weaning from mechanical ventilation. Although lorazepam or midazolam is commonly given by continuous IV infusion, intermittent IV dosing may result in more readily reversible effects, and in one recent study it was associated with shorter duration of mechanical ventilation.

Another recent study confirmed the adverse effect of continuous IV infusions of sedatives in patients on mechanical ventilation. Kress and coworkers gave ventilated patients daily interruptions of sedative infusions until the patient was awake or became distressed. For the awake patient, they stopped the agent entirely; for the distressed patient, they restarted it at a half its previous dose. Those that had the daily interruptions had significantly shorter duration on mechanical ventilation as well as shorter ICU length of stay.

Diazepam is less expensive than lorazepam or midazolam. However, because of its long half-life (~36 hours for the parent drug and >10 days for an active metabolite), sedation may persist for many days after a prolonged course of therapy. For this reason, diazepam is recommended primarily for mechanically ventilated patients who are expected to require IV sedation for longer than 2 weeks.

The minimal duration of continuous treatment associated with the development of benzodiazepine dependence in critically ill patients is unknown because drug withdrawal symptoms are particularly difficult to distinguish from other causes of irritability, anxiety, and restlessness. Under these circumstances in patients recovering from a critical illness who have received a benzodiazepine continuously for longer than 2 or 3 weeks, one should taper the dose of benzodiazepine rather than withdraw it abruptly. In some instances, tapering should continue after discharge from the hospital.

Neuroleptic Drugs and Benzodiazepines for Delirium

Neuroleptic drugs appear to calm agitated delirium in many patients. Because of its favorable hemodynamic and respiratory profile, *haloperidol* is commonly used for this purpose in the ICU (Table 4–6). Its toxicities include prolongation of the

Table 4–6. Haloperidol Dosing for Agitation in the Intensive Care Unit

INITIAL INTRAVENOUS DOSE	FOLLOW-UP DOSES	MAINTENANCE DOSAGE AND COMMENTS
5 mg IV bolus (2 mg for patients >65 years old)	Give 5–10 mg every 20 min (at a maximal rate of 5 mg/min) until the patient is calm or until corrected QT interval exceeds 480 msec	Give one quarter of the total loading dose of haloperidol by intermittent injection at 6-h intervals for the first 24–48 h; then decrease the dose by 25–50%/day

QT interval, extrapyramidal side effects, and, rarely, induction of the neuroleptic malignant syndrome (see Chapter 54).

Although small doses are sufficient in many patients, larger quantities have been given without apparent adverse effects. However, because higher doses may induce *torsade de pointe* and cardiac arrest (see Chapter 31) and provide uncertain incremental benefit, total daily doses greater than 50 mg should generally be avoided. During haloperidol administration, the patient must be monitored regularly for prolongation of the corrected QT interval and the drug should be held if the corrected QT interval exceeds 480 msec.

Benzodiazepines are preferred for the treatment of delirium associated with alcohol or sedative withdrawal. They are also effective for the prevention and treatment of withdrawal seizures, whereas, in contrast, haloperidol and other neuroleptic drugs tend to lower the seizure threshold.

Propofol for Sedation

Propofol, an intravenous anesthetic agent, is approved by the Food and Drug Administration for ICU sedation. This highly lipid, soluble drug offers one substantial advantage over other available sedating agents in terms of its short duration of action. Even after prolonged infusions titrated to deep sedation, patients regain full consciousness within 30 to 60 minutes after administration is stopped. This property is particularly useful for patients who are expected to recover quickly from respiratory failure, such as those who require mechanical ventilation for life-threatening asthma. High cost initially limited use of propofol for prolonged respiratory failure. After it becomes available generically, and its cost decreases, this drug may become more attractive for routine use.

In critically ill patients, propofol is best loaded by a step-wise continuous IV infusion rather than by bolus dosing to avoid severe hypotension (see Table 4–6). Concomitant infusion of low-to-moderate dose fentanyl or morphine provides analgesia and often limits the total required propofol dose. Because of its high lipid solubility, the agent redistributes from plasma into fat stores. Because the rate of this redistribution slows over time, the maintenance infusion rate for maintaining sedation will be less than the rate used for initially achieving sedation. It is recommended that the infusion be titrated daily to the minimally necessary sedating dose to take this into acount. Failure to reduce the maintenance dosage in this manner can result in a prolonged sedation when the agent is finally stopped.

The lipid content of total parenteral nutrition should be readjusted downwards during propofol infusion to account for the lipid emulsion in the propofol solution. Because propofol sometimes causes severe hypertriglyceridemia, serum triglyceride levels should be monitored every 2 to 3 days during its infusion. Drug administration should be sharply reduced or stopped if the serum triglyceride level is greatly elevated. Finally, there have been reports of bacteria being externally introduced into the lipid rich emulsion of propofol. Since this emulsion supports bacterial growth, some patients have developed sepsis when given contaminated solutions. Strict aseptic handling of the solution is critical and discarding the product within 12 hours of breaking the sterile seal of the bottle is recommended.

BIBLIOGRAPHY

Barr J, Donner A: Optimal intravenous dosing strategies for sedatives and analgesics in the intensive care unit. Crit Care Clin 11:827–847, 1995.
This article presents recommendations for dosing intravenous benzodiazepines and opioids based on mathematical models of blood drug levels.

Fontaine D: Nonpharmacologic management of patient distress during mechanical ventilation. Crit Care Clin 10:695–708, 1994.
This article presents alternatives to medications for improving the comfort of patients in acute respiratory failure.

Hansen-Flaschen JH, Brazinsky S, Basile C, Lanken PN: Use of sedating drugs and neuromuscular blocking agents in patients requiring mechanical ventilation for respiratory failure: A national survey. JAMA 266:2870–2875, 1991.
This article discusses which sedating drugs are used most commonly and by what methods of administration in U.S. intensive care units.

Hayden W: Life and near death in the intensive care unit: A personal experience. Crit Care Clin 10:651–658, 1994.
These are the recollections of a pediatric intensive care physician who survived intensive care for traumatic injury.

Hill L, Bertaccini E, Barr J, et al: ICU sedation: A review of its pharmacology and assessment. J Intensive Care Med 13:174–183, 1998.
This recent review includes subjective scoring schemes and objective electrophysiologic measurements to monitor level of sedation in ICU patients.

Kollef MH, Levy NT, Ahrens TS, et al: The use of continuous IV sedation is associated with prolongation of mechanical ventilation. Chest 114:541–548, 1998.
This observational study showed that giving sedation by continuous IV infusion, compared with sedation by intermittent IV boluses, was an independent risk factor for increased duration of mechanical ventilation and lengths of stay in the ICU and hospital.

Kress JP, Pohlman AS, O'Connor MF, et ai: Daily interruption of sedative infusions in critically ill patients undergoing mechanical ventilation. N Engl J Med 342:1471–1477, 2000.
This randomized, controlled clinical trial compared daily interruptions of sedative infusions followed by no further sedative therapy or therapy restarted at half the prior rate with conventional management by the ICU team. The group with planned interruptions had significantly fewer days on mechanical ventilation (median of 4.9 days vs. 7.3 days) and ICU length of stay (median of 6.6 days vs. 9.9 days).

Levine R: Pharmacology of intravenous sedatives and opioids in critically ill patients. Crit Care Clin 10:709–731, 1994.
This article presents the pharmacodynamics and pharmacokinetics of sedating drugs in patients with acute respiratory failure.

McCartney J, Boland R: Anxiety and delirium in the intensive care unit. Crit Care Clin 10:673–680, 1994.

Two experts in medical psychiatry describe the causes and manifestations of anxiety and delirium in the ICU.

Mirski M, Muffelman B, Ulatowski J, Hanley DF. Sedation for the critically ill neurologic patient. Crit Care Med 23:2038–2053, 1995.
This is a comprehensive review.

Stevens D, Edwards W: Management of pain in mechanically ventilated patients. Crit Care Clin 10:767–778, 1994.
This article describes the treatment of pain in the ICU with emphasis on local and regional anesthetic techniques.

Use of Neuromuscular Blocking Agents

··

C. William Hanson III

Neuromuscular blocking drugs (NMBDs) were initially used in the operating theater to immobilize and relax the patient and, like many other interventions, they have migrated into the ICU. Pharmacologic paralysis is now considered an important adjunct to the management of the critically ill patient in acute respiratory failure, such as acute respiratory distress syndrome (see Chapter 73). The intensivist who uses NMBDs should understand the pharmacodynamics and pharmacokinetics of the available agents, their possible interactions with other drugs, and important complications of their use in the ICU.

It is important for ICU physicians and nurses to remember that NMBDs have no intrinsic sedating or analgesic activity and that paralyzed patients must always be given sedatives concurrently, such as opioids or benzodiazepines (which also provide amnesia) or both (see Tables 4–3 and 4–4).

MECHANISM OF ACTION

Physiology of Neuromuscular Excitation

A nerve impulse initiated in the nerve body travels along the axon to the nerve terminal. The impulse is then transmitted across a synapse to a motor unit, which is composed of 15 to 1500 muscle fibers. The neuromuscular synapse consists of the nerve terminal of the neuron, the synaptic cleft (20 to 50 μm wide), and the motor end plate on the muscle. The neural signal is transmitted along the axon electrically and then across the synapse via a chemical messenger, at which point electrical transmission resumes in the motor unit.

Acetylcholine (ACH) is this chemical messenger. ACH serves as the chemical messenger not only for neural communication at the neuromuscular junction but also for some central nervous system pathways, autonomic ganglia, and postganglionic parasympathetic nerve endings. When a nerve impulse arrives at the nerve terminal of the neuromuscular junction, ACH vesicles fuse with the nerve cell membrane and are released into the synapse. Each vesicle contains 5000 to 10,000 molecules of ACH. The ACH binds to the ACH receptor on the muscle cell, causing a conformational change and increased permeability to sodium. When a sufficient number of sodium channels open, the transmembrane potential exceeds -50 mV and, as a result, the membrane depolarizes, creating an action potential that propagates to the entire motor unit and results in muscular contraction. The process requires calcium but is inhibited by magnesium.

The termination of physiologic depolarization follows diffusion of free ACH from the cleft, unbinding of ACH from the receptor, and breakdown of the ACH molecule by fixed acetylcholinesterase. ACH is hydrolyzed to acetate and choline, which are reabsorbed into the nerve terminal, reconstituted to ACH by the enzyme choline acetyltransferase, and repackaged into vesicles.

Mechanism of Neuromuscular Blocking Drugs

There are two general categories of NMBDs with effects at the neuromuscular junction.

Depolarizing Neuromuscular Blocking Drugs

Depolarizing neuromuscular blocking agents (succinylcholine, decamethonium) act as ACH analogs, binding to the nicotinic cholinergic receptors in the motor end plate. The initial effect of these drugs is depolarization followed by muscle contraction. The blockade that follows is caused by the slow hydrolysis of the drug (relative to the rapid hydrolysis of ACH). Repolarization is therefore delayed, and successive nerve impulses find the muscle refractory to depolarization. For example, succinylcholine is used to achieve rapid paralysis and control of the airway in patients who are at risk for regurgitation of gastric contents during emergent intubation. However, succinylcholine has potentially dangerous cardiac side effects that may preclude its use in the critically ill patient. Patients can experience sinus bradycardia, junctional rhythms, or even sinus arrest. Patients with chronically denervated muscle—for example, after spinal cord injury—may have a large increase in serum potassium concentration after succinylcholine administration. This results from the depolarization and potassium release from the muscle cells. In normal individuals, an increase in serum potassium on the order of 0.5 mEq/L is expected, whereas severalfold higher increases can occur in patients with extensively denervated skeletal muscle.

Nondepolarizing Neuromuscular Blocking Drugs

Nondepolarizing NMBDs (pancuronium, curare, vecuronium, and cisatracurium) do not depolarize but act by one of two alternative mechanisms. Either they bind to the ACH receptor on the motor end plate and prevent the conformational change that permits passage of sodium ions or they obstruct the sodium channel. These nondepolarizing NMBDs differ in their side effects, such as tachycardia and histamine release, and duration of action (Table 4–7). Differences in duration of action relate to differences in mechanism of drug clearance, which is particularly important in critically ill patients with organ dysfunction (see Table 4–7). Tachyphylaxis has been reported during prolonged use in the ICU setting.

Table 4–7. Nondepolarizing Neuromuscular Blocking Drugs
Used in the Intensive Care Unit

NAME OF DRUG	CLEARANCE MECHANISM	INTERMITTENT DOSAGE	INFUSION DOSAGE (~24-HR COST*)	COMMENTS
Pancuronium	Renal excretion >hepatic metabolism	Initial: 0.05–0.1 mg/kg Subsequent: 0.01–0.1 mgkg	Initial: 0.1 mg/kg/h Range: 0.06–0.4 mg/kg/h ($1–4)	Rapid onset; long-acting; boluses are likely to cause tachycardia (which may be severe) Active metabolite accumulates in renal failure
Vecuronium	Hepatic metabolism >renal excretion	Initial: 0.08–0.1 mg/kg Subsequent: 0.05–0.1 mg/kg	Initial: 1 μg/kg/min Range: 0.8–1.2 μg/kg/min ($50–80)	Rapid onset; short-to-intermediate duration of action; negligible hemodynamic effects Active 3-desacetyl metabolite accumulates in renal failure and can cause prolonged paralysis
Cisatracurium	Plasma cholinesterase; nonenzymatic degradation	Initial: 0.15–0.2 mg/kg Subsequent: 0.03 mg/kg	Initial: 3 μg/kg/min Range: 0.5–10 μg/kg/min ($30–600)	Intermediate onset; short duration of action; no effects on nicotinic, autonomic receptors, or muscarinic cardiac receptors; may cause histamine release when given rapidly in high dosage

*Costs reflect approximate hospital acquisition cost of the drug in year 2000 for a 70 kg patient.

Drug and Electrolyte Interactions

A number of other drugs (certain antibiotics and quinidine, which enhance blockage), acidosis (which enhances blockage), alkalosis (which counteracts blockage), and electrolytes (magnesium enhances blockage) may affect neuromuscular transmission. The administration of a new drug may change the degree of neuromuscular blockade significantly because of its synergistic actions at the neuromuscular junction. For example, aminoglycoside antibiotics can potentiate neuromuscular blockade by inhibition of presynaptic ACH release.

Complications of Neuromuscular Blocking Drugs

Several recent studies have shown that infusions of NMBDs for more than 24 hours have effects that were not recognized when they were used for shorter periods in the intraoperative environment. For example, NMBDs that were developed to be short acting have been shown to have active metabolites that accumulate and prolong duration of action (see Table 4–7). Conversely, patients may acquire tolerance or resistance to NMBDs when treated for extended periods and require higher than usual doses. Mechanistically, prolonged immobilization results in muscle atrophy, ACH receptor proliferation, and resistance to NMBDs.

In addition, several syndromes of prolonged weakness can follow administration of NMBDs to critically ill patients. Prolonged paralysis can be due to accumulation of active metabolites, neuropathy of critical illness, changes in the function or anatomy of the neuromuscular junction, or critical illness myopathy (see Chapter 67). NMBDs should be administered only when they are clearly necessary and with particular caution if the patient is also receiving high-dose corticosteroids, for example, to treat status asthmaticus (see Chapter 74). No method of administration or use of a certain NMBD guarantees zero risk for the development of the syndrome of prolonged weakness. Since the syndrome's recognition, however, intermittent dosing of NMBDs has become more popular compared with continuous infusion because it allows partial recovery of muscle function intermittently. During either intermittent or continuous dosing, twitch monitoring should be performed to guide NMBD dosing and to avoid loss of all twitch activity for prolonged periods.

BIBLIOGRAPHY

Behbehani NA, Al-Mane F, D'yachkova Y, et al: Myopathy following mechanical ventilation for acute severe asthma. The role of muscle relaxants and corticosteroids. Chest 115:1627–1631, 1999.
This retrospective cohort study reported that 9 of 30 (30%) patients who had received neuromuscular blocking agents (NMBAs) and corticosteroids during mechanical ventilation for severe acute asthma developed myopathy and that the risk of myopathy increases with each day of use of NMBDs.

Dulin PG, Williams CJ: Monitoring and preventive care of the paralyzed patient in respiratory failure. Crit Care Clin 10:815–829, 1994.
This article provides a wealth of details for protocol-based twitch monitoring of use of NMBDs in the ICU setting and other care of paralyzed patients.

Hanson CW III: Pharmacology of neuromuscular blocking agents in the intensive care unit. Crit Care Clin 10:779–797, 1994.
This is an in-depth review of mechanisms of action, pharmacokinetics, and clinically relevant complications of commonly used NMBDs in the ICU.

Hund E: Myopathy in critically ill patients. Crit Care Med 27:2544–2547, 1999.
This is a recent, concise review article; it has 69 references.

Larsson L, Li X, Edstrom L, et al: Acute quadriplegia and loss of muscle myosin in patients treated with nondepolarizing neuromuscular blocking agents and corticosteroids: mechanisms at the cellular and molecular levels. Crit Care Med 28:34–45, 2000.
This describes abnormalities found on muscle biopsies from seven patients who developed acute quadriplegic myopathy after receiving neuromuscular blocking agents and corticosteroids.

Raps EC, Bird SJ, Hansen-Flaschen J: Prolonged muscle weakness after neuromuscular blockade in the intensive care unit. Crit Care Clin 10:799–813, 1994.
This article reviews the differential diagnosis and mechanisms of pathogenesis of causes of prolonged weakness after exposure to NMBDs.

Saperstein A, Hurford WE: Neuromuscular blocking agents in the management of respiratory failure. Indications and treatment guidelines. Crit Care Clin 10:831–838, 1994.
This article reviews indications for the use of NMBDs and compares pancuronium, vecuronium, cisatracurium and curare for use in the ICU setting.

Topulos G: Neuromuscular blockade in adult intensive care. New Horizons 1:447–462, 1993.
This is a comprehensive review.

5 Assessment and Monitoring of Hemodynamic Function

C. William Hanson III

Pulmonary artery catheterization was first performed in 1945, and the pulmonary artery wedge (or occlusion) pressure was first measured in 1947. It was another quarter century, however, before these techniques were transplanted from the cardiac catheterization laboratory for clinical use in the intensive care unit (ICU). The advent of bedside pulmonary artery catheterization was made possible by the development of the balloon-tipped flotation catheter by Swan, Ganz, and coworkers (hence the commonly used eponym, the Swan-Ganz catheter). A purely diagnostic method was thus transformed to a physiologic monitoring tool that ICU clinicians could use to guide concurrent therapy.

Subsequent improvements in pulmonary artery catheter technology permitted measurement of right ventricular ejection fraction, pulmonary arterial oxygen saturation (mixed venous oxygen saturation), and thermodilution cardiac output. More than any other single type of technology, including mechanical ventilators, routine use of pulmonary artery catheterization and hemodynamic monitoring identifies an ICU from a non-ICU, for example, an intermediate care unit.

EFFICACY AND SAFETY OF THE PULMONARY ARTERY CATHETER

Despite its established standing as the test of "last appeal" for the assessment of hemodynamic status in the ICU, the efficacy of the pulmonary artery catheter has never been documented or even prospectively studied. As is the case for other physiologic monitors commonly employed in the ICU (radial artery catheterization, continuous pulse oximetry, and continuous electrocardiographic monitoring), which likewise have not been subjected to a rigorous prospective study of their efficacy, few questioned the utility of the pulmonary artery catheter in the ICU until recently. In 1996, a large observational study of critically ill patients found that use of a pulmonary artery catheter in the first 48 hours of ICU admission was associated with a 24% higher mortality rate as well as higher hospital cost.

This study questioning the safety of the pulmonary artery catheter reinforces the concept that risk:benefit ratio must be considered when using any invasive monitor in the ICU, including the pulmonary artery catheter. It also emphasizes the need for all invasive monitors to be used for specific indications and defined times, accompanied by frequent re-evaluations of their usefulness in each ICU patient.

Evaluation of the hemodynamic status of unstable ICU patients by physical examination is notoriously inaccurate. For example, in up to 50% of patients in whom pulmonary artery catheters are used, information obtained from the catheters redirects therapy. Pulmonary artery catheters provide ICU clinicians information about pressures as directly measured parameters and about cardiac output as a

59

derived parameter. Based on these and other clinical data, invasive monitors have been used to categorize hemodynamically unstable patients into three main subsets: cardiac pump failure states (see Chapter 6), low preload states (see Chapter 7), and low afterload states (see Chapter 8).

Although a number of clever, noninvasive devices have been developed in recent years to measure cardiac output, blood pressure, and other derived parameters, invasive catheters remain the standard of care for concurrent hemodynamic monitoring.

REVIEW OF BASIC PHYSIOLOGY

Intravascular Pressures, Volumes, and Compliance

Intravascular pressure and volume are related by compliance (Table 5–1, Equation 1). Compliance of a cardiac chamber, blood vessel, or network of blood vessels reflects its intrinsic distensibility. Vessels or chambers that are highly distensible, such as the systemic venous bed or the pulmonary vascular bed, can accommodate large changes in volume with small changes in pressure. In contrast, the systemic arterial circuit is far less compliant. Specifically, systemic veins are approximately 25 times more compliant than systemic arteries. The systemic venous circuit of a typical adult contains about 2500 mL at an average central venous pressure of about 10 mm Hg, whereas the systemic arterial circuit contains only about 750 mL at a mean pressure of about 100 mm Hg.

Table 5–1. Hemodynamic Equations

....

Equation 1. Compliance = change in volume/change in pressure ($\Delta V/\Delta P$)
Equation 2. CI = CO/BSA where
      CI = cardiac index (L/min•m²)
      CO = cardiac output (L/min)
      BSA = body surface area (m²) (derived from height and weight* or a nomogram)
Equation 3. PVR = {(mean PAP − PAWP)/CO} × 80 where
      PVR = pulmonary vascular resistance expressed traditional units (dyne sec cm⁻⁵)
      mean PAP = mean pulmonary artery pressure (mm Hg)
      PAWP = pulmonary artery wedge pressure (mm Hg)
      CO = cardiac output (L/min)
Equation 4. SVR = {(mean AP − CVP)/CO} × 80 where
      SVR = systemic vascular resistance expressed in traditional units (dyne sec cm⁻⁵)
      mean AP = mean systemic arterial pressure (mm Hg)
      CVP = mean central venous pressure (mm Hg)
      CO = cardiac output (L/min)
Equation 5. Pressure (mm Hg) = pressure (cm H_2O) × 1.36
Equation 6. The Fick Equation: CO = $\dot{V}O_2$ / (CaO_2 − $C\bar{v}O_2$) where
      CO = cardiac output (L/min)
      $\dot{V}O_2$ = oxygen consumption per minute (mL/min)
      CaO_2 = oxygen content of arterial blood (mL/L)†
      $C\bar{v}O_2$ = oxygen content of mixed venous blood (mL/L)†
[†Note: One must convert from traditional units of oxygen content (mL/dL) to mL/L]
Equation 7. Cardiac output = amount of indicator injected/area under curve

....

*See article by Mattar in Bibliography for estimating BSA from height and weight.

Compliance can vary among patients and in a given patient over time. For example, acute changes in a patient's sympathetic tone (due to drugs or disease) can have substantial effects on the compliance and, in turn, the intravascular volume of the patient's venous capacitance bed.

Pulmonary and Systemic Circulations

Both the pulmonary circulation and the systemic circulation have three essential elements arranged in series: a reservoir, pump, and resistor. For the *right* side of the circulation, the reservoir consists of the systemic veins, venules, and venous sinuses; the pump is the right ventricle; and the resistor is the pulmonary arterial bed (predominantly the pulmonary arterioles). Similarly, for the *left* side of the circulation, the reservoir is the pulmonary venous bed and left atrium, the pump is the left ventricle, and the resistor is the systemic arterial circulation (again predominantly arterioles).

To illustrate the central role of the systemic venous reservoir in maintaining hemodynamic homeostasis, 64% of the body's blood volume resides in the systemic veins. The remainder is distributed as follows: 7% in the heart, 9% in the pulmonary circuit, 13% in the systemic arteries, and 7% in the systemic capillaries. Because of its blood volume, the systemic venous reservoir can compensate for blood loss by increases in its sympathetic venous tone. Increased tone causes constriction of the venous bed, decreased compliance, and mobilization of intravascular volume to maintain cardiac preload.

Hemodynamic Pressures and Resistances

By use of a pulmonary artery catheter and systemic arterial blood pressure monitor, one can measure pressures in both circuits as well as flow through the entire circulation. Cardiac output and other hemodynamic variables are commonly corrected for variations in body size by indexing the values to the body surface area (Table 5-1, Equation 2). Body surface area is usually computed from height and weight in the ICU or, less frequently, from a nomogram. The pressure in the systemic venous reservoir is reflected by the central venous pressure (CVP) and right atrial pressure. The latter is the proximate source of right ventricular filling during diastole, that is, right ventricular preload. The tip of the pulmonary artery catheter measures the pressure in the pulmonary artery or one of its branches. The resistance in the pulmonary arterial circuit is calculated using the cardiac output, mean pulmonary arterial pressure, and pulmonary artery wedge pressure (PAWP) (Table 5-1, Equation 3). This equation represents the general hydraulic relationship in which *resistance* to fluid flow through a system equals the *pressure drop* across the system divided by the *mean flow*.

The PAWP normally reflects the pressure in the pulmonary venous reservoir, which is the source for left ventricular filling during diastole, that is, left ventricular preload. Systemic arterial blood pressure (whether monitored directly with an arterial catheter or indirectly with a sphygmomanometer), cardiac output, and CVP are used to calculate systemic vascular resistance (Table 5-1, Equation 4). The range of normal pressures is shown in Table 5–2 and the range of normal flows and calculated resistances are given in Table 5–3.

BLOOD PRESSURE AND HEMODYNAMIC MEASUREMENTS

Blood Pressure

Intravascular pressure monitoring is relatively uncomplicated using modern disposable transducers. These self-calibrating transducers are set at a reference point, typically the level of the left atrium, estimated as the midaxillary line in a supine patient. The zero point of the transducer's scale is then set to atmospheric pressure, commonly known as "zeroing." This establishes the reference value for all other pressure measurements. The mean blood pressure in a blood vessel then represents the height to which a column of blood would ascend above this zero point. Traditionally, blood pressures are typically recorded in millimeters of mercury (mm Hg), whereas certain other pressures, for example, intracranial pressures (also measured by electronic transducers), use centimeters of water (cm H_2O). (Equation 5 of Table 5–1 can be used to convert mm Hg to cm H_2O based on the specific gravity of Hg, 13.6).

Table 5–2. Normal Values of Hemodynamic Pressures (Under Unstressed Conditions)

LOCATION	MEAN (mm Hg)	RANGE (mm Hg)
Right atrium		
mean	3	1–5
Right ventricle		
peak systolic	25	17–32
end diastolic	4	1–7
Pulmonary artery		
mean	15	9–19
peak systolic	25	17–32
end diastolic	10	4–13
occlusion pressure	7	2–12
Left atrium	7	2–12
Left ventricle		
peak systolic	125	100–140
end diastolic	9	5–12
Aorta		
mean	100	70–105
peak systolic	125	100–140
end diastolic	84	60–90
Capillary	10	

From Pepine CJ, Hill JA, Lambert CR (eds): Diagnostic and Therapeutic Cardiac Catheterization. Baltimore: Williams & Wilkins, 1998.

Table 5–3. Normal Values for Selected Cardiovascular Parameters

PARAMETERS (units)	ABBREVIATION	MEAN	RANGE
Cardiac output (L/min)	CO	6	5.2–7.4
Cardiac index (L/min · m^2)	CI	3.2	2.6–4.2
Left ventricular stroke volume (mL)	LVSV	82	70–94
Left ventricular stroke volume index (mL/m^2)	LVSVI	49	30–65
Systemic vascular resistance (dyne sec cm^{-5})	SVR	1130	900–1460
Pulmonary vascular resistance (dyne sec cm^{-5})	PVR	205	100–300
Oxygen comsumption index (mL/min · m^2)	$\dot{V}O_2I$	134	113–148

From Pepine CJ, Hill JA, Lambert CR (eds): Diagnostic and Therapeutic Cardiac Catheterization. Baltimore: Williams & Wilkins, 1998.

Cardiac Output

Thermodilution Techniques

Flow through the circulation is usually determined by using an indicator dilution (indicator washout) technique. Although the indicator was originally a dye, a thermal signal (cold) is currently used in clinical practice. The indicator is injected just proximal to the right heart (in the superior or inferior vena cava) and sampled in the pulmonary artery near the tip of the pulmonary artery catheter. Rapid washout of the indicator occurs in high cardiac output states, whereas delayed washout indicates the reverse. The indicator is measured as a changing concentration over time (Fig. 5–1). The area under this "concentration versus time" curve equals the product of the mean concentration of the indicator in the blood times the duration of the curve. Calculated cardiac output is inversely proportional to the area under the curve, as expressed in Equation 7, Table 5–1.

For the thermodilution method, the amount of indicator injected is proportional to the volume injected and the difference between the baseline blood temperature and the injectate's temperature. Likewise, the area under the curve is the integral of the change in temperature below the baseline temperature times the duration of the curve (whose end is determined by extrapolation of the descending limb [Fig. 5–1] by computerized curve fitting techniques in the ICU).

Figure 5–1. Cardiac output indicator (indocyanine green or thermal indicator signal) curves for low (gray) and high (black) cardiac output. The high cardiac output curve peaks sooner (due to a shorter transit time) and has less area under the curve because of more rapid transit of the indicator past the sensor.

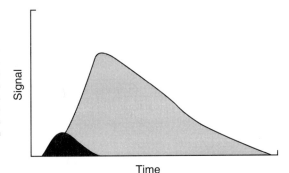

Time

Under certain circumstances, the indicator dilution method is inaccurate regardless of which indicator (dye or thermal) is used, whereas, under other circumstances, inaccuracies can occur only when a thermal indicator is used (Table 5–4). For example, if the actual injectate volume is half the value entered into the calculation, the apparent calculated cardiac output would be double the correct value. Also, tricuspid regurgitation greatly increases variability of the thermodilution technique and may result in possible errors in either direction. In patients with this disorder, the Fick method is preferred to measure cardiac output.

The Fick Method

An alternative approach to the measurement of cardiac output is the Fick method. Cardiac output is calculated using the patient's total oxygen consumption (assumed to be in a steady state) and the arterial-venous oxygen content difference across the lungs (Table 5–1, Equation 6). Like the thermodilution method, the Fick method requires the presence of a pulmonary artery catheter (to obtain the blood sample representing mixed venous blood from the pulmonary artery). Oxygen consumption per minute can be measured independently but is generally assumed to be 200 to 250 mL/min.

The Fick method is less popular than the thermodilution method for routine use in the ICU for a number of reasons. The thermodilution method is easier to use for making repeated measurements, both to follow patients over time and to

Table 5–4. Problems in Performing Thermodilution Cardiac Outputs

PROBLEM	CONSEQUENCE
Volume of injectate < "correct" volume	Overestimates true value*
Injectate is cooler than reference probe	Overestimates true value
Injectate is warmer than reference probe	Underestimates true value
Indicator injected too slowly	Overestimates true value
Large volume of intravenous fluid being given simultaneously via a central venous catheter	May overestimate or underestimate true value
Slowing of heart rate due to injection of ice-cold injectate	Underestimates true value by up to 10%
Tricuspid regurgitation with exposure of indicator to greater volume of blood	Faster washout of indicator and overestimates true value
Tricuspid regurgitation with slow release of tracer from right atrium	Prolongs descending part of injectate curve (see Fig. 5–1) and underestimates true value
Left-to-right intracardiac shunt	Early recirculation of cold blood interferes with analysis of descending limb of injectate curve
Right-to-left intracardiac shunt	Loss of indicator and overestimation of true cardiac output
Body temperature is low (33–34°C) or environmental temperature is high (−30°C)	Increased signal:noise ratio and increased variability of result
Very low cardiac output	Difficulty extrapolating descending limb of injectate curve with increased variability of result

*Gives a falsely elevated value for cardiac output.

decrease the variability of a value at a single point in time. As an example, four to six thermodilution measurements of cardiac output are routinely performed in rapid succession from which an average value is obtained. Disadvantages of the Fick method are the lack of ease in making replicate measurements, the need for obtaining blood samples, and the cost of measuring oxygen content. Furthermore, if the assumption about oxygen consumption is inaccurate (a likely possibility in a critically ill patient), the absolute value of the cardiac output by the Fick method will also be inaccurate. As noted earlier, however, the Fick method should give more accurate results than the thermodilution method in patients with moderate or severe tricuspid regurgitation.

Volumetric Methods

Volumetric methods can also measure cardiac output. Transesophageal echocardiography permits evaluation of left atrial and ventricular filling and determination of fractional area change in segments of the left ventricle between systole and diastole. Cardiac output is then extrapolated from the fractional area change. Although this technique is not currently suited to continuous monitoring in the ICU, it is conceivable that devices comparable in size to nasogastric tubes will eventually be designed for this purpose.

Arterial Catheterization

Arterial Waveforms

The pulse in the aortic root is diphasic with a systolic and diastolic phase separated by the incisura. The blood flows forward during the systolic phase as a result of cardiac ejection. The incisura represents the retrograde flow of blood during semilunar valve closure. The upstroke during diastole is due to elastic rebound of the arterial walls. The normal waveform changes as it travels distally because of multiple factors, including damping and increased impedance. One change is that the incisura evolves into the wider dicrotic notch. In general, as the arterial pressure is measured more peripherally, the greater are the systolic and pulse pressures (associated with a narrowing of the waveform). Although the *systolic blood pressures* in the periphery are higher than in central vessels, for example, the radial arterial and dorsalis pedis pressures may exceed central pressures by 15% or more, the *mean arterial pressures* measured peripherally are comparable to those measured centrally.

The character of the arterial waveform is determined to a major extent by the stroke volume and the compliance of the arterial tree and to a lesser extent by the character of systolic ejection. A "spiky" waveform with a prominent dicrotic notch in the setting of low blood pressure suggests intravascular volume depletion. A sharp systolic upstroke with a prominent pulse pressure is characteristic of a noncompliant vascular circuit, for example, atherosclerosis. These findings apply in both the pulmonary and systemic arterial circuits.

Indications

Invasive arterial catheters are used for hemodynamic monitoring in the ICU for several indications: low systemic blood pressure, evidence of end-organ hypoperfusion (e.g., lactic acidosis, low urine output). They are also used when minute-to-minute blood pressure monitoring is required, for example, in patients with unstable vital signs or receiving continuous intravenous infusions of certain vasoactive drugs. Arterial catheterization is also appropriate when frequent arterial blood samples, (e.g., four or more a day) are necessary. As with any invasive monitor, its risk:benefit ratio should be reconsidered regularly (see Chapter 9).

Central Venous Monitoring

A central venous catheter is indicated for vascular access in patients with poor peripheral venous access, for simultaneous infusion of incompatible drugs when several sites for intravenous access are needed, for infusion of fluids of high osmolality (hyperalimentation), or for determination of intravascular volume status when less invasive measures (fluid challenge) are impractical or have failed.

The CVP is a measurement of pressure that reflects the volume of blood in the systemic venous reservoir. A mean CVP less than 5 mm Hg is consistent with hypovolemia, with the caveat that variations in sympathetic tone as well as other variables can significantly affect the overall volume of the venous reservoir. The CVP is often used as a proxy for the PAWP. This assumes, however, that the right side of the heart and the pulmonary vascular bed are normal. This is valid in healthy persons, but not necessarily so in many patients with pulmonary disease or heart disease or those on mechanical ventilators (in whom increased pleural pressures due to the positive pressure may raise CVP).

Although the absolute value of the CVP gives some information, as a rule its response to infused volume is usually of greater clinical significance. If the CVP increases substantially (>30%) in response to an adequate volume challenge (e.g., 5 to 10 mL/kg of normal saline given over 30 minutes), this suggests that the systemic venous reservoir is relatively noncompliant and therefore replete. Conversely, when the CVP shows little or no response to such a volume load, intravascular volume depletion is more likely. The same inferences apply to the response of the PAWP to a volume challenge. The strategy typically followed in volume management is to infuse fluids to some predetermined end point. ICU clinicians often use a physiologic end point (systemic blood pressure, cardiac index, mixed venous oxygen saturation) or a clinical end point (urine output).

BIBLIOGRAPHY

Connors AF, Speroff T, Dawson NV, et al: The effectiveness of right heart catheterization in the initial care of critically ill patients. JAMA 276:889–897, 1996.
  This describes an observational study raising concerns about safety of the pulmonary artery catheter.

Dexter L, Haynes FW, Burwell CS, et al: Studies of congenital heart disease. I: Technique of venous catheterization as a diagnostic procedure. J Clin Invest 26:547–533, 1947.
  This is an early description of the technique of cardiac catheterization.

Dexter L, Haynes FW, Burwell CS, et al: Studies of congenital heart disease. II: The pressure and oxygen content of the right auricle, right ventricle, and pulmonary artery in control patients, with observations on the oxygen saturation and source of pulmonary "capillary" blood. J Clin Invest 26:554–560, 1947.
This is an early description of normal oxygen content and pressures in right-sided heart catheterization.

Eisenberg PR, Jaffe AS, Schuster DP: Clinical evaluation compared to pulmonary artery catheterization in the hemodynamic assessment of critically ill patients. Crit Care Med 12:549–553, 1984.
This study suggests that clinical evaluation is often inaccurate, and that right-sided heart catheterization is useful in critically ill patients.

Forrester JS, Swan HJC: Acute myocardial infarction: A physiological basis of therapy. Crit Care Med 2:283–292, 1974.
This is a classic description of the hemodynamic characteristics of acute myocardial infarction and its complications, for example, mitral regurgitation.

Mattar JA: A simple calculation to estimate body surface area in adults and its correlation with the Du Bois formula. Crit Care Med 17:846–847, 1989.
For adults, the simpler equation, BSA (m^2) = {weight (kg) + height (cm) − 60}/100, was found to correlate well with the traditional Du Bois formula for BSA.

Mimoz O, Rauss A, Rekik N, et al: Pulmonary artery catheterization in critically ill patients: Prospective analysis of outcome changes associated with catheter prompted changes in therapy. Crit Care Med 22:543–545, 1994.
This study suggests that catheter-prompted interventions lead to improved outcomes.

Pepine CJ, Hill JA, Lambert CR (eds): Diagnostic and Therapeutic Cardiac Catheterization. Baltimore: Williams & Wilkins, 1998.
This comprehensive source book was written for those who perform cardiac catheterizations and has excellent chapters of topics of importance to intensivists, such as measurement of hemodynamics.

Steingrub JS, Celoria G, Vickers-Lahti M, et al: Therapeutic impact of pulmonary artery catheterization in a medical/surgical ICU. Chest 99:1451–1455, 1991.
This article presents an analysis of accuracy of residents and attendings in predicting hemodynamics prior to right-sided heart catheterization in the ICU.

Swan HJC, Ganz W, Forrester J, et al: Catheterization of the right heart in man with the use of a flow-directed balloon-tipped catheter. N Engl J Med 283:447–451, 1970.
Initial description of the technique of right-sided heart catheterization using a balloon-tipped catheter.

Youngberg JA, Miller ED: Evaluation of percutaneous cannulations of the dorsalis pedis artery. Anesthesiology 44:80, 1976.
This study found that systolic pressures in the dorsalis pedis artery were greater than in the central arteries.

6 Cardiogenic Shock and Other Pump Failure States

Frank E. Silvestry
Irving M. Herling

Although acute circulatory shock occurs as a consequence of a wide variety of conditions, all result in inadequate oxygen delivery to the organs, tissues, and cells, relative to the oxygen requirements of their metabolic activities. The final common pathway of all shock states is an imbalance between O_2 supply and demand. The effects of inadequate tissue perfusion are initially reversible, but prolonged end-organ hypoperfusion leads to cellular hypoxia and the derangement of critical biochemical processes, including (1) cell membrane ion pump dysfunction, (2) intracellular edema, (3) leakage of intracellular contents into the extracellular space, and (4) inadequate regulation of intracellular pH. These abnormalities rapidly become *irreversible* and result sequentially in cell death, end-organ damage (multiple organ system failure), and death. As a result, the prompt recognition of shock and initiation of therapy are imperative. Despite modern aggressive treatment in the intensive care unit (ICU) setting, the mortality rates from shock remain very high—for example, mortality rates of 50 to 80% are reported for patients with acute myocardial infarction and cardiogenic shock.

Cardiogenic shock occurs when impairment of cardiac pump function results in inadequate tissue perfusion. This chapter focuses on the pathophysiology, clinical diagnosis, and approach to the patient with cardiogenic shock; Chapter 7 discusses shock resulting from low preload and Chapter 8 discusses shock resulting from low afterload. Pericardial tamponade and major pulmonary embolus, the two primary causes of "obstructive shock," are presented in Chapters 53 and 76, respectively.

PATHOPHYSIOLOGY

Determinants of Tissue Perfusion

The principal determinants of tissue perfusion are cardiac output and arterial blood pressure. Cardiac output is defined by the relationship in Equation 1 (Table 6–1). Factors that affect ventricular stroke volume include preload, intrinsic myocardial contractility, and afterload (Figs. 6–1 to 6–4). Arterial blood pressure represents the driving force for tissue perfusion and can be defined by Equations 2 and 3 (see Table 6–1). Systemic vascular resistance is principally determined by the arterioles. Shock can be caused by a variety of pathophysiologic processes that alter any of these factors, thereby reducing oxygen delivery to the tissues.

Stages of Shock

The shock syndrome is characterized by a series of physiologic stages beginning with an initial inciting event that causes circulatory compromise. Shock may

Table 6–1. Basic Hemodynamic Equations

Equation 1. **CO** **= SV × HR**
 CO = cardiac output (L/min)
 SV = ventricular stroke volume (L/beat)
 HR = heart rate (bpm)
Equation 2. **MAP** **= (CO × SVR) + CVP**
 MAP = mean arterial blood pressure (mm Hg)
 CVP = central venous pressure (mm Hg)
 CO = cardiac output (L/min)
 SVR = systemic vascular resistance
 where SVR (in units of mm Hg/L/min) × 80 = SVR (in units of dyne sec cm^{-5})
Equation 3. **MAP** **= DBP + 1/3 (SBP − DBP)**
 DBP = diastolic blood pressure (mm Hg)
 SBP = systolic blood pressure (mm Hg)

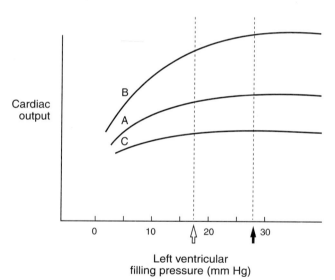

Cardiac output

Left ventricular
filling pressure (mm Hg)

Figure 6–1. "Starling curves" of ventricular function representing the relationship between cardiac output (as the dependent variable) and left ventricular filling (end-diastolic) pressure (LVEDP) (as the independent variable) for myocardial states of normal *(A)*, enhanced *(B)*, and decreased *(C)* myocardial contractility. Other important independent variables that determine cardiac output, such as afterload (Fig. 6–2), are held constant. In the intensive care unit, LVEDP is normally approximated by pulmonary artery wedge pressure (PAWP). The dashed vertical line at ~18 mm Hg *(open arrow)* indicates the PAWP at which fluid begins to accumulate in the interstitial space of the lung. The dotted vertical line at ~28 mm Hg *(closed arrow)* indicates the PAWP at which acute alveolar edema develops. Note that all curves lack "descending limbs" at high filling pressures (i.e., decreasing cardiac outputs at high LVEDP). Descending limbs of Starling curves are considered to be experimental artifacts and may have been due to development of mitral regurgitation at high distending pressures (see Elzinga G: Starling's "Law of the Heart": Rise and fall of the descending limb. News Physiol Sci 7:134–137, 1992 for more details about the descending limb.)

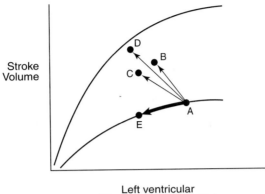

Stroke Volume

Left ventricular
filling pressure (mm Hg)

Figure 6–2. Curves relating stroke volume and left ventricular end-diastolic pressure (LVEDP) at states of normal and depressed contractility. At an elevated LVEDP on the lower curve *(point A)*, administration of an inotropic agent (e.g., dopamine) increases contractility *(point B)* and causes a modest decrease in preload (e.g., lower LVEDP). Likewise, administration of a vasodilator agent (which reduces both afterload and preload) results in improved stroke volume but with a greater decrease in LVEDP *(point C)*. Concomitant treatment with both agents produces an additional increase in stroke volume *(point D)*. In contrast, treatment with a diuretic alone decreases LVEDP with no increase in stroke volume *(point E)*. (Modified from Cohn JN, Franciosa JA: Vasodilator therapy of cardiac failure. N Engl J Med 297:27–31, 1977.)

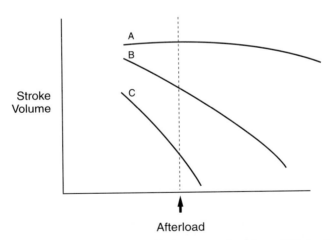

Stroke Volume

Afterload

Figure 6–3. Curves representing the relationship between stroke volume (SV) (as the dependent variable) and left ventricular afterload (as the independent variable) for states of normal myocardial function *(A)*, and moderate *(B)* and severe *(C)* myocardial dysfunction. Other variables affecting stroke volume, such as preload, are constant. When myocardial function is normal, SV is relatively preserved (curve A) as afterload increases above normal *(dashed line, closed arrow)*, but SV decreases markedly (curves B and C) when myocardial dysfunction is present. (Modified from Cohn JN, Franciosa JA: Vasodilator therapy of cardiac failure. N Engl J Med 297:27–31, 1977.)

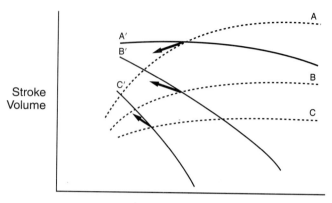

Stroke
Volume

Afterload / Left Ventricular
Filling Pressure (mmHg)

Figure 6–4. Three Starling curves *(dotted lines)* relating stroke volume and left ventricular filling pressure with normal *(A)*, moderately decreased *(B)*, and severely decreased *(C)* myocardial function are superimposed on three curves *(solid lines)* relating stroke volume and afterload for the same three states of myocardial function (normal, *A'*; moderately decreased, *B'*; and severely decreased, *C'*). Because most vasodilator agents (e.g., nitroprusside) reduce both preload and afterload, their effects on stroke volume depend on state of myocardial function. For example, when myocardial function is normal, such a vasodilator lowers stroke volume because of the predominant effect caused by lowering preload (as shown by the arrow originating at the intersection of curves A and A'). In contrast, when myocardial function is depressed, such an agent results in improved stroke volume despite a decrease in preload (arrows from the intersections of curves B and B' and curves C and C'). (Modified from Cohn JN, Franciosa JA: Vasodilator therapy of cardiac failure. N Engl J Med 297:27–31, 1977.)

subsequently progress through three stages, culminating in irreversible end-organ damage and death.

Preshock

Preshock is also known as "warm shock" or compensated shock. During this stage, the body's homeostatic mechanisms rapidly compensate for diminished perfusion. Reflex sympathetic activation leads to tachycardia and peripheral vasoconstriction, thereby temporarily maintaining blood pressure and cardiac output.

Frank Shock

During this stage, the regulatory mechanisms are overwhelmed and signs and symptoms of organ dysfunction appear, including tachycardia, tachypnea, metabolic acidosis, and oliguria. The emergence of these signs typically corresponds to one or more of the following: (1) a 25% reduction in effective blood volume in hypovolemic shock, (2) a decrease in the cardiac index to less than 2.5 L/min/M², or (3) activation of the many mediators of the sepsis syndrome.

Irreversible Shock

During this stage, progressive end-organ dysfunction leads to irreversible organ damage and death: (1) Urine output may decline and renal failure may ensue, (2) mental status may become altered, with agitation, obtundation, and eventually coma, (3) respiratory muscle fatigue may be precipitated by decreased perfusion of the diaphragms, leading to hypercapnic respiratory failure, and (4) multiple organ system failure may ensue.

DIFFERENTIAL DIAGNOSIS

In order to initiate appropriate therapy, cardiogenic shock must be differentiated from other categories of shock, such as hypovolemic shock, low afterload shock, or obstructive shock. The clinical history, physical examination, and laboratory finding should provide important clues to its origin. The use of a balloon-tipped, flow-directed pulmonary artery (Swan-Ganz) catheter can facilitate the initial categorization of the shock state as well as help to identify the individual causes of cardiogenic shock (Tables 6–2 and 6–3).

Hypovolemia, occurring as a result of blood loss or volume depletion, results in inadequate ventricular preload with resultant decreased stroke volume and cardiac output. Typically, filling pressures (such as the pulmonary artery wedge pressure) are reduced, as is cardiac output. Similarly, impaired left ventricular filling from increased intrapericardial pressure resulting from cardiac tamponade and obstruction to right ventricular outflow secondary to acute massive pulmonary embolism result in reduced left ventricular preload, stroke volume, and cardiac output. Initial treatment is with volume infusion until more definitive therapy is initiated. In patients with left ventricular systolic dysfunction, diastolic dysfunction, or right ventricular dysfunction, "normal" filling pressures may not be adequate to maintain normal cardiac output. Thus, relative hypovolemia may be present despite a "normal" central venous pressure or pulmonary artery wedge pressure. The ideal filling pressures in patients with heart failure are those that allow maximal cardiac output without producing pulmonary edema. Often, patients with chronic heart failure require a pulmonary artery wedge pressure of 16 to 20 mm Hg to maintain adequate cardiac output.

Table 6–2. Various Shock States and Typical Results of Pulmonary Artery Catheterization

CAUSE OF SHOCK	CARDIAC OUTPUT	RA AND RV PRESSURES	PAWP	SVR	MIXED VENOUS SATURATION
Hypovolemic (low preload)	↓	↓	↓	↑	↓
Distributive (low afterload)	↑, WNL, ↓	WNL, ↓	WNL, ↓	↓↓	WNL, ↑
Obstructive (major PE)	↓	↑	WNL	↑	↓
Obstructive (tamponade)	↓	↑	↑	↑	↓
Cardiogenic (LV failure)	↓	↑	↑↑	↑	↓
Cardiogenic (acute MR)	↓	WNL, ↑	↑	↑	↓
Cardiogenic (RV infarction)	↓	↑	WNL	↑	↓
Cardiogenic (acute VSD)	WNL	↑	WNL, ↑	↑	↑

RA, right atrial; RV, right ventricular; PAWP, pulmonary artery wedge pressure; SVR, systemic vascular resistance; ↓, decreased; ↓↓, markedly decreased; ↑, increased; ↑↑, markedly increased; WNL, within normal limits; PE, pulmonary embolus; LV, left ventricular; MR, mitral regurgitation; VSD, ventricular septal defect.

Table 6–3. Causes of Cardiogenic Shock

....

Myocardial Causes

Left ventricular systolic dysfunction
    Acute myocardial infarction (see Chapter 49)
    Acute myocarditis
    Cardiomyopathy
    Myocardial contusion due to trauma
    Sepsis with myocardial depression
Left ventricular diastolic dysfunction
    Hypertrophic cardiomyopathy
    Ischemic left ventricle
Right ventricular dysfunction
    Acute right ventricular infarction

Arrhythmias

Bradyarrhythmia (complete heart block) (see Chapter 30)
Tachyarrhythmia (ventricular tachycardia) (see Chapter 31)

Mechanical Problems

Acute valvular disease
    Aortic dissection with aortic regurgitation (see Chapter 50)
    Endocarditis with acute mitral regurgitation or aortic regurgitation
    Papillary muscle dysfunction, infarct, ischemia, rupture with severe mitral regurgitation
Left ventricular outflow obstruction
    Hypertrophic obstructive cardiomyopathy
Acute ventricular septal defect postmyocardial infarct

....

Shock caused by vasodilation or low afterload is termed *distributive shock* (e.g., shock caused by sepsis and anaphylaxis). Septic shock occurs as a result of endogenous and exogenous biologically active factors, which produce vasodilation and impair oxygen delivery to the tissues. Early septic shock may be associated with increased cardiac output secondary to decreased afterload and increased heart rate, but late septic shock may be associated with profound reduction in cardiac output from myocardial depression resulting from a number of factors. Late septic shock needs to be distinguished from primary cardiogenic shock because the therapy for these conditions differs significantly.

CLINICAL PEARLS AND PITFALLS

Early Diagnosis

A high index of suspicion is required to appropriately diagnose cardiogenic shock in its early stage and rapidly initiate therapy. Although cardiogenic shock is typically diagnosed when frank hypotension develops, a compensatory elevation in systemic vascular resistance may serve to maintain arterial blood pressure despite a profound reduction in cardiac output and end-organ perfusion. Thus, "preshock" should be suspected when there is evidence of low cardiac output, despite normal or near-normal systemic arterial pressures. Increasing heart rate, cool, clammy skin on the extremities with slow capillary filling (>2 sec), a decrease in urine output, and altered mental status are important clues to a reduced cardiac output that may precede frank hypotensive shock. The initial evaluation of patients with suspected cardiogenic shock should include a rapid assessment of organ perfusion and volume status (Fig. 6–5).

Pulse oximetry or arterial blood gas analysis should be done to assess oxygenation as well as a chest radiograph to assess possible pulmonary congestion. An electrocardiogram should be performed to look for evidence of myocardial infarction or dysrhythmias. An echocardiogram is extremely helpful in differentiating patients with cardiogenic shock caused by left ventricular dysfunction from those with right ventricular infarction, ventricular septal rupture, acute mitral regurgitation, and cardiac tamponade. Flow-directed pulmonary artery catheterization can

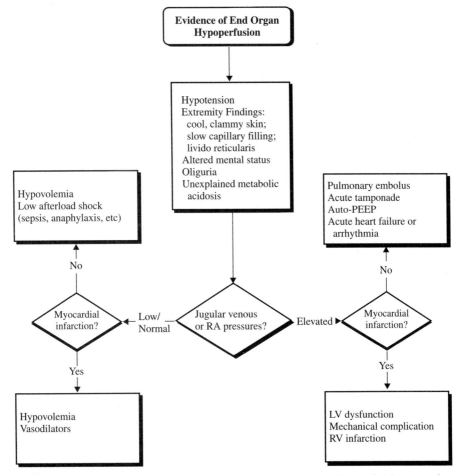

Figure 6–5. Algorithm for evaluation and management of patients with evidence of end-organ perfusion with circulatory shock. (PEEP, positive end-expiratory pressure; RA, right atrial; LV, left ventricular; RV, right ventricular.)

be used to differentiate cardiogenic shock from other categories (see Table 6–2). It can also guide volume therapy because many patients in shock require abnormally high filling pressures to maintain an adequate cardiac output.

MYOCARDIAL INFARCTION AND CARDIOGENIC SHOCK

Impaired Left Ventricular Function

The primary pathophysiologic disturbance in cardiogenic shock is compromised cardiac performance. Although a variety of processes can cause cardiogenic shock (see Table 6–3), it most often occurs as a consequence of acute myocardial infarction causing sudden severe left ventricular dysfunction. Cardiogenic shock commonly results when there is loss of a critical amount (usually >40%) of left ventricular myocardial mass. Postinfarction cardiogenic shock remains the leading cause of in-hospital mortality in those with myocardial infarction.

A large acute myocardial infarction may lead to impaired pump function with a resultant decrease in stroke volume and arterial blood pressure. Abnormalities of diastolic function occur with acute ischemia and result in elevated intracardiac pressures, pulmonary congestion, reduced left ventricular filling, and further reductions in left ventricular preload and stroke volume. Ultimately, progressive hypotension potentiates ischemia and initiates a downward vicious spiral, resulting in irreversible hypotension and death (Fig. 6–6).

Cardiogenic shock complicates 7 to 8% of all myocardial infarctions, and as myocardial necrosis progresses, shock often develops after hospitalization. In 89% of patients in whom cardiogenic shock developed in the first Global Utilization of Streptokinase and Tissue Plasminogen Activator for Occluded Coronary Arteries trial (GUSTO I) (a trial of thrombolytic strategies in acute myocardial infarction), the shock developed after hospital admission. Risk factors for the development of cardiogenic shock with myocardial infarction include advanced age, pre-existing left ventricular ejection fraction less than 35%, diabetes, and a history of a prior infarction. Mechanical complications of acute myocardial infarction, such as acute ventricular septal rupture and acute papillary muscle rupture with mitral regurgitation, typically occur 2 to 7 days after the initial event; therefore, sudden hemodynamic deterioration several days after admission should prompt a search for one of these mechanical complications.

The mortality rate for cardiogenic shock in myocardial infarction remains high when medical therapy alone is used. Revascularization procedures by percutaneous transluminal coronary angioplasty (PTCA) or coronary artery bypass grafting (CABG) are the only interventions that have yet shown improved mortality rates.

Diagnosis

Patients with acute myocardial infarction may have prolonged anginal pain, dyspnea, diaphoresis, nausea, or emesis (Chapter 49). Because cardiogenic shock usually evolves subsequent to hospitalization, the physician must be vigilant throughout the patient's hospital course for findings and symptoms that may herald its development. The physical examination may reveal tachycardia, hypotension,

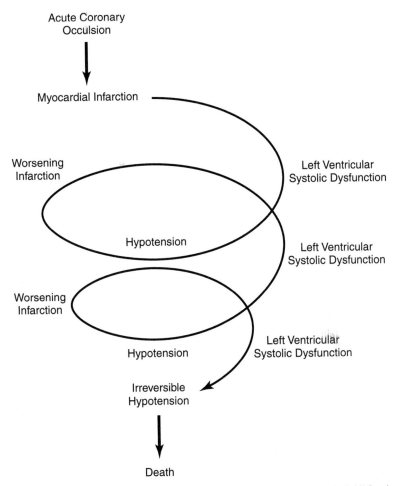

Figure 6–6. Pathophysiologic "death spiral" of cardiogenic shock in acute myocardial infarction with progressive loss of left ventricular function.

tachypnea, and signs of peripheral hypoperfusion (see Fig. 6–5), but the lack of these findings does not entirely exclude the development of the shock syndrome. There may be evidence of pulmonary congestion on auscultation of the lungs and either an S_3 or S_4 gallop on cardiac auscultation. A new murmur of mitral regurgitation suggests papillary muscle dysfunction; a precordial thrill suggests a new ventricular septal defect. The electrocardiographic signs of myocardial infarction typically include ST segment elevation in multiple leads corresponding to the distribution of the occluded coronary artery, pathologic T waves, and ST segment depression consistent with ischemia in other distributions. Patients with left main coronary artery disease may have diffuse ST segment depression in all leads, reflecting global ischemia. Assessment of jugular venous pressure or central venous pressure (see Fig. 6–5) differentiates hypotension caused by drugs or hypovolemia from hypotension resulting from left ventricular dysfunction, right ventricular infarction, or a mechanical complication of myocardial infarction.

A transthoracic echocardiogram (TTE) can distinguish primary left ventricular dysfunction from right ventricular infarction, acute papillary muscle dysfunction with mitral regurgitation, acute ventricular septal defect, or tamponade, and should be performed early in the course of complicated myocardial infarction. Preserved left ventricular systolic function by TTE in a patient with cardiogenic shock is an important clue to the presence of a mechanical complication of myocardial infarction. Transesophageal echocardiography (TEE) is especially helpful in assessing the mechanical complications of myocardial infarction such as acute papillary muscle rupture or ventricular septal defect, and should be performed if the TTE is not definitive.

General Management

Early recognition and treatment are essential to the successful management of patients with cardiogenic shock. Two critical principal therapeutic goals are to immediately stabilize the hemodynamic derangement and to restore coronary blood flow. General treatment measures include correcting the hypovolemia, hypoxemia, and acidosis; avoiding or stopping drugs that may produce hypotension or impair cardiac output (e.g., beta-blockers) is imperative. Patients with myocardial infarction should be promptly given aspirin and full-dose intravenous heparin. No randomized trial data are available on the efficacy of most modalities (intra-aortic balloon pump [IABP] counterpulsation, PTCA, and CABG) used to treat cardiogenic shock.

Drug Therapy

Sympathetic Amines

Dopamine, dobutamine, isoproterenol, norepinephrine, and epinephrine have all been used to temporarily improve cardiac performance in patients with cardiogenic shock until more definitive therapy is initiated. Although loosely categorized as beta-agonists, each agent has important differences in the degree of cardiac and peripheral beta-receptor effects, alpha-receptor effects, and effects on myocardial oxygen consumption and hemodynamics (Tables 6–4 and 6–5). Typically, drugs such as dopamine and norepinephrine are used to provide inotropic and vasopressor support when severe hypotension (e.g., mean arterial pressure < 60–65 mm Hg) is present. Because all of these drugs have the potential to increase myocardial oxygen demand and worsen myocardial ischemia, they should be used as temporizing measures to maintain adequate hemodynamics while awaiting more definitive therapy.

Vasodilators

Drugs with vasodilator properties such as dobutamine, milrinone, nitroprusside, and nitroglycerin are used to increase cardiac output by reducing afterload (see

Table 6–4. Drug Therapy for Cardiogenic Shock

DRUG	USUAL ADULT DOSE RANGE	PREDOMINANT ACTIONS
Sympathomimetic Amines		
Dopamine	3–5 μg/kg/min	Renal vasodilator
	5–10 μg/kg/min	Vasodilator and inotrope
	>10 μg/kg/min	Vasoconstrictor
Dobutamine	5–20 μg/kg/min	Inotrope > vasodilator
Isoproterenol	1–10 μg/min	Chronotropy > inotropy
Epinephrine	1–20 μg/min	Inotrope, vasodilator
	>20 μg/min	Vasoconstrictor
Norepinephrine	1–2 μg/min	Inotrope
	>2 μg/min	Vasoconstrictor
Other Agents		
Milrinone	0.25–0.75 μg/kg/min	Vasodilator > inotrope
Nitroglycerin	10–50 μg/min	Venodilator
	50–200 μg/min	Vasodilator
Nitroprusside	0.5–2 μg/kg/min	Vasodilator

Figs. 6–2 and 6–4) when frank hypotension is *not* present. In patients with systolic arterial blood pressures greater than 90 mm Hg and low cardiac output, elevated filling pressures, and elevated systemic vascular resistance, the use of vasodilators can also result in decreased pulmonary congestion. Nitroglycerin can reduce ischemia and pulmonary congestion but should only be used when systolic arterial blood pressure is more than 100 mm Hg. Profound decreases in systemic arterial pressure that occur after administration of sublingual or intravenous nitroglycerin and that do not correct with intravenous volume administration can decrease coronary perfusion and worsen myocardial ischemia. Such episodes should prompt cessation of this drug.

Intra-aortic Balloon Counterpulsation and Other Circulatory Support Devices

Intra-aortic balloon counterpulsation has been used to decrease afterload, reduce myocardial oxygen consumption, improve coronary blood flow, and improve tissue perfusion; therefore, it has been used enthusiastically in patients with acute myocardial infarction and cardiogenic shock. In the pre-thrombolytic era, however, the use of intra-aortic balloon counterpulsation did not reduce mortality. In the thrombolytic era of therapy, there is a paucity of data from randomized trials. Intra-aortic balloon counterpulsation has been shown to be helpful in initial clinical stabilization in a nonrandomized trial of 87 patients with persistent hypotension and hypoperfusion despite vasopressor therapy. Although more than 70% of these patients had normalization of urine output and acid-base status, their mortality rate remained high (83%). A randomized trial called TACTICS is currently testing whether intra-aortic balloon pump support added to thrombolytic therapy reduces mortality rate when compared to thrombolytic therapy alone. Until results from

Table 6–5. Hemodynamic Profiles of Sympathomimetic Amines

AGENT	INOTROPY	SVR	CO	HR	V̇O₂
Dopamine, low dose	↑	↓	↑	↑	↑
Dopamine, high dose	↑↑	↑↑↑	↑↑	↑↑	↑↑
Dobutamine	↑↑	↓	↑↑	↑↑	↑↑↑
Epinephrine	↑↑	↑↑	↑↑	↑↑↑	↑↑↑
Norepinephrine	↑↑	↑↑↑	↑	↑↑↑	↑
Isoproterenol	↑	↓↓	↑↑	↑↑↑	↑↑↑

SVR, systemic vascular resistance; CO, cardiac output; HR, heart rate; V̇O₂, minute oxygen consumption; ↓, decreased; ↓↓, markedly decreased; ↑, mildly increased; ↑↑, moderately increased; ↑↑↑, markedly increased.

this and other randomized trials are available, intra-aortic balloon pump counterpulsation should be considered as an adjunct to vasopressor therapy and reserved for patients with refractory cardiogenic shock or those with mechanical complications of myocardial infarction who cannot tolerate vasodilator therapy.

Newer circulatory support devices, such as left ventricular assist devices (LVADs), are available from a variety of manufacturers. For patients whose cardiogenic shock is refractory to drug therapy, a left ventricular assist device can be used as a bridge to cardiac transplantation (see Chapter 86).

Reperfusion Therapy with Thrombolytic Therapy

A number of studies have shown that arterial patency is the strongest predictor of survival in patients with myocardial infarction and cardiogenic shock. Although early thrombolytic therapy has been shown to restore arterial patency in the infarcted region, preserve myocardial function, and reduce overall mortality rate in patients with myocardial infarction, it has *not* been shown to appreciably lower mortality rate in patients with cardiogenic shock. In 80 patients with cardiogenic shock in the Italian Group for the Study of Streptokinase in Infarction (GISSI) trial, the mortality rate of patients who received streptokinase was identical to those who did not (70%). In a subgroup analysis of 322 patients with cardiogenic shock from the International Study of Infarct Survival (ISIS), the mortality rate with tissue plasminogen activator was 78% and with streptokinase was 65%; both rates were similar to those for historical control subjects. Similarly, in 315 patients with cardiogenic shock in GUSTO I, the mortality rate was 59% for patients given tissue plasminogen activator and 55% for those given streptokinase. Whether the addition of intra-aortic balloon pump counterpulsation to thrombolytic therapy improves these outcomes is currently being tested, as noted previously.

Revascularization for Cardiogenic Shock

Early revascularization in acute myocardial infarction, either by PTCA or by CABG, has been shown to restore arterial patency and to improve outcome in cardiogenic shock. There are currently 17 published studies involving 453 patients who underwent coronary angioplasty for cardiogenic shock, and those who underwent successful coronary angioplasty had lower mortality rates when compared with those with unsuccessful angioplasty. The overall success rate of coronary angioplasty in this setting was 73%, which is somewhat lower than when angioplasty is done electively.

Similarly, there are 19 studies involving 323 patients who underwent coronary artery bypass surgery during hospitalization for acute myocardial infarction and cardiogenic shock. The in-hospital mortality rate for these pooled patients is 32%, which is the lowest for any treatment modality reported. In a study of more than 200 patients, arterial patency was shown to be the strongest predictor of in-hospital mortality, whether the mechanism was spontaneous, pharmacologic, by PTCA, or by CABG. Because significant selection biases and heterogeneity exist in this literature, however, these data should be interpreted with caution.

Impaired Right Ventricular Function

Clinically important right ventricular infarction occurs in approximately 7% of inferior myocardial infarctions and is associated with a high mortality rate resulting from cardiogenic shock. Right ventricular infarction produces an acute decrease in left ventricular preload, with a resultant decrease in stroke volume and cardiac output. Right-sided filling pressures are typically very elevated. The clinical hallmarks of right ventricular infarction are elevated jugular venous pressure, hypotension, and clear lung fields on auscultation. Right-sided precordial leads may reveal ST segment elevation reflecting right ventricular infarction. These changes do not necessarily correlate with hemodynamically significant right ventricular infarction and therefore should be interpreted cautiously. The initial therapy for right ventricular infarction is rapid administration of intravenous volume, because high filling pressures (i.e., elevated right atrial and right ventricular pressures) are often required to maintain adequate left ventricular preload and cardiac output. Nitrates should be avoided because they may produce profound hypotension. Pulmonary artery catheterization is often needed for optimization of hemodynamic parameters. Patients who do not respond to volume resuscitation should be supported with inotropes such as dobutamine or milrinone if severe hypotension is not present. Drugs that increase pulmonary vascular resistance (e.g., dopamine) and therefore worsen right ventricular function should be avoided if possible. As stated earlier, prompt revascularization with either PTCA or CABG should be performed as indicated.

Acute Mechanical Complications of Myocardial Infarction

Acute mechanical complications of myocardial infarction may also result in cardiogenic shock. Papillary muscle infarction or rupture may cause acute severe mitral regurgitation. Acute ventricular septal rupture produces a left-to-right shunt with acute right-sided volume overload and an inadequate left-sided cardiac output. Physical examination of patients with papillary muscle dysfunction or rupture often reveals a holosystolic murmur of mitral regurgitation. Those with a ventricular septal defect often have a harsh systolic murmur, with an accompanying thrill across the precordium. Physical examination findings, however, may be nonspecific or even absent in patients with either complication.

TTE or TEE is particularly helpful in identifying acute mechanical complications of myocardial infarction from primary pump failure caused solely by left ventricular dysfunction. Preserved, normal, or hyperdynamic left ventricular function found on TTE in a patient with shock can be an important clue to an underlying mechanical complication and should prompt consideration of TEE if the diagnosis is not clear. Flow-directed pulmonary artery catheterization can also help differentiate severe mitral regurgitation and ventricular septal rupture from intrinsic left ventricular dysfunction (see Table 6–2). Patients with severe mitral regurgitation may have large V waves in the pulmonary artery wedge tracings, although this finding is neither sensitive nor specific for mitral regurgitation. Large V waves can also be seen in acute ventricular septal rupture as a result of the increased volume load presented to the left atrium.

Patients with acute ventricular septal rupture or mitral regurgitation and cardiogenic shock pose difficult management problems because they often benefit from afterload reduction with vasodilator drugs, but they can be profoundly hypotensive. Often, an empirical trial of low-dose vasodilators is warranted. If worsening hypotension ensues, then intra-aortic balloon counterpulsation should be considered. Definitive therapy with either surgical repair of the ventricular septal defect or replacement of the mitral valve should be undertaken promptly, because the mortality of patients who receive medical therapy alone is extremely high. The use of concomitant revascularization is controversial, but there are trends favoring improved survival rate in those who undergo ventricular septal defect repair or mitral valve replacement with CABG. The condition of some patients with acute mechanical complications of myocardial infarction may be too tenuous for them to undergo concomitant revascularization, being unable to tolerate prolonged cardiopulmonary bypass. Despite corrective surgery, mortality rates are high.

OTHER CAUSES OF CARDIOGENIC SHOCK

Disturbances of Cardiac Rhythm

Severe tachyarrhythmias or bradyarrhythmias can acutely disrupt cardiac output and result in cardiogenic shock, because heart rate is an important determinant of cardiac output and ventricular filling. Rapid supraventricular or ventricular tachycardia may be associated with marked reductions in diastolic filling time and ventricular stroke volume. Supraventricular tachycardia, such as atrioventricular (AV) nodal re-entrant tachycardia, may also be associated with simultaneous atrial and ventricular contraction, which further reduces ventricular filling. Even patients with normal ventricular function often poorly tolerate heart rates of more than 200 beats per minute. Abnormal ventricular systolic or diastolic dysfunction make it even more likely that rapid heart rates will result in hemodynamic instability. Patients with rapid tachyarrhythmias of any origin who are hemodynamically unstable should be urgently cardioverted to restore sinus rhythm (see Chapter 31 and ACLS algorithms in Appendix E).

Similarly, severe bradycardia or high-grade heart block may acutely reduce cardiac output and result in hemodynamic instability. Reduced diastolic filling may also occur as a result of asynchronous atrial and ventricular contractions, and further reduce cardiac output. Prompt treatment with transcutaneous or transvenous pacing is necessary to improve cardiac output and acutely altered hemodynamics (see Chapter 30).

Acute Myocarditis and Cardiomyopathy

Acute myocarditis can also produce cardiogenic shock through a loss of intrinsic myocardial pump function. Giant cell myocarditis, in particular, is associated with a fulminant course and rapid hemodynamic deterioration. Although certain subsets of patients may benefit from immunosuppressive therapy, no specific therapy has been shown to definitively alter mortality rates in these patients; therefore, the treatment remains supportive.

Progressive heart failure from cardiomyopathy of any cause can also result in cardiogenic shock. Chemotherapeutic agents such as doxorubicin can cause an acute toxic cardiomyopathy and result in cardiogenic shock.

BIBLIOGRAPHY

Cohn JN, Franciosa JA: Vasodilator therapy of cardiac failure. N Engl J Med 297:27–31, 254–258, 1977.
Classic review article describing importance of afterload in left ventricular function and the drugs used to modify afterload during acute and chronic cardiac dysfunction.

Forrester JS, Diamond G, Chatterjee K, Swan HJC: Medical therapy of acute myocardial infarction by application of hemodynamic subsets. N Engl J Med 295:1356–1362, 1976.
Classic description of utility of the flow-directed pulmonary artery catheter in classifying patients after acute myocardial infarctions.

Nitenberg A: Determinants of left ventricular performance. In: Pinsky MR, Dhainaut J-FA (eds): Pathophysiologic Foundations of Critical Care. Baltimore: Williams & Wilkins, 1993.
This chapter interprets changes, preload, afterload, contractility, and myocardial stiffness in terms of the left ventricle-pressure loops described by Suga.

Payen DM, Beloucif S: Acute left ventricular failure. In: Pinsky MR, Dhainaut J-FA (eds). Pathophysiologic Foundations of Critical Care, Baltimore: Williams & Wilkins, 1993.
This chapter describes the physiology underlying states of acute left ventricular failure in terms of Guyton's venous return curve and considerations of ventricular pressure-volume loops.

Suga H: Total mechanical energy of a ventricle model and cardiac oxygen consumption. Am J Physiol 236:H494–H497, 1979.
Describes the complex ventricular pressure-volume relationships during both diastole and systole that underlie current concepts of left ventricular mechanical functioning.

7 Hemorrhagic Shock and Other Low Preload States

Henry J. Schiller
Harry L. Anderson III

Simply stated, shock represents a clinical state in which blood flow to the tissues is inadequate to sustain normal metabolic function. Whereas an overt shock state may be obvious in the presence of tachycardia and hypotension, the clinical presentation may be much more subtle, reflecting end organ dysfunction secondary to hypoperfusion. Furthermore, because individual organs may be variably affected, a patient with an apparently normal blood pressure and pulse rate may manifest shock by such signs as oliguria, skin pallor, coolness of extremities, and mental confusion.

Hypovolemic shock results from a decrease in the circulating blood volume that can result from many causes (Table 7–1). Hemorrhagic shock, the most common form of hypovolemic shock, has been divided into four stages of severity by the Advanced Trauma Life Support course sponsored by the American College of Surgeons (Table 7–2). These four stages correspond to progressive loss of blood and associated physiologic responses in patients with normal cardiopulmonary systems.

Physiologic characteristics of cardiogenic shock and distributive (low afterload) shock differ from those observed in shock due to low preload, and these differences help to identify the underlying cause (see Table 6–2). In cardiogenic shock (see Chapter 6), circulating blood volume may be normal or increased but cardiac output is diminished, resulting in tissue hypoperfusion. In distributive shock, the circulating blood volume may be "normal" but becomes inadequate because of a loss of vasomotor tone in capacitance vessels. Therefore, effective circulating blood volume is insufficient, not due to loss of blood volume but because the

Table 7–1. Causes of Shock Due to Hypovolemia or Decreased Venous Return

Decreased Circulating Global Blood Volume

Gastrointestinal tract losses (vomiting, diarrhea, fistula)
Hemorrhage
Renal losses (polyuria in diabetic ketoacidosis, postobstructive diuresis)
"Third spacing" (i.e., sequestration of intravascular volume in parts of the extracellular fluid compartment, e.g., pancreatitis)

Decreased Venous Return to the Heart*

Abdominal tamponade (abdominal compartment syndrome)
Auto-PEEP (positive end-expiratory pressure)
Cardiac tamponade
Tachyarrhythmias
Tension pneumothorax
Venodilation (anaphylactic, drug-induced, neurogenic causes)

*With normal global blood volume.

Table 7–2. Four Stages of Hemorrhagic Shock

PARAMETER	CLASS I	CLASS II	CLASS III	CLASS IV
Blood loss (mL)*	Up to 750	750–1500	1500–2000	>2000
Blood loss (% blood volume)	Up to 15%	15–30%	30–40%	>40%
Heart rate (beats per minute)	<100	>100	>120	>140
Blood pressure	Normal	Normal	↓	↓
Pulse pressure (mm Hg)	Normal or ↑	↓	↓	↓
Respiratory rate (breaths per minute)	14–20	20–30	30–40	>35
Urine output (mL/h)	>30	20–30	5–15	Negligible
Mental status	Slightly anxious	Mildly anxious	Anxious and confused	Confused and lethargic
Fluid replacement	Crystalloid	Crystalloid	Crystalloid and blood†	Crystalloid and blood

From American College of Surgeons: Advanced Trauma Life Support Instructor Manual. American College of Surgeons, Chicago, 1997, with permission.

*Values are based on an adult with an ideal body weight of 70 kg.

†Ratio of administered crystalloid to blood should be 3:1.

↓, decreased; ↓↓, markedly decreased; ↑, increased.

volume required to adequately fill the vascular space increases markedly. In some patients with distributive shock due to sepsis, cardiac output can be supranormal, owing to diminished resistance to left ventricular ejection (i.e., low afterload); see Chapter 8. In other patients with sepsis, however, cardiac output can be low owing to depression of myocardial function from effects of inflammatory mediators or due to pre-existing disease.

PATHOPHYSIOLOGY OF DECREASED PRELOAD

The two determinants of cardiac output are heart rate and stroke volume; the latter, in turn, is determined by preload, afterload, ventricular elastance during diastole and systole, and myocardial contractility, as represented by ventricular ejection fraction and rate of rise of systolic pressure. Preload corresponds to the stretch placed on cardiac muscle and describes the load that the muscle fiber must contract against. As illustrated by the Starling curves, increasing preload increases the force of muscle fiber contraction and cardiac stroke volume up to a maximum after which the output plateaus (see Fig. 6–1). The term *preload* most accurately refers to left ventricular end-diastolic volume (LVEDV) rather than the left ventricular end-diastolic pressure (LVEDP), which is commonly measured in the intensive care unit (ICU). For clinical purposes, it is assumed that the LVEDP is proportional to the LVEDV, although this relationship may become nonlinear, particularly in the noncompliant, diseased myocardium. Preload is a function of the global circulating blood volume as well as venous return to the heart (see Table 7–1).

Physiologic and Pathophysiologic Changes in Hypovolemic Shock

Hypovolemic shock is characterized hemodynamically by decreased cardiac preload, which results in a decreased stroke volume. Compensatory mechanisms for low cardiac output or hypotension are mediated by means of a sympathetic adrenergic response. Cardiac contractility and systemic vascular resistance increase and tachycardia follows in an attempt to maintain cardiac output in the presence of a falling stroke volume (see Fig. 6–2). In addition, blood is shunted away from the skin and skeletal muscle and from the splanchnic and renal circulations to preserve flow to the heart and brain (the so-called "fight or flight response"). For example, renal blood flow may be only 5 to 10% of normal during acute hypovolemia.

In addition, the venous capacitance beds constrict, which tends to enhance venous blood return to the heart. The renin-angiotensin system is activated, resulting in splanchnic vasoconstriction and the release of aldosterone and arginine vasopressin (antidiuretic hormone). These enhance renal reabsorption of sodium and water, which also tends to preserve the circulating blood volume. Arginine vasopressin is also a potent vasoconstrictor. Another endocrine response leads to increased levels of plasma glucagon, cortisol, and growth hormone. Along with increased endogenous catecholamines inhibiting the effects of insulin, these hormones all tend to increase the plasma glucose level. The resulting hyperglycemia makes the plasma hyperosmolar, which, in turn, tends to mobilize fluid from the extravascular space into the intravascular space.

Nutrient blood flow is delivered to the tissues through the microcirculation. Blood pressure within the vascular bed influences microcirculatory flow, which is further regulated by precapillary and postcapillary sphincters. Sphincter tone is controlled by autoregulation of the capillary bed and by the autonomic nervous system. The former is mediated both by endothelial stretch receptors, which modulate microcirculatory tone at varying perfusion pressures, and by the concentration of various metabolites mediating local vasodilatation (e.g., nitric oxide). In contrast, the sympathetic nervous system primarily results in vasoconstriction through an increase in precapillary tone. This shunts blood away from the involved tissue.

When all these compensatory mechanisms are active, the patient may tolerate even severe fluid loss with minimal or no tissue dysfunction ("compensated shock") or with some but reversible tissue dysfunction ("progressive shock"). During these states, fluid resuscitation, if given, would promptly restore the circulation. At some point, however, the shock may become irreversible ("irreversible shock") and resistant to simple fluid resuscitation. Potential mechanisms for this irreversibility, which is characterized by loss of autoregulation of the microcirculation, are discussed at the end of the next section.

Changes in Oxygen Delivery

Systemic oxygen delivery ($\dot{D}o_2$) is equal to the product of arterial oxygen content and cardiac output (Table 7–3). Minute oxygen consumption ($\dot{V}o_2$) is dependent on the body's total metabolic activity, distribution of blood flow, and tissue extraction and utilization of oxygen. The mixed venous oxygen saturation ($S\bar{v}o_2$)

Table 7–3. Basic Equations Related to Oxygen Delivery and Uptake

Equation 1: Arterial Oxygen Content

$Cao_2 = [Hgb \times 1.39 \text{ mL } O_2/g] \times Sao_2 + [Pao_{2\text{ mm}} \times 0.0031 \text{ mL } O_2/\text{mm Hg/dL}]$
where Cao_2 = Oxygen content of arterial blood (mL/dL)
Hgb = Hemoglobin concentration (g/dL)
Sao_2 = Oxygen saturation of hemoglobin in arterial blood

Equation 2: Oxygen Delivery

$\dot{D}o_2 = Cao_2 \times CO$
where $\dot{D}o_2$ = Oxygen delivery (mL O_2/L/min)

Equation 3: Oxygen Consumption

$\dot{V}o_2 = [Cao_2 - C\bar{v}o_2] \times CO$
where $\dot{V}o_2$ = Minute oxygen consumption (mL/min)
$C\bar{v}o_2$ = Oxygen content of mixed venous blood (mL/dL)

Equation 4: Oxygen Extraction Ratio (ER)

$ER = \dot{V}o_2/\dot{D}o_2 = \{Cao_2 - C\bar{v}o_2\}/Cao_2 = \{Sao_2 - S\bar{v}o_2\}/Sao_2$
where ER = Oxygen extraction ratio
Sao_2 = O_2 saturation of arterial blood
$S\bar{v}o_2$ = O_2 saturation of mixed venous blood

is typically measured from blood taken from the pulmonary artery and is dependent on the relationship of $\dot{D}O_2$ and $\dot{V}O_2$. The oxygen extraction ratio ($\dot{V}O_2/\dot{D}O_2$) represents the proportion of delivered oxygen to that actually consumed by the tissues. Under normal conditions, the $\dot{V}O_2/\dot{D}O_2$ is approximately 1:4, which corresponds to $S\bar{v}O_2$ of about 75%. Some intensivists prefer to follow the inverse ratio, the delivery-to-consumption ratio, $\dot{D}O_2/\dot{V}O_2$, which normally is 4:1. Under normal conditions, the amount of oxygen delivered to the tissues ($\dot{D}O_2$) is far in excess of oxygen consumption ($\dot{V}O_2$), and this explains why $\dot{V}O_2$ varies independently of $\dot{D}O_2$ under normal conditions (also referred to as $\dot{V}O_2$ being "$\dot{D}O_2$ independent" or "supply independent") (Fig. 7–1).

When $\dot{D}O_2/\dot{V}O_2$ is decreased to a critical level, however, usually less than 2:1 or the equivalent, or when $\dot{V}O_2/\dot{D}O_2$ increases above 0.5, extraction of capillary oxygen by the metabolically active tissues is limited. Thus, oxygen delivery becomes inadequate to support the baseline level of oxygen consumption. As a result, the tissues affected use anaerobic metabolism for adenosine triphosphate production, and $\dot{V}O_2$ falls below baseline (see Fig. 7–1). Under these conditions, increases in $\dot{D}O_2$ can increase $\dot{V}O_2$, or, expressed in another way, $\dot{V}O_2$ becomes *dependent* on $\dot{D}O_2$ ("$\dot{D}O_2$ dependent" or "supply dependent").

By inference, when $\dot{V}O_2$ is "$\dot{D}O_2$ dependent," some tissues will be ischemic and undergo anaerobic metabolism with production of lactic acid. If ischemia is severe enough, or prolonged, cell death will occur. In uncomplicated forms of low-output shock, that is, hypovolemic and cardiogenic shock, restoration of $\dot{D}O_2$ restores the normal relationship with $\dot{V}O_2$ being "$\dot{D}O_2$ independent." However, in

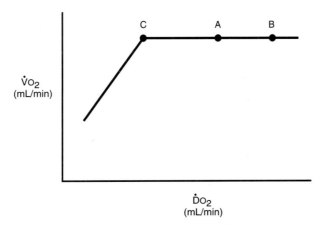

Figure 7–1. Schematic two-phase model illustrating the relationship between oxygen delivery to the whole body ($\dot{D}O_2$) and whole-body minute oxygen consumption ($\dot{V}O_2$) under normal (non–critically ill) conditions. At point A, representing a normal resting value for $\dot{D}O_2$ (e.g., when the oxygen extraction ratio, $\dot{V}O_2/\dot{D}O_2$, is 0.3, Equation 4, Table 7–3). If $\dot{D}O_2$ is increased to point B (e.g., by increasing heart rate by pacing or by transfusion), $\dot{V}O_2$ remains unchanged. In this case, $\dot{V}O_2$ is *independent* of increases in $\dot{D}O_2$ because O$_2$ delivery is already in excess of O$_2$ consumption. If $\dot{D}O_2$ *decreases* from point A, $\dot{V}O_2$ also remains unchanged (owing to increased extraction of O$_2$ from the blood by metabolizing tissues, i.e., increased $\dot{V}O_2/\dot{D}O_2$) until $\dot{D}O_2$ reaches a critical value ($\dot{D}O_2$c), at point C. Below point C, $\dot{D}O_2$ is no longer adequate to satisfy whole-body O$_2$ demand and, because oxygen extraction is maximal at this point, further decreases in $\dot{D}O_2$ result in decreases in $\dot{V}O_2$. Under these circumstances, $\dot{V}O_2$ is *dependent* on $\dot{D}O_2$.

septic shock, whether $\dot{V}O_2$ is $\dot{D}O_2$ dependent when cardiac output is normal or even supranormal remains controversial. As in low-output shock, tissue ischemia and elevated lactic acid production are also seen with septic shock but often accompanied by a high $\dot{D}O_2$, normal $S\bar{v}O_2$ (about 70%), and normal oxygen extraction ratio (about 0.30) (see Equation 4, Table 7–3). Furthermore, simply increasing global $\dot{D}O_2$ would not be expected to correct the derangements in microcirculatory blood flow or the abnormalities in oxygen extraction or utilization that have been described in septic shock. Indeed, prospective randomized clinical trials to date have not supported the efficacy of increasing global $\dot{D}O_2$ in the treatment of septic shock (see Chapter 8).

In hypovolemic shock, as in septic shock, there is activation of the inflammatory cascade, including multiple proinflammatory cytokines, such as tumor necrosis factor-alpha, interleukin-1, and interleukin-6. This development is termed *systemic inflammatory response syndrome* (SIRS). Not only does the development of SIRS increase metabolic rate, but these proinflammatory mediators can also result in tissue injury and organ failure by themselves. One likely effect is the diffuse marked cellular swelling noted earlier. This phenomenon is considered to be a major cause of loss of extracellular fluid volume seen in hemorrhagic shock. The ineffectiveness of treating hemorrhagic shock with blood alone or blood with plasma alone has been ascribed to this marked reduction in extracellular fluid volume.

Finally, reperfusion of previously ischemic organs due to hypovolemic shock can result in a reperfusion injury, usually attributed to reactive oxygen species and oxidative stress. When one takes into consideration the potential roles of these additional mediators in producing tissue injury, one can envision potential mechanisms that result in the irreversibility of shock when it is severe and prolonged.

CLINICAL MANIFESTATIONS

Hypovolemic shock is usually but not always apparent on physical examination. The skin is pallid, cool, and clammy; *livedo reticularis* may be present over poorly perfused extremities. The feet and hands are typically cooler than the torso, and capillary refill (assessed by suddenly releasing the examining finger after squeezing the distal phalanx of the middle finger, held at the level of the heart for 5 seconds) exceeds 2 seconds. Skin turgor is decreased, but only when hypovolemia is chronic. Mental status is altered by cerebral hypoperfusion. Anxiety progresses to confusion, agitation, and combativeness with increasing degrees of shock. Whereas vital signs usually reveal tachycardia and hypotension, this may be delayed in young, well-conditioned patients who can compensate for a falling cardiac output by intense vasoconstriction. Notably, the tachycardic response is blunted in patients treated with beta-blocking drugs, and a systolic blood pressure of 120 mm Hg may represent relative hypotension in an elderly patient who is normally hypertensive. The urine output decreases, due in part to renal hypoperfusion and in part to the effects of aldosterone.

The cause of hypovolemic shock can often be discerned from the patient's history and physical examination (see Table 7–1). Shock in a trauma patient is typically due to hemorrhage, although tension pneumothorax, cardiac tamponade, myocardial contusion, or neurogenic shock (due to spinal cord injury) must also be considered.

CLINICAL MANAGEMENT

The initial management of shock is dictated by well-established priorities (the "ABCs of resuscitation"). The airway (A) should be secured and adequate ventilation (breathing, B) provided. Endotracheal intubation and mechanical ventilation are appropriate in hemodynamically unstable or obtunded patients. To restore circulation (C), large-bore intravenous access should be immediately established and sources of hemorrhage controlled. Resuscitation is initiated with isotonic intravenous fluids (usually lactated Ringer's solution or normal saline) while the underlying cause of the shock state is being identified. Administration of colloid, including blood, instead of crystalloid, does not improve outcome and costs much more. Of even more concern, recent studies report worse outcomes with colloid (albumin) therapy compared with crystalloid. Fluid and blood product administration can subsequently be modified according to the clinical situation (see Chapter 15).

For hemorrhagic shock, packed red blood cell transfusion should be initiated if the patient's vital signs do not rapidly stabilize after rapid intravenous infusion of 2 L of lactated Ringer's solution. Heart rate and cardiac rhythm should be followed with a cardiac monitor. Serial blood pressure determinations should be obtained manually, with an automatic blood pressure cuff or, ideally in an unstable patient, with an indwelling arterial catheter. A urinary drainage catheter should be placed to accurately monitor urine production.

If the underlying cause of the shock state is not easily discernible or rapidly correctable, or if the patient fails to respond as expected to therapy, central venous catheterization allows monitoring of the central venous pressure as an index of the circulating blood volume. The intravascular volume status can be determined more accurately with a pulmonary artery flotation catheter, which permits measurements of cardiac output, preload, afterload, and mixed-venous oxygen saturation (see Chapters 5 and 9). This allows the titration of therapies to physiologic goals, including volume resuscitation, red cell transfusion, and inotrope or vasopressor administration. Pulmonary artery catheter placement should be strongly considered in patients with cardiac dysfunction, coronary artery disease, renal dysfunction, or multiple organ dysfunction.

Because blood is shunted away from the viscera during shock to preferentially perfuse the heart and brain, the gastrointestinal tract may remain relatively underperfused despite apparently adequate resuscitation. Gastric tonometry is a technique that may provide an indirect measurement of gastric mucosal blood flow and has been reported in several studies as a means of guiding "gut-specific" resuscitation. Widespread acceptance of this method in clinical practice in ICUs awaits confirmatory randomized controlled clinical trials.

BIBLIOGRAPHY

Chittock DR, Ronco JJ, Russell JA: Oxygen transport and oxygen consumption. In: Tobin MJ (ed): Principles and Practice of Intensive Care Monitoring, New York: McGraw-Hill, 1998, pp 317–343.

Comprehensive review, including detailed descriptions of methods to measure $\dot{V}_{O_2}$ and $\dot{D}_{O_2}$ and discussion of the controversy over whether $\dot{V}_{O_2}$ is supply dependent in patients with ARDS and other inflammatory states; with 141 references.

Holcroft JW (ed): Shock. In: American College of Surgeons: Care of the Surgical Patient. New York: Scientific American, 1996.

Le Tulzo Y, Shenkar R, Kaneko D, et al: Hemorrhage increases cytokine expression in lung mononuclear cells in mice: involvement of catecholamines in nuclear factor-kappa B regulation and cytokine expression. J Clin Invest 99:1516–1524, 1997.
This shows that proinflammatory cytokines are released during severe hemorrhage in mice and, by implication, that the same phenomena may occur in human hemorrhagic shock and perhaps shed light on the mechanism responsible for irreversible hemorrhagic shock.

Peitzman AB, Billiar TR, Harbrecht BG, et al: Hemorrhagic shock. Curr Probl Surg 32:925–1002, 1995.

Schlichtig R: O_2 Uptake, critical O_2 delivery, and tissue wellness. In: Pinsky MR, Dhainaut J-FA (eds): Pathophysiologic Foundations of Critical Care. Baltimore: Williams & Wilkins, 1993.
Clear, detailed discussion of the two-phase model of $\dot{V}_{O_2}$ and $\dot{D}_{O_2}$ with a critical review of the model's underlying assumptions when applied to critically ill patients.

8 Septic Shock and Other Low Afterload States

Scott Manaker

Septic shock is a common and important problem in the management of critically ill patients in the intensive care unit (ICU) setting. In the United States, estimates range widely from between 100,000 and 500,000 episodes of sepsis yearly. These episodes account for up to 25% of all admissions to ICUs and may result in as many as 80,000 deaths per year. Sepsis is the 13th leading cause of death in the United States and has been estimated to cost more than $10 billion yearly.

Over the past several decades, an increasing incidence of septic shock has been noted and attributed to a number of factors:

1. Corticosteroids and other immunosuppressive agents that are routinely employed to treat inflammatory diseases and to suppress organ rejection after solid-organ transplantation.
2. The use of chemotherapeutic agents in a wide variety of oncologic as well as inflammatory diseases, which predisposes these patients to infections.
3. An expanding variety of chronically implanted vascular catheters and endovascular prosthetic devices, which then can serve as an entry site for infectious agents or as a nidus for infections originating elsewhere.
4. Longer survival of populations who are at increased susceptibility of infection, such as neonates, the elderly, and those infected with human immunodeficiency virus.

Although advanced medical practices have increased both the number and the diversity of patients with sepsis, mortality from this disorder remains essentially unchanged, in the 30 to 90% range depending on subgroup studied.

CLINICAL CONSIDERATIONS

Definitions

Historically, the term *sepsis* implied the presence of a bacteremia (hence the term *septicemia*). Several epidemiologic studies, however, have found bacteremias present in fewer than half of patients with septic shock. From these observations, the concept arose that what had been called sepsis was a set of signs and symptoms reflecting the body's inflammatory response to a serious infection, but not necessarily a bacteremia. It was also realized that infection was only one of several possible triggers that could unleash this potentially deleterious state, which was termed *systemic inflammatory response syndrome (SIRS)* (Table 8–1).

Instead of resulting from direct effects of bacterial products, SIRS was found to be the result of expression of a cascade of proinflammatory mediators, such as tumor necrosis factor-alpha (TNF-α), interleukin (IL)-1, and IL-8. Consensus definitions of SIRS, sepsis, and septic shock took these observations into consider-

93

Table 8–1. Consensus Definitions of SIRS, Sepsis, and Related Terms

TERM	CRITERIA
SIRS	Presence of 2 to 4 of the following signs* of systemic inflammation: Hyperthermia (>39° C or 101.5° F) or hypothermia (<36° C or 94° F) Tachycardia (>90 or 100 beats per minute) Tachypnea (>20 breaths per minute) Elevated (or depressed) white blood cell count (>15,000 cells/μL or <2000 cells/μL)
Sepsis	SIRS criteria *plus* known or suspected presence of serious infection, including bacteremia or distant site of infection.
Severe sepsis	Sepsis *plus* evidence of end-organ dysfunction* as follows: 1. Hypotension (systolic blood pressure <90 mm Hg or >40 mm Hg fall from baseline in patients with chronic hypertension; or mean arterial pressure <60 mm Hg) 2. Oliguria (urine output <30 mL/h) 3. Hypoxemia consistent with acute lung injury (Pao_2/Fio_2 <300) 4. Change in mental status (decrease of 2 points on Glasgow Coma Scale) 5. Anion gap metabolic acidosis 6. Disseminated intravascular coagulation 7. Thrombocytopenia 8. Low systemic vascular resistance (<800 dynes·sec·cm^{-5})
Septic shock	Severe sepsis criteria including hypotension

*Without alternative explanation.

SIRS, systemic inflammatory response syndrome; criteria values are those commonly used in clinical trials for novel antisepsis agents.

ation and have provided a common nomenclature for designing clinical trials of novel antisepsis agents and for conducting and reporting epidemiologic studies. Most of the important clinical manifestations of sepsis and septic shock are also encompassed by the criteria used for these definitions (see Table 8–1).

Differential Diagnosis

A wide variety of disorders can mimic septic shock (Table 8–2). Each of these conditions not only may mimic the low afterload characteristic of septic shock but may also *coexist* with sepsis. Therefore, it is important to consider all forms of low afterload shock before concluding that hypotension in a critically ill patient is due to sepsis. Although severe anemia, hepatic failure, pregnancy, and arteriovenous shunts (from cirrhosis or a dialysis fistula) can also produce low afterload states, only rarely do they result in hypotension and organ failure.

Clinical Presentations

Sepsis presents clinically in two usual patterns, first described more than 40 years ago: (1) patients with hot, dry, flushed skin and an animated appearance manifest-

Table 8–2. Differential Diagnosis of Low Afterload Shock

....

Anaphylaxis (see Chapter 29)
Central nervous system disorders, including stroke, dysautonomias, and spinal shock (see
  Chapters 67 and 98)
Diffuse erythroderma (see Chapter 43)
Drug overdoses (see Chapter 57) and heavy metal poisonings
Effects of perispinal local anesthetics (see Chapter 85)
Endocrine emergencies, including myxedema and addisonian crisis (see Chapter 82)
Hyperthermia, including neuroleptic malignant syndrome (see Chapter 54)
Sepsis
Transfusion reactions (see Chapter 46)

....

ing "warm shock" and (2) patients with cold, clammy skin who are lethargic and hypotensive exhibiting "cold shock" (Table 8–3). Today, both warm and cold shock are regarded as representing two different manifestations within the spectrum of severe sepsis and septic shock rather than as obligatory stages of sepsis. Although some patients with "warm shock" exhibit the classic progression to "cold shock," others do not. Hours before patients with sepsis develop frank hypotension, they typically have modest decrements in blood pressure from lowered systemic vascular resistance (SVR) but for which they compensate by increasing their cardiac output. With progression of sepsis, further decreases in SVR, and limits to cardiac compensation (from development of relative hypovolemia due to capillary leakage, venodilation, or myocardial depression), patients develop frank hypotension and multiple organ system failure (MOSF), often resulting in death.

Pathophysiology

Classically, septic shock was described in the setting of infections due to gram-negative bacteria. Gram-negative bacteria contain endotoxin (lipopolysaccharide

Table 8–3. Cardiovascular and Other Profiles During Progression of Septic Shock

....

PARAMETER	PRE-SHOCK	WARM SHOCK	COLD SHOCK
Blood pressure	WNL	↓	↓
Systemic vascular resistance	↓	↓ ↓	WNL or ↑
Cardiac output	↑	↑	↓
Pulmonary artery wedge pressure	↓	↓, WNL, or ↑ *	WNL, ↑ *
Acid-base changes	Respiratory alkalosis	Respiratory alkalosis with anion gap metabolic acidosis (see Chapter 80)	Respiratory alkalosis with anion gap metabolic acidosis

....

*Pulmonary artery wedge pressure will vary depending on how much volume the patient received and myocardial functioning.
WNL, within normal limits; ↑, increased; ↓, decreased; ↓ ↓, markedly decreased.

[LPS]) in their cell wall, which promotes mononuclear cells to release of TNF-α, a highly cytotoxic agent. Both endotoxin and TNF-α also promote the release of many other proinflammatory mediators. Today, it is recognized that LPS is not specifically needed for this response and that all infectious agents, including gram-positive bacteria, fungi, viruses, and parasites, and certain noninfectious conditions, such as pancreatitis, burns, or trauma, can initiate the release of TNF-α, cytokines, and other proinflammatory mediators. Elevated levels of many proinflammatory agents, particularly TNF-α, and IL-1 and IL-6 have been demonstrated in septic patients. In experimental animals, exogenous TNF-α and other proinflammatory mediators rapidly lead to death of individual cells, MOSF, and death. After the cascade of proinflammatory mediators occurs, another network of anti-inflammatory mediators becomes activated (e.g., IL-1 receptor antagonist, IL-10). How sepsis ultimately resolves depends on whether these anti-inflammatory mediators can offset the deleterious effects of the proinflammatory mediators.

Elegant physiologic studies using infusions of endotoxin or TNF-α into normal human volunteers have reproduced much of the pathophysiology of sepsis. Endotoxin infusion produces fever, tachycardia, tachypnea, and prompt release of TNF-α. SVR falls and heart rate increases. With larger doses, arterial blood pressure can also fall. While cardiac index increases, left ventricular end-diastolic volume increases but its ejection fraction diminishes. These physiologic derangements in response to endotoxin or TNF-α administration are similar to those manifested by patients with sepsis or SIRS, thereby supporting a pathogenic role for inflammatory mediators in sepsis.

Cardiovascular Changes

The typical pattern of cardiovascular changes is presented in Table 8–3. The primary change is a decrease in SVR. The mechanism for the decreased SVR has been identified in the past decade with elucidation of the role of nitric oxide functioning as an endogenous endothelial-derived relaxing factor. The presence of LPS and proinflammatory mediators, such as TNF-α, in the blood result in the induction of a form of inducible nitric oxide synthase (INOS) in vascular endothelium. This, in turn, produces large amounts of nitric oxide, which diffuses to the nearby arteriolar smooth muscle and results in profound loss of vascular tone. Now it is clear why catecholamine infusions have limited success in reversing the hypotension of septic shock. Resistance to catecholamines is not due to down-regulation of smooth muscle adrenergic receptors or to blunting of their effects by acidosis. Rather it is due to marked increases in endogenous nitric oxide production, which is a "direct" vasodilator, independent of alpha- or beta-adrenergic receptors.

Sepsis also characteristically causes increased capillary and venular permeability, also due to effects of inflammatory cytokines. This, plus loss of vascular tone of the capacitance bed, results in a relative hypovolemia. If right-sided heart catheterization is done before fluid resuscitation, results may reflect this "natural history" of sepsis with a high cardiac output due to low afterload and tachycardia and a pulmonary artery wedge pressure (PAWP) in the low normal range (e.g., 5 mm Hg).

In addition to lower SVR and relative hypovolemia, a number of changes in left ventricular function itself have been reported in septic shock. Before fluid resuscitation, left ventricular function may be described as "hyperdynamic" with elevated heart rates combined with diastolic underfilling of left atrium and left ventricle. After volume loading, the left ventricle can dilate with its end-diastolic volume, reaching 100% greater than normal. Despite this increased left ventricular filling volume and pressure, left ventricular ejection fraction often falls below the normal range, suggesting myocardial dysfunction. Paradoxically, the ability of the left ventricle to dilate so much in septic shock has actually been found to be a good predictor for survival, whereas the contrary response, lack of ventricular dilation after volume loading in sepsis, predicts a higher risk of mortality.

In addition to left ventricular dilatation, which is associated with decreased global wall motion (decreased ejection fraction), noninvasive imaging studies of the heart in patients with septic shock have also documented *localized* left ventricular wall motion abnormalities. These findings are similar to those seen in patients with ischemic heart disease, but they disappear after recovery from sepsis; and follow-up cardiac evaluation discloses no occult coronary disease. One is left with the conclusion that regions of left ventricular myocardium are likely affected by direct actions of proinflammatory mediators, some of which have myocardial depressant effects, but without a clear understanding of how localized effects occur.

CLINICAL MANAGEMENT OF SEPTIC SHOCK

Anti-inflammatory and Novel Agents

Because of the role of inflammatory mediators in the evolution of septic shock and MOSF, a large number of anti-inflammatory agents have been studied as potential therapeutic agents. Unfortunately, administration of glucocorticoids, ibuprofen, naloxone, fibronectin, and other agents has not demonstrated efficacy in the treatment of septic patients in controlled clinical trials. Indeed, high-dose corticosteroids were associated with worse outcomes. Likewise, to date, no anti-LPS, anti-TNF, anti-IL-1 agent, or anti-inflammatory mediator, such as IL-1 receptor antagonist, has been shown to reduce mortality or morbidity (e.g., organ failure) in sepsis, nor has the removal of proinflammatory mediators by continuous hemodialysis improved outcomes in septic patients, perhaps because dialysis also removes the anti-inflammatory agents.

Discovery of the primary role of INOS as the cause of low SVR in septic shock led to the hypothesis that blunting increased INOS activity would decrease mortality. Although Phase II studies of one INOS competitive inhibitor in patients with septic shock resulted in an earlier resolution of hypotension compared with conventional vasopressor therapy, the pivotal Phase III clinical trial of the same agent was stopped prematurely because of an increased number of deaths in the treated group compared with the placebo-treated group.

Anti-infective Therapy

Because no novel anti-inflammatory or antihypotensive therapy has been shown to improve outcomes, the therapy for septic shock has remained essentially the same for the past two decades. First, appropriate antimicrobial agents are administered, often in an empirical manner (see Chapter 14), to treat the infectious cause. Infected collections are sought and, if present, drained (see Chapter 38).

Fluid Resuscitation Therapy

Fluid resuscitation to maintain intravascular volume is the first line of therapy to deal with the altered hemodynamics in septic shock (see Table 8–3). Adequate preload and cardiac output must be provided to ensure organ perfusion, such as renal perfusion to maintain urine output and central nervous system perfusion to maintain mentation. However, the maintenance of adequate preload must be balanced against volume overload with its associated risks of cardiogenic and noncardiogenic pulmonary edema. In septic patients, inflammatory mediators can produce an alveolar capillary leak syndrome, resulting in acute respiratory distress syndrome, and can depress myocardial contractility, contributing to development of cardiogenic pulmonary edema.

Studies have demonstrated variable effects of volume loading on cardiac function in septic patients. One study found that fluid administration that increased the PAWP from 7 to 12 mm Hg elevated cardiac output but there was no further benefit by increasing PAWP to 16 mm Hg. Based on these results, the study's authors recommended administration of fluids (or blood products where appropriate) to maintain PAWP at 10 to 12 mm Hg. Although this is a reasonable starting point, optimal preload therapy in septic shock is unknown because outcome studies to support the efficacy of this or other levels of PAWP are lacking. In addition, recent controversy over the safety of pulmonary artery catheterization raises questions about any recommendation for setting preload goals that can only be determined by its use.

Until outcome studies provide better guidance, fluid management should be individualized according to the clinical circumstances of each patient. For example, if severe acute respiratory distress syndrome is present, lower filling pressures (PAWP = 6 to 8 mm Hg) may be preferred to prevent worse hypoxemia. Alternatively, in the setting of depressed left ventricular contractility, higher filling pressures (PAWP > 16 mm Hg) may be desirable to improve cardiac output. Achieving optimal fluid management for an individual patient may require assessment of hemodynamics (by use of a pulmonary artery catheter, end-organ perfusion, and arterial oxygenation at several different filling pressures).

Vasopressor Therapy

In addition to volume resuscitation, vasopressor and inotrope infusions are commonly used to maintain blood pressure at a level adequate for end-organ perfusion. Understanding the physiologic use of these agents requires matching knowledge of cardiovascular pharmacology to the pharmacologic spectrum of each vasoactive agent (see Tables 6–4 and 6–5, Chapter 6).

Phenylephrine is the only vasoconstrictor without direct cardiac effects. However, its vasoconstrictive effects can paradoxically decrease cardiac output, owing to increased afterload (see Figs. 6–3 and 6–4, Chapter 6). Both epinephrine and norepinephrine also produce vasoconstriction while simultaneously stimulating cardiac output because of beta$_1$-adrenergic stimulation of the heart. Norepinephrine is a more potent vasoconstrictor because it lacks the beta$_2$-adrenergic vasodilatory effects of epinephrine, so it may decrease cardiac output more owing to increased cardiac afterload.

Dopamine has a broad spectrum of physiologic actions. At low doses (usually <5 μg/kg/min), stimulation of dopaminergic receptors produces regional vasodilation with little change in systemic arterial pressure. Moderate doses of dopamine (5–10 μg/kg/min) stimulate cardiac output by activation of beta$_1$-adrenergic receptors in the heart. Administration of dopamine in excess of 10 μg/kg/min stimulates both beta$_1$-adrenergic receptors in the heart and alpha$_1$-adrenergic receptors in vasculature to yield both increased cardiac output and vasoconstriction.

Dobutamine activates both beta$_1$-adrenergic receptors in the heart and beta$_2$-adrenergic receptors in the peripheral vasculature. By these actions, it increases cardiac output with direct inotropic and chronotropic effects on the heart and indirectly produces systemic vasodilation, with a resultant decrease in afterload. Although dobutamine administration in fluid-replete, normotensive patients can increase blood pressure indirectly owing to the increased cardiac output, it may also cause profound *hypotension* in patients with intravascular volume depletion or a limited ability to increase cardiac output due to intrinsic cardiac disease because of its vasodilatory effects.

Which vasopressor to use first in patients with septic shock remains controversial because no controlled clinical studies indicate that one agent is best. Dopamine is popular as a first agent because moderate to high dosages provide direct inotropic stimulation as well as vasoconstriction. Alternative initial choices include norepinephrine or phenylephrine. Both have also been used if high doses of dopamine prove to be ineffective or cause problematic tachycardias. Epinephrine is usually reserved as an additional agent if the patient remains hypotensive despite high doses of one or two other pressors.

In general, dobutamine should not be administered as a single agent in patients with septic shock because of its potential for producing profound hypotension. The same caution applies to epinephrine until recent concern about epinephrine as a single agent worsening splanchnic perfusion in septic shock is resolved. Finally, isoproterenol, a pure beta agonist, has no role in septic shock as a first or additional agent.

"Supercharging" Therapy for Sepsis

Several observational studies of patients with septic shock or other critical illnesses found that survivors had significantly higher values of cardiac index, oxygen delivery ($\dot{D}o_2$) and oxygen consumption ($\dot{V}o_2$) than nonsurvivors. Not only were these values higher than those of the nonsurvivors, but they were also greater than normal (deemed "supranormal"). The "supranormal" values associated with increased survival were cardiac index more than 4.5 L/min/m^2, $\dot{D}o_2$ more than 14 mL/kg/min or more than 600 mL/min/m^2, and $\dot{V}o_2$ more than 3.5 mL/kg/min or more than 170 mL/min/m^2. From these observations, it was hypothesized that using these supranormal values as *goals* of hemodynamic therapy for septic shock would improve survival.

Testing this hypothesis presents serious methodologic challenges. How should one deal with patients who are randomized to "normal" hemodynamic values but who spontaneously achieve the "supranormal" values? The same question applies to those who are randomized to the "supranormal" group but whose parameters remain at normal levels despite the experimental interventions. To date, six randomized controlled clinical trials have tested this hypothesis in a heterogeneous group of critically ill ICU patients, including many with septic shock. None found a significant difference in mortality between treated and control groups on an intention-to-treat basis. Furthermore, one of these studies was stopped prematurely because the use of dobutamine to increase $\dot{D}O_2$ may have worsened outcomes.

The results of these studies do not justify increasing $\dot{D}O_2$ or cardiac index to a certain supranormal level in patients with severe sepsis or septic shock. Titration of hemodynamic parameters to achieve end-organ perfusion in individual patients remains the basic principle of hemodynamic therapy.

Management of Other Low Afterload States

Recognition of anaphylaxis as the etiology of low afterload shock is critical because anaphylaxis should be treated differently than other forms of low afterload shock. *Epinephrine* is the agent of choice for anaphylaxis or anaphylactoid reactions. There are numerous case reports describing the unique efficacy of epinephrine in the setting of anaphylaxis when other pressors, such as dopamine or norepinephrine, were ineffective. In addition to epinephrine, other treatment includes corticosteroids (methylprednisolone 125–250 mg IV q6h), H_1 receptor antagonists (diphenhydramine 50 mg IV q6h), and H_2 receptor antagonists (e.g., ranitidine, 150 mg IV q12h).

In other forms of low afterload shock, although specific therapy depends on the inciting cause, the approach to fluid management and vasopressors in these settings parallels the management of patients with septic shock.

BIBLIOGRAPHY

Abraham E, Raffin TA: Sepsis therapy trials: Continued disappointment or reason to hope? JAMA 271:1876–1878, 1994.
  Review of the failed clinical trials of novel and cytokine therapies.

Bone RC, Balk RA, Cerra FBV, et al: Definitions for sepsis and organ failure and guidelines for the use of innovative therapies in sepsis. Chest 101:1644–1655, 1992.
  Landmark consensus conference report proposing definitions for sepsis, septic shock, and sepsis syndrome.

Casey LC, Balk RA, Bone RC: Plasma cytokine and endotoxin levels correlate with survival in patients with the sepsis syndrome. Ann Intern Med 119:771–778, 1993.
  First demonstration of elevated levels of multiple inflammatory mediators in sepsis syndrome.

Cross AS: Anti-endotoxin antibodies: A dead end? Ann Intern Med 121:58–60, 1994.
  Editorial reviewing failed clinical trials of anti-endotoxin antibodies.

Dorinsky PM: The sepsis syndrome. Clin Chest Med 17:175–350, 1996.
  Multiauthored volume comprising state-of-the-art reviews of all aspects of sepsis and sepsis syndrome.

Gattinoni L, Brazzi L, Pelosi P, et al: A trial of goal-oriented hemodynamic therapy in critically ill patients. N Engl J Med 333:1025–1032, 1995.

Randomized controlled clinical trial that compared hemodynamic therapy aiming to achieve supranormal levels for O_2 delivery but found no significant difference in outcomes.

Hinds C, Watson D: Manipulating hemodynamics and oxygen transport in critically ill patients. N Engl J Med 333:1074–1075, 1995.

Editorial accompanying the report of Gattinoni et al.

Martin C, Papazian L, Perrin G, et al: Norepinephrine or dopamine in the treatment of hyperdynamic septic shock? Chest 103:1826–1831, 1993.

Clinical trial comparing norepinephrine to dopamine for treatment of septic shock.

Meier-Hellmann A, Reinhart K, Bredle DL, et al: Epinephrine impairs splanchnic perfusion in septic shock. Crit Care Med 25:399, 1997.

Small recent case series demonstrating deleterious effects of epinephrine used alone in treatment of sepsis patients.

Packman MI, Rackow EC: Optimum left heart filling pressure during fluid resuscitation of patients with hypovolemia and septic shock. Crit Care Med 11:165–169, 1983.

This is a small study examining fluid resuscitation in sepsis syndrome.

Peters JI, Utset OM: Vasopressors in shock management: Choosing and using wisely. J Crit Illness 4:62–68, 1989.

Very practical approach to pressor choices in septic shock.

Suffredini AF, Fross RE, Parker MM, et al: The cardiovascular response of normal humans to the administration of endotoxin. N Engl J Med 321:280–287, 1989.

Physiologic classic re-creating the pathophysiology of septic shock by administration of endotoxin.

Wheeler AP, Bernard GR: Treating patients with severe sepsis. N Engl J Med 340:207–214, 1999.

Excellent recent review of the pathophysiology and management of sepsis syndrome.

9

Vascular Access Issues and Procedures

C. William Hanson III
Paul N. Lanken

Obtaining access to the arterial and venous systems is a fundamental skill and responsibility for intensivists. Arterial catheterization is used to monitor blood pressure and to obtain blood for arterial blood gas analysis and other laboratory tests. In addition, an arterial catheter is often present at admission to the surgical intensive care unit (ICU), having been inserted for intraoperative monitoring. Central venous catheterization permits determination of central venous pressure; rapid infusion of resuscitative fluids; and safe administration of certain agents, such as calcium, potassium, or hyperalimentation solutions. This chapter describes indications, techniques, and risks of cannulation of arteries, central veins, and pulmonary artery.

ARTERIAL CATHETERIZATION

Indications

Measuring blood pressure with an intra-arterial catheter is preferable to noninvasive methods when there is a need for frequent blood pressure readings (e.g., during surgical procedures or resuscitation from circulatory shock). Each of the determinants of blood pressure (blood volume, systemic vascular resistance, and cardiac contractility) can change rapidly under certain circumstances. For example, effective blood volume changes minute by minute in response to major gastrointestinal bleeding or to large increases in intrathoracic pressure (e.g., starting positive-pressure ventilation when there is a high level of associated auto-PEEP [positive end-expiratory pressure]). Systemic vascular resistance can also vary rapidly with changes in patient temperature (e.g., rewarming after surgery) or in response to vasoactive infusion. Drugs that depress cardiac contractility (e.g., beta blockers) or cardiac ischemia can also cause rapid decreases in blood pressure. In addition, arterial access may be required to sample arterial blood to determine pH, Pao_2, and $Paco_2$ frequently in patients with acute respiratory failure or acid-base disorders. Finally, the need for frequent phlebotomy by itself in the ICU patient may warrant insertion of an arterial catheter for patient comfort.

Sites

A number of superficial arteries are used for arterial catheterization in the adult, including the radial, ulnar, brachial, axillary, femoral, dorsalis pedis, and posterior tibial arteries (Table 9–1). Although the radial artery is the most commonly used site, alternative sites are often selected. For example, when the radial artery may

103

Table 9–1. Sites for Arterial Catheterization

ARTERY	ADVANTAGES	DISADVANTAGES	COMMENTS
Radial	Accessible, collaterals present	Site of prior sticks	
Ulnar	Accessible, collaterals present	Small caliber in most patients	May result in ulnar nerve injury
Brachial	Superficial	No collaterals	More difficult than radial to cannulate; may result in median nerve injury
Axillary	Collaterals present	Difficult to cannulate, deep location	Use ≥3-inch long catheter
Femoral	Good waveform fidelity, easy to cannulate, preferred site for obtaining emergency access	Highest risk of catheter-associated infection, vascular complications; patient is immobilized with limb extended	Change to another site after 48–72 hours because of infectious risk, use ≥6-inch long catheter
Dorsalis pedis	Superficial; collaterals usually present	Lower extremity must be immobilized	
Posterior tibial	Superficial; collaterals usually present	Small caliber in most patients	

not be palpable owing to systemic hypotension, previous cannulations, soft tissue swelling (e.g., fat, edema), or anatomic variation, the ulnar artery is an acceptable alternative. Indeed, it may have a larger caliber in some patients. Although some ICU clinicians perform an Allen test before radial artery cannulation to document the presence of collateral circulation, many others do not. The Allen test can be difficult to perform and interpret under common ICU situations (e.g., circulatory shock, hypothermia, or vasopressor use). In addition, the medical literature, including large series of patients receiving radial artery cannulation, has not indicated the occurrence of adverse effects attributable to omission of the Allen test. Clearly, after arterial catheterization of any site, the distal extremity must be monitored clinically for ischemia and, if it develops, it should be appropriately evaluated and treated, including removal of the catheter in question, if necessary.

Alternative sites to the radial and ulnar arteries have their own disadvantages so that the risk-to-benefit ratio should be considered before insertion and on a regular basis while the catheter remains in place. Upper extremity alternatives are the brachial and axillary arteries. The brachial artery is superficial and readily palpated, but it is somewhat difficult to cannulate and has the disadvantage of being an anatomic end-artery, lacking a collateral circulation, in contrast to the axillary artery. Some intensivists prefer the axillary to the brachial artery because it has a collateral circulation (but is more difficult to cannulate). Others prefer the brachial artery because, compared to the axillary artery, it is easier to cannulate as well as easier to repair surgically in case of dissection or thrombosis.

In the lower extremity, the femoral artery is the preferred site for arterial cannulation under emergency conditions. It is easy to access, and its arterial waveforms have good fidelity. Patients with indwelling femoral catheters, however, are difficult to mobilize from bed to chair for fear of injury to the artery. In addition, femoral catheters may cause serious complications, such as atheromatous emboli, in patients with diffuse atherosclerosis. The dorsalis pedis artery is an alternative in the lower extremity because it generally has good collateral flow and is reasonably easy to cannulate in many patients.

Insertion Methods

Cannulating an artery in the ICU setting uses one of two approaches: direct cannulation of the vessel or the modified Seldinger technique. The first approach uses a small-gauge catheter-over-a-needle. After the needle is inserted into the vessel's lumen and pulsatile arterial blood flow is identified, the catheter is gently threaded over the needle into the artery. The direct approach is used for catheterization of smaller vessels. Although the modified Seldinger technique may also be used in these vessels, it is more typically used to access larger vessels, such as the femoral artery.

The modified Seldinger technique is a multistage procedure (Fig. 9–1). The first step involves inserting a needle into the target vessel's lumen. The second step is passing a thin guide wire through the needle into the lumen. The wire typically has a flexible, often J-shaped, tip (so as not to injure the interior of the vessel). It is longer than the catheter to be placed in the vessel but small enough to pass freely through both the needle and catheter. The original needle is then removed while the operator keeps hold of the guide wire. Next, the plastic catheter is threaded over the wire into the vessel; and, finally, the wire is removed from the catheter. A complication of this technique is inadvertent loss of the wire into the

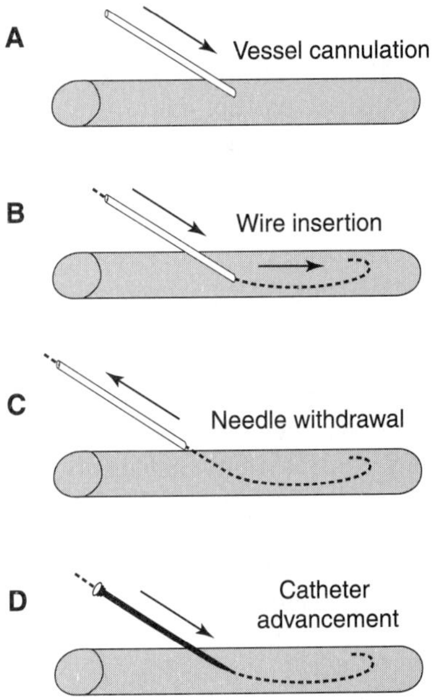

Figure 9–1. The modified Seldinger technique. *A,* Needle is inserted into the lumen of the selected vessel. *B,* Thin guide wire *(dashed line),* with flexible end first, is inserted through the needle into the vessel. *C,* Needle is removed over the wire while operator maintains control of the wire. *D,* Plastic catheter is inserted over the wire into the lumen.

vessel, which can be avoided by maintaining control of some portion of the wire throughout the procedure.

Complications

Risks of arterial catheterization include infection, thrombosis, and hemorrhage after removal of the catheter.

Infections of arterial catheters occur but are far less common than infections of central venous catheters. This is attributed to less stagnant blood flow in arteries than in the central venous circulation. Because risk of catheter-associated infection is so low and data supporting the practice are absent, one should not routinely change the catheter's site at specific intervals; nor should one routinely change arterial catheters "over a wire" (using the modified Seldinger technique with a guide wire to replace the catheter) at the same site. In addition, because arterial catheters are used so often to obtain blood for arterial blood gases or other tests, the hubs of their three-way stopcocks commonly become colonized by bacteria, such as coagulase-negative staphylococcal species. Because of this, one should never use an arterial catheter to obtain blood cultures except at the time of its first insertion.

Thrombosis of arterial lines is most likely to occur when the cannulated vessel is anatomically abnormal (calcified, narrowed) or if there is circulatory shock and impaired blood flow. Central (retrograde) embolization of air bubbles or thrombi with serious consequences can occur if an arterial catheter is flushed vigorously.

Two uncommon complications of arterial cannulation are the formation of an arteriovenous fistula or a pseudoaneurysm after removal of the catheter. These occur more frequently with larger arteries and characteristically in the setting of cardiac or diagnostic catheterization. Finally, hemorrhage can occur after removal of the catheter, especially in patients with a coagulopathy or undergoing thrombolysis. Holding pressure over the site for at least 20 minutes after removal is usually adequate to prevent this.

CENTRAL VENOUS CATHETERIZATION

Indications

The central veins are catheterized for a variety of reasons in the ICU, including pressure monitoring, administration of fluids during volume resuscitation, and hypertonic fluids. Additionally, the central veins may be the only venous access sites available in obese patients or in patients whose peripheral veins are sclerosed from prior venous cannulation or intravenous drug use. Finally, the central veins are preferable for the administration of vasoactive agents. Vasopressors can cause constriction and vessel injury when administered into small peripheral veins. Their central administration also decreases the delay between changes in dose and onset of effect because of the shorter "path length" between the drug infusion site and site of action.

Sites

The external and internal jugular, subclavian, and femoral veins are the most frequently used sites for central venous cannulation in the ICU (Table 9–2). In addition, the central circulation can also be accessed using a long catheter threaded from the basilic or axillary vein. These peripherally inserted central (PIC) catheters are becoming more popular for certain circumstances because they improve patient mobility and comfort and may lower the risk of catheter-associated infection (compared with conventional central venous catheters). Their narrow lumens (single or double) are their main limitation.

The external jugular vein is both superficial and visible in most thin patients but difficult to use for central access. Venous valves and tortuosity frequently prevent a catheter from threading into the central circulation in the thorax. The internal jugular vein is technically more difficult to access than the external because it lies deeper in the neck and adjacent to the carotid artery, which can be inadvertently punctured during catheterization attempts. Once the internal jugular vein is entered, however, the internal jugular catheter is readily advanced because the vessel is straight and lacks valves. Both the external and internal jugular veins are more difficult to cannulate in obese patients and in patients with short necks. The subclavian vein is an alternative with a relatively constant anatomic location but somewhat higher incidence of complications, such as pneumothorax and subclavian artery puncture (2 to 5%). It is also easier to maintain sterile dressings over the subclavian site than the jugular or femoral sites, and it is therefore preferred for long-term access (e.g., hyperalimentation).

The femoral vein is the least preferable site because of a higher risk of infectious complications and loss of patient mobility. Use of this site also is undesirable if one wants access for passage of a pulmonary artery catheter because it has a more convoluted route in going from the inferior vena cava to the pulmonary artery. The right internal jugular and the left subclavian veins provide the most anatomically direct routes to the heart when one is inserting a pulmonary artery catheter.

Insertion Methods

Like arterial catheters, the central venous vessels are most commonly cannulated using the modified Seldinger technique. Most intensivists access the internal jugular vein, using the middle approach (Fig. 9–2), or the subclavian vein, using the infraclavicular approach (Fig. 9–3). Other approaches to the internal jugular vein (anterior or posterior approach) are available but used less commonly. For internal jugular cannulations, one can decrease the risk of complications by using ultrasonographic guidance. Ultrasonography can be used to image the selected vessel's course and depth before the procedure (which can be marked with dots of indelible ink on the overlying skin before the skin preparation). Alternatively, ultrasonography can be used during the actual process of catheter placement by enclosing the ultrasound probe with a sterile sheath. In contrast, the subclavian vein is poorly visualized by ultrasound, which makes it a less desirable site than the internal jugular vein in coagulopathic and ventilated patients.

Table 9–2. Sites for Central Venous Cannulation

VEIN	ADVANTAGES	DISADVANTAGES	COMMENTS
External jugular	Superficial, visible, easy to tamponade bleeding	Difficult to pass catheter into central veins	Often has two valves and a tortuous course to thorax
Internal jugular	Reliable central access, no venous valves; location of vein and carotid artery can be easily identified by bedside ultrasound evaluation	Close to carotid artery, difficult to keep site dressed well, higher risk of catheter-associated infection than subclavian vein	Use right internal jugular preferably to insert pulmonary artery catheter (more direct route); right internal jugular also avoids risk of trauma to thoracic duct
Subclavian	Reliable central access	Up to 5% risk of pneumothorax and bleeding	Reposition using fluoroscopy if tip is in internal jugular vein before infusing pressors or hypertonic solutions
Femoral	Easy central access	High risk for nosocomial infection	Access of choice for emergencies
Basilic	Easy access for PIC catheter*	Catheter may become occluded if elbow is bent	Confirm proper location of tip in superior vena cava by fluoroscopy or chest radiography
Axillary	Reliable vein to use for PIC catheter	Needs ultrasound to localize; more difficult to cannulate	Requires a standard PIC catheter to be cut to proper length.

*PIC catheter, peripherally inserted central catheter.

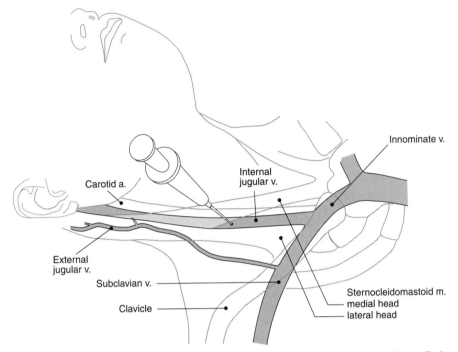

Figure 9–2. The middle approach for cannulation of the right internal jugular vein. The needle is inserted at the apex of the triangle formed by the medial (sternal) and lateral (clavicular) heads of the sternocleidomastoid muscle and the clavicle. The needle, inserted at a 45-degree angle in the direction of the ipsilateral nipple, usually enters the vein after 2 to 4 cm of insertion. (Redrawn from Preas HL, Suffredini AF: Pulmonary artery catheterization. Insertion and quality control. In: Tobin MJ [ed]: Principles and Practice of Intensive Care Monitoring. New York: McGraw-Hill, 1998, pp 773–795.)

Issues common to catheterization of all sites include use of sterile technique and prevention of air embolism, hemorrhage, and nerve injury. The site must be sterilely prepared by scrubbing widely with a povidone-iodine solution. The operator should wear sterile gown, gloves, mask, cap, and eye protection. The site should be widely draped (essentially over the entire bed) to prevent inadvertent catheter contamination. Local anesthetic is liberally infiltrated into the area around the vessel, which is then cannulated using the modified Seldinger technique (see Fig. 9–1). The electrocardiogram is monitored for arrhythmias during guide wire and catheter insertion. Vessel cannulation is facilitated by positioning the desired vessel below the level of the heart, that is, using Trendelenburg's position for the neck and thoracic vessels and reverse Trendelenburg's position for the femoral vein. These positions distend the target vessel and tend to prevent entrainment of air into the vessel when the patient inspires.

Complications

Although central venous cannulation is generally a safe procedure, it can have serious complications (Table 9–3). Careful site identification, preparation, and

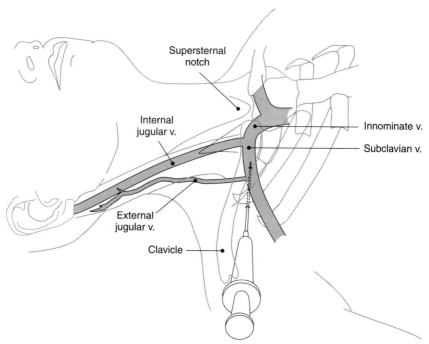

Figure 9–3. The infraclavicular approach for cannulation of the right subclavian vein. The patient should be supine with head down 30 degrees (some intensivists insert a rolled-up towel between the patient's scapulas, allowing the medial part of the clavicle to rise). The needle is inserted 1 cm below the most raised portion of the clavicle. This insertion point may be located slightly beyond the halfway point (between the medial and lateral clavicular ends) or at the junction between the middle and distal thirds of the clavicle, or in between. The needle is directed toward the suprasternal notch (which is palpated by the operator's other hand), keeping the needle parallel to the frontal plane and the undersurface of the clavicle. The bevel of the needle should be directed caudally to facilitate placement of the wire into the innominate rather than the internal jugular vein. The needle is advanced while keeping the syringe under modest suction, and it should enter the vessel after 3 to 5 cm of insertion. If there is no blood return, the needle should be slowly withdrawn while continuing to keep the syringe under suction. (Redrawn from Preas HL, Suffredini AF: Pulmonary artery catheterization. Insertion and quality control. In: Tobin MJ [ed]: Principles and Practice of Intensive Care Monitoring. New York: McGraw-Hill, 1998, pp 773–795.)

reversal of existing coagulopathies before the procedure can prevent most of these. Using the modified Seldinger technique and ensuring that the pressure in the target vessel is venous (<10–20 mm Hg) rather than arterial before threading a catheter into the vessel can minimize the risk of arterial cannulation. In difficult cases a sample of blood can be sent for Po_2 analysis to distinguish between vein and artery. In addition, the proper position of the tip is confirmed by routinely obtaining a postprocedure chest radiograph before use in most nonemergency ICU situations. The routine postinsertion chest radiograph can also identify procedure-related pneumothoraces that occur immediately, although some of these may be delayed.

A number of factors can reduce the risk of catheter-related infections and are described in Chapter 11. In addition, antimicrobial-impregnated catheters are less

Table 9–3. Complications of Vascular Catheterization

TYPE OF CATHETER	COMPLICATION
Central venous catheter	Arrhythmias (if tip or guide wire enters right ventricle)
	Arterial puncture and hemorrhage
	Catheter-associated infection (femoral risk > internal jugular risk > subclavian risk)
	Hemothorax (especially with subclavian)
	Inadvertent arterial cannulation
	Pneumothorax (subclavian risk > internal jugular risk)
	Thoracic duct injury (with left internal jugular site)
	Thrombosis
	Venous air embolism
Arterial catheter	Arteriovenous fistula (after removal)
	Distal ischemia or emboli
	Hemorrhage (during insertion attempt and after removal)
	Heparin-induced thrombocytopenia (if heparin is used)
	Nerve injury
	Pseudoaneurysm (after removal)
Pulmonary artery catheter*	Right bundle branch block (see Chapter 30)
	Pulmonary artery rupture and hemorrhage
	Ventricular arrhythmias during passage through right ventricle

*Insertion of introducer and sheath have the same complications as listed under venous catheter.

susceptible to catheter-associated infections and should be considered for high-risk patients when the catheter may be in place for more than 2 to 3 days.

As a rule, the catheter site should be changed when there are signs of local infection. Likewise, when sepsis or septic shock is present, in the absence of another source of infection, removal of the catheter with semi-quantitative culture of its tip (distal 3 cm) (see Chapter 11) is mandatory. Under less pressing clinical circumstances (e.g., recurrent fevers), the catheter can be changed "over a wire" and its tip sent for culture. If the tip culture is positive ($\geq$15 colonies), the site should then be changed. Although some studies suggest that the risk of catheter-associated infection and bacteremia increases after day 4, routine "prophylactic" catheter changes are not recommended. Controlled studies indicate that routine site changes do not decrease the rate of infections whereas they increase the rate of serious mechanical complications, such as pneumothorax. Routine "over the wire" changes are also not recommended.

PULMONARY ARTERY CATHETERIZATION

Indications

Pulmonary artery (PA) catheters are commonly used in the ICU when one wants to assess and monitor the patient's hemodynamics (see Chapter 5). These include acute myocardial infarction with congestive heart failure or shock (see Chapters 6 and 49), other types of circulatory shock (see Chapters 7 and 8), and acute cardiac and noncardiac pulmonary edema (see Chapters 51 and 73). Despite their relatively widespread use, however, controlled clinical studies to support their efficacy in any specific disorder are lacking. Furthermore, some observational studies suggest that the risks of using pulmonary artery catheters may outweigh their benefits (see Chapter 5).

Sites

Pulmonary artery catheters require prior insertion of a sheath that should be 0.5-1 Fr larger than the catheter to be used, that is, an 8.0 Fr sheath is needed for a 7.0 Fr PA catheter or an 8.5 Fr sheath is needed for an 8.0 Fr catheter. The sheath can be conveniently inserted using the "over-the-wire" modified Seldinger method with a special introducer kit if a central venous catheter is already in place in the desired vein. To do this, one uses the most distal lumen of a multilumen catheter. To avoid use of fluoroscopy in their passage, most clinicians prefer to use the right internal jugular or the left subclavian vein to provide the least tortuous route from vein to pulmonary artery.

Insertion

The PA catheter is prepared for use by attaching sterile stopcocks on its distal, right atrial, and right ventricular ports, if applicable, removing intraluminal air bubbles by filling all ports with sterile saline and attaching the distal port to a calibrated and zeroed-pressure transducer. Before insertion, one should also test the balloon for leaks. The balloon should inflate symmetrically and, when fully inflated using 1.5 mL of air, protrude beyond the tip of the catheter (to avoid damage by the catheter's tip to the right ventricular (RV) wall or the right bundle branch as it floats through the RV).

After removal of the introducer and confirmation that the distal end of the sheath lies within the lumen of the vein (by withdrawing venous blood from the sheath's side port), the PA catheter with the balloon deflated is inserted through the sheath's diaphragm and advanced toward the right atrium. This should be done while monitoring surface electrocardiographic tracings and pressure waveform tracings obtained from the distal tip of the catheter. After advancing to the vicinity of the right atrium (usually 10 to 15 cm for subclavian vein access and 15 to 20 cm for internal jugular vein access), one should confirm that the pressure tracings show the appropriate respiratory variations. If present, the balloon is inflated with 1.5 mL of air and advanced steadily through the RV and into the pulmonary artery to a wedged position. Pressure tracings should be recorded during this passage to confirm proper serial locations of the tip during its passage and to obtain measurements of right atrial (RA), RV, PA, and PA wedge pressure (PAWP) (Fig. 9–4).

Hemodynamic Measurements

Accurate measurements of the PAWP depend on the ability to recognize the pressure tracings of the wedged catheter while taking into account fluctuations in

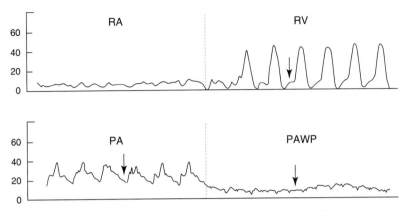

Figure 9–4. Pulmonary artery catheter pressure waveforms in a patient with ARDS receiving mechanical ventilation: right atrium (RA), right ventricle (RV), pulmonary artery (PA), and pulmonary artery wedge pressure (PAWP). One can distinguish RV from PA waveforms since RV pressure rises in diastole *(arrow)* while PA diastolic pressure falls *(arrow)*.

pleural pressure due to respiratory variations. In the ICU setting, the PAWP is measured as an end-expiratory value and not as a mean value over the entire respiratory cycle. This point is chosen to reflect the least influence of variations of intrapleural pressure on PAWP.

If the patient is receiving positive-pressure mechanical ventilation, then the end-expiratory point is the segment of tracing just before start of inspiration (Fig. 9–5). If the patient initiates inspiration with a spontaneous respiratory effort, the start of inspiration can be identified as a brief negative deflection ("trigger") before the longer positive deflection, representing the ventilator's delivery of the tidal volume to the patient. In non–spontaneously breathing patients, the start of inspiration is identified as the start of the positive deflection, representing the ventilator's positive pressure (see Fig. 9–5). There are safety concerns and no good justification for disconnecting a patient from a mechanical ventilator to try to avoid effects of positive-pressure inspirations and PEEP on these measurements. For example, even a brief disconnection may rapidly result in profound hypoxemia in patients with acute respiratory distress syndrome (ARDS). Likewise, there is no good reason (and several contraindications) to paralyze a patient just to remove effects of spontaneous breathing efforts to obtain a "true" and "accurate" PAWP.

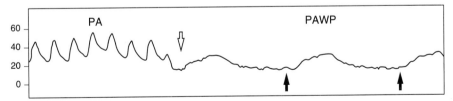

Figure 9–5. Pulmonary artery catheter waveforms from a patient receiving mechanical ventilation. The tip of the catheter resides in the pulmonary artery (PA) with the balloon deflated. The balloon is then inflated *(open arrow)*, resulting in pulmonary artery wedge pressure (PAWP) tracing. Measurement of PAWP should be made at end expiration *(closed arrows)*. The positive deflections following end-expiration reflect positive-pressure inspirations.

Complications

Interpreting the pressure tracings accurately can be challenging if there are large swings of intrapleural pressures. In addition, what appears to be the PAWP tracing may not represent left atrial pressure, such as when the tip is located in a nonperfused (Zone 1) region of the lung. In these conditions, marked increases of the apparent wedge pressure during positive-pressure inspirations often are noted. Likewise, measurements of cardiac output using the thermodilution method have the potential for several types of error (see Table 5–4).

Pulmonary artery catheters can migrate distally and cause problems. Under these circumstances, the pressure tracing on the monitor changes from a PA pressure tracing to one that resembles a persistently wedged catheter despite the balloon being deflated. If unrecognized, this may result in a pulmonary infarction.

Lesser degrees of distal migration also may occur with persistence of PA pressure tracings on the monitor. Under these conditions, catastrophic PA rupture may occur if the balloon is then inflated with the full volume of air (1.5 mL). One should always watch the PA pressure tracing when inflating the balloon and stop introducing more air immediately if it changes to a wedged tracing. If this occurs, the balloon should be deflated and the catheter withdrawn proximally. Other risk factors for PA rupture, which is often a fatal complication, include presence of coagulopathy and pulmonary hypertension. Because of these factors, some ICUs have adopted policies that prohibit routine (e.g., every 4 hours) wedging of the PA catheter in patients with one or both of these factors. In these ICUs, changes in the PA diastolic pressure are tracked as a surrogate for changes in the PAWP.

The risk of catheter-associated infections has been reported to increase dramatically after 4 days of use of a PA catheter. This has led to the consensus recommendation that PA catheters should be removed at 5 days of use. If still needed after 5 days, the site should be changed. If a PA catheter is removed, it is recommended that its associated sheath also be removed. It is poor technique to insert a triple-lumen catheter through the diaphragm on the proximal end of the sheath after removal of a PA catheter because it is no longer sterile. In addition, there have been reports of air embolism through the sheath's diaphragm.

BIBLIOGRAPHY

Agee KR, Balk RA: Central venous catheterization in the critically ill patient. Crit Care Clin 8:677–686, 1992.
General review of issues surrounding central venous catheterization in the ICU patient.

Amin DK, Shah PK, Swan HJC: The technique of inserting a Swan-Ganz catheter. J Crit Illness 8:1147–1156, 1993.
Comprehensive instructions for PA catheter insertion.

Clark VL, Kruse JA: Arterial catheterization. Crit Care Clin 8:687–697, 1992.
General review of issues surrounding arterial catheterization in the critically ill patient.

Hospital Infection Control Practices Advisory Committee: Guideline for prevention of intravascular device-related infections. Part I. Intravascular device-related infections: an overview. Am J Infect Control 24(4):262–277, 1996.
Consensus statement on the risk factors for the development of intravascular catheter-related infections.

Hospital Infection Control Practices Advisory Committee: Guideline for prevention of intravascular device-related infections. Part II. Recommendations for the prevention of nosocomial intravascular device-related infections. Am J Infect Control 24(4):277–293, 1996.
Consensus recommendations for the prevention of catheter-related infections.

Leatherman JW, Marini JJ: Pulmonary artery catheterization. Interpretation of pressure recordings. In: Tobin MJ (ed): Principles and Practice of Intensive Care Monitoring. New York: McGraw-Hill, 1998, pp 821–837.
Comprehensive review of problems interpreting PA catheter waveforms.

Linos DA, Mucha P, van Heerden JA: Subclavian vein. A golden route. Mayo Clin Proc 55:315–321, 1980.
Classic article describing subclavian vein catheterization using a "catheter-through-needle" approach.

Preas HL, Suffredini AF: Pulmonary artery catheterization. Insertion and quality control. In: Tobin MJ (ed): Principles and Practice of Intensive Care Monitoring. New York: McGraw-Hill, 1998, pp 773–795.
Comprehensive review of insertion methods and trouble shooting.

Swan HJC, Ganz W: Guidelines for use of balloon-tipped catheter. Am J Cardiol 34:119–120, 1974.
Letter to the editor by the inventors of the catheter contains a set of valuable instructions for safe use. The manufacturer also provides similar instructions with each catheter.

10 Approach to Supportive Care and Noninvasive Bedside Monitoring

Jonathan Gottlieb

Patients are commonly admitted to the intensive care unit (ICU) for four principal reasons: (1) ICU level of monitoring, (2) intensive nursing care, (3) specialized procedures, and (4) therapies that carry special requirements or risk. On ICU admission, patients have certain needs related to their admitting diagnoses such as gastrointestinal hemorrhage, septic shock, or acute renal failure. In addition, they all require special attention to several universal needs, and meeting such common needs is the collective goal of ICU supportive care.

Considering a basic checklist of supportive care for every ICU patient is important for several reasons. First, in the rush to treat a critically ill patient's acute problems, one may overlook simple but important care. Second, serious illness invariably affects remote systems not involved in the primary pathophysiologic process. Third, treatment aimed at correcting one problem may create others. Supportive care in the ICU setting conforms to the general schema of admitting orders for any hospitalized patient (Table 10–1). In addition to these, as one is writing the patient's orders, it is helpful to systematically address possible needs for each organ system ("from head to foot"), including neurologic, ophthalmologic, otolaryngologic, integumentary, endocrine, metabolic, respiratory, cardiovascular, gastrointestinal, renal, musculoskeletal, and extremities. In the head-injured patient, for example, failure to specifically address prevention of deep venous thrombosis, gastric stress ulceration, or skin injury may have serious consequences.

BODY POSITIONING

Most individuals admitted to the ICU are confined to bed for the initial part of their illness. The clinician must go far beyond the usual prescription of "bed rest" for the ICU patient, as the hospital bed becomes that patient's immediate and total physical environment. It entails risks of aspiration, pressure ulcers of skin and soft tissue, musculoskeletal problems, abnormal cerebral perfusion, increased oxygen consumption, and basic discomfort. Far from being a simple matter of placing the patient in a comfortable position, positioning has become the subject of considerable debate in recent years.

By default, most patients are placed initially in the supine position and turned regularly onto their sides to prevent prolonged exposure (>2 hours) of pressure to body protuberances and to prevent atelectasis of dependent segments. Interestingly, some patients with acute respiratory distress syndrome (ARDS) may be turned periodically in the prone position to improve oxygenation (see Chapter 73).

Also to improve oxygenation, patients with a severe unilateral pneumonia often respond favorably when the "good" (nonconsolidated) lung is "down" (in the

117

Table 10–1. Basic Orders for Patients Admitted to the ICU

BASIC ORDERS	ICU CONSIDERATIONS
Diagnosis	Are there diagnosis-specific protocols or pathways? Do the patient's characteristics match admission criteria?
Condition	All but patients admitted for monitoring should be identified as "critical."
Allergies	Extremely important to inquire and document any drug allergies.
Activity	Consider careful and explicit rationale for restraints, special beds, positioning.
Vital signs	Each ICU has its own frequency of vital signs. Specify use of noninvasive monitors, e.g., pulse oximetry; list parameters for physician notification (e.g., call physician for heart rate >120 or <60).
Diet	Specify use of nasogastric or duodenal feeding tubes where appropriate; estimate caloric requirements; consider special electrolyte or fluid needs; maintain some enteral feeding for patients receiving hyperalimentation, unless contraindicated (Chapter 13). Use nutrition consultation and special hyperalimentation order sheets. Consider measuring nitrogen balance, where appropriate.
Diagnostic procedures	Will alert nursing staff to coordinate off-site transport or to prepare the equipment for bedside procedures.
Fluids	Pay attention to decreased, insensible water loss in ventilated patients (may gain up to 500 mL/24 h).
Special considerations	Eye protection for paralyzed patients; mouth care for intubated patients.
Preventive measures	Use subcutaneous heparin or pneumatic compression devices for deep venous thrombosis prophylaxis; use enteral feeding, sucralfate, proton pump inhibitor, or H_2 blocker for stress ulcer prophylaxis if patient is in high-risk group (Table 10–2).
General medications	Assure adequate control of pain and anxiety (Chapter 4); write for a prn (as needed) sedative for sleep (Chapter 44).
Special medications	Particular care should be given to drug interactions, impaired renal and hepatic clearance, decreased blood flow in shock states (Chapter 12).

dependent position). The rationale for the latter is that gravity favors blood flow to the dependent lung and increases pulmonary blood flow to alveoli that are better ventilated. The result is improved ventilation/perfusion matching (fewer alveoli with low ventilation/perfusion) and decreased shunting through fluid-filled alveoli (whose ventilation/perfusion $= 0$). Both changes improve oxygenation.

In the case of severe hemoptysis (usually >300 mL/24 h) from a unilateral lesion, the opposite recommendation applies: the patient is turned so that the lung from which the bleeding is originating is in the dependent position. The basis for this recommendation is simply that gravity will deter blood from spilling from the lesion across the midline to the contralateral lung. This maneuver may be lifesaving in an emergent situation (see Chapter 75).

For many years, patients were routinely placed horizontally (flat) in the supine position for ease of care. Calibrating and zeroing transducers, performing routine nursing care, and keeping the patient safe from falls are all facilitated by the fully recumbent position. Unfortunately, it also increases the risk of aspiration and possibly nosocomial pneumonia. For this reason, keeping the head of the bed elevated 30 to 45 degrees, especially in mechanically ventilated patients or those receiving gastric tube feedings, has been advocated as the standard of care in the ICU. Some patients with neurologic disease may also benefit from elevating the head of the bed to 30 degrees with up to 10 mm Hg reduction in intracranial pressure. Recent studies, however, cast doubt on this recommendation as a blanket approach. For example, patients with nasogastric (NG) tubes have been shown to aspirate despite being in the semirecumbent position, although somewhat less than in the fully recumbent position. In addition, elevating the patient's upper body creates extra shear stress exposure to skin of the back, sacrum, and lower extremities, increasing the risk of skin injury and breakdown.

Without question, any special requirements for body positioning must be discussed among the entire ICU care team. Critical care clinicians tend to leave the patient in one unchanged position over prolonged periods, and the sicker the patient, the less his or her position is changed or altered. Thus, clear instructions and reinforcement must be given if any purposeful changes in position are to occur.

SKIN CARE (see also Chapter 43)

Risk Factors for Skin Injuries

The skin is the first line of the body's defense against the external environment, but multiple factors conspire to violate these defenses in the ICU patient. Whether chronically ill and debilitated or acutely and catastrophically ill, the ICU patient may have poor nutrition or poor anabolic capacity, or both. The skin becomes fragile, unable to resist normal assaults, and lacks capacity for healing. Low albumin, decreased subcutaneous fat, edema, obesity, diabetes, incontinence, extreme age, immobility, and impaired immune responses all increase susceptibility of the skin to injury. Chronic corticosteroids also exacerbate this problem. Shock and other states of hypoperfusion that decrease blood flow to the skin also impair normal healing. In addition, the skin is subject to an array of physical trauma in the ICU. This includes perforation by needles and catheters, shear stress when patients are moved over bed sheets or positioned in a nonflat position, abrasions resulting from adhesives applied for dressings and holding catheters securely in position, and pressure from orthopedic devices and other surfaces in contact with the skin.

Obviously, the first approach is to minimize physical trauma to the skin when performing procedures and applying and removing dressings. Attention must also be given to the nutritional status of the patient and to peripheral perfusion. In general, patients who are sedated with or without paralysis must be turned every 2 hours in order to avoid the development of pressure ulcers.

Specific Integumentary Conditions

Wounds. Wounds generally should be dressed with sterile dry dressings for 24 to 48 hours after surgery. After that, they may be changed for convenience as well as to protect the exposed surface and sutures. Clean healing wounds do not need any particular dressing after that time. Dressings should be changed so that the wound may be observed for signs of redness, swelling, or purulence. Contaminated wounds are generally managed "open," that is, without primary closure. Wet-to-dry dressings may be applied using normal saline, Dakin's solution, or povidone-iodine (Betadine) in 1:4 dilution.

Stomas. Stomal mucosa should at all times be warm and pink; duskiness is a sign of poor perfusion. Stomas should be framed with a ring that provides a 1/4-inch margin circumferentially. Usually, care is managed initially by an enterostomal therapist. If there are no signs of redness, ischemia, purulence, or breakdown, only infrequent changes of dressing are needed.

Drains. Drains must be left open and may be managed with frequent changes of dry dressings if the output from the drain is easily absorbed. Increased drainage may be collected into an ostomy bag or special collecting bag that is changed frequently to prevent overflow or contamination and to measure output.

Fistulas. Fistulas are some of the most difficult wounds to manage, particularly in the perineal area. They may be kept clean with frequent changes of dry dressings and observed for signs of abscess formation or skin breakdown. With copious drainage from cutaneous fistulas, it may be impossible to prevent skin breakdown, particularly if the patient is critically ill.

Pressure Ulcers. Pressure ulcers evolve through stages in response to pressure from immobility or from appliances in contact with the skin (see Table 43–1, Chapter 43). Comprehensive guidelines for the problem of pressure ulcers have been developed by the Agency for Health Care Policy and Research. (Prevention and staged treatment of pressure ulcers are described in Chapter 43.)

Superficial Fungal Infections. Superficial fungal infections frequently involve *Candida* or *Torulopsis* and may be treated with a topical mycostatin or clotrimazole cream (see Chapter 43 for more details).

Special Care Beds

Because of the frequency of pressure ulcers and other skin injury in the critical care unit, particular attention has been paid to the interface between patient and bed. This has resulted in the development of a number of specialized approaches (see Table 43–2, Chapter 43).

First, a *mattress overlay* consists of an inexpensive (several hundred dollars) surface to distribute pressure across a wider skin area. One should remember that the usual colorful but thin "egg crate" overlay mattress is inadequate to protect body protuberances against pressure injury because it "bottoms out" because of a lack of height. By doing so, it cannot distribute enough of the pressure from the body's weight away from the protuberance to prevent skin ischemia, which may occur in as short a time as *2 hours*.

A second approach combines a special pressure-reducing surface with an automatic periodic side-to-side rotation of the bed in order to alternate areas of the skin subject to pressure. This type of bed (e.g., Rotorest or Effica beds) has been used successfully for patients in traction, patients with spinal cord injury, or patients in a prone position as an adjunctive treatment for ARDS.

In a third approach, individual segments of the mattress may be inflated either concurrently or sequentially in order to distribute pressure over a wider surface area (low air-loss bed). This sequential inflation and deflation automatically rotate the points of maximal contact with the patient's skin.

A fourth approach employs air-fluidized silicon beads covered by a semiperme-able material (one example is the Mediscus brand). This bed produces a "floating" sensation and virtually eliminates concentrated pressure points on the patient's skin. In addition, the constant airflow can keep the skin dry. One drawback of this device is the requirement that the patient be in the fully recumbent position.

There is a near consensus that patients at high risk for skin breakdown benefit from one of these specialized approaches. Some studies have demonstrated cost savings and improved outcome with use of the low air-loss or air-fluidized approach compared with a standard mattress for high-risk ICU patients. Others, however, have demonstrated increased cost without significant improvements in outcome.

Malnourished ICU patients with poor skin perfusion who are subject to multiple dressing changes and puncture of the skin are at high risk for skin ischemia and pressure ulcers. These patients must be placed on an appropriate mattress overlay, low air-loss or air-fluidized bed in order to prevent serious skin breakdown. The selection of the specific product depends on local hospital and clinical practice as well as on individualized assessment. The bottom line is that these specialty beds are effective but because they are expensive to use, they should be restricted to those most in need (see Table 43–3, Chapter 43). The optimal approach to patient selection, however, has yet to be determined.

Aseptic Technique

It is noteworthy that patients with malignancy who die in the ICU do not die primarily from their cancer but rather from infectious complications. Indeed, nosocomial infection is the major cause of death in critically ill patients in general. For this reason, it is of paramount importance to observe simple but effective infection control measures (see Chapter 11).

The most common and flagrant violation of aseptic technique involves hand-washing. Numerous studies have demonstrated that resistant organisms may be carried on the hands of caregivers from patient to patient and, in some ICUs, cause epidemics of multiple drug–resistant pathogens with high mortality. Hand-washing with a germicidal solution is imperative to prevent the spread of organisms. Hands should be washed before and after contact with each and every ICU patient.

Masks and gloves should be worn for every sterile procedure performed, including thoracentesis, placement of arterial and central venous catheters, and paracentesis. The skin should be cleansed with alcohol and povidone-iodine beginning at the center and gradually increasing the cleansed area using a circular motion. Gloves should be changed after the clinician has completed the episode of patient contact and should never be worn while answering the telephone or writing in the chart. Additional use of sterile gowns during central venous and pulmonary artery catheter placement is required in many ICUs because it facilitates manipulation of equipment without losing asepsis.

As the incidence of *Clostridium difficile*, methicillin-resistant *Staphylococcus aureus* (MRSA), vancomycin-resistant enterococci (VRE or VREC), and other resistant organisms increases, compliance with infection control policies takes on critical importance in the ICU. Adherence to specific hospital policies for isolation of ICU patients with these resistant organisms is likewise of critical importance.

NONINVASIVE MONITORING

Most monitoring in the ICU is noninvasive in the sense that it does not violate the normal defense mechanisms of the patient. For example, *heart rate* can readily be taken from surface electrocardiogram electrodes, oscillometric blood pressure cuff, or pulse oximetry waveform. It may reflect adequacy of stroke volume, depth of sedation and analgesia, or the presence of pneumothorax or other problems. *Respiratory rate* may also be determined through changes in thoracic electrical impedance as the distance between standard electrocardiogram electrodes changes during respiration. Alternatively, respiratory rate is readily determined for patients connected to a mechanical ventilator by pressure or flow changes detected in the circuit. Both of these methods, however, may underestimate or overestimate the actual respiratory rate. For this reason, it is important to observe the patient and count chest excursions or inspiratory efforts to confirm the other methods.

Noninvasive determination of *temperature* may result in significant underestimation of fever. Tympanic membrane and axillary measurements, although noninvasive, may result in errors of 1 to 2° C when compared with simultaneous core or rectal temperature. For this reason, tympanic membrane measurements always need to be corrected for the discrepancy and axillary measurements should be avoided altogether in patients with shock or sepsis.

When clinicians note discrepancies between arterial catheter and cuff measurements of blood pressure, the noninvasive method is frequently mistrusted. Peripheral vasoconstriction, catheter resonance, damping, and other factors, however, may result in overestimation or underestimation of blood pressure by the catheter-transducer method, especially if a peripheral artery is cannulated. In the presence of shock or an abnormal arterial waveform, cuff blood pressure measurement by the oscillometric or ultrasonographic method may be preferable.

Noninvasive determination of arterial blood pH, Pao_2 and $Paco_2$ remains an elusive goal of critical care monitoring. *Pulse oximetry* has been found to be a valuable addition to arterial blood sampling in the ICU, although it is an imperfect replacement in the operating suite. Pulse oximetry depends on the transmission and absorbance by hemoglobin of two or three wavelengths of light through a capillary bed, usually in the fingertip or earlobe. Because hemoglobin absorbs light in relation to its saturation with oxygen, a computer can calculate hemoglobin saturation continuously. Peripheral vasoconstriction is an important cause of inaccuracy of pulse oximetry. Importantly, some patients, usually those with respiratory failure, show poor correlation between arterial blood saturation measured directly by a laboratory co-oximeter and saturation as measured by pulse oximetry. If such discrepancy is documented, one should not rely on the absolute values of pulse oximetry to guide treatment decisions but rather use changes in values as a red flag for potential problems (see also Chapter 26). One need also remember that Sao_2 by pulse oximetry tells nothing about arterial pH or $Paco_2$.

Clinicians have attempted to supplement pulse oximetry to noninvasively assess adequacy of ventilation by monitoring end-tidal Pco_2. This uses *capnography* that measures CO_2 in the patient's exhaled gas. Despite initial enthusiasm, many clinicians regard capnography in patients on ventilators as having limited value. Because most ICU patients receiving mechanical ventilation have intrinsic lung or airway disease, they have abnormal patterns of expired CO_2. This makes measurement and interpretation of an "end-tidal" P_{CO_2} problematic. Changes in this difficult to make measurement are even more challenging to interpret correctly; the same result may arise from hypoventilation, tracheal secretions, bronchospasm, pulmonary edema, or a number of other frequent complications in ICU patients. Its utility may lie in monitoring patients on ventilators who are relatively stable and free of intrinsic lung disease, such as those with respiratory failure due to neuromuscular weakness.

INVASIVE CATHETERS

See Chapter 11 for a discussion of intravascular catheters.

Urinary Catheters

Urinary catheters are frequently used to indirectly monitor renal perfusion and assist in fluid balance. They also provide a ready source of colonization and potential infection of the bladder and upper urinary tract. Traction on the catheter may produce urethral injury, particularly in patients with hemostatic disorders. In the absence of a local complication, there is no compelling reason to change the urinary catheter in an ICU patient. It should be removed as soon as the patient can assist with urination. Studies indicate that many patients in ICUs continue with these catheters beyond the appropriate time for removal.

Rectal Tubes

Rectal tubes may prevent skin breakdown and may improve the ability of nurses and others to care for patients with profuse diarrhea. However, mucosal necrosis and bleeding may occur because of the high pressure needed to maintain a rectal catheter in place. For this reason, it is advisable to deflate the balloon every 4 hours for 0.5 hour to prevent these complications. Some ICUs avoid rectal tubes completely because of these intrinsic risks in critically ill patients and use rectal "trumpets" instead.

Nasogastric Tubes

Nasogastric tubes are frequently used in intubated patients to prevent gastric distention, for ascertaining gastric pH, and for delivering food and medication. A common complication occurs when the tube is flexed upward (over the patient's forehead) to clear it from the patient's mouth, neck, and thorax. This upward angulation may produce nasal necrosis and should be avoided. Instead, one should allow the tube to follow a natural downward loop and to follow the curve laterally near the ear, where it may be redirected without causing undue pressure on the nose. When used primarily for feeding, small-diameter feeding tubes should be substituted for NG tubes.

Tracheostomy Tubes

Tracheostomy tubes are most frequently secured with adhesive tape or umbilical ties (see Chapter 24). The tape may be double-faced around the back of the neck to minimize irritation and discomfort. One finger should fit between the adhesive tape or umbilical tie and the neck to prevent excoriation of the skin. Newer Velcro and fabric fasteners have been used, but some have found that these devices are less reliable. After initial tracheostomy, a period of time (usually about 7 days) is allowed for the fistula (track) to become established, at which time a member of the surgical team that did the procedure should also do the first change of the tracheostomy tube (external cannula). After this and with the stoma and track matured, the ICU team can safely perform subsequent changes.

Endotracheal Tubes

Endotracheal tubes represent a major source of bacterial colonization of the tracheobronchial tree. Moreover, traction may produce injury or necrosis to the oral mucosa, tongue, and angles of the lips. For this reason, the tube should be repositioned at a minimum of every 24 hours, preferably alternating sides of the mouth. Mouth care should be provided regularly and the mouth should be inspected for signs of ulceration, necrosis, or injury. Once correct tube position has been determined by a chest radiograph, distance markings on the tube at the level of the maxillary teeth can be used to document tube positions after repositioning.

EYE CARE

In sedated, paralyzed, or otherwise immobile patients, particularly those connected to a mechanical ventilator, there is an increased risk of injury or infection to the eye. This problem, however, has received little rigorous investigation, resulting in a paucity of evidence on which to act.

Decreased tear protection resulting in corneal drying and ulceration may occur without appropriate interventions. For this reason, it is common practice to apply a wetting agent regularly as an ointment or liquid (e.g., Lacrilube) to the eyes to prevent drying of the cornea. Care must also be taken to prevent eye injury from falling instruments, ventilator or other tubing, or secretions. If needed, one may lightly tape simple gauze pads in place to keep eyelids closed. The eyes should be routinely examined for signs of infection, subconjunctival edema and injury, and ophthalmic consultation should be requested if there is any evidence of injury. Subconjunctival edema may result from high inspiratory ventilator pressures and does not in itself require any specific treatment.

Table 10–2. Guidelines for Stress Ulcer Prophylaxis in the ICU

....

1. Critically ill patients with coagulopathy, multisystem organ failure, head injuries, or extensive burns, or ICU patients on a mechanical ventilator are at high risk for stress ulcers and should receive prophylaxis. It should be omitted as "routine" care in low-risk groups.
2. Patients receiving gastric feeding do not need additional stress ulceration prophylaxis.
3. For patients not receiving enteral feeding, standard IV doses of H_2 blockers (e.g., ranitidine 50 mg q8h) should be administered in intermittent doses.
4. If a nasogastric tube is in place, gastric pH should be measured regularly (every 4 h) and kept >4.0 by increasing the intermittent doses or by using a constant infusion.

....

STRESS ULCER PROPHYLAXIS (Table 10–2)

In the first decades of ICU care, acute gastric stress ulceration leading to uncontrollable gastrointestinal hemorrhage was an all too frequent catastrophic complication of critical illness. Indeed, this cause of massive bleeding and associated emergent surgery was a significant contributor to ICU morbidity and mortality. However, many studies performed in the 1970s and 1980s demonstrated the benefit of prophylactic antacid or H_2-blocker administration to prevent the development of acute stress ulceration. As more experience was gained, it became clear that several alternative approaches reduced the frequency of acute stress ulceration and bleeding. These included administration of antacid (by NG tube), H_2 blockers (given in intermittent intravenous doses or by a continuous infusion), and sucralfate (by NG tube), as well as tube feeding and proton pump inhibitors (by NG tube).

After effective treatment for stress ulcer prevention became available, attention shifted from their primary effects to their potential complications. With alkalization, increased bacterial colonization of the stomach was noted. Indeed, several studies have suggested that such increased colonization may be related to an increased incidence of nosocomial pneumonia in mechanically ventilated patients treated with an H_2 blocker. Based on these studies, some have advocated the use of sucralfate in preference to histamine blockers for the prevention of stress ulceration. Even this has complications because sucralfate must be given by NG tube in the intubated and ventilated patient; its use carries the risks of sinusitis, nasal trauma associated with NG tube in those patients without other good indications for NG tubes, and violation of the gastroesophageal sphincter, possibly increasing reflux. Finally, a recent large randomized controlled clinical trial has called into question the effectiveness of sucralfate in high-risk patients.

PROPHYLAXIS FOR THROMBOEMBOLISM

A number of controlled studies document that critically ill patients are at substantial risk for venous thromboembolism and that prophylaxis for deep venous thrombosis (DVT) is effective in reducing morbidity and mortality (Table 10–3). This suggests that all critically ill patients, particularly those who are being mechanically ventilated or are immobilized, should be considered as candidates for prophylaxis for DVT.

Table 10–3. Guidelines for Prophylaxis of Deep Venous Thrombosis in ICU Patients

1. Consider all immobile, heavily sedated, or mechanically ventilated patients as candidates for deep venous thrombosis prophylaxis.
2. Begin subcutaneous heparin 5000 units q12h as prophylaxis (unless contraindicated).
3. In patients with contraindications for receiving heparin, institute pneumatic compression devices. Before using such devices in previously immobile patients, check lower extremities for presence of proximal clot by Doppler ultrasound or impedance plethysmography (Chapter 47).
4. For special high-risk groups, such as spinal cord–injured patients or trauma patients (lung ventilator dependence, multiple lower extremity fractures, major abdominal or pelvic venous injury or pelvic and lower extremity fractures), prophylactic IVC filters should be considered followed by systemic anticoagulation.

IVC, inferior vena cava.

The two most common methods for this involve subcutaneous heparin in a dose of 5000 units every 12 hours or pneumatic compression devices. The latter are usually offered for patients who initially present with active bleeding, for those with spinal cord injury, or for other neurosurgical patients.

Although subcutaneous heparin in the preceding dose may be regarded as standard care, it has been found to be inadequate in patients with major trauma. For example, in one study of this population, treatment with this regimen of heparin showed no decreased incidence of DVT detected by ultrasonography. Another group demonstrated that the placement of prophylactic inferior vena cava filters in this particularly high-risk group significantly reduced the occurrence of fatal pulmonary embolism. Some experts treat spinal cord–injured patients first with an initial period of observation using compression boots and then with adjusted-dose intravenous heparin to achieve measurable prolongation of the partial thromboplastin time in a therapeutic range.

PHLEBOTOMY

The mere presence of a patient in the ICU frequently creates a risk for excessive and unnecessary phlebotomies. Use of central venous catheters and arterial catheters increases the convenience with which large volumes of blood may be regularly drained from critically ill patients. Indeed, one study noted that for routine laboratory collections, blood drawn was 45 times in excess of the required volume. Another study examined phlebotomies in two groups of patients with similar severity of illness but only one group having arterial catheters in place. It found that although the number of blood tests and blood drawing procedures was 30% greater in the group with arterial catheters, the amount of blood volume removed was 44% greater.

The simplest and most responsible approach to this issue is to evaluate the need for each laboratory test. Daily electrolyte determinations, complete blood counts, and other studies are ordered far more frequently than required for patient management. Other approaches may be used to reduce the incidence of iatrogenic anemia. These include the use of blood-conserving devices that minimize the discarded blood volume (may be up to 50% of the total blood withdrawn) and the use of pediatric specimen tubes.

BIBLIOGRAPHY

Cook DJ, Fuller HD, Guyatt GH, et al: Risk factors for gastrointestinal bleeding in critically ill patients. N Engl J Med 330:377–381, 1994.
This important natural history study of a prospective cohort of 2252 ICU patients used as its outcome clinically important GI bleeding, defined as overt bleeding associated with hemodynamic compromise or a fall in hemoglobin and the need for blood transfusion. Multivariate analysis identified two independent risk factors: coagulopathy or requiring mechanical ventilation. Of the 1405 patients without either risk factor, only 2 had clinically important bleeding. The authors conclude that prophylaxis against stress ulcers can be safely withheld from critically ill patients without either of these risk factors.

Cook DJ, Guyatt G, Marshall J, et al: A comparison of sucralfate and ranitidine for the prevention of upper gastrointestinal bleeding in patients requiring mechanical ventilation. N Engl J Med 338:791–797, 1998.
This landmark randomized, placebo-controlled clinical trial of 1200 high-risk patients addressed the question of which agent should be used for stress ulcer prophylaxis. Patients treated with ranitidine had a significantly lower rate of clinically important GI bleeding vs. those treated with sucralfate. There were no significant differences in ventilator-associated pneumonia, length of stay in ICU, or mortality. Results suggested that sucralfate may have no effect in preventing clinically important bleeding in this patient population.

Cook D, Heyland D, Griffith L, et al: Risk factors for clinically important upper gastrointestinal bleeding in patients requiring mechanical ventilation. Crit Care Med 27:2812–2817, 1999.
This prospective cohort study (using the same group described by Cook et al, 1998) evaluated risk factors for clinically important upper GI bleeding in critically ill patients requiring mechanical ventilation for more than 48 hours. A multivariate analysis found that renal failure was an independent predictor of increased risk, whereas independent predictors of decreased risk were enteral nutrition and administration of ranitidine.

Cook DJ, Reeve BK, Guyatt GH, et al: Stress ulcer prophylaxis in critically ill patients. Resolving discordant meta-analyses. JAMA 275:308–314, 1996.
This review screened 269 articles on the effect of stress ulcer prophylaxis on GI bleeding, pneumonia, and mortality. After analyzing 63 appropriate randomized trials, the authors conclude that histamine 2 blockers decreased the incidence of GI bleeding. Sucralfate was associated with lower incidence of nosocomial pneumonia and mortality relative to antacids or histamine receptor antagonists.

Dale JC, Pruett SK: Phlebotomy—a minimalist approach. Mayo Clin Proc 68:249–255, 1993.
This study reviewed the volume of blood collected over an entire hospital stay of 113 patients in a medical ward and an ICU. The amount of blood collected was on average 45 times the required volume to perform the laboratory tests adequately.

Dennis JW, Menawat S, Von Thron J, et al: Efficacy of deep venous thrombosis prophylaxis in trauma patients and identification of high-risk groups. J Trauma 35:132–138; discussion J Trauma 35:138–139, 1993.
Of 395 patients with an injury severity score greater than 9 who survived 2 days or more, 214 were randomized to receive DVT prophylaxis and 181 were not. The risk of DVT was found to be significantly increased in those with spinal injury and head injury. The incidence of DVT was nearly 3 times greater in patients without prophylaxis than in those who received serial compression devices or subcutaneous heparin. The authors recommend consideration of vena caval filter in patients with severe neurologic injuries.

Keane MG, Ingenito EP, Goldhaber SZ: Utilization of venous thromboembolism prophylaxis in the medical ICU. Chest 106:13–14, 1994.
This survey of 152 medical ICU patients demonstrated that only a third of patients received prophylaxis, and those that did were delayed by an average of two days. Nearly half the patients had multiple risk factors for venous thromboembolism. The authors conclude that prophylaxis was underutilized in medical ICU patients.

Low LL, Harrington GR, Stoltzfus DP: The effect of arterial lines on blood-drawing practices and costs in ICUs. Chest 108:216–219, 1995.

In the absence of central venous access, arterial catheters are associated with a 29% increase in the number of blood tests and a 40% increase in phlebotomy blood volume compared to patients without arterial catheters.

Orozco-Levi M, Torres A, Ferrer M, et al: Semirecumbent position protects from pulmonary aspiration but not completely from gastroesophageal reflux in mechanically ventilated patients. Am J Respir Crit Care Med 152:1387–1390, 1995.

Using radioactive tracer, these authors suggest that semirecumbent position likely protects from pulmonary aspiration of gastric contents, but not from gastroesophageal reflux or oropharyngeal colonization.

Shannon ML, Lehman CA. Protecting the skin of the elderly patient in the ICU. Crit Care Nurs Clin North Am 8:17–28, 1996.

This is a practical consideration of issues involving skin protection of elderly patients in the ICU. It includes a good discussion of signs and symptoms as well as approach to special care beds.

Takiguchi SA, Myers SA, Yu M, et al: Clinical and financial outcomes of lateral rotation low air-loss therapy in patients in the ICU. Heart Lung 24:315–320, 1995.

This study used a retrospective design to examine the outcomes of patients on two different special care beds. They concluded that one bed was associated with statistically significant lower incidence of pneumonia, ARDS, and length of stay. The validity of these conclusions is limited by the retrospective nature of the design.

Torres A, Serra-Batlles J, Ros E, et al: Pulmonary aspiration of gastric contents in patients receiving mechanical ventilation: The effect of body position. Ann Intern Med 116:540–543, 1992.

These authors found one-third the aspirated radioactivity at one-half hour and one-tenth the radioactivity at 5 hours with semirecumbent position compared to the supine position. In addition, they noted isolation of concordant organisms from the stomach, pharynx, and endobronchial samples in 32% of semirecumbent patients and 68% of supine patients.

11 Nosocomial Infections

Jeffrey D. Edelman
Paul N. Lanken

Nosocomial infections occur 5 to 10 times more often in intensive care units (ICUs) than in non-ICU settings and significantly increase morbidity, mortality, and length of hospital stay. The risk of acquiring a nosocomial infection is influenced by numerous factors, including the patient's underlying disease; severity of illness; type of ICU; length of stay in the ICU; and number, type, and duration of invasive devices and procedures. In addition, transmission of infection from patient to patient via ICU personnel or equipment is common, making the ICU setting particularly prone to epidemic outbreaks of bacterial and viral infections. The nosocomial infections that occur most commonly in the ICU include (1) intravascular catheter–associated infections, (2) ventilator-associated pneumonias, (3) urinary tract infections, and (4) surgical site (wound) infections. These sites are discussed in detail further on. Although the resident bacterial flora vary from ICU to ICU, certain pathogens are often associated with nosocomial infections at these four sites (Table 11–1).

APPROACH TO INFECTION CONTROL IN THE INTENSIVE CARE UNIT

Infection Control Policies

Prevention of nosocomial infections requires coordination among ICU staff, infectious disease specialists, microbiologists, hospital infection control practitioners,

Table 11–1. Sites of Intensive Care Unit Nosocomial Infections and Common Associated Pathogens

BLOOD STREAM	PNEUMONIA (EARLY-ONSET) "CORE PATHOGENS"	PNEUMONIA (LATE-ONSET OR + RISK FACTOR)	URINARY TRACT	SURGICAL SITE
Coagulase-negative staphylococci	*Streptococcus pneumoniae*	*Pseudomonas aeruginosa*	*Escherichia coli*	*Enterococcus* spp.
Staphylococcus aureus	*Haemophilus influenzae*	Methicillin-resistant *S. aureus* (MRSA)	*C. albicans*	Coagulase-negative staphylococci
Enterococcus spp.	Methicillin-sensitive *S. aureus* (MSSA)	*Acinetobacter* spp.	*Enterococcus* spp.	*S. aureus*
Candida albicans	*Klebsiella pneumoniae*	"Core Pathogens" (in column to left)	*P. aeruginosa*	*P. aeruginosa*
Enterobacteriaceae	Other nonresistant enteric gram-negative bacilli	Resistant enteric gram-negative bacilli	Other enteric gram-negative bacilli	*Enterobacter* spp.

Note: Nosocomial pneumonias are commonly polymicrobial; early onset = less than 5 days in the ICU; late onset = 5 days or longer. See text for risk factors.

129

and the hospital epidemiologist. ICU physicians, nurses, and respiratory care practitioners should be familiar with the hospital's infection control policies. These include preventing transmission of infection from patient to patient and specific isolation precautions mandated by the presence of certain pathogens, such as methicillin-resistant *Staphylococcus aureus (MRSA)* and vancomycin-resistant enterococci (VREC). Policies should also establish aseptic techniques for the insertion and care of indwelling devices and standardize procedures for obtaining and interpreting culture specimens. Both regular epidemiologic surveillance and direct observation of behavior by infection control practitioners are necessary to monitor compliance, track nosocomial infection rates, and identify resistance patterns. These procedures also assess the need for changing infection control policies, increasing professional education, or enforcing existing policies more tightly. For example, although hand washing after contact with an ICU patient has been proved to be a simple, effective, and inexpensive strategy for preventing transmission of infection from patient to patient, compliance with this practice in many ICUs is often poor. Improved hand washing and disinfecting is usually the most important step in improving infection control in ICUs.

Special Infection Risks in the Intensive Care Unit

High utilization rates of invasive catheters and tubes contribute significantly to the increased risk of nosocomial infection in the ICU setting. The ongoing need for all indwelling devices should be assessed daily. Devices should be removed when their presence no longer provides the desired incremental benefit (balanced against the incremental risk of its continuation) or when one suspects that a device may be the source of infection, such as a central venous catheter infection.

There is also a high use (many would say overuse) of empirical antimicrobial agents in ICUs (see Chapter 14). This predisposes patients to superinfection by fungal organisms or multidrug-resistant bacteria. It also unnecessarily exposes patients to potential risks of side effects and drug toxicity. Before initiating empirical antimicrobial therapy, one must obtain all appropriate cultures based on suspected sources of infection and consider the known or suspected infectious agents in one's choice of antimicrobials (see Table 11–1). One should also establish a specific end point for stopping or changing antibiotics. Continuing empiric antimicrobial therapy is an issue that should be addressed daily on rounds and should be justified by culture results and the patient's clinical status (see Chapter 14).

INFECTIONS DUE TO INTRAVASCULAR CATHETERS

Definitions

Catheter-associated infections (CAIs) are defined by signs of local infection at an intravascular catheter site or the presence of 15 or more colony forming units (CFU) obtained by semiquantitative culture of the catheter tip. *Catheter-associated bacteremias* (CABs) are catheter-associated infections in which the same microorganism is isolated from the catheter tip and concurrent blood cultures. The presence

Table 11–2. Risk Factors for Central Venous Catheter–Associated Infection

Concomitant total parenteral nutrition
Duration of catheterization*
Exposure to bacteremia or distant site of infection
Insertion with less than full barrier precautions or with poor skin preparation
Repeated catheterization
Site of insertion (femoral > internal jugular > subclavian)
Type of catheter (triple lumen > single lumen; antimicrobial nonimpregnated > impregnated)

*Noted in some but not all studies

of fewer than 15 CFU by semiquantitative culture of the catheter tip is considered to be contamination.

Incidence Density Rates and Pathogens

Blood stream infections in the ICU are most often associated with central venous catheters. The rate of CAB is 5 to 15 episodes per 1000 central line days in adult medical and surgical ICUs, with the greatest frequency in burn units (a central line day is defined as each day that a central venous catheter is in place in an ICU patient). Coagulase-negative staphylococci and *S. aureus* are the organisms most commonly responsible for CAIs (see Table 11–1), although the former is more frequently isolated from catheter tip cultures and the latter more frequently causes CABs. Risk factors for CAIs are shown in Table 11–2.

Pathogenesis

Most commonly, microorganisms gain access to the blood stream by migration from the catheter insertion site along the external surface. Other mechanisms are less common. They include extension along the internal surface of the catheter from a colonized hub, contamination of the outside of the catheter during initial insertion of the catheter, or seeding the intravascular portion of the catheter from a bacteremic episode arising from an infection at a distal site.

Diagnosis

Except in clear-cut cases in which the insertion site appears inflamed or purulent, diagnosis of CAI is dependent upon removing the catheter. The technique most commonly used to detect CAI is the semiquantitative culture technique first described by Maki and colleagues in 1977. In this method, the catheter is removed using sterile forceps after preparing the surrounding skin with 70% alcohol. After removal, the distal 5 cm of the catheter tip is cut off aseptically, placed in a sterile urine container, and sent immediately to the microbiology laboratory for prompt processing (the tip should be cultured within 2 hours of removal). Growth of 15 or more CFU of a microorganism is considered to represent CAI. Since the catheter pieces are cultured by rolling on culture plates, this technique can only detect organisms on the catheter's external surface.

Less commonly, a quantitative culture technique may be used. This involves placing the tip of the catheter in broth and dislodging intraluminal and extraluminal bacteria using mechanical flushing, vortexing, or sonication. In this method, a culture yielding more than 10^3 CFU/mL indicates the presence of a CAI.

Blood cultures drawn through intravascular devices to detect bacteremia should be discouraged because they often yield false-positive results due to colonization of the catheter at the hub. If one set of blood cultures must be drawn through a central venous catheter, a second set must be drawn peripherally at the same time. Drawing blood cultures through intra-arterial catheters, which have high colonization rates of their three-way stopcocks, yields notoriously unreliable results and should rarely, if ever, be used for this purpose (the one exception is when blood cultures are taken at the time of original sterile insertion). Blood cultures obtained through intravascular catheters should be clearly marked as to their source to aid in the subsequent interpretation of a positive culture.

Prevention

All central venous catheters should be inserted using maximal barrier precautions. In a recent randomized study, this practice significantly reduced the rate of CAI and CAB. Compliance should be encouraged by making all equipment and supplies easily accessible and by requiring that all central line inserters be familiar with the institution's infection control guidelines for central venous catheter insertion and maintenance. Individual expertise, anticipated duration of cannulation, and risk factors for complications, including infection, should be considered in selecting the insertion site. On average, femoral vein sites have the highest risk of infection, followed by internal jugular vein sites, with subclavian vein sites having the least risk for infection (but also having the highest risk for mechanical complications such as pneumothorax).

The operator and attendants should wear sterile gloves, masks, caps, protective eyewear, and sterile gowns. An area at least 15 cm beyond the site of insertion should be prepped and allowed to dry for several minutes before catheter insertion. A large sterile sheet drape should be used to cover the patient, and the insertion site should be surrounded with sterile towels extending at least 5 cm within the perimeter of the sterile preparation zone.

The same precautions should be used when changing central venous catheters "over a wire" (using the Seldinger method, Chapter 9). Because catheter hubs are frequently colonized, it is preferable to cut off the hub of the distal port of a multilumen catheter and then insert the guide wire through the cut end of the tubing. When a catheter is replaced over a guide wire, the tip of the original catheter should always be sent for culture, as described earlier; the new catheter must be removed if culture of the tip of the original catheter is positive for CAI.

In most (but not all) observational studies, the risk of CAI increases with the duration of central venous catheterization with a rise in infection rates at about 4 days. A recent randomized trial, however, failed to show that "routine" scheduled replacement of central venous catheters reduces infection rates. Performing routine changes actually increased the risk of complications. The use of a new puncture site had an increased risk of mechanical complications, whereas changing lines over a guide wire had an increased risk of infection. Based on these and other results, once inserted under proper aseptic conditions, central venous catheters should remain in place as long as clinically indicated unless local signs of infection are noted or the catheter is suspected as a source of fever or sepsis. Catheters inserted emergently without the full aseptic precautions described should be removed as soon as possible and, if central venous catheterization is still necessary, another catheter should be inserted at a new site. Although their stopcocks are frequently colonized, true infections of peripheral arterial catheters are uncommon and, like central venous catheters, there is no indication for routine changes at any interval.

In contrast to conventional central venous catheters, the risk for pulmonary artery catheter infection rises dramatically at 5 days, and it is prudent to remove these catheters after this duration of use (or earlier whenever possible). If continued hemodynamic monitoring is required, both the catheter and the sheath should be replaced by using a guide wire or a new puncture site.

Treatment

As a rule, infected catheters need to be removed. In the absence of bacteremia, removal of the infected catheter is all that is usually needed. In the setting of uncomplicated CAB, however, removal of the infected catheter plus 2 weeks of appropriate parenteral antimicrobial therapy is generally sufficient. Complications such as persistent bacteremia, septic thrombophlebitis, septic emboli, or endocarditis mandate a longer treatment duration.

VENTILATOR-ASSOCIATED PNEUMONIA

Definition

Ventilator-associated pneumonia (VAP) is the most common nosocomial infection in ICU patients, accounting for about one third of the total.

Rates and Risk Factors

The National Nosocomial Infection Survey reported a range of 7 to 24 episodes of VAP per 1000 ventilator-days (number of days patients are receiving mechanical ventilation). The highest rates occur in neurosurgical, burn, trauma, and surgical ICUs. The true incidence of VAP is uncertain, however, because there is no "gold standard" for diagnosis. Patients with VAP have high mortality rates, ranging from 33 to 71%.

Specific pathogens causing VAP vary according to hospital, patient population, season, and the specific diagnostic methods employed. A period of 5 days is used to distinguish "late-onset" VAP from "early-onset" VAP with their associated differences in commonly encountered pathogens (see Table 11–1). Certain risk factors predispose to pathogens other than those listed as "Core Pathogens" in

Table 11–3. Risk Factors for Ventilator-Associated Pneumonia

Age $\geq$ 60 years
Chronic pulmonary disease
Coma, impaired consciousness, intracranial pressure monitor
H_2 blocker use, gastric colonization, and elevated gastric pH
Large-volume gastric aspiration
Mechanical ventilation $\geq$ 2 days
Organ failure
Reintubation
Supine head position
Tracheostomy

Adapted from Craven DE, Steger KA: Epidemiology of nosocomial pneumonia: New perspectives on an old disease. Chest 108:1S–16S, 1995.

Table 11–1. These include recent abdominal surgery and witnessed aspiration for anaerobes; coma, head trauma, diabetes mellitus, and renal failure for *S. aureus*; prolonged ICU (or hospital) stays, steroids, prior antibiotic therapy, and structural lung disease, such as cystic fibrosis, for *Pseudomonas aeruginosa.*

Viral agents, particularly influenza and respiratory syncytial virus (both of which can cause ICU epidemics), may be underrepresented because they are not routinely considered as causes of VAP. Factors associated with increased risk for VAP are listed in Table 11–3.

Pathogenesis

Under conditions of hospitalization for critical illness, the glycocalyx of oral epithelium undergoes changes that predispose the oropharynx to colonization by gram-negative bacilli. These are often the patient's endogenous bacterial flora. Similar colonization of gastric fluid also may occur, especially when its normal acidity is prevented or neutralized by food, antacids, or acid suppression.

In order for VAP to develop, microorganisms must reach the lower respiratory tract and overcome host defenses to cause invasive disease. Tracheal intubation provides a conduit for this to occur. The presence of a cuffed tube also impairs normal ciliary clearance of the lower airways. Pathogenic organisms enter and colonize the trachea via aspiration around the cuff, followed by distal migration and the development of pneumonia. Not only are the oropharynx, stomach, and sinuses reservoirs for these organisms, but the inner surface of the tube is also suspect. It soon becomes covered with a biofilm that may contain more than 1 million CFU/cm^2. This suggests that potential tracheal contamination may paradoxically occur during suctioning as the suction catheter passes through the catheter.

Diagnosis

The diagnosis of VAP remains a particularly vexing problem in the ICU. Having a sensitive and specific means to diagnose VAP is highly desirable to avoid the adverse effects of both undertreatment and overtreatment. Although numerous invasive and noninvasive strategies have been proposed, no one approach has been widely accepted as most reliable for diagnosis or effective in reducing morbidity and mortality. There is considerable variability in techniques, diagnostic criteria, and results in published studies. The controversy arises basically because there is no gold standard to diagnose VAP for comparison. In the absence of conclusive data, individual ICUs or hospitals should follow a consistent approach to the diagnosis of VAP based on available resources, patient population, epidemiologic surveillance, and clinical experience. Several reasonable approaches are described further on. Clinical criteria commonly used for the diagnosis of pneumonia are listed in Table 11–4. Unfortunately, most of these findings are nonspecific in mechanically ventilated patients, particularly those with acute respiratory distress syndrome. Many patients have purulent secretions in their proximal airways as a result of colonization, irritation, and localized infection in the absence of pneumonia. Furthermore, tracheal secretions may be contaminated by aspiration of secretions from above the endotracheal tube cuff. Even in the setting of pneumonia, the cultures of tracheal secretions may fail to yield the responsible pathogens, indicating an important lack of sensitivity. Quantitative cultures of tracheal aspirates with a positive threshold of greater than or equal to 10^5 (some reports use $\geq 10^6$) organisms/mL may improve specificity. Cultures of blood and pleural fluid may confirm the diagnosis of VAP under the appropriate clinical circumstances.

Compared with sputum sampling, quantitative bacterial culture of distal airways and alveoli has been reported to be more sensitive and specific for the diagnosis of VAP by a number of investigators. The two most widely used techniques are bronchoalveolar lavage (BAL) or protected specimen brushing (PSB) with quantitative cultures. The threshold for quantitative BAL is greater than or equal to 10^4 organisms/mL; the threshold for PSB cultures is greater than or equal to 10^3 organisms/mL. Both have a reported sensitivity of 70 to 100% if used before the initial administration of antibiotics (or before a change in the antibiotics present when the VAP was suspected); if used after new antibiotics are given, the sensitivity falls to less than 50%. BAL samples a much larger distal area than does PSB.

Although these procedures are generally performed using fiberoptic bronchoscopy, nonbronchoscopic techniques for blind PSB and BAL have also been de-

Table 11–4. Clinical Criteria Used for Diagnosis of Ventilator-Associated Pneumonia

CRITERIA	SENSITIVITY	SPECIFICITY
New or progressive infiltrate on chest radiograph	High	Low
Fever	Uncertain	Very low
New or increased leukocytosis	Uncertain	Very low
Purulent tracheal aspirate with >25 neutrophils per high-power field and <10 epithelial cells per low-power field	Uncertain but probably high	Low
Isolation of a pathogen (sputum or tracheal aspirate culture)	Low-moderate	Low-moderate
Isolation of a pathogen from blood or pleural fluid culture	Very low	High*

*When associated with new infiltrate on chest radiograph.

scribed with roughly comparable results. In order to ensure adequate and consistent sampling, operators must be familiar with the proper techniques for sampling and specimen processing such as the standardized bronchoscopic techniques proposed by the International Consensus Conference on the Clinical Investigation of VAP. Protected BAL using a balloon-tipped catheter may improve specificity by reducing specimen contamination from infected proximal airways. BAL fluid Gram stains may provide immediate diagnostic information and aid in initial selection of antimicrobial agents. Cytospin of BAL fluid with Wright-Giemsa staining can reveal the presence of intracellular bacteria in neutrophils, which suggests pneumonia.

Because the sensitivity and specificity of all culture techniques are reduced in the setting of recently started concurrent antibiotic therapy, all culture samples should be obtained *before* the initiation of antibiotic therapy whenever possible. In the setting of suspected superinfection in which the pathogens present are likely resistant to the current antimicrobials, sampling should be performed before new antibiotics are instituted.

Prevention

Strategies aimed at preventing VAP do not support the use of prophylactic antibiotics but rather focus on elimination of environmental sources of nosocomial pathogens and eradication of endogenous colonizing bacteria. In preventing person-to-person transmission, appropriate hand washing and glove use practices are extremely important in the ICU setting and well supported by clinical studies. Hand washing should be performed before and after patient contact and gloves and gowns should also be worn if contact with respiratory secretions or objects contaminated with respiratory secretions is likely.

Respiratory equipment is also a potential source for transmission of pathogenic bacteria, and all reusable respiratory equipment must be properly cleaned and disinfected. Disposable tubing may accumulate condensed fluids that can become colonized with bacteria usually originating from the patient's oropharynx. This condensate should be drained regularly. Despite the rapid development of tubing colonization, less frequent (every 48 hours or more) rather than more frequent (every 24 hours) routine tubing changes appear to reduce the risk of VAP.

Secretions above the endotracheal tube cuff should be cleared before deflating the cuff at the time of extubation or repositioning in the trachea. The preferred type of endotracheal suctioning system is an unresolved issue. In small studies, using a closed multiuse tracheal suction catheter system did not alter the rate of contamination or VAP. In one study, the use of a specially manufactured endotracheal tube with an extra lumen permitting continuous suctioning below the vocal cords but above the cuff significantly reduced the incidence of VAP during the first week of mechanical ventilation. This study also found that the pressure of endotracheal cuff pressures less than 20 cm H_2O was an independent risk factor for VAP in a multivariate analysis.

Probably the simplest and least expensive preventive measure is to keep the head of the patient's bed elevated at 30 to 45 degrees. This position aims to prevent gastroesophageal reflux. In addition, enteral feeding tubes and nasogastric tubes (which may affect the function of the gastroesophageal sphincter) should be removed as soon as they are no longer clinically indicated. When administering enteral nutrition, tube placement should be radiographically confirmed before starting tube feedings and later if it is suspected that the tube has moved. If possible, the head of the bed should be elevated at an angle of 30 to 45 degrees while bolus tube feedings are administered into the stomach. Intestinal mobility, abdominal girth, and residual gastric volumes should be assessed routinely. The necessity for postpyloric tube placement and the use of continuous versus intermittent feeding regimens are unresolved issues.

Stress ulcer prophylaxis with H_2 blockers, sucralfate, or antacids is a common practice in the ICU setting (see Chapter 10). Which method to use routinely for which category of ICU patient remains controversial despite multiple studies over years. It is generally accepted that ventilated ICU patients receiving antacids with or without H_2 blockers have increased gastric pH and higher gastric fluid bacterial counts. They also show a trend for an increased risk for pneumonia when compared with patients given sucralfate. Selective digestive decontamination (SDD), which prevents colonization of the oropharynx and the gut by aerobic gram-negative bacilli and *Candida* without altering the anaerobic flora, has been suggested as a means of preventing VAP. An antimicrobial paste is applied to the oropharynx and antibiotic solutions are administered enterally. Parenteral antibiotic therapy is often used with topical and enteral treatments. Although SDD appears to reduce colonization and rates of nosocomial pneumonia, ICU mortality does not appear to be reduced. Because of this, along with its cost and potential for promoting growth of resistant organisms, SDD is not recommended for this use in ICU patients. It may ultimately be useful in selected subsets of patients such as those with trauma or severe immunosuppression.

Treatment

Finally, treatment of VAP often involves the institution of empiric antibiotic therapy (see Chapter 14). The selected antibiotic must then be changed appropriately or stopped when culture results return. In selecting an empiric regimen, one must consider a number of factors (see Table 11–3), including which pathogens are likely based on national and local surveillance of nosocomial pathogens and their resistance patterns.

Tracheobronchitis without pneumonia should not, in general, be treated with aggressive broad spectrum antibiotics in the same empiric manner as VAP. Sputum Gram stains and culture results should determine antimicrobial therapy. Because of systemic toxicity, the use of aerosolized aminoglycosides to treat tracheobronchitis has been suggested. At present, however, there are little data to support this practice in the ICU setting.

URINARY TRACT INFECTION

Epidemiology, Pathogenesis, and Prevention

The urinary tract is the second most common site for nosocomial infection in the ICU, accounting for about one quarter of the total. Nosocomial urinary tract infection (UTI) is virtually always associated with urinary drainage catheter use. UTI rates range from 5 to 11 episodes per 1000 urinary catheter-days.

Table 11–5. Risk Factors for Nosocomial Urinary Tract Infection

....

Use of urinary catheter
Duration of catheter use
Open drainage and collecting system (tubes, reservoir bag, and urinometer)
Errors in catheter care
Female sex
Diabetes mellitus
Elevated creatinine

....

Bacteria may enter the bladder at the time of catheterization through the catheter lumen or, in women, via migration into the bladder from the perineum around the catheter.

Avoidance of unnecessary urinary catheterization is the primary means of preventing UTI. Other measures include proper catheter insertion using aseptic technique, use of a closed sterile drainage system and, a point that cannot be overemphasized, removal of the catheter as soon as possible. As in the case of central venous catheters, assessing the continued need for a urinary catheter, when present, should be a mandatory agenda item for daily ICU rounds. Table 11–5 lists risk factors for nosocomial UTIs.

Diagnosis

Urinalysis, urine culture, and Gram staining are used to assess for the presence of UTI. Microscopic evaluation of the urine in the setting of UTI typically shows pyuria and bacteriuria. If these findings are not present, urine culture and Gram staining should not be performed. Likewise, quantitative culture yields less than 10,000 CFU/mL represents colonization and does not warrant treatment. Gram staining and cultures are useful in determining appropriate antibiotic therapy. Blood cultures should always be obtained in the setting of systemic inflammatory response syndrome (SIRS), sepsis (urosepsis), or septic shock.

Treatment

As a rule, asymptomatic bacteriuria or bacteriuria without the presence of neutrophils does not require antibiotic treatment and usually resolves when the catheter is removed. Treatment of asymptomatic bacteriuria is indicated, however, if the cultured pathogen is associated with a high frequency of bacteremia (*Pseudomonas aeruginosa, S. aureus, Acinetobacter* spp.) or in patients who are neutropenic, immunosuppressed, pregnant, or have recently undergone urologic or penile surgery.

Except as noted earlier, catheter-associated UTIs require antibiotic therapy. Duration of treatment may range from 5 to 14 days depending on the severity of infection. Two weeks of therapy is usually administered for patients with urosepsis. When urosepsis is suspected, empiric antibiotic therapy should be instituted (see Table 14–6), with adjustments made once culture and sensitivity results are known.

Antibiotic coverage should include *Escherichia coli, Enterococcus* spp., *P. aeruginosa*, and *Klebsiella pneumoniae*. The presence of *S. aureus* in the urine should raise suspicion for hematogenous seeding from a nonurinary source.

Candiduria

Candida in the urine may reflect asymptomatic colonization, UTI, or disseminated fungal infection. The approach to candiduria remains controversial. Evaluation and treatment decisions are generally based on clinical status and risk for disseminated infection. In asymptomatic patients at low risk for disseminated infection, observation without treatment may be all that is necessary. The approach to symptomatic patients at low risk for dissemination should include (1) changing or removing the urinary catheter, (2) treatment or elimination of predisposing conditions (control of diabetes, taper or discontinuation of steroids, discontinuation of unnecessary antibiotics), (3) evaluation for urinary tract obstruction or other genitourinary abnormality, and (4) institution of antifungal therapy.

Treatment approaches in this setting are controversial. Because amphotericin B is cleared renally, and prolonged excretion after a single dose has been demonstrated, administration of a single dose of 0.3 to 1.0 mg/kg of amphotericin B may be effective in eradicating candiduria. Local irrigation with amphotericin B (generally 50 mg amphotericin B per liter of sterile water) has also been used to treat candida UTI with variable success. Systemic therapy with enteral or parenteral fluconazole may also eradicate infection due to *Candida albicans*. Other species of *Candida,* however, may not be sensitive to fluconazole. Aggressive evaluation and treatment are required for more severely ill patients with persistent SIRS or septic shock or those at high risk for disseminated fungal infection because of the presence of three or more sites of colonization (for example, urine, sputum, and wound). Despite thorough evaluation, it may be difficult to document the presence of disseminated candida infection because of the low sensitivity of current diagnostic methods. Diagnostic considerations include careful skin examination for candidal lesions, funduscopic examination for candidal retinitis (low sensitivity but highly specific), inspection of vascular access sites, and culture of central venous catheter and repeated sets of blood cultures using specific fungal isolators. Systemic antifungal therapy may be started empirically in this setting, using amphotericin B at a dose of 0.5 to 0.7 mg/kg/day. Liposomal amphotericin B is less nephrotoxic, although its efficacy has not been as well studied. Parenteral fluconazole at a dose of 400 mg/day has been shown to be equally effective with less toxicity than amphotericin B in a small number of patients with candidemia in the absence of neutropenia or severe immunodeficiency. Again, resistance of candida species other than *C. albicans* to this agent makes it less attractive in critically ill ICU patients.

SURGICAL SITE (WOUND) INFECTIONS

Surgical site infection (SSI) is the fourth most common class of nosocomial infection in the ICU, but in postoperative patients it accounts for 37% of nosocomial infections (see Table 11–1). Most SSIs occur 7 to 10 days after surgery and

Table 11–6. Criteria for Diagnosis of Surgical Site Infection

	SUPERFICIAL INCISIONAL	DEEP INCISIONAL	ORGAN OR SPACE
Degree of involvement	Only skin or subcutaneous tissue of incision	Deep soft tissues of the incision	Any area other than the incision itself that is opened or manipulated during the operative procedure
Criteria 1	Purulent drainage from the superficial incision	Purulent drainage from the deep incision but not from the organ or space component of the surgical site	Purulent drainage from a drain placed through a stab wound into the organ or space
Criteria 2	Organisms isolated from an aseptically obtained culture of fluid or tissue from the superficial incision	Deep incision dehisces or is deliberately opened when a patient has at least one of the following signs or symptoms: fever >38° C, localized pain or tenderness (unless culture of the incision is negative)	Organisms isolated from an aseptically obtained culture of fluid or tissue in the organ or space
Criteria 3	At least one of the following signs or symptoms of infection: localized pain or tenderness, swelling, redness, or heat, and superficial incision is deliberately opened (unless the culture is negative)	An abscess or other evidence of infection involving the deep incision is found on direct examination, during reoperation, or by histopathologic or radiologic examination	An abscess or other evidence of infection involving the organ or space on direct examination, during reoperation, or by histopathologic or radiologic examination

Presence of infection: patient must meet any *one* of the listed criteria.
Surgical site infections must occur within 30 days of the operative procedure (except in cases of deep incisional or organ-space infections involving foreign body in which the time limit is 1 year).

are classified as either superficial incisional, deep incisional or organ space infections (Table 11–6).

Preoperative patient-related factors increasing risk for SSI include advanced age, severity of disease, obesity, poor nutritional status, infection at distal sites, cancer, diabetes, and immunosuppression. Poor tissue perfusion and oxygenation also increase the risk for SSI. Technical risk factors for SSI include the use of a razor (as opposed to a depilatory agent) for preoperative hair removal, abdominal surgery, prolonged duration of surgery, wound contamination, intraoperative contamination, reoperation, poor hemostasis, emergent procedures, and insertion of drains or other foreign bodies. In one series, infection rates varied according to wound class (Table 11–7) from 2.1% for clean wounds, 3.3% for clean-contaminated wounds, 6.4% for contaminated wounds, to 7.1% for dirty wounds.

In general, the use of perioperative prophylactic antibiotic reduces the risk of SSI. Prophylactic antibiotics are generally administered at the time of induction of anesthesia and may need to be redosed intraoperatively and continued for a 24-

Table 11–7. Surgical Wound Classifications

CATEGORY	DESCRIPTION
Clean	Elective, primarily closed, no acute inflammation encountered, no entrance of normally or frequently colonized body cavities, and no break in sterile technique
Clean contaminated	Nonelective case that is otherwise a clean, controlled opening of a normally colonized body cavity, minimal spillage or break in sterile technique, reoperation through clean incision within 7 days, negative exploration through intact skin
Contaminated	Acute nonpurulent inflammation encountered, major break in technique or spill from hollow organ, penetrating trauma <4 h old, chronic open wounds for grafting
Dirty	Purulence or abscess encountered or drained preoperative perforation of colonized body cavity, penetrating trauma >4 h old

hour period. Clean wounds generally do not require prophylaxis unless the potential complications of infection would be disastrous (i.e., central nervous system operations, cardiac surgery requiring bypass, prosthesis placement). Prophylaxis is indicated for clean contaminated and contaminated wounds. Dirty wounds generally require preoperative antibiotics when possible with continued postoperative antibiotic treatment.

BIBLIOGRAPHY

American Thoracic Society: Hospital-acquired pneumonia in adults: Diagnosis, assessment of severity, initial antimicrobial therapy, and preventative strategies. Am J Respir Crit Care Med 153:1711–1725, 1995.
This is a consensus statement and comprehensive review.

Cobb DK, High KP, Sawyer RG, et al: A controlled trial of scheduled replacement of central venous and pulmonary-artery catheters. N Engl J Med 327:1062–1068, 1992.
This article describes a randomized, controlled trial including 160 patients.

Craven DE, Steger KA: Epidemiology of nosocomial pneumonia: New perspectives on an old disease. Chest 108:1S–16S, 1995.
Review article addressing risk factors, pathogenesis, and etiology of nosocomial pneumonia.

Fisher JF, Newman CL, Sobel JD: Yeast in the urine: Solutions for a budding problem. Clin Infect Dis 20:183–189, 1995.
This article reviews candiduria.

Maki DG, Jarrett F, Sarafin HW: A semiquantitative culture method for identification of catheter-related infection in the burn patient. J Surg Res 22:513–520, 1977.
This is the original article describing semiquantitative technique for culture of vascular catheters.

Meduri GU, Chastre J: The standardization of bronchoscopic techniques for ventilator associated pneumonia. Chest 102:557–564, 1992.
This article describes the recommendations of the 1991 Consensus Conference on the Clinical Investigation of Ventilator Associated Pneumonia and details standardized techniques for quantitative culture by PSB and BAL.

Mermel LA, Maki DG: Infectious complications of Swan-Ganz pulmonary artery catheters. Am J Respir Crit Care Med 149:1020–1036, 1994.

This article reviews studies addressing incidence, pathogenesis, epidemiology, prevention, and diagnosis of infections related to pulmonary artery catheterization.

Platt R, Polk BF, Murdock B, et al: Risk factors for nosocomial urinary tract infection. Am J Epidemiol 124:977–985, 1986.
This is a classic article on this subject.

Raad II, Hohn DC, Gilbreath BJ, et al: Prevention of central venous catheter–related infections by using maximal sterile barrier precautions during insertion. Infect Control Hosp Epidemiol 14:231–238, 1994.
This article describes a prospective randomized trial that documented efficacy of using barrier precautions.

Rex JH, Mennett JE, Sugar AM, et al: A randomized trial comparing fluconazole with amphotericin B for the treatment of candidemia in patients without neutropenia. N Engl J Med 17:1525–1530, 1994.
This article describes a prospective randomized trial.

Roy MC, Trish M, Perl MD: Basics of surgical site infection surveillance. Infect Control Hosp Epidemiol 18:659–668, 1997.
This is a review article.

Tablan OC, Anderson LJ, Arden NH, et al: Guideline for prevention of nosocomial pneumonia. Infect Control Hosp Epidemiol 15:587–627, 1994.
This article describes the Centers for Disease Control–Hospital Infection Control Practices Advisory Committee recommendations, with a comprehensive review of published studies.

12 Pharmacokinetics and Drug Interactions

Eric T. Wittbrodt
Karen J. Tietze

The pharmacokinetics of many drugs may be substantially altered in critically ill patients. Under these circumstances, appropriate dosing of a specific drug requires an understanding of how abnormal physiologic states induced by a patient's disease or by the common interventions performed in the intensive care unit (ICU) during treatment may change the drug's pharmacokinetics.

EFFECTS OF ALTERED PHYSIOLOGY ON PHARMACOKINETICS

Cardiovascular Disorders

Acute decreases in cardiac output diminish organ blood flow and may impair drug clearance. Conversely, acute hyperdynamic states may increase organ blood flow, thereby enhancing drug clearance. Absorption of orally administered drugs may also be decreased in patients with congestive heart failure.

Dialysis

Whether a drug is affected by dialysis depends on the drug's physicochemical properties and the method of dialysis. In general, highly water-soluble drugs are more dialyzable than are water-insoluble drugs. Drugs with molecular weights greater than 500 D, large volumes of distribution (>2 L/kg), and extensive protein binding are not removed by conventional intermittent hemodialysis. High-flux dialysis may remove larger molecules, whereas rapid high-efficiency dialysis may increase the clearance of small molecules.

Fluid Status Changes

Hypovolemia concentrates extracellular solutes, including drugs, and may reduce renal drug clearance. In addition, hypovolemia and shock decrease hepatic blood flow, which, in turn, reduces hepatic drug metabolism. In contrast, fluid overload lowers plasma drug concentrations, especially for highly protein-bound and water-soluble drugs.

Hepatic Dysfunction

In patients with liver dysfunction, metabolism by hepatic oxidation is usually more severely impaired than is metabolism by hepatic conjugation.

143

Malnutrition

In protein-depleted states when the total serum drug concentration is within the therapeutic range, the unbound (free) fraction of highly protein-bound drugs, for example, drugs binding to albumin, will be increased and may result in toxic effects. Thus, therapeutic levels of such a drug (reflecting the total serum concentration) will underestimate its potential for toxicity in malnourished patients.

Mechanical Ventilation

Hemodynamic depression from mechanical ventilation may impair liver and renal function, especially in patients with high levels of applied positive end-expiratory pressure (PEEP) or auto-PEEP, for example, >10 cm H_2O, and large tidal volumes, for example, >10 mL/kg. Decreases in cardiac output may occur without hypotension in some of these patients.

Renal Dysfunction

Although low molecular weight drugs (that are not highly protein-bound) are filtered at the glomerulus and then partially reabsorbed, most drugs eliminated by the kidney are secreted. The dose or interval of drugs eliminated renally by either mechanism must be changed when renal function is impaired (Table 12–1).

DOSING AND DRUG MONITORING FOR SPECIFIC DRUGS
(Table 12–2; see also Table 12–1)

Aminoglycosides

Absorption after intramuscular administration is variable because muscle perfusion may be inadequate in hypovolemia or shock. Aminoglycosides are distributed into

Table 12–1. Dosing Adjustments in Renal Impairment

| DRUG | ESTIMATED CREATININE CLEARANCE* | | |
	>50 mL/min	10–50 mL/min	<10 mL/min
Aminoglycosides	q8–12h	q12–24h	q48h or longer†
Digoxin	100% of dose q24h	50–75% of dose q24h	50% of dose q48h
Procainamide (oral)	q4–6h	q6–12h	q8–24h
Vancomycin	q12–24h	q24–72h	>q72h

*Calculate estimated creatinine clearance using ideal body weight (IBW) as follows:

Males: $\dfrac{(140 - \text{age})(\text{IBW})}{(72)(\text{serum creatinine})}$ where IBW (males) = 50 kg + 2.3 kg for each inch of height over 60

Females: $\dfrac{(140 - \text{age})(\text{IBW})(0.85)}{(72)(\text{serum creatinine})}$ where IBW (females) = 45.5 kg + 2.3 kg for each inch of height over 60

†Intervals should be individualized based on serum concentrations for more accurate dosing.
From Bennett WM: Guide to drug dosing in renal failure. Clin Pharmacokinet 15:326–354, 1988, with permission. © Adis International, Inc.

Table 12–2. Dosing Guidelines for Selected Drugs in the ICU

DRUG	LOADING DOSE	MAINTENANCE DOSE	THERAPEUTIC RANGE
Aminoglycosides	Gentamicin, netilmicin, and tobramycin: 1–2 mg/kg IV Amikacin: 5–7.5 mg/kg IV	The "loading dose" is repeated according to the intervals listed in Table 12–1	See Table 12–3
Digoxin	0.5 mg orally or IV, then 0.25 mg orally or IV q6h × 2	0.125–0.250 mg orally or IV every day	CHF*: 0.6–1.2 ng/mL (0.7–1.4 nmol/L)
Lidocaine	50–100 mg IV over 2 min	1–2 mg/min	2–6 μg/mL (6–21.5 μmol/L)
Phenytoin	15–18 mg/kg IV or orally	100 mg IV or orally q8h	10–20 μg/mL (40–80 μmol/L)
Procainamide	100 mg IV every 5 min until arrhythmia controlled or total of 1 g given	IV: 2–4 mg/min Orally: 50 mg/kg/day divided into doses given q12h (Procanbid), q6h (Procan SR), or q4h (Pronestyl)	4–10 μg/mL (P† only) (17–42.5 μmol/L) Toxicity increased if: >10 μg/mL (P only) (>42.5 μmol/L) >30 μg/mL (P + NAPA) (>127.5 μmol/L)
Quinidine	IV: Quinidine gluconate: 600 mg Orally: Quinidine sulfate: 200–300 mg q2–3h until arrhythmia controlled	Quinidine gluconate: 324–660 mg orally q6h Extended release: 324–660 mg q6–12h Quinidine sulfate: 200–300 mg orally q6–8h Extended release: 300–600 mg q8–12h	2–5 μg/mL (4.6–11.5 μmol/L) Toxicity likely if >10 μg/mL (>23 μmol/L)
Vancomycin	15 mg/kg IV	15 mg/kg IV	Peak 30–50 μg/mL Trough 5–15 μg/mL

*Congestive heart failure.
†Procainamide.
IV, intravenous; NAPA, N-acetylprocainamide.

all body fluids except cerebrospinal fluid and vitreous humor. Although small amounts are eliminated in the bile, most of the drug is excreted unchanged in the urine by glomerular filtration.

The volume of distribution increases during critical illness and then normalizes as the illness resolves. Hypotension, decreased cardiac output, renal dysfunction, and concomitant nephrotoxic drugs decrease aminoglycoside clearance. Hemodialysis, hyperdynamic shock, trauma, and vasopressors increase their clearance.

Controversy exists regarding the most effective and least toxic method of administering aminoglycosides to patients in the ICU. Traditionally, they are administered as intermittent intravenous (IV) infusions given over 60 minutes and dosed to peaks of four to eight times the minimal inhibitory concentration and troughs less than 2 μg/L (Table 12–3). The peak sample is obtained 1 hour after the end of the infusion, and the trough sample is obtained just before the next dose.

Table 12–3. Therapeutic Concentrations of Aminoglycosides*

AMINOGLYCOSIDE	PEAK	TROUGH
Gentamicin†	4–10 μg/mL	<1–2 μg/mL
Tobramycin†	4–10 μg/mL	<1–2 μg/mL
Netilmicin‡	4–10 μg/mL	<1–2 μg/mL
Amikacin§	20–30 μg/mL	<10 μg/mL

*Optimal levels for maximal efficacy and minimal toxicity have not yet been determined (see text).
†Peak 4–8 μg/mL and trough <1 μg/mL for soft tissue infections and moderately severe infections; peak 8–10 μg/mL and trough <1–2 μg/mL for severe infections (e.g., septic shock, and pneumonia).
‡Peak 12–16 μg/mL and trough <2–4 μg/mL for severe infections and pneumonia.
§Peak 20–25 μg/mL and trough 1–4 μg/mL for moderately severe infections; peak 25–28 μg/mL and trough 4–8 μg/mL for severe infections and pneumonia.
From Zaske DE: Aminoglycosides. In: Evans WE, Schentay JJ, Jusko WJ (eds): Applied Pharmacokinetics. Vancouver: Applied Therapeutics, 1992, pp 14–30.

Once-daily aminoglycoside dosing is gaining support as evidence increases regarding its safety and efficacy. This method of dosing assumes that brief drug exposure results in prolonged suppression of bacterial growth. It may be more effective and less nephrotoxic and ototoxic than traditional intermittent dosing. The best once-daily doses are not known and depend in part on concomitant antibiotic therapy. It should not be routinely used in critically ill patients with neutropenia, rapidly changing renal function, acute renal failure, cirrhosis, or cystic fibrosis, or in those undergoing dialysis. If once-daily dosing is used, a random sample should be obtained 6 to 14 hours after the first dose. Additional samples should be obtained on subsequent days to monitor the concentrations over the course of therapy.

Digoxin

Digoxin is well-absorbed orally and readily distributes into tissues. Seventy-five percent of digoxin is excreted renally unchanged; approximately 25% is metabolized. In chronic renal failure nonrenal mechanisms of digoxin clearance are up-regulated and its distribution decreases. Because oral absorption may be impaired in critically ill patients, the IV route of administration is recommended.

Digoxin is loaded over 12 hours to decrease the risk of toxicity associated with high serum concentrations. One should administer maintenance doses once daily in patients with normal renal function. In renal dysfunction, interval extension and dose reduction are necessary (see Table 12–1).

Since its serum half-life is 24 to 36 hours, one should obtain serum digoxin concentrations 5 to 7 days after initiation of therapy and at least 12 hours after administration of a dose. Although serum concentrations do not necessarily correlate with efficacy, they are often useful when assessing suspected toxicity.

Heparin

The distribution of heparin is limited to the intravascular space. The metabolism of heparin is not fully known but may involve hepatic and reticuloendothelial processes. Although heparin is usually well absorbed subcutaneously, its absorption by this route may be compromised in patients with reduced blood flow to the skin and subcutaneous tissues.

Subcutaneous (SC) heparin is used for the prevention of venous thrombosis and thromboembolism, whereas IV heparin is indicated for the treatment of venous thromboembolism. Weight-based dosing guidelines for IV heparin titrate the dose according to results of activated partial thromboplastin time (PTT) (Table 12–4). During continuous infusions, the daily PTT should be obtained at the same time of day to minimize fluctuations from circadian variation. PTT is not routinely measured for SC prophylactic heparin therapy.

Heparin (particularly low molecular weight fractions) also may be administered subcutaneously in higher than prophylactic doses for treatment of venous thromboembolism. Treatment is initiated with an IV loading dose followed by intermittent SC doses titrated to the desired PTT. As with IV heparin dosing, PTT should also be monitored daily when patients receive intermittent SC heparin for treatment.

Lidocaine

Lidocaine is well distributed into tissues and is extensively metabolized hepatically. Its two major metabolites, monoethylglycinexylidide and glycinexylidide, which have some antiarrhythmic activity, are renally excreted. Patients with hepatic

Table 12–4. Body Weight–Based Dosing of Intravenous Heparin

ALGORITHM BOX FOR HEPARIN DOSING*,†

Partial Thromboplastin Time (PTT) Result (sec)	Change in IV Infusion Rate (U/kg/h)	Additional Action Indicated
<35 (1.2 × laboratory mean for normals (LMFN))	+4	Rebolus IV with 80 units/kg Recheck PTT in 6 h
35–45 (1.2–1.5 × LMFN)	+2	Rebolus IV with 40 U/kg Recheck PTT in 6 h
46–70 (1.5–2.3 × LMFN)	0	Recheck PTT as indicated‡
71–90 (2.3–3.0 × LMFN)	−2	Recheck PTT in 6 h
>90 (>3 × LMFN)	−3	Stop infusion for 1 h Recheck PTT in 6 h

*Use 25,000 U of heparin in 250 mL D_5W and infuse through an infusion apparatus calibrated for low flow rates.
†When PTT is checked at 6 h or longer, steady-state kinetics can be assumed.
‡PTT should be checked every 6 h during the first 24 h and once each morning subsequently unless outside the therapeutic range.
From Hyers TM, Hull RS, Weg JG: Antithrombotic therapy for venous thromboembolic disease. Chest 108(Suppl):335–351, 1995.

failure, congestive heart failure, or acute myocardial infarction have reduced lidocaine clearance.

Because of its short half-life (~1 hour), an IV loading dose is necessary. Maintenance doses are administered by continuous IV infusion and titrated to control ventricular arrhythmia. Initial and maintenance doses should be lower in patients with hepatic or renal dysfunction to avoid accumulation and toxicity. Like digoxin, serum concentrations do not necessarily correlate with efficacy but may be useful for suspected toxicity.

Phenytoin

Phenytoin is well absorbed orally at a rate of about 50 mg/hour. It is highly protein-bound and is hepatically metabolized by capacity-limited enzymes. Because phenytoin binds to some proteins and calcium salts in enteral feeding products, its dose should be increased to compensate for impaired absorption. Its volume of distribution is decreased in hypoalbuminemia. Patients who are critically ill because of trauma or other disorders may have increased phenytoin clearance.

Oral loading should be accomplished by administering 5 mg/kg doses every 2 hours until the total loading dose is achieved (see Table 12–2). Rapid administration of parenteral phenytoin may induce cardiac arrhythmias, hypotension, and central nervous system depression. The infusion rate should not exceed 50 mg/minute. Small (50 to 100 mg) dosage adjustments are recommended for changing maintenance dosing. A representative non–steady-state serum drug concentration can be obtained 2 hours after IV loading. Subsequent trough samples can be obtained at 3- to 5-day intervals to determine if accumulation is occurring. Its serum half-life ranges from 75 to 125 hours.

Procainamide

Procainamide is variably absorbed orally and is rapidly distributed to body tissues. It normally has a serum half-life of about 3 hours and is hepatically metabolized to N-acetylprocainamide (NAPA). NAPA also has antiarrhythmic properties and contributes significantly to the toxicity of procainamide. It is renally eliminated with a serum half-life of 6 hours in patients with normal renal function. Since only small amounts of procainamide are cleared renally, NAPA accumulates more rapidly than does procainamide in patients with renal dysfunction.

Rapid loading with IV procainamide is used for acute management of arrhythmias, followed by continuous IV infusion or oral procainamide for maintenance therapy. The total daily dose of oral immediate- or sustained-release procainamide is approximately 17% more than the total daily IV dose. For immediate-release products, the total oral dose is divided into six equal doses and administered every 4 hours; depending on the specific sustained-release products, the total oral dose is divided into four equal doses administered every 6 hours, or into two equal doses given every 12 hours. One should check both procainamide and NAPA concentrations to assess for toxicity and therapeutic efficacy. A sample should be drawn 12 hours after the initiation of IV therapy, whereas a trough level should be obtained for oral dosing.

Quinidine

Quinidine is well absorbed from the gastrointestinal tract, is distributed into most body tissues, and is highly protein-bound. It undergoes extensive hepatic metabolism, and both the parent drug and its metabolites are excreted in the urine. The rate, but not extent, of absorption is decreased in patients with congestive heart failure, whereas liver disease may increase free drug and decrease clearance.

Loading doses may be oral or IV, but there is a risk of hypotension with IV doses. One should dilute IV doses in at least 50 mL of fluid and infuse over 20 to 30 minutes. Maintenance doses of oral quinidine vary, depending on the salt selected. Serum concentrations do not necessarily correlate with efficacy and are more useful when assessing suspected toxicity.

Vancomycin

Vancomycin is distributed into most body fluids except the cerebrospinal fluid and vitreous humor. Its elimination is mostly renal, although approximately 5% is hepatically metabolized. Changes in renal function significantly influence vancomycin clearance. Minimally cleared by conventional hemodialysis, vancomycin may be removed by high-flux membranes and high-efficiency dialysis.

Vancomycin is administered at a rate of 1000 mg/h to minimize the risk of hypotension; a loading dose is not necessary. Patients receiving standard hemodialysis may receive a dose every 3 to 7 days (since its serum half-life in anephric patients is about 7 days). Patients who are undergoing peritoneal dialysis and experience localized bacterial peritonitis (without bacteremia) due to methicillin-resistant *Staphylococcus aureus* should receive vancomycin in the dialysate (50 mg/L) for 10 to 14 days.

Controversy exists regarding the most appropriate method of monitoring vancomycin therapy. The traditional approach is to adjust the dose based on peak and trough serum concentrations. Vancomycin, however, exhibits *concentration-independent* microbial killing and the risks of ototoxicity and nephrotoxicity are minimal with currently marketed products. For these reasons, it has been suggested that optimal levels may be ensured by achieving a mean steady-state concentration of 15 μg/mL.

SIGNIFICANT DRUG INTERACTIONS

All of the drugs that have been described have clinically important interactions with other drugs that are likely to be administered concomitantly in the ICU. Table 12–5 lists some of these interactions plus those associated with theophylline (whose dosing is given in Chapter 74, Table 74–3).

Table 12–5. Drug Interactions for Selected Drugs in the Intensive Care Unit

INTERACTING DRUGS	EFFECT	MECHANISM
Aminoglycosides		
Loop diuretics (furosemide, ethacrynic acid)	↑ Auditory toxicity	Synergistic auditory toxicity
Penicillins	↓ Serum aminoglycoside level	In vivo inactivation of aminoglycoside
Neuromuscular blocking drugs	↑ Neuromuscular blockade	Synergistic activity
Digoxin		
Amiodarone, quinidine, and verapamil	↑ Digoxin level ↑ AV node block	↓ Digoxin clearance Additive effects
Antacids	↓ Bioavailability	↓ Digoxin absorption
Diuretics	↑ Kaliuresis	Hypokalemia-induced digoxin toxicity
Lidocaine		
Cimetidine	↑ Lidocaine level	↓ Hepatic metabolism of lidocaine
Phenytoin		
Allopurinol, amiodarone, chloramphenicol, cimetidine, diazepam, fluconazole, fluoxetine, isoniazid, NSAIDs, sulfonamides, trimethoprim, warfarin	↑ Phenytoin effects	↓ Phenytoin metabolism
Barbiturates, carbamazepine, theophylline, rifamycins	↓ Phenytoin effects	↑ Phenytoin metabolism
Nondepolarizing muscle relaxants	↓ Duration of paralysis	
Carbamazepine	↓ Carbamazepine level	↑ Carbamazepine metabolism
Cyclosporine	↓ Cyclosporine level	↑ Cyclosporine metabolism
Methadone	↓ Methadone effect	↑ Methadone metabolism
Primidone	↑ Primidone and phenobarbital levels	↓ Primidone and phenobarbital metabolism
Quinidine	↓ Quinidine effect	↑ Metabolism of quinidine
Sucralfate	↓ Phenytoin effect	↓ Phenytoin absorption
Valproic acid (VPA)	↑ Phenytoin effect ↓ VPA effect	↑ Metabolism of VPA
Procainamide		
Cimetidine, cotrimoxazole	↑ Procainamide level	Competes with procainamide for tubular secretion
Neuromuscular blockers	↑ Neuromuscular blockade	Synergistic activity
Quinidine		
Antacids	↑ Risk of toxicity	↓ Urinary clearance
Cimetidine, erythromycin, ketoconazole	↑ Quinidine level	↓ Hepatic metabolism of quinidine
Digoxin	↑ Digoxin level	↓ Renal or biliary clearance of digoxin
Warfarin	↑ Prothrombin time	Protein binding displacement of warfarin

Table 12–5. Drug Interactions for Selected Drugs in the Intensive Care Unit *(Continued)*

INTERACTING DRUGS	EFFECT	MECHANISM
Theophylline		
Activated charcoal	↓ Serum theophylline level	↓ Theophylline absorption
Adenosine	↓ Adenosine effect	Unknown
Nondepolarizing muscle relaxants	Dose-dependent reversal of neuromuscular blockade	Unknown
Barbiturates, rifampin	↓ Serum theophylline level	↑ Hepatic metabolism of theophylline
Nonselective beta-adrenergic blockers	↑ Serum theophylline level ↓ Theophylline effect	↓ Elimination of theophylline Pharmacologic antagonism of theophylline
Cimetidine, diltiazem, macrolides, quinolones	↑ Serum theophylline level	Inhibition of hepatic theophylline metabolism
Hydantoins (phenytoin, others)	↓ Serum theophylline level ↓ Serum hydantoin level	Each drug enhances the metabolism of the other
Vancomycin		
Nondepolarizing muscle relaxants	↑ Neuromuscular blockade	Synergistic activity

NSAIDs, nonsteroidal anti-inflammatory drugs; AV, atrioventricular
Data from Tatro DS, Olin BR, Hebel SK (eds): Drug Interaction Facts, 5th ed. St. Louis: Facts and Comparisons, 1996 *and* United States Pharmacopeial Convention: Dry Information for the Health Care Professional, 15th ed. Taunton, MA: Rand-McNally, 1995.

BIBLIOGRAPHY

Bennett WM: Guide to drug dosing in renal failure. Clin Pharmacokinet 15:326–354, 1988.
This article presents a thorough, referenced table of dosing recommendations for drugs in patients with various degrees of renal dysfunction.

Bodenham A, Shelly MP, Park GR: The altered pharmacokinetics and pharmacodynamics of drugs commonly used in critically ill patients. Clin Pharmacokinet 14:347–373, 1988.
This article provides a detailed review of previously published information regarding altered pharmacokinetics and pharmacodynamics of neuromuscular blocking drugs, benzodiazepines, anesthetic induction agents, inhalation agents, analgesics, regional analgesics, diuretics, cardiovascular drugs, theophylline, antacids, H₂-receptor blockers, and antimicrobials in critically ill patients.

Edwards DT, Zarowitz BJ, Slaughter RL: Theophylline. In: Evans WE, Schentag JJ, Jusko WJ (eds): Applied Pharmacokinetics. Vancouver: Applied Therapeutics, 1992, pp 13–15.
This chapter provides an in-depth review of theophylline pharmacodynamics, pharmacokinetics, and clinical applications.

Ferriois-Lisart R, Alos-Alminana M: Effectiveness and safety of once-daily aminoglycosides: A meta-analysis. Am J Health Syst Pharm 53:1141–1150, 1996.
This article provides a systemic overview of the use of once-daily aminoglycosides.

Hyers TM, Hull RS, Weg JG: Antithrombotic therapy for venous thromboembolic disease. Chest 108(Suppl):335–351, 1995.
Guidelines for the dosing, monitoring, and use of anticoagulants as formulated by the Fourth American College of Chest Physicians Consensus Conference on Antithrombotic Therapy are presented.

Nicolau DP, Belliveau PP, Nightingale CH, et al: Implementation of a once-daily aminoglycoside program in a large community-teaching hospital. Hosp Pharm 30:674–676, 679–680, 1995.
This article provides specific once-daily aminoglycoside dosage recommendations.

Routledge PA, Shand DJ, Barchowsky A, et al: Relationship between alpha-1-acid glycoprotein and lidocaine disposition in myocardial infarction. Clin Pharmacol Ther 30:154–157, 1981.
The authors found increased binding of lidocaine to alpha-1-acid glycoprotein in eight patients with acute myocardial infarction, which allowed accumulation of free lidocaine to occur.

Tatro DS, Olin BR, Hebel SK (eds): Drug Interaction Facts, 5th ed. St. Louis: Facts and Comparisons, Inc., 1996.
This is a standard, referenced drug interaction text.

The United States Pharmacopeial Convention: Drug Information for the Health Care Professional, 15th ed. Taunton, MA: Rand-McNally, 1995.
This is a standard drug interaction text with selected bibliographies.

Thomson PD, Melmon KL, Richardson JA, et al: Lidocaine pharmacokinetics in advanced heart failure, liver disease, and renal failure in humans. Ann Intern Med 78:499–508, 1973.
Reduction in lidocaine clearance was observed in patients with heart failure and liver disease who received intravenous lidocaine. Renal failure did not affect lidocaine clearance.

Zaske DE: Aminoglycosides. In: Evans WE, Schentag JJ, Jusko WJ (eds): Applied Pharmacokinetics. Vancouver: Applied Therapeutics, 1992, pp 14–30.
This chapter provides an in-depth review of aminoglycoside pharmacodynamics, pharmacokinetics, and clinical applications.

13   Nutritional Therapy

Nancy Evans-Stoner
James L. Mullen

Critical illness results in an well-orchestrated set of metabolic consequences encompassed by the terms *hypermetabolism* and *hypercatabolism.* The former refers to an increased expenditure of energy (which may be expressed as calories or milliliters of oxygen), whereas the latter refers to an increased destruction of existing tissues. When decreased nutrient intake and synthetic production are coupled with increased tissue catabolism, the normal anabolism-catabolism balance becomes severely negative. This leads to a rapid depletion of body tissue stores and critical protein elements, such as immunoglobulins, which is characteristic of protein malnutrition.

The *goal* of nutritional therapy in the intensive care unit (ICU) is to minimize the net negative daily protein and energy balances in critically ill patients. Over time, they accumulate and evolve into net negative tissue protein and fat store balances. Providing the appropriate type and quantity of nutritional substrate partially offsets the obligatory catabolic losses in critical illness and provides fuel needed for oxidative purposes and ongoing synthetic processes.

NUTRITIONAL AND METABOLIC ASSESSMENT

When Do You Start?

The current nutritional status of a newly admitted ICU patient is a major factor in determining when to start nutritional support. ICU patients with chronic diseases are often malnourished to a greater or lesser degree even before their ICU admission. With their tissue reserves already compromised, they are less able to tolerate subsequent further depletion of nutrient stores than patients who were previously well nourished. Despite the importance of determining the nutritional status of ICU patients, it remains a challenge to do so accurately because many of the traditional "nutritional assessment" parameters are unreliable when applied to the critically ill.

Body Weight

Although seemingly a straightforward measurement, body weights in ICU patients are often distorted by efforts at volume resuscitation and changing fluid distribution among various body compartments. Consequently, the patient's current weight should be compared with his or her "usual" as well as ideal body weight, with additional attention paid to estimating the "dry" weight of volume-overloaded patients.

Significant weight loss (>10%) before the critical illness episode should signify a patient at high risk for clinically significant malnutrition. Despite its limitations,

153

current weight, when compared with ideal body weight, can be used to estimate how the patient's fat calorie stores compare with normal and can guide the appropriate caloric prescription.

Serum Proteins

The profile of serum albumin, transferrin, and prealbumin, which normally gives a balanced composite view of the patient's serum protein status, is less reliable during periods of critical illness and vigorous intravascular fluid resuscitation. The reprioritization of the liver synthetic pathways and the increased catabolism of several of these proteins change them from good measures of nutritional status to prognostic indicators of severity of illness and systemic inflammation with good ability to predict clinical outcomes. Despite these limitations as nutritional parameters, they are traditionally followed to assess response to nutritional interventions.

Timelines for Reaching Adequate Daily Nutrition

A less objective but equally important factor in deciding which patients should receive nutritional support is the anticipated clinical course of the current illness. When will the patient again be ingesting an *adequate* oral intake? In well-nourished patients, nutrition support should be started if no oral intake is anticipated for *greater than 5 days*. In the face of pre-existing malnutrition, however, anticipation of *receiving nothing by mouth for more than 3 days* should trigger nutritional intervention. Furthermore, for major trauma patients with pre-existing malnutrition, studies suggest that nutritional therapy should start on ICU admission unless contraindicated, for example, hemodynamic instability. Some intensivists extend this practice of early nutritional therapy to other populations of ICU patients if they have pre-existing malnutrition.

Caloric Goal Delineation

Delineation of realistic clinical goals is important in order to prescribe appropriate cost-conscious prescriptions for total parenteral nutrition (TPN) or total enteral nutrition (TEN). To make a rational *caloric prescription*, one needs to know the individual patient's total energy expenditure (TEE) as well as the patient's caloric tissue goals. TEE defines the severity of hypermetabolism, and it can be estimated by indirect calorimetry in most ICU patients. In the ICU patient on bed rest, resting energy expenditure (REE) measured over approximately 30 minutes approximates TEE. After determining TEE, the caloric (or "nonprotein" energy) prescription is guided by the clinician's goal for the patient's fat stores (Table 13–1).

If the patient is being isolated for infection control purposes, indirect calorimetry to measure REE is generally not possible. Under these circumstances, REE can be estimated by using the Harris Benedict equations with "multipliers" to take into account the hypermetabolic effects of critical illness (see Table 56–2, Chapter 56).

Table 13–1. Caloric Prescriptions Based on Body Weight and Status of Fat Stores

CURRENT BODY WEIGHT VERSUS IDEAL BODY WEIGHT*	STATUS OF FAT STORES	CALORIC PRESCRIPTION
CBW <90% IBW	Subnormal	One should use sufficient energy supply to replete depleted fat stores (daily caloric supply > REE)
CBW >90% IBW and CBW <120% IBW	Normal	The caloric prescription is designed to maintain the fat stores (daily energy supply = REE)
CBW >120% IBW	Excessive	Energy supply should be designed to partially utilize the excess fat stores. To do this, some clinicians supply 800 kcal from glucose (and 2 g protein/kg/day), whereas others prefer to provide more daily kilocalories, equal to 50% of REE

*Current body weight is the best estimate of the patient's current "dry" body weight (e.g., before volume resuscitation); IBW for males = 50 + 2.3 (height [inches] − 60) and IBW for females = 45.5 + 2.3 (height [inches] − 60).

CBW, current body weight; IBW, ideal body weight; REE, resting energy expenditure, which approximates total energy expenditure in ICU patients.

Some intensivists use an even more simple "one-size-fits-all" rule, such as providing 25 kcal/kg ideal body weight (IBW)/day for males and 20 kcal/kg IBW/day for females, to which they apply the same multipliers as mentioned for the Harris Benedict equations. Even with the adjustments, these rules can still underestimate actual TEE in hypermetabolic states, emphasizing the desirability of indirect calorimetry measurements if possible and the need for regular monitoring of the patient's response to nutritional therapy as discussed further on.

Protein Goal Delineation

During critical illness, protein is mobilized from many body tissues, such as the intestinal tract, skeletal muscle, albumin mass, and the skin. This provides precursors for crucial protein synthesis, such as acute-phase plasma proteins, immunoglobulins, and wound healing and for energy if other substrates are not readily available. The magnitude of this mobilization and redistribution can be impressive, with urinary nitrogen losses of 30 to 50 g/day typically observed in patients with multiple trauma or severe sepsis or after bone marrow transplantation. *This represents a loss of greater than 1 kg of lean tissue each day* (with loss of 30 g of lean tissue being roughly equivalent to loss of 1 g of nitrogen). Although this catabolic process that is induced by inflammatory mediators cannot be reversed by providing exogenous protein (i.e., making the patient's nitrogen balance positive), the magnitude of the protein loss can be diminished by providing protein and energy substrates during periods of critical illness.

Determining how much protein to provide by nutritional therapy should, in general, be *independent* of one's total (nonprotein) caloric prescription (described earlier). How much protein to give to a critically ill ICU patient initially remains more or less an empirical decision. One acceptable approach for these circumstances is to give 2 g of protein/kg current body weight (assuming normal functioning hepatic and renal disposal systems [Table 13–2]). For sick but not critically ill ICU patients, daily protein administration on the order of 1.5 g/kg/day would be an appropriate starting point. In comparison, recommended daily protein intake for healthy, well-nourished adults is only on the order of 0.6 to 0.8 g/kg/day.

The degree of protein catabolism and effects of the daily protein prescription on this loss can be monitored by serial measurements of the patient's nitrogen balance. When calculating nitrogen balance, one should account for changes in blood urea nitrogen (BUN) and fecal nitrogen loss as shown in the equation.

$$\frac{\text{Nitrogen}}{\text{balance}} = \text{Nitrogen intake (g)} - [\text{Urinary Nitrogen (g)} + \Delta\text{BUN (g)} + 4]$$

where ΔBUN (in g) = $[0.6 \times \text{weight}] \times [\text{BUNf} - \text{BUNi}]$, BUNi and BUNf are the initial and final values of blood urea nitrogen (BUN expressed in g/L) during the measurement period, respectively, and "weight" is current body weight

Table 13–2. Adjustments to Nutrition Prescription with Organ Dysfunction

ORGAN DYSFUNCTION	ADJUSTMENTS
Cardiac	1. Avoid enteral route if vasopressors are in use for blood pressure support 2. ↓ Sodium 3. ↑ Potassium for patient on digoxin 4. Increased need for potassium, magnesium, and zinc with diuresis 5. Use maximally concentrated solutions
Hepatic	1. Provide at least 150 g (480 kcal) of glucose per day 2. Use mixed fuel system (glucose and fat) 3. ↓ Protein if encephalopathy occurs or worsens 4. Use modified amino acid (AA) formula (high branched-chain AA) if patient's encephalopathy is unresponsive to medical treatment or worsens with standard AA formula
Renal	1. ↓ Calories for patient on peritoneal dialysis or continuous arteriovenous hemodialysis (see Chapter 16) 2. ↓ Fat kilocalories with elevated triglyceride levels 3. ↓ Protein if blood urea nitrogen >100 mg/dL 4. ↓ Magnesium, potassium, and phosphorus 5. ↑ Acetate 6. Maximally concentrate all solutions
Respiratory	1. Avoid overfeeding to prevent excessive CO_2 production 2. Feed at the measured energy expenditure or at 1.1 to 1.3 times the resting energy expenditure 3. Provide 50% of calories from fat and 50% from glucose 4. Maximally concentrate all solutions

(kg) and represents the volume of distribution of the BUN. Urinary nitrogen is measured as the concentration of urea multiplied by the volume of a 24-hour urine collection.

For the purposes of the equation, 6.25 g of protein is assumed to be equivalent to 1 g of nitrogen so that nitrogen intake equals protein intake (in grams) divided by 6.25. The "4" in the equation represents normal fecal (and other nonurinary) nitrogen loss (4 g/24 hours). This may be, on the one hand, much less (close to zero) if the patient is on TPN and has no stools or, on the other hand, much more (double or triple) if the patient has diarrhea or an enterocutaneous fistula.

PROVIDING NUTRITIONAL SUPPORT

Selecting the Route of Administration

After determining that nutritional support is required, defining its goals, and writing the calorie and protein prescriptions for the patient, one must select the most appropriate route of administration. This decision, however, should not be dictated simply by what access the patient currently has available.

Enteral nutrition is strongly preferred if the gastrointestinal (GI) tract (from the jejunum distally) is functional and accessible without contraindications to its use. The potential benefits of using the GI tract relate to prevention of mucosal atrophy and its associated impairment as a barrier for bacteria and their products, the avoidance of the known and potential complications associated with TPN, and reduced cost compared with TPN.

Success in using the GI tract often depends on the intensivist's motivation and ability to assess its functional status accurately. The latter is usually based on the following five parameters: (1) stool output, (2) nasogastric tube output, (3) nausea or vomiting, (4) findings on abdominal examination, and (5) findings on radiologic examination. Enteral feedings are generally not given to patients who are in shock or are receiving vasopressors because of the risk of worsening gut ischemia during periods of compromised gut blood flow.

If enteral therapy cannot be initiated or has failed, the parenteral route should be selected. Even after parenteral therapy has started, it is important to reassess the GI tract periodically and attempt enteral feeding if feasible. *Dual modality therapy* refers to using the enteral route at a lower fraction (<20%) of daily nutrient goal to prevent mucosal atrophy while using the parenteral route to provide the majority of the daily nutrient goals.

Whatever the route, there must be constant attention to therapy tolerance and a quick response in switching patients from one route to another as necessary. The two approaches should be regarded as complementary, not competitive.

Enteral Nutrition

In general, there has been renewed interest among intensivists in providing nutritional support enterally. Improved enteral access devices and technologic advances in enteral formulas and delivery systems have resulted in improved success in meeting the patient's daily nutrient goals during critical illness.

Enteral Access

Enteral nutrition can be administered through a variety of tubes either into the stomach (tip of feeding tube is prepyloric) or into the small intestine (the tip is postpyloric). Determining which type of enteral feeding to pursue is influenced by several factors: gastric motility, continuity of the GI tract, swallowing function, and the risk of aspiration. The type of tube (temporary versus permanent) depends on the anticipated length of therapy, with temporary enteral access generally preferred if the need for nutritional support is anticipated to be less than 1 month.

Whether enteral feedings should be delivered pre- or postpylorically remains controversial and local practices tend to reflect, to a large degree, the preferences of individual ICUs and institutions. Some intensivists prefer to manage critically ill patients with postpyloric feeding to try to avoid aspiration and decrease the risk of ventilator-associated pneumonia. Although it makes good clinical sense that intragastric feedings should be avoided in patients with a high risk for aspiration, controlled clinical trials comparing pre- and postpyloric placement in ICU patients to show one or the other approach having better outcomes are lacking.

In contrast, several controlled studies of ICU patients document the benefit of elevating the head of the bed to 30 degrees for all patients receiving enteral feeding. Parenthetically, this position should also be standard ICU practice for those not receiving such feedings (unless contraindicated) because this simple maneuver has been shown to be effective in preventing aspiration and ventilator-associated pneumonia (see Chapter 11).

Placing the tip of a nasoenteral feeding tube in a postpyloric location can be aided by the use of pharmacologic agents (metoclopramide, cisapride, or erythromycin), with some series reporting successful passage rates ranging from 60 to 80% in *non-ICU patients*. Success in *ICU patients* appears to be much lower despite the use of these prokinetic agents. Because of this, most intensivists turn to radiologic placement with fluoroscopy to ensure tip postpyloric placement. This can be performed at the bedside without undue delay in most ICUs. If performed routinely, it eliminates the "down time" associated with waiting for tube passage and encourages an early start of enteral feeding.

Small-bore nasoenteral feeding tubes may become lethal weapons, however, when they are inserted with a wire stylet in vulnerable (obtunded or intubated) ICU patients because they may pass into the trachea in these patients by mistake. These tubes tend to track alongside the patient's endotracheal tube, which results in inadvertent placement into the trachea. If a tube with a stylet inadvertently passes into the lungs of intubated patients, it has sufficient stiffness to perforate the visceral pleura readily on further advancement. The resulting tension pneumothorax can have disastrous results. For this reason, some ICUs ban the use of stylets for insertion of these feeding tubes altogether. Other ICUs mandate fluoroscopic guidance (supervised by experienced physicians) during insertion of these tubes with stylets. As an additional precaution against passing the tube into the trachea, the lateral neck is viewed fluoroscopically at the bedside to confirm posterior location of the feeding tube in the esophagus.

Selection of the Enteral Formula

The selection of an appropriate enteral formula involves choosing a formula or a combination of formulas that best meets the patient's daily caloric and protein requirements.

The composition of enteral formulas has changed dramatically over the years with advances in both quantity and quality of substrate. Because the majority of critically ill patients do not have severe impairment of the digestive and absorptive functions of the GI tract, most generally tolerate formulas with intact proteins. During periods of critical illness, hypercatabolic patients benefit from formulas containing at least 50 to 60 g of protein/L. Although many specialty formulas target specific organ dysfunction, the outcomes data supporting their efficacy (and hence justifying their extra cost) are controversial. Nonetheless, the type and degree of organ dysfunction should be taken into account when providing enteral nutrition (see Table 13–2).

Delivery and Administration of Enteral Nutrition

Enteral nutrition can be administered intermittently or continuously. Intermittent infusions generally have larger volumes (150 mL to 500 mL) delivered periodically (every 4 to 6 hours) during the day. Continuous infusions deliver smaller volumes (50 mL to 150 mL/hour) over 12 to 24 hours. The position of the feeding tube tip is the major determinant of the method of administration. When enteral feeding is delivered into the small intestine, it should only be administered continuously via an infusion pump to reduce the possibility of intolerance, such as diarrhea or abdominal distention. Enteral delivery schedules during periods of critical illness are typically for 24 hours. Reducing the duration of infusion (by increasing the rate) is appropriate if there are frequent interruptions to the infusion during the day or if one wants the patient to be relatively free of the feeding apparatus during daytime activities, for example, to do physical therapy during the recovery phase.

Intermittent feeding is typical when the enteral feeding tube tip is in the stomach. Although this may be optimal for an ambulatory patient, during critical illness a slower continuous infusion may be better tolerated. It is unclear whether continuous delivery of gastric feedings reduces or increases the risk of aspiration compared with intermittent delivery in ICU patients.

Complications of Enteral Feeding

Mechanical complications relating to surgical enteral access can occur at the time of insertion or during the postoperative maintenance and care of the device. Ensuring that the tube is properly secured can prevent problems with peritubular leakage and tube migration. Tube obstruction can be minimized with attention to flushing protocols and avoidance of medications delivered via the small-bore tubes.

Using at least a 12 Fr (French) diameter tube lumen (with 14 Fr preferred) helps prevent occlusions. Avoiding the delivery of hyperosmolar medication and maintaining a closed delivery system can prevent GI complications such as diarrhea. If significant diarrhea (>500 mL/day) occurs and *Clostridium difficile* is ruled out or treated (see Chapter 35), one should provide antidiarrheal agents, such as loperamide (Imodium), on a routine schedule.

Parenteral Nutrition

Indications and Specifications

Parenteral nutrition should be used if the GI tract is nonfunctional because of dysmotility, disrupted continuity, ischemia, or obstruction or if enteral nutrition supply cannot be consistently and adequately achieved. Enteral nutrition should also be avoided if the patient is hypotensive, receiving vasopressors, or otherwise in circulatory shock.

Calories are supplied with either glucose or fat emulsions. Glucose usually provides 50 to 70% of the daily nonprotein calorie supply, but glucose should not exceed 7 g/kg ideal body weight/day. The latter is an approximation of the body's oxidative limits. Exceeding this guidepost often leads to excess CO_2 production and the storage of excess calories as fat in the liver, neither of which is desirable in ICU patients. This complication can be diagnosed by measuring the respiratory quotient (the ratio of CO_2 production to O_2 consumption measured by indirect calorimetry) and finding that it is greater than 1.0.

The other major caloric fuel is fat, which in sick patients can obviate the negative effects of excess carbohydrate infusion. Most practitioners supply 30 to 50% of the daily caloric requirement as fat and limit the total dose to 2.5 g/kg/day. The most common type of lipid used as a caloric source in TPN is long-chain triglycerides in a lipid emulsion derived from soybean or safflower oil. Long-chain triglycerides may exert negative effects on neutrophil function and macrophage phagocytosis. They also seem to result in a general impairment in the function of the reticuloendothelial system as a result of lipid particles being trapped in the reticuloendothelial cells, partially disrupting their function. The clinical relevance of these effects, however, is still controversial but emphasize that the decision to begin TPN should not be an automatic decision but should be made only after weighing the balance between potential benefits and potential harms. An alternative to long-chain triglycerides are the medium-chain triglycerides derived from palm and coconut oils and composed of mainly 8- to 10-carbon fatty acids.

The normal vehicle to supply protein is synthetic crystalline amino acid solutions available in concentrations ranging from 1 to 15% (a mix of essential and nonessential amino acids). Special-design amino acid profiles have shown metabolic improvements in patients, but it has been difficult to demonstrate improved clinical outcomes to justify their additional cost.

Vitamins and Trace Elements

During acute periods of stress and accelerated metabolic demand there may be an increased need for vitamins and trace elements, but how much of an increase is needed has not been clearly defined. If stores are depleted from a prolonged chronic illness before the onset of acute illness, deficiencies may exist even if serum levels appear normal. In addition to standard multivitamin preparations, Vitamin K (1 mg) is added daily to TPN solutions to provide maintenance needs. Giving TPN without adequate thiamine has resulted in severe lactic acidosis recently when multivitamins for TPN were in short supply in the United States.

Maintenance parenteral iron is generally not recommended during periods of critical illness because parenteral iron dextran is not compatible with lipids, preventing its being added to lipid-containing TPN solutions. Trace elements are required during periods of increased metabolic demands and can be delivered to the critically ill patient by daily addition to TPN.

Effects on Fluid and Acid-Base Balance and Glucose Homeostasis

During periods of critical illness, a multitude of factors contribute to the patient's fluid balance and electrolyte homeostasis. For example, during acute injury, there is an initial period in which there is sodium and water retention. In essence, TPN is a carbohydrate-lipid-protein–enriched fluid and electrolyte solution that can be modified appropriately to treat fluid and electrolyte disorders as well as to provide nutrition.

Maximally concentrating all solutions in the critically ill patient avoids premature discontinuation of TPN when the patient's fluid status changes quickly, for example, when he or she can no longer tolerate the same volume of fluid in the TPN prescription. Acute increments of volume can be achieved with intravenous "piggybacks."

Acid-base balance is of critical importance during periods of severe illness. The TPN solution itself contributes minimally to the disruption of acid-base balance. For example, TPN solutions designed for central venous administration generally have a pH in the range of 4 to 5. This pH is increased somewhat with the addition of lipids and any residual acidity is balanced by the addition of base in the form of acetate (as the sodium or potassium salt).

Blood glucose control can be particularly labile during periods of severe illness, and hyperglycemia may be exacerbated by TPN administration. The use of a mixed fuel system (which delivers a combination of lipid and dextrose calories) generally eases the demand for exogenous insulin. If needed, the primary route of insulin administration should be part of the parenteral nutrition solution itself. For short-term management, insulin can be given separately from the TPN solution by a "sliding scale" until the total daily insulin requirement is defined (which then can be added to the next day's TPN prescription).

Central Venous Access

Central venous access is mandatory to deliver TPN solutions safely and efficiently because these solutions are calorically dense, contain large amounts of nitrogen, and must often be prepared in a minimal volume, resulting in remarkable hypertonicity (>900 mmol/L). The catheter tip for delivery of TPN should be positioned in the superior vena cava to prevent development of thrombophlebitis as a complication.

Since the 1980s, central access catheters with multiple lumens have been used with increased frequency during periods of critical illness. Pulmonary artery catheters, when being used for hemodynamic monitoring, may also be safely used for TPN infusion. Only a proximal port of a pulmonary artery catheter, however, should be used for delivering TPN because TPN infusion via the distal port (located in the pulmonary artery) may result in pulmonary artery inflammation.

Insertion of central venous catheters using maximal barrier precautions and meticulous nursing care of the insertion site afterward is crucial to minimizing the risk of infectious complications in patients receiving TPN (see Chapter 11).

Impaired "Disposal Systems"

The "disposal systems" of the body handle the end products of metabolism. Impairments in this functional capacity of the renal, hepatic, and respiratory systems are common in the critically ill. When one or more of these systems are impaired or when there is cardiac failure, the prescription for TPN nutrients or their means of delivery or both should be adjusted (see Table 13–2).

MEASURING NUTRITIONAL GOAL ACHIEVEMENT

Serial Markers to Measure

It is important to monitor patients to determine whether the delivery of nutritional support is achieving its goals. To this end, serial measurements of body weight should be made. As a rule, body weight changes over several weeks should reflect tissue accretion or depletion, so increased "dry" body weight is an important measure of nutritional goal achievement.

To determine whether the energy prescription reflects the changing metabolic state of the patient, it is important to obtain serial measures of REE. One should also regularly assess measures of nitrogen balance and protein stores (see equation earlier). A realistic nitrogen balance goal in a critically ill patient, however, is not to achieve a positive balance but rather to *reduce* the negative nitrogen balance. Serial serum proteins, such as albumin, transferrin, and prealbumin, reflect not only changes in the visceral protein compartment over time but also their rates of synthesis and degradation, which are markedly affected by the presence of critical illness. Nonetheless, changes in these plasma proteins have considerable prognostic significance.

Reasons for Underachievement of Goals

The main reasons for not achieving nutritional goals are logistical in nature, for example, no available access, fluid restrictions, or decreased clearance through disposal systems. Most of these causes are preventable if an aggressive approach is employed to encourage a timely start and to monitor the effectiveness of parenteral or enteral therapy.

CLINICAL PEARLS AND PITFALLS

1. To add stiffness to aid in insertion of a small-bore nasoenteral feeding tube but still avoid use of a wire stylet, one can freeze the tube before insertion.
2. If a nasoenteral feeding tube ends up in the pleural space in a patient receiving mechanical ventilation, one should anticipate the development of a tension pneumothorax immediately on removal of the tube (if one is not already present).
3. Diarrhea often occurs in ICU patients receiving enteral feedings, which may or may not be due to the feedings (see Chapter 35).
4. If the patient with a nasoenteral feeding tube in place postpylorically has an episode of vomiting, one should confirm that the tip of the tube is still postpyloric because reverse peristalsis may displace it into the stomach.
5. Be aware of the "refeeding syndrome" when starting nutritional therapy in severely malnourished ICU patients (see Phosphate Disorders, Chapter 36).
6. Consider excessive production of CO_2 due to carbohydrate overfeeding while trying to wean patients with limited ventilatory capacity. If overfeeding is present, indirect calorimetry will demonstrate a respiratory quotient greater than 1.0.

BIBLIOGRAPHY

A.S.P.E.N. (American Society for Parenteral & Enteral Nutrition) Board of Directors: Guidelines for the use of parenteral and enteral nutrition in adult and pediatric patients. J Parenter Enteral Nutr 17:supplement, 1993.
These are comprehensive consensus-based and evidence-based guidelines by the professional society related to these topics. They are available online at www.clinnutr.org.

Beale RJ, Bryg DJ, Bihari DJ: Immunonutriton in the critically ill: a systematic review of clinical outcome. Crit Care Med 27:2799–2805, 1999.
This is a meta-analysis of 15 randomized controlled studies addressing whether enteral nutrition with immune enhancing components benefits critically ill patients after trauma, sepsis, or major surgery. Immunonutrition had no effect on mortality but was associated with fewer infections and a shorter length of hospital stay.

Carpentier YA, Van Gossum A, Dubois DY, et al: Lipid metabolism in parenteral nutrition. In: Rombeau JL, Caldwell MD (eds): Clinical Nutrition: Parenteral Nutrition. Philadelphia: WB Saunders, 1993.
This chapter is a review of scientific-based evidence for the use of parenteral lipid.

Cerra FB, Benites MR, Blackburn GL, et al: Applied nutrition in ICU patients. A consensus statement of the American College of Chest Physicians. Chest 111:769–778, 1997.
This is a consensus statement by a group of surgical and medical intensivists.

Eyer S, Brummit C, Crossley K, et al: Catheter-related sepsis: Prospective, randomized study of three methods of long-term catheter maintenance. Crit Care Med 18:1810, 1990.
This article reports a trial evaluating the efficacy of prophylactic changing of CVC's.

Heyland DK: Nutritional support in the critically ill patient. A critical review of the evidence. Crit Care Clin 14:423–440, 1998.
Evidenced-based review article that evaluates the strength of the scientific evidence to support current practices in ICU nutritional therapy.

Kalliagas S, Choban PS, Ziegler D, et al: Erythromycin facilitates postpyloric placement of nasoduodenal feeding tubes in intensive care unit patients: randomized, double-blinded, placebo-controlled trial. J Parenter Enteral Nutr 20:385–388, 1996.
This is a prospective, randomized controlled trial that found erythromycin to be useful in postpyloric passage of nasoenteral feeding tubes.

Matarese LE: Enteral feeding solutions. Gastrointest Endosc Clin N Am 8:593–609, 1998.
This is a review of enteral feeding solutions for general and specific therapeutic use, including discussion of their substrates, physical characteristics, and rationale for use in specific diseases (136 references).

McClaue SA, Saxton LK, Sapur DA, et al: Enteral tube feeding in the intensive care unit: factors impeding adequate delivery. Crit Care Med 27:1252–1256, 1999.
This report examines the process of prescribing and administering enteral nutrition in the ICU and delineates the factors that contribute to inadequate delivery of total enteral nutrition.

Palmblad J: Intravenous lipid emulsions and host defense: a critical review. Clin Nutr 10:303–308, 1991.
This evidenced-based review article evaluates the positive and negative effects of lipid emulsions on host defense.

Schlichtig R, Ayres SM (eds): Nutritional Support of the Critically Ill. Chicago: Year Book Medical, 1988.
This book is a concise, practically oriented textbook of nutritional therapy focused on ICU patients written by two intensivists for intensivists.

Tamada H, Nazu R, Imamura I, et al: The dipeptide alanyl-glutamine prevents intestinal mucosal atrophy in parenterally fed rats. J Parenter Enteral Nutr 16:110–116, 1992.
This is a scientific study examining the role of glutamine in supporting gut barrier function.

14 Rational Use of Antibiotics

Kathleen Brady
Jennifer Aldrich
Neil Fishman

Two major trends since the 1970s emphasize the importance for a rational approach to the use of antibiotics in the intensive care unit (ICU) patient. First, the number of antibiotics available for use in the ICU setting has risen dramatically and, second, many pathogens have become resistant to both the older antimicrobial agents and the new agents. Starting or continuing antibiotics inappropriate for the clinical situation is the main culprit for the increasing prevalence of resistant organisms. Antimicrobial-resistant pathogens now represent a major public health problem that is especially acute in the ICU setting.

EMPIRICAL ANTIMICROBIAL THERAPY

Initiating empirical antibiotic therapy requires an appreciation of the epidemiology of common nosocomial infections within one's own ICU and hospital. Although nosocomial infection rates of ICU admissions range from 3 to 31%, they vary significantly between community and university hospitals and even among types of ICUs within the same hospital. Likewise, the prevalence of specific pathogens in an ICU and their antimicrobial resistance patterns vary considerably among ICUs and over time in the same ICU.

In the ICU setting, the diagnosis of an infection can be complicated and confounded by the absence of the usual signs and symptoms. In ICU patients, even results of objective data, such as microbiologic cultures, can often be confusing. For example, a positive culture of sputum or a tracheal aspirate for a pathogenic organism does not necessarily prove the presence of a nosocomial pneumonia or even a tracheobronchitis. Likewise, a negative culture—for example, a tracheal aspirate sent the day after the start of new antimicrobials—does not confirm the absence of infection. Finally, some culture results may be uninterpretable because of an ill-considered approach to the diagnostic evaluation, such as dealing with two out of two blood culture bottles positive for coagulase-negative *Staphyloccus* species when the positive set (pair) of blood cultures were obtained from a previously inserted arterial catheter, but no blood cultures were taken from a peripheral site at the same time (see Chapter 11). If one diagnoses a bacteremia solely on the basis of the results of such cultures, many unnecessary courses of antimicrobial therapy, such as vancomycin, might ensue; the net effect would be to increase the risk of emergence of vancomycin resistance.

Initiating antibiotics in the ICU setting may be prompted by the occurrence of fever, leukocytosis, or sepsis. This is problematic because none of these signs alone, or even in combination, is highly predictive of an underlying bacterial infection. Nonetheless, these signs are often clinically important and their presence should prompt a thorough search for their cause (see Chapters 8, 11, 18, and 38).

Fever and Leukocytosis

Since fever is caused by the release of cytokines (so-called endogenous pyrogens) in response to injury, inflammation, antigenic challenge, or infection, it cannot reliably distinguish infectious from noninfectious causes. Likewise, although leukocytosis (white blood cells >15,000 cells/μL) is associated with an increased risk of bacterial infection, its specificity is low because almost half of such patients have no documentable infection.

Since no prospective studies have assessed the frequency and causes of fever specifically in ICU patients, one can only infer such data from studies of nosocomial infections in non-ICU medical and postoperative patients. Prospective studies in medical patients not in ICUs reveal that only 50% of fevers originate from an infectious cause; furthermore, a cause for the fever could be identified in only 70 to 80% of cases. Of note, 30 to 50% of febrile patients who received antibiotics had no clinical evidence for a focus of infection. These studies suggest that much antibiotic use in non-ICU patients initiated for fevers alone is unnecessary and can be eliminated without jeopardizing patient care; by inference, starting antibiotics for fever *alone* also seems suspect for ICU patients.

In addition, in a prospective study of postoperative patients, the rate of *fever* was 13.5% with no difference found among these three American College of Surgeons categories of operations: clean, clean-contaminated, or contaminated (see Chapter 11, Table 11–7). Ninety-four percent of fevers in each category had a source identified, with 62% of fevers attributed to infections. Conversely, only half the infections documented were associated with fever at all, that is, fever alone has a low sensitivity (approximately 50%) for diagnosing infections in this population. Again, starting antibiotics for fever alone seems inappropriate for postoperative patients in the ICU setting; instead, its presence should stimulate a systematic search for its cause.

Systemic Inflammatory Response Syndrome, Sepsis, and Septic Shock

The *systemic inflammatory response syndrome* (SIRS) is defined as the simultaneous presence of two or more physiologic signs that can result from systemic inflammation: (1) fever (or hypothermia), (2) tachycardia, (3) tachypnea, and (4) a neutrophilic leukocytosis. SIRS can arise from infectious or noninfectious causes. *Sepsis* has been defined as SIRS with clinical evidence (or high suspicion) of infection. *Severe sepsis* refers to the clinical situation of sepsis with evidence of (otherwise unexplained) inadequate end organ perfusion, whereas *septic shock* is severe sepsis with clinically significant hypotension. Characteristically, the hypotension in septic shock has a low afterload state as its primary hemodynamic derangement (see Chapter 8). Even though infection is common in patients with severe sepsis (present in about 90% of patients in one large prospective epidemiologic study reported by Sands and colleagues), blood stream infection (bacteremia or fungemia) was documented in only about one quarter of this group of patients overall.

ANTIBIOTIC USE AND ABUSE

One of the most common errors in antibiotic use is not the initial choice of empirical agents but rather the failure to narrow antimicrobial coverage appropriately once the results of cultures and diagnostic studies become available. The importance of limiting the use of antimicrobials, when appropriate, cannot be overemphasized. Often overlooked or minimized, the complications of antimicrobial use are important to consider at both the individual and community levels. Toxicities, such as renal failure, *Clostridium difficile* colitis, drug fever, and serious allergic reactions, all lead to further diagnostic studies with their associated morbidities as well as additional hospitalization days and increased costs of care. ICU patients given antibiotics are predisposed to colonization and eventual infection with resistant organisms such as methicillin-resistant *Staphylococcus aureus* (MRSA), vancomycin-resistant enterococcus (VREC), vancomycin-intermediate *S. aureus,* and extended-spectrum beta-lactamase–producing Enterobacteriaceae. Exposure to broad spectrum antibiotics is also a known risk factor for the development of invasive fungal infections. Infections with any of these resistant organisms or fungi lead to poor clinical outcomes for the patients as well as negative institutional and economic outcomes.

One special consideration in this regard is the development of VREC. Emergence of VREC has been associated with the overuse of vancomycin in several studies. There are concerns that this plasmid-mediated form of resistance could be transferred to other Gram-positive organisms, including *S. aureus.* Four recent cases of infection have been attributed to *S. aureus* with intermediate susceptibility to vancomycin, but the mechanism of resistance in these isolates is unknown. These concerns have led the Centers for Disease Control and Prevention to issue guidelines for the prudent use of vancomycin (Tables 14–1 and 14–2).

Obviously, one cannot make rational antibiotic choices without a better understanding of the agents themselves. This includes their mechanisms of action, spectra of activity, common adverse effects, and costs (Tables 14–3 to 14–5). Proper dosage adjustments must be made for renal or hepatic insufficiency as well as other situations known to alter pharmacokinetics (see Chapter 12).

Table 14–1. Centers for Disease Control Guidelines for the Prudent Use of Vancomycin: When Vancomycin Use Is *Appropriate*

1. Treatment of serious Gram-positive infections due to organism resistant to β-lactam antibiotics
2. Treatment of Gram-positive infections when the patient has a serious allergy to β-lactam antibiotics
3. Treatment of severe, life-threatening, metronidazole-resistant *Clostridium difficile* diarrhea
4. Endocarditis prophylaxis
5. Preoperative prophylaxis for implantation of prosthetic materials or devices, at institutions with a high rate of infections due to methicillin-resistant *Staphylococcus aureus* or methicillin-resistant *S. epidermidis.* (A single preoperative dose is sufficient unless the procedure lasts more than 6 h, at which time the dose should be repeated. Prophylaxis should be discontinued after a maximum of two doses.)

From Hospital Infection Control Practices Advisory Committee (HICPAC): Recommendations for preventing the spread of vancomycin resistance. MMWR Morb Mortal Wkly Rep 44(RR12):1–13, 1995 (also available at www.cdc.gov/ncidod/hip).

Table 14–2. Centers for Disease Control Guidelines for the Prudent Use of Vancomycin: When Vancomycin Use Is *Inappropriate* or *Discouraged*

....

1. Routine surgical prophylaxis
2. Empirical coverage in the neutropenic host (unless there is strong suspicion or evidence of an infection with Gram-positive organisms, at institutions with a high rate of infections due to methicillin-resistant *Staphylococcus aureus*
3. Treatment in response to single blood cultures growing coagulase-negative *Staphylococcus* if other contemporaneous cultures are negative
4. Continued empirical therapy after all cultures are negative for Gram-positive organisms
5. Prophylaxis (systemic or local) of infection or colonization of indwelling central or peripheral intravenous catheters
6. Decontamination of the digestive tract
7. Eradication of methicillin-resistant *S. aureus* colonization
8. Primary treatment for *Clostridium difficile* diarrhea
9. Routine prophylaxis for patients on peritoneal dialysis or hemodialysis
10. Treatment of infections with Gram-positive organisms that are sensitive to beta-lactam antibiotics, simply for convenience in patients with renal failure
11. Use of vancomycin solution for topical application or irrigation

....

From Hospital Infection Control Practices Advisory Committee (HICPAC): Recommendations for preventing the spread of vancomycin resistance. MMWR Morb Mortal Wkly Rep. 44(RR12)1–13, 1995 (also available at www.cdc.gov/ncidod/hip).

COMMON NOSOCOMIAL INFECTIONS IN THE INTENSIVE CARE UNIT SETTING (also see Chapter 11)

Nosocomial Pneumonias

Nosocomial pneumonias are common in the ICU, especially in patients receiving mechanical ventilation, with a mortality of 30 to 70% (Table 14–6). Although survival rates improve with appropriate treatment, pneumonia in the ICU patient can be particularly difficult to diagnose. Findings of new or progressing pulmonary infiltrates associated with fever, leukocytosis, and purulent tracheal secretions are neither sensitive nor specific. Radiographic changes mimicking pneumonia may be caused by many noninfectious causes, including atelectasis, atypical pulmonary edema, acute respiratory distress syndrome, hemorrhage, or chemical pneumonitis. Tracheal cultures can grow organisms because of colonization of proximal airways, making it difficult to distinguish between colonizers and true pathogens and leading to treatment on the basis of false-positive results. Quantitative cultures of distal pulmonary regions have reasonable specificity and sensitivity *before* administration of new antibiotics but, when obtained after antibiotic administration, exhibit a marked loss of sensitivity, leading to false-negative results (see Chapter 11).

Central Venous Catheter–Related Infections

Risk factors for the development of central venous catheter–related infections include length of time the catheter is in place, location of central vein used, characteristics of the patient population, and techniques used for insertion, routine dressing, and manipulation (see Table 14–6). Although a central venous catheter

Table 14–3. Penicillins: General Antibacterial Spectrum and Side Effects

ANTIBIOTIC GROUP (EXAMPLES)	COVERS	DOES NOT COVER	POTENTIAL SIDE EFFECTS AND COMMENTS
Natural penicillins (penicillin G, penicillin V)	*Streptococcus* spp. Some enterococci Anaerobes	Up to 35% of *Streptococcus pneumoniae* may be penicillin-resistant *Staphylococcus* species Most enterococci *Bacteroides fragilis, Fusobacterium* spp., and other Gram-negative anaerobes may be resistant No gram-negative coverage	Hypersensitivity reactions, interstitial nephritis, neutropenia High doses prevent platelet aggregation and increase bleeding times
Aminopenicillins (ampicillin, amoxicillin)	*Streptococcus* spp. *Enterococcus* Gram-positive anaerobes *Escherichia coli, Proteus, Salmonella, Shigella Listeria monocytogenes*	*S. pneumoniae* may be resistant Some enterococci may be resistant *B. fragilis* and other Gram-negative anaerobes may be resistant Gram-negative organisms may be resistant	See "Natural penicillins" above Ampicillin is agent of choice for *Listeria* infections
Penicillinase-resistant penicillins (methicillin, nafcillin, dicloxacillin, oxacillin)	All *Streptococcus* spp. and methicillin-sensitive *Staphylococcus aureus* (MSSA)	*Enterococcus* Methicillin-resistant *S. aureus* (MRSA) Coagulase-negative *Staphylococcus* spp. No Gram-negative or anaerobic coverage	See "Natural penicillins" above
Semisynthetic penicillins (mezlocillin, piperacillin, ticarcillin)	*Streptococcus* spp. *Enterococcus* (except ticarcillin) Anaerobes Broad Gram-negative and pseudomonal coverage	No *Staphylococcus* coverage *Enterococcus* can be resistant At least 30% of *B. fragilis* may be resistant	See "Natural penicillins" above *Usual* doses prevent platelet aggregation and increase bleeding times
Penicillins with β-lactamase inhibitors (ampicillin-sulbactam, amoxicillin-clavulanate, ticarcillin-clavulanate, pipericillin-tazobactam)	*Streptococcus* spp. *Enterococcus* (except ticarcillin-clavulanate) MSSA Broad Gram-negative and pseudomonal coverage (ticarcillin-clavulanate and piperacillin-tazobactam) Anaerobes	*Enterococcus* can be resistant MRSA Coagulase-negative *Staphylococcus* spp. No pseudomonal coverage for ampicillin-containing agents	See "Natural penicillins" above

Table 14–4. Cephalosporins: General Antibacterial Spectrum and Side Effects

ANTIBIOTIC GROUP (EXAMPLES)	COVERS	DOES NOT COVER	POTENTIAL SIDE EFFECTS AND COMMENTS
First-generation cephalosporins (cefazolin, cephalexin)	*Streptococcus* spp. Methicillin-sensitive (MSSA) *Staphylococcus aureus Escherichia coli, Proteus mirabilis*	*Enterococcus* spp. Methicillin-resistant *S. aureus* (MRSA) Coagulase-negative staphylococci *H. influenzae* Most other Gram-negative organisms, including *Pseudomonas*	Hypersensitivity reactions Interstitial nephritis 5–10% cross-reactivity between cephalosporins and penicillins in penicillin-allergic patients (see Chapter 29)
Second-generation cephalosporins (cefuroxime, cefotetan, cefoxitin)	*Streptococcus* spp. MSSA (not the preferred agent) Enterobacteriaceae *Haemophilus influenzae*	*Enterococcus* spp. MRSA, coagulase-negative staphylococci *Enterobacter* spp. frequently resistant *Pseudomonas*	See "First-generation cephalosporins" above
Third-generation cephalosporins (ceftriaxone, cefotaxime, cefixime, ceftazidime)	*Streptococcus* spp. MSSA (*only* for ceftriaxone) Gram-negative organisms *Pseudomonas* (*only* for ceftazidime) Anaerobes	*Enterococcus* MRSA Coagulase-negative staphylococci *Bacterioides fragilis* may be resistant	See "First-generation cephalosporins" above Biliary sludge formation associated with ceftriaxone
Fourth-generation cephalosporins (cefepime)	*Streptococcus* spp. MSSA Enterobacteriaceae *Pseudomonas* Anaerobes	*Enterococcus* MRSA Coagulase-negative staphylococci *B. fragilis* may be resistant	See "First-generation cephalosporins" above

infection is virtually always present when the catheter's exit site shows erythema or purulence, the lack of these signs does not exclude an infection. In fact, most infected central venous catheters show no gross evidence of infection at their exit site or along their subcutaneous portion. In response to local evidence of a catheter infection, the catheter should be removed and cultured (the distal 2 cm of its tip should be cut off using sterile technique and sent for semiquantitative culture [see Chapter 11 for more details]) and empirical antimicrobial therapy initiated. Likewise, if the ICU patient is critically ill with severe sepsis or septic shock of uncertain cause, all central venous catheters should be removed, their tips cultured, and empirical antimicrobial therapy begun.

Urinary Tract Infections

Urinary tract infections occur most frequently in ICU patients who have indwelling urinary catheters (see Table 14–6). Urine cultures from these catheters are often

Text continued on page 177

Table 14–5. Nonpenicillin and Noncephalosporin Antibiotics: General Antibacterial Spectrum and Side Effects

ANTIBIOTIC GROUP (EXAMPLES)	COVERS	DOES NOT COVER	POTENTIAL SIDE EFFECTS AND COMMENTS
Aminoglycosides (amikacin, gentamicin, netilmycin, streptomycin, tobramycin)	*Streptococcus* spp. Used for synergy (gentamicin or netilmycin) against MSSA (but not as first-line agents) Coagulase-negative staphylococci *Enterococcus* Gram-negative aerobes *Pseudomonas aeruginosa* Gram-negative anaerobes	Coagulase-negative staphylococci can be resistant Gram-positive anaerobes	Nephrotoxicity, ototoxicity, neuromuscular blockade Doses need to be individually calculated, and serum levels and renal function should be monitored (see Chapter 12) Once-daily dosing decreases nephrotoxicity
Aztreonam	Gram-negative aerobes *P. aeruginosa*	No Gram-positive coverage Anaerobes	Safe for use in penicillin-allergic patients; does not provide the synergy of aminoglycosides when used in combination with cell wall–active agents
Carbapenems (imipenem, meropenem)	*Streptococcus* spp. MSSA Enterococci Gram-negative aerobes *P. aeruginosa* Anaerobes	Coagulase-negative staphylococci Enterococci may be resistant	Seizures may occur, particularly in patients with underlying CNS pathology or renal insufficiency (less risk with meropenem), hypersensitivity, cross-reactivity between penicillin and carbapenems occurs (50%) (see Chapter 29)
Chloramphenicol	*Streptococcus* spp. ± *Staphylococcus* spp. Gram-negative aerobes Anaerobes	± *Staphylococcus* spp. *P. aeruginosa*	Dose-related, reversible bone marrow suppression; idiosyncratic dose-independent, generally fatal aplastic anemia (~1/30,000 patients who receive the drug); hemolysis in severe G6PD deficiency; its use should be restricted to clearly defined circumstances owing to its toxicity; effective second-line agent for bacterial meningitis in penicillin-allergic patients

Table continued on following page

Table 14–5. Nonpenicillin and Noncephalosporin Antibiotics: General Antibacterial Spectrum and Side Effects *Continued*

ANTIBIOTIC GROUP (EXAMPLES)	COVERS	DOES NOT COVER	POTENTIAL SIDE EFFECTS AND COMMENTS
Clindamycin	*Streptococcus* spp. MSSA Anaerobes	*Enterococcus* Coagulase-negative staphylococci Gram-negative aerobes *P. aeruginosa* *B. fragilis* may be resistant	Hypersensitivity; increased risk for *Clostridium difficile* colitis
Macrolides (erythromycin, clarithromycin, azithromycin)	*Streptococcus* spp. *Mycoplasma pneumoniae* Some MSSA *H. influenzae* and *M. catarrhalis* (*only* for azithromycin and clarithromycin) Some anaerobes *Legionella* spp. Second-line agent for *Chlamydia* spp.	Many (18–33%) *S. pneumoniae* are resistant Most MSSA Most Gram-negative aerobes *P. aeruginosa* *B. fragilis* usually resistant	GI symptoms (nausea, vomiting, diarrhea) particularly with erythromycin; thrombophlebitis with IV use; interference with hepatic metabolism of other drugs (theophylline, warfarin) Avoid use with terfenadine, cisapride, astemizole (may cause fatal arrhythmias) or with HMG-CoA reductase inhibitors ("statins") (may cause rhabdomyolysis)
Metronidazole	Gram-negative anaerobes	Everything else	Disulfiram-like reactions with alcohol ingestion; GI irritation
Quinolones (ciprofloxacin, ofloxacin, levofloxacin, sparfloxacin, trovafloxacin, grepafloxacin)	*Streptococcus* spp. (except ciprofloxacin, ofloxacin) *S. aureus* (but resistance may develop quickly) *Enterococcus* Gram-negative rods *P. aeruginosa* *Legionella* spp.	Coagulase-negative staphylococci Some enterococci may be resistant Anaerobes (except for trovafloxacin)	Mild GI symptoms; mild CNS symptoms (headache, dizziness); rash; avoid in pregnant or nursing mothers and children because of possible cartilage toxicity in infants or children; oral bioavailability similar to IV

Drug	Susceptible organisms	Resistant organisms	Adverse effects
Tetracyclines (tetracycline, doxycycline)	± *Streptococcus* spp. ± MSSA ± *Enterococcus* (VREC) ± Gram-negative rods ± Anaerobes Useful for chlamydial and rickettsial infections		Hypersensitivity; photosensitivity; gray discoloration of teeth in children (do not give to pregnant women or children <8 yr); GI irritation; increases catabolism and blood urea nitrogen
Trimethoprim/sulfamethoxazole	± *Streptococcus* spp. MSSA and some MRSA Gram-negative rods First-line agent for treatment of *Pneumocystis carinii* and *Nocardia* *Listeria* infections in penicillin-allergic patients	Pneumococcus (40%) may be resistant Group A and B streptococci always resistant *Enterococcus* *P. aeruginosa* Anaerobes	Hypersensitivity (rarely Stevens-Johnson syndrome); GI irritation; bone marrow suppression, particularly in ESRD; displacement of warfarin from albumin binding sites; aseptic meningitis
Vancomycin	*Streptococcus* spp. All *Staphylococcus* spp. *Enterococcus* Gram-positive anaerobes Oral vancomycin not absorbed but useful in treatment of *C. difficile* colitis	VREC Gram-negative aerobes *P. aeruginosa* Gram-negative anaerobes	Histamine-related flushing of face, neck, and thorax ("red man syndrome"), which may be ameliorated by slowing infusion of drug to >1 h; hypersensitivity; neutropenia and thrombocytopenia; 8th cranial nerve toxicity

CNS, central nervous system; ESRD, end-stage renal disease; GI, gastrointestinal; IV, intravenous; MRSA, methicillin-resistant *S. aureus*; MSSA, methicillin-sensitive *S. aureus*; ±, inconsistent effects; VREC, vancomycin-resistant enterococcus.

Table 14-6. Antibiotics and Their Daily Costs* for Common ICU Nosocomial Infections

INFECTION	CLINICAL SITUATION	EMPIRICAL THERAPY	COMMON ORGANISMS	DEFINITIVE THERAPY
Pneumonia	Cases *without* risk factors for *Pseudomonas* (risk factors include prior prolonged ICU, hospital, or long-term care facility stay, steroids, other immunosuppressants, prolonged antibiotics, or structural lung disease [bronchiectasis].)	Ceftriaxone ($40–50) + metronidazole ($2–3) ± gentamicin ($1) *or* Ampicillin/sulbactam ($40–50) + gentamicin ($1)	Oral flora Enterobacteriaceae *Pseudomonas aeruginosa* *Acinetobacter baumannii* MSSA MRSA See above	Ceftriaxone ($40–50) + metronidazole ($2–3) (TMP/SMX) ($3–4) + metronidazole ($2–3) Review susceptibility data Review susceptibility data Nafcillin ($5–10) *or* cefazolin ($2–4) Vancomycin ($12–15) Review hospital susceptibility data
	Cases with risk factors for *Pseudomonas* (see above)	Ceftazidime ($40–50) or cefepime ($20–60) or piperacillin ($25–35) or levofloxacin ($25) ± gentamicin ($1)		
Septic shock	Unknown site of infection; critically ill patient with central venous catheter in place but not neutropenic or immunocompromised (see Chapter 18)	Piperacillin ($25–35) or ceftazidime ($40–50) or cefepime ($20–60) + tobramycin ($11–12) or gentamicin ($1) + vancomycin ($12–15)	Gram-positive cocci MRSA Gram-negative rods *Pseudomonas*	Based on culture results
	If *Bacterioides fragilis* (abdominal site) is possible	Add metronidazole ($2–3)	*B. fragilis* Other bowel anaerobes	Based on culture results

Infection	Condition	Recommended therapy	Likely pathogens	Alternative/Comments
Urinary tract infection (UTI)	Complicated UTI (with severe sepsis, anatomic urinary tract abnormality, or urinary calculus)	Ampicillin ($2–5) + gentamicin ($1)	Enterobacteriaceae Enterococcus spp.	TMP/SMX ($3–4) or ampicillin ($2–5) ± gentamicin ($1)
	If Pseudomonas suspected (see risk factors, above)	Piperacillin ($35) + gentamicin ($1)	P. aeruginosa	Review susceptibility data
	If yeast found on urinalysis		Candida albicans	Fluconazole ($60–100)
Central venous catheter infections	Not in severe sepsis or septic shock	Cefazolin ($2–4) + gentamicin ($1)	MSSA; coagulase-negative staphylococci or MRSA Enterobacteriaceae P. aeruginosa C. albicans	Based on culture results Fluconazole ($60–100) or amphotericin B ($10)
	In severe sepsis or septic shock	Pipericillin ($25–35) or ceftazidime ($40–50) or cefepime ($20–60) + tobramycin ($11–12) + vancomycin ($12–15)	MSSA; coagulase-negative staphylococci or MRSA Enterobacteriaceae P. aeruginosa C. albicans	Based on culture results Fluconazole ($60–100) or amphotericin B ($10)
Sinusitis	If Pseudomonas not suspected	Ceftriaxone ($40–50) + metronidazole ($2–3) ± gentamicin ($1) or ampicillin/sulbactam ($20–40) + gentamicin ($1)	Enterobacteriaceae Oral flora MSSA Fungi including C. albicans	Based on culture results Fluconazole ($60–100) or amphotericin B ($10)
	If Pseudomonas is suspected (see Risk Factors, above, under Nosocomial Pneumonia)	Ceftazidime ($23–46) or cefepime ($20–60) or piperacillin ($25–35) or levofloxacin ($25) ± gentamicin ($1) ± metronidazole ($2–3)	P. aeruginosa	Based on culture results

Table continued on following page

Table 14–6. Antibiotics and Their Costs* for Common ICU Nosocomial Infections *Continued*

INFECTION	CLINICAL SITUATION	EMPIRICAL THERAPY	COMMON ORGANISMS	DEFINITIVE THERAPY
Wound infections	Postoperative GI or GU wound	Ampicillin-sulbactam ($20–40)	MSSA	Nafcillin ($5–10) or cefazolin ($2–4)
			Streptococcus spp.	Ampicillin ($2–5)
			Enterococcus spp.	Ampicillin ($2–5) ± gentamicin ($1)
			Enterobacteriaceae	TMP/SMX ($3–4)
			P. aeruginosa	Piperacillin ($25–35) ± gentamicin ($1)
	Postoperative sternotomy	Vancomycin ($12–15) + gentamicin ($1)	Anaerobes	Metronidazole ($2–3)
			MSSA	Nafcillin ($5–10) or cefazolin ($2–4)
			Coagulase-negative staphylococci	Vancomycin ($12–15)
			MRSA	Vancomycin ($12–15)
			Streptococcus spp.	Ampicillin ($2–5)
			Enterobacteriaceae	TMP/SMX ($3–4)
Clostridium difficile colitis	Uncomplicated case of colitis (see Chapters 35 and 60)	Metronidazole ($2–3)	*C. difficile*	Metronidazole (oral) ($1)
	Toxic megacolon with severe sepsis or septic shock	Vancomycin (oral) ($10) with IV vancomycin ($12–15)	*C. difficile*	If initial course of metronidazole fails, oral vancomycin ($10) Same as empirical therapy

*Approximate hospital acquisition cost (circa 1999) for the average daily dose (70-kg person with normal renal function).
GI, gastrointestinal; GU, genitourinary; IV, intravenous; MRSA, methicillin-resistant *Staphylococcus aureus*; MSSA, methicillin-sensitive *S. aureus*; TMP/SMX, trimethoprim/sulfamethoxazole.

difficult to interpret because of improper sample collection technique or frequent catheter colonization, both of which can lead to false-positive culture results. To prevent this, all urine cultures should be sent with an accompanying urinalysis to evaluate for the presence of pyuria (defined as >10 white blood cells per high-power field). A positive urine culture (>10^5 colony forming units/μL) without associated pyuria (in the absence of neutropenia) is unlikely to be caused by infection and can be attributed to colonization. Because urine infections in the ICU are usually caused by Gram-negative rods and yeasts, a Gram stain of the urine can help direct empirical therapy.

Sinusitis

The most common risk factor for nosocomial sinusitis is the presence of a nasal tube, for example, a nasogastric, nasotracheal, or nasoenteral tube (see Table 14–6). The tube not only obstructs the normal mucus drainage from the sinuses directly but also causes mucosal edema, which also blocks sinus drainage. Because clinical signs, such as purulent nasal discharge, are absent in the vast majority of cases, the diagnosis is usually made with imaging studies, such as computed tomography, in patients with persistent fever. Infections can occur with any organism colonizing the oropharynx of ICU patients, including *Pseudomonas aeruginosa,* other Gram-negative bacilli, Gram-positive organisms, such as *Staphylococcus aureus,* and fungi. Cultures of fluid obtained from the sinus or ostia, but not from the nares, are recommended to direct therapy. Successful treatment of nosocomial sinusitis depends on removal of the obstructing foreign body and an adequate course of appropriate antibiotics.

Wound Infections

The American College of Surgeons classifies categories of operative wounds by the level of their bacterial contamination (see Chapter 11, Table 11–7). The first category, a "clean" wound, is nontraumatic, with no inflammation, no breaks in sterile technique, and no entry into unsterile sites such as the respiratory, gastrointestinal, or genitourinary tracts. In the second category, "clean-contaminated" wounds, a minor break in sterile technique occurs or the respiratory, gastrointestinal, or genitourinary tracts are entered but without significant spillage occurring. The third category, a "contaminated" wound, includes fresh trauma from a relatively clean source and operative wounds with a major break in sterile technique, spillage of nonpurulent contents from the gastrointestinal tract, or an infected genitourinary tract or biliary tree.

The last category, "dirty" wound, includes encountering pus during the procedure, preoperative perforation of colonized viscous or penetrating trauma more than 4 hours old.

Postoperative wound infection rates increase stepwise from the first to the third categories. Appropriate antibiotic prophylaxis given *preoperatively* significantly decreases wound infection rates for all operative wound categories (see Table

14–6). Since adequate tissue levels of antibiotic must be present at the time of the incision in order to prevent infection, antibiotic prophylaxis must be given between 2 hours and 30 minutes *before* the start of surgery. For prolonged procedures, a second dose may be needed. In most cases, continuing antibiotics postoperatively does not decrease infection rates further.

Failure to give preoperative antibiotics *appropriately* is one significant risk factor for the development of surgical wound infections. Additional risk factors include increasing age, duration of surgery, duration of hospital stay before surgery (with ICU stays further increasing risk), presence of a malignancy, and emergency procedures. Surgical wound infections can range from an incisional cellulitis to an abscess requiring incision and drainage (see Chapter 11) or necrotizing fasciitis (see Chapter 66).

Septic Shock

In treating critically ill ICU patients with septic shock, one must remember that infection is not the only cause. However, the likelihood of infection increases with the severity of the septic response. ICU mortality due to septic shock from infections ranges from 20 to 80%, depending on the population, the type of infection, and timeliness and appropriateness of antimicrobial therapy (see Table 14–6). Because mortality is high even with appropriate antibiotics in ICU patients, the magnitude of the inflammatory response, and not the infection itself, seems to determine the outcome. Thus, continued septic shock does not necessarily imply a failure of antibiotic therapy.

Unexplained Fever, Leukocytosis, and Sepsis

In some cases in the ICU, the cause of fever, leukocytosis, or severe sepsis remains elusive and persistent despite a comprehensive diagnostic evaluation and, in cases of sepsis, empirical broad spectrum antibiotic therapy. In such instances, a therapeutic trial of antifungal therapy may be reasonable. Current microbiologic techniques, even with the best methods of culturing blood, are relatively insensitive for detecting systemic fungal infection, for example, having only 50% sensitivity. The likelihood of fungemia rises as the number of peripheral sites colonized by yeast increases, and the greatest risk is associated with three or more sites of colonization. A trial of amphotericin B is indicated in such multicolonized cases (patients who also have unexplained fevers, leukocytosis, or sepsis) at a starting dose of 0.5 mg/kg. A liposomal amphotericin B preparation may be substituted in the setting of renal insufficiency. Finally, efficacy of fluconazole after the clinical failure of broad spectrum antibiotics is currently being studied and, if proved effective, would be a less toxic alternative.

BIBLIOGRAPHY

Bates DW, Sands K, Miller E, et al: Predicting bacteremia in patients with sepsis syndrome. Academic medical center consortium sepsis project working group. J Infect Dis 176:1538–1551, 1997.

This article describes the development and validation of prediction rules for bacteremias and fungemias in patients with severe sepsis using the cohort of patients described by Sands and colleagues, listed further on.

Cunha BA, Shea KW: Fever in the intensive care unit. Infect Dis Clin North Am 10:185–209, 1996.
This is a review of the epidemiology and diagnostic approach to fever in the ICU.

Filice GA, Weiler MD, Hughes RA, Gerding DN: Nosocomial febrile illnesses in patients on an internal medicine service. Arch Intern Med 149:319–324, 1989.
This is a classic study providing a comprehensive description of nosocomial febrile illnesses arising in hospitalized internal medicine patients.

Galicier C, Richet H: A prospective study of postoperative fever in a general surgery department. Infect Control 6:487–490, 1985.
This is a classic study evaluating the etiology and outcomes of postoperative fever.

Gold HS, Moellering RC: Antimicrobial drug resistance. N Engl J Med 335:1445–1453, 1996.
This is a review of the mechanisms of resistance and issues related to the developing problems of antimicrobial resistance.

Lizan-Garcia M, Garcia-Caballero J, Asenio-Vegas A: Risk factors for surgical-wound infection in general surgery: A prospective study. Infect Control Hosp Epidemiol 18:310–315, 1997.
This article describes a prospective cohort study evaluating risk factors for the development of surgical wound infections.

Martin M: Nosocomial infections in intensive care units: An overview of their epidemiology, outcome, and prevention. New Horizons 1:162–171, 1993.
This article includes risk factors for nosocomial infections in ICUs determined by multivariate analysis of prospectively collected databases.

Nathens AB, Chu PTY, Marshall JC: Nosocomial Infections in the surgical intensive care unit. Infect Dis Clin North Am 6:657–675, 1992.
This article reviews the epidemiology of surgical ICU infections.

O'Grady NP, Barte PS, Bartlett JG, et al: Practice guidelines for evaluating new fever in critically ill adult patients. Crit Care Med 26:392–404, 1998.
This is an excellent review of the infectious causes of fever in the critically ill with clear recommendations on how an evaluation should proceed. These are official guidelines from the American College of Critical Care Medicine (also available at www.sccm.org)

Hospital Infection Control Practices Advisory Committee (HICPAC). Recommendations for preventing the spread of vancomycin resistance. MMWR 44(RR12):1–13, 1995 (also available at www.cdc.gov/ncidod/hip).
This is a comprehensive set of recommendations for preventing the spread of vancomycin resistance.

Hospital Infection Control Practices Advisory Committee. Interim guidelines for prevention and control of staphylococcal infection associated with reduced susceptibility to vancomycin. MMWR 46:626–628, 635, 1997.
These CDC guidelines relate to prevention and control of vancomycin-resistant Staphylococcus aureus.

Sands KE, Bates DW, Lanken PN, et al for the AAMC Sepsis Project Working Group: Epidemiology of sepsis syndrome in eight academic medical centers. JAMA 278:234–240, 1997.
This article describes a prospective epidemiologic study of frequency of severe sepsis in academic medical centers, 55% of which occurred in the ICU setting.

15

Rational Use of Blood Products

Addison K. May
Donald R. Kauder

Blood component therapy is an essential part of the management of patients in the intensive care unit (ICU) and, when used appropriately, saves lives. This expensive therapy is not without hazards, however, and can produce life-threatening complications. Rational use of blood products mandates a clear understanding of the risks and benefits of blood component therapy so that it can be administered appropriately, safely, and effectively.

Indications for blood component therapy can be divided into two broad categories: (1) enhancement of oxygen carrying capacity by expanding red blood cell (RBC) mass and (2) replacement of components of the coagulation system to correct deficiencies due to malfunction, loss, consumption, or inadequate production.

RED BLOOD CELL THERAPY

Until the 1980s, the decision to transfuse RBCs was based predominantly on the "10/30" rule, that is, one should transfuse if a patient's hemoglobin (Hgb) concentration fell to less than 10 g/dL and the hematocrit was less than 30%. The dogma of the "10/30" rule had not been seriously questioned for approximately 40 years. In 1988, the National Institutes of Health Consensus Conference on Perioperative Red Blood Cell Transfusions held that *no single criterion* should be used as an indication for red cell component therapy and that multiple factors related to the patient's clinical status and oxygen delivery needs should be considered in the decision to transfuse.

The delivery of oxygen to tissues can be enhanced by increasing cardiac output, arterial oxygen saturation (Sao_2), and the Hgb concentration (Table 15–1). In addition, in response to anemia (Hgb <10 g/dL), oxygen delivery to cells is

Table 15–1. Physiologic Mechanisms to Increase Oxygen Delivery in Anemia

Mechanisms That Increase Arterial Oxygen Content

Increased production of erythropoietin leading to increased Hgb synthesis and Hgb concentration
Rightward shift of Hgb saturation curve due to increased 2,3-DPG permitting increased oxygen "off-loading" at capillary Po_2 (see Appendix A, Fig. 1)

Mechanisms That Increase Cardiac Output

Increased heart rate
Increased myocardial contractility
Decreased blood viscosity leading to decreased peripheral vascular resistance (afterload)

Hgb, hemoglobin; 2,3-DPG = 2,3-diphosphoglycerate.

facilitated by a rightward shift of the oxyhemoglobin dissociation curve due to increased RBC concentrations of 2,3-diphosphoglycerate (see Appendix A, Fig. 1B). This shift permits more unloading of oxygen to cells at capillary Po_2 (estimated at 25 to 40 mm Hg depending on the metabolic rate of surrounding tissues). Despite this shift to the right to improve oxygen off-loading, oxygen loading *onto* Hgb molecules is usually preserved because Sao_2 remains greater than 90% unless Pao_2 is less than 60 mm Hg (as represented by the flat part of the oxygen-Hgb dissociation curve; see Appendix A, Fig. 1B).

Other compensatory physiologic responses to anemia include an increasing cardiac output by increasing heart rate and cardiac contractility. In addition, systemic vascular resistance decreases because of reduced blood viscosity as Hgb falls to the 8 to 10 g/dL range, which further increases cardiac output (see Chapter 6, Fig. 6–3). Overall, in response to anemia, a normal, euvolemic adult may increase cardiac output fivefold.

This increase in cardiac output, however, may be markedly restricted by the presence of cardiopulmonary disease. Both animal and human studies support the observation that Hgb levels below 10 g/dL (as low as 6 to 7 g/dL) are well tolerated in young, otherwise healthy patients undergoing surgical stress (and limited blood loss), but levels less than this are not tolerated (Table 15–2). For example, in a study of 125 Jehovah's Witnesses, Carson and colleagues demonstrated no mortality in surgical patients with preoperative Hgb between 8.1 to 10 g/dL and blood loss less than 500 mL but found that surgical patients with Hgb less than or equal to 6 g/dL sustained a 61.5% mortality. In a subsequent study of elective surgical patients, no deaths occurred among those even with hemoglobin of greater than or equal to 6 g/dL if surgical blood loss was less than 500 mL.

Numerous studies demonstrate that patients with cardiovascular disease have an increased risk of death if they undergo surgical stress with an Hgb less than 8 to 10 g/dL. Even in the *absence* of anemia, as many as one fourth of patients with known cardiac disease or cardiac risk factors undergoing noncardiac surgery demonstrate intraoperative electrocardiographic findings consistent with cardiac ischemia. Patients with a history of myocardial infarction have a 3 to 7% incidence of another perioperative myocardial infarction, and this risk is highest for those who have sustained a prior infarction within the 6 months preoperatively. As a rule, in patients with known or suspected cardiac disease, Hgb should be kept at greater than 10 g/dL (see Chapter 84).

Table 15–2. Postoperative Outcomes of Anemic Jehovah's Witnesses

PREOPERATIVE HEMOGLOBIN LEVEL	MORTALITY
<6 g/dL	61.5%
6.1 to 8 g/dL	33%
8.1 to 10 g/dL	0%
>10 g/dL	7.1%

From Carson JL, Poses RM, Spence RK, et al: Severity of anemia and operative mortality and morbidity. Lancet 1:727–729, 1988.

Table 15–3. Transfusion Guidelines in Noncritically Ill Anemic Patients Without Risk for Potential Acute Blood Loss or Acute Surgical Stress

Hemoglobin <10 g/dL
Age >65 yr
Known cardiac or pulmonary disease
Symptoms suggesting cardiac or pulmonary disease
Diabetes*
Cerebrovascular disease*
Peripheral vascular disease*

Hemoglobin ≤7–8 g/dL
Symptomatic with significant sustained compensatory mechanisms

*Included because of their high risk for coronary heart disease.

Transfusion Guidelines for Red Blood Cells

Tables 15–3, 15–4 and 15–5, which give guidelines for transfusion decision-making, are based on three clinical settings with anemia: (1) the nonbleeding and noncritically ill patient, (2) hemodynamically stable patient at high risk for bleeding or facing acute surgical stress, and (3) the unstable, bleeding patient.

In normal individuals, oxygen delivery ($\dot{D}O_2$) is in excess of tissue metabolic needs, expressed globally as oxygen consumption ($\dot{V}O_2$), and typically the $\dot{D}O_2$:$\dot{V}O_2$ ratio equals 4 to 5:1. Under these circumstances, $\dot{V}O_2$ is unaltered by modest changes in supply (see Chapter 7, Fig. 7–2). In critically ill patients, however, $\dot{V}O_2$ may become dependent on $\dot{D}O_2$.

At or near this "critical $\dot{D}O_2$" (when a decrease in $\dot{D}O_2$ begins to decrease $\dot{V}O_2$), two parameters begin to change: (1) serum lactate levels rise often creating an anion gap acidosis and (2) the oxygen extraction ratio, $\dot{V}O_2$/$\dot{D}O_2$ (also expressed as $\{SaO_2 - S\bar{v}O_2\}/SaO_2$) exceeds 0.3. An alternative expression of the second change is when the converse of oxygen extraction, the $\dot{D}O_2$:$\dot{V}O_2$ ratio, falls to less than 3:1. In critically ill patients, a $\dot{D}O_2$ less than 10 to 12 mL/kg/minute, an elevated serum lactate level, and an oxygen extraction ratio greater than 0.3 are

Table 15–4. Thresholds for Transfusion in Stable Patients at High Risk for Acute Blood Loss or Facing Acute Surgical Stress

Hemoglobin ≤10–13 g/dL

Known cardiac or pulmonary disease and estimated blood loss
  ≥1000 mL or 250 mL/h
Surgical patients with disorders of hemostasis
Surgical patients with red cell dyscrasias (e.g., sickle cell anemia)

Hemoglobin ≤8–9 g/dL

All with estimated blood loss ≥1000 mL or 250 mL/h

Hemoglobin ≤7 g/dL

All otherwise healthy patients with acute surgical stress

Table 15–5. Transfusion Guidelines for Unstable Patients Who Are Acutely Bleeding

CLINICAL SITUATION	RECOMMENDED RESPONSE
Evidence of rapid acute hemorrhage without immediate control	Transfuse PRBC*
Estimated blood loss >30–40%, presence of symptoms of severe blood loss	Transfuse PRBC*
Estimated blood loss <25–30% without uncontrolled hemorrhage (see Chapter 7, Table 7–2)	Crystalloid-colloid resuscitation, proceed to blood transfusion if recurrent signs of hypovolemia
Presence of comorbid factors	Consider transfusion with lesser degrees of blood loss
Evidence of rapid acute hemorrhage or >30–40% blood loss	Requires emergent control of bleeding source

*May require uncrossmatched or type-specific blood.
PRBC, packed red blood cells.

presumptive indicators of poor tissue perfusion and attempts should be made to increase $\dot{D}O_2$ by increasing cardiac output, Hgb saturation (if SaO_2 <100%), or Hgb concentration by RBC transfusion.

In a recent multicenter, randomized, controlled clinical trial by the Canadian Critical Care Trial Group, a restrictive strategy for RBC transfusion was compared with a liberal strategy in 838 critically ill adults who were normovolemic (excluding those with chronic anemia, pregnancy, or evidence of active bleeding). The restrictive strategy used a Hgb of less than 7 g/dL as the threshold for RBC transfusion and a Hgb of 7 to 9 g/dL as a targeted maintenance range. The liberal strategy used a Hgb of less than 10 g/dL as its threshold for transfusion with a Hgb of 10 to 12 g/dL as its targeted maintenance range. Compared with the liberal strategy group, the restrictive strategy group not only consumed significantly less RBCs (2.6 units vs. 5.6 units per patient on average) but also had a significantly lower hospital mortality rate (22.9% vs. 28.1%). Furthermore, the restrictive strategy group had fewer new cardiac events, such as myocardial infarction and pulmonary edema. On the basis of these results, it is recommended that this restrictive transfusion strategy be generally adopted for critically ill adults who are normovolemic (without chronic anemia, pregnancy, or evidence of acute blood loss). It should not, however, be applied to patients with active coronary syndromes (who were not well represented in this study) until future controlled studies in these patients confirm its safety and efficacy.

Packed RBCs are the component of choice in most clinical situations, as whole blood is rarely indicated and seldom available. Autologous blood collecting devices should be used if possible in exsanguinating patients. This includes reinfusion of blood collected via chest tubes and blood aspirated from the pleural and peritoneal cavities. Gross contamination precludes autotransfusion, but minor degrees of contamination may be acceptable in life-threatening hemorrhage. Autotransfusion systems damage cells to some degree so that autotransfusion should generally be limited to less than 10 L for mildly contaminated blood and less than 15 L for uncontaminated blood.

Recombinant Human Erythropoietin in the Acutely Anemic Patient

RBC mass is predominantly regulated by the production of erythropoietin by the kidney in response to renal hypoxia. Provided that there are adequate supplies of vitamin B_{12}, folic acid, and iron, erythropoietin stimulates an increase in red cell production by marrow and an increase in oxygen carrying capacity. In normal individuals undergoing sequential phlebotomy, RBC mass returns to steady state with a small increase in the rate of erythropoiesis. This appears to hold true for elective postsurgical patients as well. Only after major blood loss do rates of endogenous erythropoietin production and erythropoiesis increase sharply.

Erythropoietin administration is effective in increasing RBC mass in a number of chronic anemia states. In preoperative surgical patients undergoing autologous blood donation, erythropoietin has been shown to increase red cell mass. In addition, several studies have demonstrated decreased transfusion requirements in the postoperative period when patients are given erythropoietin preoperatively provided that there are adequate iron stores. Recent studies suggest that erythropoietin given postoperatively to anemic patients can increase the rate of recovery to normal Hgb levels. Unfortunately, neither its efficacy nor its safety have been determined in critically ill patients, and its routine use in the treatment of acute anemia in this population should await results of controlled clinical trials.

Massive Transfusion

Massive transfusion is defined as a volume of blood equal to, or exceeding, the patient's normal total blood volume. In general, mortality rates have correlated directly with the number of units of blood given to massively transfused patients, with a survival of only 6.6% in patients receiving greater than 25 units in one report in 1971. However, a report by Wudel and coworkers in 1991 demonstrated markedly improved survival. These authors reported a survival rate of 51% in patients receiving 20 to 30 units, 46% in those receiving 26 to 35 units, and 65% in those receiving more than 35 units. This outcome appears more likely to be related to the underlying clinical disorder that dictates the need for massive transfusion and the adequacy of that resuscitation than simply to the number of blood products received.

Appropriate management of patients needing massive transfusion requires an understanding of the specific complications that can occur. These include hypothermia, coagulopathy, acidosis, citrate toxicity, hyperkalemia (and other electrolyte disturbances), and pulmonary dysfunction.

Rapid replacement of blood products stored at cold temperatures can produce severe *hypothermia* in severely bleeding patients. This can produce cardiac irritability, peripheral vasoconstriction that limits tissue perfusion, and platelet and coagulation abnormalities (see Chapter 54).

Although *coagulopathy* may develop in these patients because of hypothermia, it may also result from varying degrees of disseminated intravascular coagulation (DIC) produced both by injured tissue and underperfused tissue. Platelet dysfunction and thrombocytopenia also develop in massively transfused patients and are believed to be clinically more important than coagulation abnormalities due to a pure loss of circulating coagulation proteins. Close attention to *acid-base status* and *electrolytes* is required. These patients are frequently acidotic secondary to inadequate tissue perfusion and can have rapid changes in serum electrolyte composition.

Citrate present in stored blood may not be adequately metabolized in these patients and *citrate-induced hypocalcemia* is not infrequent. Prophylactic administration of 1 g of calcium gluconate intravenously for every 4 to 6 units of transfused blood should be considered to prevent citrate induced hypocalcemia.

Pulmonary dysfunction in massively transfused patients ranges from mild increases in oxygen requirements to severe acute respiratory distress syndrome. Since the full extent of pulmonary dysfunction may not manifest itself for several hours to days after the transfusions have been administered, the patient's risk for alterations in pulmonary function should be kept in mind when considering extubation.

Minimizing the complications of massive transfusion mandates an almost obsessive attention to detail in patient management. Prevention or rapid correction of hypothermia should be accomplished by warming the ambient temperature to 80° C or greater, warming the inspired gases in the ventilator circuit (to 40° C), warming infused fluids with systems developed for rapid infusion, and active heating by use of warming blankets. Although prophylactic therapy with platelets and coagulation factors based solely on the amount of blood transfusion has not been shown to be of benefit, therapy of demonstrated abnormalities is essential. Thus, if a patient shows clinical signs of coagulopathy or has laboratory evidence of thrombocytopenia or a coagulopathy, correction with transfusion of platelets and fresh frozen plasma (FFP) should be continued without interruption until the abnormalities have been corrected. One must also ensure adequate volume resuscitation and tissue perfusion, as acidosis and underperfusion will aggravate DIC if present.

COAGULATION COMPONENT THERAPY

Rational use of the various components for correction of coagulopathy requires an understanding of the numerous causes of bleeding diatheses, their clinical setting, and indications for the use of each specific component.

Assessment and Management of Abnormal Bleeding

Abnormalities in clotting develop in a variety of clinical settings but are most frequently encountered in patients who have sustained trauma or major surgery (Table 15–6).

The most common cause, *hypothermia*, alters hemostasis by a number of mechanisms. Blood vessel contractility induced by direct trauma is inhibited. Platelet aggregation is reversibly inhibited by hypothermia both in vitro and in vivo, an effect ascribed to the temperature-dependent production of thromboxane B_2. In addition, the enzymatic reactions of the coagulation cascade are all slowed by decreasing temperature. The coagulopathy induced by hypothermia is **not**

Table 15–6. Causes of Abnormal Bleeding in Surgery and Trauma

Release of tissue thromboplastin	Disseminated intravascular coagulation (DIC)
Massive transfusion	Platelet dysfunction
Autotransfusion	Hypothermia

evident, however, from the patient's prothrombin time and partial thromboplastin time, since these tests are run at a standard temperature. The exact threshold of hypothermia at which clinically apparent coagulation defects occur is not clear, but current recommendations are to rewarm patients to temperatures greater than 35° C.

Both platelet deficiency and some degree of either DIC or hypocoagulability are encountered in massively transfused patients. Platelet deficiency is more common and should be considered as the most likely cause in patients with abnormal bleeding and massive transfusion. Actual deficits in individual coagulation factors are less common. Banked whole blood contains all the coagulation factors except the labile factors V and VIII. These two factors, however, are produced rapidly by the normal liver. Although both platelet deficiencies and coagulation disturbances may be encountered in massively transfused patients, as already noted, studies demonstrate that prophylactic therapy with FFP and platelets (i.e., therapy based on volume of transfusion without demonstrable defects in hemostasis) is not warranted.

Other factors that alter coagulation are frequently present in the massively transfused patient. Extracorporeal circuits such as bypass machines and autotransfusion devices injure cells and deplete coagulation factors, resulting in an elevation of the prothrombin time and partial thromboplastin time. The presence of contamination in salvaged blood increases the magnitude of this elevation. Current recommendations are to limit salvaged blood to 15 L of noncontaminated blood and 10 L when possible contamination is present. Patients sustaining head or lung injuries also experience a prothrombin time prolongation (due to the release of tissue thromboplastin from the damaged tissue). DIC may result from the combination of shock and a strong clotting stimulus. Other causes for DIC include transfusion reactions, sepsis, disseminated cancer, tissue ischemia or injury, drug reactions, and a dead fetus.

Specific Blood Components

Platelets

The indications for platelet transfusion are the prevention or control of bleeding from either thrombocytopenia or a qualitative platelet disorder (Table 15–7). Serious *spontaneous* hemorrhage seldom occurs with platelet counts greater than 20,000/μL, assuming that no disorder in platelet function exists. Several conditions and medications cause qualitative platelet disorders including uremia, the use of extracorporeal circuits and medications such as aspirin, nonsteroidal anti-inflammatory agents, antihistamines, phenothiazines, tricyclic antidepressants, and

Table 15–7. Thresholds for Platelet Transfusion in Various Clinical Settings*

....

<20,000/µL

Prophylaxis for bleeding

<60,000/µL

Active bleeding
Coagulation abnormality
Evidence of severe infection
Platelet inhibiting medication in use

<100,000/µL

Undergoing major surgery
Surgery within previous 48 h
Major trauma or brain injury within previous 48 h

Any number

Bleeding time >1.5 × upper limit of normal
Cardiopulmonary bypass
Massive transfusion with abnormal bleeding
Use of autotransfusion devices with abnormal bleeding
Abnormal bleeding with conditions or drugs that inhibit platelet function (see text)

....

*See also special clinical conditions covered in Chapters 18, 45, and 63.

certain antibiotics such as cephalosporins and penicillins (which bind to platelets when used in high doses). Adequate platelet-related hemostasis is indicated by a bleeding time that is less than one and one-half times the upper limit of normal. The recommended dose of platelets to produce an incremental increase of 5000 to 10,000/µL is 1 unit/10 kg of body weight.

Fresh Frozen Plasma and Cryoprecipitate

FFP contains all the labile and stable coagulation factors, immunoglobulins, and cholinesterases. FFP is indicated for the replacement of factors II, V, VII, IX, X, and XI when specific therapy is not available or appropriate. When fibrinogen or von Willebrand factor is needed, however, cryoprecipitate is preferred. Factor VIII deficiencies can be treated with cryoprecipitate or factor VIII concentrates, and factor IX deficiencies can be treated with factor IX complex. Antithrombin III deficiency may be treated with FFP as well as with antithrombin III preparations that are now available (Tables 15–8 and 15–9).

ALLOGENEIC TRANSFUSION RISKS

Risks from transfusions can be divided into major categories: infectious and immunologic.

Infectious Complications

Transfusion-transmitted infection remains the most common serious risk of transfusion; patients receiving a transfusion have approximately a 3 in 10,000 risk of

Table 15–8. Indications for Fresh Frozen Plasma

Emergency reversal of warfarin-induced coagulopathy
Replacement of isolated coagulation protein deficiency
Massive transfusion and documented coagulation defect
Disseminated intravascular coagulation with serious active bleeding (see Chapter 45)
Hypovolemic shock with clinical coagulation defect unresponsive to platelet transfusion
Liver disease with clinical bleeding and evidence of coagulation defect (see Chapters 19 and 59)
Thrombotic thrombocytopenic purpura (TTP) (see Chapter 63)
Replacement of clotting factors after apheresis therapy (see Chapter 67)

contracting a serious or fatal transfusion-transmitted disease. The risk of acquiring human T-cell leukemia-lymphoma virus type I or II infection is estimated at 1 in 200,000, and the risk for acquiring human immunodeficiency virus infection is estimated at 1 in 420,000 in the United States.

The most common transfusion-transmitted infection is viral hepatitis. More than 90% of post-transfusion hepatitis cases are attributed to hepatitis C virus, and about 2% to hepatitis B. Other causes include cytomegalovirus, Epstein-Barr virus, hepatitis A, and other recently identified hepatitis viruses. As many as one third of the patients who acquire hepatitis from transfusion get chronic liver disease, and cirrhosis may develop in up to 20% of these patients. Chronic liver disease due to infection with hepatitis B and hepatitis C viruses also has a strong association with hepatocellular carcinoma.

Risk of retroviral infection is small, with less than 20 cases of transfusion-related infection per year in the United States. Although current screening tests have excellent sensitivity and specificity, patients who have recently been infected by human immunodeficiency virus will not have detectable antibodies and, if they donate blood, their donations will be serologically negative (the so-called window period). Currently, all components in the United States are also tested for human T-cell leukemia-lymphoma virus type I or II antibodies. Human T-cell leukemia-lymphoma virus is endemic in southwest Japan and the Caribbean basin and can be transmitted by transfusion. In other parts of the world, transfusion-related transmission of malaria and the causative agent for Chagas' disease *(Trypanosoma cruzi)* remains a significant problem.

Immunologic Complications

Immunologic complications (see Chapter 46 for more details) include acute hemolytic reactions, delayed hemolytic reactions, febrile reactions, allergic reactions,

Table 15–9. Indications for Cryoprecipitate

Hemophilia A (factor VIII deficiency)	Dysfibrinogenemia
von Willebrand's disease	Factor XIII deficiency
Fibrinogen deficiency	Uremic platelet dysfunction (see Chapter 20)

acute lung injury, graft-versus-host disease, post-transfusion purpura, and immuno-suppression.

Acute hemolytic reaction is estimated to occur in 1 in 6000 transfusions and is fatal in one in 100,000 to 600,000 transfusions. Fatal transfusion reactions generally result from clerical errors or improperly performed type and crossmatch with the infusion of incompatible blood. Acute hemolytic reactions may present with pain at the infusion site, fever, chills, back and substernal pain, mental status changes, dyspnea, hypotension, distended neck veins, cyanosis, and bleeding diathesis. In the anesthetized or critically ill patient, these reactions may be difficult to detect but should be suspected with any unexplained hypotension, hemoglobinuria, or bleeding diathesis that occurs during or shortly after transfusion. The transfusion should be stopped immediately, the transfusion service (blood bank) notified and blood samples collected for free hemoglobin, haptoglobin, and Coombs' tests. Volume support to maintain urine output at more than 60 mL per hour should be given initially, and inotropic support and measures to improve renal clearance of Hgb (mannitol, alkalinization of urine) may also be required.

Delayed hemolytic reactions occur more frequently but are often mild and may go undetected. The incidence is estimated to be 1 per 4000 transfusions, and they affect patients with prior blood exposure (i.e., transfusion or pregnancy) who experience a rapid anamnestic response to a previously sensitized antigen. Hemolysis is generally gradual and less severe, with up to 35% of patients being asymptomatic. Symptomatic patients may acquire jaundice, hemoglobinuria, and decreasing hemoglobin concentrations. Such reactions generally need no specific therapy and do not alter compatibility of future transfusions.

Febrile reactions with elevation of core body temperature occur in up to 7% of transfusions. These reactions occur following the induction of antileukocytic antibodies induced by previous blood exposure. They are usually self-limited and patients are not at increased risk for another febrile reaction with future transfusions. Fever is also often present in acute hemolytic reactions, however, so that the presence of hemolysis must be ruled out. If hemolysis is excluded, the transfusion may be completed, with antipyretics being administered as needed.

Allergic reactions occur from the infusion of an antigen or immunoglobulin to which the patient has pre-existing antibodies; previous blood exposure is not required. Severity can range from mild urticaria and pruritus to severe anaphylaxis. In severe reactions, transfusions must be stopped immediately, and epinephrine may be required to relieve bronchospasm and support hemodynamics. Washed cells may be considered for future transfusions.

That transfusions are *immunomodulatory* is well established, but despite numerous retrospective and prospective studies, in general the clinical significance of this effect remains unclear. As early as 1973, prior history of receiving blood transfusions was found to improve allograft survival in transplant patients. Other therapeutic immunomodulatory effects include prevention of recurrent abortion and suppression of immune inflammatory disease.

Activation of latent viruses is one negative immunomodulatory effect of blood transfusions. Although other negative effects include increased infection rates and cancer recurrence rates, the clinical importance of these last two effects is controversial. Some retrospective studies have suggested that transfusions increase recurrence rates in a number of cancers, but others have not. The results of prospective studies are equivocal, with most being unable to demonstrate significant alterations related to transfusions. Moreover, some studies that found a higher risk of recurrence suggest that these alterations occur whether the patients are given autologous blood or allogeneic blood. Evidence that transfusions increase the rate of postoperative infection is stronger, however, but whether autologous blood and allogeneic blood carry equal risks remains unclear. The current consensus is that the evidence regarding infection and cancer recurrence risks is not sufficiently compelling to alter the transfusion guidelines outlined earlier.

TRANSFUSION COSTS

Increasingly, clinicians are being called on to consider the costs and cost:benefit ratios of various therapies and to limit medical expenditures without compromising patient care. Estimating the total cost versus the total benefits of various therapies is often difficult and frequently imprecise. This certainly is true for blood components.

Currently, blood component therapy is a limited resource that significantly contributes to overall health care expenditures. In the United States, approximately 12 million RBC units are transfused to nearly 4 million patients annually. Actual costs of transfusion therapy and costs of complications associated with both anemia and transfusions are unknown. Estimated hospital cost for a unit of autologous blood ranges from $250 to $750. The acquisition cost of allogenic transfusion is somewhat greater than autogenous blood but estimates vary widely. Although most place the extra cost between $250 and $350, actual costs in the clinical setting may be far greater. For example, in one study examining total transfusion costs in patients undergoing hip replacement, patients receiving allogeneic blood had incremental hospital costs of about $1000 to $1500 per unit transfused when compared with patients receiving no blood or 1 to 5 units of autologous blood.

The estimated costs of other alternatives to autologous blood transfusion are also difficult to establish. The estimated cost per patient for intraoperative cell salvage is in the range of $250 to $400. No significant decrease in the number of patients undergoing transfusion can be demonstrated until infusion volumes exceed 750 mL, and no cost savings accrue until the volume exceeds 1000 mL. Although therapy with recombinant human erythropoietin has been shown to decrease transfusion requirements in some settings, this therapy is also expensive. Decisions based on the cost and benefits of autologous blood versus its alternatives currently must be made with limited data.

Both a reduction in total blood use and substantial cost savings could result from the implementation of institutional transfusion guidelines based on the national standards and the 1999 study by the Canadian Critical Care Trials Group described earlier. For example, at one tertiary care hospital, transfusion decisions based on the former guidelines saved more than $1.5 million during a 3-year period. Thus, use of such guidelines can reduce the risks of serious complications, the cost of their treatment, and the direct costs of blood component therapy.

BIBLIOGRAPHY

Blaisdell FW: Bleeding. In: Wilmore DW, Brennan MF, Harken AH, et al (eds): Care of the Surgical Patient, vol 1, Chapter 7. New York: Scientific American, 1989.

A concise overview of mechanisms of hemostasis is provided as a guide for the preoperative assessment of bleeding risk and algorithms for the assessment and management of abnormal intra- and postoperative bleeding.

Carson JL, Poses RM, Spence RK, Bonavita G: Severity of anemia and operative mortality and morbidity. Lancet 1:727–729, 1988.
Jehovah's Witnesses undergoing surgery had no mortality if preoperative Hgb was greater than 8 g/dL and blood loss was less than 500 mL, but there was a 61.5% mortality if Hgb was less than or equal to 6 g/dL.

Consensus Conference: Fresh frozen plasma: Indications and risks. JAMA 253:551–553, 1985.

Consensus Conference: Perioperative red blood cell transfusion. JAMA 260:2700–2703, 1988.

Consensus Conference: Platelet transfusion therapy. JAMA 257:1777–1780, 1987.
These three citations present the results of the National Institutes of Health's Consensus Conference on the use of blood components. Each provides clear recommendations regarding the accepted indications for the various products.

Greenburg AG: Indications for transfusion. In: Wilmore DW, Brennan MF, Harken AH, et al (eds): Care of the Surgical Patient, vol 1, Chapter 6. New York: Scientific American, 1989.
This presents a good overview of DO_2 and red cell physiology with clinically applicable transfusion algorithms.

Hébert PC, Wells G, Blajchman MA, et al: A multicenter, randomized, controlled clinical trial of transfusion requirements in critical care. N Engl J Med 340:409–417, 1999.
Landmark multicenter study by the Canadian Critical Care Trials Group on the threshold for transfusion in the critically ill. (See text for details.)

Houbiers JG, Busch OR, van de Watering LM, et al: Blood transfusion in cancer surgery: A consensus statement. Eur J Surg 161:307–314, 1995.
A review of the risks and indications of blood products in cancer patients.

Klein HG: Allogeneic transfusion risks in the surgical patient. Am J Surg 170(6A Suppl):21S–26S, 1995.
This is an excellent review of current literature regarding the immunosuppressive effects of transfusions and conclusions based on this body of literature.

Proceedings of the Blood Management Practice Guidelines Conference. Am J Surg 170(6A Suppl), 1995.
These proceedings present consensus guidelines and several reviews regarding the use of blood products in the surgical patient. Each is replete with references. Review topics include transfusion risks, legal considerations of transfusion, risk assessment in the surgically anemic patient, erythropoiesis and strategies to avoid blood use, physiologic basis for red cell transfusion, and management of Jehovah's Witnesses as patients.

Spence RK, Carson JA, Poses R, et al: Elective surgery without transfusion: Influence of preoperative hemoglobin level and blood loss on mortality. Am J Surg 159:320–324, 1990.
Jehovah's Witnesses undergoing surgery had no deaths, even with hemoglobin as low as 6 g/dL if surgical blood loss was less than 500 mL.

Wudel JH, Morris JA Jr, Yates K, Bass SM: Massive transfusion: Outcome in blunt trauma patients. J Trauma 31:1–7, 1991.
These authors showed greatly improved outcomes for patients receiving massive transfusions.

16 Renal Replacement Therapy

Sidney M. Kobrin

Acute renal failure (ARF) is a common problem in intensive care unit (ICU) patients. When patients develop ARF, the ICU team and consulting nephrologist should work together to (1) reverse or prevent progression of ARF (see Chapter 78), (2) initiate renal replacement therapy at the optimal time, (3) choose the modality of renal replacement therapy that best suits the patient's particular circumstances, and (4) decide on the dialysis and ultrafiltration orders. This chapter reviews the thresholds for initiating renal replacement therapy and the pros and cons of available modalities.

WHEN TO START RENAL REPLACEMENT THERAPY

Most authorities would agree that certain signs and symptoms are strong indications for commencing renal replacement therapy (Table 16–1). The value of early dialysis in asymptomatic patients, however, remains unproved. Some studies have reported that prophylactic dialysis aimed at maintaining the blood urea nitrogen (BUN) at less than 100 mg/dL (35 mmol/L) reduced mortality and morbidity in patients with ARF. However, because most of these studies compared those treated with early dialysis to historical controls, unrelated improvements in ICU care may have been responsible for the observed improvement in outcomes. Two studies using concurrent controls have examined this issue, but they give contradictory results.

Despite the lack of conclusive data, many nephrologists institute early dialysis because they believe that this practice simplifies the management of ARF, reduces

Table 16–1. Indications for Acute Dialysis

Presence of the uremic syndrome
    Altered mental status (personality changes, confusion, coma)
    Anorexia, nausea, vomiting
    Asterixis, myoclonus
    Pericarditis
    Seizures
Fluid overload resistant to diuretic therapy
Metabolic acidosis
    When additional sodium bicarbonate administration would lead to volume overload
Hyperkalemia
    When unresponsive to medical therapy
Persistent bleeding secondary to platelet dysfunction
    When unresponsive to medical therapy (see Chapter 20)
Serum BUN and creatinine*
    BUN >100 mg/dL or creatinine >10 mg/dL

*These are controversial indications in the absence of uremic signs and symptoms or in the absence of their rapid rise in the preceding several days.

morbidity, and improves the well being of the patient. Conversely, two arguments can be made against the early institution of dialysis. First, recovery from ARF may be hampered as a result of hypotension and cytokine release, which often accompany dialysis. Second, early dialysis may increase costs without added benefit. In the absence of convincing studies, the decision to initiate dialysis in asymptomatic patients must be based on clinical judgment alone. For example, there is no compelling reason to commence dialysis in an asymptomatic patient with nonoliguric ARF who has a BUN of 100 mg/dL, a serum creatinine of 10 mg/dL (800 mmol/L), and a slowing in the rate of rise of these parameters over the preceding several days. Such a patient is likely to recover renal function spontaneously within a few days. However, an unstable patient with oliguric ARF and a recent rapid rate of rise in BUN and serum creatinine is unlikely to recover soon. Such a patient is said to be "hypercatabolic," generating uremic toxins rapidly and also likely to accumulate acid and potassium. Intuitively, dialysis should be started before the seemingly inevitable build-up of these dangerous chemicals.

Physicians should exercise caution when using a BUN of 100 mg/dL as a threshold for initiating dialysis. BUN can be raised out of proportion to the serum creatinine level, secondary to excessive protein administration, gastrointestinal bleeding, or tetracycline or corticosteroid use. Such patients may have a BUN exceeding the 100 mg/dL threshold but lack evidence of uremia or the need for dialysis. Alternatively, in patients with decreased urea generation due to poor nutrition or liver disease, manifestations of the uremic syndrome may appear despite the BUN being below this threshold.

AVAILABLE MODALITIES

A thorough knowledge of the efficacy, advantages, disadvantages, route of access, and cost of each modality is critical when choosing the optimal renal replacement method (Tables 16–2 and 16–3). In terms of efficacy, the major considerations are efficiency of solute clearance, volume removal (ultrafiltration), and the impact on patient survival.

Intermittent Hemodialysis

At present, intermittent hemodialysis (HD) is still the most widely used modality in the ICU to provide both dialysis and ultrafiltration. HD uses a large-diameter double-lumen central venous catheter for access. It uses a semipermeable membrane through which the patient's blood and dialysis solution flow in opposite directions. Solutes are removed largely by diffusion. Recent advances in dialysis hardware and dialysate solutions have allowed critically ill patients to tolerate this procedure better than in the past. For example, volumetrically controlled machines permit precise ultrafiltration compared with older machines. Previously, overshooting ultrafiltration goals were common and contributed to the frequent development of hypotension during dialysis. In addition, widespread use of bicarbonate rather than acetate as buffer in the dialysate has also reduced the risks of intradialytic hypotension. Despite these advances, the latter continues to occur frequently during

Table 16–2. Modalities for Renal Replacement Therapy

MODALITY	ABBREVIATION
Intermittent hemodialysis	HD
Isolated ultrafiltration	IUF
Arteriovenous methods	
Arteriovenous slow continuous ultrafiltration	AV-SCUF
Continuous arteriovenous hemofiltration	CAVH
Continuous arteriovenous hemodialysis	CAVHD
Continuous arteriovenous hemodiafiltration	CAVHD + F
Venovenous methods	
Venovenous slow continuous ultrafiltration	VV-SCUF
Continuous venovenous hemofiltration	CVVH
Continuous venovenous hemodialysis	CVVHD
Continuous venovenous hemodiafiltration	CVVHD + F
Peritoneal dialysis	PD

Table 16–3. Characteristics of Renal Replacement Modalities

MODALITY*	SOLUTE CLEARANCE (PER DAY)	ULTRAFILTRATION CAPABILITY	ANTICOAGULATION	COST†
HD	25 L	1 +	Systemic is ideal; heparin free or regional is possible	2 +
IUF	Negligible	2 +	Systemic is ideal; heparin free or regional is possible	1 +
AV-SCUF	Negligible	3 +	Systemic is ideal; regional is very cumbersome	2 +
CAVH	15–20 L	3 +	Systemic is ideal; regional is very cumbersome	4 +
CAVHD	24–36 L	3 +	Systemic is ideal; regional is very cumbersome	3 +
CAVHD + F	24–48 L	3 +	Systemic is ideal; regional is very cumbersome	4 +
Continuous venovenous modalities	Same as for analogous continuous arteriovenous modality	3 +	Same as for analogous continuous arteriovenous modality	5 +
PD	12–36 L	2 + –3 +	No systemic anticoagulation is needed	2 +

*See Table 16–2 for abbreviations.

†Cost refers to expenses accrued by Dialysis Cost Center and does not include extra work by ICU house staff or nursing staff (which would be highest for the continuous venovenous modalities).

HD, especially in hemodynamically unstable, critically ill patients receiving large volumes of intravenous fluid between dialyses. Such patients may require in the range of 4 to 6 L of ultrafiltration during a 4-hour dialysis treatment.

The cardiovascular defense mechanisms that would normally maintain blood pressure during fluid removal are often impaired or overwhelmed, or both, in critically ill patients with cardiac dysfunction or peripheral vasodilation, for example, secondary to sepsis, or liver failure. This hypotension may have many sequelae, including delayed recovery of ARF and ischemia to many organs, including the heart and intestine. Another major disadvantage of HD is that it requires that specialized dialysis nurses devote one-on-one care to the critically ill patients at the bedside in the ICU, as opposed to being able to care for three or four more stable patients in a dialysis unit.

The major advantages of HD are that most nephrologists are familiar with the technique and that it offers the most rapid clearance of solutes (including potassium) and correction of metabolic acidosis. Systemic anticoagulation is generally required to prevent clotting of the system during routine dialysis. Heparin-free regimens, however, are available and can be employed to dialyze critically ill patients with active bleeding, after recent surgery, or with suspected or proven heparin-induced thrombocytopenia.

Isolated Ultrafiltration

Isolated ultrafiltration (IUF) resembles HD and also uses a double-lumen central venous catheter for access. The major difference between IUF and HD is that dialysate is not pumped through the filter. The pressure settings across the dialyzer are programmed to remove a certain fluid volume. IUF is indicated in fluid-overloaded patients resistant to diuretics in whom there is no significant accumulation of nitrogenous wastes, hyperkalemia, or metabolic acidosis (since solute removal is negligible). IUF is less likely than conventional HD to induce intradialytic hypotension. Simultaneous ultrafiltration and fluid removal as occurs during standard HD results in a rapid decrease in intravascular osmolality, which reduces the rate of osmotically induced plasma refilling from the intracellular and interstitial compartments. In contrast, intravascular osmolality remains stable with IUF, the rate of plasma refilling is relatively rapid, and blood pressure is better maintained than during HD. In general, in the presence of peripheral edema, patients tend to tolerate ultrafiltration rates of 1.5 to 2 L/hour. However, the greater the hemodynamic instability, the less likely such rapid ultrafiltration rates will be tolerated.

Arteriovenous Slow Continuous Ultrafiltration

The equipment required for arteriovenous slow continuous ultrafiltration (AV-SCUF) is shown in Figure 16–1. Blood circulates from a catheter placed in the patient's artery (usually a femoral artery) through a filter and returns to the patient through a catheter placed in a central vein (usually a femoral vein). No pumps are used to drive blood through the system. The arteriovenous pressure gradient is the

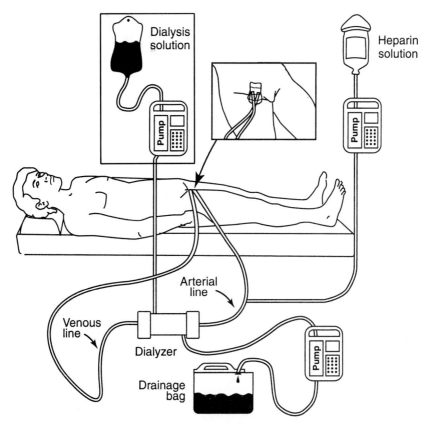

Figure 16–1. The equipment and circuit required for arteriovenous slow continuous ultrafiltration (AV-SCUF). The additional equipment required to perform continuous arteriovenous hemodialysis (CAVHD) is shown in the boxed area. (Modified from Daugirdas JT, Ing TS: Handbook of Dialysis. Boston, Little, Brown, 1988.)

driving force that moves the blood through the circuit. No diffusive dialysis takes place because no dialysis solution is used. Its limitations are similar to IUF.

The major advantage of this procedure, compared with IUF, is that fluid may be removed continuously over 24 hours, creating less stress in hemodynamically compromised patients. The ultrafiltration rate may be accurately controlled by placing a pump on the ultrafiltration line. If a pump is not available, simply elevating or lowering the ultrafiltration drainage bag may allow fairly accurate control of the ultrafiltration rate. Ultrafiltration in the range of 4 to 8 L/day is feasible with this therapy. Trained dialysis nurses are not required to be at the bedside; ICU nurses generally perform much of the procedure. The major disadvantage of AV-SCUF is the requirement for arterial access. This may be associated with considerable morbidity, especially in patients with diseased arteries (in which significant complications have been reported in up to 19% of patients). Systemic anticoagulation is also required. The nephrologist and ICU team should meet daily and decide on the goal for ultrafiltration. This is usually equal to the fluid to be administered that day plus any net ultrafiltration deemed necessary. Replacement fluid is not required, but all intravenous fluids should contain a physiologic electrolyte composition.

Continuous Arteriovenous Hemofiltration

Continuous arterovenous hemofiltration (CAVH) resembles AV-SCUF (see Fig. 16–1). The goal of this therapy is to achieve the desired volume of net ultrafiltration similar to that described for AV-SCUF while simultaneously clearing solutes. Solute clearance is purely convective. No dialysate solution is administered. Total ultrafiltration rates of 12 to 24 L/day can be achieved. The ultrafiltrate resembles that of plasma water so that if 25 L of ultrafiltrate are generated per day, approximately 25 L of blood are cleared of uremic solutes. Replacement fluid of composition similar to plasma water (e.g., Ringer's lactate) must be administered to prevent volume depletion and replace essential solutes. The net volume of desired ultrafiltration for the day is decided in advance, and the volume of replacement fluid is calculated to allow reaching this goal (Table 16–4).

The major disadvantage of this system is that large fluid shifts may occur, with potentially disastrous outcomes. Although machines are available to allow minute-to-minute microprocessor-matched replacement fluid delivery, they increase the complexity of the procedure. This, in turn, raises concern for potential errors and resultant complications. Similar clearances and net ultrafiltration can be achieved with continuous arteriovenous hemodialysis (CAVHD), which, when compared with CAVH, is simpler and safer. The only potential advantage of CAVH is theoretical in that the convective clearance may enhance middle molecule clearance (clearance in molecules in the midrange of molecular sizes, from about 5000 to 30,000 kd), including many known mediators of sepsis. However, at present there is no evidence that clearance of these mediators improves the clinical course or survival in sepsis.

Table 16–4. Dialysis Orders for Continuous Arteriovenous Hemofiltration, Continuous Arteriovenous Hemodialysis, and Continuous Arteriovenous Hemodiafiltration

ORDER*	CONTINUOUS ARTERIOVENOUS HEMOFILTRATION	CONTINUOUS ARTERIOVENOUS HEMODIALYSIS	CONTINUOUS ARTERIOVENOUS HEMODIAFILTRATION
Total ultrafiltration rate	25 L/24 h	8 L/24 h	15 L/24 h
Dialysate flow rate	None (not applicable)	17 L/24 h	10 L/24 h
Replacement fluid flow rate	17 L/24 h	None	7 L/24 h

*Orders to achieve 4 L of net ultrafiltration and 25 L of BUN clearance/24 h in a hypothetical patient receiving 4 L of maintenance intravenous fluid/day.

BUN, blood urea nitrogen.

Continuous Arteriovenous Hemodialysis

The circulatory access and equipment required for CAVHD are similar to AV-SCUF, the major difference being that dialysate is infused in a direction countercurrent to the blood flow (see Fig. 16–1). Small solutes, for example, BUN, diffuse from the blood into the dialysate and reach concentrations in the dialysate similar to those in blood. Equilibration between blood and dialysate persists, with dialysate flows up to 25 mL/min (1500 mL/hour), achieving solute clearances of up to 36 L/day. A pump placed on the dialysate outflow line allows accurate control of ultrafiltration, similar to that described for AV-SCUF. Replacement fluid is generally not required because the composition of dialysate electrolytes and minerals is equivalent to that of normal plasma so that there is a negligible net loss of these substances.

Lactate is commonly used as the base in the dialysate. Rarely, transfer of lactate from the dialysate into blood may result in acid-base disorders, particularly in patients with an ongoing lactic acidosis or liver disease in which metabolism of lactate to bicarbonate may be impaired. In these circumstances, a bicarbonate dialysate can be prepared to meet the requirements of the individual patient. The major advantage of CAVHD compared with HD is that ultrafiltration is slow and continuous and less likely to cause hypotension. The daily solute removal with CAVHD is comparable to that obtained with the usual 4-hour HD treatment (see Table 16–3).

Continuous Arteriovenous Hemodiafiltration

Continuous arteriovenous hemodiafiltration (CAVHD + F) is a hybrid of CAVHD and CAVH. Dialysate is pumped countercurrent to blood as with CAVHD, but ultrafiltration is not controlled and may reach rates of 12 to 24 L/day as with CAVH. Solute clearance is therefore by diffusion and convection and is very efficient, easily approaching 36 to 48 L/day. In contrast to CAVHD, CAVHD + F requires replacement fluid and more equipment; in addition, keeping track of fluid balance is more complex. Although CAVHD + F achieves a modest increase in solute clearance, it is rarely necessary and many clinicians believe it is usually not worth the extra effort, expense, and increased potential for human error. Orders for achieving certain levels of solute removal and ultrafiltration in CAVH, CAVHD, and CAVHD + F are illustrated in Table 16–4.

Continuous Venovenous Techniques

Continous venovenous techniques differ from the continuous arteriovenous techniques described earlier in that blood is drawn from a central vein instead of the femoral artery. The use of a roller pump is mandatory because there is no intrinsic pressure driving blood through the extracorporeal circuit (Fig. 16–2). Analogous to the continuous arteriovenous modalities, variation in the amount of ultrafiltration and use of dialysate allows for four different variations of the procedure (see Tables 16–2 and 16–3). The major advantage of the venovenous techniques is the

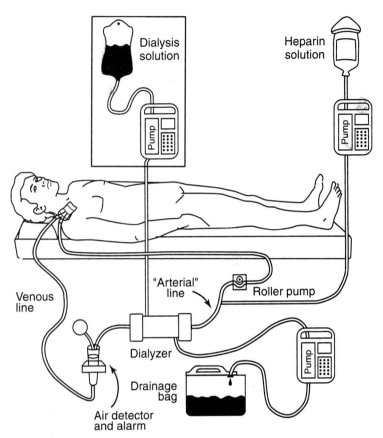

Figure 16–2. The equipment and circuit required for venovenous slow continuous ultrafiltration (VV-SCUF). The additional equipment required to perform continuous venovenous hemodialysis (CVVHD) is shown in the boxed area. The "arterial" line also normally has a pressure transducer in-line (omitted from figure) between the roller pump and the dialyzer to monitor perfusion pressure. (Modified from Daugirdas JT, Ing TS: Handbook of Dialysis. Boston, Little, Brown, 1988.)

lower morbidity associated with the venous access as compared with arterial access. Although theoretically more constant blood flow is possible and filter life may be prolonged using venovenous methods, patient survival and solute clearance appear to be similar with both modalities.

Venovenous modalities are more expensive because of the higher cost of the equipment. They also require considerably more time to train ICU nurses, given the complexity of the extra equipment. The venovenous machines are similar to HD machines with air detectors and alarms in the circuit. The "set-up" of the equipment is also labor intensive. The increased complexity of the procedure is of particular concern in large ICUs with a high turnover of nurses. If an ICU nurse rarely performs the procedure, attrition of skills will occur with periods of inactivity. These issues should be considered before an institution decides to offer venovenous techniques.

Peritoneal Dialysis

Peritoneal dialysis (PD) involves the insertion of a peritoneal dialysis catheter, either percutaneously (with or without peritoneoscopy) or surgically (using a limited "open" technique). Dialysate is then infused, allowed to dwell, and drained. Adjustment of the length of the dwell time and the glucose concentration of the dialysate results in solute removal and ultrafiltration rates similar to those of the dialytic procedures (see Table 16–3). This procedure is currently underused in the treatment of ARF. Its major advantages are that no vascular access is required, no systemic anticoagulants are needed, and fluid removal can be distributed over 24 hours. This should result in greater hemodynamic stability as compared with intermittent HD. Unfortunately, PD may not be feasible in patients with recent abdominal surgery or with severe pulmonary dysfunction because the dwelling peritoneal fluid can interfere with descent of the diaphragm and lung expansion.

FACTORS INFLUENCING SELECTION OF A SPECIFIC MODALITY

There have been no definitive randomized, controlled clinical trials comparing patient survival with the different renal replacement techniques in critically ill patients. Selection of a dialysis modality is therefore largely empirical. The presence of one or more clinical situations, however, may influence the choice of one modality over another.

Acid-Base and Electrolyte Abnormalities

Severe hyperkalemia that is unresponsive to medical therapy requires rapid correction. Intermittent HD is the procedure of choice in this situation because high potassium clearance rates on the order of 200 mL/min are possible. In contrast, the continuous extracorporeal modalities and PD are much less efficient, with maximal clearance rates of only 40 mL/min. In some circumstances, one may use a single HD treatment to achieve normokalemia and then switch to a continuous modality, such as PD or CAVHD, to maintain normokalemia and to meet additional dialysis and ultrafiltration needs. The same vascular access may be used for HD and the venous part of CAVHD or for HD and CVVHD. Potassium may be added to the dialysate or replacement fluid if hypokalemia develops.

The continuous extracorporeal therapies and PD may be ideal for management of metabolic acidosis in shock states. These patients have sustained lactic acid production. Acidosis increases between dialyses when intermittent HD is used, whereas the continuous modalities provide a steady, uninterrupted correction of acidosis. The continuous modalities may also facilitate the administration of large volumes of intravenous bicarbonate because ongoing ultrafiltration is possible.

Anticoagulation

Systemic anticoagulation is necessary while using the continuous extracorporeal therapies in order to maintain the efficacy and longevity of the filters used. Heparin is the anticoagulant of choice. This requirement for systemic anticoagulation is a potential disadvantage because many critically ill patients may have strong contraindications for heparin exposure or anticoagulation. In such patients, regional anticoagulation using protamine or citrate may obviate the need for systemic anticoagulation. These techniques, however, are relatively cumbersome. They also add another level of complexity to the procedure, which further increases the risk for human error, particularly when the technique is used infrequently. In contrast, PD and intermittent HD can both be performed without the need for systemic heparinization.

Nutrition

The continuous therapies, including PD, permit relatively large amounts of ultrafiltration compared with intermittent HD. This, in turn, results in the creation of "an intravascular space," which allows the administration of parenteral nutrition without causing fluid overload. Patients receiving these modalities tolerate this type of nutritional support better than if undergoing intermittent HD.

Amino acids and protein may be lost with continuous extracorporeal techniques and PD. Conversely, glucose may be absorbed from the dialysate used with CAVHD and PD. These losses and gains should be taken into account when nutritional orders are written. Another consequence of the glucose absorption is that carbon dioxide production may increase because of overfeeding. At times this may make it difficult to wean patients from mechanical ventilation.

Hemodynamic Considerations

Although there have been no randomized, controlled studies addressing the issue, it is intuitive that hemodynamically unstable patients receiving large volumes of intravenous fluid will better tolerate the slow rate of ultrafiltration possible with the continuous modalities as compared with intermittent HD or IUF. Although it is relatively easy to remove 3 to 5 L of fluid during a 4-hour HD treatment in a hemodynamically stable chronic dialysis patient, the same may not be possible in critically ill and unstable patients.

Vascular Access

The choice of modality is often dictated by the route of access. PD may be impossible in a patient after recent or previous abdominal surgery. The relative safety of venous access favors the use of HD or the venovenous modalities over the arteriovenous modalities, particularly in patients with peripheral vascular disease.

Choice of Membrane

Recent evidence suggests that survival of patients with ARF, as well as the time to recovery from ARF, is improved when dialysis filters composed of biocompatible membranes are used. They cause less complement and neutrophil activation than do bioincompatible cuprophane membranes. Some recommend the routine use of biocompatible membranes for the treatment of patients with ARF.

Patient Mobility

The continuous extracorporeal therapies significantly restrict patient mobility because immobility is mandatory when an arterial access is used (to prevent trauma to the artery or catheter dislodgment). Arteriovenous modalities may be problematic if the patient requires repeated procedures out of the ICU or if the patient recovers sufficiently and is capable of increased mobility or physical therapy.

Nursing and Physician Experience

The choice of modality also depends on the experience of the ICU medical and nursing team. Complicated procedures such as CVVHD should not be undertaken unless a core of dedicated and interested physicians and nurses undergo extensive training in the procedure and set up protocol manuals, support mechanisms, and quality improvement programs. Some have suggested that an institution should perform a minimum of 12 procedures annually in order to be proficient in the technique. The estimated number of procedures should be determined before starting such a program. If achieving the minimal number is unlikely, patients needing the therapy should be transferred to a center (or an ICU) with an established CVVHD program.

BIBLIOGRAPHY

Bellomo R, Boyce N: Continuous veno-venous hemofiltration compared with conventional dialysis in critically ill patients with acute renal failure. ASAIO J 39:M794–M797, 1993.
This study comparing the outcomes of patients with acute renal failure receiving continuous venovenous hemodiafiltration (CVVHD + F) with historical controls receiving hemodialysis suggested that this modality might improve survival.

Bellomo R, Parkin G, Love J, et al: A prospective comparative study of continuous arteriovenous hemodiafiltration with continuous veno-venous hemodiafiltration in critically ill patients. Am J Kidney Dis 21:400–404, 1993.
This study demonstrated similar survival, but lower morbidity, when continuous venovenous hemodiafiltration (CVVHD + F) was compared with continuous arteriovenous hemodiafiltration (CAVHD + F).

Conger JD: A controlled evaluation of prophylactic dialysis in post-traumatic acute renal failure. J Trauma 15:1056–1063, 1975.
This is the only published study that evaluated early prophylactic dialysis.

Conger JD: Intensive dialysis not routinely helpful in acute renal failure. J Crit Illness 1:10, 1986.
This is the only published study that has evaluated the impact of intensive hemodialysis on survival.

Forni LG, Hilton PJ: Continuous hemofiltration in the treatment of acute renal failure. N Engl J Med 336:1303–1309, 1997.

This is a classic and well-written review of the continuous forms of hemofiltration.

Hakim RM, Wingard RL, Parker RA: Effects of dialysis membrane in the treatment of patients with acute renal failure. N Engl J Med 331:1338–1342, 1994.

This controlled clinical trial established that synthetic dialyzer membranes should be used to treat acute renal failure.

Mehta RL, Martin RK: Initiating and implementing a continuous renal replacement therapy program: Requirements and guidelines. Semin Dial 9:80–87, 1996.

This well-written review clearly outlines the ingredients required to set up and maintain a successful continuous renal replacement therapy program.

17

Care of the Patient Infected with the Human Immunodeficiency Virus

Ian Frank

The number of human immunodeficiency virus (HIV)–infected individuals continues to increase, as does their potential for prolonged survival. Therefore, critical care specialists can expect to care for more HIV-infected patients admitted to the intensive care unit (ICU) for complications related to their HIV infection or their treatment. This chapter presents considerations regarding HIV-infected patients that may result in their admission to the ICU or that may complicate their ICU care.

Although HIV-related complications may occur throughout the entire spectrum of immunodeficiency, certain conditions are unusual until a patient's $CD4^+$ lymphocyte falls to less than a certain threshold (Tables 17–1 and 17–2). Furthermore, as the patient's $CD4^+$ lymphocyte counts continue to decline below these thresholds, the risk for these complications increases.

Table 17–1. Thresholds of $CD4^+$ Lymphocyte Counts and Disease Manifestations for Selected Pathogens

PATHOGEN	COMMON DISEASE MANIFESTATIONS	THRESHOLD OF $CD4^+$ LYMPHOCYTE COUNT*
Bacteria		
Streptococcus pneumoniae	Pneumonia, bacteremia, meningitis	500
Haemophilus influenzae	Pneumonia, bacteremia	500
Mycobacterium tuberculosis	Pneumonia	300
Salmonella	Diarrhea, bacteremia	300
Campylobacter, Shigella	Diarrhea	300
Clostridium difficile	Colitis	50
M. avium intracellulare	Cytopenias, fever, abnormal liver function test results, wasting	50
Parasites		
Pneumocystis carinii	Pneumonia	200
Giardia	Diarrhea	200
Toxoplasma gondii	Ring-enhancing CNS lesions	100
Cryptosporidium, Isospora	Diarrhea	100

*The $CD4^+$ lymphocyte count (cells/µL) when each complication may be first encountered. The risk for each complication continues to increase as the $CD4^+$ lymphocyte count declines further.

CNS, central nervous system.

205

Table 17–2. Thresholds of CD4$^+$ Lymphocyte Counts and Disease Manifestations for Selected Noninfectious Complications

COMPLICATION	COMMON DISEASE MANIFESTATIONS	THRESHOLD OF CD4$^+$ LYMPHOCYTE COUNT*
Immune thrombocytopenic purpura	Thrombocytopenia	500
Non-Hodgkin lymphoma	Adenopathy, wasting	300
Nephropathy	Nephrotic syndrome, renal insufficiency	200
Cardiomyopathy	Congestive heart failure	100
CNS lymphoma	Ring-enhancing CNS lesions	50

*The CD4$^+$ lymphocyte count (cells/μL) when each complication may be first encountered. The risk for each complication continues to increase as the CD4$^+$ lymphocyte count declines further.
CNS, central nervous system.

PULMONARY COMPLICATIONS

Bacterial Pneumonias

Pneumonias are the most common cause for hospitalization of HIV-infected patients. Acute onset of cough and fever with a lobar radiographic infiltrate suggests bacterial pneumonia. Not only do HIV-infected patients have rates of pneumonia resulting from *Streptococcus pneumoniae* that are 150-fold greater than those in the non–HIV-infected population, but they also are at higher risk for recurrences. Because immunologic response to the polysaccharide antigens is impaired at CD4$^+$ lymphocyte counts less than 500 cells/μL, pneumococcal vaccination should *not* be considered as protective in HIV-infected individuals. Furthermore, HIV-infected patients with pneumococcal pneumonia have bacteremias and other complications more often than non–HIV-infected individuals.

Likewise, *Haemophilus influenzae* pneumonia occurs 100 times more often in HIV-infected patients. Because the organisms for most of these *Haemophilus* species cannot be typed, *H. influenzae* type b vaccine is not protective. Although other pyogenic bacteria are less common causes of pneumonia in HIV-infected patients, *Pseudomonas aeruginosa* pneumonia may be seen in late stages of disease (usually associated with a CD4$^+$ lymphocyte count <100 cells/μL, cavitary lung disease, or prior treatment with broad spectrum antibiotics). Finally, despite *Legionella* pneumonia occurring infrequently, its incidence is increased 40-fold in HIV-infected patients.

Pneumocystis carinii Pneumonia

Acquired immunodeficiency syndrome (AIDS) is the most common predisposing cause of *Pneumocystis carinii* pneumonia (PCP). In the absence of chemoprophylaxis, more than 80% of patients with AIDS develop PCP in their lifetimes. Its likelihood is affected by the degree of immunologic impairment. In HIV-infected adults, this disease most commonly arises in individuals with CD4$^+$ lymphocyte counts between 50 and 75 cells/μL and is uncommon in individuals with CD4$^+$ lymphocyte counts greater than 200 cells/μL or a CD4$^+$ lymphocyte percentage greater than 20% of the absolute lymphocyte count.

Early diagnosis and therapy for PCP is associated with a more favorable outcome. Prognosis is worse if the patient has a large alveolar-arterial (A-a) oxygen difference (PA_{O_2}-Pa$_{O_2}$) at presentation, extensive infiltrates on chest radiography, neutrophilia in a bronchoalveolar lavage (BAL) specimen, elevated serum lactate dehydrogenase (LDH) levels (>500 IU/L), worse acute physiologic derangements, or chronic comorbidities.

Spontaneous pneumothorax may occur in up to 10% of patients with PCP and is the most common complication. The resulting bronchopleural fistulas may need chemical pleurodesis for closure.

Diagnostic Evaluation

PCP is rare in HIV-infected patients with CD4$^+$ lymphocyte counts greater than 200 cells/μL or greater than 20% of the absolute lymphocyte count. Elevated lactate dehydrogenase levels are present in more than 90% of hospitalized patients with PCP.

The classic PCP chest radiograph exhibits diffuse, bilateral interstitial infiltrates that extend from the perihilar region and spare the apices. More extensive disease can have an alveolar pattern. In up to 30% of cases, however, chest radiographs are normal. Moreover, in 10 to 30% of patients, atypical patterns can be seen, especially in those receiving inhaled pentamidine as PCP prophylaxis. These patterns include unilateral or asymmetric disease, single or multiple nodules, cysts or cavities, pneumatoceles, pneumothorax, hilar adenopathy, and pleural effusions.

Because it is unusual for PCP to occur in patients who are taking prophylactic trimethoprim-sulfamethoxazole (TMP-SMX) appropriately, alternative diagnoses should be sought in such patients with an illness resembling PCP. If PCP does occur in individuals receiving TMP-SMX prophylaxis, it presents atypically. For example, patients may have a protracted time course, with fever rather than cough as the predominant symptom. Conversely, in any HIV-infected patient not receiving TMP-SMX prophylaxis, PCP should be considered in the differential diagnosis of fever of unknown origin, even if the chest radiograph is normal and there is no hypoxemia. Establishing a definitive diagnosis should be attempted in all patients suspected of having PCP. This requires visualization of the organism in pulmonary secretions or a lung biopsy specimen. As many as 20% of HIV-infected individuals who present with clinical, laboratory, and radiographic evidence consistent with PCP have other diagnoses. In addition, patients who are treated empirically for PCP have a worse outcome than those in whom a definitive diagnosis is made. Therefore, empirical treatment for PCP is generally *not* recommended.

Induced sputum after ultrasonic nebulization of hypertonic saline may diagnose PCP in 15 to 90% of cases, depending on local experience and expertise. It is, however, rarely diagnosed in expectorated sputum without induction. When induced sputum testing is not available or yields a negative result, fiberoptic bronchoscopy should be performed. Specimens obtained by BAL have a diagnostic yield of 86 to 97%, especially if BAL of both lungs is performed. BAL is more sensitive than standard bronchial washing and brushing. Transbronchial biopsy has a sensitivity similar to BAL but may detect some cases missed by BAL. When combined with BAL, some centers report a sensitivity of 100%. Evidence suggests that BAL is not sufficient as a single modality to diagnose PCP in patients receiving aerosolized pentamidine for prophylaxis. In this setting, it should always be combined with transbronchial biopsy.

Treatment

Treatment for PCP that is severe enough to need admission to the ICU should be initiated with TMP-SMX administered intravenously at a dose of 15 to 20 mg trimethoprin/kg/day divided into three or four doses. Patients who are intolerant to sulfonamides should be treated with pentamidine isethionate (a single intravenous dose of 3 to 4 mg/kg/day). Survival is better in patients with severe disease (P(A-a)O$_2$ >45 mm Hg or Pao$_2$ <70 mm Hg on ambient air) treated with corticosteroids (prednisone 40 mg twice a day for 5 days followed by a taper over 15 days). Prednisone is beneficial only if it is administered within 72 hours of the initiation of antimicrobial therapy.

Some patients may experience a fall in oxygenation and a progression of infiltrates on the chest radiograph during the first 7 days of treatment. Therefore, if no improvement is evident by the end of the first week of therapy, patients who have not had a definitive diagnosis of PCP established should undergo bronchoscopy expeditiously. For patients in whom the diagnosis of PCP has been established, a second pulmonary pathogen should be sought.

Mycobacterial Infections

HIV infection is the most significant predisposing factor for reactivation of latent *Mycobacterium tuberculosis* infection. Up to 50% of HIV-infected patients who are infected with tuberculosis (TB) eventually develop active TB. It occurs most commonly when a patient's CD4$^+$ lymphocyte count is 150 to 350 cells/μL. It can, however, occur even if CD4$^+$ counts are normal. In this case, it presents in a manner similar to that in patients without HIV: subacute or chronic onset of fever, weight loss, cough, chest pain, and shortness of breath.

Patients with low CD4$^+$ lymphocyte counts also have a high risk of extrapulmonary TB (40 to 80% of TB cases). Disseminated TB and lymphadenitis are the two most common presentations of extrapulmonary disease. Disseminated disease may present acutely with hypotension and respiratory distress. TB lymphadenitis is most commonly located in cervical, supraclavicular, or axillary nodes, but intrathoracic and intra-abdominal nodes can be seen. Central nervous system (CNS) infection occurs in 5 to 10% of HIV-infected patients with TB.

Chest radiographs of active TB infection vary by level of immunosuppression. Patients with high CD4$^+$ counts often have apical cavity disease. Those with low counts infrequently have cavitation but more often have lower lobe consolidation, intrathoracic adenopathy, miliary infiltrates, and pleural effusions.

Reactivity to tuberculin skin testing is inversely related to CD4$^+$ counts. Among patients with AIDS and active TB, only 10 to 30% of patients will have a skin test reaction that is greater than or equal to 10 mm of induration. Sputum is positive by microscopy for acid-fast bacilli (AFB) in 40 to 65% of HIV-infected patients with active TB, and positive by AFB culture in 75 to 95% of patients. For patients who have not had a diagnosis made from sputum, BAL is diagnostic by AFB smear in 7 to 20% of patients and by culture in 52 to 89% of individuals, whereas transbronchial biopsy specimens result in positive AFB smears in 10 to 39% of patients and in positive cultures in 42 to 85% of individuals.

Among the nontuberculous mycobacteria, *Mycobacterium avium* complex (MAC) and *Mycobacterium kansasii* are the most common causes of pulmonary infection. Although isolated pulmonary disease can occur, MAC more commonly presents with disseminated disease as well as signs and symptoms of chronic disease (prolonged fever, weight loss, diarrhea, cytopenias, and low albumin levels). When MAC presents as pulmonary disease, the chest radiograph typically shows bilateral, interstitial-nodular infiltrates, indistinguishable from PCP. MAC may be a copathogen or colonizer in HIV-infected patients with other causes of pneumonia. Under these circumstances, the organism is often cultured from a BAL specimen as a single or rare colony and requires no treatment. *M. kansasii* infection presents primarily as pulmonary disease.

NEUROLOGIC COMPLICATIONS

During the course of disease, the majority of HIV-infected patients experience one or more neurologic complications. Some of these, for example, meningoencephalitis, seizures, and focal neurologic deficits, may lead to admission to the ICU.

Cryptococcal Meningitis

Cryptococcal meningitis, the most common manifestation of cryptococcal infection in HIV-infected patients, typically presents with headache, fever, nausea, vomiting, and no focal neurologic findings. About 10% of patients present with seizures. Cryptococcal disease starts as a pulmonary infection and then disseminates to the brain and other organs. Cutaneous disease is present in 10% of patients, typically appearing as multiple nonpigmented nodular lesions that are often mistaken for molluscum contagiosum.

The diagnosis is made by cerebrospinal fluid (CSF) analysis. The CSF white blood cell count is typically elevated, with a predominance of lymphocytes, but it may be normal in 20% of cases. CSF protein levels are also typically elevated, whereas CSF glucose levels are normal or decreased. The CSF cryptococcal antigen is positive in nearly all HIV-infected patients with cryptococcal meningitis and has a sensitivity comparable to a CSF fungal culture. Because of a high fungal burden, the India ink test produces positive results in 60 to 80% of cases. Serum cryptococcal antigen is positive in 95% of cases and can be diagnostic in the appropriate clinical setting when a lumbar puncture cannot be obtained. Imaging studies of the brain, however, are usually normal.

Amphotericin B (0.7 to 1.0 mg/kg/day) is the initial therapy. The addition of 5-flucytosine (100 mg/kg/day in four divided doses) to amphotericin B sterilizes the spinal fluid more rapidly but does not improve clinical outcome. Because patients given initial therapy with fluconazole, 400 mg/day, have a higher mortality rate during the first 7 days of therapy, it should be reserved for chronic maintenance therapy after the completion of a 2-week induction course of amphotericin B. Mortality is increased in patients who present with mental status abnormalities, cranial nerve palsies, ataxia, or elevated intracranial pressure (ICP). Treatment directed at reducing ICP, such as daily lumbar punctures, acetazolamide, and ventriculoperitoneal shunting, should be considered for asymptomatic patients with ICP greater than 32.0 cm H_2O (23.5 mm Hg) and for symptomatic patients with ICP greater than 18.0 cm H_2O (13.2 mm Hg).

Bacterial Meningitis

Acute bacterial meningitis is less common than cryptococcal meningitis in HIV-infected individuals. The most common causes are *S. pneumoniae* and *H. influenzae*. Less common are *Listeria monocytogenes*, *M. tuberculosis*, endemic fungi (histoplasmosis and coccidioidomycosis), and neurosyphilis.

Toxoplasma Encephalitis

The most common *focal* neurologic complication of HIV infection is *Toxoplasma* encephalitis. The risk of *Toxoplasma* encephalitis developing in HIV-infected patients with CD4+ lymphocyte counts less than 100 cells/μL is 20 to 30% per year in the absence of prophylaxis. It almost always results from reactivation of latent infection and presents as a subacute headache with focal neurologic findings in the majority of patients and as seizures in about 30% of patients. The diagnosis is made empirically after the detection of multiple ring-enhancing lesions on brain imaging in a patient with a positive serum toxoplasma serologic profile. A magnetic resonance imaging (MRI) study of the brain with gadolinium enhancement is the most sensitive imaging test and is preferred over a computed tomographic (CT) scan with contrast. Serologic studies are falsely negative in 10% of cases. Spinal fluid analysis is often normal and unhelpful in making the diagnosis.

The preferred treatment is pyrimethamine (100 to 200 mg loading dose and then 50 to 100 mg/day) plus folinic acid (10 mg/day) plus sulfadiazine (4 to 8 g/day). For patients who are allergic to sulfonamide, clindamycin (900 to 1200 mg intravenously or 300 to 450 mg orally), azithromycin (1200 mg/day) or clarithromycin (1 g twice per day) may be substituted for the sulfadiazine. After 2 or 3 weeks of treatment, patients should undergo repeat brain imaging. Failure to observe shrinkage of the ring-enhancing lesions suggests another diagnosis, and a brain biopsy may be indicated. Approximately 10% of patients with *Toxoplasma* encephalitis fail to demonstrate a response on imaging studies within the first 3 weeks of therapy. Assuming that a radiologic response to treatment has been observed, chronic lifelong suppressive therapy with reduced doses of drug is started after a 6-week course of induction therapy.

Other Causes of Focal Neurologic Disease

Primary central nervous system lymphoma is the second most common cause of *focal* CNS complications in HIV-infected patients. Like CNS toxoplasmosis, the presenting symptoms of CNS lymphoma depend on the neuroanatomic location of the lesions. CNS lymphoma cannot be distinguished from CNS toxoplasmosis on clinical or radiologic grounds.

The therapeutic algorithm for a patient with ring-enhancing CNS lesions begins with empirical therapy for toxoplasmosis (even in the absence of a positive serologic test result). Patients in whom a 2- to 3-week trial of anti-*Toxoplasma* therapy does not decrease the size of the ring-enhancing lesions are likely to have CNS lymphoma. However, a brain biopsy is required for a definitive diagnosis. Although primary CNS lymphoma may respond to radiation therapy, survival after diagnosis is only about 3 months. This is because a majority of such patients are severely compromised immunologically and often have other HIV-related complications.

Progressive multifocal leukoencephalopathy (PML), a disease of white matter caused by the Jakob-Creutzfeldt virus, is the third most common cause of focal CNS pathology in HIV-infected patients. PML occurs in less than 5% of HIV-infected patients. Its clinical presentation also depends on the location of the lesions. Common manifestations include seizures, and focal motor and sensory defects, including aphasia, visual field defects, and ataxia (when disease is present in the cerebellum). MRI reveals single or multiple white matter lesions without surrounding edema, but the definitive diagnosis at present requires brain biopsy. Polymerase chain reaction analysis of CSF probing for Jakob-Creutzfeldt virus DNA is being investigated as a diagnostic test. Although there is no proven therapy for PML, improvement in immunologic function after the initiation or modification of antiretroviral therapy has resulted in clinical and radiographic improvement in some patients.

DIFFERENTIAL DIAGNOSIS OF HYPOTENSION IN THE PATIENT WITH HUMAN IMMUNODEFICIENCY VIRUS INFECTION

Bacterial Causes

Bacterial sepsis is an important and underappreciated cause of death in HIV-infected patients. HIV infected patients often have neutropenia secondary to the bone marrow dysfunction of HIV infection, infectious complications or malignancies, or toxicities of several commonly used medications. Although HIV infected patients are at an increased risk of bacteremia when absolute neutrophil counts fall to less than 1000 cells/μL, their risk appears to be less than that of oncology patients with chemotherapy-induced neutropenia of the same level.

Pneumococcal bacteremia complicating pneumonia is the most common cause of bacteremia in HIV-infected patients. They also are at increased risk for staphylococcal bacteremia. This is probably the result of cutaneous complications of HIV disease providing a route for systemic entry. Staphylococcal infection also may present as pyomyositis, typically of the large muscle groups of the thigh, and should be considered the probable diagnosis in an HIV-infected patient presenting with fever and a painful or swollen leg.

Infection with *Salmonella* species (non–*S. typhi*) is another common cause of bacteremia in HIV-infected patients and can be seen in the absence of diarrhea or other symptoms related to the gastrointestinal tract. Because *Salmonella* bacteremia often recurs after discontinuation of antibiotic therapy, many authors suggest lifelong chronic suppressive therapy.

Pseudomonas bacteremia should be considered in HIV-infected patients receiving chronic antibiotic therapy for the prophylaxis of opportunistic infections or the treatment of complications such as sinusitis. Finally, as mentioned previously, disseminated TB can present with fever and hypotension.

Causes Due to Volume Depletion

Diarrhea in the HIV-infected patient may lead to intravascular volume depletion and hypotension. This may be caused by enteric bacterial pathogens *(Salmonella, Shigella, and Campylobacter)*, parasites *(Giardia, Isospora belli, Cryptosporidium, Microsporidia),* and viruses (most commonly cytomegalovirus). HIV-infected patients may have diarrhea due to *Clostridia difficile* colitis, even without a history of current or recent antibiotic use.

Although HIV patients with MAC typically present with chronic fevers and weight loss, they can appear acutely ill if they become volume-depleted because of concomitant diarrhea.

Adrenal Insufficiency

Adrenal insufficiency should also be considered in any HIV-infected patient with a low CD4$^+$ lymphocyte count presenting with hypotension and no other cause. The major risks for adrenal insufficiency in HIV-infected patients include infection with cytomegalovirus, TB, or MAC.

OTHER ORGAN SYSTEM DYSFUNCTION IN PATIENTS INFECTED WITH HUMAN IMMUNODEFICIENCY VIRUS

Cardiac Disorders

Common cardiac complications of HIV infection include valvular heart disease, pericarditis, and myocarditis. Valvular disease can be caused by infectious endocarditis, especially in intravenous drug users, or by marantic endocarditis complicating malignancies, such as Kaposi's sarcoma and lymphoma.

Pericarditis can be infectious (TB or MAC), noninfectious (lymphoma), or idiopathic. Idiopathic pericarditis often presents as tamponade and requires pericardiocentesis. However, it usually does not reaccumulate after drainage.

An increasingly common late manifestation of HIV infection is a dilated cardiomyopathy, characterized pathologically by focal myocarditis with round cell infiltration and myocardial fiber necrosis. Patients typically present in congestive heart failure. Its cause is not well understood, but, in a small percentage of cases, it may be a complication of nucleoside reverse transcriptase inhibitors. In other cases, it has improved after antiretroviral therapy was initiated.

Hematologic Disorders

Cytopenias are seen in most HIV-infected individuals. Anemia is usually normochromic, normocytic, and multifactorial, but impaired erythropoiesis is almost always a contributing factor. Although the proportion of HIV-infected patients who have positive Coombs test results increases with more advanced disease, immune hemolysis is unusual.

Granulocytopenia also increases with progressive disease. Myelotoxicity can be caused by zidovudine, sulfonamides, or ganciclovir. Filgrastim (granulocyte colony-stimulating factor [GCSF]) is indicated in patients with neutrophil counts less than 500 cells/μL.

Thrombocytopenia can be encountered at all stages of disease, independent of other cytopenias. Megakaryocytes can be infected with HIV, leading to decreased production of platelets. Immune thrombocytopenic purpura accounts for thrombocytopenia in many patients, but despite platelet counts falling to less than 10,000/μL, bleeding is rare. Effective antiretroviral therapy may improve platelet counts. Prednisone (30 to 60 mg/day) and intravenous immunoglobulin (400 mg/day for 2 to 5 days) can increase platelet counts. This lasts for 2 to 4 weeks in the majority of patients with thrombocytopenia due to immune destruction. Splenectomy produces a durable increase in platelet counts in about half the patients undergoing this procedure (see also Chapter 63).

Renal Disorders

HIV-associated nephropathy (HIVAN), which is most common in patients with low CD4$^+$ lymphocyte counts, can also occur earlier in the course of disease. Patients typically present with nephrotic syndrome or renal insufficiency. Ultrasonography often reveals large kidneys with increased echogenicity, a feature that can distinguish HIVAN from other causes of chronic renal disease in which kidney size is often small. The development of renal insufficiency is frequently rapid, especially in patients with nephrotic syndrome. The median time from presentation to dialysis is only 11 weeks.

Prospective, randomized trials investigating treatment for HIVAN are in progress. Some anecdotal reports describe improved renal function after short courses of high-dose prednisone. Initiation of antiretroviral therapy has also been reported to improve renal function.

Renal insufficiency can also be caused by several drugs that are frequently used in HIV-infected patients. Pentamidine, foscarnet, TMP-SMX, amphotericin B, sulfadiazine, and rifampin can cause acute tubular necrosis or acute tubulointerstitial nephritis.

Electrolyte Disorders

Hyponatremia is the most frequent electrolyte disturbance in hospitalized HIV-infected patients and is due to inappropriate secretion of antidiuretic hormone, hypovolemia, or adrenal insufficiency. *Hypernatremia* can be seen secondary to drug-induced nephrogenic diabetes insipidus caused by foscarnet or amphotericin B.

Hypokalemia occurs as a result of gastrointestinal losses due to diarrhea or vomiting, or urinary losses caused by drug-induced tubular acidosis (e.g., from amphotericin B). *Hyperkalemia* has been reported in association with high-dose trimethoprim adminstration used to treat patients with PCP and renal insufficiency.

Lactic acidosis, secondary to antiretroviral therapy, has been documented in the absence of tissue hypoxia in some patients with HIV infection. These patients present with gastrointestinal symptoms, subacute malaise, and hyperventilation and have an anion gap acidosis with high plasma lactate levels. Death from progressive acidosis rapidly ensues in the majority of patients.

Drug Toxicities and Drug-Drug Interactions

Many drugs used to treat HIV infection and its complications may directly cause potentially life-threatening toxicities. They also can cause toxicity from drug-drug interactions. Drug toxicity should be considered in the differential diagnosis of any condition not attributed to an HIV-related opportunistic infection or malignancy. This is especially true for patients receiving one or more HIV protease inhibitors. All these drugs inhibit one or more isoforms of cytochrome P_{450}. As a consequence, a number of other drugs are contraindicated in patients receiving protease inhibitors. Concentrations of certain drugs may become elevated and are more likely to cause toxicity. Concentrations of others may decrease and become ineffectual. Before ordering any drugs for patients continuing on a HIV protease inhibitor after admission to the ICU, one should carefully review the potential interactions of the protease inhibitor with the drug under consideration.

As a rule, antiretroviral therapy can safely be discontinued while patients are hospitalized for serious HIV-related complications. Although viral load will transiently increase, HIV resistance to the withheld antiretroviral agent does not develop, and the patient should experience the same benefit when therapy is resumed.

BIBLIOGRAPHY

Aboulafia DM, Mitsuyasu RT: Hematologic abnormalities in AIDS. Hematol Oncol Clin North Am 5:195–214, 1991.
   This a thorough review of the hematologic complications of HIV infection.

Barnes PF, Bloch AB, Davidson PT, Snider DE: Tuberculosis in patients with human immunodeficiency virus infection. N Engl J Med 324:1644–1650, 1991.
   This review includes the epidemiology, clinical manifestations, PPD testing, and treatment of tuberculosis in the HIV-infected patient.

Cheitlin MD: Cardiac involvement in the patients with AIDS. In: Broder S, Merigan TC Jr, Bolognesi D (eds): Textbook of AIDS Medicine. Baltimore: Williams & Wilkins, 1994, pp 609–615.
This reviews the cardiac complications of HIV infection, with emphasis on cardiomyopathies; it includes a section on cardiac surgery in the HIV patient.

Deeks SG, Smith M, Holodniy M, Kahn JO: HIV-1 protease inhibitors. JAMA 227:145–153, 1997.
This is a summary of the benefits and complications of the HIV protease inhibitors. For an excellent and continuously updated review of all antiretroviral therapy agents, see the DHHS guidelines for antiretroviral therapy use at: www.hivatis.org.

Frank I: Pneumocystis. In: Conn RB, Borer WZ, Snyder JW (eds): Current Diagnosis 9. Philadelphia: WB Saunders, 1997, pp 227–230.
This is a concise review of the clinical manifestations and management of pneumocystis pneumonia.

Glassock RJ, Cohen AH, Danovitch G, Parsa KP: Human immunodeficiency virus infection and the kidney. Ann Intern Med 112:35–49, 1990.
This is a classic review of the renal complications of HIV infection.

Horsburgh CR Jr: Mycobacterium avium complex in the acquired immunodeficiency syndrome. N Engl J Med 324:1332–1338, 1991.

Lane GP, Lucas CR, Smallwood RA: The gastrointestinal and hepatic manifestations of the acquired immune deficiency syndrome. Med J Aust 150:139–143, 1989.
This is an older, but still clinically current, review of the gastrointestinal and hepatic complications of HIV infection.

Moss AR, Bachetti P: Natural history of HIV infection. AIDS 3:55–61, 1989.
This is an overview of the clinical course of HIV infection prior to the era of antiretroviral therapy.

Piscitelli SC, Flexner C, Minor JR, et al: Drug interactions in patients infected with human immunodeficiency virus. Clin Infect Dis 23:685–693, 1996.
This is the first comprehensive review of drug-drug interactions potentially encountered by HIV patients. Updated versions are available on the web at: www.medscape.com/Medscape/HIV/DrugInteractions.

Price RW, Worley JM: Neurological complications of HIV-1 infection and AIDS. In: Broder S, Merigan TC Jr, Bolognesi D (eds): Textbook of AIDS Medicine. Baltimore: Williams & Wilkins, 1994, pp 489–505.
This is an excellent review of the neurologic complications of HIV infection, with 193 references.

Selik RM, Chu SY, Ward JW: Trends in infectious diseases and cancers among persons dying of HIV infection in the United States from 1987 to 1992. Ann Intern Med 123:933–956, 1995.
This CDC report describes changes in the incidence of HIV-related complications following the introduction of antiretroviral therapy.

18 Care of the Cancer Patient with Neutropenia or Thrombocytopenia

Victor M. Aviles
Kevin R. Fox

Patients with pre-existing or newly diagnosed malignancy present special challenges to the intensive care unit (ICU) provider. Among them are the wide variety of clinical presentations and treatment modalities. The latter can result in toxicities predisposing patients to potentially life-threatening events, such as infection and hemorrhage. This chapter reviews the issues surrounding management of the critically ill cancer patient with neutropenia or thrombocytopenia.

CLINICAL DISORDERS

Neutropenia

Neutropenia is generally described as *moderate* when fewer than 1000 neutrophils/μL are present and *severe* when there are less than 500 neutrophils/μL. Neutropenia may occur as a result of various oncologic conditions or their treatment (Table 18–1). Neutropenia confers an increased risk of infection and, in the setting of fever, represents a medical emergency. Both the degree and duration of neutropenia affect the risk of infection.

Among hematologic malignancies, acute myelogenous and acute lymphoblastic leukemia are most commonly accompanied by the rapid onset of systemic illness. Neutropenia in these diseases reflects suppression of normal hematopoiesis by the clonal expansion of leukemic cells in the bone marrow. Under these circumstances, neutropenia does not resolve spontaneously until the underlying condition is treated. However, the treatment itself induces a profound neutropenia generally lasting from 14 to 21 days. The most common cause of neutropenia in patients

Table 18–1. Neutropenia in the Cancer Patient: Differential Diagnosis

Decreased production (common)
    Acute and chronic leukemias
    Chemotherapy (most common)
    Infection
    Marrow infiltration by carcinoma
    Nutritional deficiency
Excess Destruction (uncommon)
    Autoimmune granulocyte destruction
    Drug toxicity

with solid tumors is the chemotherapy used to treat their disease. Conventional doses of chemotherapy given for solid tumors and malignant lymphoma typically produce a nadir in the leukocyte count between 7 and 14 days after administration, depending on the drugs. The duration of the nadir usually ranges from 3 to 10 days and is nearly always followed by full granulocyte recovery.

Thrombocytopenia

Thrombocytopenia is generally defined as fewer than 150,000 platelets/μL, but it does not contribute to clinical bleeding unless the platelet count is less than 50,000/μL. Furthermore, the risk of spontaneous bleeding events, ranging from mild mucosal bleeding, epistaxis, or petechiae, to severe events, such as fulminant gastrointestinal bleeding or intracranial hemorrhage, is not generally seen until the platelet count falls *to less than 20,000/μL*. Thrombocytopenia, like neutropenia, can be a manifestation of oncologic disease or its therapy (Table 18–2). Occasionally, bleeding in the setting of thrombocytopenia represents a hematologic disorder such as disseminated intravascular coagulation (DIC) in acute promyelocytic leukemia. Certain types of chemotherapy, for example, the nitrosoureas and mitomycin, are particularly toxic to megakaryocytes.

Bone Marrow Transplantation

The increasing use of high-dose chemotherapy programs has expanded the intensive care of cancer patients. In autologous and allogeneic bone marrow transplantation, the concept of the nadir period in the blood counts produced by conventional doses of chemotherapy is replaced by the concepts of complete *ablation* of the bone marrow and *engraftment*. In contrast to temporary bone marrow suppression, various combinations of high-dose chemotherapy and total body irradiation are intended to produce permanent ablation of the bone marrow and, it is hoped, the primary malignant disease. The bone marrow is then reconstituted through engraftment by hematopoietic elements (either bone marrow or peripheral stem

---

Table 18–2. Thrombocytopenia in the Cancer Patient: Differential Diagnosis

Decreased production
  Chemotherapy
  Hematologic malignancies
  Infiltration of bone marrow by carcinoma
Increased destruction
  Disseminated intravascular coagulation
  Drug reactions
  Immune thrombocytopenic purpura (Chapter 63)
  Sepsis
  Splenic sequestration
  Thrombotic thrombocytopenic purpura (Chapter 63)

cells) derived either from the patient before the ablative treatment (autologous) or from a compatible donor (allogeneic). After the bone marrow or stem cell rescue is delivered, a period of 1 to 3 weeks of severe granulocytopenia and thrombocytopenia occurs before the subsequent return of appreciable neutrophil and platelet counts.

DIAGNOSTIC EVALUATION

The assessment of the cancer patient with neutropenia or thrombocytopenia in the ICU begins with a thorough history and physical examination. These patients are admitted to an ICU typically for one or more of three reasons. First, septic physiology and hypotension from infections in neutropenic patients may mandate pressor support. Second, respiratory failure from complications of sepsis or opportunistic pulmonary infections, or both, may require ventilatory support. Third, uncontrolled thrombocytopenic bleeding may require an ICU level of medical care for the maintenance of hemodynamic stability via transfusion therapy. Individual patients may present with two or three of these features simultaneously. Pre-existing cancer diagnoses and the timing and types of all cancer therapies must be carefully documented, and a reasonable assessment of the likely duration of the neutropenia and thrombocytopenia should be made. Physical examination should include careful inspection of the retinas, oral mucous membranes, and the entire skin for evidence of petechiae or active bleeding. The perirectal soft tissues must be examined because they are a common site of occult infection in neutropenic patients. Subtle pulmonary findings that are as simple as mild rales, pleural rubs, or wheezing may herald an opportunistic pulmonary infection such as fungal pneumonia, for example, invasive aspergillosis. Hepatomegaly may occur in fungal or viral hepatitis, and splenomegaly should be noted. All indwelling intravenous catheter sites should be carefully inspected for local inflammation. Evidence of active dental or sinus infection should be sought as part of the routine physical examination.

Review of the peripheral blood smear is essential to confirm neutropenia or thrombocytopenia. This may provide important diagnostic clues, especially in hematologic malignancy and disorders such as thrombotic thrombocytopenic purpura. Laboratory parameters for DIC should be evaluated in cases of unexplained thrombocytopenia or bleeding. These parameters include the prothrombin time, partial thromboplastin time, fibrinogen, and fibrin split products. Bone marrow aspiration and biopsy generally are not required if the pre-existing oncologic diagnosis is known, but these procedures are mandatory if no oncologic diagnosis has been established or if the neutropenia or thrombocytopenia is unexplained.

CLINICAL MANAGEMENT

The complex issues surrounding ICU management of cancer patients with neutropenia or thrombocytopenia require close cooperation between the oncologist and the ICU providers, both to establish the goals of therapy and to execute treatment plans.

Febrile Neutropenia

Febrile neutropenia is defined as a temperature of greater than 38.0° C (100.5° F) with fewer than 1000 neutrophils/μL. Prompt evaluation and institution of antibiotics is required (Fig. 18–1). Because it may be rapidly fatal, infection with gramnegative bacteria in the setting of febrile neutropenia should *always* be assumed to be present when neutropenic patients become febrile for the first time. In the absence of an identifiable source of fever, *normotensive* patients may be treated initially with a single agent—a third-generation cephalosporin such as ceftazidime, or an extended spectrum semisynthetic penicillin, for example, piperacillin (the exact choice depends on the pattern of resistance of gram-negative bacilli in one's hospital), plus an aminoglycoside (see Chapter 14). In general, patients requiring ICU management should be considered for *double coverage* if that has not already

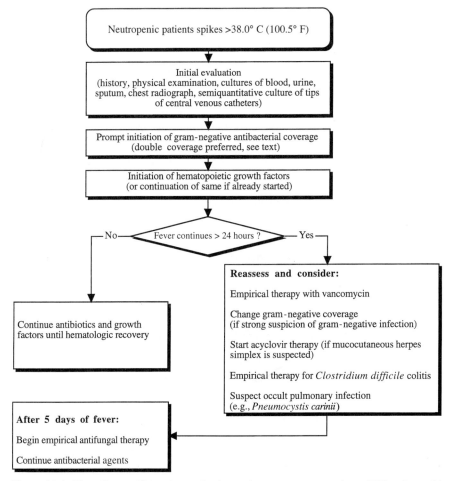

Figure 18–1. Flow diagram illustrating evaluation and management steps in an ICU patient with neutropenia and fever.

been instituted. Penicillin-allergic patients should receive a quinolone, for example, ofloxacin, in combination with an aminoglycoside. Antibacterial therapy is generally not altered until 48 hours of persistent fever has elapsed. Unstable patients require more prompt adjustments. Persistent fever (i.e., persisting for more than 48 hours) despite appropriate gram-negative coverage mandates either alteration of gram-negative coverage or the addition of agents appropriate for gram-positive or fungal infections. Ongoing re-evaluation of the persistently febrile patient is mandatory and is accomplished by frequently obtaining blood and urine cultures during febrile episodes and by repeated and thorough physical examinations. In general, the cessation of antibiotics is discouraged until the patient becomes afebrile and has full neutrophil recovery, even in the absence of an identifiable fever source. Repeated chest radiographs should be performed routinely in the persistently febrile neutropenic patient, and special studies such as computed tomograms of the chest, abdomen, and sinuses should be considered if there is a high index of suspicion of infectious sources in these sites.

The patient who remains persistently febrile despite initial gram-negative coverage poses a unique challenge to the ICU staff. The presence of gram-positive infections with skin flora is a common source of persistent fever. Vancomycin is the agent of choice for suspected gram-positive catheter infections and may obviate the need for surgical removal of an infected catheter. However, hemodynamic instability mandates prompt removal if there is an obviously infected catheter. Gram-positive coverage alone, however, does not constitute appropriate antibacterial management in a febrile neutropenic patient and should never be instituted to the exclusion of gram-negative coverage.

Metronidazole is frequently added to antibacterial regimens when diarrhea develops in persistent febrile neutropenia or if an intra-abdominal infectious source is suspected. Although anaerobic infections are relatively rare in neutropenic hosts, infection with *Clostridium difficile* should always be considered in the febrile neutropenic patient with diarrhea. It is treated with oral or intravenous metronidazole or with oral vancomycin (see Chapter 35). Finally, viral infections must be considered as a source of persistent fever, with herpes simplex mucopharyngitis a common source of fever in the leukemic or bone marrow transplant patient. Acyclovir therapy is given either orally or intravenously until full granulocyte recovery. Infections with cytomegalovirus are less common but should be considered as a possible source of unexplained fever in all patients. These infections may present as an unexplained pneumonia, hepatitis, mucoesophagitis, or cutaneous eruption.

After 5 days of persistent neutropenic fever despite broad spectrum coverage by both gram-negative and gram-positive antibacterial agents, the risk of systemic fungal infection increases markedly. The types of fungal infections seen in prolonged neutropenia vary from hospital to hospital, but species of *Aspergillus* and *Candida* are common offenders. Amphotericin B is the drug of choice and should be instituted empirically even in the absence of documented fungal infection. Empirical therapy is usually begun at a dose of 0.5 mg/kg/day, although documented fungemia or a prior history of fungal infection may require starting treatment with 1 mg/kg/day. The patient who begins empirical amphotericin B therapy should remain under close observation for a fungal infectious source, with close attention to the lungs and sinuses *(Aspergillus)* and skin and liver *(Candida)*. Ophthalmic examination for candidal retinitis has low sensitivity but high specificity. The role of oral antifungal agents such as fluconazole is primarily prophylactic and should not be considered an adequate substitute for amphotericin B.

Opportunistic pulmonary infections, such as pneumonia due to *Pneumocystis carinii*, require targeted antibiotic therapy, for example, trimethoprim-sulfamethoxazole or pentamidine. *P. carinii* pneumonia can be difficult to diagnose in the cancer patient, whose burden of organisms tends to be small but who may have rapidly progressive clinical symptoms.

Growth Factors and Other Hematologic Therapy for Neutropenia

Growth factors for neutrophils such as filgrastim (originally called granulocyte-colony stimulating factor, or G-CSF) have become critical adjuncts in oncologic care. Filgrastim has been shown to decrease the duration and severity of chemotherapy-induced neutropenia if administered *after* chemotherapy and *before* the granulocyte nadir. The drug is administered daily until greater than 1000 neutrophils/μL are present on 3 successive days. The standard dose is 5 μg/kg subcutaneously daily, although bone marrow transplant patients commonly receive higher doses after myeloablative therapy. Patients admitted to the ICU may already have been receiving growth factors before the development of neutropenia and fever, and these growth factors should be continued uninterrupted. The role of growth factors given only *after* the development of neutropenia is unclear, and several randomized studies have failed to demonstrate significant benefit to their addition in this setting. However, the critically ill patient in the ICU who has febrile neutropenia and has not yet received growth factors will suffer no additional harm from their use. Under these circumstances, it is reasonable to commence such therapy and to continue it until the neutropenia resolves.

The role of *granulocyte transfusions* has diminished greatly in this era of aggressively administered broad spectrum antibiotics. However, a patient should be considered a candidate for granulocyte transfusions if he or she meets the following criteria: (1) has a *documented* bacterial or fungal infection, (2) is failing to improve after at least 48 hours of appropriate antimicrobial therapy, and (3) is expected to remain neutropenic for 7 days or more.

Therapy for Thrombocytopenia

Platelet transfusions are commonly given in oncologic care. They are generally given empirically and in the absence of clinical bleeding under a variety of circumstances (Table 18–3). Not all cancer patients require platelet transfusions for thrombocytopenia. In certain disorders, platelet transfusions may be *contraindicated*. For instance, patients with DIC require prompt identification and treatment of reversible inciting causes, for example, sepsis or acute promyelocytic leukemia. These patients may also require measures to control the primary manifestation of the DIC (bleeding or thrombosis). Bleeding patients with DIC should receive aggressive repletion of clotting factors with fresh frozen plasma and cryoprecipitate in addition to platelets. Patients with DIC who have evidence of clotting or who continue to bleed despite factor repletion may need heparin as well.

Table 18–3. Management of Thrombocytopenia: Indications for Platelet Transfusion

Patients with *Decreased Production* as Cause of Thrombocytopenia

Platelet count <10,000–20,000/μL*
Platelet count <30,000/μL before lumbar puncture
Platelet count <40,000/μL before central venous catheter placement, dental extraction, or other
 moderately invasive procedure
Platelet count <50,000/μL before major surgery
Hyperleukocytosis in acute leukemia (blast count >100,000/μL) *and* <50,000 platelets/μL

Patients Whose Thrombocytopenia Is due to *Peripheral Destruction*

No routine transfusions unless:
There is significant ongoing bleeding, particularly intracranial bleeding
Heparin is being administered for active disseminated intravascular coagulation in acute
 promyelocytic leukemia with platelet count <40,000/μL.

*In absence of bleeding; if bleeding is present, keep platelet count >50,000/μL.

In the typical cancer patient, whose thrombocytopenia is due to chemotherapy-induced megakaryocyte suppression, platelets should be given in quantities of approximately 6 units daily to maintain a platelet count of 10,000 to 20,000/μL if there is no evidence of bleeding or a count greater than 50,000/μL if active bleeding is present (see Table 18–3). Patients receiving platelet transfusions for the first time usually receive a "random donor" product and should continue to receive this type of platelet product as long as it remains effective. The effectiveness of a given platelet transfusion is assessed by obtaining a post-transfusion platelet count, for example, one obtained 60 minutes after the transfusion is complete. An effective platelet transfusion should produce an increase in the platelet count of 60,000 platelets/μL per every 6 units of random donor platelets transfused (or per 1 unit of single-donor or HLA-matched platelets). Patients who require repeated platelet transfusions may experience alloimmunization, leading to increasing refractoriness to random donor platelets. At this juncture, close cooperation with the hospital's transfusion services becomes mandatory. Patients who are refractory to random donor platelets often receive "single-donor" platelets as the next therapeutic alternative. Once they are refractory to single-donor platelets, HLA-matched or cross-matched HLA platelets may be needed to achieve an acceptable increment in the platelet count. Alloimmunized patients typically have increments of 20,000 to 30,000/μL per platelet transfusion. Ineffectiveness of a particular platelet product is defined as two consecutive documented failures to gain increments of greater than 10,000/μL per transfusion. Once all forms of platelet transfusion become ineffective, and other causes of thrombocytopenia have been carefully excluded, a trial of intravenous immunoglobulin may be warranted, especially in the patient who continues to manifest a bleeding tendency. Intravenous immunoglobulin doses of 400 mg/kg per day for 5 consecutive days have occasionally been reported to reduce platelet refractoriness.

CLINICAL PITFALLS

Table 18–4 lists the common clinical pitfalls encountered in the neutropenic and thrombocytopenic patient in the ICU. Of these, failure to institute Gram-negative

Table 18–4. Common Pitfalls in the Management of Neutropenia and Thrombocytopenia Applicable to the Patient with Cancer in the Intensive Care Unit

....

Failure to administer empirical antibacterial therapy immediately at first fever
Failure to make timely alterations in antibacterial therapy in persistent neutropenic fever
Failure to remain vigilant for nonbacterial causes of persistent fever, e.g., fungal or viral infection, drugs, tumor
Failure to initiate antifungal therapy after 5 days of persistent fever
Failure to rule out disseminated intravascular coagulation or thrombocytopenic purpura before initiation of platelet transfusions
Failure to assess responses to platelet transfusions and subsequent failure to recognize alloimmunization

....

antibiotic coverage within an hour of the first fever in neutropenia is of the most concern. A second concern is giving platelet transfusions empirically in thrombocytopenic patients who may have thrombotic thrombocytopenic purpura or DIC, conditions in which platelet transfusions are contraindicated or ineffective.

BIBLIOGRAPHY

Fenaux P: Management of acute promyelocytic leukemia. Eur J Haematol 50:65–73, 1993.
A review of acute promyelocytic leukemia, with a concise section on the management of the coagulation disorders associated with this condition.

Lee EJ, Schiffer CA: Transfusion supportive care. In: MacDonald J, Haller D, Mayer R (eds): Manual of Oncologic Therapeutics, 3rd ed. Philadelphia, JB Lippincott, 1995, pp 438–443.
A concise review of the principles of platelet and granulocyte transfusion, with an excellent summary of alloimmunization concepts.

Maher DW, Lieschke GJ, Green M, et al: Filgrastim in patients with chemotherapy-induced febrile neutropenia. Ann Intern Med 121:492–501, 1994.
A randomized trial of considerable size, demonstrating the beneficial effects of granulocyte colony-stimulating hormone given after the development of febrile neutropenia. The benefit was most pronounced in patients with severe neutropenia.

Mayordomo J, Rivera F, Diaz-Puente M, et al: Improving treatment of chemotherapy-induced neutropenic fever by administration of colony stimulating factors. J Natl Cancer Inst 87:803, 1995.
A randomized trial of colony-stimulating factors given after the development of neutropenic fever rather than before. A small benefit in the length of hospital stay and the duration of fever is suggested.

Pizzo P, Hathorn J, Hiemenz J, et al: A randomized trial comparing ceftazidime alone with combination antibiotic therapy in cancer patients with fever and neutropenia. N Engl J Med 315:552–558, 1986.
One of the first demonstrations of the adequacy of single-antibiotic therapy of neutropenic fever in a non-ICU population of cancer patients.

Pizzo P, Meyers J, Freifeld A, Walsh T: Infections in the cancer patient. In: DeVita V, Hellman S, Rosenberg S (eds): Cancer: Principles and Practice of Oncology, 4th ed. Philadelphia, JB Lippincott, 1993, pp 2292–2337.
The definitive and exhaustive reference on all aspects of infection management in cancer patients by the recognized authorities in the field.

Care of the Patient with End-Stage Liver Disease

Frederick A. Nunes

End-stage liver disease (ESLD) is a term that encompasses the clinical manifestations associated with advanced cirrhosis. The term is used irrespective of the cause of the cirrhosis. The complications of ESLD include variceal hemorrhage, ascites, peritonitis, encephalopathy, and the hepatorenal syndrome. These conditions may precipitate admission to the intensive care unit (ICU) or complicate the stay of patients in the ICU who are admitted because of another condition. Prompt identification and effective ICU management of these complications can decrease morbidity and mortality as well as serve as temporizing measures for patients awaiting liver transplantation.

VARICEAL HEMORRHAGE

Active upper gastrointestinal (GI) bleeding in a patient with ESLD requires prompt evaluation and treatment. Up to 50% of patients with ESLD and varices who present with GI bleeding have a source of hemorrhage other than the varices. The management of variceal bleeding differs markedly from other causes of upper GI hemorrhage (Fig. 19–1 and Chapter 61). Therefore, endoscopy is critical for identifying the source of bleeding and directing appropriate treatment.

Approximately one third of patients with varices bleed from them within 2 to 5 years. Patients who have never bled from esophageal varices are candidates for nonselective beta-blockade prophylaxis. This is especially helpful in modified Child's class A and B patients (Table 19–1). Propranolol or naldolol is administered with the goal of decreasing the resting heart rate 25% to a minimum of 60 beats per minute.

The mortality rate from variceal bleeding is based on a modified Child's classification (see Table 19–1). Class A has a mortality rate of 5%, class B, 25% or less, and class C, 50% or more. The risk of recurrent variceal bleeding is increased during the first 6 weeks after the initial bleeding episode, particularly during the first several days. The goal of ICU management is to stop variceal bleeding, prevent recurrent bleeding, and avoid complications, which can include infection, decompensated liver function, aspiration pneumonia, acute renal failure, peritonitis, and encephalopathy.

Patients with ESLD who are actively bleeding should be resuscitated with intravenous fluids and blood products. Packed red blood cells are transfused to keep the patient's hemoglobin level at greater than 9.0 g/dL. Fresh frozen plasma and platelets are transfused when the patient has a coagulopathy, usually as a result of impaired hepatic synthetic function and splenic sequestration of platelets. Airway protection with intubation may be required because of massive bleeding or hepatic encephalopathy. Based on a recent meta-analysis by Bernard and coworkers, antibiotic prophylaxis, for example, ciprofloxacin 1000 mg/day for 7

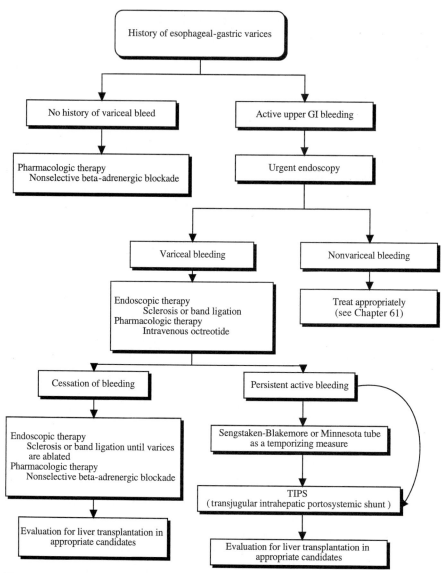

Figure 19–1. Schematic flow diagram for the management of patients with portal varices. GI, gastrointestinal.

days, should be considered for patients with cirrhosis with acute variceal bleeding (after the appropriate cultures, e.g., ascitic fluid, urine, and blood, have been obtained).

Endoscopic therapy for bleeding esophageal varices with sclerosis or band ligation is effective at stopping bleeding in more than 80% of cases. Pharmacologic therapy for bleeding esophageal varices with intravenous octreotide has supplanted the combination of intravenous vasopressin and nitroglycerin in most centers.

Table 19–1. Criteria for Points for Child-Turcotte-Pugh ("Child's") Score*

POINTS	1	2	3
Encephalopathy†	None	Grade I or II	Grade III or IV
Ascites	Absent	Slight‡	Moderate or severe
Bilirubin§ (mg/dL)	1–2	2–3	>3
Albumin (g/dL)	>3.5	2.8–3.5	<2.8
Prothrombin time (seconds prolonged)	1–4	4–6	>6
or INR	<1.7	1.8–2.3	>2.3

*Total score: class A = 1–6; class B = 7–9; class C = 10–15.
†See Table 59–2 for criteria for grades I to IV.
‡May be controlled by diuretics.
§If patient has primary biliary cirrhosis or primary sclerosing cholangitis, bilirubin of 1–4 mg/dL counts for 1 point, 4–10 mg/dL counts for 2 points, and >10 mg/dL counts for 3 points.
INR, internationalized ratio.

Octreotide is administered as a 50-μg intravenous bolus followed by a 50-μg/hour continuous infusion for 48 hours. In contrast to the cardiac complications (myocardial ischemia and infarction) of vasopressin, octreotide has minimal side effects.

A Minnesota or Sengstaken-Blakemore tube may be inserted as a temporizing measure when endoscopic and pharmacologic therapies have failed. A transjugular intrahepatic portosystemic shunt (TIPS) is a stent between branches of the portal and hepatic veins placed by a transjugular angiographic approach. The indications for TIPS placement are still evolving, but it appears useful as a treatment of initial variceal bleeding and variceal bleeding that is refractory to endoscopic and pharmacologic therapy. Hemorrhage from gastric varices is an indication for TIPS placement, as endoscopic management has limited efficacy. Complications of TIPS include encephalopathy, hepatic decompensation, hepatic capsule rupture, and intra-abdominal bleeding.

The risk of long-term rebleeding is decreased by ablating the esophageal varices with repeated banding or sclerotherapy treatments. Pharmacologic therapy alone is given to patients with varices that have not yet bled.

ASCITES

Ascites is easily diagnosed when the abdomen is distended with a large amount of fluid. In less obvious cases, abdominal ultrasonography is a sensitive means of detecting free intraperitoneal fluid. Abdominal paracentesis should be performed in all ICU patients with new-onset ascites. Ascitic fluid should be routinely sent for cell count, albumin, total protein, and bacterial culture. In the absence of disseminated intravascular coagulation or primary fibrinolysis, prophylactic transfusions of fresh frozen plasma or platelets before paracentesis are not usually necessary.

Ascites is best characterized by calculating the serum-ascites albumin gradient (SAAG) from samples obtained on the same day. The presence of portal hypertension is suggested by a SAAG greater than or equal to 1.1 g/dL.

Table 19–2. Ascites: Causes, Treatment and Pitfalls

....

Precipitating Causes

Hepatocellular carcinoma, metastatic carcinoma
Noncompliance with diuretic therapy
Noncompliance with sodium restriction
Portal vein or hepatic vein thrombosis
Spontaneous bacterial peritonitis

Treatment

Sodium restriction
Diuretic therapy
Large-volume paracentesis
Careful management of electrolytes and monitoring of renal function
Transjugular intrahepatic portosystemic shunt
Fluid restriction for low serum sodium (<130 mEq/L)
Transplantation

Pitfalls

Intravascular volume depletion
Metabolic derangements (hyponatremia, hypokalemia)
Hepatorenal syndrome

....

Multiple factors may precipitate ascites (Table 19–2). Medical management is effective in more than 90% of patients. In the ICU, it is important to avoid excessive sodium administration in intravenous fluids. For example, the volume of normal saline administered for 24 hours at a rate of 10 mL/hour, intended to keep an intravenous catheter open, contains 2.2 g of sodium chloride.

Spironolactone is the predominant diuretic used in ESLD. Because of a prolonged half-life of the drug and its metabolites, spironolactone may be administered once a day (generally initiated at a dose of 50 mg once per day). Furosemide at a dose of 20 mg once per day may be added to increase diuresis. While monitoring serum electrolytes and renal function, diuretics may be adjusted at 3- to 4-day intervals to a maximum of spironolactone 400 mg/day and furosemide 160 mg/day. If painful gynecomastia or other side effects occur from spironolactone therapy, amiloride, starting at 5 mg/day to a maximum of 40 mg/day, may be substituted. Large-volume paracentesis (4 to 6 L) may provide symptomatic relief in patients with ascites that is difficult to manage with diuretics. A TIPS procedure may improve ascites but worsen hepatic function, especially in patients with low hepatic reserve.

SPONTANEOUS BACTERIAL PERITONITIS

One must maintain a high index of suspicion with regard to spontaneous bacterial peritonitis (SBP) in ICU patients with ESLD (Table 19–3). Patients at risk for SBP include those with poor hepatic function, GI bleeding, decreased total ascitic fluid protein, and prior episodes of SBP. SBP rarely presents with severe abdominal pain or peritoneal signs. Nonspecific clinical deterioration, such as slight deterioration in mental status, chills, mild fever, mild leukocytosis, abdominal discomfort,

Table 19–3. Spontaneous Bacterial Peritonitis

Presenting Symptoms and Signs

Fever
Encephalopathy
Abdominal pain
Peritoneal signs
Worsening ascites in a stable patient
Hypotension
Renal failure
Acidosis
Peripheral leukocytosis

Diagnosis

Paracentesis (neutrophil count $>250/\mu L$ or positive bacterial
    culture for a single pathogen)

Treatment

Initial: Third-generation cephalosporin (avoid aminoglycosides)
Subsequent: As guided by culture results

or a combination of these conditions, may be its only presenting sign. A peritoneal fluid cell count greater than 250 neutrophils/μL suggests SBP. Inoculation of blood culture bottles with peritoneal fluid at the bedside is the most effective means of isolating the causative organism. The usual organisms causing SBP are streptococcal species (*Streptococcus pneumoniae*) and Gram-negative organisms (*Escherichia coli, Klebsiella pneumoniae*). A single organism is typically responsible for SBP. If multiple organisms are grown on culture medium, or if there is a marked peritoneal fluid leukocytosis, a secondary peritonitis due to an intestinal perforation or intra-abdominal abscess should be considered rather than SBP. Five to ten days of treatment with a third-generation cephalosporin is effective in controlling most episodes of SBP. Aminoglycosides should be avoided because of the increased risk of nephrotoxicity. SBP has a mortality rate approaching 30% and a 1-year recurrence rate of about 70%. Effective prophylaxis against SBP includes an oral quinolone—for example, norfloxacin, 400 mg daily—or trimethoprin (160 mg)-sulfamethoxazole (800 mg) administered 5 days per week. Prophylaxis should be considered for all patients with a prior episode of peritonitis and for those whose ascites has a low total protein level (<1 g/dL).

HEPATIC ENCEPHALOPATHY

Hepatic encephalopathy is a disturbance in cerebral function in the setting of liver disease (Table 19–4). The pathogenesis of hepatic encephalopathy is controversial but appears to be due to hepatically cleared toxins that impair brain function by poorly defined mechanisms. Altered cerebral function ranges from mild disturbances in thought or affect to deep coma. The degree of disturbance is generally graded on a four-stage clinical scale (see Chapter 59, Table 59–2).

The diagnosis of hepatic encephalopathy is usually made on clinical grounds. Serum ammonia levels are often elevated in patients with hepatic encephalopathy.

Table 19–4. Hepatic Encephalopathy in Patients with End-Stage Liver Disease: Causes, Treatment, and Pitfalls

Precipitating Causes

GI bleeding (avoid NSAIDs, aspirin)
Sepsis
Peritonitis
Toxins (acetaminophen, ethanol)
Constipation
Azotemia
Noncompliance with diet (protein restriction)
Noncompliance with medical therapy
Medications (benzodiazepines, opioids, other sedatives or tranquilizers)

Treatment

Lactulose orally (or, if not possible, by enemas)
Treat infection
Protein restriction (limit of 60–80 g/day)
Neomycin orally (in addition to lactulose in refractory cases)

Pitfalls

Do not diagnose hepatic encephalopathy based solely on the presence of elevated serum ammonia levels
Exclude other causes for a change in mental status (hypoglycemia, head trauma, meningitis, encephalitis, drug toxicity, toxins, and seizures) (see Chapter 31)

GI, gastrointestinal; NSAIDs, nonsteroidal anti-inflammatory drugs.

However, these levels correlate poorly with the degree of hepatic encephalopathy. It is important to exclude other causes for a change in mental status, such as hypoglycemia, head trauma, meningitis, encephalitis, drug toxicity, toxins (such as alcohol), and seizures.

An important goal of hepatic encephalopathy therapy is the identification and correction of precipitating causes that may occur alone or in combination. Encephalopathy may be the first clinically apparent sign of GI bleeding or sepsis. If ascites is present, a paracentesis should be performed to exclude SBP.

Treatment with oral lactulose is administered initially at high doses (30 mL every hour) until a stool is passed. Once the first stool is passed, lactulose dosage is decreased to 30 mL every 6 to 8 hours and titrated to achieve a maximum of three to four soft, formed bowel movements per day. If lactulose cannot be administered orally, it may be administered as an enema.

Dietary protein restriction is imposed until the encephalopathy resolves. Most patients can be managed with titrated lactulose therapy and modest protein restriction (60 to 80 g protein per day). Neomycin, an antibiotic poorly absorbed from the intestine, may be added in patients who do not respond to lactulose therapy and protein restriction, but ototoxicity is a potential side effect of its use.

HEPATORENAL SYNDROME

Renal insufficiency in patients with ESLD is a common problem in the ICU. It is important to avoid conditions and medications that may precipitate renal insufficiency, such as hypovolemia, nonsteroidal anti-inflammatory drugs, and aminoglycosides. When renal insufficiency develops in the ICU patient with ESLD, the most common conditions are acute tubular necrosis, prerenal azotemia, and the hepatorenal syndrome (see Chapter 37). Analysis of urine electrolytes (urine Na >10 mEq/L) and examination of the urine sediment (presence of casts) can usually differentiate acute tubular necrosis from the other two conditions. The characteristics of the urine from patients with hepatorenal syndrome are indistinguishable from those with hypovolemia. Differentiation between these two conditions depends on an assessment of intravascular status. However, this may be difficult to do in patients with ESLD. In most cases, one gives a fluid challenge and observes the response. In some cases, a pulmonary artery catheter may be needed to answer the question definitively.

The diagnostic criteria for the hepatorenal syndrome include: (1) a low glomerular filtration rate, (2) absence of infection or nephrotoxic drugs, (3) no response to fluid challenge, (4) no proteinuria and no obstruction, (5) urine volume less than 500 mL/day with urinary sodium less than 10 mEq/L, and (6) urine osmolality greater than plasma osmolality. Although the hepatorenal syndrome has a poor prognosis, it is generally reversible with liver transplantation. Diuretics should be discontinued and dialysis considered as a temporizing measure for patients awaiting liver transplantation.

CONCLUSION

Patients in the ICU with ESLD require special attention. Myriad problems may precipitate their admission to the ICU or complicate their course when admitted for another condition. Prompt identification and effective management of these problems, including variceal hemorrhage, ascites, peritonitis, encephalopathy, and the hepatorenal syndrome, can decrease their associated morbidity and mortality.

BIBLIOGRAPHY

Angeli P, Volpin R, Gerunda G, et al: Reversal of type 1 hepatorenal syndrome with the administration of midodrine and octreotide. Hepatology 29:1690–1697, 1999.
  This pilot study suggested that combined administration of midodrine and octreotide plus albumin infusions has promise in the treatment of the hepatorenal syndrome. These results need confirmation in larger, blinded clinical trials.

Arroyo V, Gines P, Gerbes A, et al: Definition and diagnostic criteria of refractory ascites and hepatorenal syndrome in cirrhosis. Hepatology 23:164–176, 1996.
  Review of the pathogenesis and treatment of ascites and mechanisms of renal dysfunction in cirrhosis.

Bernard B, Grangé J-D, Khac EN, et al: Antibiotic prophylaxis for the prevention of bacterial infections in cirrhotic patients with gastrointestinal bleeding: a meta-analysis. Hepatology 29:1655–1661, 1999.
  This meta-analysis compared 264 cirrhotic patients with gastrointestinal bleeding treated prophylactically with a broad-spectrum antibiotic(s), such as fluoroquinolone, to 270 patients who did not receive such treatment. Prophylactic antibiotics significantly improved the proportion of patients free of infections (by 32% with 95% confidence interval [CI] of 22–42%) and short-term survival (by 9% with 95% CI of 2.9–15.3%).

Besson I, Ingrand P, Person B, et al: Sclerotherapy with or without octreotide for acute variceal bleeding. N Engl J Med 333:555–560, 1995.
Sclerotherapy with octreotide is more effective in controlling acute variceal hemorrhage but does not alter overall mortality compared with sclerotherapy alone.

Chung RT, Jaffe DL, Friedman LS: Complications of chronic liver disease. Crit Care Clin 11:431–463, 1995.
This is a review directed at intensivists.

D'Amico G, Pagliaro L, Bosch J: The treatment of portal hypertension: A meta-analytic review. Hepatology 22:332–354, 1995.
This is a meta-analysis on treating portal hypertension.

Riordan SM, Williams R: Treatment of hepatic encephalopathy. N Engl J Med 337:473–479, 1997.
Practical review focused on mechanisms-directed therapy of hepatic encephalopathy in patients with ESLD.

Rossle M, Haag K, Ochs A, et al: The transjugular intrahepatic portosystemic stent-shunt procedure for variceal bleeding. N Engl J Med 330:165–171, 1994.
This is an early description of TIPS.

Runyon BA: Treatment of patients with cirrhosis and ascites. Semin Liver Dis 17:249–260, 1997.
This is an authoritative review of ascites management by an expert in the field.

Runyon B, Montano A, Akriviadis E, et al: The serum-ascites albumin gradient is superior to the exudate-transudate concept in the differential diagnosis of ascites. Ann Intern Med 117:215–220, 1992.
The serum-ascites albumin gradient accurately differentiated causes of ascites due to portal hypertension from those due to other disorders.

20 Care of the Patient with End-Stage Renal Disease

Alan G. Wasserstein

End-stage renal disease (ESRD) or its treatment influences virtually every aspect of critical care. ESRD designates advanced renal failure in which hemodialysis (HD), peritoneal dialysis (PD), or a renal allograft is required to ameliorate symptoms and prolong life. However, dialysis does not completely correct the complex derangements of uremia, and both dialysis and immunosuppressive treatment for renal transplantation introduce additional risks of their own.

COMMON PROBLEMS IN PATIENTS WITH END-STAGE RENAL DISEASE IN THE INTENSIVE CARE UNIT

Some aspects of ESRD contribute to the genesis of critical illnesses, whereas others complicate their management (Table 20–1).

Cardiovascular Complications

Fluid overload resulting from patient noncompliance with regular dialysis or from iatrogenic fluid administration should be distinguished from primary heart failure. Left ventricular hypertrophy is extremely common in dialysis patients, resulting primarily from chronic hypertension. It progresses to *diastolic dysfunction* (reduced left ventricular compliance) and ultimately to dilated cardiomyopathy with systolic dysfunction and hypotension.

Systolic dysfunction is rarely exacerbated by placement of an arteriovenous (AV) fistula (usually an upper arm fistula between the brachial artery and vein). Bradycardia during transient occlusion of an AV fistula is a specific but not sensitive marker of high-output heart failure (Branham sign). *Hypotension* complicates HD treatments in hemodynamically unstable intensive care unit (ICU) patients as well as in patients undergoing routine outpatient dialysis. This occurs because the normal homeostatic response to fluid removal, that is, vasoconstriction, is inadequate during HD. Hypotension, in turn, may result in vascular access thrombosis, usually in association with underlying stenosis of the venous anastomosis (Table 20–2).

Pulmonary edema may result from fluid overload, an episode of accelerated hypertension, or myocardial infarction, all of which are often superimposed on prior left ventricular dysfunction. Patients sometimes present with pulmonary edema caused by occult fluid overload. In these circumstances, the patient's body weight is maintained by fluid accumulation, and the loss of lean body mass is not recognized during outpatient care. *Coronary artery disease*, the leading cause of death in patients with ESRD, is due to ubiquitous hypertension and diverse

233

Table 20–1. Common Problems in Patients With End-Stage Renal Disease
in the Intensive Care Unit

....

Cardiovascular

Fluid overload with high intravenous fluid therapy
Left ventricular failure due to systolic and diastolic dysfunction
Coronary ischemia and ischemia-induced arrhythmias
Dialysis-induced hypotension

Hematologic

Anemia
Bleeding due to platelet dysfunction

Infection

Increased bacterial infections, especially at sites of dialysis access

Gastrointestinal

Bowel ischemia or obstruction
Gastroduodenitis
Pancreatitis

Neurologic

Encephalopathy
Seizures
Opioid sensitivity

Electrolyte Derangements

Hyponatremia
Hyper- and hypokalemia

Drug Dosing Problems

Excessive dosage
Inadequate dosage

....

metabolic abnormalities associated with uremia, including hyperhomocysteinemia, increased lipoprotein (a), and other abnormalities, rather than the uremia itself.

Pericarditis may precede the initiation of maintenance dialysis or it may occur in chronic dialysis patients. Although it sometimes arises in association with viral infection or a hypercatabolic state, it is most commonly due to inadequate dialysis.

Table 20–2. Treatment of Vascular Access Thrombosis

....

Perform emergency dialysis if necessary through a temporary venous catheter
In arteriovenous (AV) fistulas, clot removal (if attempted) must be performed urgently; in contrast, in
   AV grafts, removal can be delayed for up to 7–10 days
Clot is removed by surgical thrombectomy or by mechanical (wire) thrombolysis, usually by
   interventional radiologists; avoid thrombolytics if there is a bleeding risk
Thrombosed central venous catheters are treated by thrombolytic instillation or by mechanical
   thrombolysis, or replacement
After thrombectomy or thrombolysis, fistulography should be performed to detect an underlying
   vascular access stenosis

....

Pulmonary Complications

Uremic lung refers to putative increased pulmonary capillary leakiness in patients with ESRD, predisposing them to acute respiratory distress syndrome–like pulmonary edema at relatively low pulmonary capillary pressures. Clinical confirmation of this entity is lacking, and it may be due entirely to volume overload. *Pleural effusion* may be due to fluid overload, uremic serositis, tuberculosis (there is an increased incidence of reactivation of tuberculosis in ESRD patients), or diaphagmatic leak associated with PD. *Dyspnea during dialysis* can be due to dialysis-induced hypoxemia, which is generally modest (i.e., a reduction of PaO$_2$ of 10 to 15 mm Hg) but can be problematic in patients with chronic lung disease. Dyspnea can also be due to an anaphylactoid reaction to the dialyzer (first-use syndrome). Peritoneal dialysis fluid can elevate the diaphragm, especially when the patient is in the supine position, and can compromise ventilation in patients with pulmonary disease. *Sleep apnea syndrome* is also common in ESRD. These patients have an increased sensitivity to drugs that not only can worsen their sleep-disordered breathing but also can lead to respiratory depression.

Hematologic Complications

The *anemia* of ESRD is mainly due to deficiency of kidney-produced erythropoietin. Full response to recombinant erythropoietin requires 4 to 8 weeks, so it cannot be relied on to fully correct the anemia in the critically ill patient. In addition, inflammation, infection, and even minor surgery blunt the normal marrow response to erythropoietin to a remarkable degree. *Uremic bleeding* is due to defective platelet function. Measurement of bleeding time can be used to quantify bleeding risk, but its predictive power is limited. Although inadequate dialysis can increase the bleeding time, intensive dialysis may not result in complete correction. One reason is that anemia also increases bleeding time. At a hematocrit of less than 30%, platelets stream in the center of blood vessels away from the vessel wall.

Infectious Complications

Dialysis patients receiving *chronic dialysis* have decreased host defenses. For example, they have impaired granulocyte function, including chemotaxis, phagocytosis, and intracellular killing. They also have impaired lymphocyte function with defective antibody production and inadequate response to vaccines. These defects result from both the uremic state and exposure to bioincompatible dialysis membranes. Bioincompatibility connotes complement activation and cytokine release stimulated by exposure to the dialysis membrane. These changes in granulocyte and lymphocyte function in dialysis patients are manifested as increased susceptibility to common bacterial pathogens rather than to opportunistic pathogens, for example, *Pneumocystis carinii*. In contrast, patients with *renal allografts* are susceptible to both opportunistic infections and common bacterial pathogens because of the immunosuppressive therapy they receive.

Infected vascular access sites, especially central venous catheters, are the leading cause of bacteremia in dialysis patients. Offending organisms are usually staphylococci and streptococci but may include gram-negative rods. PD patients suffer from catheter-associated peritonitis, characterized by bouts of abdominal pain, an elevated peritoneal fluid white blood cell count (>100 cells/μL), and positive peritoneal fluid cultures with the same spectrum of pathogens as discussed previously. Urinary tract infections are also common in dialysis patients, including pyocystis (pus in the bladder) in anuric diabetic patients with neurogenic bladders.

Neurologic Complications

Uremic encephalopathy causes somnolence, confusion, seizures, and coma. Physical signs include hyperreflexia, asterixis, and myoclonus. Patients on maintenance HD may have unrecognized uremic encephalopathy due to access malfunction or noncompliance. Alterations in mental status may respond to intensive dialysis. *Subdural hematomas* may be spontaneous rather than traumatic. Both uremic platelet dysfunction and exposure to heparin during HD may contribute. Aluminum intoxication (dialysis dementia) and dialysis disequilibrium are now unusual with proper HD care. Metabolites of morphine or meperidine accumulate in renal failure; the latter causes seizures and its use should be avoided.

Gastrointestinal Complications

Dialysis patients have a high incidence of gastritis and nodular duodenitis. Peptic ulcer disease due to *Helicobacter pylori* is not increased. Upper gastrointestinal bleeding is usually due to superficial mucosal lesions (often drug-induced) or AV malformations rather than to gastric or duodenal ulcers. Pancreatitis is more common in ESRD patients than in nonuremic patients.

Electrolyte and Acid-Base Complications

Renal excretion of fixed acid, compensation for respiratory alkalosis or acidosis, and elimination of excess administered alkali are all absent in ESRD. Although dialysis provides alkali as acetate (HD), bicarbonate (HD), or lactate (PD) to neutralize fixed acid, ESRD patients characteristically have an elevated anion gap (16 to 20 mEq/L), but it is almost never greater than 25 mEq/L. In addition, since dialysis removes excess salt and fluid, intravenous sodium bicarbonate can be given to treat other causes of metabolic acidosis.

Hyponatremia is common in dialysis patients in the ICU because of the administration of large volumes of hypotonic fluids in the absence of renal water excretion. *Hypokalemia* may be due to malnutrition, even in anuric ESRD patients or those receiving total parenteral nutrition (TPN). It is also common in PD patients. Dialysate potassium levels must be adjusted upward to avoid hypokalemia, particularly in patients receiving digitalis. *Hyperkalemia* is treated by dialysis. Sodium bicarbonate infusion to reverse hyperkalemia transiently is ineffective in dialysis patients.

Nutritional Complications

As a rule, dialysis patients have baseline malnutrition caused by poor food intake, protein losses, and catabolism. Catabolism increases during acute illness as well. Hemodialysis increases catabolic cytokines, such as interleukin-1 and tumor necrosis factor. Hence, nutritional therapy for malnutrition is indicated early in the ICU course of patients with ESRD (see Chapter 13).

Renal Transplantation Complications

Complications of renal transplantation include opportunistic infections, malignancy, acute liver disease, and acute and chronic kidney rejection. Neoplasms are diverse but include especially squamous cell tumors of the skin and cervix and central nervous system lymphomas. Sometimes these tumors regress after immunosuppression is stopped. Acute liver disease may be due to azathioprine but more commonly arises from a flare of chronic viral hepatitis resulting from the effects of immunosuppression.

DIAGNOSTIC CONSIDERATIONS

Differential diagnoses of common problems in ICU patients are influenced if they have ESRD (Table 20–3). In addition, the manifestations of problems may be

Table 20–3. Differential Diagnosis of Common Problems in Patients with End-Stage Renal Disease in the Intensive Care Unit

PROBLEM	DIFFERENTIAL DIAGNOSIS
Chest pain	Coronary artery disease
	Gastroesophageal reflux disease
	Pericarditis
	Uremic pleurisy
	Dialyzer reaction
Bleeding	Uremia
	Platelet defect
	Heparin overdose
	Heparin-induced thrombocytopenia
Fever	Infection of vascular access
	Urinary tract infection
	Opportunistic infections of renal transplant
Obtundation	Uremia
	Opioids or other sedatives
	Sepsis syndrome
	Malignant hypertension
	Subdural hematoma or other intracranial bleeding
	Central nervous system lymphoma in renal transplant patient

altered because of ESRD. For example, fever may be less marked for a number of reasons, such as the use of steroid treatment in the renal transplant patient.

Knowledge of the cause of ESRD may also be useful, for example, is ESRD due to polycystic kidney disease, diabetes, or lupus. Associations with polycystic kidney disease include cerebral aneurysms, prolapsed mitral valve, diverticulitis, kidney stones, and infected or bleeding renal cysts.

Echocardiography is a useful diagnostic test in ESRD and may be helpful in distinguishing systolic from diastolic dysfunction and pericarditis.

Since many ESRD patients have a normal bleeding time, obtaining a bleeding time may be helpful in assessing the patient with a bleeding diathesis and a normal platelet count. With thrombocytopenia, heparin antibodies should be sought. In the patient with fever, even if anuria is present, a catheter should be inserted in the bladder for bacterial culture.

Serum enzyme levels may be altered in ESRD. For example, in ESRD without pancreatitis, serum amylase may be elevated up to three times normal levels and lipase to twice normal levels. Greater elevations than these suggest pancreatitis. Creatine kinase is elevated persistently in 10 to 50% of dialysis patients, but creatine kinase of cardiac origin (CK-MB) is persistently increased in only 5% of patients or less.

MANAGEMENT

Cardiovascular Problems

As a rule, excessive fluid administration must be avoided, but postoperative or septic patients sometimes require large amounts of crystalloid to maintain hemodynamic stability in the face of increased capillary permeability and third spacing. As capillary permeability improves, dialysis must be performed promptly to avoid intravascular fluid overload. In *hemodynamically unstable* patients, dialysis should be performed with bicarbonate rather than acetate because the latter is a vasodilator and cardiodepressant. Hemodynamic stability can be enhanced by relatively slow fluid removal, hypertonic dialysate, reduced dialysate temperature, isolated ultrafiltration, and continuous AV or venovenous HD (see Chapter 16). Adequate preload is usually critical for maintaining cardiac output in patients with diastolic dysfunction, and excessive fluid removal must be avoided in these patients. In PD, fluid removal requires an increase in frequency or tonicity of exchanges; if the PD patient has respiratory embarrassment, it is helpful to decrease exchange volume (e.g., to 1 L) and increase the frequency of exchanges.

In *angina* or *myocardial infarction* in ESRD, anemia should be corrected by blood transfusion. PD may be preferred over HD in the peri-infarction period to minimize hemodynamic stress. Percutaneous transluminal angioplasty for coronary artery disease has been disappointing in ESRD, but surgical revascularization may have a higher mortality than in nonuremic patients. In management of *arrhythmias,* it is important to avoid *hypokalemia,* especially in patients receiving digitalis. Amiodarone should be preferred to procainamide, whose metabolite NAPA may accumulate to dangerous levels in renal failure (see Chapter 12).

In *uremic pericarditis,* nonsteroidal anti-inflammatory drugs do not alter its natural history or alleviate pain. Large or symptomatic pericardial effusions should be treated with intensive dialysis and close echocardiographic monitoring. Large pericardial effusions ($\geq$250 mL or >1 cm posterior echo-free space) or pericardial tamponade requires drainage by pericardiocentesis or subxiphoid pericardiotomy.

Bleeding problems are treated by blood transfusion to achieve a hematocrit greater than 30% and by other measures (Table 20–4). Platelet transfusions are of uncertain value because transfused platelets are thought to become dysfunctional in the uremic milieu in a short time. Their use should be reserved as a therapy of last resort for patients with life-threatening active bleeding who have not responded to the other measures listed in Table 20–4.

Infectious problems are treated empirically with an antistaphylococcal agent (e.g., vancomycin to cover methicillin-resistant staphylococcal species) and an aminoglycoside pending cultures (see Chapters 12 and 14). Central venous dialysis access catheters usually should be removed during fever or bacteremia, or both, and the tip sent for semiquantitative culture (see Chapter 11). AV grafts should be observed closely and removed surgically if they manifest local signs of infection. In contrast, AV fistulas can usually be treated successfully with antibiotics without surgical intervention.

Nutritional Problems

Although dialysis patients who are only mildly catabolic may meet nutritional goals with peripheral parenteral nutrition and intradialytic parenteral nutrition, most critically ill ICU patients with ESRD require additional enteral nutrition or TPN. Use of 70% dextrose solutions minimizes the volume of administered water. In general, the daily protein goal should be increased to 1.5 g/kg. Phosphate, potassium, and magnesium should be added to the TPN solutions in normal quantities (unless their serum levels are already high) because these minerals may be shifted into cells by glucose infusion and anabolism.

CLINICAL PEARLS AND PITFALLS

1. *Residual renal function* often plays an important role in preserving the dialysis patient's quality of life, either allowing continued PD or fewer or shorter HD sessions. If a patient has significant urine output—that is, greater than 250 mL daily—an effort should be made to preserve this residual function. Radiocontrast administration, aminoglycosides, and other nephrotoxins should be avoided if feasible.

2. The *preferred* site for central venous access is the internal jugular vein *contralateral* to upper extremity vascular access. Use of the subclavian vein can cause stenosis or thombosis, precluding use of the ipsilateral arm for a future AV fistula or graft. Blood draws and intravenous catheters should be avoided in the arm with existing or intended vascular access. A central venous dialysis catheter should not be used for other infusions nor manipulated by personnel other than the dialysis staff in order to minimize risk of infection or an inadvertent infusion of heparin.

3. Probably the *most common error* in the care of ESRD patients is failure to dose medications appropriately for renal failure (see Chapter 12). A few

Table 20-4. Treatment of Bleeding in Patients with End-Stage Renal Disease in the Intensive Care Unit

TREATMENT	DOSAGE	ONSET	DURATION	COMMENT
Raise Hct to 30% by red blood cell transfusion	Variable	Immediate	Variable	Rheologic mechanism
Increase intensity or frequency of dialysis, or both	—	5–7 days	—	Variable benefit
Desmopressin (DDAVP)	0.3 µg/kg (IV over 20–30 min)	1 h	6–8 h	Tachyphylaxis after 1–2 doses (increases circulating endogenous von Willebrand factor (VWF))
Conjugated estrogens	0.6 mg/kg (IV once a day for 5 days)	6 h–2 days	14–21 days	No adverse effects
Cryoprecipitate*	10 units IV	1 h	24–36 h	Carries an infectious risk; provides exogenous von Willebrand factor
Platelet transfusion†	6 units IV	Immediate	Variable	Carries risks of transfusion reactions

*Because of its significant infectious risk, cryoprecipitate should be restricted to treatment of life-threatening active bleeding not responding to other interventions listed.
†Because transfused platelets become dysfunctional in a short period of time in uremic patients, they should only be given for active life-threatening bleeding that has not responded to the other measures listed in the table.

Hct, hematocrit; DDAVP, deamino-8-D-arginine vasopressin (desmopressin); IV, intravenous.

examples illustrate the scope of this issue: (1) magnesium- and phosphate-containing laxatives are contraindicated, (2) meperidine is contraindicated, whereas hydromorphone and fentanyl are the preferred opioids to use for analgesia, and (3) phenytoin dosing is unchanged, but the target therapeutic level of total (not free) drug is half that in nonuremic patients.

BIBLIOGRAPHY

Bennett WM, Aronoff GR, Golper T, et al: Drug Prescribing in Renal Failure: Dosing Guidelines for Adults, 2nd ed. Philadelphia, American College of Physicians, 1993.
This book is a definitive compilation.

Blumenkrantz MJ, Salehmoghaddam S, Boken, R, et al: An integrated approach to the treatment of patients with multiple organ system failure requiring intensive nutritional support and hemodialysis. Trans Am Soc Artif Intern Organs 30:468–72, 1984.
This article briefly outlines customized enteral and parenteral nutritional regimens and dialysis solutions to manage energy and protein needs, fluid overload, hyponatremia, and acidosis in patients with multiple organ system failure.

Eberst ME, Berkowitz LR: Hemostasis in renal disease: Pathophysiology and management. Am J Med 96:168–179, 1994.
This article reviews mechanisms and management approaches to the problems of bleeding and hypercoagulability in patients with ESRD.

Foley RN, Parfrey PS, Harnett JD: Left ventricular hypertrophy in dialysis patients. Semin Dialysis 5:34–41, 1992.
This is a good review of the fundamental cardiac pathophysiology in dialysis patients, including congestive heart failure and dialysis hypotension, which makes a strong recommendation for routine echocardiography.

Gennari FJ, Rimmer JM: Acid-base disorders in end-stage renal disease. Parts I and II. Semin Dialysis 3:81–5, 3:161–5, 1990.
These articles elucidate the evaluation and management of acid-base disorders in dialysis patients in whom diagnosis depends on a change of baseline serum bicarbonate rather than on a normal range or compensation.

Parfey PS, Harnett JD, Barre P: The natural history of myocardial disease in dialysis patients. J Am Soc Nephrol 2:2–12, 1991.
This is another good review of cardiovascular dysfunction in patients with ESRD.

21 Care of the Maternal-Fetal Unit

Samuel Parry
Mark A. Morgan

Care of the maternal-fetal unit in the intensive care unit (ICU) presents a number of challenges. For example, maternal physiologic changes in pregnancy and concerns for the fetus often make the diagnosis of conditions commonly seen in critical illness more difficult and their treatment more complicated. This chapter discusses maternal changes in pregnancy relevant to the ICU, how standard ICU interventions should be modified when treating pregnant patients, and when fetal monitoring should be used.

MATERNAL PHYSIOLOGIC CHANGES IN PREGNANCY

Hematologic Changes

Maternal plasma volume increases approximately 50% above baseline by 30 to 34 weeks of pregnancy. *Red blood cell mass* also increases throughout gestation but to only 18 to 30% more than nonpregnancy levels. These two phenomena result in a physiologic anemia, with the nadir of hemoglobin concentration (usually between 11 and 12 g/dL) at approximately 30 weeks of gestation. *White blood cell counts* during pregnancy may also increase (secondary to increased numbers of circulating granulocytes), with the upper limits of a pregnant woman's normal white blood cell count being in the 15,000 to 16,000/μL range. *Platelet counts* remain greater than 150,000/μL during gestation, despite increased platelet turnover and a slightly shortened platelet life span.

Pregnancy has been described as a *hypercoagulable state* for the most part due to estrogen-induced increases in hepatic production of clotting Factors I (fibrinogen), VII, IX, and X. Although pregnant patients have normal bleeding and clotting times, they are at increased risk for venous thromboembolism. This is particularly true in the puerperium when injury to large pelvic veins or venous stasis in lower extremity veins is likely to occur. Any pregnant patient in whom there is prolonged restriction to activity should be considered a candidate for prophylaxis of deep venous thrombosis. She should either be fitted with pneumatic compression stockings or receive subcutaneous heparin (5000 to 10,000 units twice per day).

Hemodynamic Changes

Blood pressure normally decreases during pregnancy secondary to decreased peripheral vascular resistance, an effect of circulating progesterone. The lowest values are seen at 24 to 28 weeks of gestation. Mean systolic blood pressure measures 5 to 10 mm Hg below baseline, whereas diastolic blood pressure falls slightly more, 10 to 15 mm Hg. Mean maternal heart rate increases at the beginning of the third trimester. Cardiac output is increased by 10 weeks of gestation secondary to increased stroke volume and later, in the third trimester, due to an increased heart rate ($+15\%$). In large part, other changes in hemodynamic parameters result from the increased plasma volume associated with pregnancy (Table 21–1).

When a pregnant patient lies supine, the gravid uterus compresses the inferior vena cava. This, in turn, decreases venous return and cardiac output. Normally, peripheral vascular resistance increases to compensate for the decreased venous return. However, in up to 10% of pregnant patients, this protective mechanism fails. These patients have *supine hypotension of pregnancy*. They become lightheaded or syncopal when supine. Maternal hemodynamics are optimized when the patient is placed in a left lateral recumbent position. Because blood pressure during pregnancy can vary with postural changes, serial blood pressure measurements should be obtained consistently with the pregnant patient in one position.

Physical Findings Attributable to Pregnancy

Pregnant patients often have dependent edema secondary to decreased colloid oncotic pressure, increased lower extremity venous pressure, and obstruction of lymphatic flow by the gravid uterus. The first heart sound is often split, and a third heart sound can be auscultated in most pregnant patients secondary to increased plasma volume. Although almost all pregnant patients have a systolic ejection murmur secondary to increased flow across the aortic and pulmonic valves, diastolic murmurs are not considered physiologic during pregnancy. Electrocardiography often demonstrates a 15-degree left axis deviation because of elevation of the heart by the gravid uterus. Echocardiography may demonstrate functional tricuspid regurgitation secondary to a dilated tricuspid valve annulus. Chest radiography typically reveals an enlarged cardiac silhouette secondary to hypervolemia.

Postpartum Hemodynamic Fluctuations

Maternal blood loss from vaginal delivery of a singleton gestation averages about 500 mL. It can be two times that for caesarean delivery. In the postpartum

Table 21–1. Hemodynamic Changes Associated with Late Pregnancy

	NONPREGNANT*	PREGNANT*
Cardiac output (L/min)	4.3 (± 0.9)	6.2 (± 1.0)
Systemic vascular resistance (dyne sec cm^{-5})	1530 (± 520)	1210 (± 266)
Colloid oncotic pressure (COP) (mm Hg)	20.8 (± 1.0)	18 (± 1.5)
Pulmonary artery wedge pressure (DCAP) (mm Hg)	6 (± 2)	8 (± 2)
COP-PAWP gradient (mm Hg)	14.5 (± 2.5)	10.5 (± 2.7)

*Means ($\pm$ standard errors).

From Clark SL, Cotton DB, Lee W, et al: Central hemodynamic assessment of normal term pregnancy. Am J Obstet Gynecol 161:1439–1442, 1989.

period, the mother mobilizes extracellular fluid, resulting in a postpartum diuresis equivalent to approximately 3 kg of weight loss. Despite the blood loss and diuresis, stroke volume and cardiac output remain elevated because of increased venous return. The clinical significance of these changes is manifested in a large subclass of preeclamptic patients as follows: (1) before delivery they have generalized vasospasm and intravascular volume depletion, (2) postpartum they mobilize their extracellular fluid as expected, (3) they often fail to diurese secondary to restricted renal blood flow, and (4) this places them at high risk for pulmonary or cerebral edema.

Respiratory Changes

Alterations in maternal lung volumes, respiratory mechanics, and arterial blood gas values precede elevation of the diaphragm due to the gravid uterus. Respiratory rate does not change during pregnancy, but tidal volume expands by 30 to 40%. This results in an increased minute ventilation beginning in the first trimester. These changes are modulated by progesterone acting on the central respiratory center. Although gravid women frequently report a mild pregnancy-associated dyspnea, their forced expiratory volume in 1 second (FEV_1) is not decreased. Arterial pH remains at 7.40 during pregnancy, whereas Pao_2 is normally elevated at 104 to 108 mm Hg and $Paco_2$ is normally decreased at 27 to 32 mm Hg (secondary to the increased minute ventilation). Increased renal excretion of bicarbonate (normal serum levels in pregnancy are 18 to 21 mEq/L) compensates for decreased $Paco_2$ and maintains the neutral pH. The lower maternal $Paco_2$ facilitates fetal-maternal CO_2 diffusion.

Renal Changes

Expanded plasma volume and decreased systemic vascular resistance result in increased renal plasma flow ($+75\%$) and glomerular filtration rate ($+30$ to 50%) during pregnancy. A normal creatinine clearance during pregnancy is 150 to 200 mL/minute, and serum creatinine values decrease to 0.5 to 0.6 mg/dL. Glycosuria is *not* abnormal during pregnancy secondary to increased filtration of glucose. It is important to consider the increased renal clearance of drugs when dosing patients during pregnancy. Although strict guidelines cannot be provided, obtaining drug levels when applicable is recommended.

Gastrointestinal Changes

The smooth muscle relaxing effects of progesterone result in delayed gastric emptying, gastroesophageal sphincter relaxation, and esophageal reflux. These predispose pregnant patients to aspiration during emergency endotracheal intubation. Portal venous compression during pregnancy increases the likelihood of portal hypertension in patients with underlying chronic liver disease. Clinical presentations of this condition range from hemorrhoids to esophageal varices.

EFFECTS OF COMMON INTENSIVE CARE UNIT INTERVENTIONS ON THE MATERNAL-FETAL UNIT

Drug Therapy

Most drugs used in critical care have not been studied extensively in the pregnant population so that little is known regarding their adverse effects on the human fetus. Although the potential risks on the fetus must be considered, as a general rule the need to treat critical illness to restore maternal well-being should far outweigh these considerations. All drugs are assigned to categories representing degrees of fetal risk (Table 21–2). These categories are indicated in parentheses for the drugs discussed in the following sections.

Dopamine (Category C)

Dopamine has been used in renal doses to augment urine output in oliguric patients with preeclampsia without adverse fetal effects. Dobutamine has not been studied in human pregnancy. A concern for both agents is whether they decrease uterine blood flow. Animal studies of dopamine have not shown any consistent effect.

Epinephrine (Category C)

Because epinephrine is a naturally occurring agent, its effects on the fetus are difficult to discern in comparison with the effects of endogenous epinephrine and a maternal disease state. In asthmatics, use of subcutaneous or endotracheal epinephrine appears to be safe. When a pressor agent is required for maternal hypotension, for example, after conduction anesthesia, ephedrine (category C) appears to be the drug of choice because it does not decrease uterine blood flow.

Antihypertensive Agents

Since swings in maternal blood pressure may cause decreased uterine blood flow and fetal compromise, pregnant patients who are being treated with intravenous antihypertensive medications require continuous fetal monitoring. In general, obste-

Table 21–2. Categories of Fetal Risk Factors Assigned to All Medications

Category A	Controlled studies in humans fail to show a risk to the fetus in the first trimester
Category B	Animal studies have not demonstrated a fetal risk, but controlled studies have not been performed in humans, *or* animal studies have shown adverse effects but those have not been confirmed in controlled human studies
Category C	Animal studies have shown adverse effects and no controlled human studies have been performed, *or* studies in animals and humans have not been performed
Category D	There is positive evidence of human fetal risk, but the benefits from use in pregnant women may be acceptable despite the risk
Category X	The drug is contraindicated based on its demonstrated capacity to cause fetal abnormalities

tricians attempt to maintain systemic blood pressure at approximately 140/90 mm Hg in hypertensive patients.

Hydralazine (category C) has been the standard antihypertensive agent in obstetrics, but its direct relaxation of arteriolar smooth muscle has been associated with maternal hypotension, decreased uterine blood flow, and transient fetal distress. Recommended dosing of hydralazine is 5 to 10 mg intravenously, which may be repeated every 20 minutes until hypertension has been controlled. That total titrated dose should then be given every 6 hours.

Labetalol (category C) has been used as an antihypertensive agent without associated decreases in human uterine blood flow. Labetalol may also augment fetal pulmonary surfactant secretion and decrease the risk of developing neonatal respiratory distress syndrome. Labetalol may be given as a 10-mg intravenous bolus with increasing boluses (20 mg, 40 mg, 80 mg) repeated every 10 minutes to a total dose of 300 mg. When desired blood pressure is attained, an intravenous labetalol drip may be instituted at 1 to 2 mg/minute and titrated accordingly.

Nitroglycerin (Category C)

The Collaborative Perinatal Project has demonstrated an increased rate of congenital malformations after exposure to vasodilators in the first trimester, but the effects of any single drug, including nitroglycerin, were not examined separately. When administered for maternal hypertension, only transient fetal heart rate abnormalities, without abnormal umbilical blood gas values or Apgar scores, have been demonstrated. Intravenous nitroglycerin has been used to correct maternal blood pressure rapidly and to treat pregnancy-induced hypertension complicated by hydrostatic pulmonary edema successfully.

Sodium Nitroprusside (Category C)

Because sodium nitroprusside has been shown to cross the placenta in animals and produce fetal cyanide levels that exceed those of the mother, one should avoid its prolonged use. Monitoring maternal serum pH and thiocyanate and methemoglobin levels has been recommended. Standard doses of nitroprusside for short periods do not pose a major risk of accumulating cyanide in the fetal liver.

Contraindicated Antihypertensive Agents

Intravenous *nifedipine* (category C) has been shown to decrease uterine blood flow in pregnant sheep. Furthermore, when given intravenously or sublingually, it may precipitate an exaggerated hypotensive response especially when used in conjunction with magnesium sulfate in the obstetric population.

As a class, angiotensin-converting enzyme inhibitors (category D), for example, enalapril and captopril, should be avoided in obstetric patients. These drugs precipitate fetal hypotension and decrease fetal renal blood flow and urine output. The resultant oligohydramnios has been associated with a variety of congenital malformations.

Diuretics

Thiazide diuretics (category D) diminish the physiologic volume expansion of pregnancy but do not alter the course of pregnancy-induced hypertension. This class of drugs is associated with decreased uterine blood flow and mild neonatal thrombocytopenia. Thiazide diuretics are recommended only for pregnant patients with cardiac disease. *Furosemide* (category C) is used commonly in pregnancy to treat pulmonary edema.

Antiarrhythmic Agents

Antiarrhythmic drugs have been used in pregnancy for both maternal and fetal indications (tachyarrhythmias, congestive heart failure). *Digitalis* (category C) dosing must be carefully monitored, as the expanded maternal volume of distribution may be associated with subtherapeutic levels. There have been no reported fetal malformations attributed to digitalis. By term, umbilical cord levels approach 85% of maternal serum levels, and digitalis has been the drug of choice for fetal indications. The following antiarrhythmic agents (all category C drugs)—*lidocaine, quinidine, procainamide,* and *flecainide*—have not been associated with fetal anomalies at therapeutic doses. Lidocaine has been used extensively as an anesthetic in obstetric patients, but high fetal plasma levels have been associated with central nervous system depression and low Apgar scores. Quinine, an optical isomer of quinidine, has been associated with cranial nerve VIII damage, and its use should be avoided. Damage to the auditory nerve has not been reported with quinidine. *Adenosine* (category C) has demonstrated no teratogenicity in animals and its short half-life (<10 seconds) precludes changes in fetal heart rate.

Sedatives, Opioids, and Neuromuscular Blocking Agents

Sedatives, opioids, and neuromuscular blocking agents do not demonstrate consistent anomalies in exposed fetuses (Table 21–3). The drugs are listed in pregnancy risk factor categories B through D, mostly because little data exist in humans or in animal models. Each of the drugs listed in Table 21–3 should be used as needed in the critically ill obstetric patient.

Modifications of Cardiopulmonary Resuscitation for Pregnant Women

No changes are recommended in closed chest compressions and dosing of pharmacologic agents. Limited information is available regarding electric shock in pregnancy, and defibrillation should be performed according to advanced cardiac life support (ACLS) algorithms (see Appendix E). Uterine displacement using a wedge or pillow will decrease aortocaval compression by the gravid uterus and enhance maternal cardiac output. Airway management may be complicated by aspiration of gastric contents before or during endotracheal intubation.

Fetal oxygenation reflects uterine venous Po_2, which is the maximal Po_2 that can be achieved by diffusion of oxygen in the placental vasculature. The increased

Table 21–3. Sedatives, Opioids, and Neuromuscular
Blocking Agents Used in Pregnancy

DRUG (FETAL RISK CATEGORY)	TERATOGENIC EFFECTS	COMMENTS
Sedatives		
Diazepam (D)	Cleft lip and palate (mice)	Rapid equilibration across the placenta
	Neurobehavioral delays (rats)	Accumulates at higher levels in the fetus than in the mother
		Neonatal withdrawal
Midazolam (D)	No teratogenicity in animal studies	Crosses the placenta less efficiently
Lorazepam (D)	or in isolated human reports	than does diazepam
		Neonatal withdrawal
Opioids		
Morphine (B)	None	Rapid placental transfer
Fentanyl (B)		Neonatal respiratory depression, withdrawal
Meperidine (B)	None	Rapid placental transfer
		Less respiratory depression, withdrawal in the neonate
Neuromuscular Blocking Agents		
Pancuronium (C)	No animal or human studies	Inefficient placental transfer
Vecuronium (C)		Alert neonatologist of potential need for ventilatory support

affinity of fetal hemoglobin for oxygen shifts the fetal hemoglobin saturation curve to the left when compared with adult hemoglobin (see Appendix A). This shift promotes oxygen loading from hemoglobin but hinders oxygen unloading. Thus, fetal oxygen saturation begins to fall rapidly if maternal arterial PO_2 falls to less than 60 mm Hg. Interventions to improve fetal oxygenation include maternal volume expansion, correction of maternal acidosis and fever, and enhanced maternal oxygen delivery (Figs. 21–1 and 21–2).

The question of whether to do a perimortem cesarean section remains controversial. Primate fetuses have demonstrated brain damage after 6 minutes of maternal asphyxia. In one large study, if the fetuses were delivered within 5 minutes of maternal cardiopulmonary arrest, 70% of neonates survived and all survivors were neurologically intact. The American College of Obstetrics and Gynecology has recommended a theoretical 4-minute limit for the performance of a perimortem cesarean section if the threshold of fetal viability (generally accepted at 24 to 26 weeks of gestation) has been reached. Importantly, cesarean delivery should not be attempted if the mother's condition is unstable.

Radiologic Studies in Pregnancy

No fetal malformations have been reported at radiation exposures less than 500 Gy (5 rad), and most investigators believe there is no serious risk to the fetus with

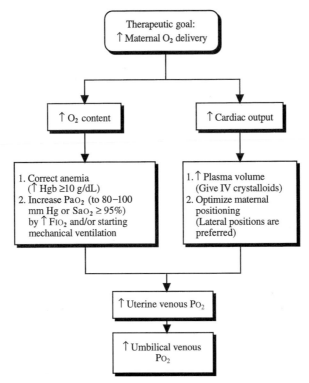

Figure 21–1. Schematic flow diagram illustrating the approach to improving fetal oxygenation by increasing maternal oxygen delivery. O_2, oxygen; Hgb, hemoglobin; PaO_2, partial pressure of arterial oxygen; SaO_2, arterial blood saturation with oxygen; FIO_2, fraction of inspired oxygen; IV, intravenous; PO_2, partial pressure of oxygen.

exposures less than 1000 Gy (10 rad). At less than 4 weeks' gestation, ionizing radiation has an all-or-none effect, potentially causing a spontaneous abortion. Organogenesis occurs during the 4th to 12th weeks of pregnancy, during which ionizing radiation may be associated with major fetal malformations, including microcephaly and growth retardation. The fetal central nervous system continues to develop rapidly up to 16 weeks of gestation, and high doses of ionizing radiation during this time may result in mental retardation. Later in pregnancy, radiation is associated with side effects similar to those in the adult, including bone marrow suppression. There may also be a 50% increase in childhood cancers, that is, an increased rate from 1 in 3000 to 1 in 2000. Radiation doses associated with various diagnostic procedures are almost universally less than 500 Gy (5 rad) (Table 21–4). One should consult with the appropriate radiologist to calculate the dose of ionizing radiation associated with a diagnostic procedure not listed.

FETAL MONITORING

For nearly 30 years obstetricians have used fetal heart rate patterns to assess fetal well-being. Importantly, an abnormal tracing is not always predictive of adverse

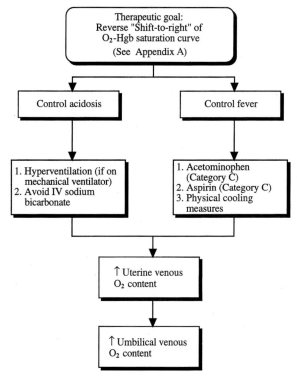

Figure 21–2. Schematic flow diagram illustrating the approach to improving fetal oxygenation by reversing the shift to the right of the oxyhemoglobin (O_2-Hgb) saturation curve induced by acidosis and fever (Appendix A). Because bicarbonate does not pass the placenta, its administration will decrease maternal hyperventilation (in a spontaneously breathing patient) and, consequently, lead to a rise in maternal and fetal Pa_{CO_2}. O_2, oxygen; Hgb, hemoglobin; IV, intravenous.

Table 21–4. Approximate Fetal Radiation Exposures During Selected Radiologic Studies

STUDY	GRAY (rad)
Chest radiograph	<0.1 (<0.001)
Abdominal radiograph (single exposure)	4 (0.04)
Barium enema	200–400 (2–4)
Abdominal CT scan (10 slices)	200 (2)
Pulmonary V/Q scan (technetium[99m])	<5 (<0.05)
Contrast venography (lower extremity)	60 (0.6)

Iodine radioisotopes are contraindicated because they accumulate in the fetal thyroid gland. Ultrasonography is not associated with any risk of fetal malformations. Magnetic resonance imaging has not been reported to cause fetal malformations.

Table 21–5. Indications for Continuous Fetal Heart Rate
Monitoring in the Intensive Care Unit

INDICATIONS	EXAMPLES
Maternal hypoxemia	Acute severe asthma attack
Maternal hypovolemia	Hemorrhage
Maternal hypertensive crisis	Severe preeclampsia
Postoperative states	Effects of anesthetic agents on fetal heart rate
	Increased risk for preterm delivery after laparotomy
Fetal indications	Preterm labor

fetal outcome. Nevertheless, in the critically ill obstetric patient, fetal heart rate patterns often reflect maternal oxygenation and the status of uterine perfusion. A nonexhaustive list of indications for continuous fetal heart rate monitoring in the ICU is given in Table 21–5.

Continuous fetal heart rate monitoring should not be instituted until the fetus has reached the threshold of viability (24 to 26 weeks of gestation in most institutions). This technology requires frequent interpretation by qualified obstetric personnel. Intermittent fetal heart rate assessment may be performed using hand-held Doppler ultrasonography after 12 weeks of gestation. Although improved fetal outcome has not been proved, intermittent electronic fetal monitoring is recommended for all hospitalized obstetric patients before 24 to 26 weeks of gestation.

BIBLIOGRAPHY

Barbour LA, Pickard J: Controversies in thromboembolic disease during pregnancy: A critical review. Obstet Gynecol 86:621–633, 1995.
This article reviews the literature concerning the epidemiology and diagnosis of thromboembolic disease (including congenital and acquired hypercoagulable states) in pregnancy. Management strategies, including choice of anticoagulants, duration of therapy, and prophylaxis in subsequent pregnancies, are discussed.

Brent RL: The effects of embryonic and fetal exposure to x-ray, microwaves and ultrasound. Clin Perinatol Teratol 13:301–330, 1988.
In this review, the author reports that exposure to low-dose ionizing radiation (fetal dose <500 Gy) is not associated with teratogenicity.

Clark SL, Cotton DB, Lee W, et al: Central hemodynamic assessment of normal term pregnancy. Am J Obstet Gynecol 161:1439–1442, 1989.
This article describes the central hemodynamic profiles of 10 carefully screened normal primiparous patients who underwent voluntary pulmonary artery catheterization between 36 and 38 weeks of gestation. The studies were repeated for comparison in the same patients between 11 and 13 weeks postpartum.

Cotton DB, Jones MM, Longmire S, et al: Role of intravenous nitroglycerin in the treatment of severe pregnancy-induced hypertension complicated by pulmonary edema. Am J Obstet Gynecol 154:91–93, 1986.
The authors describe their experience using nitroglycerin to correct the hydrostatic derangements of pulmonary edema (by reducing the mean pulmonary artery wedge pressure) in patients with severe pregnancy-induced hypertension.

Hankins GDV, Wendel GD, Cunningham FG, et al: Longitudinal evaluation of hemodynamic changes in eclampsia. Am J Obstet Gynecol 150:506–512, 1984.
In this report from Parkland Hospital in Dallas, Texas, eight primigravid women with eclampsia underwent invasive hemodynamic monitoring. Women without spontaneous postpartum diuresis had elevated postpartum mobilization of extravascular fluid in conjunction with oliguria.

Pritchard JA, Baldwin RM, Dickey JC, et al: Blood volume changes in pregnancy and the puerperium. Am J Obstet Gynecol 84:1271–1281, 1962.
The estimated blood loss associated with vaginal delivery (75 patients), caesarean section (40 patients), and caesarean hysterectomy (35 patients) is reported. The loss of blood volume from the circulation was measured by using each patient's red blood cells labeled with radiochromium.

Special resuscitation situations. JAMA 268:2242, 1992.
This report describes adaptations to ACLS protocols for cardiopulmonary arrest during pregnancy. Recommendations include left uterine displacement, strict adherence to the standard algorithms, and consideration of perimortem caesarean section.

22   End-Of-Life Care

Horace M. DeLisser
Paul N. Lanken

Advances in life-sustaining technologies have fueled the development of intensive care units (ICUs) and the demand for their services. These new technologies have made survival and recovery possible for many patients with critical illness or injury. For others, however, rather than leading to successful recovery, ICUs have only postponed their deaths. Continued use of ICU technology can make dying a prolonged process for many patients who have virtually no chance of meaningful recovery. This phenomenon has elevated competency in addressing ethical issues, particularly withholding and withdrawing life support, to a level of importance in ICU practice comparable to the management of shock or respiratory failure. ICU practitioners need to know not only which life-sustaining interventions to use and when to use them but also when it is ethical to forgo those interventions.

Ethical issues involved in decisions to limit life support often arise from conflicts between fundamental ethical principles or values. These principles or values speak to the rights of patients (autonomy), the duties of physicians (beneficence and nonmaleficence), and societal concerns for fairness and efficiency in the allocation of medical resources (distributive justice). Together, they serve as a useful framework and starting point in understanding the issues and conflicts that occur frequently in the ICU with regard to end-of-life decision-making (Fig. 22–1).

FUNDAMENTAL PRINCIPLES (VALUES) OF BIOETHICS

The Rights of Patients

Patient autonomy and self-determination have been the focus of much of the attention in contemporary medical ethics. The essence of respect for patient autonomy is that an appropriately informed adult patient with adequate decision-making capacity has the ethical and legal right to refuse any medical therapy, including life-sustaining ones. Not only has a broad ethical consensus emerged to support this principle but also both statutory law and important judicial decisions in the United States have established this as a legal right of capable patients. Under this principle, absent countervailing obligations, the physician should respect a capable and informed patient's decisions to forgo life-sustaining medical care.

Decision-Making Capacity and Informed Consent

Central to the notion of patient autonomy is the requirement that the patient be capable of making medical decisions. In other words, the patient must be able to give *informed consent* for a medical or surgical treatment (or, in the case of forgoing life support, give what might be better described as *informed refusal*). As a first step in the process of making decisions to proceed with or forgo life-sustaining therapy, the adequacy of a patient's capacity to make medical decisions

255

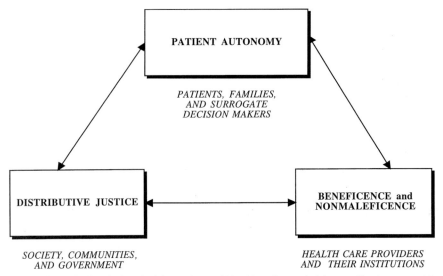

Figure 22–1. The four basic principles (values) of bioethics often underlying conflict (represented by the arrows between boxes) arising in ethical issues in withholding and withdrawing life support in ICUs. Listed below each box are the moral bodies most relevant to that principle.

should always be assessed. Having adequate decision-making capacity means that the patient meets certain specific criteria (Table 22–1). Whether a patient disagrees with the physician's recommendation should not be the only question asked. If a patient is judged to have adequate decision-making capacity, informed consent (or refusal) for a given course of medical care requires discussion of certain elements and information to make the patient's decision autonomous (Table 22–2).

Obtaining informed consent for ICU care from ICU patients remains intrinsically problematic. It is rarely possible to present, discuss, and explain the information required for informed consent if the ICU admission is unexpected and under emergency conditions. When patients unexpectedly experience an acute life-threatening illness or injury, their consent is assumed in order to preserve "life or limb." However, this implied consent may be incorrect. If so, the mistaken assumption of consent often persists because it is difficult, if not impossible, to have the same thorough and reciprocal discussion as might be possible in the outpatient setting. ICU patients often lack decision-making capacity because they are critically ill.

Table 22–1. The "Three Cs"—Three Criteria Needed
for Adequate Decision Making Capacity

1. Ability to *comprehend* information relevant to the decision
2. Ability to *compare* alternatives of the decision with personal values and goals
3. Ability to *communicate* in a consistent and meaningful manner

Table 22–2. Elements of Informed Consent Regarding
Decisions to Forgo Life-Sustaining Intervention

....

1. What are the patient's relevant medical diagnoses?
2. What is the intervention that will be withheld or withdrawn?
3. What is the purpose of the intervention and its benefits, risks, and burdens?
4. What are the likely or important consequences of withholding or withdrawing it?
5. What are the alternatives to forgoing it?
6. What are the likely or important consequences of these alternatives?
7. Is the patient free of coercion?

....

Surrogate Decision Makers

If patients lack adequate decision-making capacity, they can no longer give informed consent. They will be unable to speak for themselves when their medical care decisions need to be made. Under these circumstances, they do not lose their right to self-determination, but rather it needs to be expressed by a surrogate decision maker or health care proxy.

The *surrogate decision maker* makes the medical decisions on the basis of what the patient would have wanted in the same situation (the *substituted judgment* standard). Living wills or the patient's formal designation of an individual to make health care decisions if and when the patient loses capacity for making medical decisions (such as a durable power of attorney for health affairs), allows the patient to influence what will be decided and how he or she will be treated. In the absence of advance directives or other knowledge of what the patient would have preferred, the ICU caregivers and surrogate decision maker should decide on the basis of what would represent the best interest of the patient by weighing the benefits and burdens of specific ICU interventions (the *best interests* standard).

Unless specified by a particular state's legal hierarchy or by a patient's prior designation, the patient's attending physician should be responsible for identifying the most appropriate surrogate decision maker for the patient. Ideally this should be someone who is close to the patient and knows the patient's values, life goals, and preferences about the use of life support under different circumstances. Of course, such a person has to be willing to serve as spokesperson for the patient in making medical decisions. Usually the individual who should be the surrogate decision maker is obvious, for example, a spouse or parent or adult child. Not uncommonly, however, disputes arise as to who this should be. Some ethicists argue that those with responsibility for providing the patient's medical care, for example, the patient's attending physician, should not simultaneously serve as the patient's sole surrogate decision maker. When no one who knows the patient can be found to serve as proxy, ICU clinicians should follow their institution's policy to identify an appropriate patient representative under these conditions or seek the advice of their ethics committee.

Limits of Patient Autonomy

As in other fields of medicine, the limits of patient autonomy in the ICU need to be defined. Although autonomy gives patients the right to refuse treatment, it does not give them the unqualified right to demand treatment. Many physicians and nonphysicians alike are confused about this distinction. Patients (and their surrogate decision makers) are entitled to choose to accept or forgo medical interventions that fall within the standard of medical care. However, they do not have the unqualified right to receive medical care if it is not medically appropriate.

The Obligations of Physicians

The principles of beneficence (being of benefit to the patient) and nonmaleficence (doing no harm to the patient) have defined the fundamental obligations of physicians and other health care professionals for centuries. The scope of responsibilities of health care providers includes: (1) to promote the health and well-being of the patient (preventing and curing disease), (2) to alleviate pain and suffering (providing comfort), and (3) to do so in ways that are caring and respectful of the patient's dignity and worth as a human being (showing empathy and respect). In contemporary bioethics and medicine, being respectful of a patient's dignity includes respecting his or her right to self-determination.

In contrast to these responsibilities, the physician is *not* obligated to provide futile medical care. Although this notion has been endorsed in principle by professional organizations representing ICU practitioners, others have challenged it because of ambiguities of the term *futility* and difficulties in consistently and fairly applying it. In the ICU setting, much of the controversy surrounding using futility to justify decisions to limit life support arises from how an institution defines futile life-sustaining therapy, which may seem like a contradiction in terms. One position is that the purpose of any life-sustaining intervention should be to sustain or restore *meaningful* survival, where meaningful refers to a survival that the patient can value and appreciate. A life-sustaining intervention would be defined as futile if reasoning or experience indicate that the treatment would be highly unlikely to produce a meaningful survival for that patient.

An important question, given this definition, is how highly unlikely must an intervention be for it to be considered futile? Although no universal answer to this question has emerged, some suggest that it refer to zero successful outcomes in 100 patients in like circumstances. (Although this seems to correspond to a threshold chance of success of $<1\%$ when expressed in statistical terms, zero occurrences in 100 cases actually has a 95% confidence interval of 97 to 100%.) Success in exceptional cases does not counter the notion of futility if these successes are rare and inexplicable events in a setting of hundreds or thousands of failures.

Different ICU providers may treat the concept of futility differently. They may use a broad range of probabilities for indicating that success is highly unlikely or apply their own or what they perceive to be society's viewpoints to define what is meaningful life for the patient. Alternatively, they may consider that the potential benefit of an ICU intervention is not worth the effort of the ICU team or its financial cost. Under these circumstances, in which personal values color the definition of futility, its use is morally problematic. With this in mind, if futility is used in these decisions, it should be decided at an institutional, not an individual, level, and its application should follow an explicit institutional policy. The latter should require disclosure to the patient or surrogate decision maker of decisions made on this basis and of availability of processes for appeal and review.

Societal Concerns Regarding Fairness and Resource Allocation

Dramatic increases in the costs of health care combined with inequalities in access to health care in the United States raise questions of social justice and of the fair and efficient allocation of health care resources, including ICU resources. A number of theories of distributive justice have been proposed for allocation (some would use the term *rationing*) of valued but limited medical resources. They all require that equals be treated equally and unequals be treated unequally. However, they differ in defining which criteria are ethically significant and should be used to allocate the scarce beneficial resources. Because personal or local community values could lead to unfair covert rationing, such decisions should be made at a societal level or at an institutional level subject to public review. Decisions to allocate scarce resources can be ethical and appropriate if they involve the application of institution-wide criteria supported by a societal consensus, such as the set of national rules in the United States for allocation of scarce solid organs for transplantation. Unfortunately, the current system of U.S. medical care has no universally accepted criteria for allocation of ICU resources. Thus, the limits on ICU care that one ICU physician imposes on his or her patients will not necessarily be shared by other physicians or patients in like situations. Nor is it guaranteed that savings derived from denying marginally beneficial ICU care to some patients would be used to fund clearly beneficial health care or to improve inequities in access to medical care for others. Therefore, until the emergence of a health care system with acceptable societal criteria for deciding how to allocate scarce medical resources, including ICU beds, with provisions for fair redistribution of the savings and with public acceptance of such rationing, the physician should serve primarily as an advocate for his or her patients rather than as a steward of society's resources. Nevertheless, all ICU health care providers have an obligation to know the costs of the ICU resources that they use, to use them wisely and efficiently, and to advocate for fair and equal access to ICU and other essential health care resources for those in need.

STEPWISE APPROACH TO THE WITHHOLDING AND WITHDRAWAL OF LIFE SUPPORT

1. **Determine if the patient has adequate decision-making capacity.**
   ICU patients are often *not* capable of making medical decisions because of underlying disease, medications, or lack of ability to communicate (see Table 22–1). If this is the case, a surrogate decision maker should be identified to help make decisions on the patient's behalf. From the outset, the physician must help the surrogate decision maker or decision makers understand that their responsibility is to articulate what the patient would have wanted done based on their knowledge of the patient's goals, beliefs, deeply held values, and previously expressed preferences. In the absence of such knowledge, what is in the best interests of the patient should be jointly decided on.

2. **Establish effective communication.**
   It is essential that the ICU physicians and nurses meet early and regularly with the patient (if he or she has adequate decision-making capacity) or,

more commonly, with the family or surrogate decision maker to discuss all relevant medical issues, with particular emphasis on the patient's short- and long-range prognoses. Primary care providers, especially those with whom the patient had an established relationship prior to ICU admission, and the attending physician of record (if not the intensivist providing ICU care) should be involved as well. These meetings should be opportunities for the health care team to learn if the patient had an advance directive and to acquire a better understanding of the patient's values and goals. Meetings should be held in a setting that allows for privacy and openness of expression. These discussions should be frank, informative, consistent, and respectful. The information should be presented in language and at a level of detail that is appropriate for the patient or surrogate decision makers to understand the reality of the medical situation, analogous to presenting the elements of informed consent (see Table 22–2).

Patients and families should be encouraged to ask questions and to express their feelings. Health care team members should not respond defensively if anger or criticism is directed toward them. When large or dispersed families are involved, it is usually useful to identify one individual to serve as the family spokesperson and the conduit of information between the family and the ICU team. To attempt to limit life-sustaining interventions without having first established effective communication is to invite needless conflict and disagreement.

3. **Formulate the health care team's recommendations.**
   These must be based on a complete understanding (as much as possible) of the patient's medical condition, prognosis, and preferences regarding life-sustaining care. The patient's attending physician should actively seek input from all members of the ICU team, relevant consultants and, if available, the patient's primary care provider, in an effort to achieve a consensus about the team's recommendation. In general, a specific recommendation should *not* be presented to the patient or family until such general consensus has been achieved.

   In deciding on a course of action to recommend, the ICU team should consider the following questions:

   For this patient, at this time, is the intervention medically indicated and how likely it is to be beneficial? The aim of all medically appropriate therapy should be to preserve or restore life that the patient can appreciate and value or to alleviate suffering and pain. If an intervention is highly unlikely to accomplish such goals, it should not be offered as a defensible option, if not yet started or, if already under way, its continuation should be seriously questioned.

   If an intervention is medically appropriate and has some potential benefit, what would be the preferences of the patient? The principle of respect for patient autonomy gives the patient the right to refuse any or all therapy—even medically appropriate and beneficial interventions. Unwanted treatment should not be forced on the patient.

   When an intervention is not futile and the patient's wishes are not known, is this intervention in the best interests of the patient? Determination of the patient's best interests involves weighing the benefits and burdens of the intervention while taking into consideration how likely those benefits and burdens are. If the benefits of therapy exceed the burdens, the therapy should be offered. If the burdens outweigh the benefits, it should not.

Are there other external factors that need to be considered? Although a certain course of action may be ethically and medically correct, institutional policy or legal constraints may be in conflict. ICU clinicians must be aware of these factors in formulating their recommendations. If clarification is needed, consultation with a hospital's ethics committee or similar ethics resource, for example, a consulting bioethicist, is strongly recommended.

How should one deal with uncertainty in knowing how successful a life-sustaining therapy will be? There is no legal or ethical distinction between *withholding* and *withdrawing* treatment. This supports the rationale of a therapeutic trial when a specific intervention is of uncertain efficacy. For example, as long the intervention is not proscribed by the patient or surrogate decision maker, it should be started with the intention that it can be withdrawn at a later time if and when it proves to be nonbeneficial or too burdensome. However, one should appreciate that many clinicians and families experience greater psychologic difficulty in withdrawing life-sustaining treatments than in withholding them.

4. **Present the recommendations to the patient or family.**
   Once the decision has been made to recommend that life support be withheld or withdrawn, members of the patient's health care team should meet with the patient and family to discuss the recommendations. The attending physician is the most appropriate spokesperson. He or she should clearly and carefully outline the proposed changes in treatment, explaining the basis for the decision and how it would be carried out, and taking care to emphasize that the limitation of life support would not mean the abandonment of the patient and that intensive comfort measures would be continued. Extra efforts should be made to avoid coercion or manipulation. Patients or families, or both, should be given a reasonable amount of time to consider the ICU team's recommendations. Although some families may take more time than others to make their decision, particularly if the patient is young or was previously healthy, recommendations based on sound medical judgment and expressed empathically are almost always eventually accepted.

5. **Attempt to resolve conflicts.**
   A difficult situation arises when patients or, more commonly, their families demand ICU interventions that the patient's attending physician and other members of the ICU team do not believe would be beneficial or otherwise medically indicated. In facing this challenge, the ICU team should re-examine its recommendations to determine once again their appropriateness and to ensure that they were clearly communicated. The wish of a family to "do everything" may not reflect a desire for every conceivable medical technology, but a plea that everything be done that might make the patient feel comfortable.

   The feelings of the patient or family, or both, should also be explored. There may be unresolved and unappreciated feelings of guilt, anger, fear, or denial, particularly for family members who might have been estranged from the patient before the ICU admission. These feelings will hinder family members in their role as surrogate decision makers on behalf of the patient. Honesty, understanding, sensitivity to these issues, and a multidisciplinary approach to building trust are required of the ICU team to help patients and their families overcome these emotional road blocks. Enlisting the aid of the institution's ethics committee, a hospital chaplain, or other counseling services can often be helpful in aiding in conflict resolution. With perseverance and patience, the great majority of these conflicts are successfully resolved at a local level. Only rarely, if ever, should a conflict over forgoing life support end up in a court of law for resolution.

6. **If conflicts cannot be resolved, consider applying the futility standard, if applicable and available.**

   When agreement with a surrogate decision maker still cannot be reached despite following the preceding steps, interventions judged to be futile may be limited without the approval of the family or surrogate decision maker if institutional policy permits (the patient is not referred to here because the issue of futility almost never arises when the patient has decision-making capacity). If the patient's attending physician decides to withhold or withdraw such interventions on this basis, he or she has the responsibility to inform the family or surrogate decision maker of the decision and its rationale. When feasible, the family should be given the opportunity to transfer responsibility for the patient's care to another physician who is willing to provide the disputed intervention. This may be in the same or different institution.

   A decision to limit life support over the objections of the family or surrogate decision maker based on futility should not be made lightly. No unilateral decision by the health care providers should be made until after sincere attempts have been made to follow steps 1 through 5. It should also only be carried out after input is obtained from all members of the patient's health care team, after appropriate consultations from physicians who can independently confirm the patient's poor medical prognosis, and after consultation with the hospitals ethics committee. The latter should confirm that the decision-making process is ethically sound, that the patient meets the institution's definition of futility, and that the institutional policy is being followed properly.

7. **Withhold or withdraw life support with close attention to patient comfort and family needs.**

   Withholding or withdrawing life-sustaining therapy covers a wide spectrum of interventions that might be forgone. It can range from simply withholding cardiopulmonary resuscitation in a patient going "downhill" on maximal therapy for septic shock to complete cessation of all medical therapies except those given to ensure comfort. Individual hospitals are required by external accrediting organizations to have written policies relating to withholding and withdrawing life support (Table 22–3).

   If an intervention, such as mechanical ventilation, is to be withdrawn, the ICU team should ensure that the patient is free of pain or other suffering, such as dyspnea, during and after its withdrawal. Some ICUs prefer a rapid removal of life support, whereas others accomplish the same end incrementally over time. Ideally, the manner in which life support is with-

Table 22–3. Levels of Do Not Resuscitate Orders

LEVEL	DEFINITION OF THERAPY	DESCRIPTION AND GOALS OF THERAPY
A	All therapies but no CPR	The patient will be treated as medically indicated, including all efforts to prevent cardiac or respiratory arrest. However, if such an arrest occurs, no resuscitative efforts will be made. This order should be reviewed prior to all operative procedures and may be temporarily suspended during or immediately after such procedures based on outcome of discussions by members of the operative team and the patient (or surrogate decision maker).
B	Limited therapy; no CPR	Therapy already begun will be continued as medically indicated. However, in general, no additional treatment will be added except for providing comfort to the patient. If cardiopulmonary arrest occurs, no resuscitative efforts will be made.
C	Comfort measures only	Treatment will be limited to nursing and medical therapy appropriate for hygiene and comfort. In general, treatment needed for comfort will be given even if it depresses cardiac or respiratory function. Life-sustaining therapies already started may be discontinued by written order.

Adapted from Policy Manual of the Hospital of the University of Pennsylvania with permission.
CPR, cardiopulmonary resusitation.

drawn should reflect the preferences of the patient or family rather than simply be based on local ICU customs. The family's preferences in this regard, as well as in whether they would want to stay with the patient until the moment of death, or not, should be explored.

Sedatives and analgesics should be administered and their dose titrated to eliminate patient discomfort (see Appendix C). This is ethical and legal even if giving such agents also hastens the patient's death. Titrating sedatives and opioids to a level of patient comfort, even if given in high doses, helps avoid any impression of performing active euthanasia. The aim of palliative drug therapy is to keep patients comfortable while they are dying from their diseases. In contrast, the aim of euthanasia is to intentionally cause the patient's death by the drug's actions. If ICU nurses, respiratory therapists, or physicians are not comfortable with participating in withdrawal of life support, their preference should be respected and they should be excused. Members of ICU teams commonly need special training in how to provide high-quality palliative care to the patient and family, as well as in how to support other ICU staff in what is often an emotionally draining experience.

Unless specific exceptions are agreed on beforehand with the patient or surrogate decision maker, the patient should receive only treatments and actions consistent with the decision to forgo life support. For example, some families may authorize stopping vasopressors, antibiotics, and blood products and withholding cardiac resuscitation, but not authorize cessation of mechanical ventilation. In this case, their wishes should be respected by the ICU team. In other cases, it is the ICU team that may continue practices seemingly at odds with the goals of patient comfort and nonprolongation of the dying process. For example, are measuring arterial PO_2 and PCO_2 when mechanical ventilation is discontinued consistent with the palliative goals agreed on? Continuing medications or interventions except to provide comfort and dignity to the patient should be questioned and not continued unless specifically justified.

8. **Provide emotional support to the patient's family.**
   The withdrawal of life support and the patient's actual dying are likely to be the most stressful part for family members. They should be given ample time to stay in the room with the patient during the dying process and, if they wish, to be present at the time of death. At all times, but especially after life support is withdrawn and after the patient actually dies, the patient's family and close friends should be provided emotional support by the ICU team and other trained hospital personnel, for example, social workers or pastoral care staff.

   Unless there is another critically ill patient waiting for the dying patient's ICU bed, or if the dying process is anticipated to be long, in general the patient should not be transferred out of the ICU. This permits continuity of medical care and emotional support provided by the ICU team that already knows the patient and family well. Furthermore, titration of sedatives and opioids immediately before and after terminal extubation or weaning often requires a high level of nursing care. Often only an ICU can provide this level of care. Under extenuating circumstances, as noted earlier, the patient can be transferred to another patient care unit but only if a high level of palliative care and appropriate support for the family can be ensured.

BIBLIOGRAPHY

American College of Chest Physicians/Society for Critical Care Medicine Consensus Panel: Ethical and moral guidelines for the initiation, continuation and withdrawal of intensive care. Chest 97:949–961, 1990.

American Thoracic Society: Withholding and withdrawing life-sustaining therapy. Am Rev Respir Dis 144:726–731, 1991.
The preceding two references are consensus statements from major professional organizations of intensivists. Both endorse the principles (1) that patients or their appropriate surrogate decision maker can forgo life-sustaining therapy and (2) that physicians are not obligated to provide life-sustaining interventions that are futile.

Koch K (ed): Medical ethics. Crit Care Clin 12:1–202, 1996.
This is a comprehensive up-to-date monograph containing articles and reviews of many of the important ethical issues of critical care medicine.

Lanken PN: Ethical considerations in pulmonary intensive care. In: Fishman AP (ed): Pulmonary Rehabilitation. New York: Marcell Dekker, 1996, pp 289–308.
This chapter reviews a spectrum of ethical issues commonly encountered in respiratory intensive care but pertinent to critical care medicine in general.

Lantos JD, Springer PA, Walker RM, et al: The illusion of futility in clinical practice. Am J Med 87:81–84, 1989.
This article discusses problems with the use of medical futility as a basis for medical decision-making.

Luce JM, Fink C: Communicating with families about withholding and withdrawal of life support. Chest 101:1185–1186, 1992.
This reference as well as the Meisel reference further on include excellent discussions on withholding and withdrawing life support in the ICU.

Luce JM, Raffin T: Ethical issues in critical care. New Horizons 5:1–93, 1997.
Another recent monograph, with articles covering the span of ICU ethics, including issues related to withholding and withdrawing life-sustaining therapy.

Meisel A: Legal myths about terminating life support. Arch Intern Med 151:1497–1502, 1991.
This article is must reading for those concerned about the issue of legality of stopping life support.

Osborne ML: Physician decisions regarding life support in the intensive care unit. Chest 101:217–224, 1992.
An excellent discussion on the mechanics of withholding/withdrawal life support.

Prendergast TJ, Luce JM: Increasing incidence of withholding and withdrawal of life support from the critically ill. Am J Respir Crit Care Med 155:15–20, 1997.
This national survey of ICUs in the United States over a six-month period found that the frequency of forging life support has increased in comparison to past studies. A wide range of practice variations were found, with some ICUs reporting up to 90% of ICU deaths associated with withholding or withdrawing life support, and others reporting no deaths after withdrawal of life support.

Schneiderman LJ, Jecker NS, Jonsen AR: Medical futility: Its meaning and ethical implications. Ann Intern Med 112:949–954, 1990.
This article presents the arguments in favor of the use of medical futility as a basis for medical decision-making.

The SUPPORT Investigators: A controlled trial to improve care for seriously ill hospitalized patients: The study to understand prognoses and preferences for outcomes and risks of treatments (SUPPORT). JAMA 274:1591–1598, 1995.
This was a large prospective cohort study of preferences of seriously ill adults in academic medical centers with regard to ICU care and life-sustaining interventions. It found that many patients preferred not to undergo aggressive ICU care, but that their preferences were unknown or ignored by their attending physicians. Families also perceived that the majority of patients who died had their pain and suffering poorly controlled.

23 The Challenge to Wean Patient

Horace M. DeLisser
Kathy M. Witta

Advances in critical care medicine have resulted in more patients surviving acute catastrophic illnesses. However, a significant percentage of these patients require mechanical ventilation for an extended period. The process of weaning ventilatory support may be long and frustrating for these patients, their families, and the health care team. Fortunately, interdisciplinary approaches emphasizing consistency, continuity, collaboration, and coordination help in managing the patient who is a challenge to wean. The phrase, *challenge to wean* is preferred over the more common and pejorative label, *failure to wean.*

DEFINITION AND PREVALENCE

Patients who are a challenge to wean are defined as those who have been ventilator-dependent for more than 7 days. They are unable to breathe without assistance for more than 24 hours despite often undergoing multiple attempts at discontinuing mechanical ventilation. Although the prevalence varies with the disease, as many as 10% of all acute critically ill patients require prolonged ventilatory support. For example, after cardiac surgery, up to 20% of patients need ventilatory support beyond the third postoperative day and up to 60% of patients with chronic obstructive pulmonary disease (COPD) who experience acute respiratory failure require mechanical ventilation for more than 2 weeks.

GENERAL STRATEGIES FOR MANAGING THE CHALLENGE TO WEAN PATIENT

To manage these patients appropriately, weaning should be considered a *process* in which the goals are to promote ventilator independence, preserve functional status, and promote a high quality of life. Ventilator independence may be partial (nocturnal or noninvasive) or full. Viewed in this way, the weaning that is difficult or challenging is seen not as a *failure to wean* but as a process, often long in duration and characterized by peaks and valleys, that ultimately is usually successful.

Success with the patient who is a challenge to wean begins with a multidisciplinary team approach (Table 23–1). This approach includes not only all the relevant health care givers but also the patient and his or her family members. Consistency and continuity of care and collaboration and communication among team members are the foundation of this approach. An individualized plan should be developed based on the patient's prehospital condition, an understanding of the events and processes that have led to the patient's current state, and an appreciation of the

267

Table 23–1. Multidisciplinary Health Care Team for Weaning

Primary Care Team

Nursing staff
Respiratory care practitioners
Pulmonologist or intensivist

Consultation Team

Physical and occupational therapists
Speech therapist
Nutritionist
Other specialist consultants as medically appropriate
Physiatrist
Psychiatrist, psychologist, or psychiatric liaison nurse
Social worker, discharge planner, or clinical resource manager

natural history and prognosis of the patient's underlying disease process (Fig. 23–1). This plan should include attainable, well-defined, short-term goals and a timetable for achieving them. Accomplishment of these goals boosts the morale of the patient and staff. A "weaning sheet" kept at the bedside is helpful to facilitate and coordinate care. Those providing care must be able to recognize the subjective and objective manifestations of weaning failure and understand the strategies available for dealing with it.

THE ROLE OF WEANING PARAMETERS

Traditional predictors of weaning success (Table 23–2) have included measurement of respiratory rate, tidal volume (TV), vital capacity (VC), minute ventilation ($\dot{V}_E$), maximal inspiratory pressure (MIP) (also called negative inspiratory force [NIF]), and maximal voluntary ventilation (MVV). However, studies of patients who have undergone long-term ventilation have found these indices to be disappointing. Although somewhat predictive of a successful outcome, significant false-positive rates (successful weaning predicted, but the patient does poorly) and false-negative rates (unsuccessful weaning predicted, yet weaning was successful) have been reported. More importantly, in individual patients they have not been shown to change consistently between unsuccessful and progressive weaning periods.

The poor performance of these traditional parameters has encouraged the development of a number of integrated physiologic parameters to provide better clinical predictors of weaning. Although they appear promising, none of the new indices has emerged as a clearly superior index for assessing patients requiring prolonged mechanical ventilation. Ultimately, even the "best" index may be limited in that successful weaning depends not only on respiratory mechanics (as gauged by these weaning parameters) but also on other factors, as described further on.

The presence of "good" weaning parameters (traditional or integrated) provides objective support for proceeding with weaning, but they do not guarantee a successful outcome or lessen the need for attention to the nonrespiratory factors required to discontinue mechanical ventilation (see Table 23–2). Likewise, "poor"

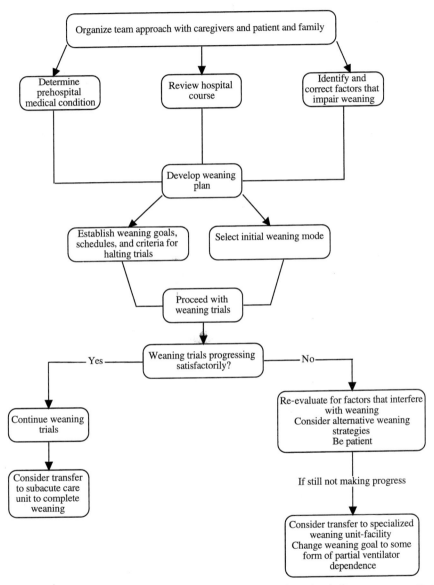

Figure 23–1. Flow diagram illustrating a comprehensive approach to the challenge to wean patient (see text for details).

Table 23–2. Criteria for Initiating Weaning from Mechanical Ventilation

··

Original indication for mechanical ventilation resolved or improved
Cardiovascular stability
Neurologic function adequate (spontaneous ventilatory efforts, satisfactory coughing and swallowing)
Adequate oxygenation (Pao$_2$ ≥60 mm Hg or O$_2$ saturation ≥90% on F$_{IO_2}$ ≤0.5%)
Adequate respiratory mechanics*

··

*Defined as one or more of the following: maximal inspiratory pressure < −20 cm H$_2$O, spontaneous respiratory rate <35/min, spontaneous tidal volume >5 mL/kg IBW, vital capacity >10 mL/kg IBW, resting minute ventilation ≤10 L/min with maximal voluntary ventilation ≥2 × resting minute ventilation.
IBW, ideal body weight (see Chapter 12, Table 12–1 for IBW formulas); F$_{IO_2}$, fractional concentration of inspired oxygen.

weaning indices should sound a note of caution about progressing and call attention to factors that might compromise the weaning process. However, they should not preclude carefully monitored attempts at withdrawing mechanical ventilation.

FACTORS THAT HINDER WEANING

Integral to the weaning plan is a careful and *ongoing* evaluation of the patient for conditions that may hinder the withdrawal of ventilatory support. Although large and diverse in number, these processes can be conveniently separated into processes that increase the work of breathing, impair respiratory muscle function, decrease the central drive to the respiratory pump, or have a psychologic or emotional basis. Typically a combination of these factors hinders weaning.

Processes that Increase the Work of Breathing

As listed in Table 23–3, the work of breathing may be increased by processes that raise airway resistance, decrease lung compliance, or stimulate respiratory drive. The role for either *N*-acetylcysteine or recombinant human deoxyribonuclease (dornase alfa) given intratracheally in mobilizing secretions in patients who are undergoing chronic ventilation has not been clearly defined. Although the exact timing of tracheostomy remains a subject of debate, a tracheostomy may be particularly beneficial in that it facilitates suctioning and enhances patient comfort. In addition, replacing an endotracheal tube with a tracheostomy tube, even of the same internal diameter, can decrease the patient's work of breathing. This is not due to the decrease in dead space in changing from endotracheal tube to tracheostomy tube, which is trivial compared with the patient's physiologic dead space (see Chapter 1). Instead, it recently has been shown that the lumen of endotracheal tube acquires an invisible *biofilm* over several weeks of use and that this markedly increases the tube's airway resistance (compared with an "off-the-shelf" endotracheal or tracheostomy tube of the same internal diameter).

The demand valve in a ventilator's circuit also contributes to airway resistance and thus increases the work of breathing. Even in assisted modes of ventilation, the work of breathing may be equal to or greater than that required for a normal spontaneous breath. Strategies for overcoming the resistance of the ventilator

Table 23–3. Factors That Increase Work of Breathing

Decreased Lung Compliance

Abdominal distention
Intrinsic PEEP (auto-PEEP)
After lobectomy-pneumonectomy
Pulmonary edema
Supine position

Increased Airway Resistance

Bronchospasm
Endotracheal tube (prolonged use)
Secretions
Small-diameter tracheal tube
Ventilator circuit

Increased Respiratory Drive

End-stage liver or renal disease
Excessive carbohydrate calories (see Chapter 13)
Fever, infection
Metabolic acidosis

PEEP, positive end-expiratory pressure.

include judicious titration of the flow rate, use of flow- rather than pressure-triggered ventilators, elimination of breathing circuit dead space, and the use of pass-over instead of cascade humidification.

Lung compliance may be reduced by abdominal distention, the presence of intrinsic positive end-expiratory pressure (auto-PEEP), or the supine position. Mild, interstitial pulmonary edema, which often is not recognized, may also be a significant factor in prolonged weaning. The transition from positive pressure ventilation to spontaneous breathing results in decreased intrathoracic pressures and increased venous return such that patients with impaired left ventricular function may develop elevated left ventricular diastolic pressure and pulmonary edema. Also the stress of weaning may precipitate coronary ischemia, resulting in ischemia-induced left ventricular diastolic dysfunction.

Processes that stimulate respiratory drive increase minute ventilation and thus the work of breathing. Some of these include fever, shivering, excess carbohydrates, and hypermetabolic states (e.g., after trauma or major surgery). One of the manifestations of an early or chronic infection may be difficulty weaning, and thus evaluation for, and treatment of, infections (particularly ventilator-associated pneumonia) are imperative in these patients. In patients with gram-negative ventilator-associated tracheobronchitis (in the absence of pneumonia), aerosolized aminoglycosides (e.g., 300 mg tobramycin given by nebulization twice a day) may control the infection without the toxicities associated with systemic aminoglycosides.

Processes That Impair Respiratory Muscle Function

A second group of processes that hinder weaning success are those that lead to respiratory muscle weakness and fatigue (Table 23–4). Causes include inadequate

Table 23–4. Factors That Impair Respiratory Muscle Function

Muscle-related Factors

Disuse atrophy
Electrolyte disturbances
Fatigue due to inadequate rest between
  weaning trials
Malnutrition
Myopathy of critical illness

Neuromuscular Junction Dysfunction

Drug-induced myasthenic syndromes

Peripheral Nerve Disease

Neuropathy of critical illness
Single or bilateral phrenic nerve injury

nutrition, electrolyte imbalances (especially calcium, magnesium, phosphorus), and inadequate respiratory muscle rest between weaning trials. True respiratory muscle fatigue may need at least 24 hours for full recovery. Diuretics and antibiotics may waste potassium and magnesium and contribute to acid-base disturbances. Recent reports have implicated the combination of steroids and paralytic agents in the development of a respiratory muscle myopathy that may last for weeks or months in critically ill ventilator-dependent patients. Several drugs, including aminoglycosides, may induce a myasthenia-like syndrome in susceptible patients. Approaches to increasing respiratory muscle strength include appropriate nutrition, careful attention to electrolytes, and a program of repetitive trials of unassisted or partially assisted breathing that avoids respiratory muscle fatigue.

FACTORS THAT DECREASE CENTRAL RESPIRATORY DRIVE

The central effects of opioids, antianxiety agents, and other sedating drugs can decrease respiratory drive and hinder weaning directly (Table 23–5). Metabolic alkalosis, for example, from aggressive diuresis and intravascular volume contraction, can result in an elevated set point for $PaCO_2$ and result in CO_2 retention. This may hinder weaning if the rise in $PaCO_2$ is misinterpreted as resulting from respiratory muscle fatigue instead of the alkalosis. Finally, pre-existing hypothyroidism or sleep-related breathing disorders, for example, obesity hypoventilation

Table 23–5. Factors That Decrease Respiratory Drive

Central sleep apnea
Hypothyroidism
Metabolic alkalosis
Opioids, anxiolytic drugs, or other sedatives
Obesity hypoventilation syndrome

syndrome or central sleep apnea syndrome (that may accompany obstructive sleep apnea), may not be appreciated as barriers to weaning unless they are specifically sought out and treated (see Chapter 77).

Psychological Factors

Psychologic factors often contribute significantly to prolonged weaning (Table 23–6). Anxiety, fear, pain, and disorientation may lead to feelings of hopelessness, powerlessness, and depression. Cognitive deficits, especially impaired short-term memory, contribute to confusion, miscommunication, and a lack of confidence in self and staff. Patients may also acquire a distorted body image in which the ventilator is viewed as an extension of self. These emotions are amplified by the inability to speak, sleep deprivation, immobility, side effects of medications, and the noise and incessant activity in the intensive care unit (ICU). These feelings lead to a vicious cycle of dyspnea, increased work of breathing, respiratory muscle fatigue, and ultimately more dyspnea.

Interventions to promote psychologic well-being include the use of assistive devices to facilitate speech (Passey-Muir valve, fenestrated or talking tracheotomy tubes [see Chapter 24]), inclusion of the patient in all decision-making, discussions of sensations that are normally experienced during weaning, frequent positive reinforcement, and liberal emotional support. A written schedule for a typical day, prominently displayed so that the patient can easily see it, provides structure and consistency, not only for the patient but also for all caregivers. A clock, a large-print calendar, and a room with a window help with orientation. Sleep deprivation is frequently experienced by ICU patients and may compromise their emotional well-being (see Chapter 44). To promote good sleep, hygiene nursing interventions should be grouped together to allow consistent sleep-wake cycles. Excessive environmental noise and light should be controlled during sleep periods. Zolpidem (Ambien) may be a useful hypnotic for the patient who is a challenge to wean because it has less suppression of stages 3 and 4 non–rapid eye movement sleep and may have less residual effects the following day compared with benzodiazepines (see Chapter 44, Table 44–6). Methods to deal with dyspnea, anxiety, and panic attacks include biofeedback, pursed lip breathing, relaxation techniques, reading, music, prayer, television viewing, and portable fans to blow air on the patient's face. A rehabilitation approach with emphasis on mobility, communication, and a sense of control is also critical in dealing with the psychologic aspects of the weaning process (see Chapter 25). When appropriate, use of

Table 23–6. Psychologic and Emotional Factors That Hinder Weaning

Anger	Fear
Anxiety	Isolation
Cognitive deficits	Pain and dyspnea
Depression	Sensory overload
Distorted body image	Sleep deprivation

anxiolytic and antidepressant drugs may prove to be helpful with the nonpharmacologic therapeutic efforts.

SPECIFIC POPULATIONS

The Patient with Chronic Obstructive Pulmonary Disease

The patient with COPD may have difficulty weaning for a number of reasons. First, clinicians often make the error of initially correcting the $Paco_2$ to a value much less than the patient's baseline when providing assisted ventilation. This causes renal excretion of bicarbonate, with the result that when the patient resumes his or her usual level of spontaneous ventilation and the $Paco_2$ rises, there is inadequate buffering to maintain the pH within the normal range. Second, COPD places the patient at risk for intrinsic PEEP (auto-PEEP). This, in turn, increases the work required to trigger the ventilator because that pressure has to be overcome before flow starts. Treatment of expiratory flow limitation (bronchospasm), adjustments in the flow rate and inspiratory:expiratory ratio, or the addition of external PEEP (to just less than the level of intrinsic PEEP) are helpful in addressing this problem. Third, the nutritional needs must be carefully addressed (see Chapter 13). Excess carbohydrate calories, that is, overfeeding resulting in a respiratory quotient (RQ) greater than 1, increase CO_2 production, minute ventilation, and the work of breathing. Conversely, malnutrition may result in diminished respiratory muscle strength and endurance. Fourth, the cardiac status of the patient with COPD must be closely evaluated. Typically, these patients have a significant smoking history that puts them at high risk for concomitant coronary heart disease. They are at risk for arrhythmias, chronic left ventricular systolic and diastolic dysfunction, and pulmonary edema from transient left ventricular dysfunction induced by ischemia. Lastly, psychologic factors may become significant obstacles to successful weaning, with patients developing strong emotional and psychologic attachments to being on their ventilator. Under these circumstances, the strategies outlined earlier for dealing with psychologic issues are helpful.

The Patient Who Has Undergone Cardiac Surgery

Congestive heart failure, related to preoperative left ventricular dysfunction or unsuccessful revascularization, is common and prolongs weaning. Also, diaphragmatic dysfunction confirmed by electromyography is reported in up to 10% of patients who have had coronary artery bypass surgery and may persist for months. This dysfunction is commonly due to phrenic nerve injury from ice slush topical cardioplegia, surgical trauma, and ischemia of the phrenic nerve from the use of the internal mammary artery as a vascular conduit. Interventions include having the patient sit in an erect position to facilitate diaphragmatic excursion and efforts to prevent or reverse atelectasis. Furthermore, the patient with a recent myocardial infarction should be weaned cautiously. These individuals may do better with a pressure support wean rather than a T-piece wean (see further on) in which the cardiovascular status can gradually adjust to the increased demands of breathing and there will be less dramatic shifts in changes in pleural pressures and venous return to the right atrium.

CHOICE OF WEANING TECHNIQUES

An important decision is the choice of weaning technique. Weaning modalities gradually allow the work of breathing to be shifted from the ventilator to the patient (see Chapter 3). The traditional methods of weaning involve (1) increasing periods of spontaneous breathing with rest modes of full ventilatory support, that is, T-piece or continuous positive airway pressure (CPAP) wean; (2) gradual removal of the support provided to each breath, that is, pressure support wean; and (3) progressive reductions in the number of fully supported breaths, that is, synchronized intermittent mechanical ventilation (SIMV) wean. Weaning can be viewed as a process of respiratory muscle training and reconditioning. From this perspective, weaning by T-piece, CPAP, or SIMV aims to strengthen respiratory muscles. Pressure support ventilation promotes respiratory muscle endurance by gradually reducing the amount of ventilator-delivered pressure to each spontaneous breath. Regardless of the technique employed, the goal is to encourage reconditioning of the respiratory muscles without inducing fatigue.

Although the merits and indications of these techniques have been the subject of numerous studies, the results have been conflicting, and no single approach has been shown to be clearly superior in the majority of chronically ventilator-dependent patients. Consequently, the decision regarding the initial weaning modality must currently be determined by the clinician's experience and the characteristics of each patient. It is recommended, however, that ventilator modes not be mixed (e.g., high levels of pressure support with high SIMV rates) and that sufficient time be allowed to judge the effectiveness of a chosen technique. At the start of the process, regardless of the approach, the weaning should be performed during the day rather than at night. At night, the respiratory muscles should be unloaded, that is, rested. The patient should not be pushed to the point of obvious respiratory muscle fatigue, for example, respiratory paradox, or severe respiratory distress. Although the optimal interval of rest is unknown, providing adequate rest is crucial. The clinician must be open and flexible to alternative strategies if the initial approach is not successful.

LACK OF PROGRESS IN WEANING

Many patients fail to make progress initially despite meticulous and appropriate care. In this setting, the ICU team needs to be patient and to maintain their focus. The patient should be continuously re-evaluated for factors that interfere with weaning, and alternative weaning strategies should be employed. Although some individuals will never be completely liberated from ventilatory support, many will with time and patience.

OPTIONS FOR THE PERSISTENTLY VENTILATOR-DEPENDENT PATIENT

Depending on the geographic region, transfer to a specialized subacute care facility that specializes in chronic respiratory care or weaning may be an option for patients who are not progressing in an acute care setting. These facilities provide a focused, multidisciplinary, consistent approach to the management of these patients. Recent studies have demonstrated that these facilities have a positive impact on cost and patient outcome.

Some patients, despite best efforts, may not be able to achieve complete independence from positive pressure mechanical ventilation. The patient with severe neuromuscular disease, high spinal cord injury, or advanced pulmonary disease, may require partial or alternative ventilatory support, such as nocturnal positive pressure ventilation, noninvasive ventilation, or negative pressure ventilation. For these patients, subacute or chronic ventilator units in long-term care facilities or home ventilation may be reasonable options. The cost of care in these facilities is one fourth to one third the cost of care in an ICU. Discharge to home on a portable ventilator may be feasible for the patient who has a dedicated family support system. A sobering statistic is that 33% of ventilator-dependent patients who were judged suitable for transfer out of the acute care setting died while awaiting placement. Consequently, the individuals responsible for discharge planning need to be notified early because the placement of these patients may be difficult.

BIBLIOGRAPHY

Burns SM, Clochesy JM, Ganneman SK, et al: Weaning from long-term mechanical ventilation. Am J Crit Care 4:422, 1995.
   This article includes a careful analysis of the problems and limitations of the currently available weaning predictors.

Criner GJ, Tzouanakis A, Kreimer DT: Overview of improving tolerance of long-term mechanical ventilation. Crit Care Clin 10:845–865, 1994.
   This article provides an excellent summary of the issues and management of patients requiring long-term ventilatory support.

DeLisser HM, Grippi MA: Phrenic nerve injury following cardiac surgery, with emphasis on the role of topical hypothermia. J Intensive Care Med 6:295–301, 1991.
   This supplies a review of the causes and management of phrenic nerve injury after cardiac surgery.

Diehl JL, El Atrous S, Touchard D, et al: Changes in the work of breathing induced by tracheotomy in ventilator-dependent patients. Am J Respir Crit Care Med 159:383–388, 1999.
   This recent intriguing study found that work of breathing in patients on pressure support was significantly decreased when tracheostomy tubes of the same diameter replaced their endotracheal tubes. Additional data presented suggest that this was due to an invisible biofilm of secretions that had accumulated on the inside surface of the endotracheal tube.

Gracey DR, Viggiano RW, Naessens JM, et al: Outcomes of patients admitted to a chronic ventilator-dependent unit in an acute-care hospital. Mayo Clin Proc 67:131–136, 1992.
   Of the 61 patients admitted to a chronic ventilator-dependent unit, 58 survived and 53 were liberated from mechanical ventilation.

Hansen-Flaschen J, Cowen J, Raps EC: Neuromuscular blockade in the intensive care unit. More than we bargained for. Am Rev Respir Dis 147:234–236, 1993.

This article reviews the data on the role of neuromuscular blocking drugs in causing acute myopathy in critically ill patients.

Hill N: Failure to wean, the chronic ventilator-dependent patient. In: Fishman AP (ed): Pulmonary Rehabilitation. New York: Marcel-Dekker, 1996, pp 577–617.
This is a comprehensive review of current approaches to the challenge to wean patient (with 112 references).

Menzies R, Gibbons W, Goldberg P: Determinants of weaning and survival among patients with COPD who require mechanical ventilation for acute respiratory failure. Chest 95:398–405, 1989.
Provided is a list of prognostic factors for mortality and failure to wean in ventilator-dependent patients with COPD.

Slutsky AS: ACCP Consensus Conference: Mechanical Ventilation. Chest 104:1833–1859, 1993.
This article is a comprehensive review of all aspects of mechanical ventilation.

Spitzer AR, Giancarlo T, Maher L, et al: Neuromuscular causes of prolonged ventilator dependency. Muscle Nerve 15:682–686, 1992.
Unsuspected neuromuscular disease was the predominant (62%) primary cause of prolonged ventilator dependency.

24

Swallowing and Communication Disorders

Andrew N. Goldberg
Melissa A. Simonian

The goal and challenge in treating intensive care unit (ICU) patients with communication and swallowing disorders is to restore two basic human functions: speaking and eating. Verbal communication and normal swallowing function can be compromised in ICU patients not only by disorders causing critical illness but also by common ICU treatments. For example, all patients with prolonged mechanical ventilation or tracheostomy are at increased risk for speech and swallowing problems. The prognosis for restoring normal speech and swallowing can be improved if one applies a multidisciplinary intervention strategy early in the course of the patient's recovery from critical illness. Three major goals of this strategy are to establish appropriate alternative methods of communication, to prevent aspiration, and to provide oral nutrition.

APPROACH TO SWALLOWING DYSFUNCTION IN THE INTENSIVE CARE UNIT PATIENT

A swallowing assessment should be made in all ICU patients as they recover from critical illness. Problems with swallowing (also called *dysphagia)* place patients at high risk for aspiration (defined as penetration of any material below the vocal cords) when they start to resume oral feeding and drinking. Dysfunction of the normal swallowing mechanism should be suspected in patients after neurologic events or surgical procedures that might affect function of the pharynx or larynx. The same suspicion should apply to all patients who have undergone tracheotomies or who have had prolonged translaryngeal intubation, or both. Similarly, one should assume that patients with endotracheal tubes in place cannot swallow food safely, and attempts at oral feeding should wait until after extubation or conversion to tracheostomy with spontaneous breathing. Consultation with a speech-language pathologist may be indicated for these ICU patients before restarting oral fluids or feeding.

THE SWALLOWING MECHANISM

The anatomic areas involved in swallowing include the oral cavity, pharynx, larynx, and esophagus. The act of swallowing is divided into three sequential phases (Table 24–1). During the *oral phase* intact labial muscles are necessary to ensure an adequate seal that prevents leakage from the oral cavity. The *pharyngeal phase* begins with triggering of the swallow reflex. This reflex comprises a series of coordinated movements crucial to successful swallowing (Table 24–2). The *esophageal phase* begins when the upper esophageal sphincter relaxes. This allows

Table 24–1. Three Phases of Normal Swallowing

PHASE	DESCRIPTION
Oral phase	The food bolus is manipulated, masticated, formed, and propelled posteriorly by lingual and buccal movements
Pharyngeal phase	The swallow reflex is triggered and the airway is closed As the food bolus moves through the pharynx, the upper esophageal sphincter relaxes
Esophageal phase	Esophageal peristalsis carries the bolus through the cervical and thoracic esophagus into the stomach

the peristaltic wave (which began in the pharynx with triggering of the swallow reflex) to continue in sequential fashion down the esophagus into the stomach.

CLINICAL ASSESSMENT FOR SWALLOWING DYSFUNCTION

A swallowing evaluation starts with a review of the patient's medical and surgical history, hospital course, and respiratory and nutritional status (Fig. 24–1). A cognitive screening and complete oral physical examination should then be performed. Patients who are not alert or who are severely cognitively impaired may not be candidates for undergoing further bedside tests to evaluate the risk of aspiration. Oxygen desaturation and copious secretions are also contraindications to these tests.

Review of Medical Record

Careful review of the medical and surgical history including medications, respiratory and nutritional status, and, if present, the reason for placement of a tracheostomy tube is important. The presence of a tracheostomy tube often contributes to aspiration and swallowing dysfunction, and this risk is often compounded by the underlying medical problem for which the tracheostomy was performed.

Table 24–2. Actions of the Swallow Reflex

Action 1	Elevation and retraction of the soft palate, with complete closure of the velopharyngeal port to prevent material entering the nasal cavity
Action 2	Initiation of pharyngeal peristalsis to carry the bolus through the pharynx
Action 3	Elevation of the larynx and its closure by the epiglottis to prevent food or fluid from entering the trachea
Action 4	Relaxation of the upper esophageal sphincter (cricopharyngeus), allowing the food bolus to pass into the esophagus

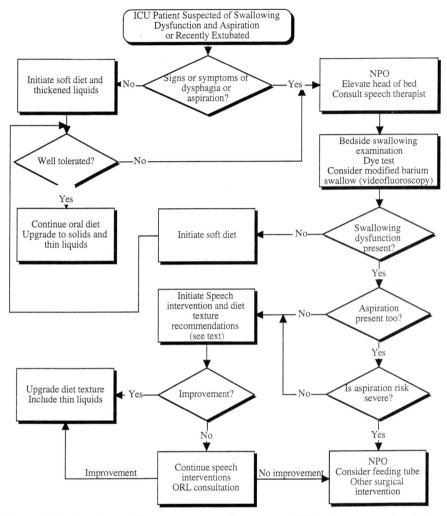

Figure 24–1. Flow diagram illustrating the general approach to ICU patients suspected of having swallowing dysfunction (see text for details).

NPO, nothing by mouth; ORL, otorhinolaryngology.

Oropharyngeal Examination

Visualizing the structural integrity of the oral cavity, the presence or absence of teeth, and the movement and coordination of the tongue, lips, mandible, and palate provides the clinician with information regarding the oral phase of the swallow as well as speech intelligibility. The presence or absence of the gag reflex should also be documented. The presence of a gag reflex alone, however, does not predict the adequacy of the swallow reflex nor, conversely, does its absence predict swallowing dysfunction.

Bedside Evaluation of Swallowing

Assessment of the *oral phase* of the swallow involves determining the patient's ability to masticate, control, propel, and clear a food bolus from the mouth without a delay. Assessment of the *pharyngeal phase* of the swallow includes observing laryngeal elevation and noting changes in vocal quality and an associated cough or throat clearing. Gurgling with speech or clearing of the throat indicates the presence of secretions pooled near the larynx. Laryngeal elevation is observed by palpating the neck to feel the larynx move superiorly and anteriorly during the swallow (Table 24–3). Assessment of the *esophageal phase* of the swallow cannot be performed at the bedside.

This approach applies to a bedside clinical evaluation for patients with or without tracheotomies. In a patient with a tracheostomy, however, the dye test is added as described in the following section.

The Dye Test

Any patient with a tracheostomy should be evaluated with the dye test to ascertain the presence of aspiration before resumption of drinking and swallowing food. Dyed food is administered while the patient is observed for manifestations of aspiration, for example, coughing or vocal quality changes. These may indicate delayed aspiration, and the patient should be encouraged to cough and clear the airway. The tracheostomy provides direct access to the lower airway via suctioning. Dyed food or fluid ingested by the patient that is subsequently deep suctioned or expectorated via the tracheostomy tube is clear evidence of aspiration.

If no aspiration is evident with the first swallowing attempts, the test continues with successive swallows of varied consistency and size of boluses. If the patient aspirates, one must decide whether to proceed or discontinue the examination. This decision rests on the patient's ability to cough and clear the material and overall respiratory condition. The patient's respiratory status should be monitored over the next 24 hours to note the presence of any additional dyed material at the tracheostomy site. Since patients aspirate intermittently, aspirate only certain consistencies of material, or aspirate silently without overt clinical signs, a video-fluoroscopic study may be needed to definitively assess the nature of the swallowing dysfunction.

Table 24–3. Overt and Covert Signs of Aspiration During Bedside Evaluation

OVERT SIGNS	COVERT SIGNS
Buccal pocketing (food retention in the cheek pouch)	Lower lobe radiographic infiltrates
Coughing with oral intake	Increased pharyngeal secretions requiring transoral suctioning
Drooling	Recurrent aspiration pneumonia
"Wet" vocal quality after eating	Significant weight loss

Videofluoroscopy

A videofluoroscopic swallowing evaluation (modified barium swallow) is a dynamic assessment of swallowing. It is used as an adjunct to the clinical bedside evaluation and the dye test. Videofluoroscopy allows observation of the dynamics of the oral, pharyngeal, and esophageal phases of swallowing, and determination of the presence and mechanism of aspiration. This study is particularly important when intermittent aspiration occurs during feeding trials or if silent aspiration is suspected secondary to sensory level deficits.

The evaluation usually begins with the administration of a thick liquid contrast bolus to swallow. This contrast provides an adequate coating of surfaces so that the structures can be well visualized. The patient should be positioned upright and encouraged to feed himself or herself, if possible. Active patient participation enables observation of the cognitive aspects that contribute to swallowing as well. If the patient tolerates a small initial bolus, larger boluses of varied consistencies are administered to stress the patient's swallowing ability.

The timing of aspiration during the swallow is important. Aspiration can occur before swallow initiation, amid the pharyngeal phase (midswallow), or after swallow completion by overflow of pooled or residual contrast material into the trachea. The timing and amount of aspiration determines which compensatory positioning maneuvers should be tried. Among these maneuvers are head turning, chin tuck, and the Valsalva maneuver. The effectiveness of each maneuver can be readily evaluated by repeated administration of contrast material.

The esophagus can also be visualized during this study, noting the presence of structural abnormalities, decreased peristaltic action, and reflux. The limitations of videofluoroscopy include radiation exposure, the need for examiner expertise, transport of the patient, and the taste of the contrast material (typically barium or meglumine diatrizoate [Gastrografin]).

Fiberoptic Evaluation

Fiberoptic endoscopic evaluation of swallowing is used in patients who cannot undergo videofluoroscopy or as an adjunct to the others tests in selected patients with complex swallowing problems. It allows the function and appearance of the pharynx and larynx to be examined and recorded. A flexible fiberoptic scope is inserted nasally and positioned to view the pharynx and larynx. With the introduction of food or liquid, the pharyngeal and laryngeal dynamics can be examined for dysfunction. Due to limited views of the structures, however, this technique does not provide a complete assessment of the oral cavity, bolus transit, or esophageal function.

MANAGEMENT OF SWALLOWING DYSFUNCTION

Management aims to improve the swallowing function to achieve adequate nutrition and to eliminate aspiration. Treatment is goal-directed, incorporating compensatory strategies, other therapeutic techniques, or surgical intervention in selected refractory cases. The preferred initial management of patients with swallowing dysfunction who are at risk for aspiration is noninvasive. The majority of ICU patients can be managed in this way.

General Approaches

For patients at risk of aspiration, reflux and aspiration precautions should be implemented. These include elevation of the head of the bed, cessation of oral feeding, and placement of a cuffed tracheostomy tube in tracheostomized patients (Fig. 24–2). Enteral or parenteral alimentation should be considered in any patient who is no longer being fed orally.

Patients intubated for 5 days or more are at increased risk for aspiration. Even patients intubated for less than 5 days may suffer from swallowing dysfunction on extubation. This is usually self-limited and, as a rule, a mechanically soft diet can be initiated in these patients without problems. Persistent dysfunction should be evaluated by a speech-language pathologist or otorhinolaryngologist, or both.

Patients intubated for more than 5 days who demonstrate swallowing dysfunction on extubation should be given no food or drink by mouth for 24 hours after extubation, followed by initiation of a soft diet. A speech pathologist or otorhinolaryngologist should be consulted to evaluate persistent dysfunction, that is, dysfunction that is still present 24 hours after extubation.

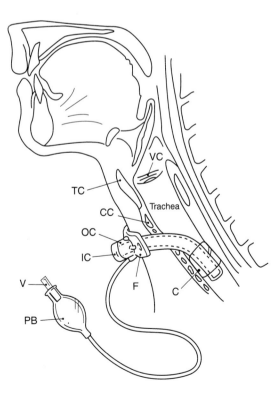

Figure 24–2. Sagittal midline view of trachea, larynx, and pharynx with an inflated cuffed tracheostomy tube in place. The tube enters the trachea via a surgical opening at the level of the second or third tracheal rings. C, cuff of tracheostomy tube (see Fig. 24–3 for details); CC, cricoid cartilage; F, flange of tube; IC, inner cannula of tube (represented by dashed lines within the outer cannula); OC, outer cannula of tube; PB, pilot balloon; TC, thyroid cartilage; V, one-way valve; VC, vocal cords. Courtesy of Voicing, Inc., Newport Beach, CA.

Noninvasive Therapies and Prosthetics

For swallowing dysfunction, the initial treatment is noninvasive, either indirect or direct. Indirect treatments include exercises to increase oral motor control, thermal stimulation of the swallow reflex, and vocal exercises to increase adduction of the vocal cords, thereby improving airway protection. Direct interventions constitute modification of swallowing technique or the bolus texture. Because thin liquids are the most difficult to control, using thick liquids and pureed solids (pudding consistency) provides a helpful early intervention in cases of mild to moderate dysfunction. Modification of head or body position by sitting the patient upright and using a Valsalva maneuver ("supraglottic swallow") are other useful techniques in managing those with mild aspiration risks.

In addition to these noninvasive therapies, selected patients with palatal dysfunction may benefit from intraoral prostheses to improve oropharyngeal swallowing functions. A palatal lift elevates the soft palate to augment velopharyngeal closure. A palatal obturator to fill or cover a defect in the hard or soft palate may be appropriate in some cases. If swallowing therapy or prosthetics are ineffective, surgical intervention focused on eliminating aspiration may be considered.

Invasive Interventions

Failure of initial treatment with conservative measures occurs for a variety of reasons. Some include severe neuromuscular dysfunction or cognitive deficits, anatomic obstruction by a scar band or tumor, and anatomic alteration by trauma or surgery. Surgical intervention may be used to provide an alternate route for alimentation, relieve a physical obstruction, or separate the air and food passages.

Tracheostomy and Feeding Tube Placement

In patients with refractory aspiration, the most common procedures employed are placement of a tracheostomy and feeding tube. There is some irony in this because a tracheostomy, as noted earlier, can actually increase one's risk of aspiration. Tracheostomy tubes do, however, provide a route for suctioning saliva, other aspirated contents, and the thick secretions characteristic of some of these patients.

Some patients benefit from inflation of the tracheostomy tube cuff, which assists in preventing aspirated material from falling into the lower respiratory tract. Tracheostomy cuff pressures must be carefully monitored to prevent mucosal and cartilage ischemia, leading to necrosis and tracheal stenosis. Balloon overinflation can also impede the flow of material down the esophagus by compression of the esophagus through the membranous posterior tracheal wall.

In other patients, the cuff may be left deflated or an uncuffed tube may be used. Placement of a Passy-Muir one-way "speaking valve" attached to the proximal adapter of the tracheostomy tube is often helpful in decreasing the risk of aspiration. For example, it restores the patient's capacity to build up intratracheal pressure (before glottic opening), which is needed for producing an effective cough.

Creation of a feeding jejunostomy is another commonly used procedure for patients who aspirate food but can tolerate their own secretions. A jejunostomy is preferred over a gastrostomy if there is considerable risk for gastroesophageal reflux and subsequent aspiration of the refluxed tube feeding. Subsequent oral feeding trials can be initiated in conjunction with a decrease in jejunostomy tube feedings until the patient is able to comfortably supply all his or her nutritional needs orally. Often a tracheostomy and jejunostomy are performed under one anesthetic in the operating room.

Upper Esophageal Sphincterotomy

Selected patients with neuromuscular dysfunction or isolated cricopharyngeal achalasia may benefit from release of the cricopharyngeus muscle (upper esophageal sphincter). This procedure carries little morbidity and can be performed selectively using local anesthesia if necessary. Its indications include a persistent, prominent, tight cricopharyngeus muscle in a patient without significant gastroesophageal reflux disease.

Surgical Separation of Air and Food Passages

For patients with severe impairment of the swallowing mechanism, life-threatening aspiration pneumonia is common. Many procedures have been attempted to separate the air and food passages, and individual preferences of the surgeon play a major role in choosing the specific operation. All procedures eliminate natural speech, although alternatives for speech and communication are available. For example, laryngotracheal separation, or the modified Lindeman procedure, definitively controls aspiration by separating the air and food passages. The procedure can be performed with low morbidity and is reversible in selected cases.

VERBAL COMMUNICATION PROBLEMS

Communication with ICU staff, family, and friends is vital for the patient's physical and psychological recovery. Adequate communication enables patients to participate in their care, which can decrease their feelings of insecurity and anxiety. In the ICU, impediments to verbal communication include the presence of an endotracheal or tracheostomy tube, abnormal function of the articulatory musculature, other neurologic impairments, and damage to the larynx.

Most ICU patients are medically unstable and require flexible, functional, and practical interventions to improve their communication. In developing an effective nonverbal system of communication, the patient's family and ICU nurses, guided by the speech-language pathologist, should consider the patient's cognitive and physical abilities as well as the basic communication needs. Commercially available computer-assisted communication systems are expensive and inappropriate for short-term use. If the patient has a tracheostomy, a modification of the tracheostomy tube or placement of a one-way valve may facilitate verbal output. There are various nonverbal (nonlaryngeal) and verbal (laryngeal) options available to achieve effective communication (Table 24–4).

Table 24–4. Nonlaryngeal and Laryngeal Approaches to Promote Communication

....

NONLARYNGEAL APPROACHES	LARYNGEAL APPROACHES
Gestural, sign, eye gaze techniques	Fenestrated tracheostomy tubes
Picture, word, alphabet boards	Tracheostomy speaking valves (Passy-Muir valves)
Lip-speaking words	Controlled tidal volume leaks*
Alaryngeal devices (e.g., electrolarynx)	Talking tracheostomy tubes

*This method uses extra-large tidal volumes, a part of which is allowed to leak around a partially deflated cuff (of a tracheostomy tube or endotracheal tube) while the patient is on the assist-control mode of mechanical ventilation. If used, the patient must have constant bedside attendance by ICU staff to ensure that adequate tidal volumes are still being delivered to the lungs.

TRACHEOSTOMY TUBES

Indications and Insertion

A tracheostomy (synonymous with tracheotomy) is commonly performed when there is a prolonged need for an artificial airway, when pulmonary toilet is needed and cannot be achieved otherwise, or obstruction of the natural airway is present. Although placement of a tracheostomy decreases dead space, this is not a justification for its placement because the decrease is almost trivial. This arises because the physiologic dead space in most ICU patients equals, and often exceeds, the anatomic dead space. Prospective studies have indicated that the main advantage in converting an endotracheal tube to a tracheostomy tube in ICU patients receiving mechanical ventilation is that the latter provides a more comfortable airway. It also provides a more secure airway for chronically ventilator-dependent patients being transferred to subacute or long-term care facilities.

Tracheostomy involves creating an opening in the trachea at the level of the second or third tracheal ring (see Fig. 24–2). The tracheostomy tube is inserted to maintain an opening after the surgical procedure. The tube must be left in place during the initial healing process to allow the skin opening and tracheal opening to form a single aligned track. The tube is generally changed on or about the seventh postoperative day after sufficient time has elapsed for this healing to occur. Before this time, the track may not be well formed. If the tracheostomy tube is inadvertently pulled out during this time, the skin and tracheal openings may become misaligned and result in potentially catastrophic loss of the airway and respiratory compromise.

Components and Types of Tracheostomy Tubes

Standard tracheostomy tubes come in a variety of sizes and types, but most have similar parts (Fig. 24–3 and Table 24–5).

Tracheostomy tubes are made of silicone, plastic, or metal. When used for ICU patients on ventilators, they are commonly cuffed and nonfenestrated. Later, during recovery from critical illness, fenestrated or cuffless tracheostomy tubes may be used (see Fig. 24–3).

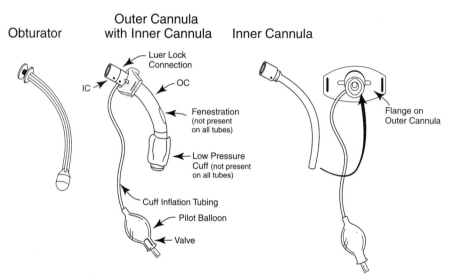

Figure 24–3. Components of cuffed tracheostomy tubes (see Table 24–5 and text for details of each part). IC, inner cannula; OC, outer cannula. Modified from Logemann JA: Evaluation and Treatment of Swallowing Disorders. San Diego: College Hill Press, 1983.

Table 24–5. Common Components of Tracheostomy Tubes

COMPONENT	DESCRIPTION AND COMMENT
Outer cannula	The outside structure of the tracheostomy tube that is inserted into, and remains in place in, the trachea; a flange attached to its proximal end is used to secure the tube to the neck with ties.
Inner cannula	A fitting that slides inside the outer cannula and can be easily removed for cleaning; most are cleaned every 8 hrs. Some tubes do not use inner cannula, predisposing them to risk of occlusion from inspissated secretions.
Obturator	A solid insert that is used to facilitate introduction of the outer cannula during replacement of tracheostomy tubes. It is removed immediately after the latter has been safely guided into the trachea.
Cap (also called a plug, cork, or button)	A small, round piece of plastic that can be placed in the tracheostomy tube (in place of the inner cannula) to occlude the proximal opening. With occlusion of the tube, patients breathe around the tube translaryngeally and not through it.
Cuff	A low-pressure, high-volume (polyvinyl chloride) balloon that is usually circumferentially fused to the lower portion of the outer cannula. It is used to occlude the trachea, analogous to an endotracheal tube's cuff.

A *cuffed* tracheostomy tube prevents air escape from the lower airway during mechanical ventilation. Having the cuff inflated also reduces the risk of aspirated material entering the trachea from the upper airway. Cuff pressures should be checked regularly at 8-hour intervals to avoid high cuff pressures that might cause ischemic injury to the tracheal mucosa; pressures should be maintained at 20 mm Hg (24 cm H_2O) or less. A cuffless tube is usually used during decannulation or when the indication for the continued presence of the tube is to provide safe access for suctioning tracheal secretions or to provide an airway when the translaryngeal route for breathing is inadequate.

A *fenestrated* tracheostomy tube has a precut opening (window) in the posterior surface of the outer cannula (see Fig. 24–3). The fenestration allows air to pass serially from the lungs, through the fenestration, through the vocal cords, and into the upper airway. They are used as adjuncts to breathing around a deflated cuff with the tube "capped" in order to enlarge the passage for air movement. An alternative to inserting a fenestrated tube is to change to the next smaller size nonfenestrated cuffed tube. This also offers a larger passageway for spontaneous breathing because its deflated cuff is much smaller than the larger tube's cuff. With occlusion of the tracheostomy tube and the cuff deflated, patients breathe around the tracheostomy tube and not through it. *Care must be taken to deflate the cuff (or use a cuffless tracheostomy tube) before capping to ensure the presence of an adequate breathing passageway around the tube.* The cap must be removed quickly if the patient experiences shortness of breath during a "capping" trial of breathing.

Fenestrated tubes generally should be avoided in patients who are at high risk for aspiration because secretions or food can easily pass through the fenestration into the airway. A fenestration may become occluded by being up against the tracheal wall or by the development of granulation tissue induced by its irregular surface rubbing on the mucosa of the posterior trachea.

Decannulation

When the tracheostomy tube is no longer indicated, it should be removed. Assessment of the patient's ability to breathe comfortably and handle respiratory secretions without aspiration are factors in the decision to decannulate. Decannulation is generally appropriate when a patient has demonstrated the ability to tolerate sustained capping of the tracheostomy tube during daytime and sleep.

Decannulation can be accomplished by removal of the tracheostomy tube, allowing the opening to close naturally. After removal of the tube, stomal closure generally occurs over a 4- to 7-day period with no additional intervention. Typically, progressively smaller tracheostomy tubes (downsizing) are used before final removal of all tubes. Capping (placing an occluding plastic cover on the proximal end of the tube's inner cannula) and one-way speaking valves are used in the decannulation process as well as to facilitate swallowing, communication, and comfort.

TRACHEOSTOMY TUBES AND COMMUNICATION

As noted earlier, tracheostomy tubes (both fenestrated and nonfenestrated) with deflated cuffs allow air from the lower trachea to pass into the upper airway. By occluding the tracheostomy tube opening with a finger or otherwise, the patient can speak using his or her larynx and vocal cords. A *tracheostomy valve* is a one-way speaking valve—for example, a Passy-Muir tracheostomy speaking valve—that obviates the need for using one's finger to close the tracheostomy. It allows air to be inhaled easily through the tracheostomy tube and then closes with exhalation so that air can be expired only through the vocal cords and oral cavity, which allows phonation. Not all patients with tracheostomies are appropriate for the use of a speaking valve however. For example, the patient must be able to tolerate cuff deflation and be off mechanical ventilation at the time. The patient should have minimal secretions as well so that the valve does not become clogged after coughing.

Talking tracheostomy tubes are designed to provide a means of verbal communication in the case of the chronically ventilator-dependent patient. Speech is produced from an independent air source flowing through a catheter that has a fenestration just **above** the tracheostomy tube cuff. These tubes provide airflow through the vocal cords, producing phonation while maintaining a closed ventilatory system. The tracheostomy cuff remains inflated with these tubes. The air port and the fenestration, however, can become clogged with secretions, affecting the vocal quality. Finally, patients must be able to synchronize their speech with the ventilator's inspirations.

BIBLIOGRAPHY

Bosma J, Donner M, Tanaka E, Robertson D: Anatomy of the pharynx pertinent to swallowing. Dysphagia 1:23–33, 1986.
   This article provides gross anatomic description of the pharynx during speech and swallowing.

Devita M, Spierer-Rundback L: Swallowing disorders in patients with prolonged orotracheal intubation and tracheostomy tubes. Crit Care Med 18:1328–1330, 1990.
   Swallowing function was tested after prolonged orotracheal intubation. It was concluded that swallowing dysfunction existed, that the deficits improved over time, and that the presence of a gag reflex did not protect against aspiration.

Dikeman K, Kazandjian M: Communication and Swallowing Management of the Tracheostomized and Ventilator Dependent Patient. San Diego, CA: Singular Publishing Group, 1995.
   This is a comprehensive text written by clinical speech-language pathologists working with tracheostomized and ventilator-dependent patients in the acute, rehabilitative, and home care settings.

Eisele DW, Yarington, CT Jr, Lindeman RC: Indications for the tracheoesophageal diversion and the laryngotracheal separation procedure. Ann Otol Rhinol Laryngol 97:471–475, 1988.
   This is a brief review of indications for tracheoesophageal diversion and includes a pertinent bibliography.

Fornataro-Clereici L, Zajac D: Aerodynamic characteristics of tracheostomy speaking valves. J Speech Hearing Res 36:529–532, 1993.
   This article presents a comparison of one-way speaking valves available for the tracheostomized and ventilator-dependent patient.

Groher ME (ed): Dysphagia: Diagnostic and Management. Stoneham MA: Butterworth-Heinemann, 1992.
   This is a comprehensive text on swallowing disorders, including anatomy and physiology, diagnosis, and treatment options.

Langmore S, Schatz K, Olsen N: Fiberoptic endoscopic examination of swallowing safety: A new procedure. Dysphagia 2:216–219, 1988.
   Fiberoptic endoscopic evaluation of swallowing provides information about the pharyngeal phase of the swallow in patients who cannot be examined by videofluoroscopy.

Logemann JA: Evaluation and Treatment of Swallowing Disorders. San Diego: College Hill Press, 1983.
Recognized as a leading authority in dysphagia research, the author provides a comprehensive sourcebook on the etiology, evaluation and treatment of dysphagia in diverse patient populations.

Mason M (ed): Speech Pathology for Tracheostomized and Ventilator Dependent Patients. Newport Beach, CA: Voicing, Inc., 1993.
This is a transdisciplinary approach to treating the tracheostomized and ventilator-dependent patient.

Nash M: Swallowing problems in the tracheostomized patient. Otolaryngol Clin North Am 21:701–709, 1988.
This article reviews the pathophysiology of aspiration with a tracheostomy.

Sonies B: Instrumental procedure for dysphagia diagnosis. Semin Speech Language 12:185–198, 1991.
This is a general review of procedures for diagnosing swallowing problems and their applications and limitations.

Yorkston J (ed): Augmentative Communication in the Medical Setting. Tuscon, AZ: Communication Skill Builders, 1992.
This book provides practical clinical techniques for alternative communication.

25   Rehabilitation Interventions

Keith M. Robinson

Recovery from critical illness does not happen automatically; rather, the process is one of gradual rehabilitation. In the intensive care unit (ICU), rehabilitation interventions treat the adverse effects of bed rest and immobility during critical illness. Rehabilitation interventions that focus on the individual patient and complement the highly technologic, lifesaving ICU therapies are essential for the patient's full functional recovery.

STARTING REHABILITATION IN THE INTENSIVE CARE UNIT

Rehabilitation is a practical, comprehensive effort integrating physical and psychosocial aspects of patient care. *Restorative* interventions reverse disabilities by applying specialized therapies, for example, physical and occupational therapy. *Maintenance* or *preventive* interventions sustain optimal function during acute illness requiring bed rest and immobility. Both types of interventions in the ICU incorporate the two basic tools of rehabilitation: functional assessment and a multidisciplinary approach.

During critical illness, the initial *functional assessment* is qualitative. The patient's current basic functional skills (Table 25–1) are compared with a preillness baseline, and changes from this baseline are then monitored during recovery. Assessing more comprehensive skills for daily life usually occurs later in the recovery process. Rehabilitative consultation facilitates the patient's transition from ICU to post-ICU to posthospital care. This approach aims for cost-efficient movement of the recovering ICU patient through successive levels of care by ongoing predischarge functional assessments and by defining the most appropriate posthospital discharge plan.

The rehabilitation team uses a *multidisciplinary approach* to achieve its goals as exemplified by the disciplines of team members (Table 25–2). Optimally, rehabilitation begins as soon as life-threatening instability has passed, although *preventive measures* can be instituted shortly after admission to the ICU to prevent the deconditioning syndrome (Tables 25–3 and 25–4). ICU physicians

Table 25–1. Basic Functional Skills During Recovery from Critical Illness

SELF-CARE	MOBILITY	COMMUNICATION AND COGNITION
Eating	Bed mobility	Hearing
Drinking	Transfers: Bed to chair	Vision
Bathing, grooming	Transfers: Chair to toilet	Orientation
Bowel, bladder control	Ambulation with or without an assistive device	Attention, memory
Toileting	Balance	Language (gesturing, talking, writing)

Table 25–2. Members of the Multidisciplinary Rehabilitation Team

TEAM MEMBER	DESCRIPTION OF ROLES AND AREAS OF EXPERTISE
Physiatrist (rehabilitation physician)	Medical specialist in disability who provides consultations regarding prognosis and rehabilitation needs, orchestrates rehabilitation services, develops and is responsible for implementation of the multidisciplinary care plan, prescribes durable medical equipment
Physical therapist	Treats basic locomotor skills (transfers, wheelchair mobility and ambulation), and teaches the use of assistive devices (canes, walkers, and wheelchairs); aids in sensory facilitation of motor control, gait, and balance training, including leg splints (orthotics) and prosthetic devices
Occupational therapist	Treats daily living skills (feeding, grooming, toileting, dressing, and homemaking) and fine motor skills of the hand, including splinting (orthotics); advises on wheelchair accessories; provides cognitive remediation (memory and visual perception) and driving evaluation
Speech and swallowing therapist	Cognitive remediation to achieve meaningful communication (attention, memory, language comprehension, conceptual organization, language production); communication enhancement in patients with endotracheal and tracheostomy tubes; performs bedside clinical swallowing evaluation, participates in videofluoroscopic evaluations (see Chapter 24)
Nutritionist	Collaborates with physicians, nurses, and therapists to establish caloric and nutritional needs during recovery; recommends nutritional support (oral, enteral, parenteral) and dietary advancement
Case manager or social worker	Identifies posthospital medical, surgical, rehabilitation, and social services based on expected recovery, treatment priorities, health insurance, and personal finances; identifies members of patient's social network to provide support, personal care, and transportation

must understand the specific skills of the nonmedical rehabilitation specialists and give precautions for specific interventions, for example, limiting range of motion and weight bearing after orthopedic procedures or specifying heart rate and blood pressure limits in patients with cardiopulmonary disease.

Rehabilitation is expensive, labor-intensive, and inefficient to perform in the ICU. Reimbursement for many of these nonmedical services is bundled into the daily costs of hospital care. Thus, the physiatrist emerges as the gatekeeper for the use of these scarce resources by defining treatment priorities. Further, therapists increasingly are assuming collaborative roles in the ICU, by directing nurses and family members to perform basic preventive and therapeutic exercise programs, coma and sensory stimulation, and graduated oral feeding. Clear communication between ICU providers and the rehabilitation team becomes essential to achieve high-quality care.

SPECIFIC REHABILITATION PROBLEMS AND THEIR INTERVENTIONS IN THE INTENSIVE CARE UNIT

Deconditioning

Deconditioning is a syndrome of reversible anatomic and physiologic effects of inactivity. These organ-specific complications of inactivity require specific preven-

Table 25–3. The Deconditioning Syndrome: Musculoskeletal and Integument Changes

PRIMARY EFFECTS ON ORGAN SYSTEM	RELATED COMPLICATIONS	PREVENTION AND TREATMENT INTERVENTIONS
Musculoskeletal		
Joint contractures	Impedes self-care and ambulation	Proper positioning of limbs, sometimes with static splinting
Muscle weakness and atrophy	Decreased strength, coordination, and balance	Passive and active range of motion exercises with terminal stretch at least twice daily
Osteoporosis	Pathological fractures	Conservative isometric and isotonic strengthening exercises
		Graduated sitting and standing protocols
Integument		
Subcutaneous tissue ischemia	Pressure sores (see also Chapter 43)	Optimize nutritional intake
Skin atrophy		Frequent repositioning
		Specialized mattresses (that distribute pressure away from bony prominences)
		Avoiding shear stress when moving patient

tive and restorative treatments (see Tables 25–3 and 25–4). Since these complications can prolong the ICU or hospital stay, early, graduated, and aggressive remobilization of the patient within the limits of medical and surgical precautions should be the current standard of practice.

Cognitive and Communication Deficits

Mental status screening tools, such as the Mini–Mental Status examination (Fig. 25–1), can quickly assess cognition during recovery from critical illness in most patients in the ICU. Other disease-specific tools, for example, the Ranchos Los Amigos Scale for use after traumatic brain injury, are available to the rehabilitation specialists for focused cognitive-behavioral screening. The consulting physiatrist generally assesses all major cognitive domains: attention, memory, language, visual perception, and executive functioning. In selected cases, further evaluation from a behavioral neurologist or neuropsychologist can be useful in the post-ICU phase of care.

Occupational therapists focus on attention, memory, and visual perception relating to basic self-care skills. Speech therapists emphasize attention, memory, and communication. Physical therapists attend to motor planning and sequencing. These therapists largely use procedural learning techniques to address deficits. These techniques incorporate behavioral learning of motor and communication skills by habituating a sequential task without factual recall of information. Multi-

Table 25-4. The Deconditioning Syndrome: Cardiovascular and Metabolic Changes

PRIMARY EFFECTS ON ORGAN SYSTEM	RELATED COMPLICATIONS	PREVENTION AND TREATMENT INTERVENTIONS
Cardiovascular		
Decreased vascular smooth muscle tone	Postural hypotension	Graduated sitting and standing protocols
Tachycardia at rest and during submaximal exercise with reduced cardiac output	Poor endurance	Strengthening exercises (low resistance, high repetition)
Hypercoaguable blood	Deep venous thrombosis (DVT) Pulmonary embolism	DVT prophylaxis
Endocrine and Metabolic		
Insulin receptor resistance	Glucose intolerance	Serum glucose monitoring
Increase in serum parathyroid hormone	Osteoporosis	Monitor serum calcium
Increased daily nitrogen loss and associated hypoproteinemia	Proteinuria	Optimize fluid and nutritional intake
Negative calcium balance with normal serum levels	Hypercalciuria	Graduated sitting and standing protocols
Decrease in total body phosphorus, sulfur, sodium and potassium primarily due to muscle atrophy	Loss of lean body mass	Progressive ambulation Conservative isometric and isotonic strengthening programs

ple, brief therapeutic encounters are preferred because patients recovering from a critical illness usually have limited attention and poor cardiopulmonary endurance.

Observations by multiple rehabilitation care providers at different times of the day validate their assessments of the patient's cognitive responses. In addition, therapists can provide specialized treatment interventions, such as coma stimulation programs, as they monitor cognitive recovery. For example, the speech therapist can suggest to other members of the rehabilitation team, ICU staff, and family specific communication strategies to enhance comprehension and speech production (see Chapter 24). Strategies include directly addressing the patient using grammatically simple language, expressing one idea at a time, embellishing verbal inputs with visual or tactile cues to enhance comprehension, and facilitating nonvocal communication approaches, such as writing, drawing, and gesturing (see also Chapter 24, Table 24-4).

Difficult Behaviors

Cognitive assessments are supplemented with qualitative behavioral observations. Agitation in the critically ill patient can elevate blood and intracranial pressure and jeopardize placement of intravenous lines, feeding tubes, endotracheal tubes,

Score *Orientation*

5 What is the (year) (season) (date) (month) (day of week)?

5 Where are we (state) (country) (town/city) (hospital) (floor)?

Registration

3 Repeat three words, for example, "ball," "flag," "tree."

Ask the patient all three after you have said them. Give one point for each correct answer.

Attention and Calculation

5 Begin with 100 and count backwards by 7 (stop after five answers). Alternatively, spell "world" backwards.

Recall

3 Ask for three words repeated above. Give one point for each correct answer.

Language

2 Show a pencil and a watch and ask subject to name them.

1 Repeat the following: "No ifs, ands, or buts."

3 A three stage command, "Take a paper in your right hand; fold it in half and put it on the floor."

Read and obey the following: (Show subject the written item).

1 CLOSE YOUR EYES

1 Write a sentence

1 Copy a design

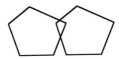 Total score possible = 30

Figure 25–1. The mini–mental status examination is used to assess cognition during critical illness or delirium. (Adapted from Folstein MF, Folstein SE, McHugh PR: "Mini-mental state": A practical guide for grading the cognitive state of patients for the clinician. J Psychiatric Res 12:189–198, 1975.)

and bladder catheters. When agitation endangers the patient in this manner, short-acting benzodiazepines should be given to control the behavior. Neuroleptic agents, such as haloperidol, generally are second-line choices to treat agitation in brain-injured patients because they may interfere with neural recovery. Haloperidol is often useful, however, when benzodiazepines are ineffective, when benzodiazepines amplify disinhibition rather than suppress it, or when the agitated patient demonstrates psychotic or delirious symptoms (see also Chapters 4 and 44). When using either benzodiazepines or neuroleptic agents, one should closely observe the patient to assess the continued need for these agents.

Observation of the patient's behaviors can identify behavioral strategies that either facilitate or impede successful task performance. Such strategies provide insights to optimize communication and cognitive remediation treatments. For example, a patient exhibiting circumlocutory speech may be encouraged to facilitate spontaneous word retrieval. An easily distracted patient may require a structured, relatively quiet treatment environment. Some recovering patients may exhibit disruptive, socially inappropriate, or aggressive behaviors. These behaviors can occur as a consequence of an underlying delirium or in response to overwhelming environmental stimuli. As with agitation, psychotropic medication to control these behaviors should be limited to dangerous situations only. Intensive behavioral management by nurses and the rehabilitation team is preferable in these situations.

Physiatrists and rehabilitation therapists can assist the ICU staff in organizing nursing-directed behavioral management programs, founded on the following four basic principles. First, difficult behaviors must be targeted. The daily patterns, specific environmental precipitants, and relationships to visual, auditory, or tactile disturbances of the targeted behavior must be identified. A detailed daily log over 24 to 72 hours (kept by the nursing staff or the patient's family) can relate behavioral patterns to medications or other interventions. Second, a highly structured, consistent, goal-oriented environment with minimal distracting influences must be created around the patient. This includes encouragement of normal sleep-wake cycles by manipulating lighting and minimizing nocturnal noise and interventions (see Chapter 44). Third, adaptive behaviors should be reinforced, usually by providing positive verbal feedback. Undesirable or dangerous behaviors should be handled neutrally because, paradoxically, negative responses may actually reinforce these difficult behaviors. Fourth, self-monitoring of a patient's own behavior should be encouraged with nonthreatening verbal feedback.

Dysphagia and Dysphonia

Dysphagia and dysphonia are discussed in depth in Chapter 24. Since oral nutrition is usually not feasible in the critically ill patient, early surgical enteral access is usually performed when the need for nutritional support is expected to be prolonged (e.g., >1 month). Because gastroesophageal reflux, gastric dysmotility, and impaired gag reflexes are common in cognitively impaired patients or those emerging from coma, jejunal access is generally preferred over gastric access for feeding. Gastrostomy should be reserved for the patient considered to be at low risk from reflux and aspiration.

Spasticity and Contractures

Spasticity is rate-related resistance to passive limb stretch and commonly occurs in patients with brain and spinal cord injuries. Spasticity and the resultant loss in joint motion can lead to contractures. Since spasticity and contractures can compromise autonomous self-care and ambulation, aggressive treatments are indicated. Both narcotic analgesics and benzodiazepines have antispasticity effects; as such, severe spasticity may not appear until these medications are tapered or discontinued.

For brain-injured patients, dantrolene sodium, a sarcoplasmic reticulum calcium blocker, is the antispasticity agent of choice because it is minimally sedating and has a peripheral site of action. Initially administered at 25 mg twice daily, the frequency of dantrolene therapy may be increased every 3 to 5 days to a maximum of four daily doses. Liver function tests should be ordered before initiating dantrolene therapy, which can produce hepatitis. Another side effect is weakness.

For spinal cord–injured patients, baclofen, an analog of gamma-aminobutyric acid, is preferred. Administered twice a day, the starting dose (5 mg) of baclofen may be increased every 3 to 5 days in 5-mg increments up to a dose of 20 mg twice a day before reconsidering the need for a higher dose. High doses of baclofen may produce sedation, whereas rapid tapering can precipitate psychosis.

Temporary use of a short-acting parenteral benzodiazepine, such as lorazepam (0.5 mg two to four times daily), should be considered for patients (previously unexposed to benzodiazepines) without oral or enteral access. The lorazepam dosage may be titrated up to 2 mg four times daily, unless sedation or disinhibition becomes limiting.

When medications produce undesirable side effects, or when spasticity and contractures are confined to two limbs or less, peripheral neurolysis is a treatment option. Diagnostic, transient neurolysis with a local anesthetic simulates permanent neurolysis with ethyl alcohol, phenol, and botulinum toxin. Physiatry consultation is essential to determine the potential utility of neurolysis and, in some centers, to perform the procedure.

Autonomic Dysreflexia

Autonomic dysreflexia is a manifestation of the disinhibited, autonomously functioning spinal cord distal to a cervical or high thoracic lesion. Any sensory stimulus (usually noxious) to the disconnected spinal cord may result in a sympathetic autonomic response and vasoconstriction resulting in severe hypertension. Common causes of autonomic dysreflexia include urinary retention, constipation, nephrolithiasis, deep venous thrombosis, pressure ulcers, acute abdominal infections, and skin infections, including ingrown toenails. Autonomic dysreflexia is treated by eliminating the offending "noxious" stimuli and demands a fastidious physical examination to search for precipitating causes. Immediate interventions should include sitting the patient up and establishing urinary outlet patency while continuing to search for other offending stimuli. Short-acting medications to control severe hypertension should be considered.

PLANNING FOR REHABILITATION AFTER LEAVING THE INTENSIVE CARE UNIT

The goal of rehabilitation in the ICU is to develop a well-organized, comprehensive, and properly timed plan for when the patient leaves the ICU and the hospital. Such a plan should be based on the patient's physiologic status, psychosocial situation, and chronic care needs.

Physiologic Status

Physiologic problems, particularly malnutrition and loss of cardiopulmonary fitness, influence functional recovery. Most critically ill patients have readily available nutritional indices, including serum protein levels, anthropomorphic measures, and supplementary nutritional requirements. Patients with poor nutritional indices who need nutritional supplementation recover slowly. Similarly, previously sedentary patients take more time to recover. Further, the more prolonged periods of bed rest are, the more they promote deconditioning and delay recovery.

Specific prognostic indicators define the natural history of some diseases. For example, loss of consciousness, post-traumatic amnesia, and anosognosia after traumatic brain injury forewarn of incomplete functional recovery, future dependence, and long-term rehabilitation and personal care needs after hospitalization. Thus, the ultimate influence of rehabilitation depends on the patient's degree of physiologic recovery. Nonetheless, rehabilitation services should not be withheld from patients with severe physiologic impairments and poor prognostic indicators. Rather, rehabilitation is important in these individuals to minimize deconditioning, educate future care providers, and optimally modify the patient's environment.

Another predictor of the future clinical course is the critically ill patient's responses to initial therapeutic rehabilitation interventions. For example, those with persistent orthostatic hypotension, tachycardia, and tachypnea during initial sitting and standing trials in physical therapy require prolonged rehabilitation. The same can be expected for those with poor tolerance for more than 10 minutes of low-level (1 to 2 METS) self-care activity in occupational therapy.

Availability of Skilled Rehabilitation Services

Most geographic areas are served by three different levels of rehabilitative care: hospital-based (acute), subacute, and community-based. These three levels of care are defined by Medicare guidelines, and other insurance systems often subscribe to these guidelines. Critically ill patients move through several levels of care during their recovery.

The most intensive and expensive programs are hospital-based, in which patients must participate in 3 hours or more of daily physical, occupational, and speech therapy. Hospital programs usually are appropriate for medically complex patients and for patients whose likely rapid recovery necessitates a short length of stay (<20 days). These patients usually require community-based services after discharge.

Subacute rehabilitation programs usually provide less than 3 hours daily of inpatient rehabilitation services, often within a skilled nursing facility. Subacute programs are appropriate for medically uncomplicated patients who require less comprehensive, intensive services for a short period, or for slowly recovering medically complex patients who are unable to tolerate a more intensive hospital-based program.

The least intensive rehabilitation services are provided in the community—in outpatient clinics or at home.

The "Informal" Care Provider

As patients recover, they depend on durable medical equipment (hospital beds, wheelchairs, walkers, commodes) and personal care provided by others. When the patient cannot manage the equipment or self-care, key family members, friends, neighbors, significant others, and volunteers must be identified as the patient's future "informal" (unpaid) care providers. Although the patient is still in the ICU, these providers should learn to participate in the patient's therapy sessions. This knowledge, experience, and teamwork optimizes the patient's and family member's competence and confidence before discharge. An informal care provider who has been well trained can help many patients be discharged home soon after medical stability is established. Otherwise, inpatient rehabilitation services should be offered until the home care providers have demonstrated their competence in providing personal care during therapy sessions. "Formal" home services are time-limited and reimbursed only for narrowly defined "skilled" nursing and therapy services. Thus, home care services only complement what the patient's extended families provide.

Few patients and families can afford personal care services beyond those reimbursed by health insurance. For patients without an informal care provider, achieving a functional level during inpatient rehabilitation to support safe home discharge becomes critical. Otherwise, a long-term care residential institution may be the only option. Ultimately, patients must depend on themselves and their "family" to return home.

Health Insurance for Rehabilitation

Insurance coverage often limits access to rehabilitation services, technologies, durable medical equipment, and home care services. Medicare provides a limited source of reimbursement for these services, and increasingly patients are insured under even more restrictive managed care plans. No consistency exists among insurers regarding which services are reimbursable. Medicaid is only available to the poor and it, too, is evolving toward managed care. To qualify for Medicaid, patients and families must "spend-down" their personal savings for non-reimbursable but necessary equipment and services.

In addition, states differ in their criteria for qualifying for Medicaid and how well Medicaid covers rehabilitation, durable medical equipment, and home care. Finally, these criteria seem to change each year. Thus, the details of each critically ill patient's health insurance become a crucial piece of the comprehensive rehabilitation plan. Consultation with a hospital-based social worker or case manager is essential in regard to sorting through these complexities.

BIBLIOGRAPHY

Applegate WB, Blass JP, Williams TF: Instruments for functional assessment of older people. N Engl J Med 322:1207–1214, 1990.
This article provides an excellent review of functional assessment tools for assessing elderly and critically ill patients.

Bassey EJ: Age, inactivity, and some physical responses to exercise. Gerontology 24:66–77, 1978.
This article reviews the classic intervention trials, documenting how simple therapeutic exercise reverses deconditioning in inactive, elderly people.

Brody EM: The aging of the family. Ann Am Acad Polit Sci Sociol 438:13–27, 1978.
This is a classic essay on the complementary relationship between "formal" and "informal" home care providers for the disabled. The major burden of caring for the disabled falls on middle-aged women or women "in the middle" of job, home, and multiple generations within a family.

Folstein MF, Folstein SE, McHugh PR: "Mini-mental state": A practical guide for grading the cognitive state of patients for the clinician. J Psychiatric Res 12:189–198, 1975.
This is a classic description of the mini–mental status test and how to use it.

Gerson MC, Hurst JM, Hertzberg VS: Cardiac prognosis in noncardiac surgery. Ann Intern Med 103:832–837, 1985.
Patients unable to complete a 1-minute, lower extremity, in-bed exercise test or achieve a heart rate greater than 99 beats per minute during the testing had reduced survival, higher complications, and longer recovery.

Heaton RK, Pendleton MG: Use of neuropsychological tests to predict adults patients' everyday functioning. J Consult Clin Psychol 49:807–821, 1981.
In chronic patients with obstructive pulmonary disease, neuropsychological tests that measured executive functioning were predictive of successful self-care performance.

Robinson KM, Siebens H: Rehabilitation. In: O'Donnell PD (ed): Geriatric Urology. Boston: Little, Brown, 1993, pp 479–491.
This chapter reviews rehabilitation functional assessment tools and their application in the acute care setting. Guidelines for the consultation of rehabilitation physicians are also provided.

Sandel ME, Robinson KM, Goldberg G, et al: Neurohabilitation. In: Cruz J (ed): Neurological and Neurosurgical Emergencies. Philadelphia: WB Saunders, 1998, pp 503–546.
This is a comprehensive review of rehabilitation interventions and functional outcome prediction in patients after head injury, stroke, or spinal cord injury.

Siebens H: Deconditioning. In: Kemp B, Brummel-Smith K, Ramsdell JW (eds): Geriatric Rehabilitation. Boston: Little, Brown, 1990, pp 177–191.
This chapter reviews the physiologic effects of deconditioning, with practical treatment advice for hospitalized patients.

26 Acute Arterial Desaturation

Barry Fuchs

Episodes of arterial desaturation (low SaO_2) or hypoxemia (low PaO_2) are frequently encountered in the intensive care unit (ICU) setting. They may result from rapid progression or a complication of the patient's disease, a recent procedure, or malfunction of the oxygen delivery system or ventilator. Fortunately, episodes of desaturation are usually discovered quickly in the ICU because of routine use of continuous monitoring by pulse oximetry. Recognition, treatment, and maintenance of adequate arterial oxygenation are essential skills in critical care medicine. This chapter briefly reviews the pathophysiology of acute hypoxemia and presents a practical approach to evaluate and manage episodes of arterial desaturation or hypoxemia in the critically ill patient.

DEFINITIONS

An episode of *hypoxemia* is the acute reduction in PaO_2 of 10% or more over a period ranging from several minutes to several hours. An episode of *arterial desaturation* occurs with an acute fall in SaO_2 of 5% or more over the same period. Such episodes should be evaluated immediately. If PaO_2 falls to less than 55 to 60 mm Hg (or SaO_2 <85 to 90%), treatment should start emergently because the oxygen content of the arterial blood (CaO_2) at these values may decrease rapidly if PaO_2 falls further. These thresholds for starting emergency treatment correspond to the start of the steep part of the hemoglobin (Hgb)-oxygen dissociation curve as PaO_2 decreases (Appendix A, Fig. 1).

Some words of caution are needed, however, in how one should react to small changes in PaO_2 in critically ill patients. Several studies have documented that small falls in PaO_2 (changes of 5 to 7%), lasting 15 minutes or less, occur frequently and are without identifiable causes or clinically relevant changes. Also, even larger transient changes in PaO_2 (on the order of 20 to 30 mm Hg) occur in many critically ill patients without clear cause or evidence of deleterious effects. These changes are ascribable only to instability of the critically ill patient's gas exchange and hemodynamics. Since falls of these magnitudes may only represent the "noise" of critical illness (rather than substantive changes in the patient's clinical status), one's response to acute drops in PaO_2 or SaO_2 should be tempered by one's clinical assessment. No change in therapy may be indicated as long as there is no evidence of an adverse clinical effect. For example, one should confirm that the decreased PaO_2 or SaO_2 is persistent before making changes in the fraction of inspired oxygen (FIO_2) or positive end-expiratory pressure (PEEP) in ventilated patients.

PHYSIOLOGIC MECHANISMS OF HYPOXEMIA

Five major physiologic mechanisms may cause acute hypoxemic episodes in the ICU setting: (1) low FIO_2, (2) hypoventilation, (3) ventilation/perfusion (V/Q) mismatch, (4) shunt, and (5) low mixed venous oxygen saturation ($S\bar{v}O_2$).

303

Reduced F_{IO_2}

A decreased F_{IO_2} results in hypoxemia by directly reducing the partial pressure of oxygen in the alveoli (P_{AO_2}) and must be considered first in all patients receiving supplemental oxygen. Examples include inadvertent disconnection of oxygen tubing or displacement of the facial oxygen device. Because a constant and predictable F_{IO_2} can be achieved only in patients who are intubated, F_{IO_2} may vary considerably in nonintubated patients receiving supplemental oxygen because of alterations in breathing pattern. For example, if the spontaneous inspiratory flow rate increases in patients, more ambient air is entrained, effectively diluting the F_{IO_2}. Under these circumstances, one needs to set less rigid thresholds for falls in P_{aO_2} (or S_{aO_2}) to trigger clinical concern and diagnostic evaluation.

Hypoventilation

Like decreased F_{IO_2}, hypoventilation also causes the P_{AO_2} to fall. In this case, however, the rate at which oxygen is taken up by blood exceeds the rate of oxygen delivery to the alveoli. In the steady state, the fall in P_{aO_2} may be predicted from the rise in P_{aCO_2} by the Alveolar Gas Equation (see Chapter 1, Table 1–1, Equation 12).

In "pure" hypoventilation, the magnitude of the fall in P_{aO_2} should be similar to the rise in P_{aCO_2}. A decrease in P_{aO_2} greater than the increase in P_{aCO_2} indicates the effects of one or more additional mechanisms responsible for the hypoxemia. Since there is no pulmonary pathology in cases of hypoventilation alone, the hypoxemia that results should be readily correctable with low concentrations of supplemental oxygen.

Ventilation/Perfusion Mismatch

V/Q mismatch is the most common cause for hypoxemia in the ICU setting. Because V/Q mismatch can result from changes in ventilation alone or changes in regional perfusion alone, it may be present without infiltrates on the chest radiograph. Examples of changes in ventilation alone include airway narrowing from bronchospasm, bronchial secretions, or edema. Pulmonary embolus can cause changes in perfusion and V/Q mismatch with a clear chest radiograph.

Baseline V/Q inequalities may be also aggravated by certain ICU interventions. Repositioning some patients may result in acute hypoxemic episodes. Since dependent lung regions receive preferential blood flow, positioning patients with unilateral lung disease—for example, atelectasis or pneumonia—such that the abnormal lung is dependent can acutely worsen the P_{aO_2}. In addition, vasodilators (especially continuous intravenous infusions of nitroglycerin, nitroprusside, or calcium channel blockers) can attenuate hypoxic pulmonary vasoconstriction and severely worsen V/Q mismatch.

Since low V/Q regions still receive some ventilation, small increments in supplemental oxygen (<0.4 F_{IO_2}) are usually effective in reversing the hypoxemia. This is because increasing the P_{O_2} of the inspired gas (P_{IO_2}) to regions with low

V/Q compensates for the reduction in bulk flow (ventilation) to that region, therefore raising the P_{AO_2} and Pa_{O_2}. This characteristic responsiveness of V/Q mismatch to small increases in F_{IO_2} plays an essential role in the diagnostic approach to episodes of arterial desaturation.

Right-to-Left Shunt

Hypoxemia due to a right-to-left shunt is characterized by a poor response to high concentrations of supplemental oxygen. Indeed, with shunt fractions greater than 30% of the cardiac output, the hypoxemia is refractory even to very high F_{IO_2}. Although patients with lungs having regions with very low V/Q ratios (<0.05 to 0.1) may also require high F_{IO_2} (>0.6) to correct their hypoxemia, they can be distinguished from patients with pure shunts by their complete response to 100% O_2 (as shown by Pa_{O_2} >550 mm Hg). In contrast, in a pure shunt, mixed venous blood bypasses the alveoli through anatomic connections (intracardiac or intrapulmonary) or through nonventilated alveoli, that is, V/Q = 0, because V = 0 and is unaffected by augmentation in inspired oxygen concentrations. Thus, the Pa_{O_2} remains less than 550 mm Hg (which reflects lower range of Pa_{O_2} in normals breathing 100% oxygen).

The most common causes of shunt physiology in the ICU setting are alveolar filling processes due to edema, blood, or exudate. These result in V/Q equal to (or approximating) zero. These patients have infiltrates on the chest radiograph and often have auscultatory findings. In fact, if shunt physiology is evident from breathing on 100% oxygen and the chest radiograph shows clear lung fields, one should suspect an intracardiac shunt. Although a newly acquired cardiac shunt is unusual, an acute increase in right-sided heart pressure, for example, after a major pulmonary embolism, may open a patent foramen ovale to create an acquired intracardiac shunt.

Low Mixed Venous Oxygen Saturation

In patients with normal lungs, an isolated reduction in $S\bar{v}_{O_2}$ (normal $S\bar{v}_{O_2} = 70$ to 75%) does not cause hypoxemia. In patients with diseased lungs, however, falls in $S\bar{v}_{O_2}$ can cause such an event. When mixed venous blood flows through well-ventilated lung (V/Q ≥ 1.0), the blood becomes fully oxygenated by the time it leaves the lung as postcapillary blood. In contrast, blood leaving an alveolus with V/Q = 0 is identical in composition to mixed venous blood. As a consequence, if $S\bar{v}_{O_2}$ falls in patients with large intrapulmonary shunts—for example, due to a fall in cardiac output—the oxygen saturation and P_{O_2} of the blood returning to the left atrium will also fall.

Reductions in $S\bar{v}_{O_2}$ can be diagnosed by sampling pulmonary artery blood using the distal port of a pulmonary arterial catheter (with the balloon deflated). Some ICUs use pulmonary arterial catheters that contain an oximeter near the distal end to continuously monitor $S\bar{v}_{O_2}$ in certain patients. Changes in $S\bar{v}_{O_2}$ may not be specific for one physiologic change, however, as illustrated in Equation 1 and Table 26–1 and thus can be difficult to interpret.

Table 26–1. Selected Physiologic Conditions That Can Alter $S\bar{v}o_2$

CONDITION	MINUTE OXYGEN CONSUMPTION ($\dot{V}o_2$) (mL/min)	HEMOGLOBIN (g/dL)	CARDIAC OUTPUT (L/min)	ARTERIAL BLOOD OXYGEN SATURATION (Sao_2) (%)	MIXED VENOUS OXYGEN SATURATION ($S\bar{v}o_2$) (%)
Normal	210	14	4.0	100	73
Arterial desaturation	210	14	4.0	90	63
High cardiac output	210	14	6.0	100	83
Low cardiac output	210	14	2.5	100	59
Hypermetabolic with high cardiac output	420	14	8.0	100	73

Note: Changes in parameters were derived from Equation 1 presented in the text.

$$S\bar{v}o_2 = Sao_2 - \dot{V}o_2 / \{10 \times Hgb \times 1.39 \times CO\} \quad \text{(Equation 1)}$$

where $\dot{V}o_2$ = minute oxygen consumption (L/min), Hgb = hemoglobin (g/dL), 1.39 = constant (mL O_2/g Hgb), CO = cardiac output (L/min).

DIAGNOSTIC EVALUATION

Hypoxemia and the Use of Pulse Oximetry

Clinical manifestations of acute hypoxemia are neither sensitive nor specific. Patients may be asymptomatic or have tachypnea, tachy- or bradyarrhythmias, or cognitive deficits. Of note, cyanosis is a late and often difficult to appreciate sign of hypoxemia. Manifestations of hypoxemia may also be overshadowed by other clinical findings. Since the sequelae of unrecognized, progressive hypoxemia can be catastrophic, culminating in cardiac arrest, continuous monitoring of Sao_2 by pulse oximetry is essential for critically ill ICU patients.

Given the importance of pulse oximetry in the ICU, it is essential to point out its pitfalls. It is insensitive to declining Pao_2 over the high-to-normal range because of the shape of the oxyhemoglobin dissociation curve (see Appendix A, Fig. 1). Inaccurate measurements can also occur. These most commonly result from poor perfusion with a reduced pulse pressure, for example, in hypovolemic or cardiogenic shock or during inflation of a blood pressure cuff on the same extremity as the sensor. Most pulse oximeters, however, provide a signal indicative of pulse pressure, alerting the clinician to this problem.

Other causes for spurious readings include dark skin pigmentation, motion artifact, bright light, dyes like methylene blue, and abnormal hemoglobins such as carboxyhemoglobin (CO-Hgb) or methemoglobin. Therefore, when an ICU patient manifests a sudden change in cardiac or respiratory status or suddenly becomes agitated or distressed, it is essential to obtain an arterial blood gas to measure Pao_2, pH, and $Paco_2$ regardless of the readings of the pulse oximeter.

Assessment of the Hypoxemic Patient

Immediate Treatment of Hypoxemia

The first step in approaching the patient with an acute episode of hypoxemia is to ensure adequate oxygenation and ventilation and to identify and manage imminently life-threatening problems. One should quickly assess the oxygen delivery system, the bedside monitor for electrocardiographic or blood pressure changes, and the physical examination for the presence of bilateral breath sounds and adequate circulatory status. For a patient in extremis, presumptive treatment may be necessary before diagnostic confirmation, for example, hypoxemia accompanied by refractory hypotension and unequal breath sounds in a patient receiving mechanical ventilation mandates emergency treatment of a tension pneumothorax (see Chapter 32).

Once the patient is stable, completion of the diagnostic evaluation can proceed less urgently by systematically considering the factors described in the following sections.

Admitting Diagnosis

Nonintubated patients with neurologic disease or altered mental status are at increased risk for aspiration. Trauma, postoperative, immobile, or peripartum patients are at the highest risk for acute pulmonary embolus (PE). Patients with acute flares of asthma or chronic obstructive pulmonary disease (COPD) are at risk for atelectasis because of mucus plugs, bronchospasm, and auto-PEEP (if on a mechanical ventilator). Finally, volume overload should be suspected in patients with renal failure or cardiac disease and in postoperative patients.

Time Since Intensive Care Unit Admission

Early after ICU admission one needs to consider progression of the presenting disorder as the cause for hypoxemia. After several days of stable or improving oxygenation, however, acutely worsening hypoxemia is likely due to a new problem or complication, such as a tension pneumothorax. If the initial condition has truly improved, the complication would likely be unrelated to the original disease process. Moreover, depending on the diagnosis, a complication may be expected to occur at different times in the course of the illness. For example, the risk of nosocomial pneumonia increases with the duration of mechanical ventilation.

Proximity to an Intervention or Procedure

Many procedures and interventions commonly performed in the ICU can precipitate acute hypoxemia, including patient repositioning, chest physiotherapy, tracheal suctioning, peritoneal dialysis and hemodialysis, thoracentesis, bronchoscopy, or endoscopy. With the exception of hemodialysis-induced hypoventilation, and pneumothorax induced by attempting to insert a central venous catheter, V/Q mismatch at the time or immediately after the procedure is the usual mechanism of the hypoxemia.

Symptoms and Signs

Pressure-like *chest pain* narrows the differential diagnosis to myocardial infarction or myocardial ischemia (see Chapter 34). *Hypotension* suggests acute hemorrhage, a drug effect, anaphylaxis, sepsis, pancreatitis, adrenal insufficiency, PE, tamponade, myocardial infarction, arrhythmia, auto-PEEP, tension pneumothorax, or a leukoagglutination reaction (see Chapter 46). Fever or an elevated white blood cell count point to a possible infectious process associated with hypoxemia as a result of sepsis-induced acute respiratory distress syndrome or nosocomial pneumonia. If accompanied by increased, purulent tracheal secretions, pneumonia may be the cause of hypoxemia. Auscultation of the neck may be an immediate clue to a cuff leak or a malpositioned endotracheal tube (cuff at or above the vocal cords), whereas absent or markedly decreased breath sounds over one hemithorax would suggest tension pneumothorax, major atelectasis, or right main stem intubation.

Investigating Physiologic Mechanisms of Hypoxemia

Assessing for a Reduced FIO_2

Problems with the oxygen delivery system, such as tubing disconnection or a displaced mask, may be discovered quickly by examination. In addition, the FIO_2 being delivered can be directly measured in the intubated patient.

Assessing for Hypoventilation

Hypoventilation is diagnosed by finding an elevation in the $PaCO_2$ (relative to the patient's baseline $PaCO_2$). In patients breathing room air there will be an approximately equal fall in PaO_2. If the fall in PaO_2 exceeds the rise in $PaCO_2$, that is, indicating an increased alveolar-arterial (A-a) gradient, an additional cause for the hypoxemia should be sought. A low respiratory rate is useful in differentiating the causes of hypoventilation, and its differential diagnosis includes administration of sedative or opioid drugs, neuromuscular blockers, and an acute neurologic event. In patients who are on supplemental oxygen, the rise in $PaCO_2$ due to hypoventilation will have less of an impact on the PaO_2. Thus, hypoventilation is usually not an important mechanism for significant hypoxemia in these patients.

Response to Supplemental Oxygen

Since low FIO_2 and hypoventilation can be easily ruled out by assessing the oxygen delivery system and measuring $PaCO_2$, the main diagnostic task is to differentiate V/Q inequality from shunt. The effectiveness of supplemental oxygen in correcting the hypoxemia may provide helpful diagnostic information in this regard. This distinction, however, cannot be applied to patients already receiving a high FIO_2.

Chest Radiography

In patients requiring an F_{IO_2} greater than 0.5 to correct the acute hypoxemic episode, the chest radiograph is the next important step in the diagnostic algorithm to determine if the lung fields are clear ("black lungs"), diffusely involved ("white lungs"), or with new focal infiltrates (focal infiltrates). For those patients with baseline infiltrates who are already receiving high concentrations of oxygen, the chest radiograph may be unchanged or show new infiltrates suggestive of either progression of the initial disease or a new process.

Black Lungs

If a pneumothorax or right main stem intubation is not apparent, one should repeat the study in several hours to rule out occult or early air space disease. If this is not suspected or does not evolve, an acute PE should be excluded (see Chapter 76). In those patients who fail to reach a 95% saturation on very high concentrations of oxygen (>0.8), one should rule out an intracardiac shunt with an echocardiographic "bubble" study. If such patients are going to undergo a perfusion lung scan to assess PE, one should alert the nuclear medicine staff and request that they scan the brain and spleen for the presence of isotope, which would also confirm the presence of an anatomic right-to-left shunt.

White Lungs

Since the new development of diffuse pneumonia (such as viral or *Pneumocystis*) or pulmonary hemorrhage would be rare in the ICU patient (except for a select few who are predisposed), findings of "white lungs" indicates the presence of pulmonary edema (cardiogenic or noncardiogenic). Prompt improvement after diuresis is probably the most useful diagnostic tool. In hypotensive patients for whom diuresis might be contraindicated, a pulmonary arterial (Swan-Ganz) catheter is indicated to measure pulmonary arterial wedge pressure and other hemodynamic parameters.

New Focal Infiltrates

Atelectasis can be distinguished from the remainder of the differential diagnoses if volume loss is also present. Absent air bronchograms in the affected lobes suggests atelectasis due to secretions obstructing the large airways. If air bronchograms are present, however, this suggests large airway patency with distal atelectasis. The latter typically occurs in patients after chest or upper abdominal procedures. Other causes include massive obesity, ascites, ileus leading to abdominal distention, head injury, or neuromuscular disease.

Without volume loss, the diagnosis of focal infiltrates depends on other clinical findings, for example, characteristics of sputum or bronchoscopic specimens. Bronchoscopy with a protected brush specimen or bronchoalveolar lavage can be performed to diagnose nosocomial pneumonia (see Chapter 11).

Prior Infiltrates

Patients recently admitted with focal infiltrates may experience worsening hypoxemia. If their prior infiltrates worsened, one should suspect progression of the initial disease as the cause of the hypoxemia. Patients with pre-existing pulmonary infiltrates manifesting shunt physiology can also acquire acute hypoxemia without any apparent changes in the baseline chest radiograph. Their differential diagnosis includes all those discussed under "Black Lungs," as well as an increase in shunt flow after a position change, administration of a vasodilator, excess PEEP, or PE. Finally, in intubated patients, worsening shunt may result from alveolar collapse due to a problem with the artificial airway or ventilator circuit.

The Intubated Patient

In the mechanically ventilated patient, a unique set of problems can occur arising from leaks from the tubing or around the cuff, obstruction of the artificial airway, or malfunction of the ventilator (Table 26–2). The ventilator alarms, peak inspiratory pressure, and the exhaled volume alarms provide essential information as to the nature of the problem (described in Chapter 48). If there is significant respiratory distress, one should manually "bag" the patient with 100% oxygen as this can help distinguish whether the problem lies in the ventilator equipment or in the patient.

When to Pursue the Diagnosis of Acute Pulmonary Embolism

The clinical findings in patients with acute PE are usually nonspecific. Since ICU patients often cannot communicate and have underlying cardiopulmonary disease, the diagnosis of PE is particularly difficult in this setting. Virtually all ICU patients are at risk for venous thromboembolism by virtue of their immobility and most have additional risk factors. Thus, patients should be evaluated for PE after any

Table 26–2. Causes of Acute Hypoxemia in the Intubated Patient

VENTILATOR-CIRCUITRY PROBLEMS	CLINICAL CLUES
ETT malposition: above vocal cords	Audible air leak, minimal resistance when bagging
ETT malposition: in right main stem	Asymmetric breath sounds
ETT obstruction	Difficulty bagging or passing suction catheter
Ventilator tubing disconnect	Audible air leak, improves with bagging
Ventilator malfunction	Improves with bagging
Tension pneumothorax	Asymmetric breath sounds, tracheal shift, hypotension, tachycardia
Auto-PEEP	Severe airways obstruction, ↑ $Paco_2$, hypotension, tachycardia, failure to trigger ventilator
Wrong ventilator setting made	Settings are different from ones ordered
Machine malfunction: low Fio_2	Improved with bagging, measured Fio_2 is reduced

ETT, endotracheal tube; PEEP, positive end-expiratory pressure.

episode of acute hypoxemia (that is not transient) in which an alternative definitive diagnosis is not apparent.

Particularly suggestive for PE is acute hypoxemia in the presence of a clear, or minimally changed, chest radiograph or in a ventilated patient when unaccompanied by changes in body position, airway secretions, or respiratory mechanics. If the patient has no serious contraindications, one should initiate anticoagulation with heparin while proceeding with the diagnostic work-up.

The V/Q scan, the cornerstone of the noninvasive diagnostic work-up, is often indeterminate (intermediate probability) in ICU patients because of pre-existing cardiopulmonary disease. Added to that is the inability to perform the ventilation part of the scan because patients are receiving mechanical ventilation. Furthermore, if the ventilated patient's chest radiograph has widespread infiltrates, the utility of even performing a perfusion scan is controversial because perfusion abnormalities are considered a given. In these cases, some intensivists recommend bypassing the V/Q scan entirely and going straight to pulmonary angiogram. Some interventional radiologists, however, prefer to review the results of the perfusion scan beforehand in order to try to minimize contrast injection, for example, injecting first into the most suspicious lobe as demonstrated by the V/Q scan. Diagnostic and therapeutic algorithms for a major PE, suspected on the grounds of acute severe hypoxemia or sudden onset of hemodynamic instability are presented in Chapter 76.

MANAGEMENT OF HYPOXEMIA IN THE NONINTUBATED PATIENT

When treating acute hypoxemia, the primary goal is to alleviate tissue hypoxia in order to preserve vital organ function. When giving supplemental oxygen, one must decide on the mode of administration, its "dosage," and the end point. In addition, if the end point cannot be reached, one must know what additional treatment options are available.

Modes of Oxygen Administration

Although divided into low- and high-flow systems, either may be used for delivering low or high concentrations of oxygen. *Low flow* refers to a delivery system that does not meet the entire inspiratory flow demands of the patient, necessitating the entrainment of ambient air. This results in variable F_{IO_2} depending on the patient's ventilatory drive. A *nasal cannula,* also called *nasal prongs,* and *simple face masks* are the two common low-flow devices used to deliver a low F_{IO_2}. The advantages of using a nasal cannula are greater patient comfort and improved compliance, but it produces nasal drying at high flows. Flows greater than 6 L/min only minimally increase F_{IO_2}.

Face masks with reservoir bags are used when a high F_{IO_2} is desired. If a blender is used to deliver a fixed F_{IO_2} to the bag, and the bag stays inflated during the respiratory cycle, it can reliably provide a high F_{IO_2}, up to 0.9. With a *partial rebreather mask,* some exhaled gas enters the bag and is then rebreathed by the patient (which may be useful if the patient is also having symptoms of hyperventilation).

Nonrebreather masks have a one-way valve to avoid rebreathing exhaled gas and a single or pair of one-way valves on the mask itself to prevent inspiring ambient air. These masks, when driven by a 100% oxygen source, can reliably deliver an FIO_2 $\geq$0.8. Because both rebreather and nonrebreather masks do not fit tightly, air entrainment still can occur so that neither can deliver FIO_2 equal to (or close to) 1.0.

High-flow systems theoretically minimize the variability in FIO_2 seen with low-flow systems; however, the common *Venturi mask system* falls short of this goal when a high FIO_2 is desired. The *high-flow humidifier system* is better in this regard because of its higher flow capacity. Unfortunately, the noise it generates is a drawback, it is more cumbersome than the low-flow reservoir masks, and it carries the risk of bacterial contamination of its reservoir.

How Much Oxygen to Administer At First

One can begin with a low FIO_2 and titrate upward to the desired goal or start high and titrate down. The selection should depend on how much oxygen, if any, the patient is already receiving, whether the patient has COPD and chronic CO_2 retention, and the severity and cause of the acute hypoxemia. Patients who should initially be treated with high oxygen concentrations are those already receiving an FIO_2 greater than 40%, those with severe hypoxemia or shock, those believed to have shunt physiology, and those needing imminent airway intubation.

The problem with using this approach of starting with a high FIO_2 for all patients is that some have admitting diagnoses for which a high FIO_2 may be deleterious. This includes patients with COPD and baseline CO_2 retention who present with an acute flare of their COPD. The fear is that these patients will have a worsening of their respiratory acidosis. Recent studies have shown that respiratory acidosis does worsen in about two thirds of such patients, in half of whom it may be severe and require noninvasive or invasive ventilation. Recent studies have demonstrated that this oxygen-induced hypoventilation results predominantly from an increased V/Q mismatch (i.e., increased dead space ventilation due to reversal of hypoxic vasoconstriction) and displacement of CO_2 from hemoglobin by O_2 (the Haldane effect) rather than simply suppression by oxygen of the patient's hypoxic drive to breathe.

In those patients with COPD who become somnolent after oxygen administration of any type, noninvasive or invasive mechanical ventilation should be instituted rather than oxygen withdrawal. Fortunately, a low FIO_2 is usually adequate to correct the hypoxemia in this patient population. If the end point of adequate saturation is not achieved, higher concentrations should be given only with close monitoring.

Goals of Oxygen Therapy

The therapeutic goal depends on the patient's diagnosis, whether there are marked fluctuations in oxygenation, and how refractory the hypoxemia is to high FIO_2. Generally one should aim to correct the PO_2 to approximately 60 to 70 mm Hg, which corresponds to SaO_2 greater than or equal to 90%. Values greater than this do not significantly raise the oxygen content because of the shape of the oxyhemoglobin dissociation curve (see Appendix A). Furthermore, at this level of oxygenation the symptoms, signs, and morbidity of hypoxemia are usually eliminated. Exceptions to this guideline include patients with myocardial ischemia, pregnancy, or rarely those with signs of persistent tissue hypoxia in which even the small amount of additional oxygen content may be critical for organ function. In these settings, titrating to a PaO_2 of 90 to 100 mm Hg (or greater) is reasonable. Also, in patients who demonstrate wide fluctuations in PaO_2, it is prudent to maintain them at higher values, thus creating a "buffer" for their next episode of desaturation.

In general, equilibration in a patient's PaO_2 requires only 5 to 10 minutes after a change in FIO_2. This usually allows one to establish oxygenation goals within a half hour when titrating FIO_2 up or down, for which pulse oximetry can usually be used.

Finally, because many intensivists believe that any FIO_2 greater than 0.6 can cause lung injury, patients with higher oxygen requirements may need other treatment modalities to avoid exceeding this "safe" upper limit for extended periods. These include noninvasive means, such as use of a continuous positive airway pressure (CPAP) mask or noninvasive ventilation, as well as invasive ventilation. If the patient has received certain drugs that predispose the lung to the development of oxygen toxicity, of which bleomycin is the most thoroughly studied, the lowest FIO_2 should be sought by applying adjunctive interventions as discussed in the following section.

Adjuncts to Oxygen Therapy

Patients who fail to respond to mask oxygen delivery systems or ventilated patients requiring high FIO_2 need alternative therapies. Since the majority of these patients have diffuse airspace filling disorders, the application of positive airway pressure can be helpful. CPAP can be given to the nonintubated patient by face mask or a noninvasive ventilator (see Chapter 77). CPAP can also be applied through a mechanical ventilator following intubation. When CPAP is used in conjunction with a ventilatory support mode, for example, assist control, it is referred to as PEEP (see Chapter 73).

PEEP and CPAP reduce the right-to-left shunt fraction primarily by recruiting collapsed and poorly ventilated alveoli. Up to 10 cm H_2O of CPAP may be applied noninvasively with a tight fitting mask or via noninvasive ventilation for several days in appropriate patients. This group includes those who are expected to improve quickly, for example, those with acute congestive heart failure, and those whose airway secretions are controllable by coughing. Invasive ventilation is preferred in patients with circulatory shock because mechanical ventilation can improve distribution of cardiac output by decreasing the blood flow requirements of the respiratory muscles.

BIBLIOGRAPHY

Gibson RL, Comer PB, Beckham RW, et al: Actual tracheal oxygen concentrations with commonly used oxygen equipment. Anesthesiology 44:71–73, 1976.
This article demonstrates the principle that FIO_2 is sensitive to inspiratory flow rate in patients on supplemental oxygen.

Glauser FL, Polatty RC, Seeler CN: Worsening oxygenation in the mechanically ventilated patient: causes, mechanisms, and early detection. Am Rev Respir Dis 138:458–465, 1988.
This article presents a complete differential diagnosis for this patient population with an emphasis on the mechanisms of hypoxemia.

Hanning CD, Alexander-Williams JM: Pulse oximetry: A practical review. Br Med J 311:367–370, 1995.
This is a practical review of the applications and limitations of pulse oximetry.

Kacmarek RM: In-hospital administration of oxygen. In: Kacmarek RM, Stoller JK (eds): Current Respiratory Care. Toronto: BC Decker, 1988.
This is a review of the oxygen supplementation devices.

Marcey TW, Marini JJ: Respiratory distress in the ventilated patient. Clin Chest Med 15:55–77, 1994.
This article presents a thorough review of a related topic stressing the pathophysiology and management.

Remolina C, Khan AU, Santiago TV, Edelman NH: Positional hypoxemia in patients with unilateral lung disease. N Engl J Med 304:523–525, 1981.
This article illustrates an important pathophysiologic mechanism that is both a cause and a treatment for the hypoxemia in patients with unilateral infiltrates.

Thorson SH, Marini JJ, Pierson DJ, Hudson LD: Variability of arterial blood gas values in stable patients in the ICU. Chest 84:14–18, 1983.
This article demonstrates that marked variability in Pa_{O_2} occurs even in stable patients with a constant FI_{O_2}.

Wood LDH, Hall JB: A mechanistic approach to providing adequate oxygenation in acute hypoxemic respiratory failure. Respir Care 38:784–799, 1993.
This is a outstanding review of the comprehensive treatment of hypoxemia.

Zwillich CW, Pierson DJ, Creagh CE, et al: Complications of assisted ventilation: a prospective study of 354 consecutive episodes. Am J Med 57:161–170, 1974.
Useful for evaluating the incidence of complications related to mechanical ventilation that may cause hypoxemia.

27 Acute Hypercapnic Episodes

Cynthia B. Robinson

Acute hypercapnic episodes are episodes of alveolar hypoventilation. They are defined as acute elevations of $Paco_2$ greater than 45 mm Hg (or greater than the patient's baseline $Paco_2$, if elevated) accompanied by a decrease in arterial pH less than 7.35. By this definition, diagnosing an acute hypercapnic episode requires performing an arterial blood gas determination. Likewise, as a rule in the intensive care unit (ICU) setting, monitoring arterial oxygen saturation alone is inadequate to detect a hypercapnic episode. This limitation is illustrated by the ICU patient who has an episode of hypercapnia but whose saturations by pulse oximetry remain high because the patient is also receiving supplemental oxygen. The oxygen therapy blunts the arterial desaturation that, in its absence, would have accompanied the hypercapnic episode as predicted by the Alveolar Gas Equation (see Chapter 1, Table 1–1, Equation 12).

PHYSIOLOGIC EFFECTS OF HYPERCAPNIA

The major physiologic effects of acute hypercapnia occur on the central nervous system (CNS) and are manifested initially by lethargy and stupor, which can progress to coma with increasingly higher levels of $Paco_2$. Effects on the CNS occur with acute elevations of $Paco_2$ in the range of 15 to 20 mm Hg. Some patients who have severe underlying pulmonary disease and are receiving oxygen therapy, however, may have chronic elevations of $Paco_2$ greater than 100 mm Hg without any apparent disturbance of consciousness. Patients with chronic elevations in $Paco_2$ and nocturnal exacerbations of hypercapnia may complain of morning headaches or conjunctival redness.

Hypercapnia produces *vasodilation* of systemic arterioles that tends to increase local blood flow. The clinical effects of vasodilation are most evident in the CNS, where two important regulators of cerebral blood flow are $Paco_2$ and Pao_2. Increases in $Paco_2$ of 15 mm Hg are associated with a cerebral blood flow increase of approximately 33%. Conversely, hyperventilation decreases cerebral blood flow, which is the rationale to use hyperventilation in the therapeutic approach to elevated intracranial pressure (see Chapter 42).

Acute hypercapnia also produces *disturbances in acid-base balance*. Extreme changes can predispose the patient to cardiac dysrhythmias or heart failure. Likewise, acidosis causes a transient hypercalcemia (particularly increasing ionized calcium because of the decreases in protein binding) that may exacerbate changes in mental status and worsen respiratory and cardiac function. Lastly, hypercapnia stimulates renal bicarbonate production, usually in conjunction with enhanced sodium absorption. The process of renal compensation for an episode of continuing hypercapnia begins within hours but takes several days to achieve its compensatory end point.

Correct interpretation of arterial blood gas measurements is critical to the diagnosis and management of hypercapnia. The arterial blood gas determination helps to distinguish among acute and chronic respiratory acidoses, hypoventilation representing respiratory compensation for a metabolic alkalosis, and mixed disturbances (see Appendix D). For example, to compensate for a primary metabolic alkalosis, patients may hypoventilate to a moderate degree (usually $Paco_2$ ≤ 55 mm Hg), whereas arterial pH remains elevated (>7.45).

Determining whether hypercapnia is acute or chronic assists in the differential diagnosis and the subsequent management. *Acute hypercapnia* generally causes arterial pH to decrease by 0.08 for every 10 mm Hg rise in $Paco_2$. In *chronic hypercapnia,* the arterial pH decreases by 0.03 for every 10 mm Hg rise in $Paco_2$, reflecting the buffering effects of prior renal bicarbonate retention. Intrinsic renal disease compromises the capacity of the kidney to compensate for hypercapnia, which exaggerates the acidosis.

Simple chronic hypercapnia (primary respiratory acidosis with elevated serum bicarbonate due to chronic renal compensation) must be distinguished from mixed acid-base disturbances with hypercapnia (primary acute or chronic respiratory acidosis with a primary metabolic alkalosis). Combined respiratory acidosis and metabolic alkalosis commonly occur together in patients with chronic obstructive pulmonary disease (COPD) after volume contraction from diuresis. Similarly, excessive ventilation of COPD patients with a chronic respiratory acidosis that decreases $Paco_2$ to a modestly elevated range, as sometimes occurs inadvertently with initiation of mechanical ventilation (see Chapter 2), can produce a transient (posthypercapnic) metabolic alkalosis combined with a mild chronic respiratory acidosis.

DIFFERENTIAL DIAGNOSIS OF ACUTE HYPERCAPNIC EPISODES

Mechanistically, hypercapnia can result from dysfunction of one of the four components of the respiratory system: the CNS; the chest "bellows," including the peripheral nervous system and the respiratory muscles; the airways; and the alveoli (see Chapter 1).

Central Nervous System Component

CNS abnormalities can lead to acute hypercapnia through a failure to sense a potent stimulus to breathe or to generate an adequate neural output sufficient to activate the chest "bellows." The control of breathing is a complex neural system within several brainstem respiratory nuclei that are stimulated by peripheral and central chemoreceptors. They generate a respiratory rhythm and determine the overall "set point" of the respiratory system (see Chapter 1, Fig. 1–1). Localized lesions of these brainstem respiratory nuclei account for less than 0.1% of all cases of central hypoventilation. Rather, most hypercapnia commonly results from a raised set point for $Paco_2$ or an inadequate motor response to an adequate neural output.

Patients with primary central hypoventilation usually have a normal sensorium during wakefulness but have disturbed respiratory patterns during sleep. The

Table 27–1. Central Nervous System Depressant Drugs Causing Acute Hypercapnia

Anxiolytics (benzodiazepines)	Tricyclic antidepressant overdose
Opioids	Epidural opioids and local anesthetics
Sedatives and hypnotics	Magnesium toxicity (iatrogenic)
Barbiturates and other antiseizure drugs	

classic "pickwickian" patient with obesity-hypoventilation syndrome has daytime hypersomnolence and manifests hypercapnia that worsens with sleep (see Chapter 77). The diagnosis of obesity-hypoventilation syndrome requires $Paco_2$ measurements that rise more than 10 mm Hg when going from wakefulness to sleep. These patients also have a characteristic pattern of desaturation on polysomnography (see Chapter 77, Fig. 77–1*B*).

Although obesity-hypoventilation syndrome is not uncommon, a more frequent cause for central hypoventilation in the ICU is global CNS depression caused by drugs, either given for sedation or analgesia or taken as an overdose (Table 27–1).

Chest Bellows Component

The stimulus to breathe must be converted into a mechanical response to ensure adequate ventilation and prevent hypercapnia. Conversion of a neural stimulus into motor contraction involves peripheral nerves, motor end plates, neurotransmitters, and myofibrils. Abnormalities in any of these elements of the chest bellows can produce respiratory muscle weakness and acute hypercapnia (see Chapter 1).

Respiratory muscle weakness and fatigue may occur well before abnormalities in arterial blood gases. *Respiratory muscle fatigue* is evident from abnormal breathing patterns in a supine patient. *Respiratory alternans* occurs when supine patients preferentially contract their thoracic inspiratory muscles while maintaining only tonic activity in their diaphragms, thereby "resting" them. When the thoracic inspiratory muscles begin to fatigue, diaphragms are used for ventilation and the thoracic muscles are then "rested." Clinically, one usually observes first chest movements in isolation and then abdominal movements in isolation.

When the fatigue becomes more pronounced, the patient experiences a breathing pattern termed *respiratory paradox*. In this case, the fatigued muscle cannot contract to resist the pull of the other set of respiratory muscles, and a peculiar rocking motion of the chest and abdomen ensues. Instead of their normal parallel movements (in which both the chest and anterior abdominal wall move anteriorly), the chest and abdominal walls alternate moving forward. This pattern is classically produced by diaphragmatic fatigue but can occur in other states when the patient is breathing against high mechanical loads, such as severe airway obstruction. Regardless of the cause of the respiratory muscle fatigue, incipient respiratory failure is often manifested by respiratory paradox.

Both the vital capacity and the negative inspiratory force (also referred to as the *maximal inspiratory pressure*) reflect respiratory muscle function and may be measured in the conscious, cooperative patient, even while intubated. In general, accurate measurements of both depend on the patient's cooperation. In addition, the vital capacity maneuver depends on lung compliance and airway resistance. The negative inspiratory force depends on inspiratory muscle strength as well as cooperation. Patients with profound respiratory muscle fatigue may not be able to generate a negative inspiratory force more negative than -20 cm H_2O. Serial vital capacity or negative inspiratory maneuvers are generally more informative than a single measurement. Muscle fatigue may also manifest itself as a pattern of recurrent shifting lobar atelectasis on chest radiographs.

The neural pathways involved in respiration include the phrenic nerves, the intercostal nerves, and the nerves innervating the sternocleidomastoid and other strap muscles of the neck. Phrenic nerve injuries or dysfunction commonly occur after cardiac surgery. Postoperatively, these can cause hypercapnia and prolonged ventilator dependence if the injury is bilateral or if other respiratory impairments are present. The mechanisms of phrenic nerve injury include stretching, transection, and cooling.

Diagnosis of *phrenic nerve injury* in the ICU is difficult. Bilateral diaphragmatic paralysis is not detectable with plain radiographs, particularly when the patient is receiving positive pressure ventilation. Unilateral diaphragmatic paralysis can be revealed by performance of a quick inspiratory maneuver (or "sniff") while observing the movement of both hemidiaphragms simultaneously under fluoroscopy. The paralyzed and flaccid hemidiaphragm moves cephalad because it does not resist the forceful negative inspiratory pleural pressure. Successful performance of this subjective test requires unilateral paralysis in a cooperative, spontaneously breathing patient.

More precise, albeit invasive, are phrenic nerve conduction studies with diaphragmatic electromyograms (EMGs) (see Chapter 67). These studies can detect slowed nerve conduction velocities indicating unilateral or bilateral phrenic nerve dysfunction, even in patients on ventilators. Total lack of detection of a diaphragmatic electromyographic signal, however, is difficult to interpret because it can result either from phrenic nerve transection or from the recording electromyographic electrode not being located on the surface of the chest wall directly opposite the hemidiaphragm.

Other neuromuscular disorders can lead to acute respiratory failure on occasion in the ICU setting (Table 27–2). Before starting the diagnostic evaluation for neuromuscular weakness in the ICU (see Chapter 67), one must first eliminate the

Table 27–2. Neuromuscular Problems Causing Acute Hypercapnic Episodes

Respiratory muscle fatigue (most common by far)
Respiratory muscle weakness due to effects of neuromuscular blockers (see Chapter 4)
Exacerbation of effects of neuromuscular blocker by other drugs (see Chapter 4)
Respiratory muscle weakness due to local anesthetics in epidural analgesia (see Chapter 85)
Myasthenic crises (see Chapter 67)
Worsening myasthenia due to untoward effects of other drugs (see Chapter 67)
Acute spinal cord injury or ischemia (see Chapter 98)
Acute respiratory muscular weakness due to electrolyte disorders, such as hypokalemia or hypophosphatemia (see Chapter 36)
Respiratory muscular weakness due to critical illness myopathy or neuropathy (see Chapter 67)
Spasm of truncal muscles, as a reaction to intravenous opioids, dystonic reactions to phenothiazines, or other rare causes (neuroleptic malignant syndrome)

Table 27–3. Airway Problems Causing Acute Hypercapnic Episodes

Acute bronchospasm (asthma, COPD, transfusion reaction, allergic reaction)
Artificial airway problems (see Chapter 28)
    Obstruction (tube kinking, biting tube, secretions in lumen, concretions or clots at tip)
    Loss of tidal volume (leaking cuff, cuff at or above vocal cords, high peak pressures)
    Displacement of tip of tracheostomy tube (into subcutaneous tissues)
Upper airway obstruction postextubation
    Edema of false cords and supraglottic tissues
    Laryngospasm
    Tracheal obstruction (hematoma, intraluminal mass, mediastinal mass)
    Tracheomalacia

COPD, chronic obstructive pulmonary disease.

CNS as a cause by excluding all sedatives or similar acting agents (see Table 27–1) and then conduct both a motor and sensory examination. A "pure" myopathy suggests the myopathy of critical illness, polymyositis, or myasthenia gravis, whereas mixed motor and sensory disorder suggests Guillain-Barré syndrome, the polyneuropathy of critical illness, or spinal cord injury.

Airways Component

Mechanical problems in the upper airway, particularly in mechanically ventilated patients, can also lead to acute hypercapnic episodes in the ICU (Table 27–3). Endotracheal tube obstruction by blood or mucus, tube kinking, hypoventilation due to a leak around the tracheal cuff, or inadvertent main stem bronchus intubation can cause acute hypercapnia (see Chapter 28). However, hypercapnia is, as a rule, a late sign of these mechanical problems, and alarms for high peak inspiratory pressures, low exhaled tidal volumes, or low exhaled minute ventilation should alert the ICU staff long before the $Paco_2$ becomes elevated (see Chapter 48).

After extubation, about 5% of patients develop acute upper airway obstruction and stridor. Some require reintubation. The upper airway obstruction may result from supraglottic edema, reflex vocal cord closure (laryngospasm), or tracheal lumen compromise due to compression by a hematoma or tracheomalacia. Upper airway obstruction results in stridor only if the patient has adequate airflow, but otherwise it may only produce progressive hypercapnia, hypoxemia, bradycardia, and paradoxical breathing. To treat postextubation stridor due to supraglottic edema, racemic epinephrine (or neosynephrine) is commonly given as a nebulized aerosol with the rationale that its alpha-agonist properties can reduce swelling by vasoconstriction. Steroids are generally also given as an antiedema agent.

In the case of laryngospasm after extubation (which usually occurs within seconds after extubation), the initial therapy includes manual bagging and oxygenation with a resuscitation bag. If the obstruction persists and manual bagging cannot ventilate or oxygenate the patient, pharmacologic paralysis and reintubation is indicated.

No risk factors have been identified to predict the population at risk for the development of postextubation stridor (except for patients whose initial indication for intubation was upper airway obstruction). For example, the endotracheal tube size, the number of intubation attempts, and the duration of intubation are not predictive. As a result, all newly extubated patients should be monitored carefully for this complication over the first hour or so after extubation.

Probably the most common cause of hypercapnia in the ICU is chronic airflow obstruction from asthma or COPD (see Chapter 74). Hypoxemia accompanied by hypercapnia in the asthmatic patient is an ominous sign, denoting incipient respiratory failure and the need for mechanical ventilation. Although hypoxemia can be relieved with administration of oxygen, hypercapnia can be difficult to treat in the intubated asthmatic patient. Achieving a normal Pa_{CO_2} in a severely obstructed asthmatic patient on a ventilator often requires heavy sedation and pharmacologic paralysis. Paralyzing patients in status asthmaticus lost popularity after it was reported that the combination of neuromuscular blockade and high-dose corticosteroid therapy was a risk factor for prolonged weakness from a diffuse myopathy (see Chapter 67). As a result, the strategy of allowing the Pa_{CO_2} to rise, known as *permissive hypercapnia,* has gained popularity and widespread acceptance.

Exacerbations of COPD are frequently accompanied by increasing hypercapnia and worsening hypoxemia. Oxygen administration in COPD patients experiencing an exacerbation can often increase Pa_{CO_2}. A mild rise that then plateaus occurs in about one third of such patients, whereas a severe rise in Pa_{CO_2} that continues upward occurs in another third. Previously, these elevations in Pa_{CO_2} were ascribed to suppression of hypoxemic ventilatory drive. However, increases in Pa_{CO_2} can occur even with a baseline Pa_{O_2} greater than 55 to 60 mm Hg when little or no hypoxic drive exists. Furthermore, studies have revealed that the mechanism of oxygen-induced hypoventilation is predominantly due to increased dead space and altered V/Q relationships (occurring when the supplemental oxygen relieves hypoxic vasoconstriction) and oxygen-induced displacement of CO_2 from the hemoglobin molecule (Haldane effect). Oxygen should *never* be withheld from hypoxemic COPD patients, even if their Pa_{CO_2} rises further. Rather, if the elevation in Pa_{CO_2} results in severe acidemia, obtundation or severe respiratory distress, one should begin noninvasive or invasive mechanical ventilation.

In a patient with chronic hypercapnia and an acute exacerbation of COPD, an arterial blood gas measurement is required to determine the relative proportion of acute hypercapnia and chronic hypercapnia. This distinction is important because current treatments can reverse the acute hypercapnia but do not correct the chronic hypercapnia of advanced lung disease. This situation occurs in the ICU when a patient with chronic CO_2 retention is mechanically overventilated, completely correcting the Pa_{CO_2} to the normal range. Such patients with diminished pulmonary function cannot maintain a Pa_{CO_2} at 40 mm Hg and an acute respiratory acidosis will result when one attempts to wean them from the ventilator (see Chapter 3).

Alveolar Failure

Patients with cardiogenic pulmonary edema (see Chapter 51) or acute respiratory distress syndrome (ARDS) (see Chapter 73) frequently manifest hypercapnia with hypoxemia when they initially present in respiratory distress. A worsened V/Q mismatch, leading to increased ventilation to nonperfused units (increased dead space ventilation), increased work of breathing (from high respiratory rates and low lung compliance), leading to increased CO_2 production and the onset of respiratory muscle fatigue contribute to the hypercapnia in these disorders.

Patients with cardiogenic pulmonary edema and hypercapnia should be treated initially with noninvasive ventilation, which has been reported to have better outcomes than conventional invasive ventilation (see Chapter 51). Patients with ARDS, however, need invasive ventilation but can be ventilated with low tidal volumes and low distending alveolar pressures. Although this method may result in permissive hypercapnia, it is an accepted method for ventilating patients with ARDS and has resulted in improved outcomes (see Chapter 73).

TREATMENT OF ACUTE HYPERCAPNIA

The first step in treating an acute hypercapnic episode is to assess the urgency of the clinical situation. Next is to determine its cause because treatment focuses on the underlying disease. Initially, all patients with hypercapnia should be assessed for hemodynamic stability and for level of CNS functioning.

Noninvasive mechanical ventilation can be used to treat spontaneously breathing patients with reversible causes of hypoventilation, such as those with respiratory muscle fatigue postextubation, cardiogenic pulmonary edema, or a COPD flare. In many ICUs, noninvasive mechanical ventilation has become the initial therapy of choice for these problems. Noninvasive ventilation is less successful, however, in patients who require prolonged ventilatory support, in patients who cannot cough up secretions, or when a high risk of aspiration prohibits the use of a tight-fitting face mask.

A similar approach can be used to evaluate an acute hypercapnic episode in mechanically ventilated patients. First, the patient should be assessed for hemodynamic instability and mechanical problems with the artificial airway, and tension pneumothorax should be ruled out. Problems with the artificial airway can generally be identified by noting increased peak airway pressures, decreased tidal volumes, or decreased expired minute ventilation (see Chapter 48). If peak airway pressures exceed their baseline values, one should suspect partial obstruction of the artificial airway and verify the patency of the endotracheal tube by manual bagging and suctioning. Once the tube is confirmed to be free of obstruction and pneumothorax has been ruled out, one should assess for the presence of bronchoconstriction. If the problem is worsened bronchospasm, more aggressive bronchodilator therapy is indicated (see Chapter 74). In the setting of diffuse airway obstruction, ventilator treatment of acute hypercapnia is accomplished by increasing the tidal volume or allowing permissive hypercapnia to occur. If one suspects the problem is likely due to decreased respiratory compliance, such as in pulmonary edema, management is to preferentially increase respiratory rate or allow permissive hypercapnia.

For spontaneously breathing patients with altered mental status, mechanically ventilated patients with normal peak inspiratory pressures, or patients who are being weaned from the ventilator, the management of acute hypercapnia is based on determining the cause. In all cases, therapy should be directed against the underlying pathophysiologic abnormality. For example, one should observe the patient's breathing efforts. If respiratory paradox is present, respiratory muscle fatigue is likely and the patient should be given more ventilatory support.

BIBLIOGRAPHY

Cheng EY, Woehlck H, Mazzeo AJ: Capnography in critical care medicine. J Intensive Care Med 12:18–32, 1997.
This is a thorough review of capnographic devices, capnograms and clinical uses of capnography for monitoring ICU patients. It has 67 references.

Cohen CA, Zagelbaum G, Gross D, et al: Clinical manifestations of inspiratory muscle fatigue. Am J Med 73:308–315, 1982.
This is a classic description of the changes in respiratory pattern that occur during weaning from mechanical ventilation, including the predictive value of respiratory paradox. Increasing respiratory rate is the earliest and most sensitive index but it lacks specificity. Respiratory paradox, which develops before changes occur in arterial blood gases, is an accurate predictor of an unsuccessful extubation trial.

Goldberg M, Green SB, Moss ML, et al: Computer-based instruction and diagnosis of acid-base disorders: A systematic approach. JAMA 233:269, 1973.
This is a classic presentation of single and multiple acid-base disorders in a user-friendly graphic format (see Appendix B).

Hillberg RE, Johnson DC: Noninvasive ventilation. N Engl J Med 337:1746–1752, 1997.
This article reviews the methods, indications, and limitations of this modality as applied to patients with a variety of cardiorespiratory disorders.

Kramer N, Meyer TJ, Meharg J, et al: Randomized prospective trial of noninvasive positive pressure ventilation in acute respiratory failure. Am J Respir Crit Care Med 151:1799–806, 1995.
Compared with standard care, noninvasive ventilation in patients with acute respiratory failure decreased the need for intubation from 73 to 31%. The results were even more striking with COPD patients: only 9% (1 of 11) needed intubation with noninvasive ventilation compared with 63% (8 of 12) with standard care.

Weinberger SE, Schwartzstein RM, Weiss JW: Hypercapnia. N Engl J Med 321:1223–1231, 1989.
This is a comprehensive review of the mechanisms that contribute to hypercapnia, its clinical causes and manifestations, and its treatment.

28 Airways and Emergency Airway Management

Elizabeth Cordes Behringer
Erica R. Thaler

One of the essentials of care in the intensive care unit (ICU) is to establish and maintain a secure airway. This should permit adequate gas exchange and pulmonary toilet, protect against aspiration of orogastric contents, and allow administration of drugs and humidified gases. In some instances, the patient's natural airway meets these needs.

AIRWAY MANAGEMENT SKILLS

Airway assessment is a mandatory skill of an intensivist. In nonintubated ICU patients, this begins with a physical examination of the patient's natural airway to ascertain the ease of conventional endotracheal intubation. Assessing respiratory status and the need for tracheal intubation is the next essential step. Finally, adequacy of gas exchange and security of the patient's airway must be continuously reassessed. For example, because restlessness and combativeness may be symptoms of hypoxia or a compromised airway, sedatives should not be administered until these conditions have been ruled out (see Chapters 4, 26, and 27).

The intensivist must also be skilled with the basics of emergency airway management. This includes knowledge of the indications for endotracheal intubation, familiarity with the equipment and standard techniques of basic airway management, and the drugs available to facilitate such maneuvers. The intensivist also should be familiar with methods of advanced airway management such as fiberoptic bronchoscopic intubation, the laryngeal mask airway (LMA), and surgical methods for obtaining airway access.

The intensivist must also know how to recognize and manage common and potentially life-threatening airway complications, such as mainstem intubation, esophageal intubation, cuff herniation, and inadvertent extubation. Equipment, drugs, and monitors necessary for basic and advanced airway management of these complications should be readily available in the ICU.

As a rule, emergency airway management in the ICU setting is more technically difficult and hazardous than airway management in the setting of elective surgery. The *difficult airway* has been defined as the clinical situation in which a skilled operator experiences difficulty with mask ventilation or tracheal intubation, or both. The most common problem is difficult direct laryngoscopy giving only a limited view of the glottic opening.

USEFUL DRUGS FOR EMERGENCY AIRWAY MANAGEMENT

Local anesthetics, benzodiazepines, opioids, barbiturates, and muscle relaxants are examples of drugs commonly used during emergency airway management. All should be readily available in the ICU.

323

Local Anesthetics

Topical anesthetics, sometimes used in conjunction with vasoconstrictors, facilitate awake intubation by the orotracheal or nasotracheal route. Techniques available for applying topical anesthetics include the use of sprays, atomizers, and nebulizers. A metered-dose delivery system permits the application of precise doses of the drug. Translaryngeal injection of lidocaine anesthetizes the tracheal mucosa and the inferior aspect of the larynx. An alternative method to anesthetize the vocal cords and trachea is the "spray as you go" technique, often used during bronchoscopy.

The safety of local anesthetics depends on proper dosage and appropriate administration. Topical anesthesia impairs swallowing and blunts protective reflexes. Excessive doses of local anesthetic also lower the seizure threshold.

Anticholinergic Agents

Anticholinergic drugs, such as atropine, glycopyrrolate, and scopolamine, are used to help dry secretions and facilitate awake intubation. Atropine and glycopyrrolate are both antisialagogues devoid of sedative properties (but atropine may cause tachycardia). Scopolamine has antisialagogue as well as sedating properties.

Hypnotic Agents Used for Rapid Sequence Intubation

A number of hypnotic agents, commonly used to induce general anesthesia in the operating suite, can also be used to facilitate rapid-sequence endotracheal intubation in the ICU (Table 28–1). They are generally used in conjunction with a neuromuscular blocking agent (Table 28–2). Because these hypnotic agents can worsen hypotension in critically ill patients who are in shock, receiving pressors, or are severely hypovolemic, other agents, such as fentanyl or midazolam, are commonly used alternatives in these clinical circumstances (see Table 28–1).

GASTRIC ASPIRATION PRECAUTIONS

Patients requiring urgent intubation in the ICU may have a full stomach, and precautions should be taken against the aspiration of orogastric contents. Simple maneuvers include holding oral or gastric feedings in patients who are considered at high risk for needing urgent intubation and suctioning a nasogastric tube, if present, to empty the stomach. During induction of anesthesia, one can exert pressure on the cricoid cartilage with the thumb and index finger to occlude the esophagus (the Sellick maneuver). Some clinicians also administer nonparticulate antacids, such as a solution of sodium citrate and citric acid (Bicitra), or H_2 histamine–receptor antagonists, such as cimetidine and ranitidine, to raise gastric pH prophylactically. Metoclopramide, a dopaminergic antagonist that increases lower esophageal sphincter tone and stimulates upper gastrointestinal motility, may also be used to promote gastric emptying.

Table 28–1. Selected Agents to Facilitate Endotracheal Intubation in the Intensive Care Unit

AGENT	CLASS	DOSE	COMMENTS
Sodiumthio-pental	Hypnotic (barbiturate)	1–5 mg/kg	Dose-dependent effects of myocardial depression and peripheral vasodilation; causes hypotension; contraindicated in patients with even mild volume depletion, shock, or congestive heart failure
Etomidate	Hypnotic (benzyli-midazole)	0.3 mg/kg (0.3–0.6 mg/kg range)	Has less hemodynamic effects than sodium thiopental; provides no analgesia; suppresses cortisol release; myoclonus occurs in approximately 30%; contraindicated in patients with moderate volume depletion or pregnancy
Propofol	Hypnotic (alkylphenol)	1–2.5 mg/kg	Give only half the dose for elderly, debilitated or critically ill patients; it may cause profound hypotension in these vulnerable populations when given in anesthetizing doses; avoid in hypotensive or hypovolemic patients
Ketamine	Dissociative anesthetic	1–2 mg/kg	Depresses myocardium but can preserve blood pressure by sympathetic stimulation; emergence reactions occur in approximately 12%; preserves pharyngeal and laryngeal reflexes; contraindicated in patients with moderate volume depletion or increased intracranial pressure
Fentanyl	Opioid	1–3 μg/kg	Provides sedating effects without amnesia; may cause hypotension; does not blunt hypertensive reflex to endotracheal intubation; patients previously exposed to opioids will generally need higher doses
Midazolam	Benzodiazepine	2–10 mg	Can cause hypotension when given in high doses, with other agents, (opioids) or in hemodynamically unstable patients; patients previously exposed to this class of agent will generally need higher doses

Table 28–2. Neuromuscular Blocking Agents Used for Endotracheal Intubation in the Intensive Care Unit

AGENT	CLASS	DOSE	COMMENTS
Succinylcholine	Depolarizing	1–2 mg/kg	Profound paralysis lasting 5–10 min in normal individuals. Releases potassium from skeletal muscle (serum potassium rises by 0.5–1.0 mEq/L in normal individuals). Severe hyperkalemia with cardiac arrest may occur in patients with massive trauma, burns, lower extremity paralysis or denervated states (multiple sclerosis), or muscular dystrophies.
Pancuronium	Nondepolarizing	0.1 mg/kg	Rapid onset; long acting; likely to cause tachycardia (may be severe). Active metabolite accumulates in renal failure and can cause prolonged paralysis.
Vecuronium	Nondepolarizing	0.1 mg/kg	Rapid onset; short-to-intermediate duration of action; negligible hemodynamic effects. Active 3-desacetyl metabolite accumulates in renal failure and can cause prolonged paralysis.
Cisatracurium	Nondepolarizing	0.15–0.2 mg/kg	Intermediate onset; short duration of action; no effects on nicotinic, autonomic receptors or muscarinic cardiac receptors; may cause histamine release when given rapidly in high dosage.

Modified from Chapter 4, Table 7.

EQUIPMENT FOR EMERGENCY AIRWAY MANAGEMENT

The equipment used during emergency airway management includes oral and nasal airways, bag, mask, suction apparatus, stylets, endotracheal tubes, and laryngoscopes. All should be immediately available in the ICU.

The ability to deliver ventilation by use of a *mask* may be lifesaving. This is a mandatory but often underemphasized skill for intensivists. The ideal face mask is clear plastic (to monitoring for vomiting) and constructed with a cushioned rim to help prevent air leaks during mask ventilation. Bags for ventilation should include the traditional anesthesia bag and the self-inflatable bag, also called the manual resuscitation bag.

Oropharyngeal and *nasopharyngeal airways* are useful adjuncts to mask ventilation. Oropharyngeal airways prevent upper airway obstruction caused by the collapse of the tongue on the palate or posterior pharynx. A nasopharyngeal airway bypasses obstruction from the nares to the hypopharynx; it should be lubricated before insertion to avoid trauma and bleeding. Like nasotracheal tubes, nasopharyngeal airways are contraindicated in patients with coagulopathies or basilar skull fractures.

Several types of *laryngoscopes* are commercially available. The most commonly used are the Miller and MacIntosh blades. The Miller blade is straight, long, rounded on the bottom, and slightly curved at the tip. It was designed to allow for a minimum of mouth opening and greater anterior movement of the mandible. The MacIntosh blade is curved and was designed to be introduced into the right side of the mouth so that the tongue is displaced to the left during endotracheal intubation. Both blades are used during direct laryngoscopy. Newer rigid, indirect fiberoptic laryngoscopes, such as the Bullard laryngoscope, are available as well.

Most *endotracheal tubes* are polyvinyl chloride and have a low-pressure, high-volume (floppy) cuff that is fused to the tube (Fig. 28–1). They are classified according to their internal diameter (ID). The choice of an appropriately sized endotracheal tube is important for the mechanically ventilated ICU patient because small endotracheal tubes (≤6 mm ID) increase airway resistance and work of breathing during weaning. Small endotracheal tubes also make it difficult or impossible to perform fiberoptic bronchoscopy through their lumens.

In general, one should use a 7.0- to 7.5-mm ID endotracheal tube for adult females and a 7.5- to 8.0-mm ID tube for adult males. Endotracheal tubes smaller than these are required for certain pathologic conditions such as laryngeal edema. The correct depth of insertion of an endotracheal tube is important in ICU patients because changes in head position may occur. An endotracheal tube can move up to 2 cm toward the carina with neck flexion and another 2 cm away from the carina with full neck extension. In general, the tip of the tube should be placed about 3 cm above the main carina with the neck in the neutral position.

Endotracheal tubes have also been designed for special indications. These include preangled nasal and oral tubes designed to prevent kinking and interference with the surgical field. Another has a finger-activated cable that directs the tip of the tube anteriorly. Double-lumen endotracheal tubes can ventilate each lung independently and are occasionally used in the ICU to permit single-lung ventilation or simultaneous ventilation of each lung via separate ventilators, for example, after single-lung transplantation when the patient's old and new lungs have markedly different compliances.

Endotracheal stylets are pliable, firm wire-like devices that facilitate curvature of an endotracheal tube before insertion. Specialized stylets, such as the lightwand,

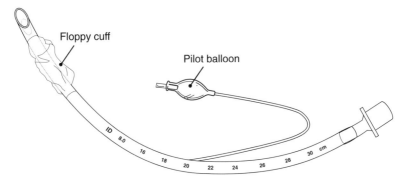

Figure 28–1. Typical polyvinyl chloride endotracheal tube with a high-volume, low-compliance ("floppy") cuff connected to a pilot balloon. Distance from the tip of the tube is marked in centimeters; these can guide the depth of initial tube placement (in the range of 22 to 24 cm for adults) and subsequently when the tube is moved and resecured in the mouth.

are also available to facilitate endotracheal intubation. No stylet, however, should extend beyond the endotracheal tube.

The *LMA* is a unique airway device with a fenestrated aperture surrounded by a cuff. It is inserted blindly into the pharynx and the cuff is inflated. The LMA forms a low-pressure seal around the laryngeal inlet to permit positive pressure ventilation. The insertion technique is simple and relatively easy to learn. The LMA has several advantages notable in the ICU environment. It can be inserted with little sedation. The LMA can function as an adjunct to blind or fiberoptic intubation because an endotracheal tube can be threaded over a fiberoptic bronchoscope or stylet, through the channel of LMA, and then through the vocal cords and into the trachea.

OBTAINING A SECURE AIRWAY

Endotracheal Intubation

Several indications warrant placement of an endotracheal airway in the ICU setting. In general, intubation is indicated to deliver positive pressure ventilation for the treatment of respiratory failure, to limit the likelihood of aspiration of gastric contents, or to perform diagnostic procedures safely, such as fiberoptic bronchoscopy. Noninvasive ventilation may be a reasonable alternative in some circumstances and should always be considered before intubating patients in respiratory distress.

Clinical signs such as symmetric breath sounds over the chest, absence of gastric insufflation, symmetric chest excursion, and respiratory gas moisture on the inner surface of the endotracheal tube are consistent with endotracheal intubation. The presence of CO_2 in exhaled gas generally confirms endotracheal intubation (although there may be a false-positive CO_2 detection from the first or even second breath from an esophageal intubation).

Nasotracheal intubation may be a suitable alternative to orotracheal intubation in the spontaneously breathing patient. Limited mouth opening resulting from arthritis or fractures of the maxilla or mandible is an indication for nasal intubation, whereas coagulopathies, nasal polyps, and known or suspected basilar skull fractures are contraindications.

Emergent Surgical Airway

Indications for *emergent surgical airway* include multiple failed attempts at endotracheal or nasotracheal intubation complicated by sudden or rapidly progressive upper airway compromise due to bleeding or edema, tumor, infection or trauma. Options include cricothyroidotomy, emergent tracheotomy, and needle cricothyroidotomy.

Cricothyroidotomy

Although cricothyroidotomy has largely been abandoned as an elective procedure because of the unacceptably high rate of subglottic stenosis, it is the emergency procedure of choice to secure the airway in an emergency situation. This is primarily because of the ease of determining anatomic landmarks while performing the procedure.

The thyroid cartilage is stabilized and an incision is made through skin and subcutaneous tissue overlying the cricothyroid membrane below the inferior aspect of the thyroid cartilage. The cricothyroid membrane is then opened with a stab incision, and an endotracheal or tracheostomy tube is inserted. Alternatively, one can use a Seldinger technique to dilate the cricothyroid membrane and place the cricothyrotomy tube. Commercial cricothyrotomy kits are available, containing all the appropriate components, including the adapter to permit hand ventilation.

Needle cricothyroidotomy is a temporary measure to ensure oxygenation. This involves insertion of a 14-gauge needle through the cricothyroid membrane. Since one cannot adequately ventilate an adult through this bore airway, even with positive pressure ventilation, it should be regarded only as a temporizing step until a cricothyrotomy kit can be obtained or an emergent tracheotomy performed.

Emergent Tracheotomy

Emergent tracheotomy is less desirable than cricothyrotomy because it is slower, requires additional steps, and has a greater potential for bleeding. It is performed by first making a vertical incision in the neck overlying the trachea and cricoid cartilage (the vertical incision minimizes bleeding). Next, skin and soft tissue are divided with a scalpel through the platysma and the midline raphe of the strap muscles. The thyroid isthmus, if encountered, is retracted inferiorly or clamped and divided, exposing the first few tracheal rings. A horizontal incision is made between the first and second tracheal rings, and the tube is introduced into the trachea.

Elective Tracheotomy

Tracheotomy is often used in securing the airway in ICU patients with prolonged dependency on mechanical ventilation. Indications include the need for prolonged ventilation, bypass of an obstructed upper airway, and pulmonary toilet especially if the patient is to be transferred out of the ICU. There are two acceptable tracheotomy techniques: traditional (surgical) tracheotomy (described in Chapter 24) and percutaneous tracheotomy.

Percutaneous Tracheotomy

Originally conceived of during World War II (but abandoned because of a high rate of complications), percutaneous tracheotomy was reintroduced in the mid-1980s as an alternative to traditional tracheotomy. Although the method varies somewhat among institutions, one approach to percutaneous tracheotomy includes the following steps:

1. It is performed at bedside under bronchoscopic guidance.

2. A guide wire is passed via needle through the skin of the anterior neck into the tracheal lumen.
3. Correct intratracheal location of the guide wire is confirmed by bronchoscopy.
4. A 2-cm horizontal incision is made in the skin at the site of guide wire insertion.
5. Sequential percutaneous dilators are used to form a track from skin to upper trachea.
6. The appropriate sized tracheostomy tube is inserted into the trachea.
7. Correct placement of the tracheal tube is confirmed bronchoscopically.

As with any "new" surgical procedure, percutaneous tracheotomy has its advocates and detractors. Several studies suggest that it is a reasonable alternative to conventional tracheotomy. They have similar (low) complication rates, while the percutaneous tracheotomy has a cost advantage (since no time in the operating room is needed). Random controlled trials comparing conventional and percutaneous techniques, however, have not established the superiority of one method over the other. Percutaneous tracheotomy is contraindicated for the patient with an obese neck, enlarged thyroid, coagulopathy, or cervical spine instability.

Tracheotomy Complications

Complications of both emergent and elective tracheotomy can occur early in the postoperative period and after some delay. Common early complications include hemorrhage, displacement of the tracheostomy tube, and pneumomediastinum or pneumothorax. Rare early complications include recurrent laryngeal nerve trauma and tracheoesophageal fistula. Delayed complications include tracheal stenosis, tracheocutaneous fistula, tracheoinnominate artery fistula, and tracheomalacia. Since a tracheoinnominate artery fistula is a catastrophic complication whose development may be heralded by slight tracheal bleeding, any bleeding from an established tracheotomy requires prompt and thorough diagnostic evaluation.

Tracheotomy Timing

The appropriate timing for placement of a tracheostomy tube is controversial. The development of compliant cuffs for endotracheal tubes and cuff pressure monitoring has decreased the frequency of tracheal injury from prolonged endotracheal intubation. Surgical tracheostomy is indicated for patients in whom lengthy periods of mechanical ventilation are anticipated or when the patient's ability to clear the airway of secretions is impaired. Tracheotomy tubes and parts are described in detail in Chapter 24.

Problems with Artificial Airways

The intensivist may encounter several common problems with endotracheal tubes (Fig. 28–2). Loss of tidal volume and minute ventilation can occur for several

Figure 28–2. Schematic representation of endotracheal tube inserted through the mouth into the trachea. Common problems with the tube arise at various points along its length, as designated by the numbers on the figure. *1,* Teeth (or gums) can occlude the tube (and tube can erode corner of mouth by pressure necrosis if not moved daily). *2,* Tongue can push the tube out. *3,* Tube can kink at posterior pharynx. *4,* Cuff can deflate because of a leak or, if overinflated, can damage tracheal mucosa. *5,* Tip of tube (and its side opening) can be occluded by secretions or blood, or tip can be located too distally, that is, in the right main bronchus. *6,* Pilot balloon or its one-way valve can cause leaks.

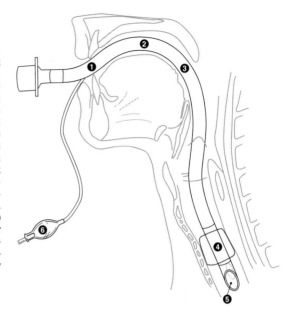

reasons. One is that the endotracheal tube is positioned incorrectly above the vocal cords. Another is that the cuff may be deflating due to air leaks that can occur anywhere from the pilot balloon's one-way valve to the cuff itself. In addition, high intratracheal pressures due to very high peak pressures can exceed the ability of the cuff to seal the trachea during inspiration.

Changing Endotracheal Tubes

The intensivist may need to change an endotracheal tube for one of several reasons, including a persistent cuff leak, the need for a larger endotracheal tube, partial obstruction of the endotracheal tube with blood or mucus, and the need to change from a nasotracheal to an oral tube because of sinusitis or nasal erosion. Common approaches include elective extubation and reintubation by using conventional laryngoscopy or using a *"tube changer"* as a stylet over which the tubes are exchanged (some tube changers can provide oxygen during the change via a lumen within the tube itself). A fiberoptic bronchoscope loaded with a new endotracheal tube can also be maneuvered alongside the existing endotracheal tube before tube exchange. Finally, if the endotracheal tube has a small enough diameter, an LMA can be inserted over an existing endotracheal tube. The original endotracheal tube is then withdrawn and a new one inserted while the LMA is left in place.

BIBLIOGRAPHY

Benumof JL: Management of the difficult adult airway. With special emphasis on awake tracheal intubation. Anesthesiology 75:1087–110, 1991.
   This is an extensive review of the difficult airway by the foremost expert in the field.

Berrouschot J, Oeken J, Steniger L, et al: Perioperative complications of percutaneous dilational tracheostomy. Laryngoscope 107:1538–1544, 1997.
This is a review article about the technique and its complications with and without bronchoscopic assistance.

Blosser SA, Stauffer JL: Intubation of critically ill patients. Clin Chest Med 17:355–378, 1996.
This is a review of modern techniques, devices, guidelines, intubation versus tracheostomy, and medicolegal issues surrounding airway management in the critically ill.

Cullen DJ, Bigatello LM, DeMonaco HJ: Anesthetic pharmacology and critical care. In: Chernow B (ed): The Pharmacologic Approach to the Critically Ill Patient, 3rd ed. Baltimore: Williams & Wilkins, 1994, pp 291–308.
This article provides a scholarly, comprehensive review of induction agents and neuromuscular blocking agents and their use in ICU patients.

Kovac AL: Controlling the hemodynamic response to laryngoscopy and endotracheal intubation. J Clin Anesth 8:63–79, 1996.
This is a review of the pharmacologic management of intubation.

Pennant JH, White PF: The laryngeal mask airway—its uses in anesthesiology. Anesthesiology 79:144–163, 1993.
This article reviews the use and application of the LMA.

Rose DK, Cohen MM: The airway: Problems and predictions in 18,500 patients. Can J Anaesth 41:372, 1994.
This article details a large study of risk factors and airway characteristics associated with difficult intubation.

Williamson JA, Webb RK, Szelky S, et al: Difficult intubation: An analysis of 2000 incident reports. Anesth Intensive Care 21:602, 1993.
This article provides an analysis of common problems associated with airway management.

Wilson DJ: Airway appliances and management. In: Kaczmarek RM, Stoller J, Decker BC (eds): Current Respiratory Care. St. Louis: CV Mosby, 1988, p 80.
Airway appliances are discussed and compared.

Wood DE: Tracheostomy. Chest Surg Clin North Am 6:749–764, 1996.
This is a surgical description of the complications associated with tracheostomy.

29   Allergies To Antibiotics

Liza C. O'Dowd
Paul Atkins

Adverse drug reactions are responsible for 2 to 5% of all hospitalizations in the United States. In addition, an estimated 30% of patients experience an adverse drug reaction during their hospital stay. Allergic reactions account for 5 to 10% of these adverse drug reactions, and one of every 25 to 50 of these reactions is severe and life-threatening. Immediate hypersensitivity allergic reactions are listed as type I reactions in the four traditional types of immunologic reactions, based on the Gell and Coombs classification system (Table 29–1). This chapter focuses on the evaluation and prevention of these potentially life-threatening reactions.

EVALUATION OF PATIENTS WITH A HISTORY OF ALLERGY TO PENICILLIN AND OTHER BETA-LACTAM ANTIBIOTICS

History of Allergic Reactions

Beta-lactam antibiotics are among the most frequent and clinically important causes of allergic reactions. Critical to the evaluation of an allergy is a carefully obtained history of previous drug reactions to this class of antibiotics. If the initial reaction was immediate, that is, occurring within 30 minutes of drug administration, the patient is considered to be at *high risk* for a potentially life-threatening immediate hypersensitivity reaction such as anaphylaxis. *Anaphylaxis* is an immediate, immunologically mediated, systemic reaction to antigen and is characterized by smooth muscle contraction and capillary dilatation due to release of mediators from mast cells and basophils. Hypotension, shock, and bronchospasm are its common manifestations.

Reactions occurring more than 2 hours after drug administration and that are limited primarily to the skin are much less likely to have been anaphylactic in nature. Patients with a history of isolated cutaneous symptoms are at *low risk* for an immediate hypersensitivity reaction.

The time interval since the previous adverse drug reaction is also significant: Reactions that happened within the last year are more likely to recur on challenge with the antibiotic than are reactions that took place more than 5 to 10 years in the past. Patients are at *intermediate risk* for a life-threatening allergic reaction if they have only a remote (>10 years prior) history of anaphylaxis.

Skin Testing

Skin testing is the most reliable method of determining if the patient with a prior allergic history to beta-lactam antibiotics is truly at risk for an immediate hypersensitivity reaction to penicillin or other beta-lactam antibiotics. This procedure is performed using reagents containing the major antigenic determinant as

333

Table 29–1. Classification of Allergic Reactions (Gell and Coombs)

TYPE	DESCRIPTION	MECHANISM	CLINICAL FEATURES
I Immediate reaction (30–60 min) Accelerated reaction (1–72 h)	Immediate hypersensitivity	IgE-mediated degranulation of mast cells and basophils	Anaphylaxis Angioedema Bronchospasm Urticaria (hives)
II	Antibody-mediated cytotoxicity	Antigen binds to cell; IgG or IgM combines with antigen and with complement to destroy cell	Hemolytic anemia Interstitial nephritis
III	Immune complex disease	Antigen and IgG or IgM form complexes that deposit in tissue, fix complement, and cause local inflammation and injury	Serum sickness
IV	Delayed hypersensitivity	Lymphocyte-mediated	Contact dermatitis
V (>72 h)	Idiopathic	Uncertain	Maculopapular rash Stevens-Johnson syndrome (exfoliative dermatitis)

IgE, immunoglobulin E; IgG, immunoglobulin G; IgM, immunoglobulin M.
Modified from Weiss ME, Adkinson NF: Immediate hypersensitivity reactions to penicillin and related antibiotics. Clin Allergy 18:515–540, 1988.

well as the minor antigenic determinants of penicillin. Patients with a positive skin test result have a wheal and flare reaction to the major or minor determinants greater than or equal to the reaction induced by concomitantly placed control reagents. The most severe anaphylactic reactions occur in patients who have positive skin test results to the *minor determinants.*

The prevalence of drug-specific immunoglobulin E (IgE), determined by performing skin tests in a population of patients *without* a history of previous allergic reaction to penicillin, is 4%. If subsequently given penicillin, these skin test–positive patients are at risk for the development of an immediate hypersensitivity reaction. Conversely, only 10 to 20% of patients with a history of a previous allergic reaction to penicillin have positive skin test results to the drug.

Predictive Value of Skin Testing

The *negative predictive value* of a negative skin test to both major and minor determinants, representing the percent of patients with negative skin test results who will tolerate beta-lactam therapy without an immediate allergic reaction, is 97%. In addition, those patients with negative skin tests who do react on challenge with penicillin tend to have mild reactions. It should be noted, however, that negative penicillin skin test results have no predictive value for the development of non-IgE–mediated reactions such as serum sickness, Stevens-Johnson syndrome, hemolytic anemia, maculopapular rashes, drug fever, or interstitial nephritis. Patients may also experience urticarial eruptions late in the course of therapy despite an initial negative skin test result.

The *positive predictive value* of the penicillin skin test, signifying the number of patients with positive skin tests who will experience anaphylactic reactions on receiving beta-lactam antibiotics, is estimated to be 40 to 73%. Thus, the likelihood ratio of a positive test result compared with a negative skin test result is 13 to 25; that is, if challenged, a patient with a positive skin test result is *13 to 25* times more likely to have an anaphylactic reaction than is a patient with a negative skin test result.

Indications for Skin Testing

Skin tests are indicated for any patient with a history of penicillin allergy who requires a beta-lactam drug to treat *a life-threatening condition* when *no other alternative antibiotic is appropriate*. Skin tests should be avoided in those patients at *high risk* for an anaphylactic reaction as determined by history as described previously. These patients should be desensitized to penicillin if the drug must be given. *Contraindications* to skin testing include the lack of a suitable site to perform the test (e.g., secondary to rash), the use of antihistamines and the tricyclic antidepressant doxepin in the 6 weeks before the test, and the lack of a positive reaction to skin test controls.

Skin test results to penicillin may remain negative up to 6 weeks after an allergic reaction to beta-lactam antibiotics. Skin testing should therefore be repeated after this interval if it is initially negative and the test is clinically indicated. A history of penicillin-induced exfoliative dermatitis, that is, Stevens-Johnson syndrome or toxic epidermal necrolysis (see Chapter 43), is *an absolute contraindication* to skin testing as well as the administration of beta-lactam antibiotics. The approach to a patient with a history of a beta-lactam allergy is summarized in Figure 29–1.

Although most investigators feel that penicillin skin tests are predictive of reactions to other semisynthetic penicillins, controversy does exist. It is recommended that patients who have a history of a recent and severe reaction to a semisynthetic penicillin (i.e., they are at high risk for an anaphylactic reaction) continue to avoid the specific antibiotic that caused the reaction, even if penicillin skin test results are negative.

The risk of having an adverse reaction to the skin test reagents is less than 1%, but systemic and fatal reactions occur. The risk of becoming sensitized to beta-lactam antibiotics as a result of penicillin skin testing is also less than 1%. However, after a course of penicillin therapy, 16% of patients with a history of beta-lactam allergy but initially negative skin test results have positive results on repeat testing. Thus, patients with a history of penicillin allergy should have a repeat skin test evaluation immediately before any subsequent courses of beta-lactam antibiotic therapy.

EVALUATION OF ALLERGIES TO CEPHALOSPORINS AND OTHER NON–BETA-LACTAM ANTIBIOTICS

Patients with positive skin test results to penicillin have a fourfold increased risk of an allergic reaction to cephalosporins, especially to first- and second-generation

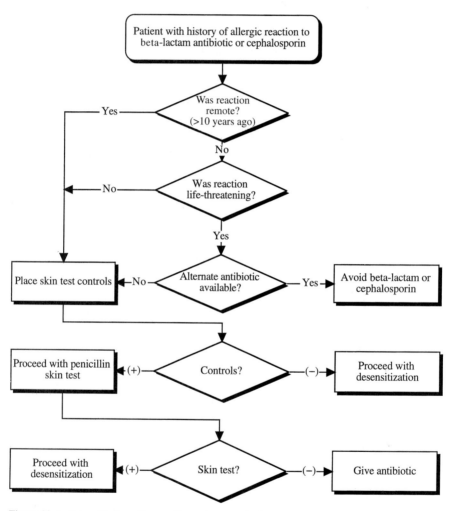

Figure 29–1. Schematic flow diagram illustrating steps in the evaluation of a patient with a history of allergy to penicillin, other beta-lactam antibiotics, or a cephalosporin.

agents, compared with those who are skin test negative. Because no reliable, validated cephalosporin skin test reagents are commercially available, if a patient has a history of a cephalosporin allergy but a negative penicillin skin test result, one should administer a penicillin, *not* a cephalosporin.

No clinically significant cross-reactivity among the monolactam, aztreonam, and penicillin has been demonstrated. Thus, patients with positive skin test to penicillin can be given this drug safely. However, aztreonam does cross-react with ceftazidine, so patients allergic to either antibiotic should avoid both. Imipenem, a carbapenem that cross-reacts with penicillin, should not be given to patients with positive penicillin skin test results unless they undergo desensitization.

Reliable skin tests to other classes of antibiotics, such as vancomycin or sulfonamide-type drugs, are not commercially available. A detailed history is critically important for appropriate evaluation of allergic reactions to these medications. The specific drug in question should be avoided unless life-threatening infections demand its use. Desensitization would then be necessary.

MANAGEMENT OF PATIENTS WITH POSITIVE SKIN TEST RESULTS TO PENICILLIN

If a patient with a positive penicillin skin test result requires therapy with a beta-lactam or cephalosporin to treat a life-threatening infection because no other effective alternative antibiotic is available, desensitization can be attempted. Patients who cannot undergo skin testing or who do not react appropriately to controls should also be desensitized if beta-lactams are required. Desensitization with other antibiotics, such as vancomycin and trimethoprim-sulfamethoxazole, has also been performed successfully in patients who were at high risk for an anaphylactic reaction to these drugs. As previously indicated, *an absolute contraindication to desensitization* is a history of exfoliative dermatitis to the chosen antibiotic.

Successful desensitization induces immunologic tolerance and significantly reduces the risk of anaphylaxis to the drug, but has no effect on the incidence of other non-IgE–mediated reactions. This tolerance to the specific antibiotic persists only while the patient continues to receive it. Once therapy ceases for a period greater than 24 hours, the patient is again at risk for an immediate, IgE-mediated reaction and therefore would require desensitization again.

Desensitization can be performed both orally and parenterally. However, because the oral route is often difficult or impossible to use in the patient in the intensive care unit (ICU), intravenous desensitization is the preferred method of desensitization. Approximately 30% of patients have an allergic reaction during desensitization or during the treatment course that follows. Although most are mild, serious reactions have been reported. Late immunologic reactions such as serum sickness may also occur.

A variety of different methods of desensitizing patients parenterally have been reported in the literature. Protocols for desensitization (Table 29–2) and managing adverse reactions during this procedure (Table 29–3) are adapted from these methods.

Table 29–2. Desensitization Protocol

....

Before Beginning Desensitization

1. Transfer the patient to an ICU or intermediate care unit so that a physician is immediately available at all times and can evaluate the patient for any reaction (wheeze, hives, change in vital signs) before each sequential dose of antibiotic is administered.
2. Monitor and record vital signs every 15 minutes. Monitor peak flows between doses in patients with bronchospastic pulmonary disease.
3. Provide adequate intravenous (IV) access (preferably 2 IV lines 16-gauge or larger). Optimize the patient's hemodynamic status and avoid use of beta-blockers.
4. Ensure that epinephrine, IV diphenhydramine and methylprednisolone are at the bedside. Equipment and drugs for tracheal intubation should be readily accessible.
5. Obtain informed consent from the patient or appropriate surrogate decision maker.
6. Do *not* premedicate the patient with antihistamines or steroids.

Preparation of Dilutions

After the specific antibiotic and dose (e.g., ceftriaxone 1g) is decided on and the desired final dose is calculated, serial 10-fold dilutions of that dose in 50 mL of normal saline should be made:

Dilution 1: 1×10^{-6} concentration of the final dose in 50 mL normal saline
Dilution 2: 1×10^{-5} concentration of the final dose in 50 mL normal saline
Dilution 3: 1×10^{-4} concentration of the final dose in 50 mL normal saline
Dilution 4: 1×10^{-3} concentration of the final dose in 50 mL normal saline
Dilution 5: 1×10^{-2} concentration of the final dose in 50 mL normal saline
Dilution 6: 1×10^{-1} concentration of the final dose in 50 mL normal saline
Dilution 7: Full strength final dose in 50 mL normal saline

Administration of Dilutions

1. 50 mL of each dilution, starting with dilution 1, should be administered intravenously over 20 minutes.
2. After completion of the dose, the patient should be observed for 15 minutes and be evaluated by a physician.
3. If no reaction has occurred, the next dose can be given in the same manner.
4. If a reaction occurred, follow recommendations in Table 29–3.

....

Adapted from Weiss ME, Adkinson NF: Immediate hypersensitivity reactions to penicillin and related antibiotics. Clin Allergy 18:515–540, 1988.

Table 29–3. Management of Adverse Reactions During Desensitization

REACTION SEVERITY	SYMPTOMS AND SIGNS	MANAGEMENT
Mild	Mild urticaria *without* hemodynamic instability, respiratory distress, or angioedema	The last dilution tolerated *without* difficulty should be repeated and the protocol continued if no further reaction occurs.
Moderate	Chest tightness, diffuse hives, but no hemodynamic or airway compromise	Administer 0.3 mL 1:1000 epinephrine (0.3 mg) subcutaneously. If the patient's symptoms resolve within 30 min, the last dilution tolerated *without* a reaction should then be repeated and the protocol continued if no further reaction occurs.
Moderate to severe	Diffuse wheezes, throat tightness	Administer epinephrine as described above. Epinephrine can be repeated every 15 min if required. If the reaction is severe, 0.5–1.0 mg of 1:10,000 epinephrine can be given IV every 5 min. If the symptoms subside quickly and if the antibiotic is considered to be *absolutely necessary* to adequately treat the patient, *one-half* the dose of the last tolerated dilution should be given with a physician at the bedside.* Desensitization can then be continued if this dose is tolerated without reaction.
Severe	Hypotension, laryngeal edema with or without urticaria	Treat with epinephrine as above, and give IV: 50 mg diphenhydramine, a histamine H_2 receptor blocker, and corticosteroids (60 mg of methylprednisolone). The desensitization protocol must be discontinued.

*For example, if dilution 4 (1×10^{-3} concentration of the final dose) in Table 29–2 was the last tolerated dose, administer 0.5×10^{-4} concentration of the final dose in 50 mL normal saline.

Adapted from Sheffer AL, Pennoyer DS: Management of adverse drug reactions. J Allergy Clin Immunol 74:580–588, 1984.

CONCLUSION

The approach presented allows the ICU physician to evaluate and manage patients with histories of beta-lactam allergy. A carefully obtained history combined with appropriate skin testing can identify patients at risk for an anaphylactic reaction to beta-lactam therapy. When properly performed, desensitization may allow the administration of antibiotics to patients at risk for life-threatening allergic reactions.

BIBLIOGRAPHY

Absar N, Daneshvar H, Beall G: Desensitization to trimethoprim/sulfamethoxazole in HIV-infected patients. J Allergy Clin Immunol 94:1001–1005, 1994.
This study evaluated the efficacy and safety of oral desensitization to trimethoprim-sulfamethoxazole.

Anderson JA: Allergic reactions to drugs and biological agents. JAMA 68:2845–2857, 1992.
This article presents a general overview of allergic drug reactions, with attention to selected drugs.

Borish L, Tamit R, Rosenwasser LJ: Intravenous desensitization to beta-lactam antibiotics. J Allergy Clin Immunol 80:314–319, 1987.
This study evaluated the efficacy of intravenous desensitization to beta-lactam antibiotics.

Deswarte RD: Drug allergy—Problems and strategies. J Allergy Clin Immunol 74:209–221, 1984.
This article presents a general overview of allergic drug reactions.

Green GR, Rosenblum AH, Sweet LC: Evaluation of penicillin hypersensitivity: Value of clinical history and skin testing with penicilloyl-polylysine and penicillin G. J Allergy Clin Immunol 60:339–345, 1977.
This was a landmark study evaluating the utility of penicillin skin tests.

Lin RY: A perspective on penicillin allergy. Arch Intern Med 152:930–937, 1992.
This article presents an excellent review of penicillin allergy.

Sheffer AL, Pennoyer DS: Management of adverse drug reactions. J Allergy Clin Immunol 74:580–588, 1984.
This is a review of the management of allergic as well as other types of adverse drug reactions.

Shepherd GM: Allergy to β-lactam antibiotics. Immunol Allergy Clin North Am 11:611–633, 1991.
This article presents a review of beta-lactam allergy, with an excellent synopsis of the evaluation of nonpenicillin beta-lactam allergy.

Sullivan TJ, Yecies LD, Shatz GS, et al: Desensitization of patients allergic to penicillin using orally administered β-lactam antibiotics. J Allergy Clin Immunol 69:275–282, 1982.
This was one of the original studies evaluating the efficacy of oral desensitization to penicillin.

Weiss ME, Adkinson NF: Immediate hypersensitivity reactions to penicillin and related antibiotics. Clin Allergy 18:515–540, 1988.
This article presents a detailed review of penicillin allergy, its diagnosis, and management.

Winbery SL, Lieberman PL: Anaphylaxis. J Allergy Clin Immunol 15:447–475, 1995.
This is a review of definitions, incidences, and risk factors.

Wong JT, Ripple RE, MacLean JA, et al: Vancomycin hypersensitivity: Synergism with narcotics and "desensitization" by a rapid continuous intravenous protocol. J Allergy Clin Immunol 94:189–194, 1994.
This study evaluated the efficacy and safety of desensitization to vancomycin.

30 Arrhythmias (Bradycardias)

Brian H. Sarter
David J. Callans

Bradyarrhythmias occur commonly in patients treated in the intensive care unit (ICU). The majority are transient and asymptomatic and do not require acute or chronic intervention. When bradyarrhythmias occur in patients without intrinsic heart disease, they are usually associated with a high vagal state or the use of cardioactive drugs. Because these arrhythmias usually resolve spontaneously or after the removal of the offending agent, cardiac pacing is rarely required. Bradyarrhythmias in patients with pre-existing heart disease, however, are more ominous and should prompt additional considerations, as discussed later. This chapter presents a concise but comprehensive approach to ICU patients in whom bradyarrhythmias develop (bradyarrhythmias in acute myocardial infarctions are discussed in Chapter 49).

CLASSIFICATION OF BRADYARRHYTHMIAS

Sinus Node Dysfunction

Bradyarrhythmias may result from dysfunction of the sinus node or disturbances of atrioventricular (AV) conduction. The spectrum of sinus node dysfunction encompasses sinus pauses, sinus arrest, sinus bradycardia, sinus node exit block and the tachycardia-bradycardia syndrome (sick sinus syndrome). All these result in bradycardia (ventricular rate <50 beats per minute) or pauses caused by the lack of impulse formation or propagation from the sinus node. Occasionally, not only does the sinus node fail, but "back-up" subsidiary pacemakers (atrial and junctional) may also fail, and appropriate heart rate is not maintained.

Causes of sinus node dysfunction in ICU patients are listed in Table 30–1. It is important to recognize that sinus bradycardia is commonly seen in young athletic patients, during sleep, and during conditions associated with high vagal tone (pain, nausea, vomiting, endotracheal manipulation, bowel movements). These episodes are almost uniformly transient and asymptomatic. Treatment should be considered only if the bradycardia persists, is symptomatic, or results in hemodynamic compromise.

In patients with *pre-existing heart disease*, sinus node dysfunction may present with significant hemodynamically compromising bradyarrhythmias, particularly in the ICU setting. Ischemia, electrolyte abnormalities, drugs, hypoxia, and metabolic and endocrinologic derangements may all precipitate significant bradycardia in patients with chronic, previously stable sinus node disease. Patients with severe left ventricular systolic dysfunction are at high risk of significant sinus bradyarrhythmias, particularly in the setting of worsening heart failure. Furthermore, because inappropriately slow sinus rates may be causally related to heart failure symptoms, permanent pacing has a role in the management of these patients.

Intrinsic sinus node dysfunction can occur in the elderly patient without evi-

Table 30–1. Common Causes of Bradyarrhythmias in Intensive Care Unit

Extrinsic causes
  Carotid sinus hypersensitivity
  Drugs
    Antiarrhythmic agents (procainamide, propafenone, amiodarone)
    Beta-adrenergic blockers
    Calcium channel blockers
    Digoxin
    Morphine
    Tricyclic antidepressants
  Elevated intracranial pressure
  Electrolyte abnormalities (hyperkalemia, hypokalemia, hypocalcemia, hypermagnesemia)
  High vagal tone (mechanical ventilation, myocardial ischemia-infarction, nausea, vomiting, pain, sleep, vasovagal reflex)
  Hypothermia
  Hypothyroidism
  Hypoxia
  Obstructive sleep apnea
Intrinsic causes
  Collagen vascular disease (systemic lupus erythematosus, rheumatoid arthritis, scleroderma)
  Conduction system disease
  Congenital heart disease (e.g., atrial septal defect)
  Hypertensive heart disease
  Infections (endocarditis, Lyme disease, viral myocarditis, diphtheria)
  Infiltrative cardiomyopathy
  Intrinsic sinus node disease
  Myocardial ischemia or infarction
  Sarcoidosis
  Valvular heart disease (aortic stenosis, aortic insufficiency, mitral annular calcification)

dence of other significant cardiac abnormalities. More often, these patients present with the tachycardia-bradycardia syndrome in which symptoms may be related to the tachy- or bradyarrhythmia. Tachycardia-bradycardia syndrome is characterized by periods of atrial tachyarrhythmias (atrial flutter, atrial tachycardia, or atrial fibrillation [see Chapter 31]) interspersed with periods of sinus bradycardia, sinus pauses, or sinus arrest associated with a junctional escape rhythm. This syndrome is typically seen in older patients with some evidence of atrial disease or long-standing hypertension, or both. The most common manifestations of this disease are paroxysmal atrial fibrillation and sinus bradycardia. Frequently, there is a prolonged pause (>3 seconds) after spontaneous termination of the atrial fibrillation ("offset pause"), which may result in syncope. Since symptoms can be due to both the tachycardia and the bradycardia, combination therapy including medication and permanent pacing may be required in these patients.

Atrioventricular Conduction Disturbances

Disturbances of propagation of electrical impulses from the atria to the ventricles are classified as first-, second-, and third-degree AV block. This classification is based on the electrocardiographic pattern of the conduction disturbance and not the underlying anatomic substrate. Block occurring in the AV node generally signifies a more benign prognosis than does block due to disease of the infranodal structures (e.g., His-Purkinje disease); therefore, it is important to use information from the electrocardiogram (ECG) to identify the anatomic site of the conduction disturbance. Although intrinsic cardiac disease can lead to AV conduction disturbances, reversible extrinsic causes should be investigated and eliminated before chronic intervention is considered (see Table 30–1). Regardless of the cause or site of conduction block, acute intervention (pharmacologic or pacing) should be reserved for those patients who are acutely symptomatic or hemodynamically compromised. The anatomic site of block is important in defining which patients should receive a permanent pacemaker.

First-Degree Atrioventricular Block

First-degree AV block, defined as a PR interval greater than 0.20 seconds, rarely results in symptoms or significant hemodynamic compromise. It is most often due to delay of the electrical impulse as it traverses the AV node, although disease of the His-Purkinje system can occasionally prolong the PR interval. Since every impulse originating in the sinus node propagates to the ventricle, first-degree AV *delay* is a more accurate description of this phenomenon.

Second-Degree Atrioventricular Block

Second-degree AV block is divided into Mobitz I block (Wenckebach) and Mobitz II block. *Wenckebach block* is characterized as progressive prolongation of the PR interval until a P wave fails to propagate to the ventricle (Fig. 30–1). Since the increment of PR prolongation decreases with each consecutive beat, the RR intervals progressively shorten during Wenckebach. The presence of Wenckebach block generally indicates that the site of block is in the AV node, and this portends a more benign prognosis. Wenckebach block can rarely occur in the infranodal structures, but intracardiac recordings are required for this diagnosis. Permanent pacemaker implantation is indicated only in the rare patient in whom Wenckebach block has clearly been demonstrated to cause symptoms.

Mobitz II block is defined as the sudden failure of conduction of an impulse from the atria to the ventricles and manifests on the ECG as unexpected block of a P wave without preceding prolongation of the PR interval. Mobitz II block

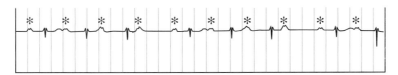

Figure 30–1. Atrioventricular Wenckebach (second-degree atrioventricular [AV] block, Mobitz I) with 4:3 AV conduction. P waves marked with *. Note progressive prolongation in PR interval before blocked P wave. This pattern localizes the site of block to the AV node and implies no risk of progression to complete heart block.

signifies infranodal disease and often is associated with other electrocardiographic signs of conduction system disease (i.e., bundle branch block, intraventricular block). Although a permanent pacemaker is not absolutely indicated for patients with asymptomatic Mobitz II block, most clinicians elect to implant pacemakers in all patients with Mobitz II block (in whom reversible causes have been ruled out) given the relative high risk (40 to 80%) of progression to higher grade AV block.

Patients with 2:1 AV block cannot be classified as either Mobitz I or II block because there is no opportunity for the PR interval to become prolonged (Fig. 30–2). The site of block in these patients may be AV nodal or infranodal. Clues on the ECG that suggest an infranodal site include block that occurs at faster heart rates, a wide QRS (>120 msec) on the conducted beats, and a normal PR interval on the conducted beats. An infranodal site of block is also suggested by worsening degrees of heart block as the sinus rate increases. These findings should prompt consideration of placement of a temporary pacemaker in the acutely symptomatic patient and permanent pacemaker in those without a definite reversible cause.

Third-Degree Heart Block

Third-degree heart block, or complete heart block, defined as the complete absence of impulse propagation between the atria and ventricles, may be intermittent or persistent. The electrocardiographic manifestation of complete heart block includes AV dissociation, a regular junctional or ventricular escape rhythm, and an atrial rate that is faster than the ventricular rate. All three of these criteria need to be present in order to diagnose complete heart block. In the absence of reversible

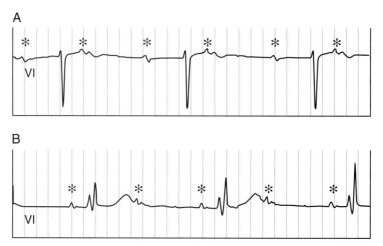

Figure 30–2. 2:1 Atrioventricular block. P waves marked with * *A,* Block at the level of the AV node. Note narrow QRS and long PR interval on conducted beats. Block in the AV node is usually mediated by autonomic tone and does not imply a risk of progressive block. *B,* Block at the infranodal level (His-Purkinje). Note wide QRS (right bundle branch block) signifying significant distal conduction system disease, and normal PR interval on conducted beats. Patients with infranodal 2:1 block have a significant risk for the development of higher degree AV block.

causes, complete heart block indicates severe conduction disease and, with rare exception, implantation of a permanent pacemaker should be performed.

Electrophysiologic evaluation with intracardiac recordings from the His bundle should be performed in patients in whom the site of conduction block is ambiguous. Specific measurements during this evaluation (e.g., HV interval, response to rapid atrial pacing) may provide additional information that is helpful in identifying patients who require permanent pacing.

BRADYARRHYTHMIAS UNDER SPECIAL CIRCUMSTANCES

After Cardiac Surgery

Patients are at high risk for the development of both tachyarrhythmias and bradyarrhythmias during the early postoperative period after cardiac surgery. Transient postoperative conduction disturbances have been reported in up to half of patients undergoing cardiac surgery with most of these being isolated right bundle branch block. Because of the high occurrence of these conduction disturbances, temporary epicardial pacing wires are routinely placed in all these patients during the surgery. These wires are typically removed 3 to 7 days after surgery, provided that the patient is stable.

The development of postoperative conduction disturbances appears to be related to multiple preoperative and intraoperative factors. *Clinical characteristics* associated with their development include advanced age, hypertension, specific coronary anatomy, left ventricular function, use of digoxin, and the presence of pre-existing conduction abnormalities. *Intraoperative factors* include the number of bypass grafts, duration of aortic cross-clamp time, concomitant valve surgery, and the type of cardioplegia used. Specifically, the use of cold cardioplegia intraoperatively has been shown to have a dramatic impact on the development of postoperative conduction disturbances. A significantly higher incidence of conduction abnormalities at hospital discharge has been found in patients who had received cold compared with warm cardioplegia (19.6% versus 1.7%, respectively). Furthermore, these defects persisted in 17.4% and 1.7% of patients, respectively, at late follow-up. Complete AV block developed in 3.8% of the patients who had received cold cardioplegia and in none of the patients who received warm cardioplegia.

Fortunately, the majority of postoperative conduction disturbances resolve spontaneously, and permanent pacemaker insertion is rarely required. In a large cohort of 1645 patients who underwent coronary artery bypass grafting (CABG), only 13 patients (0.8%) required permanent pacemaker implantation for persistent complete AV block (8 patients) or symptomatic sinus node dysfunction (5 patients). These pacemakers were implanted at a mean of 10.5 ± 6.5 days after surgery.

It is unclear whether the development of fascicular conduction disturbances postoperatively (bundle branch block, fascicular block, or intraventricular block) is associated with decreased long-term survival. Early reports demonstrated a significantly higher mortality in patients who developed left bundle branch block (LBBB), left anterior fascicular block (LAFB), or intraventricular block after CABG compared with patients in whom these abnormalities did not develop. Subsequently larger studies failed to confirm these findings. Although development of high-grade AV block postoperatively does appear to be associated with a higher mortality, these patients also have a higher incidence of perioperative myocardial infarction and low cardiac output states. Therefore, it may be that high-grade AV block is merely a marker of severe cardiac dysfunction.

Patients in whom symptomatic bradyarrhythmias develop in the early postoperative period should be supported acutely with pacing via the temporary epicardial wires placed during the operative procedure. Placement of temporary pacing wires should be considered in patients who are truly pacemaker-dependent. Discontinuation of agents that depress the cardiac chronotropic response (digoxin, beta-blockers, calcium channel blockers, and the antiarrhythmic drugs listed in Table 30–1) should be considered. Determination of the pacing threshold should be performed daily. Since most of the conduction disturbances are transient, daily assessment of the patient's native rhythm should be performed as well. Generally, 5 to 7 days should be allowed for recovery of function before a permanent pacemaker is considered.

ENDOCARDITIS

Bacterial endocarditis is frequently seen in the ICU setting. The development of conduction disturbances in a patient with endocarditis is an ominous sign and suggests deep invasion of the infection into the perivalvular tissue. Conduction disturbances occur in approximately 10% of patients with endocarditis, of whom 80 to 90% have perivalvular abscesses. Disturbances in AV conduction most often complicate infection of the aortic valve and carry a significantly higher mortality. The development of a new conduction disturbance in a patient with documented or suspected endocarditis should prompt immediate evaluation with a transthoracic or transesophageal echocardiogram, or both. Urgent surgical consultation is indicated, and valve replacement should be strongly considered. Surgery should not be delayed, even in patients with "active" infection, as most studies have demonstrated better survival and a low reinfection rate with earlier surgical intervention.

OBSTRUCTIVE SLEEP APNEA

Nocturnal arrhythmias are seen in up to 50% of patients with obstructive sleep apnea (see Chapter 77). These arrhythmias are often discovered serendipitously in the ICU during routine cardiac monitoring of these patients and frequently prompt cardiac evaluation. The spectrum of arrhythmias associated with obstructive sleep apnea includes isolated premature venticular contractions, nonsustained ventricular tachycardia, sinus bradycardia, sinus pauses, and second-degree AV block (Mobitz I and II). With rare exception, they are seen only during episodes of hypoxemia while the patient is asleep. The mechanism of these arrhythmias is unknown, but autonomic nervous system imbalance and arterial oxygen desaturation are thought to be important factors. Prolonged sinus pauses (>10 seconds) and severe sinus bradycardia (<30 beats/minute for >10 seconds) can be seen in these patients, and this frequently leads to consideration of permanent pacemaker implantation. Unless there is evidence of significant cardiac disease or documented symptomatic bradycardia while the patient is awake, permanent pacing is rarely indicated because these arrhythmias almost universally resolve with appropriate treatment of the sleep apnea.

DIGOXIN TOXICITY

Digoxin toxicity can present with both cardiac and extracardiac signs and symptoms. Cardiac manifestations of toxicity result both from decreased conduction and increased automaticity (Table 30–2). Generally, patients *without* structural heart disease present with arrhythmias due to depressed impulse conduction, whereas patients *with* pre-existing heart disease exhibit arrhythmias because of abnormalities of both impulse conduction and generation. Unfortunately most of these arrhythmias are not specific for digoxin toxicity and therefore the development of one of these arrhythmias in a patient taking digoxin is suggestive but not diagnostic of toxicity.

Atrioventricular conduction block, of various degrees, is the most common manifestation of toxicity, occurring in 30 to 40% of patients. Although digoxin can increase the frequency of ventricular ectopy, it only rarely causes a wide complex, regular monomorphic ventricular tachycardia. The development of this arrhythmia should prompt consideration of other causes, most commonly chronic coronary artery disease. Specific arrhythmias that are uncommon but specific for digoxin toxicity include atrial tachycardia with variable AV block, accelerated junctional rhythm resulting in the apparent "regularization" of atrial fibrillation (Fig. 30–3), and fascicular tachycardia. The development of any of these arrhythmias should heighten the suspicion of toxicity from digoxin, regardless of the serum digoxin level.

The extracardiac manifestations of digoxin are nonspecific but invariably present to some extent in all patients with toxicity. Nausea, vomiting, and anorexia, the most common symptoms, are seen in almost half of patients presenting with toxicity. Other symptoms include dizziness, fatigue, abdominal pain, and headache. Visual disturbances characterized by halos around bright objects and changes in color perception have been classically described with digoxin toxicity but actually occur in less than 10% of patients.

The incidence of digoxin toxicity has dramatically decreased since the availabil-

Table 30–2. Arrhythmias Associated with Digoxin Toxicity

....

Nonspecific arrhythmias
  Sinus bradycardia
  Sinus exit block
  AV conduction disturbances
  Ventricular ectopy
  Ventricular fibrillation
Specific arrhythmias (see Chapter 31)
  Atrial tachycardia with variable AV block
  Accelerated junctional rhythm (regularization of atrial fibrillation)
  Fascicular tachycardia

....

AV, atrioventricular.

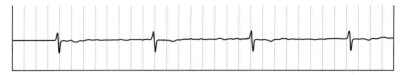

Figure 30–3. Digoxin toxicity. Baseline rhythm is atrial fibrillation (undulating baseline consistent with fibrillatory activity) with complete heart block and junctional escape rhythm at 30 beats per minute. The ventricular response during atrial fibrillation is always irregular. The sudden "regularization" of the ventricular response during atrial fibrillation is highly suggestive of digoxin toxicity, particularly if the heart rate is slow, as in this case.

ity of digoxin bioassays. Studies conducted in the 1960s and 1970s estimated that approximately 20% of patients receiving maintenance digoxin therapy acquired signs or symptoms of toxicity at some point in their clinical course. A more recent prospective trial of 563 patients admitted to the hospital with heart failure who were taking digoxin found definitive evidence of toxicity in only 4 patients (0.8%). Despite the dose-related therapeutic and toxic effects of digoxin, the correlation between specific digoxin serum levels and clinical toxicity is poor and varies considerably from patient to patient. Risk factors for the development of toxicity include advanced age, depressed renal function, acid-base abnormalities, hypo- and hyperkalemia, hypomagnesemia, hypercalcemia, and concurrent use of other drugs that affect the pharmacokinetics of digoxin, such as quinidine, verapamil, and amiodarone (see Chapter 12).

The first step in successful treatment of digoxin toxicity is its early recognition. Once toxicity is suspected, a careful history regarding dosage and frequency of digoxin use should be obtained. Laboratory tests, including blood urea nitrogen and creatinine concentrations, digoxin serum level, and electrolyte levels should be included in the initial evaluation. Cardiac monitoring should be performed in all patients with suspected toxicity. Both hypokalemia and hypomagnesemia should be corrected, with close monitoring to avoid excessive supplementation. Because of the extensive tissue distribution of digoxin, hemodialysis or hemoperfusion is generally ineffective for treatment of advanced toxicity. These modalities should be reserved for the patient with advanced renal dysfunction in whom acute digoxin intoxication may result in hyperkalemia.

Specific antiarrhythmic therapy should be considered in patients with hemodynamically compromising arrhythmias. Atropine is transiently effective in digoxin-induced bradyarrhythmias and can be used as a temporizing measure until more definitive therapy can be instituted. A temporary pacing wire should be used in patients with compromising bradyarrhythmias. Lidocaine and phenytoin have demonstrated efficacy in the treatment of digoxin-induced tachyarrhythmias. Both of these drugs have little effect on either sinus nodal or AV nodal tissue at therapeutic concentrations and therefore are least likely to potentiate any conduction disturbances associated with toxicity.

Clearly, the preferred therapy for significant digoxin toxicity is digoxin-specific antibodies (Fab antibody fragments). The Fab antibody fragments bind to digoxin and the antibody fragment–digoxin complex is rapidly cleared. The use of digoxin-specific Fab antibodies is associated with a partial or complete response in 74 to 90% of patients with digoxin toxicity. The response to therapy is rapid (mean time to initial response = 19 minutes) and associated with few significant side effects

(0 to 8%). Frequent monitoring of serum electrolytes, particularly potassium, is required, as administration of these antibody fragments frequently leads to significant hypokalemia. Widespread use of this therapy has been limited by its relative high cost; however, given its efficacy and short onset of action, Fab antibody fragments may prove to be the most cost-effective management of patients with serious digoxin toxicity.

Digoxin-specific antibodies should be used in patients with clear evidence of toxicity and hemodynamically compromising arrhythmias. Older patients, patients with renal dysfunction, and patients with a large acute ingestion of digoxin, presenting with tolerated arrhythmias, should also receive digoxin-specific antibodies because they are at risk for progression to more serious arrhythmias. Additionally, ingestion of large quantities of digoxin (>3 mg) associated with marked elevation in serum digoxin levels ($\geq$5 ng/mL) warrants treatment with digoxin-specific antibodies before arrhythmias develop.

ELECTROLYTE DISTURBANCES

Electrolyte abnormalities are an infrequent cause of bradyarrhythmias and, when present, are predominantly related to potassium imbalances. Hyperkalemia raises the resting membrane potential in cardiac cells, which results in inactivation of ion channels responsible for impulse conduction. Sinus exit block, atrial quiescence, and high-degree AV block can result from significant elevation of the serum potassium concentration. Severe hyperkalemia can lead to a slow, wide complex rhythm. This terminates in cardiac arrest when potassium depolarizes ventricular tissue to a level at which the fibers are nonexcitable (Fig. 30–4).

Hypokalemia promotes the appearance of atrial and ventricular premature depolarizations and atrioventricular conduction disturbances. Hypocalcemia, by itself, does not result in significant arrhythmias but may exacerbate the conduction disturbances of hyperkalemia. Cardiac conduction is depressed in severe hypermagnesemia, but respiratory depression occurs at lower serum levels and therefore usually dominates the clinical picture.

HEART BLOCK INDUCED DURING PULMONARY ARTERY CATHETERIZATION

Right bundle branch block (RBBB) occurs in up to 6% of patients who undergo pulmonary artery catheterization using a balloon-tipped, flow-directed catheter (Swan-Ganz catheter). The RBBB is caused by local trauma to the right bundle as the catheter is advanced from the right atrium through the right ventricular outflow tract into the pulmonary artery. Almost all cases of catheter-induced RBBB in

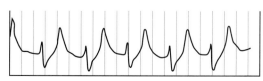

Figure 30–4. Hyperkalemia. Note characteristic loss of atrial activity (absent P waves), peaked T wave, loss of ST segment, and QRS widening.

patients without pre-existing LBBB are asymptomatic and transient. The development of RBBB in patients with pre-existing LBBB is problematic, and several case reports have described complete heart block occurring because of pulmonary artery catheterization in these patients. This led to the recommendation by some authors that a prophylactic temporary pacing catheter should be placed in all patients with LBBB before insertion of a pulmonary artery catheter. Two large studies have demonstrated that the risk of complete heart block in patients with pre-existing LBBB undergoing pulmonary artery catheterization is actually low. Shah and colleagues noted complete heart block in only 1 of 113 patients (0.8%) with chronic LBBB who had undergone pulmonary artery catheterization before surgery. Morris and associates demonstrated that complete heart block complicating pulmonary artery catheterization was seen in only 2 of 47 patients with pre-existing LBBB undergoing 82 catheter insertions (2.4%). Both of these patients had developed LBBB in the setting of an acute myocardial infarction complicated by congestive heart failure, hypotension, or cardiogenic shock, or a combination of these conditions. Complete heart block did not occur during insertion of the pulmonary catheter in either of these patients but after the catheter had been in place for at least 1 day.

Based on this information and the inherent risks associated with pacing catheter insertion, prophylactic temporary pacing with a percutaneous pacing wire does not appear to be justified in patients with chronic LBBB undergoing pulmonary artery catheterization. Transcutaneous pacing with a Zoll pacemaker (see later) can be performed noninvasively and should be available for the rare patient who does acquire high-grade AV block. Patients in whom new LBBB develops during an acute myocardial infarction are at higher risk for progression to high-grade AV block, and therefore placement of a temporary pacing catheter in these patients before pulmonary artery catheterization is indicated (see Chapter 49).

THERAPY

Acute Management

Bradycardia causing significant symptoms (altered consciousness, syncope, dizziness, light-headedness) or significant hemodynamic compromise requires acute therapy, regardless of the cause. Early cardiologic consultation can be helpful for acute and chronic management decisions in the acutely symptomatic patient, the patient in whom reversible causes cannot be identified, and the patient with pre-existing heart disease.

The approach to the patient with acutely symptomatic bradycardia should follow the standard advanced cardiac life support (ACLS) guidelines (Fig. 30–5). Atropine (up to 3 mg) may be efficacious in treating any bradyarrhythmia that is associated with inappropriately high vagal tone. Particular care should be taken in patients with infranodal block, as atropine may paradoxically worsen the block as the sinus rate increases (e.g., 2:1 block may become 3:1 or 4:1). Transcutaneous pacing (e.g., with a Zoll pacemaker) can be effective in the acute management of the patient with bradycardia. Transcutaneous pacing is performed through two large surface electrode pads that are placed over the cardiac apex on the anterior chest wall and over the right posterior scapula. The output of the Zoll pacemaker is

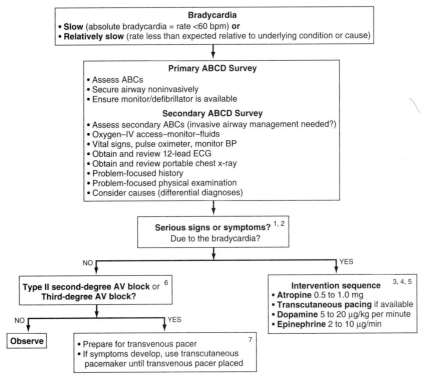

Figure 30–5. Algorithm for the management of acute bradycardia. **(1)** If the patient has *serious signs or symptoms,* make sure they are related to the slow rate. **(2)** Clinical manifestations include: *symptoms*—chest pain, shortness of breath, decreased level of consciousness; *signs*—low blood pressure, shock, pulmonary congestion, congestive heart failure. **(3) If the patient is symptomatic, do not delay transcutaneous pacing while waiting for IV access or for *atropine* to take effect. (4)** *Denervated transplanted hearts* will not respond to *atropine.* Go at once to pacing, *catecholamine* infusion, or both. **(5)** *Atropine* should be given in repeat doses every 3 to 5 minutes up to a total of 0.03 to 0.04 mg/kg. Use the shorter dosing interval (3 minutes) in severe clinical conditions. **(6)** Never treat the combination of *third-degree heart block* and *ventricular escape beats* with *lidocaine* (or any agent that suppresses ventricular escape rhythms). **(7)** Verify patient tolerance and mechanical capture. Use analgesia and sedation as needed. (Reproduced with permission. © *Guidelines 2000 for Cardiopulmonary Resuscitation and Emergency Cardiovascular Care, 2000.* Copyright American Heart Association.)

increased until reliable ventricular capture is achieved. Because of the intervening skin, subcutaneous fat, muscle, and visceral structures, high outputs are often required for reliable capture, particularly in larger patients. Consistent ventricular capture is unpredictable, often difficult to achieve, and associated with significant discomfort in the awake patient. In light of these limitations, the Zoll pacemaker should be used as a temporizing measure only.

If a Zoll pacemaker is not available or is ineffective, isoproterenol can be used to increase the heart rate temporarily. Isoproterenol is a pure beta-adrenergic agonist with predominantly chronotropic cardiac effects. High doses of isoproterenol can precipitate tachyarrhythmias, both supraventricular and ventricular, and ischemia in patients with pre-existing heart disease and should be used with extreme caution in this population, if at all.

Any significant bradyarrhythmia that is not acutely reversible mandates placement of a temporary ("hardwire") pacing catheter. These catheters are introduced transvenously—preferably through the right jugular, left subclavian, or left brachial vein—and positioned in the right ventricular apex. An experienced operator should place these catheters, as this procedure is associated with significant risks, including vascular injury, cardiac tamponade, ventricular tachycardia, thrombosis, bleeding, and infection. Some Swan-Ganz catheters have a port through which a pacing catheter can be passed into the right ventricle. Adequate positioning of the pacing catheter at the right ventricular apex is often difficult to achieve through these ports, and therefore consistent ventricular capture is unreliable. Consequently, the use of these pacing port Swan-Ganz catheters is not recommended for patients with serious bradyarrhythmias.

Chronic Management: Indications for a Permanent Pacemaker

The sole treatment option for chronic symptomatic bradycardia is permanent pacemaker implantation. The indications for permanent pacing have been the subject of considerable debate, mostly because of the difficulty in providing a secure definition of *symptomatic* bradycardia. Clinically relevant manifestations of the low cardiac output state may be fairly vague, particularly in the elderly patient. Occasionally, mild personality changes or signs of apparent dementia are the only clues of the need for intervention; often, the benefit can be recognized only retrospectively. One avoidable pitfall is the assumption that end-organ perfusion is adequate if the blood pressure is maintained, independent of the heart rate.

In the ICU, the typical indications for permanent pacing are similar to those discussed for temporary pacing interventions. Disorders resulting in symptomatic bradycardia that are not transient in nature are appropriately treated with pacemaker implantation. As noted earlier, these disorders are caused either by sinus node dysfunction or disorders of AV conduction. In addition, pacing is also considered for asymptomatic patients at high risk for the development of complete heart block (such as patients with bifascicular block complicating acute myocardial infarction; see Chapter 49) or patients with symptomatic bradycardia caused by medications that are required for treatment of other conditions. The latter is often seen in patients with the tachycardia-bradycardia syndrome. A comprehensive set of guidelines, classified as well-accepted (class I), controversial (class II), and unnecessary (class III) indications for permanent pacing, has been published by an American College of Cardiology/American Heart Association joint task force.

Before pacemaker implantation, it is extremely important to exclude active infection that might contaminate the intravascular pacing wires. The risk of infection in a population of ICU patients may be considerable. Once established, pacemaker infection usually cannot be resolved by antibiotic therapy and requires removal of both the generator and the intracardiac lead system. In situations in which pacing is required but ongoing infection is a concern, as in the ICU, temporary transvenous pacing should be used until permanent implantation can be performed safely.

Pacemaker Troubleshooting

Modern pacemaker generators are extremely reliable and much of the component failure observed in the early days of pacing, such as sudden failure of output or "run-away pacing" (ultrarapid delivery of pacing stimuli), is no longer observed. However, pacemaker malfunction, relating to either failure to pace (capture) or failure to sense, does occasionally occur. Causes of transient or sustained pacemaker malfunction include the following: (1) lead fracture or migration, (2) generator battery depletion, and (3) improper programming. In addition, apparent malfunction can often be explained by appropriate programmable behaviors (hysteresis, safety pacing) that may be different in devices manufactured by different vendors. Because of the complexity involved, cardiologic consultation should be obtained for evaluation of suspected pacemaker malfunction.

One important bedside intervention that can be rapidly employed for pacing malfunction is magnet application. Applying a magnet over the top of the pacemaker generator causes suspension of sensing function, resulting in single- or dual-chamber asynchronous pacing. This can be helpful when the pacing rate is inappropriately slow because of *oversensing*. An important extension of this phenomenon is the more general consideration that pacemaker function can be adversely effected by exposure to high-intensity electromagnetic sources. External cardioversion, surgical electrocautery, and lithotripsy often inhibit or reset the programming of pacemaker generators. Magnetic resonance imaging can have more profound and unpredictable effects on permanent pacemaker function and is generally contraindicated.

BIBLIOGRAPHY

American Heart Association Task Force: Guidelines for implantation of cardiac pacemakers and antiarrhythmia devices. Circulation 84:455–67, 1991.
These are the recommendations of the 1991 American College of Cardiology/American Heart Association Task Force evaluating indications for permanent pacemaker implantation.

Antman EM, Wenger TL, Butler VP, et al: Treatment of 150 cases of life-threatening digitalis intoxication with digoxin-specific Fab antibody fragments. Circulation 81:1744–1752, 1990.
This article describes a randomized trial examining the efficacy and safety of digoxin-specific Fab antibody fragments in the treatment of serious digoxin toxicity.

DiNubile MJ, Calderwood SB, Steinhaus DM, et al: Cardiac conduction abnormalities complicating native valve active infective endocarditis. Am J Cardiol 58:1213–1217, 1986.
This study analyzed the incidence of conduction abnormalities in a cohort of patients presenting with native valve endocarditis.

Dreifus LS, Michelson EL, Kaplinsky H: Bradyarrhythmias: Clinical significance and management. J Am Coll Cardiol 1:327–338, 1983.
A review and classification of bradyarrhythmias resulting from sinus node, AV node, and infranodal dysfunction.

Flack JE, Hafer J, Engelman RM, et al: Effect of normothermic blood cardioplegia on postoperative conduction abnormalities and supraventricular arrhythmias. Circulation 86(Suppl II):II-385–II-392, 1992.
The study compared the effect of warm versus cold cardioplegia during cardiac surgery on the subsequent development of conduction system disturbances and supraventricular arrhythmias.

Guilleminault C, Connolly SJ, Winkle RA: Cardiac arrhythmia and conduction disturbances during sleep in 400 patients with sleep apnea syndrome. Am J Cardiol 52:490–494, 1983.

This study examined the frequency of cardiac arrhythmias and conduction disturbances during 24-hour Holter monitoring of 400 patients with sleep apnea.

Kelly RA, Smith TW: Recognition and management of digitalis toxicity. Am J Cardiol 69:108G–119G, 1992.
This is a review of the signs, symptoms, and risk factors for the development of digoxin toxicity. It provides a comprehensive review of the management of digoxin toxicity.

Mahdyoon H, Battilana G, Rosman H, et al: The evolving pattern of digoxin intoxication: Observations at a large urban hospital from 1980 to 1988. Am Heart J 120:1189–1194, 1990.
This was a large observational study of 717 patients who had received digoxin-specific Fab antibody fragments for the treatment of digoxin toxicity.

Morris D, Mulvihill D, Lew WYW: Risk of developing complete heart block during bedside pulmonary artery catheterization in patients with left bundle-branch block. Arch Intern Med 147:2005–2010, 1987.
This study examined the frequency of complete heart block complicating pulmonary artery catheterization in 47 patients with pre-existing left bundle branch block.

Pires LA, Wagshal AB, Lancey R, et al: Arrhythmias and conduction disturbances after coronary artery bypass graft surgery: Epidemiology, management, and prognosis. Am Heart J 129:801–808, 1995.
This study analyzed the incidence of conduction disturbances in a large cohort of patients after coronary artery bypass graft surgery.

Shah KB, Rao TLK, Laughlin S, et al: A review of pulmonary artery catheterization in 6245 patients. Anesthesiology 61:271–275, 1984.
This is a review of the complications associated with pulmonary artery catheterization in a large cohort of patients undergoing a surgical procedure.

31 Arrhythmias (Tachycardias)

Dina R. Yazmajian
Francis E. Marchlinski

Management of tachyarrhythmias in the intensive care unit (ICU) requires a systematic approach to evaluation, electrocardiographic (ECG) diagnosis, and treatment. Whereas some tachycardias are transient in nature, a result of drug toxicity or electrolyte imbalance, others require further cardiac evaluation and long-term management. This chapter presents a general approach to the evaluation of the ICU patient with a tachyarrhythmia, reviews the differential diagnosis and describes ECG clues for both narrow and wide complex tachycardias, and details options related to acute treatment. Specific clinical situations are also described, such as digoxin toxicity, ventricular tachycardia (VT) in the absence of structural heart disease, the Wolff-Parkinson-White (WPW) syndrome, and acute management of the patient with an implantable cardioverter-defibrillator (ICD).

GENERAL APPROACH TO TACHYARRHYTHMIAS IN THE ICU SETTING

Overview

Recommendations for acute treatment can come only after a rapid but accurate assessment of the arrhythmia, its consequences, and its potential causes (Table 31–1). Whereas the hemodynamic consequences of the tachycardia dictate the urgency of treatment, timely assessment of multiple other factors is also essential.

In fact, most tachyarrhythmias in the ICU setting are precipitated or potentiated by metabolic and hemodynamic derangements, electrolyte imbalances, or drug effect. These include sinus tachycardia, atrial fibrillation, atrial flutter, multifocal

Table 31–1. Checklist for Rapidly Assessing Patients with Tachyarrhythmias

1. Hemodynamic status: perform emergency cardioversion if unstable ("When in doubt, knock it out," see text)
2. Cardiac status: check for angina and heart failure symptoms
3. Volume status: consider hypovolemia, blood loss, or volume overload
4. Body temperature: evaluate for fever or hypothermia
5. Medications: note both dosage and time of administration, especially
   Aminophylline
   Catecholamine infusions
   Digoxin
   Antiarrhythmic agents
6. Serum electrolyte levels: especially K^+, Mg^{2+}, and Ca^{2+}
7. Oxygen saturation and hemoglobin level
8. Acid-base balance
9. Pain control status

atrial tachycardia, automatic atrial and junctional tachycardias, and polymorphic VT. In contrast, sustained monomorphic VT, atrioventricular (AV) nodal reentrant tachycardia (AVNRT), reentrant atrial tachycardia, and macro-reentrant tachycardia (also called AV reentrant tachycardia [AVRT] which uses the atria, AV nodal tissue, ventricles, and an accessory pathway), occur in the setting of a predisposing structural substrate. Even with such a substrate, however, a metabolic or hemodynamic factor may be responsible for the initiation and maintenance of the tachycardia. Furthermore, reversal of such underlying abnormalities may control the tachycardia and prevent its recurrence.

Diagnostic Tools

The appropriate intervention for a tachyarrhythmia depends on obtaining adequate information to arrive at the correct ECG diagnosis (Table 31–2). A reference or baseline 12-lead ECG during sinus rhythm should be sought immediately. This

Table 31–2. Differential Diagnosis of Sustained Supraventricular Tachycardia*

RHYTHM (FIGURE NO.)	KEY FEATURES	RESPONSE TO ADENOSINE OR VAGAL MANEUVER
Sinus tachycardia (31–2A)	Upright P wave in II, III, aVF; inverted P wave in aVR	No effect or transient slowing
Atrial fibrillation (31–2B)	No repetitive organized atrial activity; irregularly irregular ventricular response	Transient slowing of ventricular response
Atrial flutter (31–2C)	P wave activity 260–300 beats per minute; ventricular response 2:1, but higher grade AV block possible	Transient slowing of ventricular response with unmasking of flutter waves (see Fig. 31–1)
Multifocal atrial tachycardia (31–2D)	Multiple (≥3) discrete P wave morphologies with isoelectric interval between P waves	No effect or transient AV block
Atrial tachycardia (31–2E)	P wave morphology distinct from sinus P wave; may have variable AV block	Transient AV block; termination of tachycardia is possible
Atrial tachycardia of digoxin toxicity	Upright P wave in II, III, aVF, V_1; typically with variable AV block and ventriculophasic effect	Transient AV block
Junctional tachycardia of digoxin toxicity	Regular RR interval; no association between P wave and QRS complex	No effect
AV nodal reentrant tachycardia (31–2F)	P wave may only be visible at the end of the QRS complex (pseudo R wave in V_1; pseudo S wave in II, III, aVF)	Termination of tachycardia
AV reentrant tachycardia (31–2G)	P wave is seen after the QRS complex; inverted P wave in II, III, aVF	Termination of tachycardia after the P wave

*Ranked in order of frequency of occurrence in ICU patients.
AV, atrioventricular.

may provide important information regarding underlying heart disease, conduction abnormalities, and baseline P wave morphology. A 12-lead ECG during the tachycardia provides further information regarding the AV relationship during tachycardia, morphologic features of the QRS complex, and P wave morphology. Long telemetry rhythm strips are also helpful in determining the AV relationship, regularity of the ventricular response, and initiation and termination of the tachycardia (Table 31–3). Additional information regarding the AV relationship may be obtained by recording directly from epicardial pacing leads in the postoperative cardiac patient or from permanent endocardial pacing leads.

Many tachycardias are short-lived or require immediate cardioversion, making it difficult to obtain a 12-lead ECG during the event. In these cases, telemetry recordings from the appropriate leads are crucial. The V_1 precordial lead is the most helpful lead in assessing bundle branch block (BBB) morphology and suspected VT. Based on morphologic criteria, V_1 may also be useful in localizing the arrhythmia and guiding pharmacologic and ablative treatment. It is important to note that V_1 and MCL_1 recordings are not equivalent. Although the two leads may appear identical during sinus rhythm, they may be very different during wide complex tachycardias.

As a rule, the inferior limb leads (II, III, aVF) are good starting points for supraventricular tachycardias because P waves and atrial flutter waves are often well seen in these leads. If the telemetry system allows simultaneous monitoring of two leads, V_1 and an inferior limb lead provide the greatest amount of informa-

Table 31–3. Electrocardiographic Clues from Initiation and Termination of Supraventricular Tachycardias

RHYTHM	INITIATION PHASE	TERMINATION PHASE
Sinus tachycardia	"Warm up" in atrial rate	Atrial rate slows gradually without an abrupt stop
Atrial flutter	Transient AV block may reveal flutter waves (see Fig. 31–1)	
Atrial tachycardia	Warm up in atrial rate with changing PR interval; transient degree of AV block during which P waves appear	Oscillations in PP interval precede changes in RR interval; terminates after QRS complex
Junctional tachycardia	No APC triggering the tachycardia	
AV nodal reentrant tachycardia	APC followed by a significantly prolonged PR interval and then supraventricular tachycardia; BBB only transient following initiation	Terminates after P wave with adenosine
AV reentrant tachycardia	APC and slightly prolonged PR interval; late coupled VPC; persistent BBB; fixed RP relationship	Oscillations in RR interval precede changes in PP interval; terminates after P wave with adenosine; may terminate after a single, especially late coupled, VPC

AV, atrioventricular, APC, atrial premature contraction; BBB, bundle branch block; VPC, ventricular premature contraction.

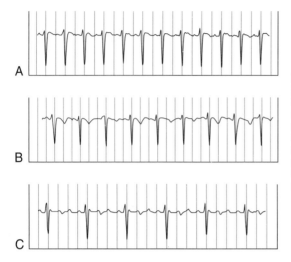

Figure 31–1. *A,* Regular supraventricular tachycardia at a rate of 150 beats/min. *B,* Pharmacologic slowing of atrioventricular (AV) nodal conduction results in variable AV block suggesting atrial flutter. *C,* After slowing conduction through AV node even more, the P waves of atrial flutter (conducted at 4:1) become clearly evident.

tion. If only one lead can be monitored at a time, lead selection should be based on the arrhythmic information sought for an individual patient.

Interventions during tachycardia can also provide useful information. Slowing AV nodal conduction with vagal maneuvers or pharmacologic agents can reveal previously masked flutter waves or the P waves of atrial tachycardia (Fig. 31–1). Adenosine, an endogenous nucleoside, interacts with specific receptors on the extracellular membrane acutely slowing AV conduction. Because adenosine has a half-life of only 0.5 to 5 seconds, doses (6 mg and then 12 mg) must be given in a rapid bolus injection followed by a flush. Even administration through a peripheral intravenous line can attenuate its effects. The short-lived adverse effects of adenosine include facial flushing, chest pain or pressure, bronchospasm, and dyspnea. By briefly but effectively blocking the AV node, adenosine is capable of terminating AVNRTs. Adenosine is not a perfect diagnostic tool, however, because it may also terminate some episodes of atrial tachycardia and VT.

The "When in Doubt, Knock it Out" Rule

Severe hemodynamic instability due to a tachycardia warrants prompt electrical cardioversion. Before cardioversion, however, one needs to consider that the tachycardia may be sinus tachycardia or multifocal atrial tachycardia, neither of which responds to electrical cardioversion. In addition, the hemodynamic instability may be due to a separate cause, such as blood loss or sepsis, and the tachyarrhythmia is just a secondary event. Once the decision is made to perform electrical cardioversion, patient comfort should be ensured by administering a short-acting intravenous benzodiazepine, such as midazolam (see Chapter 4).

One must choose a mode of delivery (synchronous or asynchronous) and an energy level. Delivery of shock energy for ventricular fibrillation (VF) and polymorphic VT should be performed in the asynchronous mode. For all other arrhythmias, energy should be delivered in the synchronous mode to decrease the risk of causing arrhythmia acceleration or VF. For any rhythm with dire hemodynamic consequences, energy output should begin at 200 joules and then increased to 300 joules followed by 360 joules if the initial attempts fail (see Appendix E for ACLS algorithms). Only in the stable patient should lower energy levels be attempted.

One always should anticipate adverse consequences when performing electrical cardioversion or defibrillation. Even in the stable patient, synchronous cardioversion can precipitate VF. Because bradycardia and significant sinus pauses are not unusual after cardioversion, intravenous atropine should always be immediately available and ready access to an external pacing unit is desirable.

NARROW COMPLEX TACHYCARDIAS

Supraventricular tachycardia (SVT) is a commonly used but imprecise term. By definition, all narrow complex tachycardias, including sinus tachycardia, are supraventricular in origin because only depolarization over the His-Purkinje system through the AV node results in a narrow QRS. The frequency of the different SVTs occurring in the ICU setting differs from that seen in the emergency department or outpatient office (Fig. 31–2 and see Table 31–2). Underlying diseases, heightened sympathetic tone, and use of medications, such as inotropes, aminophylline, or digoxin, can precipitate these tachyarrhythmias. Clues to their ECG diagnosis can be found in rhythm strip analysis with recording of the onset and termination of tachycardia (see Table 31–3). More detailed recommendations of pharmacologic and nonpharmacologic management strategies for specific SVTs are discussed next.

Sinus Tachycardia

The most common SVT encountered in the ICU is sinus tachycardia (ST), which occurs in response to underlying conditions, such as pain, fever, infection, anemia, pulmonary embolism, thyrotoxicosis, myocardial ischemia, and congestive heart failure (CHF) (see Fig. 31–2A). Autonomic dysfunction may also play a role, particularly in certain neurologic disorders, such as Guillain-Barré syndrome. The clinical challenge lies in making the diagnosis of ST and recognizing its significance as a secondary problem. It should be viewed as a warning sign of underlying abnormalities and prompt a thorough evaluation. Treatment is directed toward the underlying cause ("treat the patient, not the heart rate").

Atrial Fibrillation and Atrial Flutter

Atrial fibrillation and atrial flutter are sister arrhythmias that occur commonly in the ICU (Fig. 31–2B and C). Risk factors for the development of atrial fibrillation include CHF, coronary artery disease (CAD), advanced age, pulmonary disease, thyrotoxicosis, and diabetes. Acute respiratory failure and high sympathetic tone, particularly in patients with other risk factors, can precipitate a paroxysm of atrial fibrillation or flutter. On the 12-lead ECG, atrial fibrillation is marked by the replacement of organized atrial activity with an undulating baseline. At times, the

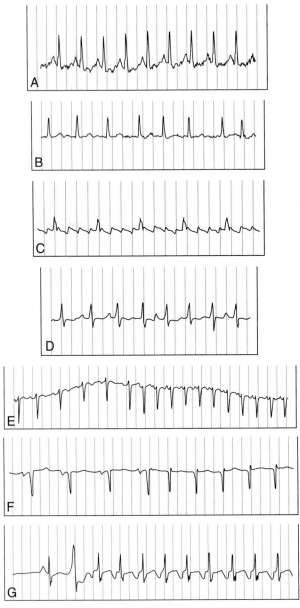

Figure 31–2. *A,* Sinus tachycardia. *B,* Atrial fibrillation. *C,* Atrial flutter (AVNRT). *D,* Multifocal atrial tachycardia. *E,* Atrial tachycardia. *F,* Atrioventricular nodal reentrant tachycardia. *G,* Atrioventricular reentrant tachycardia (AVRT). See Tables 31–2 and 31–3 and text for diagnostic features of each tachycardia.

undulations may be coarse and mimic atrial activity. These coarse waves are not truly cyclical, and the RR interval is always irregular.

In contrast, atrial flutter is due to a reentrant mechanism within the atria and results in regular flutter waves (typically at a rate of 260 to 300 beats per minute (bpm)) on the 12-lead ECG. In the absence of medications, the ventricular rate is typically regular, with 2:1 conduction of flutter waves, resulting in a ventricular rate of 150 bpm. In fact, when encountering a narrow complex tachycardia at the rate of 150 bpm, one should always first consider the diagnosis of atrial flutter. Flutter waves can be easily overlooked, and blocking conduction in the AV node can help unmask them (see Fig. 31–1). If atrial wires (temporary or permanent) are present, direct recordings from these wires can clarify the diagnosis.

Acutely, these arrhythmias can result in a rapid ventricular rate, loss of effective atrial contraction, and hypotension. In this situation, the treatment is electrical cardioversion. If the patient is stable, management is directed at controlling the ventricular rate, converting the arrhythmia to sinus rhythm, maintaining sinus rhythm, and preventing embolic sequelae.

A number of pharmacologic agents are available to control the ventricular response during atrial fibrillation and flutter (Table 31–4). Once the rate is controlled and the patient is hemodynamically stable, cardioversion to sinus rhythm can be pursued on an elective basis. The timing of elective cardioversion is largely determined by the need to reduce the risk of thromboembolic complications. The lack of organized atrial activity associated with atrial fibrillation can lead to circulatory stasis within the atria, formation of atrial thrombi, and embolism into the systemic circulation. Even in new-onset atrial fibrillation, there is some embolic risk. If a patient has no contraindications, anticoagulation should be started as soon as possible, certainly within 24 to 48 hours if spontaneous conversion to sinus rhythm has not occurred. If a patient cannot receive anticoagulation, prompt cardioversion within 24 to 72 hours should be considered.

Table 31–4. Treatment of Atrial Fibrillation and Flutter: Ventricular Rate Control

MEDICATION	ADMINISTRATION*	ADVANTAGES	DISADVANTAGES
Propranolol	IV bolus or oral	Shorter half-life, especially effective for thyrotoxicosis	Frequent dosing required for control
Metoprolol	IV bolus or oral	Longer half-life	
Esmolol	IV infusion	Half-life of 9 min	Needs close monitoring
Verapamil	IV bolus or infusion or oral		Acute control lasts only 30 min after IV dose; negative inotrope
Diltiazem	IV bolus or infusion or oral	Short half-life	Less negative inotropic effects than verapamil
Digoxin	IV bolus or oral	Positive inotropic effect	Delayed onset of action Narrow therapeutic window

*For specific doses, see Table 34–4 (beta-blockers) and Table 34–5 (calcium channel blockers) in Chapter 34.

When the duration of atrial fibrillation is unclear, one must assume that it has been present for more than 72 hours. In this case, conventional therapy has consisted of anticoagulation for 4 to 6 weeks before cardioversion. A transesophageal echocardiogram can be used to rule out the presence of thrombus located in the left atrial appendage, but the absence of thrombus does not preclude the need for immediate postcardioversion heparin therapy and anticoagulation for several weeks thereafter. Anticoagulation is essential during this period because atrial stunning may lead to thrombus formation despite sinus rhythm. Patients with atrial flutter are also at risk for embolic phenomenon and should also receive anticoagulation, especially because atrial fibrillation frequently coexists with flutter.

Once the decision is made to proceed to cardioversion, several options exist, particularly for atrial flutter. Because atrial flutter is a reentrant arrhythmia, overdrive pacing by means of a permanent or temporary pacing wire or an esophageal electrode can terminate the tachycardia. Overdrive pacing, however, can result in atrial fibrillation rather than sinus rhythm.

Atrial fibrillation and flutter respond to the same antiarrhythmic drugs outlined in Table 31–5. In fact, atrial fibrillation frequently organizes into stable atrial flutter on these medications. It is common, however, for these arrhythmias to resist pharmacologic interventions and require electrical cardioversion. Despite this, the use of antiarrhythmic agents before electrical cardioversion is indicated because drug treatment may help maintain sinus rhythm after cardioversion. In patients whose condition is stable, electrical cardioversion of atrial fibrillation typically begins at 200 joules, but higher doses of energy may be required. It is always performed in the synchronous mode. Cardioversion of atrial flutter requires significantly lower energies, usually 50 to 100 joules, and, again, should always be delivered in the synchronous mode. An amnestic agent, such as midazolam, should always be given beforehand.

Some patients have a clear precipitating factor for atrial fibrillation, such as pulmonary embolism or pneumonia, and do not require long-term medical management. Spontaneous conversion to sinus rhythm may occur as the patient recovers from the acute insult. Other patients who have underlying risk factors remain at risk for recurrence and may require chronic antiarrhythmic management and anticoagulation. The patient with atrial fibrillation and the WPW syndrome is discussed later.

Multifocal Atrial Tachycardia

Multifocal atrial tachycardia (MAT) (see Fig. 31–2D), also referred to as chaotic atrial tachycardia, occurs exclusively in the setting of a serious underlying disease, typically a chronic obstructive pulmonary disease (COPD) flare, other types of acute respiratory decompensation, pulmonary embolism, or CHF. The presence of MAT has been associated with a high in-hospital mortality rate, which correlates with the severity of the underlying disease rather than with the hemodynamic consequences of the tachycardia. The atrial rate in MAT tends to be 100 to 150 bpm but can be higher. The ECG generally reveals at least three P wave morphologies with marked variation in the PP intervals and frequently the PR intervals (see Table 31–2).

The most effective treatment for MAT is treatment of the underlying condition

Table 31–5. Treatment of Atrial Fibrillation and Flutter: Conversion to Sinus Rhythm

MEDICATION	ADMINISTRATION*	ADVANTAGES	DISADVANTAGES
Procainamide	IV bolus and infusion or oral	IV bolus usually tolerated; first choice for medical treatment of atrial fibrillation over a bypass tract (see text)	Hypotension with IV; long-term use limited by side effects; proarrhythmia
Quinidine	IV bolus or infusion or oral	No negative inotropic effects	Proarrhythmia; vagolytic effect may cause increase in heart rate; hypotension with IV; gastrointestinal side effects common
Disopyramide†	Oral	Twice-a-day dosing	Anticholinergic effect; negative inotropic effect
Flecainide†	Oral	Twice-a-day dosing	Proarrhythmia, especially in congestive heart failure and coronary artery disease; negative inotropic effect; teratogenic
Propafenone†	Oral	Beta blocking adds to rate control	Negative inotropic effect
Sotalol†	Oral	Beta blocking adds to rate control	Proarrhythmia
Amiodarone†	IV or oral	More effective in maintaining sinus rhythm; once-daily dosing; long half-life (2–15 wk) after prolonged therapy	Variety of side effects, most reversible; rare but potentially fatal lung fibrosis

*See Chapter 12 for dosing guidelines for procainamide and quinidine.
†Consider cardiology consultation before using these agents.

and cessation of potentially exacerbating drugs, such as aminophylline. Some patients may have concomitant electrolyte disturbances, such as hypokalemia and hypomagnesemia, and magnesium administered intravenously has been reported to control MAT in such patients. In general, electrical cardioversion, class IA antiarrhythmic agents, and digoxin are ineffective. Occasionally, when the rate is very rapid, it becomes important to control the ventricular response. Calcium channel blockers and beta blockers have been used with variable success, but, unfortunately, the use of beta blockers, even cardioselective agents, is often limited due to concomitant bronchospastic disease.

AV Nodal Reentrant Tachycardia

AV nodal reentrant tachycardia (see Fig. 31–2F) is a common mechanism of SVT, although it occurs less often in the ICU than the tachycardias discussed earlier. AVNRT can occur at any age, is unrelated to pre-existent heart disease, and depends only on the presence of two functionally dissociated AV nodal pathways. The reentry circuit also occurs within the AV node and results in near simultaneous depolarization of both the atrium and ventricle (see Table 31–2). The tachycardia rate ranges from 100 to over 200 bpm with regular RR intervals. Hemodynamic consequences are due to increased heart rate and the loss of sequential AV contraction. Patients with normal left ventricular function generally tolerate it, but substantial hypotension can result. Treatment is directed at slowing conduction within the AV node, thereby terminating the tachycardia. Maneuvers that increase vagal tone such as a Valsalva maneuver, gagging, or carotid sinus massage are often effective. Likewise, drugs such as adenosine, calcium antagonists, and beta blockers are useful. Despite its AV nodal blocking effects, digoxin is usually ineffective as acute therapy. A variety of agents, including calcium antagonists, beta blockers, digoxin, and class IA and IC drugs, can all be used to prevent recurrences. Radiofrequency catheter ablation, a curative procedure, is the therapy of choice to prevent recurrent AVNRT in the symptomatic patient.

AV Reentrant Tachycardia over a Bypass Tract

AV reentrant tachycardia is an SVT that uses the AV node and bypass tract as the two limbs of the reentrant pathway (Fig. 31–2G). Like AVNRT, AVRT may occur at any age and is not associated with underlying heart disease. The baseline 12-lead ECG may reveal pre-excitation over the bypass tract (Fig. 31–3) or may be normal (so-called concealed accessory pathway). The AVRT circuit can result in (1) a narrow complex tachycardia when the AV node serves as the antegrade limb and the ventricle is depolarized over the His-Purkinje system or (2) a wide complex tachycardia when antegrade conduction occurs over the bypass tract. Because both the atrium and ventricle are necessary components to the circuit, a 1:1 AV relationship exists and retrograde P waves are typically discernible on the 12-lead ECG (see Table 31–2). During a given tachycardia, the RP intervals remain constant, which can help differentiate it from an atrial tachycardia. The RP interval, however, depends on the individual characteristics of the bypass tract and can be short or long.

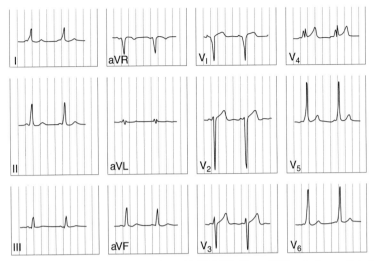

Figure 31–3. Normal sinus rhythm in a patient with Wolff-Parkinson-White syndrome. Note the short PR interval (<0.12 sec) and slurred onset of QRS complexes, the hallmark of preexcitation.

Treatment is directed at slowing conduction within the AV node, usually the most vulnerable limb of the circuit, which results in termination of the SVT. Adenosine is the drug of choice, although calcium antagonists and beta blockers may be used. If the patient has a surface ECG manifesting WPW syndrome during sinus rhythm and is predisposed to developing atrial fibrillation, verapamil should be avoided. Although antiarrhythmic agents such as procainamide or flecainide, which can slow conduction over the bypass tract, and calcium antagonists or beta blockers, which slow conduction over the AV node, can be used to prevent recurrences, radiofrequency catheter ablation is the most effective method to prevent recurrences.

Other Atrial Tachycardias

In the ICU setting, atrial tachycardia generally occurs in patients with underlying heart disease, COPD, pneumonia, pericarditis, or digitalis toxicity (see Figs. 31–2E). Atrial rates are commonly 150 to 200 bpm with P wave morphology on the 12-lead ECG distinct from the sinus P wave (see Table 31–2). The ventricular response may be 1:1, 2:1, or variable AV conduction block, such as Wenckebach (Mobitz I) block.

Treatment of atrial tachycardia consists of ventricular rate control with AV nodal blocking agents and suppressive therapy with antiarrhythmic drugs. The tachycardia is often resistant to electrical cardioversion. Reversible underlying conditions, such as digitalis toxicity, pericarditis, or respiratory decompensation, should be aggressively treated if present. Otherwise, class IA agents such as procainamide, administered intravenously, are appropriate in an ICU setting. Class IC agents, such as flecainide, or class III agents, such as sotalol or amiodarone, can also be very effective but should be used with caution in patients with underlying cardiac disease.

Accelerated Junctional Rhythm

The AV junctional pacemaker typically fires at a rate of 40 to 60 bpm. Junctional tachycardia with rates above 100 bpm occurs in certain clinical situations such as digitalis intoxication, rheumatic fever, myocardial ischemia, and postoperatively after cardiac surgery, especially after valvular procedures. Atrial activity may be sinus P waves with AV dissociation or inverted P waves reflecting retrograde activation. Frequently, there is a 1:1 AV relationship. This differentiates it from the junctional tachycardia of digoxin toxicity, which has some degree of AV block or frank dissociation. In addition, an automatic junctional tachycardia often exhibits acceleration in rate that can differentiate it from AVNRT. Loss of sequential AV contraction, especially in patients with poor left ventricular function, can have adverse hemodynamic effects. In the postoperative cardiac surgery patient, temporary atrial wires can often overdrive pace the junctional rhythm. Otherwise, management is supportive and directed toward the precipitating factor.

Atrial Fibrillation in Patients with Wolff-Parkinson-White Syndrome

Patients with the WPW syndrome have muscular connections between the atrium and ventricle, commonly called Kent bundles, which are responsible for the pre-excitation seen on the ECG. Typically, the ECG during normal sinus rhythm reveals a short PR interval (less than 120 msec) and a wide QRS complex (exceeding 120 msec) with a slurred upstroke (delta wave) (see Fig. 31–3). These patients are predisposed to developing a number of SVTs, including atrial fibrillation. Because the ventricular response during atrial fibrillation can be very rapid over the bypass tract with heart rates well over 200 bpm, these can degenerate into VF (Fig. 31–4). If the patient's condition is hemodynamically unstable, immediate cardioversion should be performed.

Of note, standard AV nodal blocking regimens can actually increase the ventricular response in the patient with WPW syndrome and result in VF. For example, digoxin can directly increase the ventricular rate by accelerating antegrade conduction over the bypass tract. Verapamil can also result in a faster ventricular response through vasodilatation and reflex sympathetic stimulation. Therefore, if the pa-

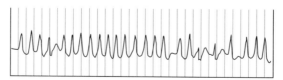

Figure 31–4. Atrial fibrillation in the same patient as Figure 31–3. Note the irregularity of the RR intervals and the bizarre and changing morphologies of the QRS complexes. The shortest RR intervals occur at 300 beats per minute and could result in degeneration into ventricular fibrillation.

tient's condition is stable, conversion to sinus rhythm with procainamide or electrical cardioversion with adequate sedation is the treatment of choice.

WIDE COMPLEX TACHYCARDIAS

A wide complex tachycardia that is monomorphic, that is, all QRS morphologies are identical, can pose a diagnostic dilemma because a wide QRS complex may be due to VT or SVT with BBB. The patient's hemodynamic response also cannot be used to differentiate between the two mechanisms: some patients with VT can be minimally symptomatic whereas some with SVT can have hemodynamic collapse. When the patient's condition is unstable, regardless of mechanism, he or she should be immediately cardioverted or defibrillated. If initial cardioversion or defibrillation is unsuccessful, repeated high-energy defibrillation should be delivered and cardiopulmonary resuscitation initiated. If the tachycardia remains refractory or VF occurs, standard therapy is recommended using repeated high-energy shocks and lidocaine administration (see Appendix E for ACLS algorithms).

If the patient's condition is stable, however, a precise diagnosis should be pursued. VT carries a very different prognosis from SVT and requires different long-term management. Because the clinical scenario cannot definitively differentiate between diagnoses, ECG data are critical. Whenever possible, one should obtain a 12-lead ECG during tachycardia to evaluate QRS morphology and the AV relationship (Table 31–6). The presence of AV dissociation (ventricular activity independent of atrial activity) is diagnostic of VT. Conducted sinus beats in the form of capture beats (QRS complex identical to baseline morphology) or fusion beats (distinct QRS morphology) also confirm the diagnosis of VT (Fig. 31–5).

Morphologic features of the QRS complex are also important because they

Table 31–6. Electrocardiographic Support for Diagnosis of Ventricular Tachycardia

....

1. Atrioventricular dissociation
2. Right superior QRS axis in the frontal plane (positive in aVR and negative in I and aVF)
3. QRS duration >140 msec in the absence of antiarrhythmic drug therapy
4. Evidence of Q wave myocardial infarction pattern on baseline ECG
5. Bundle branch block (BBB) pattern during wide complex tachycardia different from BBB pattern on baseline ECG
6. QRS complex narrows during tachycardia
7. Morphologic characteristics:
   a. RBBB tachycardia:
      (1) Duration of QRS onset to nadir of S wave in any precordial lead >100 msec
      (2) Monophasic R or QR pattern in V_1
      (3) When a triphasic R wave is present in V_1, a left "rabbit ear" taller than the right. (*Note:* A taller right "rabbit ear" does not indicate supraventricular tachycardia with aberration)
      (4) QRS complexes pointing in the same direction, either positive or negative
      (5) RS or QS pattern in V_6
   b. LBBB tachycardia:
      (1) An R wave in V_1 or V_2 >30 msec duration
      (2) A duration >60 msec from the onset of the QRS to the nadir of the S wave in V_1 or V_2
      (3) Notching on the downstroke of the S wave in V_1 or V_2
      (4) Any Q wave in V_6

....

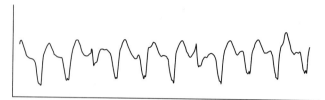

Figure 31–5. Rhythm strip during ventricular tachycardia. The intermittent narrower beats represent fusion beats of ventricular tachycardia and sinus capture beats.

reflect how the ventricles have been activated. If the morphology is similar to the BBB pattern on the baseline sinus rhythm ECG or during times of rate-related BBB (e.g., during clear sinus tachycardia or an exercise test), it is very likely to be SVT with aberration. During VT, the QRS complex may be very wide and oddly shaped, with a bizarre axis reflecting a ventricular focus. Typically, wide complex tachycardias are divided into left bundle branch block (LBBB) tachycardias when there is a dominant (and usually terminal) Q or S wave in V_1 (Fig. 31–6) and right bundle branch block (RBBB) tachycardias when there is a dominant (and usually terminal) R wave in V_1 (Fig. 31–7). Morphologic characteristics of VT have been observed in each BBB pattern (see Table 31–6).

It may not always be possible to distinguish between SVT and VT, particularly if information is limited to that from an isolated rhythm strip. When the diagnosis is unclear, it is always safer to assume a diagnosis of VT, especially in the presence of underlying heart disease. Intravenously administered verapamil, an effective treatment for SVT, can precipitate severe hypotension and loss of consciousness in patients with VT. Adenosine, with its very short half-life, is unlikely to cause the hemodynamic collapse found with verapamil. Therefore, when a supraventricular

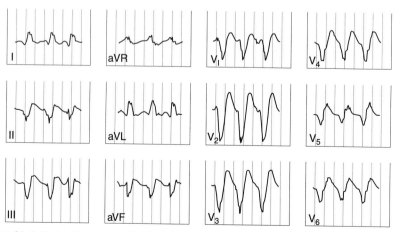

Figure 31–6. Ventricular tachycardia of a left bundle branch morphology. Leads V_1 and V_2 reveal the characteristic slurred and slow downstroke, and V_6 has a clear Q wave.

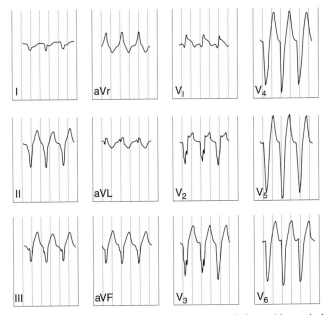

Figure 31–7. Ventricular tachycardia of a right bundle branch morphology with a typical right superior axis and wide QRS complex. The QR pattern in V_1 is a characteristic morphology and suggests a prior anteroseptal myocardial infarction.

mechanism is suspected, adenosine can be administered with relative safety. Termination of the tachycardia with adenosine does not definitively rule out VT. Adenosine should not be used, however, in the presence of active bronchospasm or myocardial ischemia. Intravenously administered procainamide, which can terminate many episodes of VT and SVT, is a general first-line therapy when the diagnosis is unclear.

Monomorphic Ventricular Tachycardia

The majority of sustained monomorphic VTs occur in the setting of CAD, previous myocardial infarction, and left ventricular dysfunction. Many of these patients have a history of myocardial infarction complicated by CHF, BBB, or hypotension, which reflects extensive myocardial damage. Any patient who presents with VT, therefore, should receive an evaluation for ventricular function and CAD. Sustained VT also occurs in patients with other types of structural heart disease, such as dilated cardiomyopathies or repaired congenital heart abnormalities. Although their long-term treatment may differ, acute therapy is essentially the same.

Acute management of VT is dictated by hemodynamic status as outlined earlier. Intravenous administration of lidocaine and procainamide is standard therapy for tolerated VT, with procainamide probably being more efficacious (Table 31–7).

Table 31–7. Acute Drug Therapy for Ventricular Tachycardia

DRUG	DOSAGE*	ADVERSE EFFECTS
Lidocaine	*For cardiac arrest:* initial bolus: 1–1.5 mg/kg *If persists:* additional bolus (0.5 mg/kg) every 10 min as needed; maximum dose: 3 mg/kg; infusion: 2–4 mg/min	Reduced clearance in congestive heart failure and acute myocardial infarction (decrease dose) Reduced volume of distribution in patients older than 70 years (decrease dose) Central nervous system effects include agitation, lethargy, and seizure Large doses can induce heart block
Procainamide	Loading: 17 mg/kg over 1 h Infusion: 1–4 mg/min	Hold infusion if QRS complex widens >50% Vasodilatation and hypotension Negative inotropic effects
Amiodarone	Oral: 800–1600 mg/day for 2 weeks, then 200–400 mg/day Intravenous: 1050–1200 mg over 24 h	Vasodilatation Negative inotropic effects with intravenous preparations Bradycardia and heart block
Bretylium	*For cardiac arrest:* bolus: 5 mg/kg *If persists:* additional bolus: 10 mg/kg every 15 to 30 min; maximum dose: 30 mg/kg *For ventricular tachycardia:* initial bolus: 5–10 mg/kg over 10 min *If persists:* 5–10 mg/kg in 1–2 h and then every 6–8 h or continuous infusion of 1–2 mg/min	Postural hypotension Nausea and vomiting in conscious patients May exacerbate digoxin toxic ventricular arrhythmias
Epinephrine	*For cardiac arrest:* bolus: 1 mg every 5 min Give through endotracheal tube if no intravenous access is available	Profound inotropic effects can precipitate ischemia Can exacerbate digoxin toxic ventricular arrhythmias

*See Chapter 12 for more dosing guidelines and drug-drug interactions for lidocaine and procainamide.

Procainamide, which has vasodilating properties, can lead to acute hypotension, making close monitoring and adequate intravenous access essential. Fortunately, the hypotension usually responds to slowing or discontinuing the infusion or giving intravenous fluids. Other adverse effects include negative inotropic effects, which can lead to decompensation in individuals with poor ventricular function and heart block in patients with underlying His-Purkinje disease. Amiodarone, available in both oral and intravenous forms, can also be used for refractory VT. Like procainamide, amiodarone has vasodilating effects and intravenous preparations can have negative inotropic effects (see Table 31–7). Acute treatment options for VT include overdrive pacing through a temporary pacing wire, an epicardial wire, or a pre-existing ICD. Because attempts at overdrive pacing can result in tachycardia acceleration or VF, a defibrillator should always be readily available. Long-term therapy for monomorphic VT in patients with underlying heart disease includes antiarrhythmic drugs, therapy with an ICD, and radiofrequency catheter ablation.

A foreign body within the ventricle can also cause VT, although it is typically nonsustained. For example, brief runs of VT during placement of a guide wire, Swan-Ganz catheter, or temporary pacing wire within the right ventricle are common. The etiology is usually clear because the VT is temporally related to catheter placement and terminates with its removal or repositioning.

Ventricular Tachycardia in the Absence of Structural Heart Disease

It is well known that ventricular ectopy can occur in normal hearts. Although the exact incidence is not clear, sustained VT in the normal heart is probably underrecognized. This VT is marked by monomorphic morphologies, which can arise from either the left or the right ventricle. The LBBB morphology VT arises from the right ventricular outflow tract (Fig. 31–8) and is precipitated by exercise and catecholamines. It can be terminated by adenosine, verapamil, beta blockers, and even vagal maneuvers. It is also amenable to catheter-based ablation procedures.

There is also RBBB morphology, which arises from the apical posterior portion of the left ventricular septum. Like the LBBB VT, it can be initiated with exercise (although less frequently) and responds to verapamil.

Polymorphic Ventricular Tachycardia

Although often lumped together, patients with polymorphic VT represent a spectrum of underlying pathologic processes. When approaching the patient with polymorphic VT, one should begin with examination and careful measurement of the QT interval of the 12-lead ECG and rhythm strip in sinus rhythm.

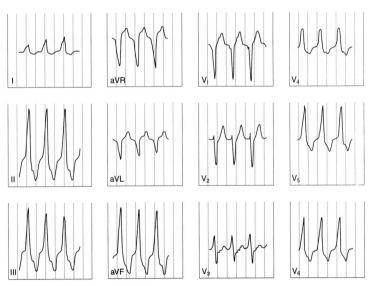

Figure 31–8. Idiopathic ventricular tachycardia originating from the right ventricular outflow tract. Note the typical left bundle branch morphology and inferior QRS axis.

Polymorphic VT with Normal QT Duration

If the QT duration is normal, then myocardial ischemia is the most likely precipitating factor. In the scenario of active ischemia, intravenous infusion of lidocaine often has a stabilizing effect. Refractory polymorphic VT and VF may respond to intravenous infusion of bretylium or amiodarone. Treatment of active ischemia with beta blockers, nitrates, antiplatelet therapy, and anticoagulation is important to the treatment of the electrical instability. Patients with suspected ischemia should receive a prompt cardiac catheterization and revascularization when appropriate. Revascularization alone may not provide adequate protection against recurrence of polymorphic VT, however, and an ICD may be required for long-term management.

Polymorphic VT with Prolonged QT Duration

If the QT duration is prolonged in the setting of polymorphic VT, then it falls into a separate category, referred to as "torsades de pointes" (or "torsades" for short). Classically, the QRS complexes exhibit a phasic "twisting" around the isoelectric line. Phasic variation in QRS amplitude and polarity should be observed in two or more leads because variation in a single rhythm strip may be misleading. The QT prolongation may be idiopathic (referred to as congenital long QT) or acquired in the setting of medications and electrolyte derangements. Typically, there is baseline sinus bradycardia, which adds to the absolute QT interval prolongation and predisposes to the generation of premature beats (Fig. 31–9). Torsades has even been noted in patients with a normal baseline QT who have a prolonged pause (i.e., from sinus node arrest or complete heart block), followed by a beat with a significantly prolonged QT coupled with a premature ventricular beat.

In the ICU, acquired long QT occurs frequently. Many drugs used in the ICU, especially haloperidol, can precipitate QT abnormalities and torsades (Table 31–8). Other underlying conditions that may set the stage for torsades include electrolyte imbalance, particularly hypokalemia and hypomagnesemia, hypothyroidism, intracranial events, myocardial ischemia, starvation, and anorexia nervosa. Some investigators suggest that patients with congenital long QT are susceptible to the acquired forms of torsades de pointes. Torsades de pointes may occur in self-terminating salvos, which may be asymptomatic or result in syncope. It is critical

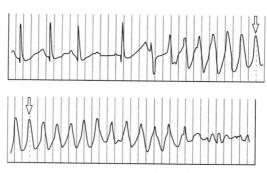

Figure 31–9. The top tracing initially shows sinus rhythm with a long QT interval followed by onset of torsades de pointes after an atrial premature contraction. The two open arrows indicate the same QRS complex on this continuous tracing.

Table 31–8. Drugs Associated with Torsades de Pointes

....

Class IA antiarrhythmic agents (quinidine, procainamide, disopyramide)
Class III antiarrhythmic agents (sotalol, d-sotalol, amiodarone, bretylium, dofetilide, sematilide)
Other agents with antiarrhythmic properties (bepridil, encainide, propafenone, ajmaline, aprindine)
Psychotherapeutic drugs
    Haloperidol
    Phenothiazines (chlorpromazine, thioridazine)
    Serotonin reuptake antagonists (fluoxetine, paroxetine)
    Tricyclic and tetracyclic antidepressants
Antihistamines (terfenadine, astemizole)
Antimicrobials (erythromycin, trimethoprim-sulfamethoxazole, pentamidine)
Poisons (organophosphate insecticides, arsenic)
Miscellaneous (chloral hydrate, cisapride,* lidoflazine, prenylamine, probucol, terodiline)

....

*Especially when given with macrolide antibiotics, antifungals, such as fluconazole or ketoconazole, and HIV (human immunodeficiency virus) protease inhibitors, such as indinavir or ritonavir.

to consider drug-induced torsades in any patient with runs of polymorphic VT and a prolonged QT interval. When such episodes are correctly identified, appropriate treatment may prevent a cardiac arrest. Initial therapy involves discontinuation of precipitating agents and correction of electrolyte and metabolic abnormalities. When an arrest has occurred, direct cardioversion is at least transiently effective. An intravenous bolus of magnesium may have stabilizing effects during resuscitation or long runs of polymorphic VT. Because acquired torsades is predominantly bradycardia or pause dependent, interventions also aim to increase heart rate. Isoproterenol infusion at doses of 2 to 10 μg/min is a readily available method of increasing sinus rate but can be potentially hazardous in patients with CAD and left ventricular dysfunction. Temporary pacing (both atrial and ventricular) is an effective method, but its use is dependent on availability of trained personnel. Atropine can be used as third-line management when other treatment modalities are unavailable.

In contrast, first-line therapy for patients with congenital long QT is with beta blockers, titrated to the maximum tolerated dosage. Beta blockers also serve to blunt the sympathetic response, which can trigger an episode of torsades. It is critical to avoid any medications that can further prolong the QT interval and precipitate episodes of tachycardia. Some patients, particularly resuscitated sudden death survivors, require ICDs.

SPECIAL CONSIDERATIONS

Ventricular Fibrillation

Ventricular fibrillation in the ICU setting may occur either in patients with underlying heart disease, particularly ischemic heart disease, or as the end result of profound hypoxemia, acidosis, electrolyte derangements, and hypotension from noncardiac causes. In these latter situations, ultimate recovery depends on adequate oxygenation, tissue perfusion, and resolution of underlying disease. Successful resuscitation depends on prompt defibrillation, and several high-energy defibrillation attempts may be necessary. Boluses of epinephrine and lidocaine may aid in resuscitation attempts when repeated defibrillation attempts are initially unsuccessful (see Appendix E for ACLS algorithms).

Digoxin Toxicity

Digoxin is a commonly prescribed drug in patients with left ventricular dysfunction and atrial arrhythmias, but toxic levels can be life threatening. Unfortunately, the first signs and symptoms of digoxin toxicity are easily overlooked. The extracardiac manifestations are relatively nonspecific: fatigue, anorexia, nausea, headache, confusion, and visual symptoms. Factors associated with increased risk for toxicity include renal insufficiency, electrolyte derangements (especially hypokalemia and hypomagnesemia), advanced pulmonary disease, and concomitant treatment with agents that increase serum digoxin levels such as quinidine or amiodarone. Patients receiving digoxin in the ICU are clearly at increased risk for toxic side effects.

Digoxin affects all types of cardiac tissue. Typically, in sinus rhythm, digoxin at therapeutic levels can slow the heart rate through decreased adrenergic tone without significant effects on atrial tissue. At toxic levels, however, it can increase automaticity of atrial tissue, resulting in atrial tachycardia with upright P waves in the inferior limb leads and V_1. Toxic levels may also result in increased automaticity of AV junctional tissue, resulting in a junctional tachycardia (see Table 31–2). When there is underlying atrial fibrillation, this junctional tachycardia results in a paradoxical regularization of RR intervals. AV conduction is slowed by digoxin, however, and may result in advanced AV block at toxic levels (see Chapter 30). Digoxin toxicity should be suspected whenever the combination of increased automaticity and depressed AV conduction is observed. Digoxin also affects ventricular tissue, primarily through enhanced automaticity and triggered activity. The most common manifestation is frequent ventricular premature beats. Sustained bidirectional VT and fascicular tachycardia (Fig. 31–10) are highly sensitive markers of digoxin toxicity.

Effective treatment of digoxin toxicity depends on prompt recognition. When the manifestations do not result in hemodynamic consequences, drug withdrawal and electrolyte correction suffice. VT, however, demands more aggressive management. F(ab) fragments of digoxin-specific antibodies are the treatment of choice for life-threatening digoxin toxic rhythms. Most patients show some response within 20 minutes after their infusion. Their most prominent adverse effect is the rapid development of hypokalemia, presumably due to sodium pump reactivation. When Fab fragments are unavailable or an immediate response is required for VT, the most useful drugs are lidocaine and phenytoin, both of which have little effect on AV conduction. Beta blockers can further depress AV conduction but may

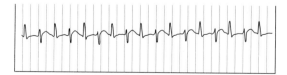

Figure 31–10. Bidirectional ventricular tachycardia in the setting of digoxin toxicity. The alternating morphologies reflect the alternating foci of the left posterior fascicle and the left anterior fascicle.

prove effective in reducing automaticity. Overdrive pacing can result in tachycardia acceleration and should not be attempted.

Tachycardias That Do Not Require Immediate Intervention

Not all tachycardias require immediate intervention. It is not unusual to observe self-limited paroxysms of tachycardia that are not hemodynamically significant in the ICU. Patients with pulmonary or cardiac disease, for example, may have paroxysms of atrial tachycardia that are entirely asymptomatic. Suppression of such self-limited episodes with antiarrhythmic agents may cause significant side effects and is not indicated. Nonsustained VT is also common in patients with cardiac disease. Although nonsustained VT is a marker of risk for sudden death and may require further evaluation, suppression of self-limited ventricular ectopy is not indicated. In fact, suppression of ventricular ectopy with antiarrhythmic medications may be associated with increased mortality.

Postoperative Cardiac Patients

Patients experience a variety of atrial and ventricular tachyarrhythmias after open-heart surgery, typically within the first 72 postoperative hours. Inflammation of the pericardium and trauma to the atria during surgery, plus digitalis toxicity, may precipitate atrial fibrillation, flutter, and atrial tachycardias. AV junctional tachycardia occurs frequently secondary to trauma during surgery. When the type of SVT is not clear, recordings from the temporary epicardial wires can help identify atrial activity and clarify the AV relationship. Atrial wires also permit overdrive pacing of atrial flutter, atrial tachycardia, and junctional tachycardias.

Because most arrhythmias in the immediate postoperative period are exacerbated by high sympathetic tone, a beta blocker is the logical first-line agent in patients without contraindications. Prophylactic use of beta blockers has been shown to decrease the incidence of postoperative SVT. Although it is still frequently used, digoxin poorly controls ventricular response to atrial arrhythmias. Circulating catecholamines overwhelm its vagomimetic effects, and the large doses that are necessary to achieve adequate control often result in toxic levels.

Nonsustained VT also occurs postoperatively in up to 50% of cardiac surgery patients. Typically, it occurs within the first 12 to 24 hours and is limited to short runs. Electrolyte disturbances, perioperative myocardial ischemia, and beta blocker withdrawal can increase the frequency of the VT. Correction of precipitating causes is the mainstay of therapy for nonsustained VT. In contrast, sustained VT or long runs of nonsustained VT that are hemodynamically significant require further evaluation and management. Standard cardioversion and antiarrhythmic therapy as discussed earlier can be used acutely. Temporary ventricular pacing wires may be used to overdrive pace VT, but there is always a risk of accelerating the tachycardia and precipitating VF.

Implantable Cardioverter-Defibrillators

ICD technology has rapidly evolved. Today, the devices are smaller in size, easier to implant, and associated with a reduced operative morbidity and mortality. Likewise, the indications for implantation are expanding with increasing numbers of patients receiving them. The majority of patients with an ICD have underlying heart disease as well as a host of comorbid conditions, any of which may result in an ICU admission. There are some important basic facts to remember when caring for these patients in an acute setting. First, the presence of an ICD does not preclude external defibrillation. If a patient has a hemodynamically unstable tachycardia and the ICD is not effectively terminating it, one should not hesitate to perform standard external defibrillation. Likewise, if a patient requires it, one should not hesitate to perform cardiopulmonary resuscitation. Touching the patient while the device is charging or delivering a shock results only in a buzzlike sensation. One will *not* be shocked.

Inappropriate, and possibly incessant, device discharges for sinus tachycardia, SVT, or even well-tolerated VT may also be encountered. Current ICDs recognize ventricular rate only and cannot discriminate between an SVT and a VT. In the event that the ICD is delivering inappropriate shocks, placing a magnet over the generator can temporarily disable it. Newer-generation ICDs are deactivated only while the magnet remains in position over the generator. Securing a magnet over the ICD may also be used in the operating suite if a patient requires emergency surgery. The device must be inactivated before electrocautery (and electromyographic studies) to avoid spurious discharges. Finally, patients with an ICD should not undergo magnetic resonance studies.

BIBLIOGRAPHY

Buxton AE, Marchlinski FE, Doherty JU, et al: Hazards of intravenous verapamil for sustained ventricular tachycardia. Am J Cardiol 59:1107–1110, 1987.
Emphasizes the danger of using verapamil in the setting of a wide complex tachycardia of unknown etiology.

Desai AD, Chun S, Sung RJ: The role of intravenous amiodarone in the management of cardiac arrhythmias. Ann Intern Med 127:294–303, 1997.
This is a review of the electropharmacology, clinical applications, side effects, and hemodynamic profile of intravenous amiodarone.

Drew B, Scheinman M: ECG criteria to distinguish between aberrantly conducted supraventricular tachycardia and ventricular tachycardia. Practical aspects for the immediate care setting. PACE 18:2194–2208, 1995.
A practical algorithm for approaching the differential diagnosis of a wide QRS complex tachycardia.

El-Sherif N, Beheit S, Henkin R: Quinidine-induced long QTU interval and torsades de pointes. Role of bradycardia-dependent early afterdepolarizations. J Am Coll Cardiol 14:252–257, 1989.
A case report that illustrates the pathophysiology underlying quinidine-induced torsades de pointes.

Josephson M, Wellens HJJ: Differential diagnosis of supraventricular tachycardia. Cardiol Clin 8:411–442, 1990.
A very clear and thorough discussion of the electrocardiographic criteria and differential diagnosis for the various mechanisms of supraventricular tachycardias. Replete with figures and tracings. Highly recommended.

Kelly R, Smith T: Recognition and management of digitalis toxicity. Am J Cardiol 69:108–119, 1992.
An excellent overview of the manifestations and treatment of digitalis toxicity.

Kindwall KE, Brown J, Josephson M: Electrocardiographic criteria for ventricular tachycardia in wide complex left bundle branch block morphology tachycardia. Am J Cardiol 61:1279–1283, 1988.
Recommended as additional reading for those interested in furthering their ability to diagnose a wide complex tachycardia with a left bundle branch block morphology.

Lerman BB, Belardinelli L: Cardiac electrophysiology of adenosine. Basic and clinical concepts. Circulation 83:1499–1509, 1991.
A review of adenosine's pharmacokinetics, spectrum of electrophysiologic effects, therapeutic uses, and role as a diagnostic tool.

Stanton MS, Prystowsky EN, Fineberg NS, et al: Arrhythmogenic effects of antiarrhythmic drugs. A study of 506 patients treated for ventricular tachycardia or fibrillation. J Am Coll Cardiol 14:209–215, 1989.
This is a clinical study of proarrhythmic effects of antiarrhythmic drugs.

Zipes DP: Specific arrhythmias. Diagnosis and treatment. In: Braunwald E (ed): Heart Disease: A Textbook of Cardiovascular Medicine. Philadelphia, WB Saunders, 1992, pp 667–725.
A comprehensive textbook chapter that covers tachyarrhythmias and their management in a well-organized format.

32 Barotrauma and Chest Tubes

Lori J. Morgan
Michael B. Shapiro

Barotrauma is defined as iatrogenic lung injury due to mechanical ventilation. Usually resulting from high alveolar pressures due to large tidal volumes or dynamic hyperinflation (see Chapters 2 and 74), it is manifested as extra-alveolar gas. Barotrauma complicates mechanical ventilation in up to 40% of patients, depending on the population studied. Its clinical effects can vary from trivial to lethal.

MANIFESTATIONS OF EXTRA-ALVEOLAR GAS

Barotrauma results from overdistention and rupture of alveoli. A pressure gradient at the common border of the vascular sheath and the alveolar base causes alveolar rupture (Fig. 32–1). Once the peribronchiolar sheath is disrupted, air can dissect along any plane and result in a variety of clinical manifestations (Table 32–1).

Pulmonary interstitial emphysema, subpleural air cysts, and *subcutaneous emphysema* are benign conditions usually requiring no specific therapy. They indicate, however, that alveolar disruption with an air leak has occurred and that the patient is at risk for progression to the more serious conditions. Progression in some patients may be avoided by decreasing alveolar pressure or tidal volume or both. Prophylactic insertion of chest tubes is generally *not* recommended because their risks generally outweigh their benefits.

Although pneumomediastinum and pneumopericaridium are also usually benign, they can cause severe hemodynamic instability and, thus, require close monitoring. If persistent cardiovascular instability develops, pericardiocentesis or other drainage of the pericardial air may be necessary. *Pneumoperitoneum* and *pneumoretroperitoneum* from extra-alveolar gas leakage are likewise usually benign, but it is

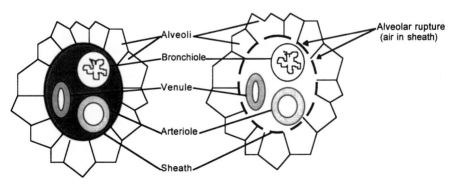

Figure 32–1. Schematic diagram of the alveoli and peribronchiolar sheath: intact and ruptured. Once an alveolus is ruptured, air can dissect along any of the structures. (Adapted from Maunder RJ, Pearson DJ, Hudson LD: Subcutaneous and mediastinal emphysema. Arch Int Med 144: 1447, 1984.)

Table 32–1. Spectrum of Clinical Manifestations of Extra-alveolar Gas

Benign end of spectrum	Pneumoperitoneum
Pulmonary interstitial emphysema	Pneumoretroperitoneum
Subpleural air cysts	Pneumothorax
Subcutaneous emphysema	Tension pneumothorax
Pneumomediastinum	Systemic gas embolization
Pneumopericardium	*Life-threatening end of spectrum*

essential to establish that the air is not from an intra-abdominal source. In a critically ill patient, this may necessitate an abdominal computed tomographic scan or even an exploratory laparotomy.

Most simple pneumothoraces (including small ones) occurring in patients receiving positive-pressure ventilation should be treated with immediate tube thoracostomy. Even a small or localized pneumothorax can impair ventilation and oxygenation and compromise the patient's hemodynamic status. It can also develop rapidly into a tension pneumothorax.

A *tension pneumothorax* is one of the most serious complications of mechanical ventilation; if untreated, it can be life-threatening. If one is suspected and the patient is hemodynamically unstable, treatment including tube thoracostomy should proceed *without* prior confirmation by a chest radiograph. The hallmarks of a tension pneumothorax are rapid deterioration in gas exchange and hemodynamic instability. Peak inspiratory pressures and "plateau" (end-inspiratory) pressures increase (see Chapters 2 and 48). The patient becomes progressively more difficult to ventilate as the volume of air in the pleural space increases.

If suspected, a tension pneumothorax can be decompressed initially with a 14-gauge catheter-over-a-needle. This catheter-over-a-needle is placed through the chest wall anteriorly in the midclavicular line at the second intercostal space. If breath sounds are diminished on one side relative to the other, that hemithorax should be decompressed first. If there is no improvement or if no rush of air is appreciated, the other hemithorax is also decompressed. The needles are removed and the catheters are held firmly in position (usually attached to a saline-filled syringe that acts as a water seal) until tube thoracostomy (required after needle decompression) is performed.

Systemic gas embolization is another potentially lethal manifestation of alveolar rupture. This is primarily described in the neonatal population but can occur in any patient and cause cerebral infarction, seizures, or myocardial injury.

Barotrauma can also cause more general damage to lung parenchyma called *diffuse lung injury* (some refer to this as *volutrauma* because the damage is due to alveolar overinflation and not the applied pressure per se). In animal models, diffuse lung injury is manifested by the development of noncardiogenic pulmonary edema after ventilation with high peak inspiratory pressures or excessive tidal volumes. It is thought to result from overdistention of alveoli, injury to the alveolar-capillary basement membrane, and a consequent increase in microvascular permeability. Mechanical ventilation at high pressures also decreases surfactant production and function. The changes in surfactant and the development of pulmonary edema result in decreased lung compliance. This makes the lung more susceptible to barotrauma and can lead to a cycle of more severe lung injury.

The clinical relevance of the results of these animal experiments remains to be established. Likewise, the thresholds and conditions for the occurrence of this type of barotrauma actually to occur in ventilated patients, particularly those who already have stiff lungs, such as acute respiratory distress syndrome, remain incompletely defined (see Chapter 73).

CHEST TUBE SELECTION, INSERTION, AND MANAGEMENT

Selecting a Chest Tube for Different Indications

Chest tube placement is generally a straightforward and safe procedure when performed for the proper indications and with careful preparation. Although there are many indications for chest tube placement in the intensive care unit (ICU) (Table 32–2), pneumothorax is the most common. The indication for the chest tube and the size of the patient determines the size and placement location of the tube. For average-sized adults, a 36 French (Fr) chest tube is standard. This is a good choice for draining both air and fluid. If one is draining a hemothorax, the smallest tube that one should use is 36 Fr, with a 40 Fr tube preferable. If the goal is to drain a pneumothorax only, a 20 Fr tube is adequate. If it is a spontaneous pneumothorax, a 16 Fr anterior chest tube may be sufficient.

Insertion Technique

Chest tube placement is usually well tolerated by patients with proper preparation. The patient is placed supine and should always be pretreated with sedation and opioids unless hemodynamically unstable. The ipsilateral arm is raised over the patient's head or abducted away from the body (e.g., in cases of recent upper arm fracture or shoulder dislocation). If the patient has large breasts, the breast near the insertion site should be pulled to the contralateral side and taped into position to reduce the amount of tissue over the thoracostomy site. The procedure is performed in a sterile manner with the operator wearing a cap, gown, mask, and sterile gloves. The chest is prepared and draped in a sterile manner from midline

Table 32–2. Indications for Tube Thoracostomy in the Intensive Care Unit

Pneumothorax	Bronchopleural fistula
Barotrauma	Chylothorax
Iatrogenic	Empyema
Spontaneous	Penetrating chest injury
Traumatic	Postoperative thoracotomy
Hemothorax	After needle decompression
Iatrogenic	Prophylactic (in patients with rib fractures prior
Traumatic	to starting positive-pressure ventilation)
Hydrothorax	
Malignant	
Sympathetic	

to the bed sheets and clavicles to umbilicus, including the axilla. The nipple should be draped into the field if possible because it is a good landmark for the location of the fifth intercostal space.

Once prepared and draped, a local anesthetic is injected into the skin and subcutaneous tissue at the fifth intercostal space in the anterior axillary line. A 2-inch skin incision is made over the sixth rib (a larger skin incision may be necessary in obese patients). This is carried through the subcutaneous tissue either with scissors or a scalpel down to the level of the rib. More anesthesia may be required as the dissection proceeds. Hugging the top of the rib, one then inserts a hemostat through the intercostal muscles and gently spreads to form the insertion tract. A finger is placed through this tract into the chest and is gently swept around the thoracic cage to push the lung away and free up any adhesions. The chest tube is then pushed through the tract, generally aiming superiorly and posteriorly. All the drainage ports on the tube must be within the thorax for proper function, but a tube should not be forced into the chest against resistance. If there is resistance, the tube is withdrawn and redirected. Because the tips of chest tubes are especially rounded to prevent lung injury, cutting the distal ends of chest tubes places the patient at higher risk for lung laceration and is not recommended.

When the tube seems to be located in a good intrathoracic position, it should be attached to a drainage system (see further on) and sutured into position with heavy suture. Dressings are applied and all connections of the tubing are secured with tape. A chest radiograph is then obtained to evaluate tube placement and its therapeutic effect. Chest tubes that are kinked but functioning should be repositioned only if this can be performed without pulling the ports extrathoracically. Chest tubes that are not functioning must be repositioned or replaced. If there are ports outside the thoracic cavity, the tube needs to be replaced and should not simply be pushed in further.

Complications of chest tube placement occur commonly and range from bleeding to infection (Table 32–3). Most are easily treated but can be problematic if unrecognized or not corrected properly.

Drainage Systems

Three-Bottle System

Immediately after placement, chest tubes are attached to a drainage apparatus. Classically, a three-bottle system or its equivalent is used (Fig. 32–2A). With this

Table 32–3. Complications of Tube Thoracostomy

Hemorrhage (due to laceration of intercostal artery, muscle, or vein)
Lacerated lung
Bronchopleural fistula
Cardiac injury
Subcutaneous tube placement
Intraperitoneal placement (with or without hepatic or splenic injury)
Infection (cellulitis, empyema)
Allergic reactions (from local anesthetics, skin preparation, or tape)
Damage to intercostal nerve

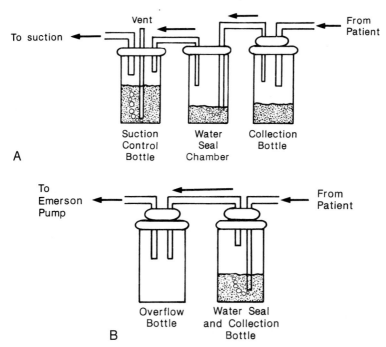

Figure 32–2. *A,* Classic three-bottle chest evacuation system (see text for description). The depth of the "vent" tube in the suction control bottle determines the negative pressure exerted on the water seal chamber and collection bottle. The fluid in the collection bottle comes from the chest tube; the fluid in the other two bottles is supplied by the operator. Arrows indicate flow of gas through tubing from patient to suction source. Bubbles in the water seal bottle indicate an air leak proximal to that bottle (i.e., in the connecting tubing, chest tube, or a bronchopleural fistula). Bubbles from the vent tube in the suction control bottle indicate that there is suction being applied to the system. *B,* Two-bottle system (using Emerson pump). When setting up the system, the operator puts some fluid in the water seal and collection bottle to establish a water seal; to this is added fluid draining from the chest tube. Excess fluid is suctioned into the overflow bottle. (Arrows as in 2A).

system, the chest tube drains into a collection chamber that is marked for accurate recording of its output.

The collection chamber is connected in series to a water seal chamber. This second chamber has several functions. First, it serves as a one-way valve for air to exit from the pleural space. It also can be used as a manometer to measure the amount of negative pressure in the chest cavity. Additionally, it is the location that one should examine for an air leak and patency of the chest tube. Air leaks are seen as a stream of bubbles in the chamber that increases when intrathoracic pressure rises such as during a cough, performing a Valsalva maneuver, or getting positive-pressure breath from a mechanical ventilator. Continuous air leaks indicate a large rent in the lung parenchyma, a bronchopleural fistula, or a leak from the apparatus (usually due to a loose connection). Patency of a chest tube is evaluated with the tube on water seal (suction off). A patent tube demonstrates fluctuations in the water seal chamber fluid level with respirations ("tidaling"). A nonpatent tube should be removed because it serves no purpose and carries a risk of infection.

The water seal chamber is attached in series to the suction control bottle. The amount of water in the suction control bottle determines the amount of negative pressure in the pleural space. This is most commonly set at -20 cm H_2O as a start. The suction bottle is vented to the atmosphere to prevent the transmission of excessive negative pressure to the pleural space. An increase in wall suction makes the suction chamber bubble more briskly but does not increase the negative pressure transmitted to the pleural space. The increase in bubbling actually increases evaporation in this chamber and eventually results in a decrease in the transmitted pressure.

Pleuravac

Most institutions now use some type of disposable one-piece plastic apparatus, for example, a Pleuravac, for the initial drainage of chest tubes. These are designed to approximate the three-bottle technique. The collection and water seal chambers are in a compact form, and the suction chamber is usually controlled with a valve instead of water. The principle of the three-bottle method remains the same, but the apparatus is more portable with fewer and more secure tubing connections.

Emerson Pump

There is also a two-bottle system, for example, an Emerson pump (Fig. 32–2B). This is typically used when a high negative pleural pressure is required. It can deliver the equivalent of 60 cm H_2O or more of suction. This two-bottle system uses the first bottle as both water seal and collection bottle. The second bottle is generally not used as a suction control bottle but rather as an overflow bottle. It is hooked to the pump and the desired amount of negative pressure is set on the pump itself. Emerson pumps are usually used only after lower levels of suction have failed to evacuate the chest. This may be seen with empyemas or large air leaks.

Heimlich Valve

Another option for drainage of the chest cavity is the Heimlich valve. This is almost exclusively used to treat patients with pneumothoraces that are amenable to outpatient treatment. Their most common use is for spontaneous pneumothorax. A small chest tube (14 to 16 Fr) is inserted and attached to the device, which consists of a one-way flutter valve encased in a clear plastic cover. The "one-way" valve allows the egress of air while preventing its influx. It is appropriate only for drainage of a pneumothorax. If there is any fluid to be drained from the chest cavity, a standard drainage system must be used.

Monitoring Chest Tubes

Once chest tubes are in position, they should be monitored carefully to ensure that they are working properly and achieving the desired therapeutic end. The presence or absence of an air leak and the character of the fluid and the amount drained per day are assessed. The tube site must also be monitored for local cellulitis. The position of the chest tube, the fluid content of the pleural space, and the expansion of the lung should be followed by regular chest radiographs. Chest tube function

Table 32–4. Troubleshooting Chest Tube Problems

PROBLEM	CAUSE	INTERVENTION
Lung not re-expanded	Subcutaneous tube	Remove tube and place new tube in proper position
	Intraperitoneal tube	Remove tube and place new tube in proper position; assess for intra-abdominal injury
	Side port of tube is subcutaneous	Remove tube and place new tube in proper position
	Plugged tube	Remove tube and place new tube in proper position
	Plugged bronchus	Bronchoscopy
	Large air leak	Check all connections; increase suction; consider Emerson pump; place second chest tube
	Entrapped lung secondary to empyema	Operative decortication
Fluid in chest not drained	Tube located too high	Place second chest tube closer to the diaphragm and posteriorly
	Clotted hemothorax	Operative debridement
	Loculated fluid	Computed tomography–guided placement of new tube or operative drainage
	Fluid too thick (empyema)	Emerson pump or operative drainage
Continuous air leak	Large parenchymal leak	Place second tube; evaluate for bronchial injury
	Side port of tube is subcutaneous	Remove tube and place new tube in proper position
	System leak	Tighten all tubing connections; replace leaking tube
	Bronchopleural fistula	Decrease ventilator pressures; operative intervention; use Emerson pump
Water seal chamber not "tidaling"	Chest tube is clotted or kinked	Replace tube
	Lung is fully re-expanded	Remove tube
	Tube is on suction	Remove suction temporarily
	High PEEP on ventilator	Decrease PEEP if possible (Note: Problem may be a nonfunctional tube instead of high PEEP)

PEEP, positive end-expiratory pressure.

should be continuously monitored for problems, which, if they arise, should be addressed appropriately (Table 32–4).

Removing a Chest Tube

When to remove a chest tube is often a complex decision based on objective data combined with the experience of the management team. In general, before chest tube removal is entertained, *all* the following criteria should be met:

1. The fluid draining from the chest is less than 100 to 150 mL/day.

2. The lung is seen to be fully re-expanded on chest radiograph.
3. No air leak is noted in the water seal chamber.

Chest tubes are usually removed in a two-step process. First, the chest tube is taken off suction, that is, the tube is placed "on water seal" (after there is no active air leak while on suction). In the absence of an air leak, the water seal chamber maintains negative intrathoracic pressure. However, if an air leak occurs, it provides a one-way valve to prevent a tension pneumothorax. After the patient's chest tube is on water seal for 6 to 24 hours without a recurrent pneumothorax, it is generally safe to remove the tube. If the patient experiences hemodynamic or respiratory instability while on water seal, the tube should immediately be placed back on suction.

Another technique to evaluate how well a patient will tolerate the removal of a chest tube is to clamp the tube. This maneuver is considered riskier than the water seal method because there is no safety mechanism automatically available for decompression of the chest if a tension pneumothorax develops. Thus, this method should be used only if medical personnel who understand the potential danger of clamping the tube are immediately available to unclamp the tube if hemodynamic or respiratory instability occurs.

If the trial of being on water seal (or clamping) is tolerated by the patient, the chest tube can be removed. The key to safe chest tube removal is to have all the necessary supplies at hand for tube removal. The procedure is explained and the patient is usually premedicated with opioids and sedatives. The patient is placed in a supine position with the arm over the head or abducted. All tube dressings are removed. One should prepare a dressing of petrolatum gauze under a 4 × 4 inch gauze pad or use the backing from a thick hydrocolloid (DuoDerm) 4 × 4 inch square. One should note if a pursestring suture was placed at the time of chest tube insertion in order to use it to close the skin after removal of the tube. After ensuring that the chest tube is not on suction, one should cut the chest tube sutures. The patient is instructed to inhale deeply and hold his or her breath and then the chest tube is pulled out of the chest in a rapid, smooth motion. As the tube is removed, the dressing of choice is used to cover the wound quickly. If a pursestring suture is present, it should be tied first and the dressing then applied. Finally, a chest radiograph is obtained to ensure that a pneumothorax did not occur from air entry into the pleural space via the chest tube path during chest tube removal.

The preceding technique is used for chest tubes placed to remove air, fluid, or blood from the chest cavity. One manages tubes placed for drainage of an empyema ("empyema tubes") differently. These tubes are left in position for a long time while the patient is treated with antibiotics. After the pleural cavity is drained of purulent material, the empyema evolves into an abscess cavity that gradually heals by granulation. The chest tubes are left in the chest with their tips in this cavity and are disconnected from the suction and drainage system. They are cut close to the skin and a bag is placed over the tubes to collect any ongoing drainage. The tubes are gradually backed out of the chest over a period of weeks to months. If they are removed abruptly, their tracks may form new undrained, localized collections of pus.

BIBLIOGRAPHY

Jantz M, Pierson D. Pneumothorax and barotrauma. Clin Chest Med 15:75–91, 1994.
This article presents a discussion of the causes of pneumothorax and barotrauma.

Kirby T, Ginsberg R: Management of the pneumothorax and barotrauma. Clin Chest Med 13:97–112, 1992.
This article presents a review of the causes and complications of pneumothorax and barotrauma.

Macklin MT, Macklin CC: Malignant interstitial emphysema of the lungs and mediastinum as an important occult complication in many respiratory diseases and other conditions: An interpretation of the clinical literature in light of laboratory experiments. Medicine 23:281–358, 1944.
This is the original paper discussing the clinical implications of alveolar rupture and the development of extra-alveolar gas.

Marcy T: Barotrauma: Detection, recognition and management. Chest 104:578–584, 1993.
This is a good review of the manifestations and management of barotrauma.

Parker J, Hernandez L, Peevy K: Mechanisms of ventilator-induced injury. Crit Care Med 21:131–143, 1993.
This article presents a review of the causes of barotrauma and a definition of the primary risk factors for its development.

Schnapp L, Chin D, Szaflarski N, Matthay M: Frequency and importance of barotrauma in 100 patients with acute lung injury. Crit Care Med 23:272–278, 1995.
This is a report on the frequency of barotrauma in patients with acute respiratory distress syndrome.

Quigley R: Thoracentesis and chest tube drainage. Crit Care Clin 11:111–126, 1995.
This is a review of the indications and procedure for chest tube placement.

33 Change in Mental Status or New-Onset Seizures

James W. Teener
Eric C. Raps

Changes in mental status or new-onset seizures are common reasons for neurologic consultation in the intensive care unit (ICU). Although each has a broad differential diagnosis, the cause can usually be determined by applying a systematic diagnostic approach to the problem.

CHANGES IN MENTAL STATUS

Changes in mental status range in severity from mild confusion to coma. Alterations in consciousness can arise by two mechanisms: (1) disruption of function in the brainstem reticular activating system or, more commonly, (2) through processes affecting both cerebral hemispheres. Severe dysfunction produces *coma* defined as an unresponsive and unarousable state. Less severe dysfunction produces an acute confusional state in which the patient may be sleepy, disoriented, or inattentive but responds to some stimuli in a purposeful manner. This acute confusional state encompasses changes in mental status: acute delirium, acute encephalopathy, obtundation, lethargy, or psychosis. The term *delirium* refers to a floridly abnormal mental state, often with visual hallucinations or agitation (see also the "ICU Syndrome" in Chapter 44).

Differential Diagnosis

Acute confusional states must be differentiated from dementia, aphasia, or psychiatric decompensation. An acute confusional state lasts for hours to days; in contrast, *dementia* has a much longer time course and is associated with fewer fluctuations in attention and perception. *Aphasia* can be detected by careful examination of language function. *Psychiatric conditions* that can mimic an acute confusional state include schizophrenia, depression, mania, autism, and dissociative states. *Seizures* can also produce a confusional state during the period of actual epileptic discharge or for minutes to hours during the immediate postictal period.

Causes of acute confusional states are numerous (Table 33–1). Indeed, almost any severe medical or surgical illness may cause delirium in a patient in the ICU, and many such patients have more than one risk factor (Table 33–2). In younger patients, drug abuse and alcohol withdrawal are the most common causes; in contrast, in the elderly, metabolic disturbances, infection, stroke, and iatrogenic drug effects predominate.

Metabolic Disturbances

Because many of these disorders are potentially life-threatening or may cause permanent damage, their early identification is critical. Laboratory screening tests

389

Table 33–1. Differential Diagnosis: Acute Confusional States in Patients in the Intensive Care Unit

Electrolyte Disorders

Hypo-, hypernatremia
Hypo-, hypercalcemia
Hypo-, hyperphosphatemia
Hypermagnesemia

Endocrine and Metabolic Disorders

Hypo-, hyperglycemia
Hypo-, hyperthyroidism
Wernicke encephalopathy

Neurologic Disorders

Seizure-related
  Ictal
  Interictal state
  Complex partial status
  Postictal state
  Medication effects
Strokes
  Any location for first 48 h
Strokes in specific locations
  Right parietal
  Bilateral occipital
  Septal region
  Cingulate gyrus
Other vascular disorders
  Hypertensive encephalopathy
  Vasculitis
  Subarachnoid hemorrhage
Other neurologic causes
  Intracranial hemorrhage
  Acute hydrocephalus
  Demyelinating disease
  Paraneoplastic disorders

Drug Related

Ethanol withdrawal
Sedative effect or withdrawal
Opioids (systemic or perispinal)

Anticholinergic agents
Sympathomimetic (cocaine) withdrawal
Corticosteroids
Lidocaine toxicity
Digitalis
Antiarrhythmic agents (procainamide, quinidine)

Nosocomial Infections

Bacterial meningitis (*Listeria*)
Fungal meningitis (*Candida*)
Severe sepsis or septic shock
Systemic inflammatory response (with urinary tract infection; pneumonia)
High fever of any cause

Organ System Failure

Hepatic encephalopathy
Uremia
Dialysis disequilibrium syndrome
Acute hypercapnia
Hypoxemia

Perioperative Causes

Hypoxemia
Hypotension
Psychological stress
Residual anesthesia effects

Miscellaneous

Hypo-, hyperthermia
Circulatory shock or other low cardiac output states
Major bone fractures (with fat emboli syndrome)
ICU syndrome (see Chapter 44)
Blood dyscrasias
  Thrombotic thrombocytopenic purpura
  Disseminated intravascular coagulation

Table 33–2. Risk Factors for the Development of Delirium in the Intensive Care Unit

Dementia
Advanced age
Severe illness
Visual impairment
Dehydration
Electrolyte changes (see Table 33–1)
Malnutrition

Trauma
Drug effects (see Table 33–1)
Infection (see Table 33–1)
Hip or other major bone fractures
Loss of circadian clues (day-night)
Sleep deprivation (see Chapter 44)
Sleep fragmentation (see Chapter 44)

identify most metabolic disturbances. Although the actual level of an electrolyte may be found to be abnormal, rapid changes in electrolyte levels may also cause delirium or a change in mental status. Organ failure, particularly liver and kidney failure, is a frequent cause of confusion. Endocrine dysfunction may also cause delirium, frequently accompanied by prominent affective symptoms. Many toxins also produce metabolic disturbances and delirium. The most important nutritional metabolic disturbance is *thiamine deficiency.* Thiamine must be given prophylactically to alcoholics to prevent precipitating Wernicke encephalopathy with the administration of glucose.

Drugs

Drug intoxication and withdrawal commonly cause delirium and other acute confusional states. Drugs work in an additive fashion, and a combination of medications may result in an acute confusional state when an individual drug alone would not. Drugs with anticholinergic properties, including over-the-counter cold preparations, antihistamines, tricyclic antidepressants, and neuroleptic agents, are frequent offenders. Other important medications to consider include sedatives and hypnotics, opioids, and H_2-histamine receptor blockers. High-dose corticosteroids may induce an acute toxic psychosis.

Many drugs, including barbiturates, benzodiazepines, sedatives and hypnotics, amphetamines, cocaine, and alcohol can induce drug withdrawal syndromes. The classic alcohol withdrawal syndrome, delirium tremens, begins 72 to 96 hours after alcohol withdrawal. It is characterized by profound agitation, tremulousness, diaphoresis, tachycardia, fever, and visual hallucinations.

Infections

Systemic infections as well as infections involving the central nervous system frequently produce a change in mental status. The main offenders in patients in the ICU are urinary tract infections, pneumonia, and intravenous catheter–associated bacteremias. Nosocomial central nervous system infections, such as those caused by *Listeria monocytogenes* or fungi, should be considered in the setting of immunosuppression.

Strokes

Any acute stroke may transiently result in confusion, which typically clears within 48 hours. Strokes involving the right middle cerebral artery distribution, however, often cause prolonged changes in mental status. This has also been reported after infarcts in the posterior cerebral artery distribution that cause either bilateral or left-sided occipitotemporal lesions, as well as with lesions of the anterior cingulate gyrus and septal regions. These lesions may occur after anterior communicating artery aneurysm repair or rupture. Other cerebrovascular causes include hypertensive encephalopathy, subarachnoid hemorrhage, and central nervous system vasculitis.

Seizures

Both seizures and their treatment are potential causes of changes in mental status. After generalized or complex partial seizures, patients often are confused for minutes to hours. Occasionally, patients in nonconvulsive status epilepticus may appear confused without other seizure manifestations. Many anticonvulsant medications can also induce changes in mental status because of their sedative properties.

Perioperative Causes

Patients recovering from surgery often experience acute delirium (see Chapter 83, Table 83–5). There are numerous possible causes, many of which have already been discussed. Additional factors to consider include residual effects of anesthetic agents, perioperative hypoxia or hypotension, psychological stress, and sleep fragmentation or deprivation. Postoperative delirium typically develops around the third postoperative day and lasts several days.

Miscellaneous Causes

Many other disturbances occasionally produce change in mental status. For example, in some studies, 50% of elderly patients admitted with hip fractures experienced delirium, which was likely multifactorial in origin.

The ICU syndrome is a delirium that may result from the multiple stressors in the ICU, including sleep deprivation, immobilization, unfamiliarity, fear, and sensory overstimulation or deprivation (see Chapter 44 for more details).

CLINICAL APPROACH TO CHANGE IN MENTAL STATUS

Diagnostic Evaluation

Diagnosis requires the recognition that a change in mental status has occurred as well as identification of the cause of the confusional state (Fig. 33–1). Since the clinical characteristics of impaired attention, disorganized thinking, fluctuating course, altered level of consciousness, perceptual disturbances, disturbed sleep-wake cycle, altered psychomotor activity, disorientation, and memory impairment are common to all causes of delirium, making the correct diagnosis relies primarily on history, physical examination, and laboratory assessment.

The diagnostic evaluation begins with a careful history. Particular attention should be paid to the presence of risk factors (see Tables 33–1 and 33–2). The history and physical examination may also identify some of the signs and symptoms that may suggest a specific cause for the delirium (Table 33–3). Laboratory studies are often necessary to confirm the cause (see Fig. 33–1).

Two specific tests, the electroencephalogram (EEG) and lumbar puncture, deserve special comment. The EEG is useful not only in identifying specific causes

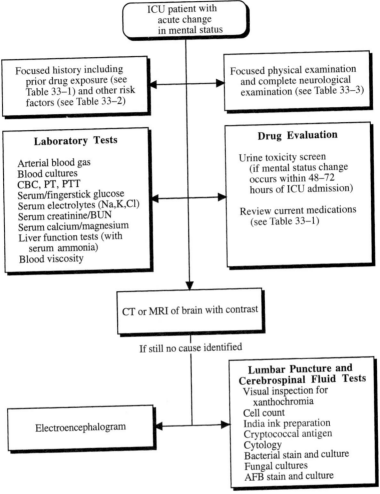

Figure 33–1. Flow diagram illustrating elements of the diagnostic evaluation for an acute change in mental status in a patient in the intensive care unit (ICU) (see text for details). CBC, complete blood count; PT, prothrombin time; PTT, partial thromboplastin time; BUN, blood urea nitrogen; CT, computed tomography; MRI, magnetic resonance imaging; AFB, acid-fast bacilli.

of delirium but also in differentiating delirium from dementia or psychiatric abnormalities. EEG changes are *always* present in delirium. Generalized slowing and disorganization are the most common changes. The degree of slowing correlates with the degree of delirium. Specific electroencephalographic patterns also suggest specific causes. For example, low-voltage fast activity is present in patients who are withdrawing from sedatives or ethanol. Focal slowing, asymmetric delta activity, paroxysmal discharges, or periodic lateralizing epileptiform discharges (PLEDs) suggest a structural lesion. In contrast, triphasic waves may be seen in many metabolic disturbances but most commonly with hepatic or uremic encephalopathy.

Table 33–3. Signs and Symptoms Helpful in Determining Change in Mental Status

SIGN-SYMPTOM	ASSOCIATION
Asterixis	Metabolic encephalopathy
Ataxia	Ethanol or sedative intoxication, Wernicke encephalopathy
Bradycardia	Hypothyroidism, cholinergic drug
Constricted pupils	Opioid intoxication
Dilated pupils	Head trauma, anticholinergic or sympathomimetic drug intoxication, ethanol or sedative withdrawal, postictal state
Fever	Infection, anticholinergic drug intoxication, ethanol withdrawal, neuroleptic malignant syndrome
Headache or meningismus	Meningitis, subarachnoid hemorrhage
Hypertension	Hypertensive encephalopathy, anticholinergic or sympathomimetic drug intoxication, ethanol or sedative withdrawal
Hyperventilation	Central neurogenic hyperventilation, hepatic encephalopathy, hyperglycemia with diabetic ketoacidosis, sepsis, uremia
Hypothermia	Sedative intoxication, hepatic encephalopathy, hypoglycemia, hypothyroidism, sepsis, uremia
Hypoventilation	Sedative or opioid intoxication
Nystagmus or ophthalmoplegia	Ethanol or sedative intoxication, Wernicke encephalopathy, vertebrobasilar ischemia, phenytoin
Papilledema	Hypertensive encephalopathy, intracranial mass, acute hydrocephalus
Rigidity	Neuroleptic malignant syndrome, opioid reaction, dystonic reaction
Seizures	Ethanol or sedative withdrawal, theophylline toxicity, hypoglycemia, severe alkalosis
Tachycardia	Anticholinergic or sympathomimetic drug intoxication, ethanol or sedative withdrawal
Tremor	Sympathomimetic drug intoxication, ethanol or sedative withdrawal, thyrotoxicosis

Lumbar puncture should be performed when the cause of delirium remains uncertain or in patients who have fever, meningismus, or any other feature suggestive of a central nervous system infection. The lumbar puncture should, however, be preceded by a brain imaging study.

Treatment

Once the cause or causes of the change in mental status are identified, attempts should be made to reverse or eliminate them. If the delirium is severe or persistent, however, additional treatments may be needed. In all cases, the sensory environment should be controlled. Sensory overstimulation or deprivation should be avoided by limiting ambient noise and visitation or by providing a radio or television set, eyeglasses, and hearing aid if a hearing disorder is present. The room should include a calendar, clock, family picture, and some personal items. Frequent family visits should be encouraged, and a full-time bedside companion may be needed. A regimen to promote good sleep hygiene should be initiated (see Chapter 44 for more details).

Pharmacologic treatment should be employed only when the patient's behavior is dangerous, interferes with medical care, or causes the patient severe distress (see Chapters 4 and 44). Haloperidol and lorazepam are commonly employed medications. These drugs should be started at the lowest possible dose. Sedatives, such as chloral hydrate, zolpidem, or benzodiazepines, may be useful in promoting a normal sleep-wake cycle. Physical restraints should be avoided as much as possible because they often seem to aggravate the problem.

Prognosis

In general, delirium and other acute confusional states clear when the causative factors are corrected. Even in the elderly, in whom delirium may be prolonged and have residual deficits, it typically lasts only days to weeks. It is likely that improved recognition of delirium and its early treatment will limit sequelae.

NEW-ONSET SEIZURES

A seizure is an alteration of brain function due to excessive or oversynchronized discharges of cerebral neurons. The presence of new-onset seizures implies that the central nervous system has been affected either directly or indirectly by disease.

Diagnostic Evaluation

Many medical and surgical disorders can cause new-onset seizures (Table 33–4). The occurrence of seizures, however, should not be confused with the diagnosis of epilepsy. The latter implies recurrent, spontaneous seizures. Many patients in the ICU have seizures related to metabolic derangements that will not recur if their medical illness is treated. Some patients with epilepsy, however, present with their first seizure during a medical illness.

Abnormal movements that could be confused with seizures may arise in critically ill patients. *Myoclonic jerks* are probably more common than seizures. *Decorticate* or *decerebrate posturing* may rarely be confused with seizure activity. Some movements so closely resemble seizures that neurologic consultation and a formal electroencephalographic evaluation for seizures are indicated.

The evaluation of a patient with new-onset seizures is similar to the evaluation of a patient with an acute confusional state (Fig. 33–2). In critically ill patients, metabolic derangements and withdrawal from chronically used substances, such as alcohol or benzodiazepines, account for nearly two thirds of new-onset seizures.

Table 33–4. Causes of New-Onset Seuzures

Electrolyte and Metabolic Disturbances

Hyponatremia
Hypoglycemia
Hyperglycemia
Hypocalcemia
Hyperosmolar states
Severe acute alkalosis

Organ System Failure

Uremia
Hepatic encephalopathy
Central nervous system vasculitis
Thrombocytopenic purpura

Drugs

Drug overdose (multiple)
Drug withdrawal (alcohol, barbiturates and
  benzodiazepines)
Drug toxicity (meperidine use in renal failure, cyclosporine,
  theophylline)

Neurologic Disorders

Neurosurgical procedures
Idiopathic epilepsy
Head trauma
Stroke
Vascular malformations
Hypertensive encephalopathy
Eclampsia
Global cerebral ischemia (hypoxia)

Infections

Meningitis
Encephalitis
Fever

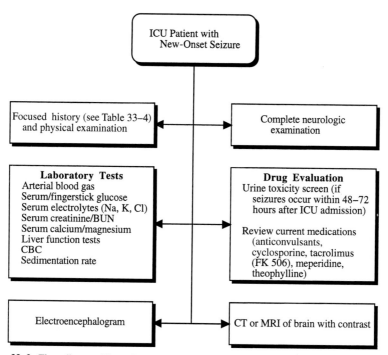

Figure 33–2. Flow diagram illustrating elements of the diagnostic evaluation for new-onset seizures in a patient in the ICU (see text for details). BUN, blood urea nitrogen; CBC, complete blood count; CT, computed tomography; MRI, magnetic resonance imaging.

Hyponatremia is the most frequently identified metabolic derangement. Previously unrecognized structural abnormalities are occasionally identified in patients with new-onset seizures in the ICU. In general, a high-quality computed tomographic scan or, preferably, a magnetic resonance imaging scan of the brain with contrast injection should be performed in every patient with new-onset seizures.

Management

A single seizure need not always be treated with anticonvulsant medication. If no readily correctable underlying cause is identified or numerous seizures occur, however, treatment is indicated. The most common anticonvulsant agents used for new-onset seizures include phenytoin (Dilantin) and carbamazepine (Tegretol).

Phenytoin can be given intravenously or by mouth. If an oral load is used, approximately 1000 mg should be given in two to four divided doses over 12 to 24 hours. An intravenous load consists of 18 mg/kg infused intravenously at a rate not exceeding 50 mg/min. Hypotension is a frequent complication and blood pressure should be monitored continuously during the infusion. Typical maintenance doses of phenytoin are 300 to 400 mg per day. The daily dose of phenytoin intravenously should be given every 8 hours in equal amounts. If given orally, a single daily dose can be used. If phenytoin is given by feeding tube, one should be aware that enteral feedings decrease absorption of phenytoin; therefore, they should be held for 2 hours before and after the drug is administered.

Carbamazepine is not available in an intravenous preparation and must be given orally or by nasogastric tube. It must be loaded more slowly than phenytoin. A typical beginning dose is 200 mg twice a day. The dose can be increased by 200 mg per day to a typical dose of 600 to 1200 mg per day given three times a day.

Drug treatment of status epilepticus is a special consideration and is discussed in detail in Chapter 70.

BIBLIOGRAPHY

Arieff AI, Griggs RC (eds): Metabolic Brain Dysfunction in Systemic Disorders. Boston: Little, Brown, 1992.
  This book includes chapters by a large number of experts who describe the basic science and clinical aspects of all important causes of metabolic encephalopathy.
Bleck TP, Smith MC, Pierre-Louis S, et al: Neurological complications of critical medical illnesses. Crit Care Med 21:98–103, 1993.
  An excellent prospective study that defines the frequency of neurologic complications in the medical ICU.
Cascino GD: Epilepsy: Contemporary perspectives on evaluation and treatment. Mayo Clin Proc 69:1199–1211, 1994.
  An excellent review of epilepsy evaluation and management in the 1990s.
Plum F, Posner JB: The Diagnosis of Stupor and Coma, 3rd ed. Philadelphia: FA Davis, 1982.
  This classic text should be read by all physicians caring for critically ill patients. Chapters 1, 7, and 8 are particularly applicable to ICU practitioners.
Strub RL, Black FW: The Mental Status Examination in Neurology. Philadelphia: FA Davis, 1985.
  This is an in-depth guide to the evaluation of all aspects of cognition. Useful for those who wish to go beyond the "mini–mental status" examination.
Wijdicks EFM, Sharbrough FW: New-onset seizures in critically ill patients. Neurology 43:1042–1044, 1993.
  A 10-year study of the etiology of new-onset seizures in the ICU.

34
Chest Pain and Myocardial Ischemia

Bruce D. Klugherz
Daniel M. Kolansky

Evaluation of chest pain and recognition of myocardial ischemia in patients in intensive care units (ICUs) are essential skills of intensivists. Increased myocardial blood flow in response to increased myocardial metabolic demand precipitated by critical illness is dependent on patency of the coronary arteries. Any fixed stenosis ($\geq$75% of lumen) in an epicardial vessel may limit this augmentation of myocardial blood flow, upsetting the normal supply/demand balance and precipitating ischemia. In the ICU setting, fever, pain, and endogenous or exogenous catecholamines promote tachycardia, increased myocardial contractility, and generation of higher systolic wall tension, all of which increase myocardial oxygen demand. Furthermore, oxygen-carrying capacity may be reduced as a consequence of hypoxemia or anemia, both of which can impair myocardial oxygen supply.

In the postoperative patient, this oxygen supply may be also diminished as a result of intraoperative blood loss or anesthetic- or opioid-related hypotension. Like critical illness, recovery from major trauma or surgical interventions places extra demands on the myocardium by increasing total-body minute oxygen consumption (see Chapter 84). Finally, oxygen supply/demand balance may also be offset by pharmacologic interventions. For example, the vasoconstrictor pitressin (used to treat variceal gastrointestinal bleeding, see Chapter 61) can induce coronary spasm and must be administered in conjunction with nitroglycerin to avoid myocardial ischemia.

Symptoms of ischemia or myocardial infarction may be difficult to discern in the critically ill patient because of comorbid illnesses and sedative medications. Even when patients have the capacity to communicate, nearly 20% of those with acute myocardial ischemia or infarction will not develop chest discomfort. In this case, ischemia is "silent," that is, manifest only as objective signs in the absence of patient awareness. Recognition of ischemia in the ICU therefore requires careful scrutiny of hemodynamics, targeted physical examinations, and careful review of electrocardiographic (ECG) changes from baseline.

CLINICAL PRESENTATION OF ANGINA AND CHEST PAIN

Symptoms

Typical angina may range from a minor discomfort to severe pain. The discomfort is often described as pressure, heaviness, or indigestion. If "pain" is present, it is frequently described as crushing, squeezing, or burning. Classically, angina is located substernally and radiates to the left arm, neck, or jaw. Superficial discomfort is less likely to be caused by myocardial ischemia. Moreover, the chest

399

discomfort of myocardial ischemia does not begin suddenly at maximal intensity but rather crescendos in intensity.

Three different anginal syndromes are recognized. *Provokable* angina generally results from transient changes in myocardial supply and demand balance in the setting of a stable, flow-limiting atherosclerotic plaque. *Unstable* angina differs anatomically from provokable angina. It results from rupture of a previously stable plaque with a superimposed thrombus. A significant proportion of patients with unstable angina can progress to acute myocardial infarction, reflecting complete occlusion of a coronary artery. *Variant*, or *Prinzmetal's*, angina, attributed to coronary vasospasm, is neither provokable nor due to plaque rupture and generally occurs at rest.

The differential diagnosis of chest pain in the ICU patient is extensive and includes a number of cardiovascular and noncardiovascular causes (Table 34–1). Esophageal pain shares some features with classic angina; it is typically retrosternal and frequently relieved with nitroglycerin. If pain is aggravated by lying down, as in gastroesophageal reflux, or by movement, as in musculoskeletal causes, it is less likely due to myocardial ischemia. The description of chest pain may be most helpful in differentiating other cardiopulmonary causes. For instance, the chest pain of pericarditis is typically sharp and pleuritic, relieved by leaning forward. The chest pain of aortic dissection is typically "tearing" in quality, reaches maximal intensity instantaneously, and radiates to the back or flanks. The chest pain of pulmonary embolism, when present, is more often sharp and associated with dyspnea, hypoxemia, or hemoptysis in the absence of other signs of left-sided heart failure.

Although chest discomfort remains the most common complaint of patients with cardiac ischemia, certain *associated symptoms* often support the diagnosis. Patients frequently experience *dyspnea* as a result of increased interstitial pulmonary edema and *diaphoresis* resulting from autonomic instability. *Nausea* and *vomiting* due to gastric dilatation may ensue as a consequence of cardiac sensory receptor stimulation. *Syncope* may accompany ischemia or infarction, typically either vasovagally mediated or due to tachyarrhythmias or bradyarrhythmias.

Physical Findings

Physical signs of myocardial ischemia are frequently nonspecific in the critically ill patient. Agitation, tachypnea, diaphoresis, and hemodynamic instability may be unrecognized as manifestations of ischemia if the examiner's index of suspicion is low. When tachycardia is present and accompanied by a thready pulse, compromised cardiac output must be suspected. Alternatively, bradycardia may be seen due to excessive vagal tone or sinoatrial or atrioventricular nodal ischemia; in association with poor peripheral perfusion this is suggestive of right ventricular ischemia or infarction. Hypertension may accompany ischemia, secondary to excessive catecholamine release, whereas relative hypotension may also occur on the basis of impaired cardiac output. Peripheral signs of ischemia include ashen skin due to peripheral vasoconstriction, or cyanosis, slow capillary filling, and livedo reticularis due to poor cardiac output. Jugular venous pressure may be elevated if right ventricular failure is present. When ischemia is accompanied by left ventricular heart failure, auscultation of the lungs may reveal crackles, resulting

Table 34–1. Differential Diagnosis of Chest Pain in the ICU Patient

CARDIOVASCULAR	PULMONARY	GASTROINTESTINAL	MUSCULOSKELETAL
Aortic dissection	Pleurisy	Cholecystitis	Chest tube(s)
Cardiomyopathy	Pneumonia	Esophageal reflux	Costochondritis
Infarction	Pneumothorax	Esophageal spasm	Incision(s)
Ischemia	Pulmonary embolus	Esophagitis	Post-CPR trauma
Pericarditis		Hepatic capsular distention (e.g., hematoma)	Trauma
Postcardiotomy syndrome		Pancreatitis	
(Dressler's syndrome)		Peptic ulcer	
		Subdiaphragmatic abscess	

CPR, cardiopulmonary resuscitation.

from opening of fluid-filled alveoli, or wheezes, due to reflex bronchoconstriction. Examination of the heart may reveal a new S3 or S4 gallop from acute systolic or diastolic dysfunction.

Electrocardiographic Abnormalities

Repolarization Abnormalities

Most commonly, myocardial ischemia is accompanied by changes in the T waves or ST segments on the standard 12-lead ECG. These include transient T-wave inversion or ST-segment depression. Right coronary artery ischemia is best visualized in leads II, III, and aVF; circumflex artery ischemia in leads I, aVL, V_5, and V_6; and left anterior descending artery ischemia in the precordial leads, V_1 to V_4. Leads V_1 and V_2 may also reflect posterior wall ischemia or infarction by recording electrical forces opposite in direction to the forces of anterior ischemia. This is attributable to ischemia of the right coronary artery or the left circumflex artery (whichever is dominant).

The classic ECG manifestation of ischemia is downward displacement of the ST segment (Fig. 34–1). Although less specific, flattening of the ST segment with increased angulation at the ST-segment/T-wave junction is also suggestive of ischemia (Fig. 34–2). When associated with precordial ST-segment depression, precordial inversion of the U wave implies left coronary artery ischemia. With resolution of ischemia, ST segments typically return to baseline. When ST segments remain depressed, subendocardial myocardial infarction should be suspected. ST-segment elevation is consistent with acute transmural myocardial infarction and is often followed by T-wave inversion and the appearance of Q waves. Less often, ST-segment elevation reflects transient myocardial ischemia secondary to vasospasm (Prinzmetal's angina) or, if it is widespread, may be secondary to pericarditis.

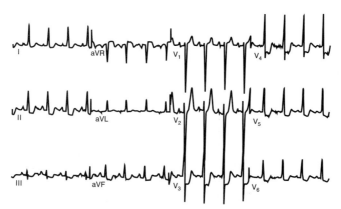

Figure 34–1. Twelve-lead electrocardiogram from a 76-year-old diabetic, hypertensive man with excellent exercise tolerance, who developed asymptomatic ECG changes on the first postoperative day after total hip replacement. He ruled in for myocardial infarction and developed heart failure; cardiac catheterization revealed left main and three-vessel disease. Note ST-segment depression in leads I, II, III, aVF, and V_3 through V_6, with reciprocal ST-segment elevation in lead aVR.

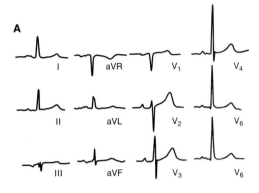

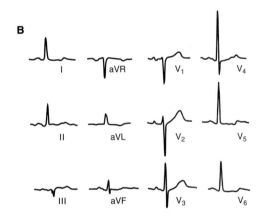

Figure 34–2. Twelve-lead electrocardio-grams from a 67-year-old man with pe-ripheral vascular disease who underwent carotid endarterectomy. When compared with the preoperative ECG *(A)*, the ECG from the first postoperative day *(B)* shows flattening of the ST segment with exagger-ated ST-T wave angulation in leads I, aVL, V₅, and V₆, consistent with lateral ische-mia.

Interpretation of T-wave changes in the absence of ST-segment changes is more difficult, owing to lack of specificity. T-wave inversion is most suggestive of ischemia when deep and symmetric in several leads; less specific are T waves that invert asymmetrically, with a gentle downslope and a rapid upslope. Such T-wave morphologies are typical of repolarization abnormalities seen in association with ventricular hypertrophy or bundle branch block. In patients whose baseline ECG demonstrates inverted T waves, ischemia may result in pseudonormalization of T waves to the upright position.

In the ICU, postural adjustments, hyperventilation, neurologic events (e.g., subarachnoid hemorrhage), and anxiety can produce T-wave changes identical to those precipitated by ischemia. A number of pharmacologic agents often used in the ICU may also produce T-wave changes, including digitalis, antiarrhythmic drugs, sympathomimetic and sympatholytic agents, tricyclic antidepressants, barbi-turates, lithium, and insulin. A variety of reversible extracardiac illnesses fre-quently seen in the ICU have also been implicated in T-wave changes, including allergic reactions, hemorrhage, viral infections, hypothyroidism or hyperthyroid-ism, adrenal insufficiency, hypokalemia, strokes, pulmonary embolism, and intra-abdominal diseases, such as acute pancreatitis or acute cholecystitis.

Arrhythmias

Arrhythmias are additional ECG manifestations of myocardial ischemia or infarction. Sinus tachycardia, due to pain, anxiety, or heart failure, and sinus bradycardia are the most common supraventricular arrhythmias. Sinus bradycardia is usually seen in the setting of inferior ischemia, as a result of the high concentration of vagal efferents in the inferoposterior wall and sinus node. Less frequent supraventricular arrhythmias include atrial tachycardia, atrial flutter, and atrial fibrillation (see Chapter 31). The underlying causes of these arrhythmias are atrial ischemia and increased left atrial pressure due to pump failure, pericarditis, or excess catecholamines. Isolated ventricular premature contractions are also quite common. Although these are usually of little concern, they may be harbingers of more serious ventricular arrhythmias, such as polymorphic ventricular tachycardia (VT) or ventricular fibrillation (VF) (see Chapter 31).

Treatment of atrial arrhythmias depends on the patient's hemodynamics and degree of systolic dysfunction. If a patient in atrial fibrillation or flutter is actively ischemic and/or hemodynamically unstable, synchronized electrical cardioversion should be performed immediately. If otherwise stable, these patients may be treated first with an atrioventricular nodal blocking agent to slow ventricular response, such as intravenous beta blockers or calcium channel blockers, followed by attempted cardioversion, either chemically or electrically.

The treatment of ventricular dysrhythmias is also determined by patient stability (see Chapter 31). Patients with unstable VT or with VF should also be electrically cardioverted immediately. Patients with sustained VT who are not actively ischemic or hemodynamically unstable may be initially treated with intravenous lidocaine or procainamide. Parenteral amiodarone is an alternative antiarrhythmic agent for patients with VT that is recurrent or refractory to other therapy. If long-term antiarrhythmic therapy becomes necessary, use of type IA (e.g., procainamide, quinidine) or type III (e.g., amiodarone, sotalol) medications or an implantable cardioverter-defibrillator may be appropriate. Cardiologic consultation and electrophysiologic study should guide this therapy.

Conduction Blocks

Conduction block may be another manifestation of ischemia in the ICU (see Chapter 30). Atrioventricular nodal blockade is most often evident in *inferior* ischemia or infarction, owing to excessive vagal tone or to hypoperfusion by means of the atrioventricular nodal branch. First-degree, second-degree (Mobitz type I), or third-degree block may occur. Conduction block from inferior ischemia is self-limited and usually does not portend a poorer prognosis; transvenous pacing is warranted if hemodynamic instability, symptoms, or bradycardia-dependent ventricular arrhythmias accompany inferior ischemia. Right bundle branch block or left posterior hemiblock may also occur in this setting, because branches from the posterior descending artery perfuse both the proximal third of the right bundle and the left posterior fascicle.

In *anterior* ischemia or infarction, conduction block carries a poorer prognosis. The left anterior descending artery supplies blood to the distal right bundle, the main left bundle, and the left anterior fascicle. Block due to hypoperfusion in the left anterior descending arterial distribution is more typically infranodal than in inferior ischemia and is manifest as Mobitz type II second-degree heart block, left or right bundle branch block, or third-degree heart block. Transvenous pacing is usually warranted under these circumstances (see Chapters 30 and 49).

Chest Radiography

In the setting of myocardial ischemia, chest radiographs frequently demonstrate evidence of interstitial or alveolar edema. When it appears in an interstitial pattern, edema manifests as haziness among pulmonary vascular markings, owing to pulmonary venous engorgement as well as peribronchial cuffing. This is accompanied by thickening of interlobular septa with engorged lymphatic vessels, known as Kerley B lines, which appear as short, horizontal, linear densities at the lung periphery. If interstitial fluid accumulates rapidly, it may flood alveoli, resulting in confluent opacification, usually in a perihilar or "batwing" distribution. Unilateral or bilateral pleural effusions may also accompany acute ischemic cardiac failure.

DIAGNOSTIC EVALUATION

Cardiac Enzymes

Myocardial injury results in the release of a variety of intracellular biochemical markers, including creatine kinase (CK), lactate dehydrogenase (LDH), transaminases, and troponins I and T (Table 34–2). The most commonly measured detectable abnormality after infarction is elevation of total serum CK and the dimeric isoform CK-MB (isoenzyme of creatine kinase with muscle and brain subunits). Typically, postinfarction CK rises within 4 to 8 hours and peaks within 12 to 24 hours. As a result of faster clearance, CK-MB usually returns to baseline before total CK. Measurement of CK and its isoenzymes is very sensitive, but trace

Table 34–2. Characteristics of Serum Myocardial Protein Assays

ASSAY	TIME TO PEAK	RETURN TO BASELINE	OTHER SOURCES
Creatine kinase	12–24 h	3–4 d	Muscle, liver, lung, GI tract, brain, kidney, spleen
Creatine kinase-MB	12–20 h	2–3 d	Muscle, uterus, GI tract, thyroid, prostate, urethra
Lactate dehydrogenase	3–6 d	8–14 d	Ubiquitous
Aspartate aminotransferase	18–36 h	3–4 d	Muscle, liver, lung
Troponin I	8–24 h	4–8 d	None
Troponin T	10–18 h	10 d	Muscle*
Myoglobin	4–8 h	1–2 d	Muscle

GI, gastrointestinal.
*Recent reports of skeletal muscle expression and unexplained elevations in uremic patients.

amounts of CK-MB are also found in a number of other tissues, so care must be taken in interpreting rises in CK-MB after surgery or trauma.

LDH is a tetrameric enzyme, composed of subunits M (for muscle) and H (for heart). The subunits combine to form five isoenzymes, which are numbered in the order of electrophoretic migration. LDH 1 and 2 are predominantly found in the heart, but LDH 1 is also concentrated in brain, stomach, and pancreatic tissue. Because of its later peak, measurement of LDH may not be necessary if CK isoenzyme levels are sent promptly. A ratio of LDH 1/LDH 2 greater than 1.0 has a specificity greater than 90% and a sensitivity of 80 to 90% for myocardial infarction.

More recently acknowledged markers of myocardial injury include the troponins (T and I). Unlike CK and LDH, troponins T and I are not usually detectable in serum in the absence of myocardial injury. Because of the rapidity of the immuno-assay for troponin I and its specificity, measurement of this marker is rapidly becoming the test of choice for perioperative and ICU patients. Because elevations in troponin I in the setting of severe unstable angina have been shown to be associated with future adverse outcomes, some have advocated the use of troponin I to triage these patients.

Echocardiography

Left ventricular systolic dysfunction is an important prognostic indicator in ische-mic heart disease. Echocardiography, by virtue of its capacity to assess global and regional ventricular function, has become a useful bedside tool in the evaluation of patients with coronary artery disease. Regional function analysis includes an assessment of both wall thickening and motion toward the left ventricular center. Segmental abnormalities of wall thickening or motion suggest the presence of scarred or chronically hypoperfused myocardium. When coexisting with areas of normally contractile myocardium, such regional asynergy is highly suggestive of ischemic heart disease. Two-dimensional echocardiography is also quite accurate in the detection of regional myocardial dysfunction during transient ischemia (although similar changes may occur in severe sepsis, which resolve completely if the patient survives). In conjunction with either exercise or dobutamine-enhanced contractility, echocardiography has a predictive value for detecting coronary artery disease approaching that of traditional single-photon emission computed tomogra-phy (SPECT) perfusion imaging.

Nuclear Imaging

SPECT myocardial perfusion imaging with sestaMIBI labeled with either thallium-201 or technetium-99m is very sensitive for the diagnosis of coronary artery disease. When thallium is injected intravenously, it accumulates in well-perfused myocardium. In the presence of flow-limiting coronary arterial stenosis, initial planar or tomographic images demonstrate a regional decrease in radiotracer uptake. Shortly after initial uptake, redistribution to hypoperfused myocardium occurs. Ischemia is represented by reversibility of a regional defect on delayed images, whereas fixation of the perfusion defect implies the presence of scar.

SPECT can be performed in conjunction with exercise or dipyridamole, adenosine, or dobutamine infusion to identify zones of myocardium where augmentation of coronary blood flow is limited by arterial stenosis. Recent interest has also been generated in using SPECT imaging to assist in the diagnosis of acute coronary syndromes. In the ICU setting, injection of radiotracer during or after suspected ischemia identifies both the location and severity of disease, thus offering unique prognostic information.

Pulmonary Artery Catheterization

Right-sided heart catheterization may be extremely helpful in guiding therapy for ICU patients with ischemia. Flow-directed (Swan-Ganz) catheterization of the pulmonary arterial circulation allows rapid measurement of central venous, right ventricular, pulmonary arterial, and pulmonary artery wedge pressure. The latter approximates left ventricular end-diastolic pressure, which is often elevated in the setting of ischemia. Large V waves appearing on the wedge pressure tracing suggest mitral regurgitation, possibly due to ischemic papillary muscle dysfunction or rupture. Measurement of both pulmonary artery wedge pressure and cardiac output is useful in guiding pharmacologic intervention. Right-sided heart catheterization in the setting of myocardial infarction can also be helpful in the recognition of right ventricular infarction and rupture of the ventricular septum. Pulmonary artery catheterization should be considered whenever suspected myocardial ischemia is associated with hemodynamic changes.

Coronary Arteriography

Coronary arteriography remains the gold standard for delineating the anatomic severity of coronary artery disease. Among patients in the ICU, coronary arteriography is generally reserved for patients who are failing medical therapy to help guide more aggressive therapy, such as angioplasty or coronary artery bypass grafting. It may also be useful in assessing cardiac risk preoperatively for noncardiac procedures in these patients.

MANAGEMENT OF ISCHEMIA AND INFARCTION

The goal of therapy for suspected myocardial ischemia in the ICU is to restore the oxygen supply/demand balance. Therapy should include supplemental oxygen for all patients, diuretics for hemodynamically stable patients with pulmonary edema, and the addition of antithrombotic and antianginal agents.

Nitrates

Initial therapy for suspected ischemia should include nitrates (Table 34–3). In addition to venodilation, which results in reduced end-diastolic pressures, nitrates cause arteriolar dilation, which reduces systemic arterial pressure and ventricular

Table 34–3. Dosing and Pharmacology of Nitrates

NITRATE	RECOMMENDED DOSE	ONSET	DURATION
Sublingual NTG	0.3–0.4 mg	2–5 min	10–30 min
NTG patch	0.1–0.3 mg/h	30–60 min	8–14 h
NTG ointment	0.5–2 inches q6h	20–60 min	3–8 h
Intravenous NTG	10–200 μg/min	0.25–2 min	5 min
Isosorbide mononitrate	10–60 mg bid	30 min	6–8 h
Isosorbide dinitrate	10–60 mg tid	15–30 min	3–6 h

NTG, nitroglycerin.

afterload. They can also reverse coronary arterial spasm, generating an early increase in myocardial blood flow. Because of their effect on preload, nitrates are especially valuable in patients with elevated left-sided filling pressures, as in congestive heart failure. The most significant adverse effect of nitroglycerin is hypotension, which can exacerbate myocardial ischemia. Therefore, nitrates should be avoided in the setting of profound hemodynamic compromise or severe aortic stenosis. Sublingual nitroglycerin may be administered with close monitoring of hemodynamics. If angina or ECG abnormalities persist, additional doses of sublingual nitroglycerin may be given 5 minutes apart, as long as they are tolerated hemodynamically. For more precise control, continuous intravenous nitroglycerin may be initiated and titrated until symptoms are controlled or until mean arterial pressure falls by at least 10% in normotensive patients or by at least 25% in hypertensive patients. Nitrate tolerance may result from prolonged intravenous infusion, resulting in recurrence of symptoms or relative hypertension. Long-term nitrate therapy can be delivered effectively with oral isosorbide dinitrate or mononitrate, or with nitroglycerin paste or patches, allowing a nitrate-free period each day to avoid tolerance. Nitrate-induced headaches are a common side effect, but they are usually mild, can be managed with analgesics, and subside within a week.

Beta Blockers

Beta blockers are the cornerstone of therapy for acute myocardial ischemia (Table 34–4). Indeed, like thrombolytic agents and unlike most other agents commonly used, they have been found to be efficacious in reducing mortality acutely in the setting of acute myocardial infarction. By reducing heart rate, blood pressure, and contractility, beta blockers effectively reduce myocardial oxygen demand. Additionally, the negative chronotropic effect of beta blockade results in prolongation of diastole with concomitant augmentation of coronary blood flow. All patients with ischemia, especially those with reflex tachycardia or coexisting hypertension, are potential candidates for beta blockers unless they have signs of heart failure or significant bradycardia or another contraindication to beta blockade, such as reactive airways disease. Other relative contraindications to beta blocker usage include severe aortic stenosis, atrioventricular conduction defects, and peripheral

Table 34–4. Dosing and Pharmacology of Beta Blockers

BLOCKER	INITIAL DOSE	MAINTENANCE DOSE	HALF-LIFE
Metoprolol	5 mg IV or 12.5 mg PO q6h	50–100 mg PO q12h	3–4 h
Propranolol	10 mg PO q6h	40–80 mg PO q6h	3.5–6 h
Esmolol	500 μg/kg over 1 min	50–300 μg/kg/min	9 min
Labetalol	50 mg PO q12h or 10 mg IV q6h	100–400 mg PO q12h	6 h

arterial disease. Bronchospasm may be minimized with the use of beta$_1$-cardioselective drugs, such as atenolol, esmolol, or metoprolol. At higher doses, these agents become less selective and may reduce expiratory flows through blockade of airway beta$_1$ receptors. Some beta blockers, such as propranolol, metoprolol, and labetalol, have *membrane-stabilizing* or quinidine-like activity. Such type I antiarrhythmic effects are unrelated to their beta-blocking properties. Their overall effect is a prolongation of the effective refractory period relative to the action potential duration, which may be beneficial in patients prone to ischemia-induced ventricular tachyarrhythmias. *Metoprolol* is an appropriate first-choice beta blocker because of its cardioselectivity and membrane-stabilizing activity.

Calcium Channel Blockers

Calcium channel antagonists are also effective antianginal agents and should be considered second-line therapy for ischemia in the ICU. A variety of calcium channel blockers are available, each different in its effect on contractility or atrioventricular conduction (Table 34–5). When administered orally, calcium channel blocker therapy should be initiated at low doses and titrated as tolerated. Verapamil, diltiazem, and nicardipine may also be administered as continuous intravenous infusions. The efficacy of calcium channel blockade in unstable coronary syndromes is unproven by randomized, controlled clinical trials. These agents are most useful for patients with continued ischemia despite therapy with nitrates and beta blockers. In many patients with *stable* angina, the combined use of beta blockers and calcium channel blockers is more effective than monotherapy. Some agents, such as the dihydropyridines, can cause reflex tachycardia, which is potentially detrimental in patients with ischemia. Relative contraindications to calcium channel blockers include severe aortic stenosis, atrioventricular conduction defects, congestive heart failure, and hypotension. Additional drugs often used in the ICU that may interact with calcium antagonists include amiodarone (potentiates atrioventricular conduction defects), cimetidine (increases bioavailability of calcium antagonists), neuromuscular blockers (action potentiated by calcium antagonists), cyclosporine and digoxin (increased plasma levels), quinidine (decreased plasma levels), and phenobarbital and rifampin (decreased hepatic enzyme induction).

Table 34–5. Dosing and Pharmacology of Calcium Channel Blockers

NAME	INITIAL DOSE	MAINTENANCE DOSE	HALF-LIFE	VASODILATION	NEGATIVE INOTROPY OR CHRONOTROPY
Verapamil	40 mg PO q8h	80–120 mg PO q8h	3–7 h	+	+++
Diltiazem	30 mg PO q8h	60–120 mg PO q8h	3.5–6 h	++	++
Amlodipine	2.5 mg PO qd	10–20 mg PO qd	35–50 h	+++	+
Nifedipine	10 mg PO q8h	30–90 mg PO q24h	2–5 h	+++	+

+, mild effect; ++, moderate effect; +++, strong effect.

Analgesia

In addition to traditional antianginal therapy with nitrates, beta blockers, and calcium channel blockers, effective analgesia should be administered to reduce myocardial oxygen demand. Opioids, such as morphine sulfate, fentanyl, and meperidine, are especially useful and have modest vasodilatory capacity in addition to their analgesic effects. Morphine (2–5 mg IV q10–30 min) and fentanyl (25–50 μg IV q5–30 min) are considered first-line therapy, except in patients with documented allergies. In patients with inferior ischemia, meperidine may be particularly helpful as a result of its vagolytic properties. With cumulative doses of opioids, care must be taken to avoid respiratory depression, which may precipitate hypoxemia and exacerbate ischemia.

Antithrombotic and Antiplatelet Agents

Antiplatelet agents and anticoagulants are key components of therapy for myocardial ischemia. In patients with unstable angina, aspirin alone, heparin alone, or a combination of the two is effective at reducing in-hospital cardiac events. Aspirin exerts its beneficial effect through inhibition of cyclooxygenase and hydroperoxidase reactions, thus limiting the production of thromboxane A_2, a potent vasoconstrictor and promoter of platelet aggregation. Heparin exerts its beneficial effect primarily through disruption of the coagulation cascade but also through inhibition of platelet aggregation. In the ICU patient, these agents may increase the risk of gastrointestinal bleeding. For acute myocardial ischemia, aspirin therapy should be initiated immediately with 325 mg administered orally or rectally. Intravenous heparin is best administered on a weight basis, with a bolus of 70 units/kg, followed by a continuous infusion at a rate of 18 units/kg/h (see Chapter 12). Heparin requirements are variable, and optimal therapeutic benefit with minimization of bleeding complications is best accomplished when the activated partial thromboplastin time is maintained at 2.0 to 2.5 times control.

Novel antithrombotic agents have also been investigated, and there is growing evidence for their efficacy in unstable angina. In particular, inhibitors of the platelet IIb/IIIa receptor have been shown to reduce adverse coronary events in patients with unstable angina both during medical therapy and in conjunction with coronary angioplasty. These are emerging as important agents in this syndrome, and their exact role is still evolving. Low molecular weight heparins (LMWH) have also been shown to be at least as effective as unfractionated heparin and can be used in these patients. Potential advantages to use of LMWH include the ease of administration by subcutaneous injection and the elimination of need for laboratory monitoring of the partial thromboplastin time with these agents. Direct thrombin inhibitors, such as bivalirudin (Hirulog) and hirudin, may also be useful alternatives.

Considerations for the Infarcting Patient

When ECG evidence of myocardial infarction is present, immediate consideration must be given to therapy directed at re-establishing coronary patency. Intravenous thrombolytic therapy is administered when there is definite recent (within 6 hours) ST-segment elevation and no contraindications, such as active bleeding, recent stroke, persistent hypertension, recent surgery or trauma, retinopathy, or significant comorbidity. There is no evidence that patients with ST-segment depression alone will benefit from thrombolytics. Primary angioplasty in acute myocardial infarction is an alternative, and evidence suggests that immediate percutaneous transluminal coronary angioplasty (PTCA) is associated with higher early patency rates and lower risk of reinfarction, death, and frequency of intracranial hemorrhage when compared with thrombolytic therapy (see Chapter 49).

Considerations for the Patient Undergoing Noncardiac Surgery

Not infrequently patients in the ICU develop a need for noncardiac operative intervention. The risk for perioperative cardiac morbidity or mortality among patients who are actively ischemic is extraordinarily high. All efforts should be made to risk-stratify patients with suspected ischemia using a combination of clinical signs and symptoms and a noninvasive study such as stress SPECT. These assessments may indicate a need for coronary angiography and/or revascularization with PTCA or coronary artery bypass grafting before noncardiac surgery. If patients require urgent operative intervention, prophylaxis against cardiac events should include judicious use of intravenous beta blockers and nitrates perioperatively, as well as pulmonary arterial catheterization for hemodynamic monitoring (see Chapter 84). Serial ECGs and myocardial enzymes should be obtained postoperatively, and aspirin therapy should be resumed as soon as bleeding risk is believed to be low enough from a surgical standpoint.

BIBLIOGRAPHY

Abrams J, Pepine CJ, Thadani U: Medical Therapy of Ischemic Heart Disease. Boston: Little, Brown & Co, 1992.
This text provides an exhaustive account of the mechanisms of action and clinical utility of nitrates, beta blockers, and calcium antagonists.

Galvani M, Ottani F, Ferrini D, et al. Prognostic influence of elevated values of cardiac troponin I in patients with unstable angina. Circulation 95:2053–2059, 1997.
This study of 106 patients admitted for unstable angina showed that elevated troponin I levels predicted adverse short- and long-term outcomes (death and nonfatal myocardial infarction).

Ganz P, Swan HJC, Ganz W: Balloon-tipped flow-directed catheters. In: Grossman W, Baim DS (eds): Cardiac Catheterization, Angiography and Intervention, 4th ed. Philadelphia: Lea & Febiger, 1991, pp 91–102.
This chapter offers a complete review of pulmonary arterial catheter construction, insertion technique, applications, and complications. The significance of large V waves is specifically addressed.

Hamm CW, Heeschen C, Goldmann B, et al. Benefit of abciximab in patients with refractory unstable angina in relation to serum troponin T. N Engl J Med 340:1623–1629, 1999.
Elevated troponin T levels identify a high-risk group that benefits from abciximab before and during percutaneous transluminal coronary angioplasty.

Oler A, Whooley MA, Oler J, Grady D: Adding heparin to aspirin reduces the incidence of myocardial infarction and death in patients with unstable angina: A meta-analysis. JAMA 276:811–815, 1996.
Meta-analysis of six randomized trials found that heparin plus aspirin reduced the risk of acute myocardial infarction or death by 33% versus aspirin alone (but with a P value of 0.06).

Marriott HJL: ECG/PDQ. Baltimore: Williams & Wilkins, 1987.
This is an exceptional introductory book of electrocardiography with helpful illustrations and a myriad of examples of arrhythmias, conduction block, and patterns of ischemia.

Rutherford JD, Braunwald E: Chronic ischemic heart disease. In: Braunwald E (ed): Heart Disease: A Textbook of Cardiovascular Disease. Philadelphia: WB Saunders, 1992, pp 1295–1297.
The referenced pages provide a thorough discussion of the host of disorders that can mimic anginal discomfort. In the same chapter the various interventions useful in the treatment of myocardial ischemia are fully described.

Zaret BL, Wackers FJ: Nuclear cardiology. N Engl J Med 329:775–782, 1993.
The authors have provided an up-to-date reference discussing the technical aspects of single photon emission computed tomography, stress imaging protocols, and the variety of clinical applications of perfusion stress imaging.

35 Diarrhea Developing in the Intensive Care Patient

Gary R. Lichtenstein

Diarrhea is an important nosocomial disorder in hospitalized patients and occurs, on average, in up to one third of patients in the intensive care unit (ICU). It has potentially debilitating consequences in these patients, consisting of (1) perineal and sacral skin ulcers with secondary superinfection, (2) decreased absorption of enterally administered medications, and (3) abdominal discomfort and the urge to defecate. Severe diarrhea can also cause intravascular volume depletion with its associated electrolyte abnormalities. These place the patient in the ICU at risk for other complications, such as azotemia and cardiac arrhythmias. Furthermore, with moderate to severe diarrhea, patients may lose weight and lean body mass resulting, in part, from decreased oral or enteral intake.

Diarrhea is defined as an increase in the fluidity, volume, and frequency of daily stool output. Typically, daily stool volume output greater than 200 mL (or >200 g in weight) is considered diarrhea for an adult.

PATHOPHYSIOLOGY

Four major mechanisms can produce diarrhea: (1) secretory, (2) osmotic, (3) inflammatory, and (4) motility-related (Table 35–1).

Secretory Diarrhea

Active chloride secretion is the basic mechanism leading to secretory diarrhea. There are many known stimuli for this, including toxins, peptides, amines, and derivatives of arachidonic acid. These substances exert their action through intracellular mediators that stimulate active chloride secretion. Secretory diarrhea occurs even when the patient fasts because the secretory process is independent of enteral intake or the absorptive process (see Table 35–1). Active secretion of chloride anion creates an osmotic gradient in favor of moving water passively from plasma

Table 35–1. Major Types of Diarrhea and Their Response to Fasting

TYPE	EXAMPLE	RESPONSE TO FASTING
Secretory	Medications	None
Osmotic	Tube feedings	Resolves within 1 day
Inflammatory	*Clostridium difficile* toxin	Decreased volume
Altered intestinal motility	Small bowel bacterial overgrowth	Decreased volume

415

and interstitial space into the intestinal lumen. The osmolality of the secreted fluid is iso-osmolar to plasma and is nearly equal to that calculated by its electrolyte concentrations.

Osmotic Diarrhea

An osmotic agent causing diarrhea is (1) soluble in water, (2) cannot be absorbed by the small intestine, or (3) may be metabolized by bacteria and converted to substances with smaller molecular weight in the distal intestine. On a per gram basis, a smaller molecular weight substance is a more effective osmotic agent than is a larger molecular weight substance. Osmotic diarrhea is the result of consuming nonabsorbable solutes by mouth or by nasogastric or nasoenteral tube. Thus, this type of diarrhea resolves once the osmotic load is eliminated, that is, after the patient is fasting (see Table 35–1).

Inflammatory Diarrhea

Inflammatory (leaky membrane) diarrhea is usually associated with a damaged intestinal lining. Exudation via the damaged mucosa plus a decrease in absorption is the underlying mechanism. There are several clinical characteristics of leaky membrane diarrhea, including (1) mucosal damage that can be detected by endoscopy, (2) the presence of fecal leukocytes, (3) diarrhea that persists after fasting, and (4) diarrhea that often worsens after feeding (see Table 35–1).

Motility-Related Diarrhea

Decreased Motility

Gastrointestinal motility disorders such as scleroderma, diabetes, and pseudo-obstruction result in less effective clearance of bacteria from the intestine. Under these conditions, chronic small bowel bacterial overgrowth can occur. Although both anaerobes and aerobes overgrow, anaerobes produce most of the clinical problems. Many clinical manifestations may occur. Deconjugation of bile salts by bacterial enzymes results in free bile acids in the proximal small intestine. Bile acids not only are toxic to mucosal cells but also can promote secretion. Both effects can cause diarrhea. In addition, impaired micelle formation due to reduced conjugated bile salt concentrations may cause fat malabsorption and steatorrhea. Unconjugated bile salts, bacterial infection, or fatty acids may induce malabsorption because of mucosal damage. Protein malnutrition may be exacerbated because proteins are catabolized by bacteria, and transluminal transport of amino acids and peptides may be decreased because of mucosal defects.

Increased Motility

Motility disturbances such as postgastrectomy dumping syndrome is an example of increased motility of the small intestine relevant to the ICU population. This condition typically results in a decreased contact time of chyme with the absorptive surface areas.

DIFFERENTIAL DIAGNOSES (Table 35–2)

Antibiotic-Associated Diarrhea

Antibiotic-associated diarrhea is frequently seen in patients in the ICU. Diarrhea may occur in up to 25% of patients receiving antibiotics. Antibiotic therapy predisposes the patient to the development of at least two separate types of diarrhea: (1) osmotic diarrhea due to altered colonic salvage of carbohydrates and (2) secretory diarrhea due to *Clostridium difficile* toxin. Administration of oral or systemic antibiotics reduces the normal competitive flora, impairs colonic fermentation of carbohydrates, and increases the risk for the development of *C. difficile* strains. In patients with antibiotic-associated diarrhea (without *C. difficile* toxin), ingested carbohydrate that is unabsorbed in the small intestine enters the colon. There, it is not metabolized as normally occurs and can induce an osmotic diarrhea. Stool studies are typically normal in these individuals, and diarrhea resolves once the offending antibiotics are discontinued.

However, when an individual acquires diarrhea after the antibiotics are discontinued, one should suspect the development of *C. difficile*–related diarrhea. One third of the cases of *C. difficile*–related diarrhea occur *after* the antibiotics have been discontinued. It may be several weeks or longer between discontinuing antibiotics and the onset of the diarrhea. *C. difficile* is the pathogen in one third of cases of antibiotic-induced diarrhea. However, it is also present in many hospitalized patients with diarrhea unrelated to *C. difficile* toxin. Those who harbor the organism without the demonstration of symptoms are not at increased risk for the development of subsequent clinical illness, for example, pseudomembranous colitis. However, they are capable of transmitting the organism to other patients through person-to-person contact and environmental contamination.

Intestinal Ischemia

Intestinal ischemia is another cause of diarrhea in patients in the ICU. Risk factors include hypotension, hypoxemia, or sepsis. Ischemia limited to the colon, that is,

Table 35–2. Common Causes of Diarrhea in the ICU Patient

··

> Antibiotic–associated diarrhea
> *Clostridium difficile* toxin–related diarrhea
> Drugs (see Table 35–3)
> Enteral feeding–related diarrhea
> Fecal impaction
> Hypoalbuminemia
> Fecal incontinence
> Intestinal ischemia
> Intestinal pseudo-obstruction
> Lactose ingestion in a lactase-deficient individual

··

ischemic colitis, often presents with an abrupt onset of lower abdominal cramping, rectal bleeding, vomiting, and fever. The finding of fecal leukocytes indicates colonic involvement. Individuals with underlying atherosclerotic disease are especially vulnerable, as are those who have an abdominal aortic aneurysm repair (during which the inferior mesenteric artery may be compromised) (see Chapter 91). Ischemic colitis may also result from vasculitis, a ruptured abdominal aneurysm, collagen vascular disease (e.g., systemic lupus erythematosus, rheumatoid arthritis, polyarteritis nodosa, scleroderma), or colorectal cancer. The clinical presentation may vary from mild to severe diarrhea, with or without substantial abdominal discomfort. Ischemia involving the small bowel, that is, mesenteric ischemia, is a more serious problem than is ischemic colitis because of its higher associated mortality.

Diarrhea Related to Enteral Feeding

Another cause of diarrhea occurring in the ICU is enteral feeding because of poor tolerance to the constituents of enteral feeding formulas. A multitude of causes has been proposed, including a high osmolality of the solution (e.g., up to 690 mOsm/kg in some preparations), high rate of delivery, bacterial contamination of the feeding solution, malabsorption due to partial villous atrophy of small bowel mucosa from prolonged fasting, previous malabsorption, and motility alterations with rapid intestinal transit.

Drug-Related Diarrhea

Many medications given alone or in combination may result in diarrhea. Medications suspended in sorbitol, such as elixir of theophylline, may cause profuse diarrhea, for example, greater than 1 L/day. This diarrhea is osmotic in nature and thus it resolves on discontinuation of the medication. The amount of sorbitol is not specified on labels of elixirs because it is considered to be an inactive ingredient. There are no fecal leukocytes present, no blood in the stool, and the patient is afebrile in the prototypic case. Many drugs may cause diarrhea in hospitalized patients (Table 35–3).

Lactose intolerance is common in the general population and occurs in about 10 to 15% of individuals. Other populations have an even higher prevalence for this disorder, for example, as high as 60 to 70% in African Americans, Jews, Hispanics, southern Europeans, and east Asians, and as high as 90% in Native Americans. Diarrhea occurs when a lactase-deficient individual ingests products containing lactose. Many medications (and foods) contain lactose because it is often used as a binder in certain medications. When such medications are given to patients in the ICU who have acquired temporary lactase deficiency due to fasting, diarrhea may result.

Other Causes of Diarrhea

Fecal impaction is a common cause of diarrhea in hospitalized or institutionalized patients and may occur in patients admitted to the ICU for other reasons. This disorder tends to occur more commonly in patients who have dementia or psycho-

Table 35–3. Selected Medications Associated with Diarrhea in Hospitalized Patients

Magnesium-containing medications (antacids, $Mg(OH)_2$, Milk of Magnesia)
Sorbitol-containing products (elixirs, sugar-free gums or mints, or from pears, peaches, prunes, and orange juice)
Quinidine, quinine
Lactulose
Antineoplastic agents
Digitalis
Colchicine
Para-aminosalicylic acid
Diuretics (furosemide, thiazides)
Cholinergic drugs (glaucoma eye drops, bladder stimulants)
Prokinetic agents (metoclopramide and cisapride)
Prostaglandin analog (misoprostol)
Gold preparations
Theophylline
Thyroid hormone
Cholinesterase inhibitors
Mesalamine derivatives (Asacol, olsalazine, Azulfidine, Pentasa)
Antihypertensive medications (angiotensin-converting enzyme inhibitors)
Laxatives with phenolphthalein, anthraquinones, senna, aloe, ricinoleic acid (castor oil), bisacodyl

sis. A rectal examination and a flat plate of the abdomen should be performed to rule this out.

It has been suggested that a *low serum albumin* level is an independent risk factor for the development of diarrhea in the ICU setting. Some report that patients in the ICU with an albumin level of less than 2.5 g/dL consistently experience diarrhea when given full-strength tube feedings. In contrast, patients with a serum albumin level greater than or equal to 2.6 g/dL do not experience diarrhea under the same conditions. Hypoalbuminemia may predispose the patient to the development of diarrhea by several mechanisms, including decreased submucosal oncotic pressure and mucosal edema in the intestinal tract. The latter is more likely to occur in individuals who experience hypoalbuminemia in association with a hypercatabolic state. Hypoalbuminemia per se does not always lead to diarrhea because many individuals with nephrotic syndrome and other causes of hypoalbuminemia never acquire diarrhea.

Incontinence, defined as the involuntary release of rectal and bladder contents, may result in a clinical situation that is difficult to differentiate from diarrhea. It is thus termed *pseudodiarrhea.* It is associated with the release of solid feces. This may occur alone or in association with another cause of diarrhea. A digital rectal examination can estimate the rectal tone as well as the patient's ability to generate a rectal squeeze response. In individuals with this disorder, the stool weight is less than 200 g daily. Incontinence may also result from anal fistulas and fissures, tears from childbirth, diabetic neuropathy, trauma, anal intercourse, or neuromuscular diseases.

DIAGNOSTIC EVALUATION

In the evaluation of diarrhea in the patient in the ICU, the first determination to make is whether or not the patient actually has diarrhea. An accurate description of the diarrhea is helpful for appropriate diagnosis and treatment. In particular, one should ascertain the duration of the suspected diarrhea, the stool volume, color, consistency, and relationship to feedings. Also, it is important to identify any underlying illnesses, travel history, systemic symptoms, and current medications.

The *history* can help differentiate small bowel from large bowel diarrhea. Classically, patients with diarrhea due to a small bowel cause have high-volume diarrhea (several liters daily) with periumbilical cramping. The stools may be greasy or watery or contain particles of undigested food. In large bowel–related diarrhea, the patient classically passes small volumes of diarrhea, frequently with mucus and occasionally with blood. The patient may have a sense of urgency or tenesmus. If abdominal pain is present, it is typically localized to the lower abdomen, pelvis, or sacral region. The finding of blood in the diarrhea (either macroscopic or occult) should suggest inflammatory, vascular, neoplastic, or infectious causes.

The *physical examination* should evaluate for the presence of intravascular volume depletion and a rash suggestive of a vasculitis. Several findings may be of help in the evaluation of an individual with diarrhea, including the presence of a goiter, abdominal bruit, arthritis, uveitis, peripheral neuropathy, orthostatic hypotension, perianal disease (fistula, abscess, mass), or fecal impaction.

Several *diagnostic tests* have proved useful in evaluating the patient with diarrhea in the ICU (Fig. 35–1). They include a complete blood count with differential, serum electrolytes, blood urea nitrogen, and creatinine determinations. A chemistry profile and urinalysis may also help assess for the presence of systemic diseases. Several tests on the stool itself can help to determine the cause of the diarrheal disorder.

Fecal leukocytes are found in several infectious conditions. Typically, fecal leukocytes are present in *Shigella, Campylobacter,* and invasive *Escherichia coli,* whereas they may be present variably in *Salmonella, Yersinia enterocolitica, Vibrio parahaemolyticus, C. difficile,* or antibiotic-associated diarrhea. They may also be present in inflammatory bowel disease or ischemic colitis. One should note that it would be unusual for an infectious bacterial cause (other than *C. difficile*) to be responsible for *nosocomial* diarrhea.

The *absence of fecal leukocytes* suggests a nonbacterial, noninvasive process involving the intestinal tract. Several examples of this include viral infections, giardiasis, and medication-associated diarrhea. However, absence of fecal leukocytes (false-negative results) does not exclude the possibility of ischemia or other disorders in which they typically are present.

The presence of *gross or occult blood* in the stool is suggestive of severe mucosal inflammation, a neoplasm, ischemic bowel disease, radiation enteritis, or amebiasis. One should remember that upper gastrointestinal mucosal disease, for example, peptic ulcer disease, may cause stools to be positive for occult blood, (i.e., false-positive results).

Measurement of *stool osmolality* can help differentiate osmotic from secretory diarrhea (Fig. 35–2). In addition, high stool sodium concentration (>90 mmol/L) suggests secretory diarrhea (or osmotic diarrhea caused by ingestion of Na_2SO_4 or Na_2PO_4), whereas a low stool sodium concentration (<60 mmol/L) suggests osmotic diarrhea.

Bacterial pathogens (other than *C. difficile*) and *parasitic organisms* may cause disease that results in patients being admitted in the ICU. However, such infectious

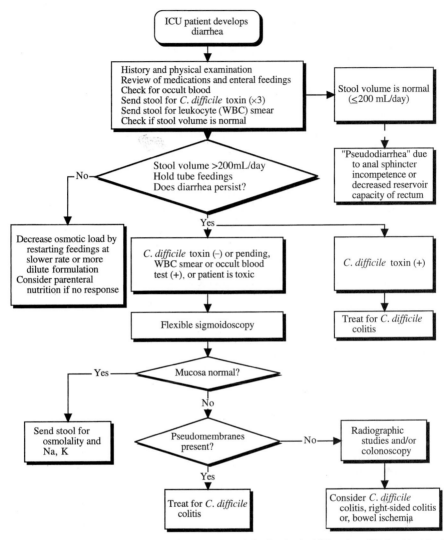

Figure 35–1. Schematic flow diagram for evaluation of diarrhea in the ICU patient. WBC, white blood cell; Na, sodium; K, potassium.

causes would rarely cause diarrhea with an onset more than 2 days after hospitalization (especially when the patient had no symptoms before admission). Under such conditions, stool cultures for bacterial pathogens should *not* be requested but, instead, a *C. difficile* toxin assay performed.

Flexible sigmoidoscopy is a helpful procedure and can be performed without any preparatory enemas or with normal saline enemas. During the test, stool samples can be obtained via suction if further testing is indicated. Sigmoidoscopy is especially helpful for the evaluation of patients in whom pseudomembranous colitis is suspected.

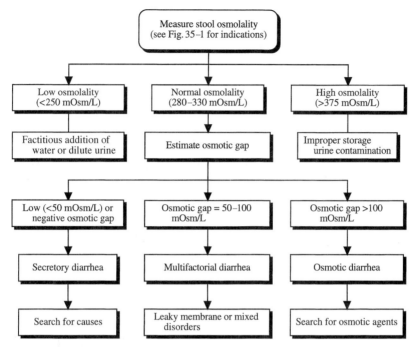

Figure 35–2. Flow diagram for measuring stool osmolality in the evaluation of diarrhea in the ICU patient. The osmotic gap equals the measured minus the calculated stool osmolality. Calculated stool osmolality = 2 × {stool [Na] + stool [K]} where [Na] is sodium concentration (mEq/L) and [K] is potassium concentration (mEq/L).

Radiographic studies may be helpful but usually are not necessary if the preceding studies have been performed. A plain radiograph of the abdomen may show thumbprinting suggestive of mucosal disease (e.g., inflammatory bowel disease or ischemic bowel disease). Computed tomography of the abdomen may show similar changes and help establish a specific diagnosis, for example, ischemic bowel disease.

MANAGEMENT AND TREATMENT

Treatment of diarrhea depends on its specific cause (see Table 35–2 and Fig. 35–1). However, a careful review of medications (especially antibiotics, elixirs, and magnesium-containing antacids) and probable causes is recommended as the first step for all patients. A physical examination, including a rectal examination, should be performed to exclude an impaction and to search for occult blood.

In a patient receiving enteral nutrition in the ICU who experiences diarrhea, several strategies can help eliminate this as its cause. They include decreasing the rate of feeding, increasing the dilution of the feeding, or stopping the enteral feedings and changing to parenteral feeding temporarily if not contraindicated. The fecal osmotic gap in patients with an osmotic diarrhea due to enteral feedings is typically greater than 100 mOsm/kg (see Fig. 35–2).

If *C. difficile* is suspected, patients should have three separate stool samples tested for *C. difficile* toxin. If the patient appears toxic, a sigmoidoscopy or colonoscopy, looking for pseudomembranes, should be urgently performed. When searching for ischemia, one should look for occult blood in stool. Sigmoidoscopy (or possibly colonoscopy) or radiographic studies (computed tomography, barium studies, or plain abdominal radiographs) may be needed to search for changes of ischemia. If ischemia is found, one should maintain adequate blood flow and oxygen delivery to the gastrointestinal tract, that is, transfuse if necessary and increase cardiac output as well as decrease its metabolic demands by "resting" the bowel (fasting). Surgery is indicated in severe cases or in recurrent prolonged colonic disease. Mortality is high (50%) for small bowel ischemia.

The treatment of infectious diarrhea is divided into several categories, including (1) symptomatic therapy (fluid and electrolyte replenishment and use of antidiarrheal agents) and (2) specific antimicrobial treatment. In all patients, the degree of intravascular volume depletion should be determined and patients rehydrated with intravenous fluids.

For the treatment of *C. difficile* toxin–related diarrhea, the use of metronidazole (500 mg orally every 8 hours for 7 to 14 days) is the preferred initial treatment. If patients have an ileus, the use of intravenous metronidazole (500 mg every 8 hours for 7 to 14 days) has been demonstrated to be equally efficacious. Metronidazole should be the initial drug of choice for the treatment of *C. difficile* because of the higher cost of treatment with vancomycin and concern that the overuse of vancomycin predisposes to resistant organisms, such as enterococci or staphylococci. When used, vancomycin is effective only when administered orally or via nasogastric tube, that is, intravenous vancomycin is *ineffective*. Vancomycin is given at a dose of 125 mg every 6 hours for 10 days. Approximately 15 to 20% of patients relapse after treatment with vancomycin, which sometimes occurs 1 to 5 weeks after completion of therapy. Retesting for *C. difficile* toxin is the preferred method of diagnosis (or detection of pseudomembranes on flexible sigmoidoscopy or colonoscopy when necessary). Eradication of the toxin from the stool occurs in about 80% of individuals within 5 days of initiation of therapy using vancomycin. The use of agents to slow intestinal motility, for example, loperamide, should not be used in individuals who have diarrhea caused by *C. difficile* toxin. Their use in this disorder may precipitate toxic megacolon. Similarly, the use of opioids and anticholinergics are *not* recommended in these individuals.

CLINICAL PEARLS AND PITFALLS

The following imperatives can serve as general guidelines:

1. Look carefully at the medications that the patient is receiving, especially elixirs that may contain sorbitol.
2. Check stool for *C. difficile* toxin three times.
3. Perform a rectal examination to exclude impaction.
4. Assess for tube feeding–related diarrhea.
5. Look for complications of systemic diseases.
6. Look for evidence of ischemic bowel disease.
7. Avoid antimotility agents until diarrhea due to *C. difficile* toxin is excluded.

8. Avoid empirical antibiotics to treat *C. difficile* unless indicated by demonstration of its toxin or the patient is toxic.

BIBLIOGRAPHY

Baubut F, Corthier G, Charpak Y, et al: Prevalence and pathogenicity of *Clostridium difficile* in hospitalized patients: A French multi-center study. Arch Intern Med 156:1449–1454, 1996.
This is an excellent study evaluating the prevalence of C. difficile *in hospitalized patients.*

Eastwood GL, Avunduk C: Diarrhea. In: Manual of Gastroenterology. Boston: Little, Brown, 1988, pp 148–158.
This is a simple to read review of the work-up and evaluation of diarrhea.

Fine KD, Krejs GJ, Fordtran JS: Diarrhea. In: Scharschmidt BF, Feldman M (eds): Gastrointestinal Disease: Pathophysiology, Diagnosis, Management. Philadelphia: WB Saunders, 1993, pp 1043–1072.
This is an outstanding, comprehensive review of the subject matter and is extremely well written.

Greenberger NJ: Chronic diarrhea: How should we approach the diagnosis? In: Barkin JS, Rogers AI (eds): Difficult Decisions in Digestive Diseases. Chicago: Yearbook Medical, 1989, pp 307–325.
This volume presents a well-written, problem-oriented approach to common, yet difficult to manage problems.

Krejs GJ: Diarrhea. In: Wyngaarden JB, Smith LH, Bennett JC (eds): Cecil Textbook of Medicine. Philadelphia: WB Saunders, 1992, pp 680–687.
This is a well-written review of general principles.

Powell DW: Approach to the patient with diarrhea. In: Yamada T, Alpers DH, Ouyang C, et al: Textbook of Gastroenterology. Philadelphia: JB Lippincott, 1995, pp 813–863.
This is an outstanding reference textbook with encyclopedic review of subject matter.

36 Electrolyte Disorders

Charles H. Rodenberger
Fuad N. Ziyadeh

Electrolyte disorders are common in the intensive care unit (ICU), both on admission to the ICU and as complications of ICU treatment. Anticipation and prompt recognition of these disorders and understanding their pathogenesis are mandatory skills for intensivists. Optimal therapy takes into account both the laboratory abnormalities and the patient's clinical state (see Chapter 81 for serum sodium disorders).

POTASSIUM DISORDERS

Although potassium concentration is typically measured in *serum* (from coagulated blood in a red-topped tube), *plasma* potassium is the active extracellular component. Although the normally small difference between the two concentrations (<0.5 mEq/L) is not clinically important, *pseudohyperkalemia* arises when measured *serum* values are in the hyperkalemic range despite *plasma* being normokalemic. Causes include hemolysis during phlebotomy, thrombocytosis ($>10^6/\mu L$) or leukocytosis ($>10^5/\mu L$).

Hyperkalemia

Table 36–1 lists common acute causes of hyperkalemia relevant to the ICU setting. As a general rule, multiple causes are necessary, especially chronically, to overcome the multiple mechanisms protective of extracellular [K$^+$].

Clinical Manifestations and Treatment

Hyperkalemia is toxic because of its effect on the membrane potential of excitable cells. This is manifested primarily as cardiac conduction changes (Table 36–2), but neuromuscular weakness may also occur. The toxicity of any given level of hyperkalemia varies widely among patients and is partly dependent on coexistent electrolyte abnormalities. Hypocalcemia, hypomagnesemia, acidemia, and hyponatremia all *increase* the toxicity of hyperkalemia.

Treatment of hyperkalemia requires treatment of reversible conditions, including eliminating offending medications and restricting potassium intake. Potassium excretion can be accelerated with intravenous (IV) saline, diuretics, or a cation exchange resin, such as sodium polystyrene sulfate (Kayexalate). In *severe* hyperkalemia (serum [K$^+$] >6.5 mEq/L), or electrocardiographic changes more severe than peaked T waves (see Table 36–2), the goals of therapy are (1) stabilizing cell membranes, (2) shifting extracellular potassium to the intracellular space, and (3) reducing total body potassium. Continuous electrocardiographic monitoring is mandatory throughout therapy.

Table 36–1. Causes of Acute Hyperkalemia in the ICU Setting

. . . .

Excess intake
    Excessive IV or oral potassium load
    Blood products
    Cardioplegia or transplant organ baths
Intracellular-to-extracellular shift of potassium
    Beta-adrenergic blockers
    Digitalis toxicity
    Hypertonicity (hyperglycemia, hypernatremia, mannitol)
    Insulin deficiency
    Malignant hyperthermia (see Chapter 54)
    Metabolic acidosis (especially acute hyperchloremic acidosis)
    Severe hemolysis
    Succinylcholine (due to fasciculating muscles) (see Chapter 4)
    Tissue necrosis (rhabdomyolysis, tumor lysis syndrome, organ ischemia)
Inadequate excretion
    Acute renal failure
    Effective arterial volume depletion (hypovolemia, congestive heart failure, liver failure)
    Obstructive uropathy
Pseudohyperkalemia (see text)

. . . .

IV, intravenous.

Membrane Stabilization

If the electrocardiogram discloses a widened QRS, 10 mL of 10% calcium gluconate (one ampule contains 90 mg elemental calcium) is given IV over several minutes. By raising the threshold potential of excitable cells, calcium counters the toxic membrane effects of high extracellular potassium. Within seconds to minutes, the widened QRS should narrow and P waves return. Although its effects are transient, the same dose of calcium may be repeated every 5 minutes as needed if electrocardiographic changes recur. Calcium chloride, a less desirable alternative because of its sclerosing properties, may be used if the gluconate salt is unavailable, but only one quarter of the dose is needed (one-quarter ampule or 2.5 mL of 10% calcium chloride provides the same 90 mg elemental calcium). Intravenous calcium must be used cautiously when digitalis is present, as it can induce digitalis toxicity.

Table 36–2. Progressive Electrocardiographic Manifestations of Acute Hyperkalemia

. . . .

Peaked T waves
P-R widening
Flattening of QT interval
QRS widening
Loss of P waves
Sine wave
Asystole

. . . .

See also Fig. 30–4, Chapter 30.

Extracellular-to-Intracellular Shift of Potassium

A rapid pharmacologic shift of potassium into cells mitigates toxicity until potassium can be excreted. *Regular insulin* (10 U given as an IV bolus) stimulates Na-K-ATPase, which drives potassium into cells. Hypoglycemia is prevented by giving an IV bolus of 50 to 75 mL of 50% dextrose (D_{50}), followed by a continuous infusion of 10% dextrose (D_{10}) or 20% dextrose (D_{20}) while making frequent blood glucose determinations. Glucose may be omitted, however, if the serum glucose exceeds 300 mg/dL before insulin administration. Insulin lowers potassium by approximately 0.5 to 1.0 mEq/L, starting within 15 to 30 minutes, peaking at 60 minutes, and lasting several hours.

Bicarbonate therapy buffers extracellular H^+. *Sodium bicarbonate* (one 50-mL ampule of 7.5% solution contains 44 mEq of HCO_3^-) given IV over several minutes causes extrusion of intracellular H^+, which is then exchanged for extracellular K^+. A fall in serum potassium concentration usually occurs within 30 to 60 minutes. Bicarbonate is less effective in lowering potassium than is insulin and is most effective in the presence of a metabolic acidosis. Hypertonic sodium bicarbonate solution is ideal for hyperkalemic patients with hyponatremia but must be given cautiously with congestive heart failure or renal failure.

Beta-adrenergic agonists also stimulate Na-K-ATPase activity and drive potassium into cells, thus lowering the serum potassium concentration. Inhaled albuterol (20 to 40 mg nebulized, a dose 8–10 times the typical doses to treat asthma) lowers potassium within 0.5 hour but should be used only to supplement bolus insulin therapy. Inhaled albuterol is contraindicated with ischemic heart disease. Epinephrine should be avoided because its alpha-agonist activity transiently worsens hyperkalemia.

Reduction of Total Body Potassium

Definitive treatment of hyperkalemia requires elimination of excess potassium. In patients with adequate renal function, isotonic saline infusions followed by a loop or thiazide diuretic enhances urinary potassium excretion. Cation exchange resins (Kayexalate) are used when renal excretion is suboptimal. Oral Kayexalate, 15 g in 60 mL sorbitol solution (to prevent constipation), typically binds approximately 15 mEq potassium and may be repeated every several hours. Alternatively, Kayexalate enemas (50 to 60 g in a 70% sorbitol solution) retained for an hour typically bind only 0.5 mEq potassium for each gram of Kayexalate. Gastrointestinal obstruction, ileus, or recent abdominal or transplant surgery precludes resin use because colonic necrosis has been reported in these patients. Since these resins can add 2 to 3 mEq Na^+ for each mEq K^+ removed, the sodium load can be problematic in patients with renal or cardiac failure.

Rapid and definitive potassium removal is achieved by dialysis, with hemodialysis being more effective than peritoneal dialysis (see Chapter 16).

Hypokalemia

Clinical Manifestations

Hypokalemia (Table 36–3) refers to serum $[K^+]$ less than 3.5 mEq/L; serum $[K^+]$ less than 4.0 mEq/L represents relative hypokalemia in the setting of cardiac

Table 36–3. Causes of Hypokalemia in ICU Patients

Shifts in internal potassium balance
  Insulin (endogenous or exogenous)
  Beta-adrenergic agonist (albuterol, epinephrine, or other catecholamine)
  Hypothermia (produces hypokalemia until frank tissue necrosis ensues)
Excess potassium loss
  Gastrointestinal losses (vomiting, nasogastric suction, fistulas, diarrhea)
  Renal potassium wasting
    Acute tubular necrosis
    Diuretics (except potassium-sparing diuretics)
    Magnesium depletion with hypomagnesemia, usually drug-induced (amphotericin B,
      aminoglycosides, high-dose carbenicillin [a physiologic, not toxic effect])
    Malignant hypertension
    Osmotic diuresis (e.g., glycosuria)
    Saline diuresis
    Renal tubular acidosis, type I or II

ischemia, arrhythmias, or liver failure. Symptoms include constipation, ileus, and muscle weakness, whereas profound hypokalemia can produce paralysis or rhabdomyolysis. Although early electrocardiographic findings (U waves and flattened T waves) are clinically unimportant, more problematic electrocardiographic changes can occur with worsening hypokalemia and include ST-segment depression, decreased QRS amplitude, slowed atrioventricular node conduction, and multiple atrial and ventricular arrhythmias. Mild hypokalemia alone should not produce clinically relevant arrhythmias in young patients with healthy hearts. In contrast, in elderly patients, patients receiving digitalis with a tendency to arrhythmias or with acute myocardial ischemia, [K^+] less than 4.0 mEq/L is associated with more frequent arrhythmias. Patients with this degree of hypokalemia also have increased myocardial damage during ischemia.

Hypokalemia has important noncardiac effects. For example, hypokalemia impairs insulin release, which aggravates hyperglycemia. It can cause metabolic alkalosis and stimulate production of ammonia, which may contribute to worsening encephalopathy in patients with advanced liver disease. Finally, hypokalemia impairs the renal concentrating mechanism, causing polydipsia and polyuria.

Differential Diagnosis

Shifts in internal potassium balance generally produce only transient falls in extracellular potassium. These are seldom of clinical importance unless superimposed on total body potassium depletion, as in the chronically malnourished or alcoholic patient. Hypertension-associated potassium wasting is characterized by functional hyperaldosteronism, whereas K^+ wasting without hypertension is usually due to renal tubular defects. The hypokalemia seen with vomiting or continuous nasogastric suction is secondary to the associated metabolic alkalosis and volume depletion. The resulting bicarbonaturia and hyperaldosteronism produce large renal potassium losses.

The diagnosis of hypokalemia usually rests on potassium determinations (see Table 36–3). In the setting of hypokalemia and normal renal function, spot urine potassium concentration should be less than 10 mEq/L and 24-hour urine potassium less than 20 mEq. Levels exceeding these values suggest renal potassium wasting, thus focusing the diagnostic search.

Treatment

Treatment of hypokalemia should combine identification and management of specific underlying causes with potassium supplementation. Serum [K$^+$] is monitored frequently during therapy to avoid hyperkalemia. The total body potassium deficit averages 200 to 400 mEq for every 1.0 mEq/L decrement in serum [K$^+$]. This relationship becomes nonlinear at very low serum concentrations. For example, this deficit can be greater than 1000 mEq when serum [K$^+$] is less than 2.0 mEq/L. However, critically ill patients, even those with large total body potassium deficits, cannot rapidly move large extracellular loads of potassium into cells, so the rate of deficit repletion must be slow to avoid extracellular hyperkalemia.

Enteral therapy is safest. One gives 40 to 80 mEq of potassium every 4 hours until serum potassium is corrected. When enteral therapy is not possible, potassium is given intravenously, typically no faster than 10 to 20 mEq/hour, as 40 to 60 mEq K$^+$/L of IV fluid. Potassium replacement to correct hypokalemia should not be given in dextrose-containing solutions because dextrose stimulates insulin release, further lowering serum [K$^+$]. In emergencies with life-threatening or myocardial-threatening hypokalemia, potassium can be given at 40 mEq/hour, rarely faster. For example, in one study, single infusion of 40 mEq of potassium chloride in 100 mL 0.9% sodium chloride over 1 hour was found to be safe in 11 ICU patients with serum [K$^+$] less than 3.0 mEq/L. High rates of infusion require electrocardiographic monitoring and frequent serum potassium measurements to avoid potentially fatal transient hyperkalemia. Delivery in fluid more concentrated than 60 mEq/L may be necessary, but this requires large veins to avoid sclerosis. Use of central venous catheters with their distal tips in the superior vena cava or right atrium are best avoided because delivery of concentrated potassium solutions to the heart can precipitate hyperkalemic arrhythmias.

Potassium chloride is most effective in rapidly raising the extracellular potassium concentration, especially in patients with volume contraction. Potassium phosphate can be given to phosphate-depleted patients and potassium citrate can be given to acidemic patients.

CALCIUM DISORDERS

Laboratories routinely measure total serum calcium concentration (normal range = 9.0 to 10.2 mg/dL or 2.25 to 2.55 mmol/L). Although this correlates well with the ionized calcium concentration (normal 1.0 to 1.3 mmol/L) in healthy patients, only the latter is physiologically active. In ICU patients, various factors (hypoalbuminemia, acute or chronic renal failure, acid-base disturbances, and circulating calcium chelators, such as citrate, phosphates, lipids) can alter the fraction of total serum calcium found in the ionized form. In the presence of these factors, total serum calcium concentration is a poor proxy for ionized calcium concentration.

A low serum albumin concentration is common in ICU patients. This results in

Table 36–4. Signs and Symptoms of Acute Hypercalcemia

··

      Cardiovascular: hypertension, shortened QT interval
      Gastrointestinal: constipation, nausea, vomiting, ileus, pancreatitis
      Mental status: psychiatric symptoms, confusion, obtundation
      Renal: acute renal failure, salt wasting, loss of concentrating function

··

less protein-bound calcium at any given ionized calcium level, making total serum calcium concentration lower in states of hypoalbuminemia. One can correct for this by adding 0.8 mg/dL to the total calcium concentration for each 1.0 g/dL in albumin concentration less than 4.0 mg/dL.

Plasma pH also affects the fraction of free calcium. Like hypoalbuminemia, acidemia (a fall in plasma pH) also results in an increased fraction of free calcium because of less binding of calcium to albumin. Conversely, as pH rises, albumin binds more free calcium, lowering the relative fraction of ionized calcium.

Direct measurement of ionized calcium should be made with a calcium-sensitive electrode in patients with signs or symptoms of hypercalcemia (or hypocalcemia) when these or other comorbid conditions confound the interpretation of total serum calcium.

Hypercalcemia

Signs and symptoms of hypercalcemia depend on the ionized calcium level (Table 36–4). The clinical history, examination, and routine laboratory data generally resolve the differential diagnosis (Table 36–5).

Treatment

Acute treatment of hypercalcemia requires volume repletion with 1 to 2 L of isotonic saline solution, antihypercalcemic agents (Table 36–6), and correction of

Table 36–5. Causes of Hypercalcemia in the ICU

··

Adrenal insufficiency
Secondary hyperparathyroidism (especially in patients with end-stage renal disease who are taking vitamin D and calcium supplements)
Immobilization (especially in young patients)
Lithium intoxication
Malignancy-associated hypercalcemia*
Recovery from rhabdomyolysis-induced acute renal failure
Thiazide diuretics
Thyrotoxicosis
Total parenteral nutrition

··

*Due to release of PTH-related peptide, local production of bone-resorbing cytokines, or unregulated 1,25-dihydroxyvitamin D (calcitriol) production.
PTH, parathyroid hormone.

Table 36–6. Drugs to Reduce Serum Calcium

CLASS OF AGENTS	MECHANISM OF ACTION, DOSE, AND COMMENTS
Bisphosphonates (etidronate, pamidronate)	Inhibit osteoclast-mediated bone resorption; their onset of action takes several days, but their effect lasts weeks. Pamidronate is given as 60–90 mg IV once over 4 to 24 h (give only 30–60 mg if renal failure is present).
Salmon calcitonin	Increases osteoblast and decreases osteoclast activity, thus decreasing bone calcium release. Although effective within several hours, it is short-lived. The dose of 4 U/kg SQ or IM should be repeated every 12 h until slower acting agents take effect. Tachyphylaxis typically develops after several doses.
Glucocorticoids	Effective only in hypercalcemia caused by granulomatous diseases or hematologic malignancies. They act by direct toxicity to offending cells, thereby decreasing calcitriol production and inhibiting calcitriol-mediated calcium absorption in the gut. Doses of 30–60 mg/day of prednisone or equivalent are used.

IV, intravenous; SQ, subcutaneously; IM, intramuscularly.

the underlying abnormality, if possible. A *loop* diuretic (e.g., furosemide 20 to 40 mg IV) can be added but only *after* the initial saline loading has replaced intravascular deficits. Saline infusions should be continued (100 to 250 mL/hour) to increase urinary calcium excretion. They are contraindicated, however, in renal failure, congestive heart failure, and other edematous states.

In patients with renal failure, hemodialysis may be effective in lowering the serum calcium concentration (see Chapter 16). In severe hypercalcemia (>12 mg/dL), especially when caused by malignancy or hyperparathyroidism, specific calcium-lowering therapy is necessary (see Table 36–6). The preferred therapy for severely hypercalcemic patients is a combination of calcitonin (for its rapid effect) and pamidronate (for its prolonged effect), along with normal saline with or without furosemide.

In severe, life-threatening hypercalcemia with obtundation or cardiovascular collapse, direct calcium chelation with ethylenediaminetetra-acetic acid (EDTA) or IV phosphate is indicated. Both of these, however, can induce severe *hypocalcemia*. Phosphate administration is contraindicated in the presence of hyperphosphatemia, as calcium-phosphate precipitation in tissues will occur. Hemodialysis may be the treatment of choice in severe, life-threatening hypercalcemia, whereas emergent surgical parathyroidectomy may be warranted in a parathyroid crisis.

Hypocalcemia

Clinical Manifestations

True hypocalcemia (low ionized calcium concentration) occurs in up to 40% of ICU patients, usually due to defects in mobilization of bone calcium reserves rather than inadequate intake or excessive loss of calcium. Hypocalcemia may contribute to left ventricular dysfunction, decreased cardiac output, and lowered systemic vascular resistance due to decreased resistance vessel tone. Electrocardiographic signs of hypocalcemia include QT prolongation, bradycardia, and heart block. Severe hypocalcemia can lead to neuromuscular excitability, including numbness, tingling, the Chvostek and Trousseau signs, twitching, laryngeal spasm, and, finally, generalized tetany and seizures.

The cause of hypocalcemia can usually be determined from the clinical history, examination, routine laboratory testing, and medication review (Table 36–7). *Serum phosphate and magnesium concentrations should be measured in all cases.*

Treatment

Acute treatment of symptomatic hypocalcemia (ionized calcium level <0.8 mmol/L) is controversial and based on minimal clinical data. Tetany and seizures related to hypocalcemia are treated with IV calcium, such as one or two ampules (10 to 20 mL) of 10% calcium gluconate (90 to 180 mg elemental calcium) over 20 minutes, followed by 0.5 to 1.0 mg/kg/hour elemental calcium IV in D_5W or isotonic saline solution. Therapy also requires frequent monitoring of ionized calcium levels. Because animal data suggest that supplemental calcium may worsen tissue damage in sepsis or circulatory collapse, treatment is reserved for cardiovas-

Table 36–7. Causes and Mechanisms of Acute Hypocalcemia

CAUSES	MECHANISM AND COMMENTS
Calcidiol deficiency	Inadequate calcitriol production due to end-stage liver disease or anticonvulsant drugs, e.g., phenytoin
Calcitriol deficiency	Inadequate gut calcium absorption and impaired PTH action on bone resorption due to renal failure
Chelation, endogenous	Acute pancreatitis (peripancreatic chelation of calcium by locally produced free fatty acids)
Chelation, exogenous	Citrate in blood products and during apheresis, calcium-poor albumin, foscarnet therapy (can cause severe falls in ionized calcium despite normal total calcium levels; concurrent use of IV pentamidine increases this risk)
Hungry bone syndrome	Rapid bony uptake of calcium (and phosphate and magnesium) immediately after surgical treatment of severe, prolonged hyperparathyroidism
Hyperphosphatemia	Produces calcium-phosphate precipitation in situ, such as that due to rhabdomyolysis, tumor lysis syndrome, phosphate enemas, or renal failure
Hypertriglyceridemia	Binding calcium in situ, such as with total parenteral nutrition or drugs, like propofol
Hypomagnesemia	Impedes release and the calcemic action of PTH
Renal failure	1. Hyperphosphatemia with resulting serum calcium binding and precipitation 2. Impaired renal calcitriol production 3. Uremia-induced skeletal resistance to PTH action
Septic shock, toxic shock syndrome	Mechanism poorly understood

PTH, parathyroid hormone; IV, intravenous.

cular compromise refractory to volume expansion and pressors. Because IV calcium corrects hypocalcemia only transiently, oral therapy with enteral calcium or vitamin D supplements, or both, must be started expeditiously if the underlying condition cannot be corrected.

Calcium-containing IV solutions should not be given with bicarbonate, phosphate, blood, or some drugs because precipitation will occur. Electrocardiographic monitoring is needed during IV calcium infusion and is especially important for patients taking digitalis. Intravenous calcium should not be given to hypocalcemic patients with hyperphosphatemia, as calcium-phosphate tissue precipitation will occur. Hemodialysis can be used instead in this setting to raise calcium and lower phosphate.

Simultaneous correction of *hypomagnesemia* is imperative to treat hypocalcemia effectively. Correction of magnesium deficits alone will frequently restore calcium homeostasis. In patients with acidemia and true hypocalcemia, the hypocalcemia must be corrected before rapidly correcting a coexistent acidemia. Otherwise, raising the plasma pH will bind more ionized calcium to albumin and aggravate the hypocalcemia.

MAGNESIUM DISORDERS

Normal serum magnesium concentration is 1.8 to 2.4 mg/dL (1.5 to 2.0 mEq/L or 0.75 to 1.0 mmol/L). Hypermagnesemia is rare in the ICU patient and is often iatrogenic, for example, due to magnesium sulfate treatment of pre-eclampsia (see Chapter 72). In contrast, total body magnesium deficiency with or without overt hypomagnesemia occurs frequently with potentially grave clinical consequences.

Hypomagnesemia

Clinical Signs

Hypomagnesemia (Table 36–8) is present in up to 65% of patients in the ICU. Most cases are mild ($[Mg^{2+}]$ between 1.2 and 1.8 mg/dL) and without pathophysiologic significance. More severe hypomagnesemia ($[Mg^{2+}]$ <1.2 mg/dL) produces neuromuscular excitability (tremors, twitching, seizures, and tetany) and muscle weakness (including respiratory muscles). Hypomagnesemia can be associated with refractory ventricular and supraventricular arrhythmias, especially in the setting of digitalis therapy or myocardial ischemia.

Associated Hypokalemia and Hypocalcemia

Hypokalemia and hypocalcemia often accompany hypomagnesemia because of common underlying causes and impaired magnesium-dependent homeostatic mechanisms. Because magnesium depletion induces renal (loop of Henle) potassium wasting, hypokalemia cannot be corrected until magnesium is repleted. Magnesium depletion also impairs parathyroid hormone secretion and interferes with the calcemic effect of parathyroid hormone on bone. Again, correction of hypocalcemia first requires repletion of magnesium. Hypocalcemia or hypokalemia, how-

Table 36–8. Causes of Hypomagnesemia in the ICU

Renal losses
 Alcoholic intoxication
 Diuretic phase of acute tubular necrosis
 Hypercalcemia
 Interstitial nephritis
 Loop or thiazide diuretics
 Nephrotoxic drugs (aminoglycoside antibiotics,
  cisplatin, carboplatin, amphotericin B,
  cyclosporine A, and pentamidine)
 Persistent volume expansion
 Postobstructive and osmotic diuresis
Gastrointestinal losses
 Chronic diarrhea, steatorrhea, or malabsorption
 Malnutrition with obligate stool magnesium loss

Massive tissue magnesium uptake
 Acute respiratory alkalosis
 Hungry bone syndrome after
  parathyroidectomy
 Refeeding following starvation
Chelation of magnesium
 Acute pancreatitis
 Massive blood product transfusion
Combined causes
 Alcoholism and alcohol withdrawal
 Diabetes mellitus and diabetic
  ketoacidosis

ever, should *not* be blamed on mild hypomagnesemia ($[Mg^{2+}] = 1.2$ to 1.8 mg/dL).

Treatment

Treatment of hypomagnesemia is dictated by the degree of hypomagnesemia and magnesium depletion, related symptoms, and renal function. Patients with $[Mg^{2+}]$ greater than 1.2 mg/dL and minimal symptoms are repleted orally. Symptomatic magnesium deficiency typically results from a 0.5 to 1.0 mmol/kg magnesium deficit.

Intravenous repletion is more rapid than oral (although 50% of the IV administered magnesium may be excreted in the urine if renal function is intact). The following regimen has been shown to be safe and effective:

1. Over the first 3 hours, give 12 mL of 50% magnesium sulfate (24 mmol elemental magnesium) diluted in 1 L D_5W.
2. Over the next 21 hours, give 20 mL of 50% magnesium sulfate (40 mmol elemental magnesium) in 2 L of D_5W.
3. Over subsequent days, give 12 mL of 50% magnesium sulfate (24 mmol elemental magnesium) per day.

Life-threatening symptoms, such as convulsions or ventricular arrhythmias, require 8 to 16 mmol 50% magnesium sulfate (4 to 8 mL), given IV in 100 mL D_5W over 10 minutes, followed by a continuous infusion of 12 mL of 50% magnesium sulfate in 1.0 of D_5W. Repletion is continued until normomagnesemia persists. Magnesium therapy is especially effective for torsades de pointes and digitalis-induced arrhythmias stemming from hypomagnesemia (see Chapter 31).

Frequent serum magnesium measurements and clinical assessments (checking deep tendon reflexes, mental status, cardiovascular status, and respiratory function) should guide replacement therapy. Since excess serum magnesium cannot be excreted, cautious repletion is required in patients with any degree of renal insufficiency.

PHOSPHATE DISORDERS

The body contains about 1000 g of phosphorus, of which approximately 85% resides in bone and most of the remainder is intracellular. Of the total plasma inorganic phosphorus, 10% is protein-bound, 5% is complexed, and the rest is in the form of orthophosphates. Serum inorganic phosphate (P_i) is measured as elemental phosphorus and thus "phosphate" and "phosphorus" concentrations are, by convention, synonymous. Normal P_i concentrations are 3.0 to 4.5 mg/dL (1.0 to 1.5 mmol/L or 1.8 to 2.7 mEq/L) at pH 7.4. Since extracellular P_i represents only 0.5% of total body phosphate, changes in serum P_i concentration do not necessarily reflect changes in total body phosphate.

Hypophosphatemia

Clinical Manifestations

Hypophosphatemia with or without total body phosphate depletion occurs in 10 to 25% of ICU patients. Moderate hypophosphatemia (1.5 to 2.5 mg/dL) is problematic only when symptoms are present or in the setting of severe total body phosphate depletion. The latter, however, can only be inferred from the clinical presentation.

Severe hypophosphatemia (<1.5 mg/dL) generally implies coexistent total body phosphate depletion. Occasionally, very low serum phosphate levels are found with minor or no total phosphate depletion, especially when due to acute respiratory alkalosis or diabetic ketoacidosis. In these cases, specific treatment is usually not needed.

Signs and symptoms of severe hypophosphatemia (Table 36–9) generally result from depletion of intracellular adenosine triphosphate or from decreases in erythrocyte 2,3-diphosphoglycerate. Decreases in 2,3-diphosphoglycerate impair release of oxygen from hemoglobin, and the resulting shift to the left in the oxyhemoglobin dissociation curve may compromise oxygen delivery to tissues (see Appendix A, Fig. 1).

Table 36–10 lists common causes of hypophosphatemia relevant to ICU patients. Multiple mechanisms may contribute to the phosphate depletion and hypophosphatemia, including poor intake, usual or accelerated gastrointestinal losses, inappropriate renal P_i loss (urinary P_i excretion should approach zero with hypophosphatemia), and internal losses (extra- to-intracellular redistribution). The clinical history and examination generally pinpoint its cause or causes.

Table 36–9. Symptoms and Signs of Severe Hypophosphatemia and Phosphate Depletion

Cardiac arrhythmias	Metabolic acidosis
Cardiomyopathy with decreased ventricular function	Proximal muscle weakness
Hemolysis (if Pi < 0.5 mg/dL)	Respiratory muscle weakness
Impaired platelet and leukocyte function	Rhabdomyolysis
Mental status changes	

Table 36–10. Causes of Severe Hypophosphatemia in the ICU

· ·

Burns
Chronic alcoholism
Chronic diarrhea or malabsorption
Chronic obstructive pulmonary disease with malnutrition
Chronic total parenteral nutrition
Decompensated diabetes mellitus
Drugs (ifosfamide, cyclophosphamide, aminoglycosides)
Hungry bone syndrome (after parathyroidectomy)
Major surgery
Malignancy (elevated PTHrP, oncogenic osteomalacia, acquired vitamin D–resistant osteomalacia)
Neuroleptic malignant syndrome
Phosphate binders (aluminum-, magnesium-, or calcium-containing antacids)
Refeeding syndrome
Respiratory alkalosis

· ·

PTHrP, parathyroid hormone–related peptide.

Chronic Alcoholism and Phosphate Depletion

Chronic alcoholism is an important cause of phosphate depletion and hypophosphatemia. Inadequate nutrition alone is usually insufficient to generate hypophosphatemia because bone mineral mobilization and tissue catabolism release phosphates to the circulation. In chronic alcoholics, however, the "empty" calories of alcohol attenuate tissue catabolism so that the hypophosphatemia related to poor intake can become manifest. Furthermore, frequent use of phosphate-binding antacids and vomiting further reduce intake from dietary sources, whereas diarrhea and malabsorption (from pancreatic insufficiency) increase phosphate losses. In addition, alcoholism-associated proximal tubular toxicity and hypomagnesemia promote renal P_i loss. Thus, even if the serum P_i is normal, the majority of individuals with chronic alcoholism will have total body phosphate depletion.

On admission to the hospital, many alcoholics are given IV saline for volume expansion, which accelerates renal P_i losses. Administration of supplemental glucose, insulin, and calories stimulates rapid shifts of phosphate into cells. Both the respiratory alkalosis and the catecholamine discharge of alcohol withdrawal worsen this transcellular shift. As a result, the alcoholic typically becomes severely hypophosphatemic after several days of hospitalization. Severe symptoms, including rhabdomyolysis, can result without phosphate repletion. This diagnosis can be masked, however, because of supervening renal failure and release of tissue phosphate (from rhabdomyolysis), which can quickly raise serum phosphate concentrations to normal or even high levels.

Diabetes and Phosphate Depletion

In patients with diabetic ketoacidosis, total body phosphate depletion is generally present but to a lesser degree than in chronic alcoholism. Although the serum P_i level can fall precipitously in patients with diabetic ketoacidosis after admission with therapy, generally only those patients who are frankly hypophosphatemic at admission may benefit from phosphate repletion.

Refeeding Syndrome and Phosphate Depletion

As noted earlier, chronically malnourished patients have total body phosphate depletion but may have nearly normal serum phosphate concentrations because of the release of phosphates from bone mineral mobilization and tissue catabolism. Refeeding, especially with carbohydrate, results in rapid anabolism, which has a high tissue requirement for P_i to generate adenosine triphosphate and other phosphate-requiring substances. As a result, phosphate stores are rapidly consumed. In addition, intracellular shift of P_i caused by insulin release worsens the situation so that severe, symptomatic hypophosphatemia may ensue.

Hypophosphatemia may also occur in ICU patients when total parenteral nutrition is administered chronically without phosphate supplementation; 10 to 15 mmol P_i is indicated normally for each 1000 Kcal of total parenteral nutrition.

Treatment

Treatment of hypophosphatemia is indicated when signs or symptoms of hypophosphatemia develop and when serum P_i level is less than 2.0 mg/dL. Treatment should also be given when hypophosphatemia is severe (<1.0 to 1.5 mg/dL) or when the clinical presentation (e.g., chronic alcoholism) implies significant phosphate depletion despite less severe hypophosphatemia (1.5 to 2.5 mg/dL). In ICU patients with mental status changes of uncertain cause, or in patients with respiratory muscle weakness or those preparing to be weaned from the ventilator, treatment of moderate hypophosphatemia should also be considered.

A typical patient with phosphate depletion needs 1 to 2 g of elemental phosphorus orally per day for 7 to 10 days to replace total body deficits. Serum P_i concentration cannot be used to estimate total body phosphate deficit, so treatment is empirical and guided by serial measurements of serum P_i concentration. Oral therapy is preferred but frequently limited by diarrhea.

Intravenous therapy is appropriate for patients unable to take oral therapy or those with severe, symptomatic presentations. Many different IV repletion regimens have been proposed: 0.08 mmol (2.4 mg) per kg of elemental phosphorus over 6 hours is generally safe. A dose of 15 mmol (450 mg) sodium phosphate given over 2 hours in 100 mL 0.9% sodium chloride with serum P_i less than 2.0 mg/dL has been reported to be safely tolerated without complication in surgical ICU patients. Serum phosphate and calcium should be checked every 6 to 12 hours to guide therapy.

The choice of agent is dictated by clinical condition. Most preparations contain significant potassium, which must be avoided in the presence of hyperkalemia and renal failure. Others contain sodium, which demands judicious use in patients with volume overload. One should avoid phosphate repletion in hypercalcemic patients because an elevated $[Ca] \times [P_i]$ product risks metastatic tissue calcification. Phosphate repletion with any preparation must be cautious in patients with renal failure because hyperphosphatemia can develop precipitously.

Phosphate depletion may also occur with hypocalcemia and hypomagnesemia, especially in alcoholics. Under these circumstances, phosphate repletion alone tends to worsen hypocalcemia and may precipitate tetany. Correcting the magnesium deficit (usually the proximate cause of hypocalcemia) and the phosphate deficit simultaneously is preferred.

Hyperphosphatemia

Causes and Clinical Manifestations

Although there are multiple causes of hyperphosphatemia, renal failure is most common (Table 36–11). Reduction of the glomerular filtration rate to less than 30 mL/min impairs phosphate excretion despite marked degrees of secondary hyperparathyroidism. Trauma and rhabdomyolysis often lead to further elevations in serum phosphate concentration in acute renal failure.

Redistribution of phosphate commonly causes hyperphosphatemia. For example, states of rapid catabolism with increased destruction of body tissues are associated with hyperphosphatemia. Similarly, severe hyperphosphatemia, hyperkalemia, hypocalcemia, and hyperuricemia (tumor lysis syndrome) occasionally follow administration of cytotoxic drugs or radiotherapy to patients with leukemia or lymphoma. Renal insufficiency in these patients is often caused by acute urate nephropathy but may also result from deposition of calcium-phosphate complexes in the kidney. Rhabdomyolysis after trauma, thermal injury, heat stroke, or opioid overdose may result in marked hyperphosphatemia caused by massive release of phosphate from intracellular sites. Finally, respiratory acidosis may cause hyperphosphatemia, presumably through shifts of intracellular phosphate into the extracellular fluid.

Clinical manifestations of hyperphosphatemia are primarily related to associated disorders of calcium metabolism, such as secondary hypocalcemia and ectopic soft tissue calcifications. The chances of ectopic calcification increase when the [Ca] × [P_i] product in the serum exceeds 70.

In most situations, the cause of hyperphosphatemia is easily identified by the clinical situation. A reduction in the glomerular filtration rate to less than 30 mL/min is the most common cause. Even if the renal failure is severe, however, the serum level of phosphate rarely exceeds 12 mg/dL, unless excessive amounts of phosphate are added to the circulation.

Treatment

Treatment of acute hyperphosphatemia with symptomatic hypocalcemia can be approached as follows: If renal failure is not present, urinary phosphate excretion

Table 36–11. Causes of Hyperphosphatemia

....

Decreased renal excretion
    Renal failure (acute or chronic)
    Increased tubular reabsorption of phosphate (thyrotoxicosis, bisphosphonate therapy, sickle cell anemia)
Exogenous phosphate load
    Acute intravenous phosphate load
    Gastrointestinal sources (phosphate-containing enemas or laxatives, vitamin D overdose)
Increased cellular release
    Rhabdomyolysis
    Tumor lysis syndrome
    Malignant hyperthermia
    Transfusion of stored blood
    Respiratory acidosis

....

can be increased with the use of isotonic saline or sodium bicarbonate, 1 to 2 L over 2 hours, and acetazolamide, 500 mg every 6 hours. When renal failure is present, institution of hemodialysis can promptly remove substantial amounts of phosphate and correct both the hyperphosphatemia and hypocalcemia. When very rapid control is required, glucose and insulin infusions promote cell phosphate uptake and may ameliorate hyperphosphatemia until dialysis is begun. The chronic hyperphosphatemia seen in chronic renal failure or hypoparathyroidism is treated primarily by a low-phosphate diet and calcium-containing antacids.

BIBLIOGRAPHY

Adrogue HJ, Lederer ED, Suki WN, Eknoyan G: Determinants of plasma potassium levels in diabetic ketoacidosis. Medicine (Baltimore) 65:163–172, 1986.
The ketoacidemia and hyperglycemia in diabetic ketoacidosis result primarily from insulin deficit and are the main determinants of increased plasma potassium levels. Renal dysfunction, by enhancing hyperglycemia and reducing potassium excretion, also contributes to hyperkalemia.

Al-Ghamdi SM, Cameron EC, Sutton RA: Magnesium deficiency: pathophysiologic and clinical overview. Am J Kidney Dis 24:737–752, 1994.
Hypomagnesemia produces a wide variety of clinical presentations, including neuromuscular irritability, cardiac arrhythmias, and increased sensitivity to digoxin. Refractory hypokalemia and hypocalcemia can be caused by concomitant hypomagnesemia and can be corrected with magnesium therapy. The dose and route are dictated by the clinical presentation, the degree of magnesium deficiency, and the renal function.

Allon M: Hyperkalemia in end-stage renal disease: mechanisms and management. J Am Soc Nephrol 6:1134–1142, 1995.
This review discusses known mechanisms for hyperkalemia in patients with end-stage renal disease, including less appreciated causes such as prolonged fasting and the use of nonselective beta-adrenergic blockers. The results of studies on the acute treatment of hyperkalemia are summarized, confirming the efficacy of intravenous insulin while raising doubts about the utility of intravenous bicarbonate. The beta-adrenergic agonist albuterol appears to be a useful adjunct to insulin for acutely lowering plasma potassium in some patients.

Buell JF, Berger AC, Plotkin JS, et al: The clinical implications of hypophosphatemia following major hepatic resection or cryosurgery. Arch Surg 133:757–761, 1998.
A retrospective study in a university referral center found that the overall incidence of hypophosphatemia was 67% with a mortality rate of 3%. The occurrence of hypophosphatemia correlates with an increased incidence of postoperative complications.

Collins MT, Skarulis MC, Bilezikian JP, et al: Treatment of hypercalcemia secondary to parathyroid carcinoma with a novel calcimimetic agent. J Clin Endocrinol Metab 83:10833–10838, 1998.
The first of a new class of calcimimetic compounds with activity at the calcium-sensing receptor has been used to effectively control hypercalcemia in a patient with parathyroid carcinoma. During 2 years of treatment, no adverse clinical effects were observed.

Fatemi S, Singer FR, Rude RK: Effect of salmon calcitonin and etidronate on hypercalcemia of malignancy. Calcif Tissue Int 50:107–109, 1992.
The authors administered etidronate, 7.5 mg/kg/day intravenously and salmon calcitonin, 100 U subcutaneously, every 12 hours for 3 days in 9 patients with hypercalcemia associated with malignancy. This regimen more effectively lowers the serum calcium concentration than the use of either agent alone because it combines the rapid hypocalcemic effects of calcitonin with the more delayed effect of bisphosphonate.

Fine A, Patterson J: Severe hyperphosphatemia following phosphate administration for bowel preparation in patients with renal failure: two cases and a review of the literature. Am J Kidney Dis 29:103–105, 1997.
Repeated doses of phosphate bowel preparations/purgatives can be dangerous in patients with renal impairment because of severe hyperphosphatemia and hypocalcemia.

Gucalp R, Theriault R, Gill I, et al: Treatment of cancer-associated hypercalcemia. Double-blind comparison of rapid and slow intravenous infusion regimens of pamidronate disodium and saline alone. Arch Intern Med 154:1935–1944, 1994.

A 4-hour infusion of pamidronate disodium, 60 mg, was as safe and effective as a 24-hour infusion, and both were superior to saline alone in lowering corrected serum calcium concentrations in patients with cancer-associated hypercalcemia.

Hande KR, Garrow GC: Acute tumor lysis syndrome in patients with high-grade non-Hodgkin's lymphoma. Am J Med 94:133–139, 1993.

The syndrome is characterized by increase in the serum phosphate, potassium, uric acid, and urea nitrogen concentrations, and a decline in the serum calcium concentration. Patients with a high serum lactate dehydrogenase level or renal insufficiency are at increased risk for metabolic complications after chemotherapy and should be closely monitored.

Kruse JA, Carlson RW: Rapid correction of hypokalemia using concentrated intravenous potassium chloride infusions. Arch Intern Med 150:613–617, 1990.

Data are presented that endorse the relative safety of using concentrated (200-mEq/L) potassium chloride infusions at a rate of 20 mEq/h via central or peripheral vein to correct hypokalemia in patients in the intensive care unit.

Larner AJ: Pseudohyperphosphatemia. Clin Biochem 28:391–393, 1995.

The author reviews instances of spurious elevation of inorganic phosphate measurements due to interference with analytic methods, including paraproteinemia (probably the commonest), hyperlipidemia, hemolysis, and hyperbilirubinemia.

Weisinger JR, Bellorin-Font E: Magnesium and phosphorus. Lancet 352:391–396, 1998.

This is a summary of new findings regarding alterations of magnesium and phosphorus metabolism. Alterations in serum concentrations of these ions are frequently observed in acutely ill patients. Correction of the abnormalities must be done early in the course of the alterations.

37 Falling Urine Output and Rising Creatinine Levels

Ashraf A. Elshami
Scott Manaker

A fall in urine output with the accumulation of creatinine, urea, and other metabolic wastes are the hallmarks of acute renal failure (ARF). ARF is a common complication in hospitalized patients and may occur in up to one third of patients in the intensive care unit (ICU). The development of ARF prolongs hospitalizations and increases costs. However, even severe ARF is potentially fully reversible with proper management. For these reasons, a rational diagnostic and therapeutic approach to ARF is necessary (Fig. 37–1).

DEFINITIONS

ARF is acute renal dysfunction characterized by the accumulation of nitrogenous wastes. It is detected clinically by a rise in the blood urea nitrogen (BUN) or serum creatinine level, or both. Urea nitrogen is formed in the liver as a result of protein metabolism. Creatinine is a hydrolysis product of creatine and is normally released at a relatively constant rate from muscle. ARF occurs over hours to days and may be superimposed on pre-existing chronic renal failure. The precise pathogenic pathway leading to ARF depends on the interaction of several processes that decrease glomerular filtration, including vascular, glomerular, and tubular factors. The final common pathway of these processes is a sudden decline in the glomerular filtration rate, which prevents the kidney from maintaining a normal chemical environment.

A falling urine output is important because it is often the first sign of ARF. *Oliguria* is defined as a urine output that is insufficient to excrete the daily osmolar load (generally <400 mL/day). *Anuria* is often defined as a urine output less than 50 mL/day, and it is frequently associated with urinary tract obstruction. Renal dysfunction also occurs in the presence of a normal urine output. In fact, the majority of cases of ARF are *nonoliguric*.

Acute tubular necrosis (ATN) denotes the clinical syndrome of reversible intrinsic ARF in the absence of renovascular, glomerular, or interstitial disease.

DIFFERENTIAL DIAGNOSIS

ARF most commonly presents with both oliguria and azotemia. However, decreased urinary output confers little diagnostic sensitivity or specificity. Adequate urine output (≥1 L/day) is *not* a reliable indicator of adequate renal function. Conversely, in the anuric patient with no urine output there is most likely an obstructive cause (although renal artery occlusion, rapidly progressive glomerulonephritis, or ATN uncommonly cause anuria). *Polyuria* (>3 L of urine daily) may

441

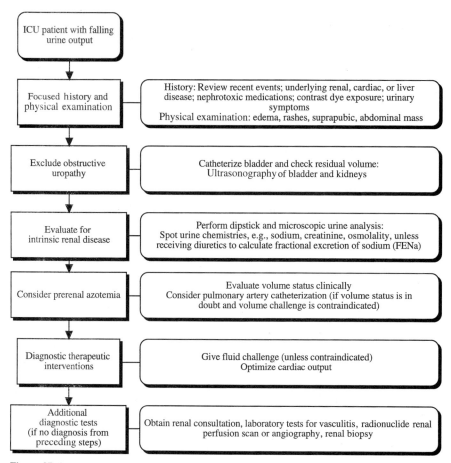

Figure 37–1. Schematic flow diagram that illustrates the general diagnostic approach to the development of acute renal failure or oliguria in ICU patients.

represent a less severe form of renal failure, with preservation of small amounts of glomerular filtration despite tubular damage. Patients with partial urinary obstruction frequently have polyuria.

As a rule, in the absence of glomerular filtration, serum creatinine levels should rise by only 1 to 2 mg/dL per day. However, serum creatinine levels may also rise with normal renal function (Table 37–1). Likewise, in the absence of urine formation, the serum BUN should rise about 10 to 20 mg/dL per day. It may rise more than 30 mg/dL per day in catabolic states or with excessive protein loading. Because of variability in its hepatic synthesis and potential renal tubular reabsorption in low urine flow states, the BUN is a less reliable indicator of the glomerular filtration rate than is the serum creatinine level. An increased ratio of BUN:serum creatinine (which is normally 10:1) suggests various pathologic conditions (see Table 37–1). A ratio of less than 10:1 may be seen with decreased urea nitrogen

Table 37–1. Differential Diagnoses for Elevated Creatinine and
Increased Blood Urea Nitrogen-to-Creatinine Ratio

ELEVATED SERUM CREATININE LEVEL	ELEVATED BLOOD UREA NITROGEN: CREATININE RATIO (>20 : 1)
Rhabdomyolysis	Excessive protein loading (e.g., >1.5 g protein/kg/day)
Drugs that interfere with tubular secretion of creatinine (cimetidine and trimethoprim)	Increased catabolism (glucocorticosteroids, tetracyclines)
Drugs that interfere with laboratory assay for creatinine (serum ketones, cefoxitin)	Intravascular volume contraction with low urine flow states
Renal failure	Gastrointestinal bleeding (with digested blood causing disproportionate rise in BUN)

BUN, blood urea nitrogen.

synthesis (e.g., protein malnutrition, advanced liver disease), disproportionate reductions in BUN, or increases in creatinine levels.

CLASSIFICATION OF ACUTE RENAL FAILURE

The formation of urine begins with the ultrafiltration of blood in the glomerulus,
followed by tubular reabsorption and secretion, and culminates in urine outflow
through the ureters, bladder, and urethra. ARF can arise when disease processes
act at any of these different sites: (1) prerenal (decreased renal perfusion), (2)
intrinsic (renal parenchymal injury), and (3) postrenal (obstruction to urine outflow). (Refer to Chapter 78 for a complete list of causes within each of these
categories.)

Prerenal Azotemia

In general, the most common and readily reversible cause of ARF is prerenal
azotemia resulting from a decrease in renal perfusion. Decreased renal perfusion
may result from hypotension, hypovolemia, a reduction in effective (functionally
depleted) intravascular volume, renovascular disease, or drugs, such as nonsteroidal
anti-inflammatory drugs (NSAIDs) and angiotensin-converting enzyme (ACE) inhibitors. Classically, these patients have a high BUN:serum creatinine ratio (>20:1)
and renal conservation of salt and water, resulting in low urine sodium concentration and high urine specific gravity or osmolality. However, measurement of urine
sodium and osmolality are of little value in the presence of diuretic therapy.
Untreated prerenal azotemia may progress to tubular damage and ATN.

Intrinsic Renal Disease

ARF may result from damage to any part of the kidney from primary renal disease
or an underlying systemic illness. Such disorders may affect the renal vasculature,

glomeruli, interstitium, or tubules. Of these, tubular injury (ATN) is the most common cause of intrinsic renal disease. Nearly 60% of all cases of ATN occur in surgical and trauma patients, 38% occur in a medical setting, and 2% are pregnancy-related. ATN often occurs after renal ischemia or nephrotoxic drug exposure, such as intravenous contrast for radiographic studies or pigmenturia due to hemoglobin or myoglobin.

Acute interstitial nephritis results from a generalized allergic reaction. The drugs most often implicated include antibiotics, diuretics, and NSAIDs. Although a skin rash occurs in a minority of patients, eosinophilia is common (but often transient), while eosinophiluria occurs in up to 95% of cases.

Postrenal Azotemia

The most common cause of acute urinary obstruction in the ICU arises from obstruction of indwelling bladder catheters. Other causes include prostatic enlargement (especially in the presence of drugs that can cause acute urinary retention), neurogenic bladders in noncatheterized patients and, rarely, papillary necrosis. Both kidneys must be involved to result in azotemia except in patients with a single functioning kidney or underlying chronic renal disease. A precipitous fall in urine output or complete anuria should suggest obstruction.

DIAGNOSTIC EVALUATION

Appropriate management of ARF requires identifying the cause or causes. However, in most cases of ICU-acquired renal failure, there are multiple factors contributing to renal injury. For example, ARF often occurs concomitant with the failure of other organ systems. Sepsis is the most common predisposing condition for ARF. Other common renal insults in the ICU include hypotension, nephrotoxic medications, and congestive heart failure. Under these circumstances, it may not be possible to classify renal failure neatly into prerenal, intrinsic, and postrenal categories, but using this general approach is often helpful (see Fig. 37–1).

History and Physical Examination

The history and physical examination should focus on pre-existing renal, cardiac, or hepatic disease; recent events (hypotension, hemorrhage, fever); prior ingestion of nephrotoxic drugs, such as acetaminophen or lithium; and any urinary tract symptoms. A medication review may reveal exposure to other nephrotoxins, including aminoglycosides, radiocontrast agents, or diuretics. The physical examination should assess volume status, possible obstructive uropathy (the presence of abdominal or pelvic masses), vascular compromise (abdominal aortic aneurysm), and rashes (drug-induced interstitial nephritis, palpable purpura associated with vasculitis, nonpalpable purpura associated with thrombotic thrombocytopenic purpura, and livedo reticularis in atheroembolic disease or vascular insufficiency).

Hypovolemia may be indicated by a review of daily weights and fluid balance or by overt or orthostatic hypotension. Invasive hemodynamic monitoring, a volume challenge or echocardiography to assess left ventricular diastolic filling may be required for some patients, for example, those in hepatic failure, whose intravascular volume status is unclear.

Rule Out Urinary Obstruction

The exclusion of urinary obstruction is a critical step because ARF may be easily reversible with rapid relief of an obstruction. Bladder catheterization should be performed first. If it shows a residual volume greater than 100 mL, the presence of bladder outlet obstruction is suggested, requiring catheter drainage. If the residual volume is low, a noninvasive scan may be necessary to rule out obstruction of the ureters, particularly if the history and physical examination suggest obstructive uropathy. Ultrasonography is the test of choice to exclude obstruction. However, false-negative results with renal ultrasonography may occur with extensive retroperitoneal disease. In this instance, computed tomography or magnetic resonance imaging may be useful.

Urinalysis

The urine sediment should be examined in all cases of ARF. Although prerenal and postrenal causes of ARF are usually not associated with an abnormal sediment, rare granular or hyaline casts may be seen with prerenal azotemia and hematuria; pyuria or crystals may be seen with postrenal azotemia. Many cells, casts, and protein suggest intrinsic causes of renal failure. ATN often has granular casts, pigmented granular casts, and renal tubular epithelial cells. Pyuria, leukocyte casts, eosinophils, and casts of eosinophils suggest interstitial nephritis. A special stain (Hansel's stain) is usually needed to distinguish eosinophils from neutrophils. Eosinophils may also be seen with vascular disorders, but red cells are more characteristic. Erythrocytes and erythrocyte casts, as well as abundant proteinuria, suggest glomerulonephritis. A positive result from the urine dipstick test for blood, along with a negative microscopic examination for erythrocytes, suggests pigmenturia.

Urine Electrolytes

In the absence of diuretics, urine electrolytes are useful for distinguishing prerenal azotemia from ATN. In prerenal azotemia, spot urine sodium concentration is usually less than 30 mEq/L and the fractional excretion of sodium (FENa = ([urine sodium/plasma sodium]/[urine creatinine/plasma creatinine]) $\times$ 100) is less than 1%. However, other conditions that cause renal vasoconstriction (radiocontrast agents, myoglobinuric ARF, early sepsis, the hepatorenal syndrome, NSAID therapy) may also result in low urine sodium excretion and an FENa less than 1%.

In contrast, ATN is characterized by urinary sodium levels greater than 30 mEq/L and an FENa greater than 1%. Diuretic therapy in the prior 12 to 24 hours, glycosuria, or pre-existing chronic renal failure with a concentrating deficit may result in an FENa greater than 1% even with prerenal azotemia. Finally, urine sodium levels and FENa are not helpful in the evaluation of postrenal azotemia or renal azotemia resulting from vascular disorders, glomerulonephritis, or interstitial nephritis.

Laboratory Tests

Standard laboratory tests may provide additional clues. Thrombocytopenia and microangiopathic hemolysis may indicate thrombotic thrombocytopenic purpura, intravascular hemolysis due to an acute transfusion reaction, or the presence of vasculitis. Eosinophilia may be seen with allergic interstitial nephritis or cholesterol emboli. An elevated creatine kinase level (skeletal muscle fraction, CK-MM) indicates rhabdomyolysis. Tumor lysis syndrome can be associated with hyperuricemia, hyperphosphatemia, and high levels of lactate dehydrogenase. Specific serologic studies and other tests may be indicated in vasculitides (antineutrophilic cytoplasmic antibody for Wegener's vasculitis, antiglomerular basement membrane antibody for Goodpasture's syndrome, and complement levels and antinuclear antibody for systemic lupus erythematosus).

Volume Challenge

In prerenal azotemia, a careful volume challenge may be both diagnostic and therapeutic. Intravenous infusion of 500 to 1000 mL of normal (0.9%) saline over 1 to 2 hours is usually sufficient. However, patients with volume overload but functionally depleted (ineffective) intravascular volume, (e.g., patients with congestive heart failure, cirrhosis with ascites or nephrotic syndrome) should not be treated with extra fluids, but rather with therapy directed at the underlying disorder. For example, the patient with congestive heart failure should receive inotropes and vasodilators to optimize cardiac output.

Additional Diagnostic Tests

If the cause of ARF remains unknown, seek renal consultation. Further tests may be indicated. Radionuclide renal scans may reveal decreased renal blood flow, suggesting vascular occlusion. Intravenous pyelography is rarely indicated and is best avoided because of the radiocontrast dye load. Percutaneous renal biopsy is reserved for patients suspected of intrinsic renal disease, such as acute glomerulonephritis, interstitial nephritis, or vasculitis.

MANAGEMENT

The management of ARF depends on the underlying cause (Table 37–2). As noted previously, patients in the ICU often have multiple factors predisposing to ARF. Efforts should be directed at the maintenance of euvolemia and renal perfusion, discontinuing and avoiding nephrotoxic drugs, treating infections, and correcting electrolyte derangements.

Table 37–2. General Approach to the Management of Acute Renal Failure

MANAGEMENT STEPS	DESCRIPTION
Correct prerenal factors and maintain renal perfusion	Fluid challenge or inotropic agents, or both
Establish urine output	High-dose loop diuretic or low-dose dopamine, or both
Address biochemical complications	Measure electrolytes daily; correct electrolyte and acid-base abnormalities
Prevent further renal injury	Avoid nephrotoxins; volume expansion diuresis for crystalluria, pigmenturia, significant trauma, major vascular surgery, radiocontrast agents, amphotericin B, cisplatin
Fluid and electrolyte management	Maintain euvolemia, limit daily potassium and sodium intake, avoid magnesium-containing antacids, give phosphate binders enterally
Provide adequate nutrition	Minimize negative nitrogen balance
Monitor drug therapy	Adjust dosing; measure drug levels
Hemodialysis or ultrafiltration	Indicated for severe uremia, fluid overload that is unresponsive to conservative measures, intractable hyperkalemia, acidemia, or bleeding

Diagnosis and Treatment of Postrenal Obstruction

Unless an initial volume challenge clearly indicates a prerenal cause, bladder catheterization should be followed by renal ultrasonography to evaluate for ureteral obstruction. Ureteral stents or percutaneous nephrostomy may be required to relieve obstruction. A postobstructive diuresis may result after decompression and should be treated aggressively with fluids and electrolytes to prevent hypovolemia, hypotension, and electrolyte derangements.

Maintain Renal Perfusion

Maintenance of renal perfusion is central to the management of ARF. If it is unclear whether ARF is prerenal or due to intrinsic renal disease, it is advisable to perform a fluid challenge while monitoring urine output and creatinine levels. Pulmonary artery catheterization is indicated when renal failure and oliguria occur in the setting of an uncertain intravascular volume status after there has been no response to volume challenge or in the presence of persistent hypotension. Other indications for central hemodynamic monitoring include patients with hepatic failure and possible hepatorenal syndrome and patients with increased total body fluid in whom intravascular volume depletion is suspected. The pulmonary artery (Swan-Ganz) catheter may be used to optimize intravascular volume by maintaining pulmonary arterial wedge (occlusion) pressure at greater than 10 mm Hg and to guide vasoactive therapy to maintain adequate cardiac output. In some cases (e.g., chronic congestive heart failure), higher filling pressures (pulmonary arterial wedge pressure = 16 to 18 mm Hg) may be necessary.

In certain clinical settings, intravascular volume expansion and high urine flow rates may prevent ARF. In several retrospective studies, patients undergoing major cardiac and vascular surgery with maintenance of adequate intravascular volume and Swan-Ganz catheter monitoring had fewer cases of postoperative ARF. Volume expansion is also thought to be useful in myoglobinuria or hemoglobinuria in which alkalinization of the urine may solubilize the urine pigments. Therefore, in patients with rhabdomyolysis (e.g., in patients who have had a crush injury), forced alkaline diuresis until the urine is no longer dipstick-positive for blood (but negative for red blood cells by urinalysis) is a reasonable approach. In crystalluria resulting in renal tubular obstruction, a high urine output prevents nephrotoxicity. Crystalluria can occur in tumor lysis syndrome or hyperuricemia or when high doses of methotrexate or acyclovir result in their intratubular precipitation. Finally, patients should routinely receive volume expansion before and after exposure to intravascular contrast media.

Eliminate Nephrotoxic Drugs

Commonly used nephrotoxins include aminoglycosides, NSAIDs, ACE inhibitors, and radiographic contrast agents (see Tables 78–1 and 78–3). Patients with hypotension, underlying renal disease, or volume depletion or patients with bilateral renal artery stenosis are at increased risk for nephrotoxicity from NSAIDs or ACE inhibitors. Patients at greatest risk for contrast-induced nephropathy include those with diabetes, chronic renal insufficiency, volume depletion, heart failure, or multiple myeloma, those who receive large contrast loads, or those with a combination of these conditions. Simultaneous exposure to other nephrotoxins also increases the risk of contrast-induced ARF. Risk factors for aminoglycoside nephrotoxicity include patients who are elderly, those with decreased renal perfusion or liver disease, and those who receive other nephrotoxins concomitantly, or high-dose and long-duration aminoglycoside therapy. In these patients, aminoglycoside dosage should therefore be carefully adjusted by following drug levels (see Chapter 12). In addition, serum creatinine measurements should be followed, other nephrotoxins should be avoided, and adequate renal perfusion should be maintained.

Maintain Urine Output

If the nonobstructed, euvolemic patient with ARF remains oliguric, many clinicians attempt to make the patient nonoliguric. Although it is unproved that this shortens the duration of ARF, achieving adequate urinary flow makes ARF easier to manage. High-dose loop diuretics (bolus or continuous infusion) or renal vasodilators, or both, may be used. Continuous intravenous infusion of furosemide (0.5 to 1.0 mg/kg per hour) or bumetanide (1.0 mg/hour) may be used after trials of intermittent boluses of high doses are unsuccessful. Anecdotal data support the use of low-dose dopamine (≤ 2.5 μg/kg per minute) combined with loop diuretics in oliguric ARF. Diuretics must be given early in the course of ARF because the likelihood of a response diminishes the longer the oliguria persists.

Fluid and Electrolyte Management

Patients with ARF are usually catabolic and lose an average of 0.3 kg of lean body mass daily. Therefore, weight gain is usually due to salt and water retention. Total daily sodium and potassium intake (dietary and intravenous) should not exceed measured 24-hour urinary losses of these electrolytes. Magnesium-containing drugs should be avoided. If the serum phosphate concentration exceeds 6.0 mg/dL, oral phosphate-binding antacids, for example, aluminum hydroxide, should be given. If acidemia is severe (serum bicarbonate levels <15 mEq/L), sodium bicarbonate or equivalent base should be administered. Many drug doses require adjustment in renal failure. However, because creatinine is often not at steady state in ARF, it is impossible to calculate appropriate drug doses based on the patient's creatinine levels, and serum drug levels must be monitored.

Adequate calories and protein should be provided to minimize negative nitrogen balance. Severe ARF in the ICU requires approximately 30 to 60 Kcal/kg per day, but no more than 50 to 60% of the nonprotein calories should be fat. Protein is given at 0.5 to 1.0 g/kg per day orally or 10 to 20 g/day intravenously (if the patient is receiving total parental nutrition).

Dialysis

Dialysis is indicated for the management of fluid overload unresponsive to conventional therapy, intractable acidemia or hyperkalemia, or severe uremia. Dialysis is discussed in detail in Chapters 16 and 78.

CLINICAL PEARLS AND PITFALLS

1. ICU-related ARF results from more than one renal insult. Sepsis, hypotension, aminoglycosides, and radiocontrast exposure are the most common causes in the ICU.
2. Urine volume is not a reliable indicator of renal function, particularly with the use of diuretics.
3. As a rule, anuria suggests an obstructive uropathy.
4. Pre- and postrenal azotemia may be readily reversible and should be excluded early in the diagnostic evaluation.
5. A prerenal cause of ARF is suggested by:
   a. a normal urinary sediment (also seen in postrenal causes)
   b. an elevated serum BUN to creatinine ratio (>20:1)
   c. FENa <1.0%
   d. development after exposure to NSAIDs or ACE inhibitors
6. In the absence of obstruction, a careful volume challenge may distinguish prerenal from renal causes of ARF.
7. An attempt should be to convert oliguric to nonoliguric ARF to make management easier.

BIBLIOGRAPHY

Hock R, Anderson RJ: Prevention of drug-induced nephrotoxicity in the intensive care unit. J Crit Care 10:33–43, 1995.
This article reviews the risk factors, clinical course, and prevention of nephrotoxicity after exposure to aminoglycosides, anti-inflammatory drugs, and radiographic contrast agents. It lists 75 references.

Jochimsen F, Schafer JH, Maurer A, Distler A: Impairment of renal function in medical intensive care: Predictability of acute renal failure. Crit Care Med 18:480–485, 1990.
Acute and chronic risk factors for the development of acute renal failure by prospective analysis are identified.

Mandal AK, Visweswaran RK, Kaldas NR: Treatment considerations in acute renal failure. Drugs 44:567–577, 1992.
This article presents a review of the therapeutic strategies for prerenal, intrinsic renal, and postrenal causes of ARF.

Miller TR, Anderson RJ, Linas SL, et al: Urinary diagnostic indices in acute renal failure. Ann Intern Med 88:47–50, 1978.
This is a classic prospective study of the value of urinary indices (e.g., urine sodium, osmolality, fractional excretion of sodium) in ascertaining the cause of acute renal failure.

Molina MF, Riella MC: Nutritional support in the patient with renal failure. Crit Care Clin 11:685–704, 1995.
The various metabolic alterations and nutritional support in the setting of acute renal failure are reviewed and 83 references are listed.

Shilliday I, Allison ME: Diuretics in acute renal failure. Renal Failure 16:3–17, 1994.
This article reviews studies on the ability of loop diuretics, mannitol, dopamine, and atrial natriuretic peptide to ameliorate or reverse acute renal failure. It lists 73 references.

Thadhani R, Pascual M, Bonventre JV: Acute renal failure. N Engl J Med 334:1448–1459, 1996.
Acute renal failure is reviewed and 143 references are listed.

38

Fever, Hypothermia, or a Rising White Blood Cell Count

Ashraf A. Elshami
Scott Manaker

Fever and leukocytosis are common problems in the intensive care unit (ICU). Because they are frequently due to acute infection, aggressive diagnostic efforts should be made to identify their cause. Imaging studies are important because many intra-abdominal, pulmonary, cerebral, and musculoskeletal causes of infection and fever can be subtle, particularly in heavily sedated, paralyzed, or immunocompromised patients. Because many noninfectious processes can also cause fever in patients in the ICU and must be distinguished from infections, the evaluation of fever should be systematic and thorough. This chapter provides a general diagnostic and therapeutic approach to the patient in the ICU with fever (or hypothermia) or with a rising white blood cell count.

DEFINITIONS

Classic teaching defines *fever* as a core body temperature exceeding 38° C (100.4° F). In normal subjects, many factors affect body temperature, including age, physical activity, emotion, eating, pregnancy, and diurnal variation (with an evening peak and a morning trough). Thus, fever may be best defined on an individual basis by following temperature trends.

Several methods can be employed to measure body temperature. In the ICU, pulmonary artery and bladder thermistor catheters give highly reliable core temperature measurements. Rectal temperatures, however, are used more frequently and closely approximate core temperature. Oral temperature measurement, although convenient in adults, is not commonly used in the ICU, where patients may be intubated or uncooperative. Oral readings tend to be 0.30 to 0.65° C lower than rectal values. They are unreliable indicators of fever, with spuriously low readings in certain conditions. Tympanic membrane temperature is usually 0.05 to 0.25° C less than rectal temperature, but the measuring device can correct for this difference in its output display. Axillary and skin temperatures in patients in the ICU are unreliable because of variations in peripheral perfusion.

Hypothermia is defined as a core temperature less than 35° C. Its occurrence is important because some patients exhibit a hypothermic rather than febrile response to infection. The clinical syndrome of hypothermia is discussed in greater detail in Chapter 54.

PATHOPHYSIOLOGY

The hypothalamus regulates body temperature by controlling heat gain and heat loss mechanisms. Fever is a disorder of thermoregulation resulting from upward

451

displacement of the temperature set point. A family of endogenous fever-inducing substances (pyrogens) act on receptors in the hypothalamus to raise this set point. Leukocytes and macrophages produce these endogenous pyrogens (including interleukin-1, tumor necrosis factor, platelet-activating factor, interleukin-6, and interferon) in response to microorganisms, toxins, or other immunologic mediators. Interleukin-1 is regarded as the prototypic endogenous pyrogen. Although these cytokines are important in activating the immune and inflammatory systems, their adverse effects may be observed in other body systems, for example, as increased metabolic rate and oxygen consumption.

Heat stroke, malignant hyperthermia, and neuroleptic malignant syndrome, which have distinct pathophysiologic mechanisms, are discussed in Chapter 54.

DIFFERENTIAL DIAGNOSIS

Infectious Causes of Fever

The most common and serious cause of fever in patients in the ICU is acute infection. Symptoms of acute infection include chills, rigors, hemodynamic parameters indicating low afterload, or leukocytosis with a shift in the differential count to a higher percentage of granulocytes and immature white blood cell forms ("left shift"). Although these nonspecific findings may occur with noninfectious causes of fever, empirical therapy for infection may still be warranted until the source of fever is found. This is usually the case if the patient becomes hypotensive and appears to be in septic shock. Although fever patterns may provide clues to the diagnosis in certain conditions, such patterns are generally unhelpful in the ICU, where the use of antipyretics, antibiotics, steroids, and other medications may alter the course of the underlying disease and the daily fever curve.

Common infections encountered in the ICU setting are listed in Table 38–1. The use of invasive devices and the general debility of critically ill patients predispose them to nosocomial infections. Invasive devices used for monitoring or therapy bypass normal host defenses. For example, tracheal intubation facilitates entry of organisms into the lower respiratory tract, with resultant pneumonia. Nasal

Table 38–1. Infectious Causes of Fever in the Intensive Care Unit

Abdominal, gastrointestinal	Acalculous cholecystitis; appendicitis; diverticulitis; intra-abdominal, pelvic, or retroperitoneal abscess; liver abscess; mesenteric infarction; peritonitis; pseudomembranous colitis; viral hepatitis (transfusion-related)
Nosocomial infections	Intravascular catheter–related infection (phlebitis, cellulitis, bacteremia-fungemia, endocarditis or septic thrombophlebitis, or both), pneumonia, sinusitis, systemic candidiasis, tracheobronchitis, urinary tract infection
Surgical	Deep operative infection, infected prosthesis, retained surgical sponge, wound infection

catheters obstruct sinus drainage, producing sinusitis and occult fever in intubated patients. Indwelling urinary catheters allow entry of organisms into the urinary tract, resulting in infection. Intravenous catheters, arterial catheters, temporary transvenous pacemakers, and intra-aortic assist devices can also be sources of bacteremia in the ICU. The vast majority of nosocomial infections are bacterial and involve the urinary tract, surgical wounds, lower respiratory tract, or intravascular catheters (see Chapter 11).

Respiratory Tract Infections

Nosocomial pneumonia is often a difficult diagnosis to make in the ICU. Fever may be present in 50% of patients with atelectasis and no pneumonia, and positive sputum cultures may represent colonization rather than infection. The diagnosis in the setting of the acute respiratory distress syndrome is even more difficult because of the radiographic changes seen in this condition. Patients with fever, leukocytosis, purulent sputum, new radiographic infiltrates, air bronchograms, asymmetric or segmental infiltrates, or ipsilateral pleural effusion have a higher probability of having pneumonia. However, new infiltrates and fever may also be of noninfectious origin, for example, atelectasis, pulmonary embolism, or progression of underlying parenchymal pulmonary disease. Some authors advocate the use of bronchoscopy with quantitative culture of bronchoalveolar lavage or a protected specimen brush (see Chapter 11), especially before initial antibiotics are started or, in the case of patients already on antibiotics, before new antibiotics are begun.

Abdominal Infections

Another common source of infection and fever is the abdomen. Acute cholecystitis frequently causes sepsis in critically ill patients. In the general population, most cases of acute cholecystitis are associated with gallstones, whereas acalculous cholecystitis accounts for only 5 to 10% of cases. In the ICU setting, however, *acalculous cholecystitis* accounts for up to 47% of postoperative cases of acute cholecystitis, commonly associated with trauma, burns, diabetes, or hyperalimentation. The diagnosis of abdominal causes of fever or leukocytosis is often delayed because patients are frequently obtunded or unresponsive. Mesenteric infarction occurs in elderly patients with generalized atherosclerosis, hypotension, or atrial fibrillation. Pseudomembranous colitis due to *Clostridium difficile* is associated with antibiotic use and may occur even in the absence of diarrhea.

Postoperative Causes

In the postoperative patient, the temporal appearance of fever may give clues to the diagnosis (see Fig. 88–1). Fever within the first 24 hours is ordinarily of pulmonary origin resulting from atelectasis. Rarely, fulminant wound infections also cause fever within the first 24 hours. *Third-day fever* refers to infection of indwelling catheters and deep venous thrombosis (DVT) at postoperative day 3. Wound infection, pulmonary embolism, and pneumonia are common culprits when fever occurs at postoperative days 5 or 6. Intra-abdominal abscesses become evident at postoperative days 6 to 8. Urinary tract infections and acalculous cholecystitis may occur anytime postoperatively.

Fungal Causes

Occult fungal infections are an increasing problem in hospitalized and immuno-compromised patients. Broad spectrum antibiotics, corticosteroids, immunosup-pression, diabetes, burns, and intravascular catheters have been associated with systemic candidal infections. The diagnosis can be difficult to make because fungemia is not always present. Skin lesions are present in only 10% of patients with candidal sepsis, and biopsy of these lesions may reveal *Candida* about half the time. Candidal endophthalmitis on ophthalmic examination (a highly specific sign but with low sensitivity) or liver lesions on abdominal scanning are important clues to disseminated candidal infection (see Chapter 11).

Other Causes

Transfusion of blood products commonly results in a fever (see Chapter 46). Only rarely, however, is this due to bacterial contamination of the transfused product.

Febrile patients with a malignancy who are receiving cytotoxic medication or irradiation have a complicated differential diagnosis (see Chapter 18). Possibilities include common and opportunistic infections, the underlying malignancy, compli-cations of the malignancy (perforation, hemorrhage, obstruction), or complications of antitumor therapy (radiation pneumonitis, cytotoxic lung injury).

Noninfectious Causes of Fever

Noninfectious illnesses are an important cause of fevers in the ICU (Table 38–2). Other chapters in this volume discuss many of these conditions in greater detail. Drug reactions commonly occur in the ICU and are often manifested by fevers and skin rashes (see Chapter 43). Patients on bed rest may acquire fever from DVT or pulmonary embolism (see Chapter 47), or both. Patients with myocardial infarction (see Chapter 49), aortic dissection (see Chapter 50), or subarachnoid

Table 38–2. Noninfectious Causes of Fever in the Intensive Care Unit

Inflammatory	Allergic drug reaction, allograft rejection, aspiration pneumonitis, atelectasis, crystalline arthritis (gout, pseudogout), neoplasm, pancreatitis, postpericardiotomy syndrome, transfusion reaction, vasculitis
Metabolic	Alcohol and sedative withdrawal, hypoadrenalism, malignant hyperthermia, neuroleptic malignant syndrome, thyrotoxicosis
Neurologic	Aseptic meningitis, dysautonomias, spinal cord injury (C4 and C5), subarachnoid hemorrhage, thermoregulatory disorders resulting from hypothalamic injury (e.g., after cardiac arrest or head trauma)
Vascular	Aortic dissection, deep venous thrombosis, myocardial infarction, pulmonary embolism, hemorrhage

hemorrhage (see Chapter 71), as well as those who have just undergone cardiotomy (see Chapter 86) may be febrile without infection. Organ transplantation can result in fever from organ rejection.

Another important cause of fever is alcohol withdrawal, which is often associated with muscle tremors, agitation, hallucinations, or seizures. Withdrawal from chronic use of sedatives (e.g., barbiturates or benzodiazepines) is also a frequently overlooked cause of fever. Similarly, withdrawal from corticosteroids or surgery in patients receiving chronic corticosteroid therapy may unmask adrenal insufficiency with fever and hypotension resembling sepsis. However, before fevers are attributed to withdrawal of these medications, infection must always be ruled out.

Hypothermia

Acute infection may also present with hypothermia. Patients predisposed to this response include those who are elderly, debilitated, or in chronic renal or hepatic failure. Hypothermia is often related to noninfectious causes as well. Postsurgical patients, patients receiving large volumes of unwarmed fluid or blood intravenously or by gastric lavage, and burn patients may also become hypothermic in the ICU.

Leukocytosis

Although leukocytosis often signifies acute infection, it also accompanies many of the noninfectious conditions listed in Table 38–2. In addition, leukocytosis may result from drugs (e.g., corticosteroids), "stress" (trauma, burns, critical illness), myeloproliferative disorders, or leukemoid reactions. One common diagnostic problem occurs in patients receiving corticosteroids who acquire leukocytosis. In this case, an increase in the percentage of immature band forms on differential blood cell count analysis suggests an infectious cause.

DIAGNOSTIC EVALUATION

When the patient in the ICU experiences fever, a timely assessment with an organized and logical approach is necessary. The *initial step* should be examination of current and previous records, particularly the list of current medications. One should review the medical record and interview the patient or family members about localizing complaints. Although signs on physical examination can help direct the diagnostic approach to fever, these findings are often unclear in the critically ill individual. Serial examinations are important and may reveal localizing signs not initially present. In patients receiving immunosuppressive agents or analgesics, with advanced age or altered sensorium the absence of abnormal findings in an abdominal examination can be particularly misleading.

A diagnostic algorithm for the laboratory work-up of fever is presented in Figure 38–1. Initial studies should include two sets of blood cultures (both sets should preferably be obtained from separate peripheral venipuncture sites or, less preferably, one from such a site and one from a central venous catheter). Blood culture specimens should **not** be drawn from arterial catheters (except at the time

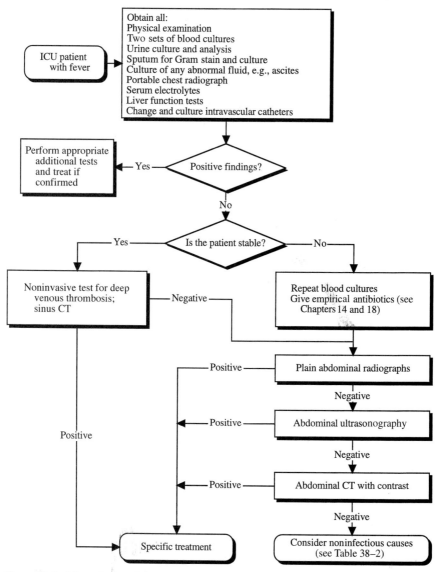

Figure 38–1. Schematic flow diagram to evaluate fever in ICU patients. CT, computed tomography.

of their initial insertion). A high false-positive rate due to colonization of their hubs makes results uninterpretable.

Also, one should obtain urine for urinalysis and culture and sputum or tracheal aspirate for culture and Gram stain. A chest radiograph should also be obtained. Gram staining of sputum is critical for later interpretation of sputum cultures because most patients in the ICU have Gram-negative bacterial colonization of the oropharynx within a few days of admission. Demonstration of many polymorphonuclear leukocytes with few or rare epithelioid cells on sputum Gram stain may help distinguish infection from colonization as well as guide initial antibiotic therapy. If sputum is not available and pneumonia is still suspected, nasotracheal suctioning or induced sputum with nebulized saline should be considered in the unintubated patient. Bronchoscopy with bronchoalveolar lavage or protected specimen brush for quantitative culture may be useful in patients receiving mechanical ventilation (see Chapter 11). In the patient with nosocomial diarrhea, initial studies should include stool testing for *C. difficile* toxin in the setting of current or recent (past month) antibiotic use. In addition, any abnormal fluid collections (e.g., pleural or joint effusions, ascites) should be sampled and sent for culture and cell counts. However, small pleural effusions occurring in patients with volume overload or after thoracic or abdominal surgery need not be tapped. In the absence of meningeal or focal neurologic signs, cerebrospinal fluid sampling is usually not indicated because nosocomial meningitis is rare. Exceptions are neurosurgical patients and patients with head trauma, unexplained sudden changes of mental status, or bacteremia with virulent organisms that may involve the meninges. Another exception is the inability to evaluate the neurologic status (due to drugs, sedatives, or neuromuscular blockade).

In the stable patient with fever, central venous catheters can be exchanged by the Seldinger technique (over a wire) if the site does not appear infected as long as one sends the tip (distal 3 cm) of the catheter for semiquantitative culture (see Chapter 11). If the patient is hemodynamically unstable or neutropenic, one should insert a new catheter at a new site, remove the original catheter, and send its tip for culture.

Further studies to consider initially include serum creatine phosphokinase (CPK) determination (if myocardial infarction or neuroleptic malignant syndrome are suspected), immunologic studies (if connective tissue diseases are suspected), and serologic studies for suspected viral and other infections as clinical circumstances dictate.

For patients with localizing signs on initial examination, more focused diagnostic testing is indicated. If results of these evaluations are unrevealing, or if no localizing signs are present, one should next rule out common sources of infection in the ICU such as an unrecognized urinary or vascular catheter infection, sinusitis, or occult DVT.

If these investigations are unrevealing, further imaging studies should be performed, particularly in the hemodynamically unstable febrile patient. Ultrasonography (US) or computed tomography (CT) are often the initial tests of choice as rapid and effective modalities. However, US appears to be advantageous as an initial diagnostic screening test in the ICU setting because it is relatively inexpensive, noninvasive, and portable. Disadvantages of US include restricted field of view because of wound dressings, and interference by bowel gas.

Suspected Abdominal Infection

A frequent source of sepsis of unknown origin in critically ill patients is the gallbladder and biliary tract. US, a sensitive detector of gallbladder and biliary tree pathology, is the initial method of choice for imaging of the right upper quadrant. US is useful in the diagnosis of acute cholecystitis, gangrenous cholecystitis, biliary obstruction, and hepatic pathology, including abscesses and candidiasis.

The sensitivity of US for gallstones is about 95% (CT is somewhat less sensitive). Because a significant number of patients harbor asymptomatic gallstones, other criteria have been developed to increase the accuracy of US for diagnosing acute *calculous* cholecystitis. They include focal gallbladder wall tenderness during scanning (ultrasonographic Murphy's sign), gallbladder wall thickening, pericholecystic fluid, sludge, and gallbladder distention. CT offers complementary findings to US in the evaluation of the gallbladder and biliary tree but is superior to US when imaging of the entire abdomen is indicated.

For the diagnosis of acute cholecystitis, however, cholescintigraphy showing nonvisualization of the gallbladder after intravenous administration of technetium-99m iminodiacetic acid derivative utilizing the method of morphine augmentation is probably the best test, with 95% sensitivity and 85% specificity versus 85% sensitivity and 60% specificity of US.

For the clinical diagnosis of *acalculous* cholecystitis, US and CT are less sensitive and depend on the presence of the relatively nonspecific findings mentioned earlier in the absence of gallstones. This clinical diagnosis is based on both imaging results and clinical findings.

Other abdominal sources for infection that can be easily detected by US and CT include ascites, intra-abdominal abscesses, and acute pancreatic inflammatory diseases. CT with opacification of the bowel by contrast is the method of choice for localizing abscesses in the abdomen or pelvis. Percutaneous abscess drainage is an alternative treatment to surgical drainage in most cases. CT-guided aspiration or catheter placement is preferred by most radiologists over bedside ultrasonographic guidance if the patient can be transported safely. For splenic abscesses, both US and CT are sensitive, although CT is better at delineating the left upper quadrant and the remaining abdomen. For acute appendicitis, both may show nonspecific periappendiceal fluid or stranding in the surrounding fat. CT is more useful for the detection of appendiceal abscess or phlegmon. For diverticulitis, CT detection is only 77% sensitive but increases with complications such as perforation, abscess, colovescical fistula, or ureteral obstruction. For diagnosing a small pneumoperitoneum due to intestinal perforation, CT is more sensitive than conventional portable erect chest or abdominal radiographs. CT may also give direct or indirect evidence of intestinal infarction, although angiography remains the procedure of choice.

Although CT and US are the initial tests of choice for the evaluation of abdominal or pelvic infections, indium-111 leukocyte scintigraphy is suited for patients without localizing signs when whole body imaging is desired or if a diffuse inflammatory process is suspected. In some series, it has a diagnostic accuracy similar to CT and US for abdominal pathology. It can also be useful for suspected Tenckhoff's tunnel infections or vascular graft infections.

Renal and Retroperitoneal Pathology

Both CT and US can be useful for diagnosing renal, perinephric, and retroperitoneal pathology. CT scan is more sensitive than US at detecting small renal abscesses, acute nephritis, or air within the collecting system. Occult retroperitoneal hemorrhage, abscess, tumor, or lymphadenopathy may also be sources of fever that are best detected by CT scanning.

In the febrile renal transplant patient, renal scintigraphy is useful in identifying acute rejection, renal artery thrombosis, and urinary leaks. For the evaluation of postoperative abscesses or hematomas, US and CT are the procedures of choice.

Pulmonary Infections

The routine chest radiograph is the initial imaging procedure for infections of the lung or pleural space. In the ICU setting, portable films make it difficult to identify pleural collections or lung abscesses. US and CT can be useful as secondary modalities in these settings. As a result of its portability and sensitivity for fluid collections, US is frequently used in the ICU to localize pleural effusions and empyemas before diagnostic or therapeutic thoracentesis. For complicated or loculated pleural effusions and empyemas, and before surgical intervention, CT is the preferred mode of imaging.

In the detection of septic pulmonary emboli, CT is more sensitive than is plain radiography. It may show multiple small pulmonary nodules with or without cavitation or pleural effusion even before septic emboli are suspected clinically or radiographically.

In the evaluation of pulmonary infections in the ICU, indium-111 leukocyte scintigraphy is not useful because of nonspecific uptake. Bronchoscopy remains the test of choice to confirm the diagnosis of opportunistic pulmonary infections. In patients with ventilator-associated nosocomial pneumonia, bronchoscopy with bronchoalveolar lavage or protected specimen brush with quantitative culture may also be helpful but should be done before a start or change in antibiotics to achieve good sensitivity.

Osteomyelitis

Plain radiographic findings in acute osteomyelitis may be normal in the first 10 to 14 days of infection. In the acutely ill patient, radionuclide scans are helpful for early detection of bone inflammation. Indium leukocyte scintigraphy is most helpful in acute infections and in the appendicular skeleton, whereas gallium scanning is more useful for the axial skeleton and chronic osteomyelitis.

Deep Venous Thrombosis and Pulmonary Embolism

A frequent cause of fever of unknown origin in the ICU setting is DVT. This condition commonly occurs in the lower extremities, although intravenous catheter–related thromboses may occur in any vein. Thromboses may cause fever in the absence of infection or they may become secondarily infected. Color flow Doppler techniques or impedance plethysmography are appropriate as initial noninvasive modalities for the detection of DVT of the lower extremity above the knee (see Chapter 47). Venography, however, remains the gold standard test. Lung ventilation/perfusion (V/Q) scanning is the preferred initial test when pulmonary embolism is suspected as a source of fever. Pulmonary angiography may be necessary when results of the V/Q scan are equivocal or when clinical suspicion is high in the setting of a low-probability scan. Newer magnetic resonance imaging techniques are also currently under investigation for the noninvasive evaluation of DVT and pulmonary embolism, although availability is limited to only a few centers.

Sinusitis

Portable sinus films, especially in intubated patients, are likely to be of poor quality. Sinus CT is more sensitive for soft tissue changes in the evaluation of sinusitis. It is recommended for patients with nasal catheters who are febrile without other localizing sources of infection.

MANAGEMENT

Appropriate primary therapy for the underlying disease process should be the highest priority in the management of fever. In addition, to reduce the risk of nosocomial infections and aid in the therapy of established infections in the ICU, it is advisable to remove intravenous catheters, urinary catheters, and nasogastric tubes as soon as clinically feasible.

Many physicians take measures to lower the patient's temperature. Fever increases basal metabolic rate, insensible water losses, heart rate, and oxygen consumption (by 13% for every 1° C increase greater than 37° C). Supportive measures include adequate fluids and nutritional support and, in many cases, maneuvers to lower the body temperature. Fever reduction is somewhat controversial, as fever itself may play a beneficial role in the defense against disease. However, it is generally accepted that fever reduction is indicated for fevers higher than 39° C (102° F) in patients who have underlying cardiovascular or pulmonary disease, in fever due to head injury or other central nervous system disease, in pregnancy, and in severe hyperthermia.

In general, acetaminophen is the antipyretic of choice for fever reduction. Aspirin is less desirable because of its effects on platelet function and the gastric mucosa and its potential for toxicity and worsening of bronchospasm in some asthmatic patients. Both aspirin and acetaminophen work by lowering the hypothalamic temperature set point toward normal. External cooling is a less physiologic approach that may be necessary in cases of more severe temperature elevation.

BIBLIOGRAPHY

American College of Critical Care Medicine: Practice parameters for evaluating new fever in critically adult patients. Crit Care Med 26:392–408, 1998.
   This comprehensive statement by experts in critical care medicine, infectious diseases, and surgery describes how an intensivist should respond to a patient with a temperature ≥ 38.3° C. The fever should trigger a clinical assessment in all cases but not an automatic battery of laboratory or radiological studies. This reference is also available at htpp://www.sccm.org.

Cabana MD, Alavi A, Berlin JA, et al: Morphine-augmented hepatobiliary scintigraphy: a meta-analysis. Nuclear Med Commun 16:1068–1071, 1995.
This systematic review of use of cholescintigraphy with or without morphine augmentation to detect acute cholecystitis found that morphine augmentation significantly improved the test's specificity from 68% (95% confidence interval [CI] of 61–75%) to 84% (95% CI of 75–94%). Both scans had sensitivities in the 95% range.

Davis LP, Fink-Bennett D: Nuclear medicine in the acutely ill patient. Crit Care Clin 10:383–400, 1994.
This is a good review of nuclear medicine evaluation of sepsis and the detection of pulmonary, abdominal, pelvic, and skeletal infections.

Fagon JY, Chastre J, Hance AJ, et al: Detection of nosocomial lung infection in ventilated patients: Use of a protected specimen brush and quantitative culture technique in 147 patients. Am Rev Respir Dis 128:110, 1988.
In mechanically ventilated patients suspected of having nosocomial pneumonia, stepwise logistic regression analysis of 16 clinical variables failed to find any combination that was useful in identifying patients with bacterial nosocomial pneumonia.

Guze BH, Baxter LR: Neuroleptic malignant syndrome. N Engl J Med 313:163–166, 1985.
This is a concise but thorough description of this rare but important syndrome.

Merrell RC: The abdomen as source of sepsis in critically ill patients. Crit Care Clin 11:255–272, 1995.
This is a good review of the most common gastrointestinal emergencies seen in the ICU and presents a general diagnostic and therapeutic algorithm for abdominal sepsis.

Pizzo PA: Management of fever in patients with cancer and treatment-induced neutropenia. N Engl J Med 328:1323–1332, 1993.
This is a review article that is useful for the management of cancer patients with neutropenia. Discusses use of empirical antibiotics and hematopoietic growth factors.

Raad II, Bodey GP: Infectious complications of indwelling vascular catheters. Clin Infect Dis 15:197–208, 1992.
This article reviews nosocomial blood stream infections related to intravascular catheters.

Romano WM, Platt JF: Ultrasound of the abdomen. Crit Care Clin 10:297–319, 1994.
This article reviews the utility and accuracy of ultrasonographic imaging in the ICU for abdominal pathologic conditions.

Washington JA II, Ilstrup DM: Blood cultures: Issues and controversies. Rev Infect Dis 8:792–802, 1986.
This article reviews the variables affecting yields, including volume and number of cultures needed.

Zingas AP: Computed tomography of the abdomen in the critically ill. Crit Care Clin 10):321–339, 1994.
The utility and accuracy of CT in the ICU for abdominal pathologic conditions is reviewed.

39 Hypertensive Episodes

Daniel H. Sternman
Scott Manaker

Hypertension is defined as an elevation in the arterial blood pressure. Distinguishing between normal and abnormal systemic blood pressure, however, remains somewhat arbitrary. Normal blood pressure for an adult is typically considered a systolic pressure less than 140 mm Hg associated with a diastolic blood pressure less than 90 mm Hg. Systolic pressures of 140 to 159 mm Hg are regarded as "borderline" hypertension, whereas pressures of greater than 160 mm Hg signify definite systolic hypertension. Diastolic pressures greater than 120 mm Hg are characterized as *severe* hypertension. On noninvasive blood pressure monitoring, elderly patients often present with isolated systolic hypertension, which appears to resolve after obtaining intra-arterial measurements. This phenomenon is attributed to the stiffening of the arterial wall associated with advanced age, causing alterations in the timing of the Korotkoff sounds.

CLINICAL CONTEXT AND DEFINITIONS

In the intensive care unit (ICU), episodes of elevated blood pressure can be encountered in an array of clinical situations, but most are secondary to other causes. In some, hypertension arises concurrently with another serious medical problem, such as acute renal failure, congestive heart failure, aortic dissection, or cerebrovascular hemorrhage. In others, elevated blood pressure occurs in *response* to other problems, for example, inadequate sedation or pain control, hypoxemia, or dyssynchrony between patient and mechanical ventilator. Since giving antihypertensive agents without addressing the primary cause of the hypertensive episode may produce dire results, distinguishing between primary and secondary causes of hypertension is critically important in the ICU.

Primary hypertensive episodes in the ICU can be subdivided into hypertension without urgency, urgent hypertensive episodes ("accelerated" hypertension), and hypertensive emergencies ("malignant" hypertension). In hypertension without urgency, systolic or diastolic pressures, or both, are mildly to moderately elevated without evidence of acute end-organ damage. *Urgent* hypertensive episodes manifest *severe* elevations in blood pressure (diastolic pressures >120 mm Hg or systolic pressures >180 mm Hg) but no signs of end-organ damage. *Hypertensive emergencies* are defined as severe blood pressure elevations, as in an urgent hypertensive episode, but *with* end-organ damage (focal neurologic deficits, pulmonary edema, cardiac ischemia, retinal hemorrhage, or acute renal failure) (see Chapter 52).

BLOOD PRESSURE MEASUREMENTS

Evaluating episodes of elevated blood pressure in the ICU starts with confirming the presence and severity of hypertension. Several available modes of blood

463

pressure measurement and monitoring are available, and each has advantages and drawbacks. No precipitous clinical action should be taken until the measurement is repeated and the elevated pressure confirmed.

Indirect Methods

Manual Sphygmomanometer

This classic modality employs a pneumatic cuff, manometer, and stethoscope in the Korotkoff auscultatory method for indirect arterial blood pressure measurement. Such measurements typically *underestimate* the *systolic* pressure. Underestimates commonly occur with rapid release of the air from the pneumatic cuff or inadequate cuff inflation before complete vascular occlusion. Furthermore, these measurements may be highly inaccurate in patients with arrhythmias.

Underestimation of systolic pressures can also occur when cuffs too large for arm circumference are used (i.e., using standard adult cuffs for children or thin adults). Standard adult cuffs are designed for arm circumferences between 24 and 32 cm (standard cuffs *overestimate* systolic blood pressure when limb girth exceeds 33 cm). Other situations in which sphygmomanometry underestimates central arterial pressure include marked peripheral vasoconstriction (due to severely attenuated limb flow) and severe aortic insufficiency.

Automatic Cuff Methods

Automated pneumatic cuff systems are common in ICUs, emergency departments, and operating suites. These systems retain the disadvantages and inaccuracies of the manual pneumatic cuff but can record blood pressure variations and trends. They also incorporate high- and low-pressure alarms. Since cuff inflations are performed at defined intervals, this method may be inadequate when treating patients with infusions of rapidly acting drugs (e.g., nitroprusside). In addition, ulnar neuropathy and venous stasis can occur with repeated, frequent cuff inflations.

Oscillometric Method

Continuous, noninvasive pressure waveform monitoring may be performed in many critical care settings with oscillometric techniques. Automated oscillometric devices also underestimate systolic and mean pressures, particularly when arterial pressures are high.

Direct Methods

Intra-arterial Catheter

Measuring blood pressure by an intra-arterial catheter has two significant advantages over indirect techniques: increased accuracy and blood sampling capability, particularly for arterial blood gas analyses. Direct blood pressure monitoring requires an intra-arterial catheter, a stopcock or stopcocks, appropriate connecting tubing, a continuous-flush device, a pressure transducer, and a pressure monitor with display screen and high and low alarms.

Improper zeroing is the most important source of error in direct pressure monitoring systems. These systems should be zeroed frequently, especially before altering therapy. Proper zeroing requires opening the stopcock to the atmosphere and aligning the resulting fluid-air interface point at the midaxillary line (approximating the left atrial position in the supine patient). The most common cause for improper zeroing is changing the patient's position relative to the pressure transducer without rezeroing.

Calibration problems with direct pressure measurements can be minimized by employing disposable pressure transducers. These transducers are precalibrated, durable, reliable, and cost-effective. They also remove the risk of potential transmission of infection to the patient via contaminated reusable pressure transducers. This was a significant issue when such transducers were commonly used.

Comparison of Central and Peripheral Blood Pressure Measurements

Since the peak of the arterial pulse increases as it moves peripherally, systolic pressure measured by peripheral arterial catheters may exceed systolic pressure in the central arterial system by 15 mm Hg or more (see Chapter 5). However, *mean* pressures, whether measured peripherally of centrally, are normally the same. Because of this and because it is mean blood pressure, not systolic blood pressure, that determines flow to the brain, liver, and kidneys, many intensivists recommend titrating vasoactive agents and other interventions to *mean* rather than systolic blood pressure (e.g., see treatment of strokes in Chapter 71). Central arterial catheters (e.g., femoral arterial catheters) are uncommonly used under routine circumstances in the ICU because of increased risk of complications compared with peripheral catheters (see Chapter 9).

EVALUATION OF A HYPERTENSIVE EPISODE

The most important considerations in evaluating a hypertensive episode are whether the elevated blood pressure is secondary or primary and whether it is causing end-organ damage. End-organ damage defines the presence of a hypertensive emergency and necessitates immediate medical intervention. Assessment of the critically ill patient with an acute episode of hypertension should follow the standard assessment of any patient event in the ICU, which requires a thorough medical history and focused physical examination.

Medical History

The pertinent medical history should include reviewing the medical record and, if possible, communicating directly with the patient or his or her family. Current symptoms that might be contributing to blood pressure elevations should be an immediate focus. A previous history of hypertension, including duration, severity, and compliance with a medical regimen, must be identified. Pre-existent neurologic, cardiac, renal, and ocular diseases should be reviewed and the current medical regimen, including over-the-counter medications (e.g., decongestants), must be determined. Finally, one should identify any coexisting acute or chronic medical or surgical condition (e.g., pregnancy, postoperative state). Special attention should be paid to possible precipitating causes of secondary hypertension in the critically ill patient (Table 39–1).

Physical Examination

The focused physical examination combines a systematic evaluation with attention to those end-organs most susceptible to hypertensive damage: brain, heart, kidney, and eye.

The neurologic examination seeks to detect an altered mental status or focal neurologic deficit. Altered mental status may indicate hypertensive encephalopathy, uremia, or cerebral dysfunction caused by poor perfusion. Focal neurologic deficits may represent cerebral hemorrhage or a postictal state. A neurologic examination should be performed early and repeated frequently to document any changes.

Performing a careful funduscopic examination is critical. Retinal hemorrhages,

Table 39–1. Causes of Secondary Hypertensive Episodes in the Intensive Care Unit

Anxiety
Cardiovascular disease
    Acute myocardial infarction (without pump failure)
    Aortic dissection
    Congestive heart failure
    "Flash" pulmonary edema due to ischemia
Endocrine disease
    Thyroid storm (systolic hypertension with widened pulse pressure)
    Myxedema
    Pheochromocytoma (may also have hypotensive episodes)
    Hypercalcemia
Neurologic disease
    Subarachnoid bleeding
    Head injury (with increased intracranial pressure)
    Autonomic hyperreactivity in spinal cord injury or Guillain-Barré syndrome
Pain
Preeclampsia, eclampsia
Renal disease (systolic and diastolic hypertension)
    Acute renal failure
    Renal infarction
    Renovascular stenosis
    Scleroderma renal crisis
Ventilator, respiratory problems
    Inadequate ventilation or oxygenation
    Obstructive sleep apnea episodes
    Patient-ventilator dyssynchrony

exudates, cotton-wool spots, and papilledema reflect the severity of the hypertension and may provide clues to its underlying cause. For example, severe retinopathy is common with renovascular hypertension. Hard retinal exudates are often in a "macular star" configuration. Arterial microaneurysms, flame hemorrhages, and chorioretinal atrophy are common. Retinal detachment, vitreous hemorrhage, neovascularization, and central or branch occlusion of retinal vessels occur more rarely. Arteriovenous nicking and arteriolar sclerosis ("copper wiring") are associated with chronic hypertension and are typically bilateral. Unilateral hypertensive retinopathy suggests a carotid artery occlusion on the side of the normal eye, with the blockage sparing the ipsilateral retina from the effects of the elevated pressure.

Performing thorough chest and cardiac examinations is also crucial. Dullness to chest percussion (indicating a pleural effusion) or auscultation of diffuse inspiratory rales (associated with pulmonary edema) are signs found in congestive heart failure or fluid overload from renal insufficiency. A loud fourth heart sound suggests left ventricular hypertrophy due to chronic hypertension, whereas a third heart sound signifies the presence of ventricular dilatation and fluid overload. A new diastolic murmur of aortic insufficiency may be present in acutely hypertensive patients with proximal aortic dissections dilating or disrupting the aortic annulus (see Chapter 50).

Examination of the abdomen and back may reveal the presence of unilateral or bilateral renal artery bruits, the most reliable physical sign of renovascular hypertension. Palpation of a large pheochromocytoma may exacerbate the underlying hypertension and help establish the diagnosis. A pulsatile midabdominal mass may represent an enlarging abdominal aortic aneurysm—a potential complication of uncontrolled hypertension. Finally, femoral pulse delay and normotensive pulses in the lower extremity can be seen in patients with coarctations. Diminished lower extremity pulses can also signify poor perfusion attributable to aortic and peripheral vascular disease.

Diagnostic Laboratory Evaluation

A thorough laboratory examination assists in the diagnosis and management of hypertension in the critically ill patient. Increased serum blood urea nitrogen and creatinine levels may indicate severe renal damage from hypertension or other causes. Elevated potassium and decreased bicarbonate concentrations may occur in hypertensive renal disease. Cardiac dysfunction associated with increases in the MB fractions of creatine phosphokinase, serum troponin I, or T levels suggests myocardial ischemia or infarction (see Chapter 34). Anemia may reflect decreased erythropoietin production from chronic renal disease or the presence of microangiopathic hemolytic anemia (see Chapter 63).

Urinalysis in patients with chronic hypertension typically demonstrates the presence of significant proteinuria. However, finding gross or microscopic hematuria with red cell casts suggests acute glomerular injury from hypertensive renal crisis or acute glomerulonephritis.

Electrocardiography may also be revealing in patients with an acute hypertensive episode in the ICU. ST-segment elevations or depressions, T-wave inversions, or new Q waves can reflect ongoing or recent myocardial ischemia (see Chapter 34). Tall R waves in leads aVL, III, V_2, and V_3 suggest left ventricular hypertrophy from chronic hypertension. Peaked T waves may signify early ischemia or hyperkalemia from renal disease. Diffuse upsloping ST-segment elevations suggest acute pericarditis, which may result from uremia, transmural myocardial infarction, or retrograde aortic dissection with leakage of blood into the pericardial space. Diffuse low voltage and electrical alternans may suggest pericardial tamponade (see Chapter 53). Diffuse deeply inverted T waves can be seen in some patients with cerebral edema and stroke as well as in the late stages of pericarditis.

Radiographic studies can aid in the evaluation of hypertensive episodes. Standard chest radiography may demonstrate pulmonary edema, bilateral pleural effusions, or enlargement of the cardiac silhouette (from congestive heart failure); mediastinal widening (from thoracic aortic aneurysms or dissections); or a globular cardiac enlargement (from pericardial effusion due to pericarditis). In patients with focal neurologic abnormalities or depressed mental status, noncontrast computed tomography of the brain may document intracranial bleeding or edema.

Special Clinical Situations in the Intensive Care Unit

Patients admitted to the ICU can have significant anxiety, pain, or other reactions that cause hypertension by increasing systemic catecholamine levels and sympathetic tone. Appropriate treatment of elevated blood pressure in this setting includes anxiolytic agents (e.g., benzodiazepines) or analgesics (e.g., opioids) rather than antihypertensive medications.

Endotracheal intubation in patients admitted to the ICU reflexly induces acute hypertension. Paralyzed intubated patients may be hypertensive and tachycardiac because of inadequate sedation. Patient-ventilator dyssynchrony may produce elevated systolic and diastolic pressures and requires increasing sedatives or, preferably, changing ventilator settings. Insufficient ventilatory support (hypercapnia) or inadequate oxygenation (hypoxemia) may also result in hypertension.

On occasion, new-onset hypertension in patients in the ICU represents withdrawal from therapeutic or illicit drugs (Table 39–2). A previously prescribed oral antihypertensive medication may have inadvertently been stopped on the patient's arrival to the ICU. *Clonidine* is a prime example of an antihypertensive medication

Table 39–2. Drug Effects Precipitating Hypertensive Episodes in the Intensive Care Unit

··

Drug ingestion
   Antidepressants (tricyclics, monoamine oxidase [MAO] inhibitors)
   Sympathomimetics (cocaine)
Drug withdrawal
   Alcohol, nicotine, or other drugs (cocaine, benzodiazepines)
   Antihypertensive agents (clonidine and beta-blockers)
Drug interactions
   MAO inhibitors and meperidine
Inadequate drug effects
   Insufficient analgesia for pain
   Therapeutic paralysis without adequate sedation or analgesia
   Undersedation for anxiety

··

that can cause significant rebound hypertension if stopped abruptly. *Acute alcohol withdrawal* can also present with hypertension and tachycardia, sweating, fever, tremulousness, and seizures. Similar withdrawal signs may occur in *chronic opioid* or *sedative users* (benzodiazepines and barbiturates). *Nicotine* withdrawal also occurs frequently and may result in hypertension.

MANAGEMENT OF HYPERTENSION IN THE INTENSIVE CARE UNIT

If the medical history, focused physical examination, and laboratory studies demonstrate severe hypertension with evidence of significant end-organ dysfunction (otherwise not explainable), one should suspect the presence of a hypertensive emergency and institute immediate intravenous therapy (see Chapter 52). Severe hypertension in the critically ill patient also requires immediate attention to forestall further end-organ damage. Intravenously administered agents, such as labetalol, esmolol, and nitroprusside, have the advantage of being short-acting and are useful for close titration of blood pressure. Mild or moderate pressure elevations in of blood pressure in the ICU should prompt a search for previously unrecognized causes of transient hypertension (see Tables 39–1 and 39–2).

In general, the intravenous route for antihypertensive therapy is preferred. Although one can treat nonemergent hypertension sublingually or orally, via nasogastric or nasoenteral tubes, or topically, these other routes may be problematic when used in patients in the ICU. Despite their rapid onset, sublingually delivered antihypertensive drugs, such as nifedipine, should be avoided. They may drop blood pressure below desired levels and induce coronary or cerebrovascular ischemia. Enteral antihypertensive agents typically decrease blood pressure slowly, and they have relatively long half-lives making their titration difficult. In addition, critically ill patients may have altered gastrointestinal mucosa and acid production, both of which may inhibit drug absorption. Blood pressure control via topical medications, such as nitroglycerin ointment or a clonidine patch, may have unpredictable absorption secondary to subcutaneous edema or poor skin perfusion. If titration is attempted with topical medications, one should note that removal of the paste or patch may not eliminate the drug effect because of subcutaneous tissue deposition.

CLINICAL PEARLS AND PITFALLS

1. Elderly patients often have isolated systolic hypertension on noninvasive blood pressure monitoring. This may resolve after obtaining intra-arterial measurements.
2. It is important to distinguish between primary and secondary causes of hypertension in patients admitted to the ICU because treatment of the elevated blood pressure without addressing the primary disorder may result in serious adverse consequences.
3. Standard cuffs *overestimate* systolic blood pressure when limb girth exceeds 33 cm.

4. Improper zeroing of the transducer is the most important source of error in direct pressure monitoring systems. This commonly results from a change in the patient's position without rezeroing.
5. Special attention should be paid to recognizing possible iatrogenic precipitating causes of acute hypertension in the critically ill patient (see Tables 39–1 and 39–2).

BIBLIOGRAPHY

Abramowicz M (ed): Drugs for hypertension. Med Lett 37:45–50, 1995.
This is an excellent review of oral antihypertensive agents useful for chronic hypertension.

Calhoun DA, Oparil S: Treatment of hypertensive crisis. N Engl J Med 123:1177–1183, 1990.
This is a superb, comprehensive review of approaches to severe hypertension, including physical examination findings.

Gramm HJ, Zimmermann J, Meinhold H, et al: Hemodynamic responses to noxious stimuli in brain-dead organ donors. Intensive Care Med 18:493–495, 1992.
This article reviews physiologic responses in patients with brain death, including a discussion of the cause of elevated blood pressure.

Kiselak J, Clark M, Pera V, et al: The association between hypertension and sleep apnea in obese patients. Chest 104:775–780, 1993.
This article describes an association between sleep apnea and systemic hypertension.

Zeigler MG: Advances in the acute therapy of hypertension. Crit Care Med 20:1630–1631, 1992.
This article reviews the proper evaluation and pharmacological approaches to hypertension.

40

Hypotensive Episodes or Falling Hemoglobin

Jonathan Zuckerman
Scott Manaker

Critical care physicians are frequently challenged to evaluate and manage patients with hypotensive episodes or falling hemoglobin (Hgb) or both. Since there are many causes of hypotension (Table 40–1), one important challenge is to separate those patients who have iatrogenic causes for their hypotension, such as a drug effect, from those in circulatory shock. This chapter presents approaches to the evaluation and management of episodes of hypotension and decreases in Hgb or hematocrit (Hct), with particular emphasis on hemorrhagic shock.

DEFINITIONS AND PATHOPHYSIOLOGY OF HEMORRHAGIC SHOCK

Shock is a pathophysiologic condition characterized by inadequate tissue perfusion. Three categories of shock describe the mechanisms of the compromised circulation: (1) preload-dependent (hypovolemic) shock (see Chapter 7), (2) cardiogenic shock (see Chapter 6), and (3) low afterload shock (see Chapter 8). Hypovolemic shock can result from multiple causes, such as internal plasma losses (severe acute pancreatitis), reduced venous return (tension pneumothorax) or gastrointestinal fluid loss (severe vomiting or diarrhea). However, hypovolemic shock is most commonly due to hemorrhage.

Responses to acute, limited blood loss have been well studied. There appear to be three sequential hemodynamic phases of hemorrhagic shock (Table 40–2): (1) compensated shock (class I and II), (2) uncompensated but reversible shock (class III), and (3) irreversible shock (class IV).

Table 40–1. Selected Causes of Hypotensive Episodes in the Intensive Care Unit

Acute transfusion reaction
Allergic reactions
Autonomic instability (Guillain-Barré syndrome)
Auto-PEEP (Positive end-expiratory pressure)
Cardiogenic causes (acute ischemia, pericardial tamponade)
Drug effects (IV opioids, benzodiazepines, and many others)
Epidural anesthesia (see Chapter 85)
Hemorrhage
Hypovolemia due to overdiuresis or fluid shifts
Sepsis
Tachyarrhythmia or bradyarrhythmia
Tension pneumothorax
Volume removal by dialysis or apheresis

IV, intravenous.

Table 40–2. Classification of Progressive Hemorrhage

CLASS	CLINICAL SIGNS	INTRAVASCULAR VOLUME LOSS
I	Slightly anxious Tachycardia Urine output >30 mL/h	15%
II	Anxious Orthostatic hypotension Urine output 20–30 mL/h	15–25%
III	Confused Supine hypotension Urine output 5–15 mL/h	25–40%
IV	Confused and lethargic Circulatory collapse Urine output minimal	>40%

Adapted from Alexander RH, Proctor HJ: Advanced Trauma Life Support Course for Physicians: Shock. Chicago: American College of Surgeons, 1993, pp 75–110.

With mild acute blood loss, the Hgb concentration initially remains unchanged, whereas systemic responses maintain arterial blood pressure and support tissue oxygen delivery. Increases in catecholamine release lead to precapillary arteriolar vasoconstriction and increased heart rate and contractility. Secretion of renin, angiotensin, aldosterone, and antidiuretic hormone increases vascular tone and limits renal sodium and water loss. On physical examination, these early responses are manifested by tachycardia and a narrowed pulse pressure. Within 2 hours of the hemorrhage, fluid mobilizes from the interstitial space, decreasing the blood Hgb concentration. This mobilization of interstitial fluid can continue for days until intravascular volume is restored.

Progressive intravascular volume depletion leads first to orthostatic changes in heart rate and then in blood pressure. When blood loss exceeds 40%, compensatory responses are overwhelmed, precipitating circulatory collapse (see Table 40–2). In this setting, cardiac output is limited by reduced preload so that increases in heart rate and vascular tone do little to restore tissue perfusion.

The general principles of tissue oxygen delivery and consumption apply to the hemorrhaging patient (see Chapter 7). However, the red cell contribution to arterial oxygen content (Cao_2) and oxygen delivery ($\dot{D}o_2$) transport, described by Equations 1 and 2, commands more attention than in other shock states:

$$Cao_2 = [Hgb \times 1.39 \times O_2\text{-Hgb saturation}] + [0.003 \times Pao_2] \quad \text{(Equation 1)}$$

$$\dot{D}o_2 = Cao_2 \times \text{cardiac output} \quad \text{(Equation 2)}$$

The terms in Equation 1 are the oxygen content attributable to the Hgb concentration (approximately 1.39 mL of oxygen binds to each gram of Hgb) and the much smaller amount of unbound oxygen, which is dissolved in serum. The second term is generally ignored except when high-tension inspired oxygen is being administered, such as in hyperbaric oxygen therapy. During vigorous volume resuscitation with crystalloid solutions in the bleeding patient, hemodilution occurs and may significantly hinder oxygen delivery despite maintenance of the cardiac output.

Significant hemorrhage also leads to impairment of the immune system and may be associated with sepsis syndrome, even in the absence of major tissue trauma. Increased serum levels of proinflammatory cytokines, such as tumor necrosis factor-alpha and interleukin-1, accompany progressive circulatory compromise. Elevated levels of these mediators are associated with an increased risk of subsequent infection, acute respiratory distress syndrome, multiple organ system failure, and death.

DIFFERENTIAL DIAGNOSIS OF FALLING HEMOGLOBIN RELEVANT TO PATIENTS IN THE INTENSIVE CARE UNIT

Often the clinical scenario associated with a falling Hgb permits a confident diagnosis of significant hemorrhage, such as in the case of a visible site of active bleeding. However, many other circumstances may cause an acute or a subacute drop in Hgb (Table 40–3). Dilution by intravenous infusion of large fluid volumes is a common cause even in the absence of bleeding. Sample collection error should always be considered, particularly in a patient receiving aggressive fluid resuscitation for hypotension. Specimens drawn from multilumen catheters or from a percutaneous venipuncture site proximal to an intravenous crystalloid infusion can be diluted by the infusate, resulting in a falsely low measured Hgb. A concomitant decrease in platelet and white blood cell counts, along with a change in serum electrolyte concentrations toward the composition of the infusate, suggests collection error. Massive hemolysis (acute hemolytic transfusion reaction, hemolytic anemia) is usually associated with circulatory instability (see Chapters 46 and 62). However, this diagnosis is usually evident on clinical grounds and can be confirmed by examination of the blood smear, urinalysis, and laboratory measurement of reticulocyte count, appropriate circulating antibodies, bilirubin, and haptoglobin.

DIAGNOSTIC EVALUATION

Both the evaluation and treatment of the hemorrhaging patient need to proceed concurrently. Important historical factors in the initial patient survey include

Table 40–3. Causes of Falling Hemoglobin in the Intensive Care Unit

Acute hemolytic transfusion reaction
Blood loss due to frequent phlebotomies (subacute fall in Hgb)
Factitious anemia due to sample collection error
Hemodilution due to IV crystalloids
Hemolytic anemia
Hemorrhage or blood loss from known source
Occult hemorrhage

Hgb, hemoglobin concentration; IV, intravenous.

previous episodes of bleeding or coagulopathy; use of anticoagulant, antiplatelet, or thrombolytic medications; recent invasive procedures or trauma; and intoxication (which may limit the usefulness of symptoms and physical signs). The physical examination should rapidly assess cardiopulmonary function and intravascular volume status and try to identify the source of bleeding. Special challenges to the physical examination often arise. The immobilization of trauma patients limits orthostatic measurements. Intoxicated patients who have sustained blunt trauma may deny pain despite significant internal bleeding. Diagnostic peritoneal lavage may prove lifesaving in this setting (see Chapter 94). Life-threatening blood loss in trauma patients with fractures or penetrating wounds may not be immediately apparent (e.g., pelvic fracture, ruptured spleen, liver laceration, or hemothorax). Since later chapters in this volume present how trauma patients should be surveyed for bleeding, the remainder of this discussion is directed to the diagnostic evaluation of nontraumatic hemorrhagic shock.

The most common source of nontraumatic bleeding is the gastrointestinal (GI) tract. Thus, if another source of bleeding is not evident in the hypotensive patient with or without a falling Hgb, the upper and lower GI tract should be quickly investigated by nasogastric tube aspirate and rectal examination, respectively (Fig. 40–1). Directed endoscopy may prove useful in selected patients in whom bleeding has ceased (see Chapters 60 and 61).

Two important clinical points should be emphasized about upper GI bleeding. First, aspiration of clear, nonbilious or even bilious fluid from the stomach does not exclude an upper GI bleeding source. In these cases, a postpyloric bleeding source may be present but not evident on gastric aspirate. For example, occasionally duodenal ulcer disease may lead to stricture formation in the postpyloric bulb, preventing reflux of blood into the stomach when the ulcer bleeds. Second, patients with bright red blood in the rectal vault may have an upper GI source of brisk bleeding associated with rapid GI transit. These patients may demonstrate marked hemodynamic compromise from rapid bleeding and intravascular volume depletion.

Upper GI bleeding should be evaluated by esophagogastroduodenoscopy (EGD). Even patients with a previously diagnosed source of hemorrhage, such as esophageal varices, may have a different bleeding site. Endoscopically, the source of upper GI bleeding can usually be identified and treated simultaneously (see Chapter 61).

The evaluation of lower GI bleeding is often frustrating and difficult (see Chapter 60). Frequently, the bleeding is intermittent in elderly patients in whom repeated invasive diagnostic procedures are poorly tolerated.

If the source of bleeding is not the GI tract and is not related to a recent invasive procedure, consideration should be given to the possibility of retroperitoneal or groin hemorrhage. These diagnoses are readily confirmed by computed tomography.

TREATMENT OF HEMORRHAGIC SHOCK

Early endotracheal intubation and mechanical ventilation should be considered in all patients with shock, particularly if surgical intervention is anticipated. Progressive circulatory deterioration often alters mentation and increases the risk of pulmonary complications. Assisted ventilation significantly reduces oxygen con-

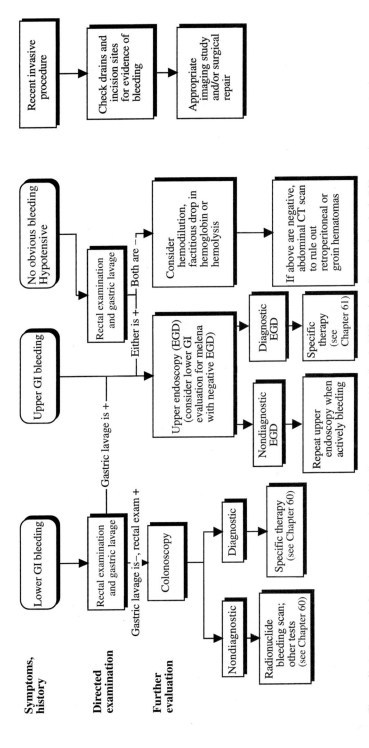

Figure 40–1. Schematic flow diagram to evaluate bleeding or suspected bleeding in ICU patient. GI, gastrointestinal; EGD, esophagogastroduodenoscopy.

sumption in unstable or agitated patients by reducing the work of breathing and permitting safe sedation.

Selection of the Intravenous Site and Catheter Size

Intravenous catheter insertion is discussed in detail in Chapter 9. Flow rate through a catheter varies directly with the fourth power of the radius of its lumen and inversely with its length and the viscosity of the infused liquid. The relevance of optimal catheter length and internal radius is underscored in the patient with hemorrhagic shock who requires replenishment of intravascular volume and tissue oxygen delivery as rapidly as possible. Short, large-bore catheters (so-called trauma lines) are therefore preferable to long, multilumen central venous catheters, which have a relatively small internal diameter (18 or 20 gauge) for each port. Trauma lines have 8 French (Fr) or 8.5 Fr internal diameters like the sheathed introducers used for insertion of pulmonary artery catheters. Special large-bore intravenous (IV) tubing and three-way stopcocks should be used in configuration with a trauma line (or equivalent) to treat severe cases of hemorrhaging. The use of these large-bore delivery systems has obviated the need to use pressurized cuffs on the IV bags or to decrease the viscosity of the infusate.

Fluid Administration

The optimal amount and composition of resuscitation fluid for hemorrhagic shock patients remains hotly debated. Rapid volume expansion can be achieved with smaller volumes of colloids than with isotonic crystalloid solutions. Conversely, crystalloid solutions rapidly infused through large-bore catheters restore intravascular volume and concomitantly replenish the interstitial fluid deficit. Numerous randomized clinical trials have failed to establish convincingly the superiority of either colloid or crystalloid resuscitation. Table 40–4 lists advantages and disadvantages of crystalloid and colloid preparations that are currently available for volume resuscitation.

The four categories of hemorrhagic shock (see Table 40–2) allow formulation of a general approach to fluid resuscitation. Usually, patients with class I hemorrhage respond to crystalloids and do not require infusion of blood products. More advanced hemorrhage can be treated initially with intravenous crystalloid while awaiting blood products. In an individual patient, however, signs and symptoms of shock may not identify a specific hemorrhage class and may not reflect the degree of intravascular volume depletion. Response to therapy is more important than the initial hemodynamic parameters. Furthermore, standard clinical measures of cardiac function and organ perfusion—such as blood pressure, pulse rate, urine output, and mentation—remain important therapeutic end points. Patients with class III hemorrhage may show a transient response followed by deterioration. Lack of improvement in hemodynamics after a rapid fluid challenge of 1000 to 2000 mL of crystalloid suggests class IV hemorrhage.

Table 40–4. Common Crystalloid and Colloid Resuscitation Fluids

FLUID	CLASS	ADVANTAGES	DISADVANTAGES
0.9% saline ("normal" saline)	Crystalloid	Inexpensive Easy storage No risk of viral infection	May lead to hyperchloremic acidosis Less effective volume expander when compared with colloids
Ringer's lactate	Crystalloid	Inexpensive Easy storage No risk of viral infection	May lead to hyperkalemia Lactate levels may increase in patients with liver disease Less effective volume expander when compared with colloids Incompatible with a number of medications
Hypertonic saline (7.5% saline)	Crystalloid	Smaller infusion volume needed when compared with 0.9% saline or Ringer's lactate solution May increase left ventricular contractility May increase intracranial pressure less than isotonic fluids No risk of viral infection	May produce hypernatremia, hyperchloremia, and hyperosmolarity Volume expansion is transient unless combined with colloid
Albumin	Colloid	Rapid volume expansion	Expensive Allergic reactions
Dextran (Dextran-40, Dextran-70)	Colloid	Rapid volume expansion	Expensive Large volumes associated with coagulopathy May cause renal failure Allergic reactions
Hydroxyethyl starch (Hetastarch)	Colloid	Rapid volume expansion Longer activity than albumin	Expensive Hyperamylasemia (does not indicate pancreatitis) Allergic reactions

Red Cell Transfusions

Another area of long-standing controversy is when to transfuse blood products. Transfusion of blood products bears short- and long-term health risks and complications (see Chapters 15 and 46). However, investigators have been unable to identify a critical Hgb above which patients can be safely supported with cell-free fluids. The commonly cited goal of 10/30 (Hgb [g/dL]/hematocrit [%]), although easy to remember and often straightforward to achieve with transfusions, has not been substantiated as the most desirable end point by controlled clinical trials. Although Equations 1 and 2 predict that oxygen delivery will increase directly with Hgb levels, in reality changes in tissue oxygen metabolism after transfusion are more complex. The cardiac index may be adversely affected by increased afterload because of higher blood viscosity, particularly in the setting of hypothermia and vasoconstriction. Banked blood contains Hgb with higher than normal oxygen affinity because of decreased levels of 2,3-diphosphoglycerate (2,3-DPG) and therefore does not release bound oxygen as efficiently as does host blood (see Appendix A). The decision to transfuse an individual patient should start with the patient's Hgb determination but should also take into account the patient's age, comorbid disease, duration of anemia, intravascular volume status, and adequacy of tissue oxygenation.

Uncrossmatched type O-negative packed red blood cells may be used to resuscitate exsanguinating patients for whom immediate transfusion is necessary. Type O *whole* blood should be avoided because it will contain anti-A and anti-B antibodies, which can react with the recipient's blood cells and any subsequently transfused type-specific blood. During large-volume infusions, packed cells should be mixed with an equal volume of isotonic saline and infused through a warming device to improve fluid viscosity and prevent hypothermia. If blood warmers are not immediately available, the blood may be immersed in warm water before infusion. If time allows, particularly for patients demonstrating at least a transient response to cell-free infusions, type-specific or fully crossmatched blood should be used.

Other Blood Products

Unfortunately, there is a lack of data to guide clinical decisions in the use of platelets and fresh frozen plasma (FFP) during aggressive resuscitation of hemorrhagic shock. Current guidelines are based on the recommendations from the most recent National Institutes of Health Consensus Development Conferences on transfusion medicine. Platelets should be transfused to actively bleeding patients who have received antiplatelet therapy (e.g., aspirin or nonsteroidal anti-inflammatory agents) or in whom comorbid disease affects platelet function (e.g., uremia). During massive transfusion (5 units of blood within 1 hour or 10 units of blood within 24 hours) platelet counts may drop significantly. Therapy should be guided by the serial platelet counts and not empirically by the number of units of blood given. Transfusion is recommended for platelet counts less than 50,000/μL. Colloidal blood products, such as FFP or cryoprecipitate, should not be used as primary volume expanders given their infectious risk and expense. Prophylactic FFP therapy has been shown to be of no benefit during massive transfusion of blood products, but therapy for documented coagulation abnormalities is essential.

CLINICAL PEARLS AND PITFALLS

1. One should ask oneself early in the course of the evaluation and management of the bleeding patient whether surgical intervention is necessary and revisit this question if bleeding continues despite appropriate medical therapy.
2. One should not become complacent when IV access is secured and fluids are being administered. Hemorrhagic shock can progress despite vigorous volume resuscitation and can lead to catastrophic consequences.
3. Intracranial bleeding does not result in hypovolemia or a decreased Hgb (unless the integrity of the cranial vault is violated).

BIBLIOGRAPHY

Bickell WH, Pepe PE, Wall MJ, et al: Immediate versus delayed fluid resuscitation for hypotensive patients with penetrating torso injuries. N Engl J Med 331:1105–1109, 1994.
This article describes a provocative randomized clinical study of 598 adults, showing improvement in survival with delayed fluid resuscitation before the time of surgery in this trauma patient population.

Ellison N, Silberstein LE: A commentary on three consensus development conferences on transfusion medicine. Anesthesiol Clin North Am 8:609–625, 1990.
This is a cogent commentary on the three major National Institutes of Health consensus conferences that published guidelines for the use of red blood cells, platelets, and fresh frozen plasma in the late 1980s. It highlights many areas for which there remains little scientific data.

Griffiths WJ, Neumann DA, Welsh JD: The visible vessel as an indicator of uncontrolled or recurrent gastrointestinal hemorrhage. N Engl J Med 300:1411–1413, 1979.
This article describes an important study of 317 consecutive patients, showing that a visible vessel at the time of endoscopy is predictive of rebleeding.

Moore FD: The effects of hemorrhage on body composition. N Engl J Med 273:567–577, 1965.
This was a landmark study describing the physiology of controlled hemorrhage in humans.

Ogden JE, Parry ES: The development of hemoglobin solutions as red cell substitutes. Int Anesthesiol Clin 33:115–129, 1995.
This is a well-written overview of the state of the art and outlines the approaches being explored in the design of better red cell substitutes.

Shippy CR, Appel PL, Shoemaker WC: Reliability of clinical monitoring to assess blood volume in critically ill patients. Crit Care Med 12:107–112, 1984.
This well-designed study based on more than 1500 measurements in critically ill patients shows that clinical monitoring does not correlate well with measured blood volume and also demonstrates the relative changes in blood volume resulting from crystalloid and colloid infusions.

Spence RK, Costabile J, Norcross ED, et al: Perfluorocarbons as blood substitutes: The early years. Experience with Fluosol DA-20% in the 1980s. Artif Cells Blood Substit Immobil Biotechnol 22:955–963, 1994.
This review of perfluorocarbon use supports the safety but lack of efficacy of this agent in major hemorrhage.

Wilcox CM, Alexander LN, Cotsonis G: A prospective characterization of upper gastrointestinal hemorrhage presenting with hematochezia. Am J Gastroenterol 92:231–235, 1997.
This prospective study conducted over a 4-year period examined the clinical characteristics of over 700 patients with upper gastrointestinal tract bleeding, 14% of whom presented with hematochezia. Interestingly, patients with hematochezia had an initial hemodynamic profile similar to those with melena. However, transfusion requirements, need for surgery, and mortality rates were worse in the hematochezia group.

Velanovich V: Crystalloid versus colloid fluid resuscitation: A meta-analysis of mortality. Surgery 105:65–71, 1989.
This article describes a meta-analysis of eight previously published randomized clinical trials. The analysis suggests small mortality rate benefits for both colloid and crystalloid solutions, depending on the patient population studied.

41

Ileus

Gary R. Lichtenstein

Ileus refers to an inhibition of gastrointestinal motility. It commonly occurs in patients in the intensive care unit (ICU). It can be seen as a physiologic response—for example, after abdominal surgery—or it may be pathologic. The presence of ileus may be associated with significant morbidity because it restricts individuals from using the gastrointestinal tract. Because of its high prevalence and potentially adverse effects, the recognition and management of ileus is important in the care of patients in the ICU.

Ileus (also called adynamic ileus) is defined as the functional inhibition of propulsive bowel activity, irrespective of pathogenic mechanism. This differs from other gastrointestinal motility disorders resulting from structural abnormalities, for example, small bowel obstruction. *Postoperative ileus* is the uncomplicated ileus that follows surgery and usually resolves spontaneously within 2 to 3 days. The term *postoperative paralytic ileus* refers to a postoperative ileus that lasts longer than 3 days. Ileus of the colon with sudden massive dilatation is called *acute colonic pseudo-obstruction* or *Ogilvie's syndrome. Toxic megacolon* is another form of colonic ileus in which inflammation involves all colonic tissue layers and that results in systemic toxicity.

PATHOPHYSIOLOGY

A multitude of pathologic phenomena are associated with the presence of an ileus. An *impairment of intestinal blood flow* (arterial or venous) can lead to an ileus. Conversely, the presence of a simple ileus itself does not lead to the impairment of intestinal blood flow. Analogous to that which occurs in states of mechanical bowel obstruction, a *change in bowel flora* may also occur during ileus. This can lead to stasis, overgrowth of bacteria, and subsequent malabsorption. There may also be a *change in the bowel contents* similar to that which occurs in distended loops of bowel during intestinal obstruction. Under these circumstances, fluid inside the bowel lumen increases because of intestinal secretion plus a failure of absorption. Intestinal gas also contributes to the abdominal distention, and the gas-filled loops of intestine are routinely seen on the abdominal radiographs of a patient with ileus. In the case of ileus, this gas results primarily from swallowed air.

Significant *changes in motility* occur in both the small and large intestine in the presence of ileus. Unfortunately, the mediators of these changes have not yet been identified, even in postoperative ileus (the best studied type of ileus to date). Although it has been suggested that adrenergic mediation is responsible, this does not explain why the ileus persists for several days. Also, evidence suggests that mechanisms other than spinal reflexes play a role because the use of epidural anesthesia (which blocks efferent sympathetic nerves) does not shorten the duration of ileus. Although damage to cholinergic nerves from hypoxemia or from surgical manipulation could explain some cases of ileus, activation of the nonadrenergic noncholinergic inhibitory nerves is the most likely cause for most cases of ileus.

481

Table 41–1. Intra-Abdominal Causes of Ileus

Infectious disorders	Ischemic disorders
Peritonitis	Local arterial insufficiency
Diverticulitis	Local venous insufficiency
Cholecystitis	Mesenteric arteritis
Appendicitis	Strangulated obstruction
Tubo-ovarian abscess	Retroperitoneal disorders
Inflammatory disorders	Nephrolithiasis
Pancreatitis	Pyelonephritis
Perforated viscus	Hemorrhage
Toxic megacolon	
Intraperitoneal bleeding	
Peritonitis	
Radiation	

CAUSES OF ILEUS IN THE INTENSIVE CARE UNIT

Common intra-abdominal and extra-abdominal causes of ileus that would be relevant for patients in the ICU are listed in Tables 41–1 and 41–2. Likewise, intra-abdominal and extra-abdominal conditions associated with acute colonic pseudo-obstruction or Ogilvie's syndrome (a nonobstructive, acute massive dilatation of the colon that is temporary and reversible) are listed in Tables 41–3 and 41–4.

DIAGNOSTIC EVALUATION OF THE ICU PATIENT WITH ILEUS

Initial steps include evaluation for electrolyte disturbances (measuring serum sodium, potassium, chloride, and bicarbonate levels) and searching for evidence of infection or inflammatory disorders (obtaining a white blood cell count with differential) is often carried out. In ischemic or infarcted bowel, the presence of other laboratory abnormalities may be found, including elevated levels of serum

Table 41–2. Extra-Abdominal Causes of Ileus

Drug-induced	Reflex inhibition
Anticholinergic medication	Myocardial infarction
Opioids	Pneumonia
Chemotherapy	Pulmonary embolus
Ganglionic blocking agents	Burns
Metabolic disturbances	Fractures of the pelvis, ribs, or spine
Electrolyte abnormalities	
Sepsis	
Uremia	
Diabetic ketoacidosis	
Sickle cell anemia with painful crisis	
Hypothyroidism	

Table 41–3. Intra-Abdominal Disorders Associated with
Acute Colonic Pseudo-Obstruction

Inflammatory disorders
  Acute pancreatitis
  Acute cholecystitis
  Inflammatory bowel disease
  Radiation colitis
Infectious disorders
  Herpes simplex or herpes zoster infection
  Spontaneous bacterial peritonitis
Ischemic disorders
  Inferior mesenteric artery insufficiency

Retroperitoneal disorders
  Neoplasms
  Bleeding
Reflex inhibition
  Trauma
  Cholecystectomy
  Urologic operations
  Cesarean section

amylase, alkaline phosphatase (ALP), creatinine phosphokinase (CPK), aspartate aminotransferase (AST), alanine aminotransferase (ALT), and lactate dehydrogenase (LDH) as well as an anion gap metabolic acidosis. However, all these laboratory abnormalities are nonspecific.

In patients with suspected ileus, it is important to obtain an obstruction series, that is, abdominal radiographs (supine and upright views), to help localize the abnormality and to exclude free intraperitoneal air. Chest radiographs can indicate the presence of associated pulmonary disease as an extra-abdominal cause of the ileus. When an ileus is present, intestinal gas and fluid are present in various amounts throughout the intestinal tract. In contrast, in acute colonic pseudo-obstruction, only the large bowel becomes dilated throughout its extent. However, it is typically the cecum that is greatest in diameter. Computed tomography (CT) can be helpful in assessing the presence of thickened bowel loops (suggestive of ischemia), abscesses, pancreatic disease, venous thrombosis, and other similar disorders. CT should be considered only if plain radiographs are inconclusive.

Differentiating ileus from mechanical obstruction may be difficult and require a barium enema, colonoscopy, or small bowel contrast radiography. However, care

Table 41–4. Extra-Abdominal Disorders Associated with
Acute Colonic Pseudo-Obstruction

Medication-related
  Phenothiazines
  Chemotherapy
  Laxative abuse
  Tricyclic antidepressants
Metabolic disorders
  Systemic infection
  Chronic obstructive pulmonary disease with acute exacerbation
  Ethanol
Reflex inhibition
  Bone fractures
  Coronary artery bypass graft surgery
  Valvular heart surgery

should be taken to avoid administration of barium proximal to an area of obstruction because it can become trapped, inspissated, and impacted. Magnetic resonance imaging with venography or angiography has been used with increasing frequency in selected patients. In these cases, plain abdominal radiographs are not revealing, and either pancreatic disease or venous disease (such as mesenteric venous thrombosis) is suspected or CT is not performed because of contrast allergy.

Endoscopy, colonoscopy, or enteroscopy may be of value if the bowel mucosa must be visualized or biopsied. However, these procedures should be avoided if a perforated viscus or an acute abdomen is present. When an ileus is associated with ascites without a clear cause, a paracentesis should be performed to search for several abnormalities, including those of blood and bile, as well as high amylase levels, infection, and malignant cells.

MANAGEMENT AND DISCUSSION OF THERAPIES

The initial management should entail establishing the presence of obstruction or ileus and whether there are associated fluid, electrolyte, or acid base disorders. If the bowel is distended, initiation of nasogastric suction with low intermittent suctioning is appropriate because bowel distention can result in nausea, vomiting, and an increased risk of aspiration. One should avoid, if possible, the use of opioids and other agents (see Table 41–2) that may slow down bowel motility.

Acute bowel obstruction is a surgical emergency. Surgery is also necessary in some patients with ischemic small bowel disease. The use of intraoperative Doppler ultrasonography and fluorescein dye injection helps localize the obstruction and tests patency of other mesenteric vasculature. After restoring mesenteric circulation, the use of the hand-held Doppler is helpful in assessing remaining blood flow. In contrast to ischemic small bowel disease, ischemic colonic disease has a low mortality. Thus surgery should be contemplated only when symptoms persist or if the bowel is suspected to be infarcted. The therapy for ileus should be directed primarily toward the treatment of its underlying cause. In the postoperative period, an ileus is expected and typically resolves within a few days. If there is evidence of bowel obstruction after resolution of the ileus, appropriate therapy should be initiated.

In patients with acute colonic pseudo-obstruction, appropriate management of fluid and electrolytes is of key importance. Patients are usually kept fasting and treated with intravenous (IV) fluids and a nasogastric (NG) tube with low intermittent suction. When resolution is slow with the use of a NG tube alone, a rectal tube should be placed to low intermittent suction. Opioids and other antimotility agents should be withdrawn, and efforts to correct any underlying associated condition should be made. If conservative care fails, giving 2 mg IV neostigmine has recently been reported as being highly effective. If the colonic diameter becomes large (usually >12 cm in maximal transverse dimension), ischemia, perforation, and sepsis may ensue. Even in the case of a massively dilatated colon, conservative management via NG tube, rectal tube, avoidance of antimotility agents, and neostigmine should be attempted initially. This is usually successful, but more aggressive decompression may be needed either by colonoscopy or surgical cecostomy.

CLINICAL PEARLS AND PITFALLS

Several key points can be summarized in the following general guidelines:

1. Look at medications and discontinue antimotility agents (see Table 41–2).
2. Check obstruction series and chest radiograph.
3. Check electrolytes, complete blood count with differential and thyroid status.
4. Consider colonoscopic or endoscopic procedures.
5. Look for complications of systemic diseases.
6. Look for evidence of ischemic bowel disease.
7. Consider CT examination to search for a cause for ileus.
8. In acute colonic pseudo-obstruction, follow obstruction series and attempt decompression via nasogastric tube, rectal tube and, if needed, colonoscopy or surgical cecostomy while attempting to reverse the associated cause (see Tables 41–3 and 41–4).

SUMMARY

It is common for a patient to acquire an ileus during a stay in the ICU. The presence of an ileus can lead to significant morbidity and possibly mortality. A rapid and efficient search for the cause of the ileus is critical to reduce this morbidity and to restore enteral nutrition promptly.

BIBLIOGRAPHY

Benson MJ, Wingate DL: Ileus and mechanical obstruction. In: Kumar D, Wingate D: An Illustrated Guide to Gastrointestinal Motility. New York: Churchill Livingstone, 1993, pp 547–582.
This describes a comprehensive and complete review of the work-up and evaluation of ileus.

Livingstone AS, Sosa JL: Ileus and obstruction. In: Haubrich WS, Schaffner F, Berk JE: Bockus Gastroenterology. Philadelphia: WB Saunders, 1995, pp 1235–1248.
This is an outstanding review of ileus and obstruction, with emphasis on causes and principles.

Ponec RJ, Saunders MD, Kimmey MB: Neostigmine for the treatment of acute colonic pseudo-obstruction. N Engl J Med 341:137–141, 1999.
This prospective randomized trial of 21 patients with acute colonic pseudo-obstruction showed that 2 mg neostigmine given IV decompressed the colon rapidly. Side effects included abdominal pain, excess salivation, and vomiting; two patients developed symptomatic bradycardia, which responded to atropine. See also follow-up comments about this study in N Engl J Med 341:192–193, 1999 and 341:1622–1623, 1999.

Schuffler MD, Sinanan MN: Intestinal obstruction and pseudo-obstruction. In: Scharschmidt BF, Feldman M: Gastrointestinal Disease: Pathophysiology, Diagnosis, Management. Philadelphia: WB Saunders, 1993, pp 898–916.
This is an outstanding, comprehensive review of the subject matter. It is extremely well written.

Silen W: Acute intestinal obstruction. In: Wilson JD, Braunwald E, Isselbacher KJ, et al: Harrison's Principles of Internal Medicine. New York: McGraw-Hill, 1991, pp 1295–1298.
This is a well-written review of general principles.

Summers RW, Lu CC: Approach to the patient with ileus and obstruction. In: Yamada T, Alpers DH, Owyang C, et al: Gastroenterology. Philadelphia: JB Lippincott, 1995, pp 796–812.
This is an outstanding reference textbook with encyclopedic review of the subject matter.

42

Increased Intracranial Pressure

Todd M. Lasner
Eric L. Zager

Treatment of acute increases in intracranial pressure (ICP) may be among the most urgent and dramatic interventions in the intensive care unit (ICU), akin to other life-threatening situations such as acute respiratory failure, cardiac dysrhythmias, or hemorrhagic shock. Elevated ICP in adults is defined as a pressure *greater than 20 mm Hg* as measured by lumbar puncture or an ICP monitor. Intracranial hypertension may also be inferred from the clinical examination along with magnetic resonance imaging (MRI) or computed tomography (CT) (showing hydrocephalus or a mass lesion with midline shift). Therapies directed at lowering ICP affect the contents of the cranium, that is, the cerebrospinal fluid (CSF), blood, and cerebral (or neoplastic) tissue. This chapter focuses on the pathophysiology of elevated ICP, its acute clinical presentation and differential diagnosis, and the selection of medical and surgical interventions for the management of elevated ICP. Discussion of traumatic brain injury can be found in Chapter 96.

PATHOPHYSIOLOGY

Anatomic Considerations

The intracranial space is a closed compartment with a relatively fixed volume that accommodates hemorrhage or other acute expansive processes poorly. It is divided by the tentorium, a dural reflection that separates the cerebral convexities and the diencephalon from the posterior fossa (brainstem and cerebellum). The midbrain is located at the tentorial incisura and bridges these two spaces. Pressure differentials between these separate regions may lead to herniation of tissue through the tentorial notch, causing compression of the midbrain. Transtentorial herniation may thus cause contralateral hemiparesis (from compression of the ipsilateral cerebral peduncle) and loss of consciousness (from compression of the reticular activating system in the brainstem). In addition, the oculomotor nerve abuts the uncus of the temporal lobe at the level of the tentorial incisura. Thus, as a consequence of uncal herniation, compression of the third cranial nerve may develop, causing a dilated pupil ipsilateral to the mass lesion. A mass lesion in the temporal lobe, because of its proximity to the midbrain, would be more likely to cause transtentorial herniation than would a lesion of similar size in the frontal or occipital lobe.

There may be herniation of cerebellum upward across the tentorium or downward through the foramen magnum (so-called tonsillar herniation) due to a lesion in the posterior fossa. The latter causes compression of the cervicomedullary junction, with ensuing coma and cardiorespiratory dysfunction. Because of the smaller volume of the posterior fossa than of the supratentorial space, lesions of

487

the cerebellum may lead to brainstem compression more rapidly than would a similar-sized lesion in the cerebrum.

The brain is covered by three layers of meninges (from superficial to deep): the dura mater, the arachnoid, and the pia mater. Traumatic hematomas may occur in the epidural space (usually from a skull fracture with or without an injury to the middle meningeal artery), in the subdural space (from tearing of veins bridging the cortex to the dura), or in the brain parenchyma (from a direct contusion). Trauma is the most common cause of subarachnoid hemorrhage, which may also be caused by a ruptured cerebral aneurysm or arteriovenous malformation.

The brain may accommodate large, slowly expanding lesions, such as tumors, or chronic subdural hematomas before symptomatic elevated ICP occurs. In contrast, rapidly expanding masses (e.g., hematomas) usually become symptomatic at much smaller volumes. However, even when there is an acute mass lesion, there is little increase in ICP if the mass is small. Once the mass reaches a certain threshold volume, there is an *exponential rise* in ICP. Patients with intracranial hypertension and incipient cerebral herniation may acquire the Cushing's triad (systemic hypertension, respiratory arrest, and bradycardia), which results from medullary compression and ischemia. This is usually a preterminal event and not generally seen until severe intracranial hypertension occurs.

Regulation of Cerebrospinal Fluid

Obstruction of the flow or absorption of CSF causes dilatation of the ventricular system (hydrocephalus) and thus elevates the ICP. CSF is produced in the choroid plexus within the ventricular system, the majority of which is in the lateral ventricles. CSF flows from the lateral ventricles through the foramen of Monro, bilaterally, into the third ventricle. From there, it proceeds through the aqueduct of Sylvius into the fourth ventricle and then through the foramina of Luschka and Magendie into the subarachnoid space. CSF is reabsorbed into the venous system through the arachnoid granulations that abut the dural venous sinuses. There may be a blockage of CSF at any point along this pathway. This will cause a dilatation of the ventricular system proximal to the obstruction (obstructive or noncommunicating hydrocephalus). For instance, space-occupying lesions of the posterior fossa may compress the fourth ventricle or aqueduct, causing dilatation of the third and lateral ventricles. Meningitis or subarachnoid hemorrhage may cause symmetric dilatation of the ventricular system because of a failure to reabsorb CSF through the arachnoid granulations (communicating hydrocephalus).

Regulation of Cerebral Blood Flow

Cerebral blood flow is tightly regulated in the normal brain to maintain a cerebral perfusion pressure (CPP) between 50 and 150 mm Hg. CPP is defined as the difference between mean arterial pressure and ICP. Within this range of CPP, perfusion is sufficient for the metabolic needs of the brain. Higher CPP may cause breakdown of the blood-brain barrier, which normally prevents leakage of proteins and other components of plasma into the brain. Clinical studies of patients with traumatic brain injury have shown that maintenance of CPP at greater than 60 mm Hg improves patient outcomes.

Clinical Presentation and Differential Diagnosis

The time course of neurologic deterioration is important in arriving at the appropriate diagnosis. For instance, vascular events such as strokes and hemorrhage frequently present with profound deficits at the time of the vascular event. Patients with ruptured cerebral aneurysm or hypertensive hemorrhages often experience the acute onset of headache, loss of consciousness, or seizure. However, tumors generally have a subacute presentation, with a progressive neurologic deficit evolving over weeks or months. Nonetheless, patients with vascular, neoplastic, infectious, or traumatic processes may all present acutely with seizures as the initial manifestation.

Patients with cerebral hematomas also may vary in their presentations. Individuals with acute traumatic *epidural hematomas* classically have a loss of consciousness at the time of the injury and may subsequently awaken—the lucid interval—before deterioration into coma. Conversely, patients with *subdural hematomas* often have an underlying cerebral contusion and therefore have no interval of consciousness. Because therapeutic decisions depend on the patient's level of consciousness, any paralytic agents, benzodiazepines, or opioids that are used must be short-acting and pharmacologically reversible to allow frequent neurologic examinations. It is also important to note that the maximal amount of cerebral edema occurs *3 to 4 days* after an acute event (trauma, infarction, or hemorrhage). The patient may deteriorate during this time as the ICP increases. Differential diagnoses for causes of intracranial hemorrhage and mass effect are illustrated in Figure 42–1.

APPROACH TO CLINICAL MANAGEMENT

Initial Approach

Patients with head trauma and altered consciousness should be appropriately stabilized before further evaluation (the ABCs of resuscitation—airway, breathing, and circulation) with endotracheal intubation, if necessary, to protect their airway. After a directed neurologic examination, CT of the brain should be performed immediately. CT is preferable to MRI because it can be performed more rapidly and reveals acute hemorrhage better than MRI. The decision to operate depends on both the neurologic examination and the computed tomographic findings. Generally, if the patient has a Glasgow Coma Scale (GCS) score less than 9 (see Table 96–1 for GCS scoring) and does not have an operative lesion, an ICP monitor should be placed. Medical management of elevated ICP should be instituted to maintain the CPP at greater than 60 to 70 mm Hg. If the ICP becomes refractory to medical management, CT should be repeated and surgery should be considered (Fig. 42–2). Additionally, in some centers, a catheter may be inserted retrograde from the internal jugular vein to the skull base to determine the cerebral oxygen extraction and monitor for global cerebral ischemia (see Chapter 96).

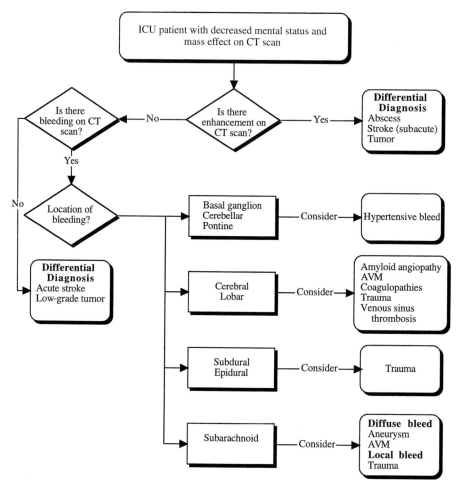

Figure 42–1. Schematic flow diagram of differential diagnosis in ICU patient with decreased mental status and mass effect on head computed tomography (CT). AVM, arteriovenous malformation.

Standard Intracranial Pressure Monitors

Standard ICP monitors are designed to be placed in the various regions of the intracranial space that were outlined previously. All these devices may be placed under sterile conditions at the bedside with only a small opening in the calvarium. *Epidural monitors* are fiberoptic devices and have the least reliability, as they require pressure to be transmitted across the dura. The *intraparenchymal fiberoptic monitor* is placed a few millimeters into the brain parenchyma. It is highly reliable because it is not dependent on an intact fluid column to function and is not prone to occlusion. *Intraventricular monitors* are the only monitoring devices that may be used to lower ICP directly by draining CSF, which may be beneficial even in the absence of hydrocephalus. The *subarachnoid bolt* uses a column of CSF,

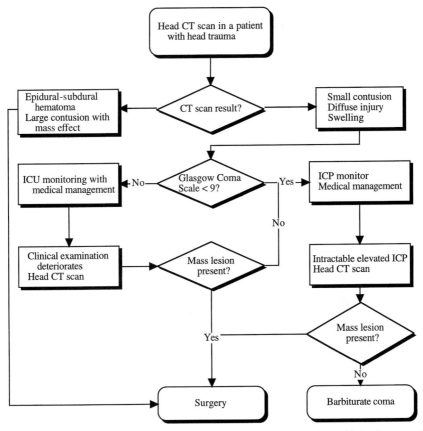

Figure 42–2. Schematic flow diagram outlining management of ICU patient with head trauma depending on findings on head computed tomography (CT). ICP, intracranial pressure.

formed by a small opening in the dura, that is linked to a pressure transducer. This device gives more dampened pulse pressures over time and is more inaccurate than the fiberoptic monitor and ventricular catheter. Frontal monitors are not useful for the management of masses in the posterior fossa. They also may not predict impending herniation in lesions of the mesial temporal lobe. Thus, neurologic deterioration or signs of impending herniation may be more important in these clinical circumstances.

Finally, *lumbar puncture* (LP) may reflect ICP only if the ventricles are not obstructed and if there is not a cerebral or spinal mass lesion. In the latter two instances, however, LP is contraindicated because it may precipitate cerebral herniation or increase spinal cord dysfunction, respectively. In the pre-CT era, LP was thought to be safe if the patient did not have papilledema. This was erroneous because papilledema may *not* develop acutely in response to elevated ICP. Current practice mandates that a MRI or computed tomographic scan be performed first to rule out a mass lesion that may contraindicate LP.

Surgical Therapy

Intracranial Bleeding

Patients with intraparenchymal lobar hematomas from an arteriovenous malformation or aneurysm may benefit from acute evacuation of the clot. If either is suspected, a preoperative arteriogram is preferred if the patient's clinical status permits. Patients with a subarachnoid or intraventricular hemorrhage may require a ventriculostomy acutely to treat symptomatic hydrocephalus (Fig. 42–3). For a spontaneous hemorrhage or stroke in the cerebellum, patients benefit from prompt craniectomy and removal of clot and infarcted tissue if there is mass effect and symptomatic brainstem compression.

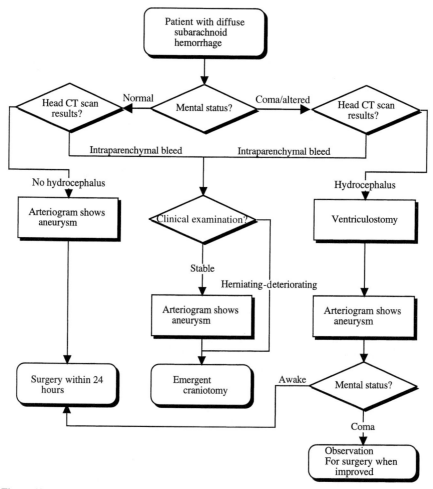

Figure 42–3. Schematic flow diagram outlining management of ICU patient with diffuse subarachnoid hemorrhage on head computed tomography (CT).

The management of patients with a hypertensive hemorrhage into the basal ganglia is controversial. Studies suggest that craniotomy and evacuation of putaminal and thalamic hematomas do not improve outcome. Generally, if the patient is otherwise healthy, is deteriorating into coma despite optimal medical management, and the lesion is in the nondominant hemisphere, an operative approach may be indicated. Otherwise, medical management of ICP may be appropriate. In elderly patients with massive hemorrhages or thromboembolic strokes, comfort measures alone should be recommended, particularly when the stroke is in the dominant hemisphere, because of a poor prognosis.

Hemispheric Strokes

Decompressive craniectomy for swelling associated with large hemispheric strokes has not been demonstrated to improve outcome in a randomized, controlled trial (although anecdotal reports of satisfactory recoveries after surgery continue to appear). As indicated previously, maximal swelling occurs 3 to 4 days after the stroke. Despite an overall poor prognosis, it may be appropriate to recommend instituting medical therapies, depending on the anticipated severity of the neurologic sequelae and the patient's previously expressed preferences for aggressive care in the face of grim prognosis for recovery of cognitive function. Early intravenous administration of tissue plasminogen activator improves long-term morbidity and mortality in patients with acute nonhemorrhagic stroke but does not affect short-term morbidity from swelling. It is also associated with a 6% risk of hemorrhage into the infarct. Therefore, patients who receive thrombolytic therapy for strokes should be closely monitored clinically for potential hemorrhage into the infarct (see Chapter 71).

Tumors and Abscesses

Tumors generally do not require an emergent operation to control ICP, as the intracranial space has sufficient time to accommodate to a relatively slowly growing mass, and patients often respond well to steroids and diuresis. However, because of its small volume, tumors in the posterior fossa can rapidly cause brainstem compression and the development of hydrocephalus.

Ring-enhancing lesions may be either tumors or abscesses. Because abscesses do not always present with fever or leukocytosis, there may be some preoperative diagnostic uncertainty. A stereotactic aspiration or an open procedure will confirm the diagnosis of abscess and allow a drain to be placed into the abscess cavity at the same time. Appropriate intravenous antibiotics should be administered for several weeks, with serial CT or MRI to confirm progressive shrinkage of the lesion. Some abscesses may require craniotomy for resection.

Hydrocephalus

Patients with hydrocephalus may be managed acutely, if necessary, with a ventriculostomy, which drains to an external reservoir, or with an internalized shunt. If the patient has hydrocephalus from an acute subarachnoid or intraventricular hemorrhage, a ventriculostomy is placed so that pressure may also be monitored. Many of these patients do not require a shunt after the hemorrhage resolves.

Malfunctioning Shunts

Patients with malfunctioning chronic ventricular shunts ideally should have antero-posterior and lateral views of the skull, neck, and chest, plus abdominal plain radiographs (a shunt series) to diagnose disconnection or malposition of the shunt, followed by a computed tomographic scan of the head. After these studies, the shunt reservoir should be palpated and aspirated to determine whether the obstruction is proximal or distal, to measure the ICP with a manometer, and to sample the CSF for routine laboratory analysis. When this is performed outside the operating room, there is a 5 to 8% risk of infecting the shunt. If the shunt is malfunctioning, it is usually revised in the operating room. An infected shunt usually requires externalization of drainage, appropriate intravenous antibiotics, and shunt replacement once the CSF is sterile.

Medical Therapy (Table 42–1)

Elevation of the head of the bed to 30 degrees lowers ICP by improving venous drainage. It also decreases ICP while not affecting CPP, cerebral blood flow, or cerebral oxygen extraction. The neck should be placed in a neutral (nonrotated) position to prevent kinking of the jugular veins and obstruction to cerebral venous return.

The ICP is normally tightly regulated by the $Paco_2$. As the $Paco_2$ decreases, the capacitance vessels in the cerebral circulation constrict (and vice versa). In intubated patients, *hyperventilation* can be used to decrease the cerebral blood volume and ICP. Its effect is almost immediate, and several breaths in rapid succession may be given to achieve this result. Hyperventilation, however, is only

Table 42–1. Medical Management of Elevated Intracranial Pressure

....

Anticonvulsant (phenytoin) for seizure prophylaxis
Barbiturates with electroencephalographic monitoring to achieve burst suppression
Control agitation (with continuous ICP monitoring) by use of:
  Benzodiazepines
  Opioids
  Neuromuscular blocking agents
  Diuresis (mannitol, furosemide) to serum osmolality of 315–320 mmol/L
  Elevate head of bed to 30 degrees and place head of patient in nonrotated position
  Hyperventilate to $Paco_2$ 30 mm Hg with mechanical ventilation (for $Paco_2$ < 30 mm Hg, consider
    jugular venous monitoring)
ICP monitoring
Isotonic intravenous fluids
Maintain normoglycemia, normal electrolyte levels, and coagulation profiles
Mild hypothermia ($\approx$34° C)
Steroids (only for tumors)

....

  ICP, intracranial pressure.

effective down to a $PaCO_2$ of 20 mm Hg. Lowering $PaCO_2$ to less than 20 mm Hg not only is ineffective in decreasing ICP further but also may increase cerebral arteriolar resistance and induce cerebral ischemia. In some centers, jugular venous monitoring is used if $PaCO_2$ is lowered to less than 30 mm Hg.

Corticosteroids are effective for decreasing edema in patients with cerebral tumors. They are ineffective, however, in the treatment of edema from cerebral trauma, stroke, or hemorrhage.

Fluid management is also critical in the management of intracranial hypertension. Normal saline is an appropriate maintenance fluid for the initial management of most head-injured patients. Hyponatremia, which may be associated with the syndrome of inappropriate antidiuretic hormone or cerebral salt wasting, must be avoided, as it increases cerebral edema and ICP.

Hyperglycemia has been shown to increase tissue injury in the ischemic brain in animal studies and to worsen outcomes in cases of acute cardiac arrest in humans. Although it has not been demonstrated to influence the functional outcome or survival in patients with ischemic infarction, it seems reasonable to maintain *normoglycemia* in patients with strokes (who have ischemia around the infarcted core) and patients with severe brain injuries (who likely have areas of focal or diffuse ischemia).

Diuretics may also be used to lower ICP acutely. Diuretics lower ICP by increasing serum osmolality and causing water to diffuse out of the brain into the intravascular space. Mannitol lowers the ICP over several minutes, whereas furosemide takes somewhat longer. Osmotic therapy is generally effective up to an osmolarity of 320 mmol/L, but there is a high incidence of renal failure beyond this point.

Mannitol is recommended as a first-line therapy because it works more rapidly than furosemide. Mannitol is administered at a dose of 0.5 to 1 g/kg intravenous push to lower ICP acutely. It is subsequently administered in 25-g intravenous boluses as required, with frequent monitoring of electrolytes and renal function. Since there is no blood flow into the infarcted core in infarction, hyperosmolar therapy is directed at the surrounding edematous brain. It may be of limited benefit, however, in controlling ICP because of increased permeability to small solutes due to the breakdown in the blood-brain barrier.

If an ICP monitor is employed, *opioids, paralytic agents,* and *benzodiazepines* can be used safely for agitation. In the agitated patient, these drugs decrease the ICP as well as undesirable patient movement and dyssynchrony with mechanical ventilation. Because seizures may cause hypoxia and elevate ICP, they can exacerbate the brain injury. Therefore, *anticonvulsants* should be used for prophylaxis of early seizures.

Intentional mild hypothermia to 34° C decreases the brain's metabolic demand and protects parts of the brain with marginal blood flow while lowering ICP. Temperatures below this point can cause cardiac dysfunction and coagulopathy. A randomized clinical trial is in progress to assess the effect of moderate hypothermia on outcome in patients with head injury.

Finally, *barbiturates* may be used to treat intractable ICP elevations when other methods have failed. Although the complete mechanism of the effect of barbiturates on ICP is unclear, it is known that they decrease the brain's metabolic demand. Because patients in barbiturate coma have no neurologic examination to follow, an ICP monitor must be employed. An electroencephalogram is used to titrate the dose to achieve burst-suppression at 1:3 (see Chapter 70). Initially, 1 g of pentobarbital is administered intravenously at a rate that avoids hypotension. Additional 100-mg intravenous boluses are used to achieve burst-suppression. A continuous intravenous infusion or intermittent boluses should be administered to maintain the burst-suppression state.

Because barbiturates depress cardiac contractility, an arterial catheter should be inserted, and a central venous catheter or Swan-Ganz catheter should be placed to monitor intravascular volume status. Patients with known cardiac ischemia or dysfunction are poor candidates for barbiturates. During barbiturate therapy, CPP should be maintained at greater than 60 to 70 mm Hg, with pressors if necessary, particularly during the initiation of therapy. Since the half-life of most barbiturates is long, it may take several days to reverse their effects. Serum levels may be monitored when therapy is withdrawn. Propofol and etomidate are also effective in achieving burst-suppression. Because of short half-lives, their pharmacologic effects are short-lived. Clinical experience in the management of ICP with propofol and etomidate, however, is limited.

BIBLIOGRAPHY

Batjer HH, Reisch JS, Allen BC, et al: Failure of surgery to improve outcome in hypertensive putaminal hemorrhage. A prospective randomized trial. Arch Neurol 47:1103–1106, 1990.
This randomized trial of surgery versus medical management for hypertensive basal ganglion hemorrhages demonstrated that surgery failed to improve outcome in these patients.

Changaris DG, McGraw CP, Richardson JD, et al: Correlation of cerebral perfusion pressure and Glasgow Coma Scale to outcome. J Trauma 27:1007–1013, 1987.
This study demonstrated that cerebral perfusion pressure >60 mm Hg and higher Glasgow Coma Scale scores are associated with improved neurologic outcome following severe head injury.

Delashaw JB, Broaddus WC, Kassell NF, et al: Treatment of right hemispheric cerebral infarction by hemicraniectomy. Stroke 21:874–881, 1990.
This small anecdotal series suggested that decompressive craniectomy may be a lifesaving procedure in certain patients following large right hemispheric infarction.

Eisenberg HM, Frankowski RF, Contant CF, et al: High dose barbiturate control of elevated intracranial pressure in patients with severe head injury. J Neurosurg 69:15–23, 1988.
This randomized clinical trial demonstrated that high-dose barbiturate therapy is useful in aborting otherwise medically refractory elevations in ICP following severe head injury.

Feldman Z, Kanter MJ, Robertson CS, et al: Effect of head elevation on intracranial pressure, cerebral perfusion pressure, and cerebral blood flow in head-injured patients. J Neurosurg 76:207–211, 1992.
This clinical study demonstrated that head elevation in patients with traumatic brain injury is effective in lowering the ICP without reducing the CPP or cerebral blood flow.

Hornig CR, Rust DS, Busse O, et al: Space-occupying cerebellar infarction. Clinical course and prognosis. Stroke 25:372–374, 1994.
This anecdotal series demonstrated that surgical evacuation of cerebellar infarctions and hemorrhages may be lifesaving.

Hurst RW, Raps EC, Zager E, et al: Selective intra-arterial thrombolysis in acute stroke: Implications for emergency management. J Stroke Cerebrovasc Dis 4:30–35, 1994.
This anecdotal series demonstrated that acute intra-arterial thrombolysis for bland cerebral infarction may reverse stroke symptoms.

Marler JR, Brott T, Broderick J, et al: Tissue-plasminogen activator for acute ischemic stroke. N Engl J Med 333:1588–1593, 1995.
This randomized controlled study demonstrated that intravenous thrombolysis with t-PA for acute nonhemorrhagic cerebral infarction improved clinical outcome at 3 months.

Matchar DB, Divine GW, Heyman A, Feussner JR: The influence of hyperglycemia on outcome of cerebral infarction. Ann Intern Med 117:449–456, 1992.
This prospective cohort study failed to demonstrate an association of admission serum glucose level and neurologic outcome following cerebral infarction.

Shackford SR, Zhuang J, Schmoker J: Intravenous fluid tonicity: Effect on intracranial pressure, cerebral blood flow, and cerebral oxygen delivery in focal brain injury. J Neurosurg 76:91–98, 1992.
This laboratory investigation of a focal porcine brain injury demonstrated that the administration of hypertonic fluids improves cerebral compliance and increases cerebral blood flow compared with the infusion of hypotonic fluid.

Shiozaki T, Sugimoto H, Taneda M, et al: Effect of mild hypothermia on uncontrollable intracranial hypertension after severe head injury. J Neurosurg 79:363–368, 1993.
This randomized controlled study demonstrated that mild hypothermia significantly reduced the ICP and increased the CPP in patients with severe head injury.

Temkin NR, Dikmen SS, Wilenski AJ, et al: A randomized, double-blind study of phenytoin for the prevention of post-traumatic seizures. N Engl J Med 323:540–542, 1990.
This randomized double-blind study demonstrated that phenytoin is effective in preventing early post-traumatic seizures, but is not effective in preventing late seizures.

43

Skin Rashes and Pressure Ulcers

Christen M. Mowad
David J. Margolis

Multiple dermatologic illnesses or complications occur in the intensive care unit (ICU) setting. The focus of this chapter is to describe a variety of benign and serious skin problems, including pressure ulcers, that are relevant to ICU patients.

COMMON BENIGN SKIN RASHES

Candidal Infections

Candidiasis is caused by *Candida albicans* and occasionally by other candidal species. *C. albicans* is a yeast that can often be found in the gut, oral mucosa, vagina, and occasionally on the skin. Commonly it results in infection of mucous membranes and skin and, less commonly, in disseminated systemic infection.

Although *C. albicans* is not considered to be a permanent resident of the normal skin flora, colonization—that is, positive cultures—frequently occurs in areas in close proximity to the gastrointestinal tract where it is a colonizer and in intertriginous areas where moisture and maceration encourage its proliferation. Candidal intertrigo occurs commonly and can involve any skin fold, especially when an individual is overweight.

When mucous membranes are involved, creamy, well-demarcated curd-like debris on an erythematous base is typically seen on the tongue, buccal mucosa, gums, and palate. In severe cases, it can extend to the esophagus and pharynx. Intertriginous sites develop erythematous, macerated plaques with satellite papules and pustules that extend beyond the body fold. The skin lesions are pruritic or painful.

Oral candidiasis is treated with anticandidal troches (Mycelex) and intertriginous disease with topical creams (ketoconazole, econazole) twice daily, soaks (25% acetic acid or saline compresses), and keeping the area dry.

Contact Dermatitis

Contact dermatitis occurs from the interaction of a chemical on the skin. There are two major forms: irritant and allergic. Irritant contact dermatitis accounts for 80% of cases and results in damage to the skin via a toxic effect. Common irritants in the ICU are soaps, and those caused by stool and urinary incontinence. Allergic contact dermatitis, a type 4 cell-mediated delayed hypersensitivity immune response (see Chapter 29), accounts for the other 20% of cases. It is agent (antigen)-specific and the reaction requires prior sensitization. In the ICU, patients may

499

become sensitized to a variety of topical preparations, such as iodine, topical antimicrobials, or the adhesives used in tape.

Generally, contact dermatitis appears as a well-demarcated, erythematous, pruritic, eczematous patch in a geometric pattern corresponding to where the agent was applied to the skin. Detection of the causative allergen can be determined by patch testing. Treatment is avoidance of the causative allergen or irritant and midstrength topical steroids, such as triamcinolone ointment 0.1%, for mild cases and more potent topical steroids, such as clobetasol propionate ointment 0.05% or betamethasone dipropionate 0.05%, for severe reactions. Topical treatment is twice daily for 10 to 14 days. Rarely, systemic steroids are required for extensive severe contact allergy.

Herpes Simplex Virus Skin Infections

Herpes simplex virus (HSV) is a common acquired infection caused by HSV type 1 or 2. Clinically, it appears as recurrent grouped vesicles on an erythematous base especially in the perioral or genital areas, which may be accompanied by enlarged lymph nodes. The infection is acquired and often recurs after trauma, illness, or stress. Patients describe burning, itching, or stinging before or coincident with each attack. Diagnosis is by Tzanck smear, which reveals multinucleated giant cells, or by culture.

Treatment is symptomatic with compresses. Oral acyclovir, 200 mg five times daily for 7 to 10 days, may decrease viral shedding, pain and crusting, and duration of disease if initiated early in the course of illness. Newer antiviral agents, such as famciclovir and valaciclovir, may also be used.

Herpes Zoster

Herpes zoster, also known as shingles, is a vesicular eruption that occurs in a dermatomal distribution and is due to varicella zoster virus (VZV). Clinically, vesicles are seen on an erythematous base, distributed unilaterally in a dermatome, most commonly on the trunk (see Appendix F for sensory dermatomes). Occasionally the lesions become hemorrhagic. Burning, stinging, itching, or pain often precedes the lesions. Up to 20 to 50 lesions can be found outside the dermatome, and adjacent lymph nodes can be enlarged and tender.

Treatment is symptomatic in immunocompetent patients. Oral acyclovir, 800 mg five times daily for 7 to 10 days, can be used in an attempt to decrease viral shedding, pain, and duration of the disease course. Therapy should be instituted within 48 hours of the onset of the rash. Intravenous therapy is occasionally necessary for the immunocompromised patient. The newer antiviral agents, for example, famciclovir, can be used as well. Some suggest the adding of prednisone. Patients can experience postherpetic neuralgia in the affected dermatone. This can be treated with topical capsaicin 0.025% or topical or intralesional steroids. Occasionally, nerve blocks or amitriptyline are needed for severe pain.

Miliaria

Miliaria results from obstruction of eccrine sweat ducts at various levels of the epidermis and dermis; as a result, sweat is retained in the skin. Clinically, lesions appear as pruritic, discrete, inflammatory papules and occur after repeated episodes of sweating, usually on the patient's hot, moist, occluded back. Miliaria is fairly common in ICU patients confined to bed with fevers.

The cause of the obstruction is not clear. The condition resolves within days and treatment is symptomatic, keeping the area dry and unoccluded. Topical antibiotics, such as erythromycin or clindamycin, are also used, given the possible role of microorganisms.

Seborrheic Dermatitis

Seborrheic dermatitis is a common, benign papulosquamous disease. It affects sebaceous-rich areas such as the scalp, eyebrows, nasolabial folds, and central chest. Clinically, it appears as erythematous macules and plaques with associated scale that can be pruritic.

The cause is unclear, but *Pityrosporum ovale,* a yeast found on normal skin and increased in seborrheic dermatitis, has been implicated. Seborrheic dermatitis flares in ill individuals and is associated with neurologic conditions such as Parkinson's disease. Patients with acquired immunodeficiency syndrome not only have a higher incidence of the disease but also have manifestations that are more extensive, severe, and resistant to therapy. The disease is chronic with a waxing and waning course. Treatment is with topical antifungal agents, such as ketoconazole cream twice daily, low-potency steroids, (hydrocortisone ointment 1 or 2.5%) as needed, and medicated shampoos.

DRUG REACTIONS

Cutaneous reactions to drugs present in many different patterns, including relatively benign morbilliform eruptions as well as more serious forms such as erythema multiforme minor and major, toxic epidermal necrolysis, and vasculitis.

Morbilliform Drug Rash

The most common drug reaction seen is a morbilliform eruption, particularly in hospitalized patients on numerous drugs. It is an erythematous maculopapular eruption that proceeds in a cephalocaudal progression. In patients confined to bed, however, the eruption can begin in dependent areas. Mucosal surfaces should be examined for evidence of a more serious drug reaction.

The patient's medications should be scrutinized and the suspected agent discontinued. Because it is difficult to identify the inciting agent accurately, any nonessential drugs should be discontinued. Daily cutaneous examinations should be performed to watch for progression. Drugs, such as penicillin, phenytoin, and those containing "sulfa" (sulfonamide-like chemical structures), are common causes of drug eruptions.

After a suspected drug is discontinued, the rash can persist for up to 2 weeks and can even worsen for a few days. Symptomatic treatment of pruritus with topical midstrength steroids (triamcinalone ointment 0.1%) and lubricants (petroleum jelly, Absorbase) are helpful as many patients experience mild superficial exfoliation as the rash resolves.

Erythema Multiforme

Erythema multiforme (EM) is a serious drug reaction characterized by targetoid lesions; however, the eruption can occur as macules, papules, vesicles, or bullae. The targetoid lesion is described as a "bull's eye," with peripheral erythema and a central bulla or dusky necrotic center. It can be classified as minor or major. EM minor is usually an acute self-limited syndrome without mucosal involvement. In EM major, there is significant mucosal involvement, in which case it is known as Stevens-Johnson syndrome.

Reported causative factors include infections, drugs, and neoplasms. The most common causes, however, are drugs (sulfa, penicillin, and phenytoin) and infections, such as herpes simplex or *Mycoplasma*. Occasionally, EM is recurrent and, when this clinical pattern occurs, herpes simplex is often the cause.

Therapy for both forms is supportive, with wound care to prevent infection. Pruritus can be treated with topical steroids or antihistamines. In EM major, painful eroded mucosal surfaces need attentive wound care and can be treated symptomatically with oral preparations such as lidocaine. Removal of suspected drugs or treatment of associated infections or neoplasms is also necessary. EM minor heals without sequelae, except hyper- or hypopigmentation often occurs. Conversely, in EM major with mucosal involvement involving the eyes, esophagus, trachea, and urethra, serious scarring can sometimes occur, leading to blindness and strictures. Ophthalmic consultation is advised. Other organ systems can also be involved, such as the hepatic, pulmonary, and renal systems, resulting in significant morbidity and mortality. The use and effectiveness of systemic corticosteroids remains controversial.

Toxic Epidermal Necrolysis

Toxic epidermal necrolysis results in extensive epidermal loss and is believed to be a drug hypersensitivity reaction. Sulfonamides, penicillin, and anticonvulsants have most frequently been associated with toxic epidermal necrolysis.

Clinically, patients experience burning and painful skin that is erythematous and edematous, occasionally with target lesions. The skin is fragile with flaccid blisters that extend with pressure, known as the Nikolsky's sign, resulting in extensive detachment of the epidermis. Frozen section of the skin provides rapid confirmation of the suspected clinical diagnosis and reveals full-thickness necrosis of the epidermis.

Mucosal involvement is also present in the majority of patients. Ophthalmic consultation should evaluate ocular lesions to prevent scarring and blindness.

Dysphagia and painful micturation are other complications. Treatment should ensure adequate nutrition and prevention of strictures. Visceral involvement can be seen in the gastrointestinal tract, upper respiratory tract, kidneys, or hematologic system.

Mortality is high, often due to secondary infection and sepsis. Transfer to a specialized burn unit for treatment should be considered, with special attention to fluid replacement, nutrition, infection, meticulous wound care, and removal of suspected causative agents. The use of corticosteroids is controversial, with proponents arguing they help treat the hypersensitivity reaction and opponents arguing they increase the risk of sepsis, delay re-epithelialization, and enhance protein catabolism. The skin generally re-epithelializes in several weeks with hyper- and hypopigmented areas; however, there can be high morbidity with mucosal scarring and blindness.

Vasculitis

Cutaneous vasculitis is associated with numerous causes, and drugs are one of many. Vasculitis secondary to drugs most often appears as palpable purpura on the lower extremities. Diagnosis is confirmed by skin biopsy. Other organ systems such as the kidney, liver, or brain can be involved. Appropriate testing should be conducted to evaluate these systems. Several drugs have been reported to cause vasculitis and, although the exact mechanism is unknown, drug-induced vasculitis is felt to be an immune mechanism. Discontinuation of the drug generally results in resolution of the clinical findings.

LIFE-THREATENING DISORDERS AFFECTING THE SKIN

Purpura Fulminans

Purpura fulminans is an uncommon but severe condition that results in hemorrhagic infarction and necrosis of large areas of the skin. The cause is unknown, but it is associated with infections and is related to major disturbances in clotting. The organisms involved are bacteria such as group A streptococci, meningococci, staphylococci, or pneumococci and occasionally viruses such as varicella. Other associated conditions include obstetric complications, neoplasms, and major tissue damage. Disseminated intravascular coagulation and depletion of coagulation factors are common associated findings.

Patients acquire large, well-demarcated ecchymoses, with hemorrhagic bullae located symmetrically on the extremities and pressure areas. A rim of erythema can be seen surrounding these areas. Minor or insidious courses of purpura fulminans reveal petechiae, purpura, acral cyanosis, and hemorrhagic bullae. The patient appears extremely ill with high fevers, tachycardia, and sometimes shock. Laboratory studies reveal elevated white blood cell counts and changes indicative of disseminated intravascular coagulation (increased prothrombin time and partial thromboplastin time, decreased fibrinogen, and increased fibrin split products).

Mortality is high. Therapy includes treatment of infection or the underlying condition and sometimes replacement of clotting factors or plasma. Treatment with heparin to prevent clotting is occasionally used.

Ecthyma Gangrenosum

Ecthyma gangrenosum is an uncommon cutaneous finding that results from *Pseudomonas* sepsis and often occurs in immunocompromised individuals. Its lesions appear as round, indurated erythematous to purpuric macules or plaques or as cellulitis. A central vesicle or hemorrhagic bulla that ulcerates or forms an eschar can be seen. These lesions are often painless and may be a form of vasculitis. Punch biopsy and culture make the diagnosis.

PRESSURE ULCERS

Pressure ulcers commonly afflict individuals who receive acute or long-term care. It has been estimated that 11% of all hospital admissions and 25% of all nursing home patients have one or more pressure ulcers. A similar percentage—that is, as many as 25% of all ICU patients who are also "at risk"—may acquire pressure ulcers.

Definition

A pressure ulcer is described as a pressure-induced disruption of normal anatomic structure and function of the soft tissues. More generally speaking, ulcers (wounds) of the skin disrupt the epidermis and dermis, resulting in the loss of barrier function. In a pressure ulcer, the anatomic disruption often includes the underlying subcutaneous fat, muscle, tendon, or bone. A pressure ulcer is due to unrelieved pressure resulting in damage of tissue subjected to the pressure. The pressure load is usually a force external to the body that is perpendicular to the skin and parallel to a bony surface. Forces between 32 and 480 mm Hg are believed to be necessary to cause an ulcer. The combination of the external force and a bony surface compresses blood vessels, which, in turn, results in tissue hypoxemia, ischemia, and ultimately necrosis. Although excessive external pressures may commonly be present over bony prominences (e.g., in a seated position the ischial tuberosities commonly develop an external force of 150 to 500 mm Hg), these forces are generated for only short periods. Usually they are relieved by body movement, which allows reperfusion of the pressure-bearing soft tissues. The length of time required for an unrelieved external force to result in significant human tissue ischemia and a clinically relevant ulcer is not known exactly under all circumstances. It has been estimated, however, that moderate force—for example, 60 mm Hg—applied to the skin for only 1 to 2 hours is sufficient. After a pressure insult, a clinically relevant cutaneous wound may take 2 to 7 days to develop.

External forces other than direct pressure may also cause tissue destruction. Both frictional forces (moving the patient while the skin rubs against the sheet) and shearing forces (positioning a patient at a 45-degree angle produces a shear stress on the skin in contact with the sheet, even when there is no movement) have been implicated in the formation of pressure ulcers. Furthermore, the deleterious effects of both of these forces are exacerbated by tissue maceration. Finally, the combination of a shearing and direct pressure force act synergistically to form a pressure ulcer.

Location and Stages

Pressure ulcers usually occur at sites of bony prominence: the iliac crest, sacrum, ischial tuberosities, gluteal folds, trochanters, heels, Achilles' tendons, medial and lateral knees, medial and lateral malleoli, scapulas, elbows, and occiput. Of these, the trochanters and sacrum are involved most commonly. Pressure ulcers are staged according to the National Pressure Ulcer Advisory Panel system (Table 43–1).

Prevention and Treatment

Preventing the occurrence of a pressure ulcer depends on both identifying those individuals at risk and diminishing the effects of external forces on the skin.

At-Risk Patients

Two risk assessment scales are currently in wide use, the Norton and Braden scales. Both are based on an assessment of the patient's activity and mobility. The Norton scale also assesses physical and mental condition and continence, whereas the Braden scale additionally assesses nutrition, sensory perception, skin moisture, and friction and shear forces to the skin. These parameters are weighted and tabulated.

Individuals with scores indicative of a higher risk for the development of pressure ulcers tend to be less aware of their environment, unable to ambulate, incontinent, and poorly nourished. Population studies of individuals in high-risk environments who have pressure ulcers tend to agree with the dimensions of these assessment tools. For example, in a cross-sectional study of 2803 nursing home residents, those with a pressure ulcer were more likely to have these risk factors: inability to walk (Parkinson's disease or paraplegia), diabetes, frequent inconti-

Table 43–1. Stages of Pressure Ulcers

STAGE	DESCRIPTION
I	Nonblanchable erythema of intact skin
II	Partial-thickness skin loss involving epidermis or dermis, or both
III	Full-thickness skin loss involving, but not including, tissues as deep as the fascia
IV	Full-thickness skin loss involving tissues as deep as muscle, tendon, and bone

From Bergstrom N, Bennett MA, Carlson CE, et al: Treatment of Pressure Ulcers. Clinical Practice Guideline No. 15. Rockville, MD: Agency for Health Care Policy and Research (AHCPR), 1994. (AHCPR Publication No. 95–0652, December, 1994.)

nence, and previous hospital admissions. They were also more likely to be under-weight (malnourished), older (which increases risk by 1% per year), male, and in need of assistance for feeding.

Pressure-Reducing Mattresses and Beds

To prevent a pressure ulcer in a patient at high risk or to treat a pressure ulcer, sources of pressure must be removed or minimized. Patients should be mobilized as soon as clinically feasible, and those who are immobile should be repositioned at least every 2 hours. When moving a patient, however, one should take care not to cause a friction or sheer injury unintentionally.

Appropriate mattress overlays, replacement mattresses, low-air-loss mattresses and air-fluidized beds (see Chapter 10) can be used to relieve pressure to most body sites (Table 43–2). The use of these special interventions should be consistent with the level of need of the patient and how well each functions for a particular patient. If signs of mattress failure occur (e.g., blanchable erythema, stage I pressure ulcer, poor healing of existing pressure ulcers), the next higher level of pressure-reducing mattress or bed should be selected (while being cognizant that each higher level generally costs considerably more than those at lower levels).

Since these pressure-reducing mattresses all relieve pressure on the heels poorly, devices such as pillows and ankle-foot orthotics should be considered. Since most ICU patients are frequently immobile, as a rule all these patients should be considered at risk and receive a pressure-relieving mattress for prevention of pressure ulcers. For those already with pressure ulcers, consultation with the person serving as the local institutional resource is recommended regarding which specialty mattresses and beds are available.

Table 43–2. Performance Characteristics of Support Surfaces to Prevent or Treat Pressure Ulcers

	TYPE OF SUPPORT SURFACE (COMMERCIAL EXAMPLE)					
PERFORMANCE CHARACTERISTICS	Standard Mattress	Foam Overlay Mattress	Low-Air-Loss Bed (Soft-Care)	Alternating Air (SPR+)	Static Flotation (Rik)	Air-Fluidized Bed (Clinitron)
Increased support area	No	Yes	Yes	Yes	Yes	Yes
Low moisture retention	No	No	Yes	No	No	Yes
Reduced heat accumulation	No	No	Yes	No	No	Yes
Shear reduction	No	No	?	Yes	?	Yes
Pressure reduction	No	Yes*	Yes	Yes	Yes	Yes
Dynamic	No	No	Yes	Yes	No	Yes
Cost per day	Low	Low	Low-medium	Low-medium	Medium	High

*Pressure reduction is lost if less than 1 inch of support material between anatomic site and mattress ("bottoming out").

Modified from Bergstrom N, Bennett MA, Carlson CE, et al: Treatment of Pressure Ulcers. Clinical Practice Guideline No. 15. Rockville, MD: Agency for Health Care Policy and Research (AHCPR), 1994.

Skin Care

Good skin care is also important and especially includes preventing problems due to bladder and bowel incontinence. Incontinence can cause skin maceration and irritation of tissue. The skin should be cleansed gently. In order to protect the skin, moisturizer—for example, petroleum jelly—or skin sealant should be applied. If these interventions are not adequate, devices to contain feces and urine should be considered.

Nutrition

Adequate nutrition is also important both to prevent the occurrence of and aid in the healing of a pressure ulcer. All patients at risk for, or with, a pressure ulcer should have a comprehensive nutritional assessment (see Chapter 13). If the patient is judged to be malnourished, one should request nutritional consultation and appropriate nutritional therapy should begin.

Agency for Health Care Policy and Research Guidelines

The treatment of pressure ulcers has been summarized in guidelines (Table 43–3) in the early 1990s by the Agency for Health Care Policy and Research (AHCPR). As mentioned earlier, the use of pressure-relieving mattresses and beds, good skin care, and adequate nutrition are approaches to be used for both the prevention and the treatment of pressure ulcers.

Treatment

Treatment also includes wound débridement, wound cleansing and moist wound care (dressings). *Wound débridement* is essential to remove devitalized and infected tissue and can be surgical, mechanical, enzymatic, or autolytic. In contrast, *wound cleansing* is not débridement but rather involves the gentle removal of foreign material, usually by a liquid (e.g., saline) between wound dressing changes. Wound cleansing should be minimally traumatic to the healing tissues. Several clinical and laboratory studies have demonstrated the superiority of moist *wound care*. This can be achieved by frequent dressing changes using gauze soaked in saline or in one of many commercially available products. The goal of both liquids is to cover the wound and help to establish a moist wound environment. The commercial products have the advantage of needing less frequent dressing changes than saline. If an appropriate treatment plan has been instituted, improvement of a pressure ulcer should occur within 2 to 4 weeks. If it fails to improve, one must carefully re-evaluate the treatment plan. Surgical consultation is indicated as part of the management of severe (stages III and IV) pressure ulcers. Several surgical options—for example, skin grafts or skin flaps—can be considered to achieve ultimate closure of these wounds.

Table 43–3. AHCPR Recommendations for Managing Tissue Loads in Patients with Pressure Ulcers

While in bed:

1. Use a *pressure-reducing surface* for ICU patients with existing ulcers who remain at risk for developing more pressure ulcers. Avoid positioning patients on a pressure ulcer.
2. Use a *static support surface* (see Table 43–2) if a patient can assume a variety of body positions without bearing weight on an existing pressure ulcer and without "bottoming out."
3. Use a *dynamic support surface* (see Table 43–2) if the patient cannot assume multiple positions without bearing weight on an existing pressure ulcer, if the patient bottoms out, or if the pressure ulcer does not show evidence of healing.
4. If a patient has large Stage III or IV pressure ulcers on multiple turning surfaces, a *low-air-loss bed* or an *air-fluidized bed* (see Table 43–2) may be indicated. No studies have compared the effectiveness of these two types of beds, but clinicians generally prefer a low-air-loss bed for these individuals for a variety of practical reasons.

While sitting:

1. Position the sitting patient (without a pressure ulcer on a sitting surface) so that the points under pressure are shifted at least every hour. Patients who are able should be taught to shift their weight every 15 minutes.
2. A patient who has a pressure ulcer on a sitting surface should avoid sitting unless the pressure on the ulcer can be *totally* relieved.
3. Avoid using a *ring-cushion* ("donut") for sitting since it is more likely to *cause* pressure ulcers than *prevent* them in at-risk patients.

From Bergstrom N, Bennett MA, Carlson CE, et al: Treatment of Pressure Ulcers. Clinical Practice Guideline No. 15. Rockville, MD: Agency for Health Care Policy and Research (AHCPR), 1994.

BIBLIOGRAPHY

Bergstrom N, Allman RM, Carlson CE, et al: Pressure Ulcers in Adults: Prediction and Prevention. Rockville, MD: Agency for Health Care Policy and Research, 1992, pp 1–63.

Bergstrom N, Bennet MA, Carlson CE, et al: Pressure Ulcer Treatment. Rockville, MD: U.S. Department of Health and Human Services, Public Health Service, Agency for Health Care Policy and Research, 1994, pp 1–54.
  The preceding two references are the Agency for Health Care Policy and Research–sponsored guidelines based on a comprehensive review of the literature and consensus process by expert clinicians.

Dinsdale SM: Decubitus ulcers: Role of pressure and friction in causation. Arch Phys Med Rehabil 55:147–152, 1974.
  This early study explored factors involved in experimental pressure ulcers.

Greene S, Su D, Miller S: Ecthyma gangrenosum: Report of clinical, histopathologic, and bacteriologic aspects of eight cases. JAAD 1984; 11:781–787.
  Eight cases of ecthyma gangrenosum are reported, with a review of histopathologic features, clinical presentation, bacteriologic features, and systematic approach to diagnosis and therapy.

Inman KJ, Sibbald WJ, Rutledge FS, Clark BJ: Clinical utility and cost effectiveness of an air suspension bed in the prevention of pressure ulcers. JAMA 269:1139–1143, 1993.
  This study nicely demonstrates the effectiveness of pressure relief for pressure ulcer prevention in high-risk ICU patients.

Kosiak M: Etiology and pathology of ischemic ulcers. Arch Phys Med Rehabil 40:62–69, 1959.
  This was a landmark study on the cause of pressure ulcers.

Margolis DJ: Management of unusual causes of ulcers of the lower extremity. J Wound Ostomy Continence Nurs 22:89–94, 1995.
  Unusual causes of leg ulcers, including ecthyma gangrenosum and purpura fulminans, are briefly reviewed.

Marks JG, DeLeo VA: Contact and Occupational Dermatology. St. Louis: CV Mosby, 1992.
This book provides complete coverage of irritant and allergic contact dermatitis, including the pathophysiology and common allergens associated with both.

Roujeau JC, Stern RS: Severe cutaneous reactions to drugs. N Engl J Med 331:1272–1285, 1994.
This is an extensive discussion of numerous adverse reactions to drugs covering differential diagnosis as well as treatment.

Spector WD: Correlates of pressure sores in nursing homes: Evidence from the National Medical Expenditure survey. J Invest Dermatol 102:42s–45s, 1994.
This article provides a case-controlled analysis of risk factors for patients who acquired pressure ulcers in subacute and chronic care facilities.

Spicer TE, Rau JM: Purpura fulminans. Am J Med 26:566–571, 1976.
This is a brief review of the clinical course and causes of this relatively uncommon syndrome.

Versluysen M: How elderly patients with femoral fracture develop pressure sores in hospital. Br Med J 292:1311–1313, 1986.
This article presents a prospective analysis of the incidence of pressure ulcers in a high-risk population.

44 Sleep Disturbances in the Intensive Care Unit

Neil Freedman
Richard J. Schwab

Adequate quantity and quality of sleep are essential for health maintenance, but achieving either is universally difficult for patients in the intensive care unit (ICU). As a consequence, these patients commonly suffer from sleep deprivation and associated sleep disturbances. The latter can be some of the most challenging clinical problems in the ICU. In response, critical care clinicians must be aware of the causes of sleep deprivation and fragmentation, their adverse effects, and both pharmacologic and nonpharmacologic methods to improve sleep in patients in the ICU.

NORMAL SLEEP

Sleep is a complex process characterized by a variety of physiologic, behavioral, and electroencephalographic changes. It has two distinct major states: (1) nonrapid eye movement sleep (NREM) and (2) rapid eye movement sleep (REM). The initiation of sleep occurs through NREM sleep. This is subdivided into four stages that together normally make up about 75% of a person's sleep per night. Each subsequent (higher number) stage of NREM sleep represents a deeper sleep state so that arousal thresholds are lowest in stage 1 and highest in stage 4 (delta sleep). Although variability exists, normal adults pass through stages 1 through 3 and enter stage 4 about 35 minutes after the onset of sleep.

Dreaming occurs primarily during REM sleep. This stage of sleep is characterized by increased central nervous system metabolic activity, skeletal muscle atonia, episodic rapid eye movements, and an electroencephalographic pattern (low-amplitude fast waves) similar to wakefulness. Periods of REM and NREM sleep normally alternate throughout a person's night of sleep. REM sleep cycles occur every 90 to 110 minutes and typically last 10 to 30 minutes. The duration of REM sleep cycles increases as one progresses through one's normal period of sleep. During a normal 8-hour period of sleeping, REM sleep usually occurs in four to six separate episodes that make up about 25% of one's total sleep.

The physiologic function of sleep remains unknown. However, evidence suggests that it may be needed for normal growth and repair of body tissues. For example, in most tissues, peak rates of protein synthesis and cell division coincide with sleep. Hormones that inhibit protein synthesis, such as cortisol and catecholamines, remain low during most of the night (when there is a normal circadian variation). Sleep is the normal stimulus for the release of the majority of growth hormone. In contrast, degradative metabolism is greater during wakefulness, and prolonged sleeplessness promotes a catabolic state. Animal studies have shown that 2 to 3 weeks of total sleep deprivation ultimately leads to death. In summary, it is suspected, but not proved, that sleep deprivation impairs healing and recovery.

POLYSOMNOGRAPHIC STUDIES OF SLEEP IN THE INTENSIVE CARE UNIT

Polysomnography (which includes electoencephalography and respiration-related monitoring) is the best validated method to determine sleep patterns in patients in the ICU. Polysomnographic studies of patients in medical and surgical ICUs have demonstrated severe sleep deprivation (decreased total duration of sleep per 24 hours) and profound sleep fragmentation (loss of normal sleep "architecture," which is the normal sequence and cycles of sleep stages) (Table 44–1). These changes have been demonstrated in a wide range of patients in ICU settings, for example, after myocardial infarction, general surgery, or open heart surgery. Repeated arousals (awakenings or changes in sleep states to very light sleep) have been found to occur on average of every 20 minutes. They disrupt the normal continuity of sleep stages and prevent attainment of the deepest stages of sleep (delta sleep and REM sleep). Clearly, most patients in the ICU are at high risk for being sleep-deprived. In addition, the normal circadian variation in which most sleep occurs during the nighttime hours is disrupted. For example, only 50 to 60% of sleep in patients in the ICU occurs during nighttime hours. In order to compensate for sleep deprivation at night, they often sleep during the day.

Although polysomnography is the gold standard for determining sleep in the ICU, it may be difficult to perform in an ICU setting. Furthermore, REM sleep and wakefulness may be difficult to distinguish with polysomnography alone in paralyzed patients.

CONSEQUENCES OF SLEEP DEPRIVATION

Why should ICU clinicians be concerned about sleep deprivation? Although much remains to be discovered about the function of sleep, as mentioned previously it is likely necessary for normal growth and body repair. Furthermore, there are important adverse physiologic effects of sleep deprivation. For example, its effects on the respiratory system may contribute to hypoventilation, respiratory muscle weakness, and prolongation of mechanical ventilation (Table 44–2).

The effects of sleep deprivation on host defenses and the immune system appear contradictory. Earlier studies suggested that it induced slight decreases in cell-mediated immunity and leukocyte phagocytic activity. Sleep loss was also associated with increased levels of interferon and suppressed antibody responses. However, more recent studies demonstrate significant increases in white blood cell

Table 44–1. Types of Sleep Disturbances Common in the Intensive Care Unit

Prolonged time (latencies) to sleep onset
Frequent arousals, resulting in sleep fragmentation and increased wakefulness
Increased stage 1 sleep (lightest level of sleep)
Decreased time in stage 4 sleep (deep sleep)
Decreased time in REM sleep

REM, rapid eye movement.

Table 44–2. Adverse Effects of Sleep Deprivation on the Respiratory System

Decreased forced vital capacity
Decreased maximal voluntary ventilation
Decreased ventilatory response to hypercapnia
Decreased ventilatory response to hypoxia
Decreased inspiratory muscle endurance
Increased upper airway collapsibility (predisposing to obstructive sleep apnea)

counts as well as granulocyte, monocyte, and natural killer cell activity at the peak of sleep deprivation. The leukocytosis and increased natural killer cell activity returned to normal after 2 nights of recovery sleep. These results suggest that sleep deprivation may suppress some elements of the host defenses while stimulating others.

Sleep deprivation may be a major cause of the *ICU syndrome*. This is defined as a reversible confusional state attributable to hospitalization in the ICU (Table 44–3). It resembles the syndrome of nocturnal delirium (sundowning). Experimental sleep deprivation in normal individuals reproduces the same set of mental status changes as seen in the ICU syndrome. These signs and symptoms of psychosis resolve if the sleep-deprived but otherwise normal individuals are allowed 1 night of normal sleep. Likewise, as a rule, the symptoms of the ICU syndrome resolve several days after patients are transferred out of the ICU. The ICU syndrome potentially hinders clinical recovery and may increase the length of stay in the ICU. Treatment of the ICU syndrome should start by focusing on its prevention and then using nonpharmacologic means (see Table 44–3). For example, since delirium is twice as common in ICUs without windows, day-night light orientation in the patient's room can be both an important preventive and a therapeutic maneuver.

Table 44–3. The Intensive Care Unit Syndrome

Definition:
   Reversible acute confusional state occurring in ICU patients with no other
     identifiable cause
Time course:
   Onset is usually on the third to seventh day after an ICU admission
   Usually resolves within 48 h after ICU discharge
Clinical manifestations:
   Emotional states: anxiety, depression, fear
   Mental status changes: delirium, disorientation, hallucinations
Treatment:
   Nonpharmacologic:
     Decrease sensory stimulation to encourage sleep
     Orient to day-night, place and time
     Increase communication with patient
   Pharmacologic:
     Benzodiazepines for anxiety (but may exacerbate confusion)
     Haloperidol for delirium (agitated confusion) (see Chapter 4)

CAUSES OF SLEEP DEPRIVATION

Sleep disturbances in patients in the ICU are caused by a variety of conditions. Patient- and disease-related, ICU personnel– and medical care–related, and environmental factors may act independently or additively (Table 44–4).

Patient-Related and Disease-Related Factors

Commonly used medications contribute to sleep disturbances. For example, opioids and barbiturates suppress REM sleep, whereas benzodiazepines suppress stage 3 and stage 4 sleep. Withdrawal from these medications can also cause rebound insomnia as well as other symptoms of withdrawal. Neuroleptics, for example, haloperidol, reduce slow wave (stage 4) sleep at therapeutic doses. Cimetidine increases slow wave sleep in healthy individuals, but it can lead to daytime drowsiness in patients with impaired renal and hepatic function. Lipophilic beta-receptor antagonists, such as propranolol, metoprolol, and pindolol, have been associated with difficulty falling asleep, which is measured by increased sleep latencies (how long it takes a person to fall asleep) and increased awakenings after falling asleep. Little is known about the effects on sleep of angiotensin-converting enzyme inhibitors, calcium channel blockers, or intravenous vasopressors as well as a host of other drugs commonly used in the ICU.

Pain and fever may cause frequent arousals from sleep. Fear, anxiety, and

---

Table 44–4. Selected Causes of Sleep Deprivation in the Intensive Care Unit

Patient- and disease-related factors
  Underlying disease (infections)
  Medications
    Drugs that suppress REM sleep (opioids, barbiturates, tricyclic antidepressants)
    Drugs that suppress NREM stages 3 and 4 sleep (benzodiazepines, haloperidol)
    Medication withdrawal (rebound insomnia)
  Other disease-related factors (pain, fever, pruritus)
  Psychologic stress (due to being restrained, pharmacologic paralysis, fear, anxiety)
Intensive care unit personnel– and medical care–related factors
  Diagnostic testing and invasive procedures (chest radiographs, phlebotomy, vascular or urinary catheter insertion)
  Nursing interventions (obtaining vital signs, administrating medications, repositioning patient's body)
Environmental factors
  Continuous high-intensity lighting
  High noise levels (for example, 75 dB is as loud as a cafeteria at noon)
    Mechanical devices including ventilators and alarms (45–76 dB)
    Background noise
      Nursing or respiratory care (55–83 dB)
      Nebulizer (50–80 dB)
      Beepers (70–84 dB)
      Intercom (60–83 dB)
      Conversations between hospital staff (60–74 dB)

REM, rapid eye movement; NREM, non–rapid eye movement.

psychologic stress all contribute to sleep disruption. The loss of a patient's independence, from a variety of causes, including pharmacologic paralysis and restraints, may exacerbate the patient's inability to achieve quality sleep.

As noted earlier, sleep deprivation influences host defenses, while the presence of infectious disease may affect a patient's sleep architecture. For example, animal studies demonstrate that infections increased NREM sleep and decreased REM sleep. Similarly, bacterial wall products and proinflammatory cytokines alter sleep patterns in experimental animals.

The underlying acute or chronic disease may adversely affect sleep quality and architecture. For example, patients with class III and class IV stable congestive heart failure have decreased total sleep time and slow wave sleep, a greater proportion of stage 1 sleep, and a high number of sleep stage changes and arousals. Cheyne-Stokes respiration (periodic breathing characterized by sine wave–type cycles of rapid breaths that alternate with slow breathing and apneas) in patients with congestive heart failure predominantly occurs during sleep stages 1 and 2. It may be associated with severe oxygen desaturation. Individuals with chronic obstructive pulmonary disease (COPD) exhibit similar alterations in sleep architecture. They have poor sleep quality at baseline, with maximal oxygen desaturation occurring predominantly in REM sleep. The correlation between severity of acute illness and sleep disturbances has not been studied, but sleep fragmentation likely increases as disease severity worsens.

Factors Relating to Intensive Care Unit Personnel and Medical Care

ICU physicians and nurses disrupt sleep patterns. Each invasive procedure, diagnostic test, or nursing intervention can cause arousals from sleep. For example, one study found that after cardiotomy, patients were interrupted from sleep an average of 59.5 times on their first postoperative night. Their longest uninterrupted period of sleep was only 43 minutes on postoperative day 1. These parameters improved on subsequent hospital days. Thus, as preventive therapy, all procedures and interventions should be minimized while the patient is sleeping and especially between 11:00 PM and 7:00 AM unless they are clearly essential.

Environmental Factors

Environmental stimuli are likely to be the most disruptive factors in achieving high-quality sleep in the ICU. Constant environmental light alters normal circadian patterns of light and darkness. If this disturbs a patient's normal circadian rhythm, the patient's ability to follow weaning programs during the day may be compromised. Light levels in ICU settings often reflect a pattern of 24 hours of daylight instead of a day-night pattern.

Although light is important, the environmental stimulus most likely to disturb sleep in the ICU is *noise*. The Environmental Protection Agency recommends that hospital noise levels not exceed 45 decibels (dB) during the day and 35 dB at night. However, noise levels in ICUs often exceed these recommended limits. For example, the mean noise level over a 24-hour period made in the center of one ICU was 58 dB, with a range from 50 to 76 dB. Even worse was the mean noise level of 66 dB at the head of a typical ICU bed. Peak ICU sounds can exceed 82 dB.

Although noise levels were greatest between 12 noon and 6 PM, they were not significantly reduced during the nighttime hours.

Noise levels of less than 35 to 40 dB are generally required for a patient to fall asleep, whereas bursts of loud noise may arouse patients from sleep. Two polysomnographic studies specifically demonstrated that ICU noise significantly decreased total sleep time and total REM sleep time while increasing REM latency and the number of arousals per 24 hours.

Table 44–4 describes various causes for noise in the ICU and the range of decibel levels corresponding to these sounds. No studies relate mechanical ventilation directly to sleep disruption. However, decibel levels for ventilators and their alarms have ranged from 60 to 76 dB. These loud noise levels likely cause severe sleep fragmentation and poor sleep quality.

Other common sources of noise in the ICU include ambient noise (telephones, beepers, radios, televisions) and staff communication. The latter may be one of the most disturbing noises in the ICU because sounds with meaning may be more disruptive to sleep than meaningless mechanical sounds. Clearly, prevention of sleep disturbances begins with noise control. This must be attempted in every ICU, especially during the nighttime hours when sleep should be encouraged.

TREATMENT OF SLEEP DISTURBANCES

Many interventions have been proposed to improve sleep in the ICU. However, few data demonstrate a relationship between these specific interventions and sleep improvement. Despite lack of outcomes data, certain "common sense" recommendations can be made (Table 44–5).

Environmental Modifications

Single-patient ICU rooms should be provided and conversation minimized in close proximity to these rooms especially at night. Locating monitor and ventilator

Table 44–5. Treatment of Sleep Disturbances in the Intensive Care Unit

Nonpharmacologic
    Reduce environmental noise
    Maintain or reestablish normal light-dark cycles and circadian rhythm (sleeping during night, being awake during day)
    Decrease interruptions while patient is asleep
    Obtain a thorough sleep history to better define patient's baseline sleep patterns
    Expose patient to white noise or ocean sounds
Pharmacologic (see Table 44–6)
    Consider using zolpidem, short-acting benzodiazepines, or other hypnotics
    Avoid diphenhydramine for sedation or for sleep

alarms outside the patient's room can alert the staff to potential medical problems while reducing sleep disruptions. Noisy bedside devices, especially those with alarms, such as intravenous infusion pumps or nebulizers, should not be placed near the head of the bed. Periodic measurements of ICU noise levels should be made as a quality control measure.

Promotion of Normal Light-Dark Cycles and Circadian Rhythm

Normal light-dark cycles and circadian rhythms may be achieved by designing each ICU patient room with a window (to maximize natural lighting) and having a lighting system for each patient's room with dimmers so that lighting can be reduced during the night. One should decrease patient interruptions by planning procedures and interventions (including baths and bed changes) to maximize uninterrupted sleep time. Obtaining "routine" vital signs that waken stable sleeping patients throughout the night or obtaining routine chest radiographs and performing phlebotomy between 5:00 AM and 6:30 AM should be discouraged. Similarly, oral medications should be administered during sleep only when absolutely necessary.

Pharmacologic Treatment of Sleep Disturbances in the Intensive Care Unit

Nonpharmacologic interventions are difficult to implement in the ICU, and patients often require a hypnotic in order to sleep (Table 44–6). Hypnotics are drugs that are used primarily to promote sleep. Although they often shorten sleep onset or reduce nocturnal wakefulness, the ideal hypnotic does not yet exist. An ideal hypnotic would have (1) a short half-life so that its sedating effects would not last beyond the normal sleep period, (2) few drug interactions, (3) minimal effects on the cardiovascular or respiratory system, (4) no influence on normal sleep architecture, (5) absence of tolerance to its continued administration, and (6) no rebound insomnia on its cessation.

Chloral hydrate is a rapidly acting hypnotic that seldom causes excitement or hangover. However, high doses cause both central nervous system and respiratory depression, and patients often become tolerant to it after several continuous nights of use. Furthermore, hepatic and renal clearance of chloral hydrate mandates avoiding its use in patients with renal or hepatic dysfunction.

Diphenhydramine (Benadryl) should not be used as a hypnotic, especially in the elderly, because of its long half-life and prominent anticholinergic side effects. The latter may predispose patients to development of the ICU syndrome.

Benzodiazepines are probably the hypnotic most commonly administered to patients for sleep. They also induce amnesia, anxiolysis, sedation, and muscle relaxation. Temazepam (Restoril), triazolam (Halcion), midazolam (Versed), and lorazepam (Ativan) are some of the most frequently used benzodiazepines to promote sleep in the ICU. Unfortunately, all benzodiazepines have deleterious effects on sleep architecture and the control of respiration. Although they have little effect on REM sleep, benzodiazepines suppress stages 3 and 4 NREM sleep while increasing stage 2. Furthermore, even effects of short-acting benzodiazepines may linger into the next day or night. Benzodiazepines at recommended doses

Table 44-6. Commonly Prescribed Medications for Sleep

MEDICATION (TRADE NAME)	HALF-LIFE (h)	DOSING	SIDE EFFECTS	CONTRAINDICATIONS
Zolpidem* (Ambien)	2.5	5–10 mg orally (PO) 5 mg in elderly or those with hepatic disease	Drowsiness Diarrhea	End-stage liver disease (ESLD)
Triazolam* (Halcion)	1.6–5.4	0.125–0.25 mg PO Decrease by 50% with erythromycin	Early morning insomnia Amnesia	Sleep apnea
Chloral hydrate	8–11	500–1000 mg PO or rectally	Gastrointestinal irritation Respiratory depression Leukopenia	Marked hepatic or renal dysfunction Esophagitis, gastritis, or peptic ulcer disease Concurrent IV furosemide Use with caution with warfarin
Diphenhydramine (Benadryl)	2.4–9.3 (↑ in ESLD)	25–50 mg PO or IV	Anticholinergic effects	Hepatic dysfunction Acute angle-closure glaucoma Bladder, gastric outlet obstruction
Lorazepam (Ativan)	10–20	0.5–1 mg PO, IV, IM	Hypotension, especially when given IV Amnesia	Sleep apnea
Temazepam (Restoril)	10–20	15–30 mg PO		End-stage renal or hepatic disease Sleep apnea

Note: All hypnotics can cause central nervous system depression and altered mental status.
*Denotes hypnotics of choice.
PO, by mouth; IV, intravenous; IM, intramuscular.

may exacerbate underlying hypercapnia in patients with obesity hypoventilation syndrome, or COPD. Finally, they exacerbate sleep-disordered breathing because of their depressive effects on respiration and by causing upper airway muscle hypotonia. Because they increase the frequency and length of apneic events, they are contraindicated for nonventilated patients with obstructive and central sleep apnea syndromes.

The hypnotic zolpidem (Ambien) holds promise for use in patients in the ICU. Zolpidem is an imadazopyridine hypnotic. Although chemically unrelated to benzodiazepines, it binds selectively to one of the benzodiazepine receptors. This selective binding may explain the paucity of muscle relaxant, anxiolytic, and anticonvulsant effects. Unlike benzodiazepines, zolpidem alters sleep stages minimally. It preserves stages 3 and 4 and REM sleep. Fewer next-day residual effects and less cognitive impairment and memory loss is observed with zolpidem compared with benzodiazepines. No significant differences in arterial oxygen saturation have been demonstrated between zolpidem and benzodiazepines in COPD, but it may cause hypercapnia in individual patients. Dosing of zolpidem is 5 to 10 mg before sleep in adults (5 mg in the elderly). However, it is currently limited to enteral administration, plus it is much more expensive than generic benzodiazepines. Further controlled studies comparing it with benzodiazepines and other hypnotics in patients in the ICU are needed to further define its advantages and limitations before it can be endorsed as the hypnotic of choice in these patients.

BIBLIOGRAPHY

Aurell J, Elmqvist D: Sleep in the surgical intensive care unit: Continuous polygraphic recording of sleep in nine patients receiving postoperative care. BMJ 190:1029–1032, 1985.
   Nine noncardiac, postoperative, extubated patients demonstrated decreased total sleep time, stage 3 and 4 sleep, and REM sleep. Sleep as judged by clinical observation was grossly overestimated.

Easton C, MacKenzie F: Sensory-perceptual alterations: Delirium in the intensive care unit. Heart Lung 17:229–237, 1988.
   This article describes the ICU syndrome and includes a discussion of its prevention and treatment.

Krachman S, D'Alonzo G, Criner G: Sleep in the intensive care unit. Chest 107:1713–1720, 1995.
   This is a review discussing the effects of medical illness, surgery, medications, and environmental influences on sleep in the ICU.

Langtry HD, Benfield P: Zolpidem: A review of its pharmacodynamic and pharmacokinetic properties and therapeutic potential. Drugs 40:291–313, 1990.
   This article is an overview of zolpidem with emphasis on its pharmacokinetics, therapeutic uses, and potential side effects.

Meyer T, Eveloff S, Bauer M, et al: Adverse environmental conditions in the respiratory and medical ICU settings. Chest 105:1211–1216, 1994.
   Light and sound levels and frequency of interruptions were continuously monitored in a medical ICU, respiratory care unit, and standard patient care unit over a 7-day period. Light levels in rooms with windows reflected a normal day-night cycle, overall peak sounds were high in all areas, and interruptions occurred at least hourly around the clock in the ICU.

Richards KC, Bairnsfather L: A description of night sleep patterns in the critical care unit. Heart Lung 17:35–42, 1988.
   This decribes a nocturnal polysomnographic study of 10 male patients with cardiovascular disease that revealed decreased total sleep time, stage 2 sleep, and REM sleep when compared with normal controls.

Topf M, Davis JE: Critical care unit noise and rapid eye movement (REM) sleep. Heart Lung 22:252–258, 1993.
   This study of 70 women who were exposed to audiotapes of critical care unit night time sounds showed that the ICU noise induced significantly decreased REM activity.

45 Thrombocytopenia

Marc J. Kahn

Platelets are cell fragments derived from megakaryocytes in the bone marrow. They initiate hemostasis by adhering to damaged vessels, forming a plug, and providing a surface for the coagulation cascade. Their counts normally vary between 150,000/μL and 450,000/μL. Platelet counts significantly less than this range constitute *thrombocytopenia*. Its differential diagnosis includes disorders that have (1) increased platelet destruction (on an immune basis or on a nonimmune basis), (2) decreased platelet production, and (3) sequestration of circulating platelets (Table 45–1).

Before any therapeutic or management decisions regarding thrombocytopenia are made, a careful review of the peripheral blood smear should exclude *pseudothrombocytopenia*. This occurs when platelets clump in the presence of the anticoagulant used in the blood collection tube. Although its estimated incidence is only 0.1%, it is the most common cause of a falsely low platelet count. These platelet clumps are not counted by automated cell counters, resulting in a fictitiously low reported platelet count. Pseudothrombocytopenia is most common in samples anticoagulated with ethylenediaminetetra-acetic acid (EDTA), but it also occurs with anticoagulants, such as heparin or citrate. The true platelet count can be correctly estimated with a manual count on a finger-stick blood sample. Alternatively, an automated count on blood anticoagulated in substances other than EDTA

Table 45–1. Differential Diagnosis of Thrombocytopenia

Disorders of increased platelet destruction
  Non–immune-mediated destruction
    Thrombotic thrombocytopenic purpura (TTP)
    Disseminated intravascular coagulation (DIC)*
    Drug-induced (see Table 45–2)*
    Infections*
    Sepsis syndrome
  Immune-mediated destruction
    Idiopathic (immune) thrombocytopenic purpura (ITP)*
    Drug-induced (e.g., heparin)*
    Post-transfusion purpura (PTP)*
Disorders of decreased platelet production
  Marrow infiltration
  Drugs suppressing hematopoiesis*
  Aplastic anemia
  Viral infections
Disorders due to splenic sequestration of platelets
  Hypersplenism*
  Hypothermia

*In the differential diagnosis of thrombocytopenia that develops while a patient is in the ICU.

may be attempted. The condition is of clinical importance only as a source of confusion with true thrombocytopenia.

DISORDERS OF INCREASED PLATELET DESTRUCTION BY NONIMMUNE MECHANISMS

Thrombotic Thrombocytopenic Purpura

The prototypic disease for nonimmune platelet destruction is thrombotic thrombocytopenic purpura (TTP) (see Chapter 63). Patients with TTP present with the clinical pentad of fever, renal abnormalities, central nervous system disorders, thrombocytopenia, and microangiopathic hemolytic anemia (MAHA). MAHA is characterized by the presence of fragmented red cells, or schistocytes, caused by erythrocyte destruction in the microvasculature. The disorder, hemolytic uremic syndrome (HUS), shares pathologic features with TTP but manifests a preponderance of renal abnormalities. The primary treatment for the thrombocytopenia associated with TTP is plasmapheresis, accompanied by glucocorticoids. Patients with TTP become thrombocytopenic from activation of platelets, leading to intravascular aggregation and ultimately their clearance from the circulation. Platelet transfusions in TTP have been associated with fatal outcomes, presumably from microthrombosis, and are therefore contraindicated except for life-threatening bleeding. Fortunately, patients with TTP rarely bleed. Thrombocytopenia with MAHA in other conditions usually responds to treatment of the underlying condition or removal of the offending drug (Table 45–2; see also Chapter 63). Again, as with classic TTP, there should be a reluctance to transfuse platelets in all but the most serious bleeding episodes.

Table 45–2. Drugs Commonly Associated with Thrombocytopenia

Drugs Inducing an Immune-Mediated Thrombocytopenia

Amrinone	Phenytoin
Aspirin	Procainamide
Cimetidine	Quinidine
Gold salts	Quinine*
Heroin	Ranitidine
Heparin	Rifampin
Indomethacin	Sulfonamides

Drugs That Induce a Non–Immune-Mediated Thrombocytopenia

Increased destruction (HUS-like syndrome)
    Cyclosporine
    Mitomycin C
Decreased production
    Many chemotherapeutic agents

*Also produces a condition identical to HUS (hemolytic-uremic syndrome).

Disseminated Intravascular Coagulation

Disseminated intravascular coagulation (DIC) is another disorder of platelet destruction. In fact, the most common laboratory abnormality in DIC is thrombocytopenia. DIC results from various causes, including Gram-negative and Gram-positive bacterial infections, trauma, snake bites, brain injury, and burns. In DIC, the generation of thrombin occurs without its subsequent neutralization, which is normally carried out by coagulation pathway inhibitors. Since thrombin promotes the conversion of fibrinogen to fibrin, microvascular thrombosis occurs. This results in tissue ischemia along with consumption of coagulation components such as platelets, fibrinogen, and prothrombin. DIC is often identified clinically by skin hemorrhage in the form of petechiae and ecchymoses. Shock, organ dysfunction, and frank hemorrhage may occur as well. Other laboratory findings in DIC include prolongation of the prothrombin time, partial thromboplastin time and thrombin time, a decrease in the fibrinogen level, and an increased level of fibrin degradation products (FDP), also known as fibrin split products or FSP. *D-Dimers* result from the degradation of cross-linked fibrin by plasmin, and their levels also increase in DIC. Primary fibrinogenolysis, a rare condition that results when plasmin is generated in the absence of DIC, is characterized by normal levels of D-dimers despite a low fibrinogen level.

One common clinical problem is differentiating DIC from the coagulopathy resulting from liver disease. In both, the fibrinogen level is low, clotting times are prolonged, and fibrin degradation products are increased. Measuring levels of *Factors VII and VIII* can help in distinguishing one from the other. Patients with DIC have consumption of all clotting factors and decreased levels of both Factors VII and VIII. In contrast, since Factor VIII is not synthesized solely by the liver, patients with liver failure have low Factor VII levels but may have normal levels of Factor VIII. Although schistocytes can be seen on the peripheral smear in patients with DIC, this finding is inconsistent.

The treatment of DIC is more an art than a science because of the paucity of randomized, controlled trials in the literature. The primary therapy remains treatment of the underlying disorder. For bleeding complications, platelet transfusions should be used in the setting of thrombocytopenia. Although concern exists about promoting the coagulopathy of DIC by transfusing blood components, there is little evidence from controlled clinical trials that blood components "fuel the fire" in DIC. Therefore, in actively bleeding patients with DIC, 8 units of cryoprecipitate should be infused for fibrinogen levels less than 100 mg/dL and fresh frozen plasma administered to correct a prolonged prothrombin time. Other therapies, including heparin, antithrombin III, and serine protease inhibitors, have been used to treat DIC anecdotally, but insufficient data exist to recommend their routine use.

Other Causes

Several drugs can cause platelet destruction on a nonimmune basis. Two such drugs, cyclosporine and mitomycin C, induce a condition identical to HUS. (On an immune basis, quinine-dependent antibodies can also induce an HUS-like syndrome). Treatment is simply the removal of the offending drug.

Thrombocytopenia can complicate a variety of infections, even in the absence of DIC. Bacterial infections and sepsis syndrome can be associated with platelet aggregation and destruction. Rickettsial infections can cause vasculitis, leading to platelet adhesion and destruction. Malaria commonly presents with thrombocytopenia. These infection-associated thrombocytopenias resolve with treatment of the infection.

DISORDERS OF INCREASED PLATELET DESTRUCTION BY IMMUNE MECHANISMS

Heparin-Induced Thrombocytopenia

Although immune (idiopathic) thrombocytopenic purpura (ITP) (see Chapter 63) is the paradigm disorder that results in thrombocytopenia from immunologically mediated platelet destruction and it may on occasion lead to admission to the intensive care unit (ICU), ITP probably should be at the bottom of the list of causes of decreased platelets occurring de novo in patients in the ICU. In contrast, immune-mediated thrombocytopenia due to drugs should be high on the ICU clinician's list of causes of thrombocytopenia under such circumstances (see Table 45–2).

The most common drug associated with thrombocytopenia is *heparin*. This agent causes a mild and reversible decrease in the platelet count in 5% of patients during the first 4 days of exposure to the drug. Severe thrombocytopenia (platelet counts $<50,000/\mu L$) occurs in 1% or less of patients receiving heparin, usually after 6 to 12 days (with a range of 3 to 22 days) of exposure to heparin. However, if the patient had previously been exposed to heparin, the heparin-induced thrombocytopenia (HIT) may occur within hours of re-exposure.

Platelet factor 4 (PF4) is a protein contained in platelet alpha granules; it binds heparin. HIT results from antibody formation to heparin-PF4 complexes, which, in combination, are able to induce platelet aggregation. After aggregation, the platelets are usually cleared from the circulation, but in about 20% of cases, they also cause venous or arterial thrombosis. The patient's blood can be assessed for HIT in the laboratory by demonstrating the presence of heparin-PF4 antibodies by enzyme-linked immunosorbent assay or by demonstrating the release of the granule contents of normal platelets on exposure to therapeutic concentrations of heparin.

Heparin-Induced Thrombotic Thrombocytopenia

A high index of suspicion is needed to suspect HIT and its more life-threatening related condition, heparin-induced thrombotic thrombocytopenia (HITT). For example, any arterial clot occurring in a patient receiving heparin in the ICU should be suspected as being caused by HITT (which may occur with or without a detectable fall in platelets). This so-called white clot syndrome (reflecting the unusual gross appearance of the clot in occluded arteries) carries high morbidity and substantial mortality (28% mortality in one large series). The suspicion for HITT should arise when a patient receiving heparin acquires a venous clot distinct from the one that triggered the heparin therapy or a drop of 50% in the platelet count or a drop in platelet count to less than 100,000/μL.

Other warning signs of HITT are the development of heparin resistance, skin necrosis (especially at sites of prior subcutaneous heparin injections) and abdominal or limb pain. The most common sites of arterial thrombosis in HITT are the distal aorta and ileofemoral arteries. Others especially at risk include native coronary vessels, coronary bypass grafts, and spinal and cerebral arteries. Previously injured vessels, for example, at sites of prior catheter insertions, seem predisposed to HITT clots.

Treatment of Heparin-Induced Thrombocytopenia and Heparin-Induced Thrombotic Thrombocytopenia

Treatment of HIT and HITT consists of the prompt removal of all sources of heparin. Even the smallest amount of heparin, such as the heparin coating of some intravascular catheters, can induce and exacerbate HIT. After removal of heparin, most patients recover spontaneously in several days.

Repeat exposure to heparin in patients with HITT may lead to recurrent arterial clots and death. Platelet transfusions in HIT are also contraindicated because the infused platelets may aggregate and cause thrombosis. Should the patient require anticoagulation, options include aspirin, heparinoids (e.g., danaparoid), ancrod, or fibrinolytic agents such as urokinase or hirudin. There is risk to giving low molecular weight heparin because it shows significant cross-reactivity to heparin when tested by heparin-induced antiplatelet antibodies.

Post-transfusion Purpura

A rare cause of thrombocytopenia is post-transfusion purpura (PTP). This condition is characterized by severe thrombocytopenia occurring 7 days after a blood transfusion. PTP most commonly occurs in the 10% of patients whose platelets lack the Pl^{A1} antigen, a polymorphism of glycoprotein IIIa. Such patients acquire alloantibodies to Pl^{A1}. On exposure to transfused platelets possessing the Pl^{A1} antigen, alloantibodies to Pl^{A1} destroy both transfused platelets and also native platelets. Treatment for PTP includes plasmapheresis to remove the offending antibody or circulating antigen, or both. One must avoid platelet transfusions in PTP because the transfused platelets are likely to be Pl^{A1}-positive again, and they may cause life-threatening transfusion reactions. Patients with PTP should receive blood only from individuals known to be negative for Pl^{A1}. PTP should be considered in all cases of severe thrombocytopenia that occur 7 days after a blood transfusion.

DISORDERS OF DECREASED PLATELET PRODUCTION

Thrombocytopenias resulting from decreased platelet production are characterized by thrombocytopenia with a decrease in the number of megakaryocytes in the bone marrow. A major group of acquired diseases that result in platelet hypoproduction in the marrow are infiltrative diseases, such as leukemias, myelofibrosis, or metastatic tumors. In all of these conditions, the peripheral smear reveals thrombocytopenia with erythrocytes that are teardrop-shaped, called dacrocytes. In addition, a leukoerythroblastic picture may be present, characterized by nucleated red blood cells and early myeloid forms. Definitive diagnosis of these conditions is made by reviewing the bone marrow biopsy and aspirate results.

Aplastic anemia is characterized by a reduction in the marrow production of all cell lines. Amegakaryocytic thrombocytopenia is a variant of this condition and is characterized by the absence of megakaryocytes, with preservation of other cell lines. Thrombocytopenia is part of both of these disorders.

Viral infections commonly result in decreased platelet production. Mumps, varicella, parvovirus, cytomegalovirus, Epstein-Barr virus, and others are associated with thrombocytopenia that is usually mild. These usually self-limited disorders and the resultant thrombocytopenias require no therapy.

DISORDERS OF PLATELET SEQUESTRATION

Normally, one third of the body's total number of platelets is pooled in the spleen. This sequestration can be exaggerated in cases of liver cirrhosis, portal venous hypertension, or splenomegaly. Splenomegaly can result from hemoglobin C or SC disease, hemoglobin SS in children, thalassemias, Gaucher's disease, myelofibrosis, and various infectious diseases. All have been associated with thrombocytopenia. In these conditions, platelet production is normal and the total body content of platelets may be normal with an increased fraction of platelets pooled in the spleen. Thrombocytopenia resulting from splenic sequestration usually results in platelet counts greater than $50,000/\mu L$. Since circulating platelets function normally and platelets can be mobilized from the spleen if needed, splenic sequestration usually requires no therapy.

Thrombocytopenia has also been reported transiently in hypothermic patients,

Table 45–3. Treatment of Thrombocytopenia in Various Disorders

DISORDER	TREATMENT
DIC	Treat underlying cause; transfuse platelets only if actively bleeding
Drug-induced	Remove offending drug
Hypothermia	No treatment needed
Hypersplenism	No treatment needed
ITP	Glucocorticoids, IVIG, splenectomy (see Chapter 63)
Massive transfusion	Fresh frozen plasma
Production problems	Platelet transfusions if actively bleeding or if platelets $<5,000/\mu L$ (see Chapter 18 for other thresholds for transfusions)
PTP	Plasmapheresis
TTP	Plasmapheresis, glucocorticoids, *avoid* platelet transfusions (see Chapter 63)

DIC, disseminated intravascular coagulation; ITP, immune thrombocytopenic purpura; IVIG, intravenous immunoglobulin; TTP, thrombotic thrombocytopenic purpura; PTP, post-transfusion purpura.

presumably from platelets pooling in the spleen. On rewarming, platelet counts usually return to normal.

PLATELET TRANSFUSION THERAPY

Since the development of plastic tubing in the 1960s, platelets have been available for transfusion. Platelet transfusions are often given to improve the thrombocytopenia associated with the preceding disorders of platelet production (see Chapter 18). However, the exact platelet count requiring prophylactic platelet transfusion is controversial. The first study to address this question was published in the early 1960s. This study evaluated patients with thrombocytopenic leukemia and looked for evidence of both cutaneous bleeding and gross hemorrhage. Although the study concluded that no "threshold level" existed below which hemorrhage was more likely to occur, others have misinterpreted the results to assume a threshold level of 20,000 platelets/μL for prophylactic transfusion of platelets. More recent data suggest that for the afebrile, nonbleeding patient, a level of 5000 platelets/μL is a more reasonable threshold for prophylactic transfusion. In the patient who is

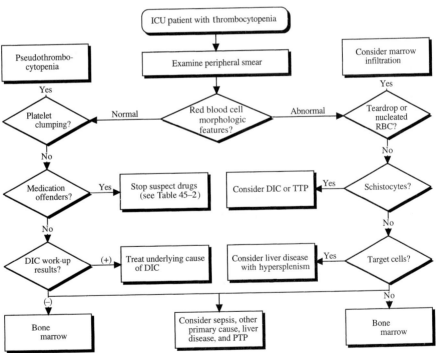

Figure 45–1. Schematic flow diagram outlining the diagnostic evaluation of an ICU patient who acquires or presents with thrombocytopenia. DIC work-up includes measurement of fibrinogen, fibrin degradation products, and prothrombin and partial thromboplastin times. RBC, red blood cell; DIC, disseminated intravascular coagulation; TTP, thrombotic thrombocytopenic purpura; PTP, post-transfusion purpura.

febrile, bleeding, or with other complicating factors, a higher threshold such as 10,000 to 15,000 platelets/μL appears reasonable (see Chapter 18).

The surgical literature maintains that preoperative platelet counts should be at least 50,000/μL for most procedures and at least 100,000/μL for neurologic or ophthalmic procedures. A threshold platelet count of 50,000/μL also appears reasonable for most ICU procedures, including insertion of central venous catheters, lumbar puncture, thoracentesis, paracentesis and other minor surgeries, including incision and drainage and chest tube insertion.

CLINICAL PEARLS

1. Avoid platelet transfusions in TTP, HUS, HIT, HITT, or PTP unless there is life-threatening hemorrhage.
2. In disorders of platelet production, transfuse platelets prophylactically if the platelet count is less than 5000/μL. If an invasive procedure is planned, platelet counts should be at least 50,000/μL.
3. If a patient becomes thrombocytopenic in the ICU, first think about drugs such as heparin.
4. Remember that HIT can also cause arterial or venous thrombosis.
5. In many disorders causing thrombocytopenia (Table 45–3), one must treat the underlying cause and not simply transfuse platelets.
6. Review of the peripheral smear can provide clues to the pathogenesis of thrombocytopenia and should be the first step in the approach of any thrombocytopenic patient (Fig. 45–1).

BIBLIOGRAPHY

Beutler E: Platelet transfusions: The 20,000/μL trigger. Blood 81:1411, 1993.
This is a carefully researched article on the data available for prophylactic platelet transfusion.

Bussels JB, Schreiber AD: Immune thrombocytopenic purpura, neonatal alloimmune thrombocytopenia, and post-transfusion purpura. Hemostasis Thrombosis 70:1485–1504, 1993.

Bussels JB, Schreiber AD: Thrombocytopenia due to platelet destruction and hypersplenism. Hemostasis Thrombosis 70:1505–1513, 1993.
Both of the Bussels and Schreiber references provide many details of mechanisms, diagnosis, and therapy for various types of immune-mediated and non–immune-mediated thrombocytopenias.

Gaydos LA, Freireich EJ, Mantel N: The quantitative relation between platelet count and hemorrhage in patients with acute leukemia. N Engl J Med 266:905, 1962.
This was the first attempt to identify a threshold for prophylactic platelet transfusion; the conclusion was that no threshold level exists below which bleeding tendencies increase substantially.

Griffiths E, Dzik WH: Assays for heparin-induced thrombocytopenia. Transfus Med 1:1–11, 1997.
This review discusses the laboratory diagnosis of HIT, which remains an inexact science (with 54 references).

Kelton JG, Warkentin TE: Heparin-induced thrombocytopenia. Diagnosis, natural history, and treatment options. Postgrad Med 103:169–171, 175–178, 1998.
This is a concise review of HIT and treatment options.

Magnani HN: Heparin-induced thrombocytopenia (HIT): An overview of 230 patients treated with orgaran (Org 10172). Thrombosis Hemostasis 70:554–561, 1993.
This is a description of the most successful use of danaparoid (a mixture of "heparinoids"-

glycosaminoglycans other than heparin) on compassionate open label use for anticoagulation in patients with HIT.

Rutherford CJ, Frenkel EP: Thrombocytopenia, issues in diagnosis and therapy. Med Clin North Am 78:555, 1994.
This article provides a thorough review of thrombocytopenia.

Shorten GD, Comunale ME: Heparin-induced thrombocytopenia. J Cardiothorac Vasc Anesth 10:521–530, 1996.
This is a comprehensive review of HIT, including a detailed consideration of the issue of anticoagulation while the patient with HIT is undergoing cardiopulmonary bypass.

Warkentin TE: Heparin-induced thrombocytopenia. Pathogenesis, frequency, avoidance and management. Drug Safety 17:325–341, 1997.
This is a comprehensive review of HIT including treatment with danaparoid (with 111 references).

46   Transfusion Reactions

Steven R. Sloan
Leigh Jefferies

Although precautions are taken during collection, processing, and administration of blood to ensure that blood components transfused to patients are safe, adverse reactions still occur. One particularly severe type of adverse reaction (acute hemolytic transfusion reaction) is usually due to clerical errors, such as mislabeling of blood specimens sent to the blood bank. Other serious as well as mild reactions are inevitable on occasion, even if all procedures are followed appropriately. This chapter summarizes the approach to *acute* transfusion reactions. The conclusive diagnosis of such a reaction often requires additional laboratory testing. This is primarily coordinated by the blood bank (transfusion service), which should be notified of all suspected transfusion reactions and consulted if questions arise.

A *transfusion reaction* is defined as any adverse consequence of transfusion of blood products. Blood products include, but are not limited to, red blood cells (RBCs), fresh frozen plasma (FFP), and platelets. This chapter is concerned principally with acute reactions, that is, those that occur during or soon after transfusions. Acute adverse effects of massive transfusion of blood products, including hypothermia, hypocalcemia, and other metabolic abnormalities, are discussed in Chapter 15. Uncommon transfusion reactions that occur under specialized conditions are discussed in Chapters 38 and 62.

DEFINITIONS AND PATHOPHYSIOLOGIC MECHANISMS

Acute Hemolytic Transfusion Reactions

The patient has antibodies that destroy the donor RBCs. Hemolytic antibodies that are capable of causing acute hemolytic transfusion reactions are usually directed against antigens of the red cell ABO system. The presence of these antibodies accounts for approximately 80% of all fatal acute hemolytic transfusion reactions. The latter are usually due to transfusion of ABO-incompatible blood. Activation of the complement and coagulation systems, plus a neuroendocrine response, contributes to mechanisms potentially leading to hypotension, renal failure, disseminated intravascular coagulation, and death.

Febrile Transfusion Reactions

Red blood cell units and platelet products are contaminated with leukocytes. A patient's antibodies can bind to these donor leukocytes, resulting in their releasing cytokines that may cause fever or chills, or both. These antibodies are also known as *leukoagglutinins*.

Allergic Reactions

Patients can have antibodies to plasma proteins in the donor unit. These can cause mild allergic reactions or severe anaphylactic reactions. Some cases of severe anaphylactic reactions are observed in IgA-deficient patients who have high titers of anti-IgA antibodies.

Septic Reactions

Bacteria can contaminate blood products. This can lead to a febrile response in the patient. Also, endotoxins associated with Gram-negative bacteria can be in the donor unit, possibly resulting in septic shock. A small but important (5 to 10%) fraction of transfusion reaction deaths is due to septic reactions.

Nonimmune Hemolysis

Transfusion of RBCs diluted inappropriately with solutions other than 0.9% saline can lead to lysis of RBCs because of osmotic pressure. In addition, malfunctioning blood warmers, the use of extracorporeal circuits, the administration of drugs into administration sets, and transfusion through small-bore needles can lead to excessive hemolysis.

Volume Overload

Blood products have significant volume and oncotic pressure, which can lead to hypervolemia that is manifested clinically as left-sided congestive heart failure.

Transfusion-Related Acute Lung Injury

Acute respiratory distress syndrome (ARDS) may result from immune-mediated destruction of a patient's white blood cells by donor antibodies, antibodies in the patient's circulation reacting with donor leukocytes, or transfusion of cytokines accumulated in the stored blood. Recently, reactive lipid products in stored blood have been implicated in the pathogenesis of these reactions. Transfusion-related acute lung injury is estimated to be the cause of about 15% of transfusion-associated deaths.

Cytokine Reaction

A variety of vasoactive and pyrogenic mediators of inflammation, including IL-1, IL-6, tumor necrosis factor-alpha (TNF-alpha), can be released from contaminating donor leukocytes during storage of blood products and cause fever, hypotension, chills, and rigors. Activation of complement, kinin, and killikrein systems may result in production of C3a, C5a, and bradykinin, which can result in hypotension, flushing, bradycardia, and dyspnea. These reactive substances of anaphylaxis may also be generated following exposure to negatively charged surfaces of extracorporeal circuits during hemodialysis (see Chapter 16) or apheresis (see Chapter 67). Patients receiving angiotensin converting enzyme (ACE) inhibitors are at increased risk for adverse effects from these reactions since ACE is important for the degradation of bradykinin.

DIFFERENTIAL DIAGNOSIS

If a patient experiences changes in vital signs or acquires new symptoms during or soon after (within 4 hours) transfusion of a blood product, those changes may be due to a transfusion reaction. Table 46–1 shows the frequency of the most serious and most common acute transfusion reactions. Fortunately, the most severe reactions are the least frequent.

A variety of signs and symptoms may occur during the transfusion or within 2 to 4 hours after transfusion (Table 46–2). Because transfusion reactions have variable presentations, the lack of a specific sign or symptom *cannot* exclude a particular reaction type. For instance, chills and fever alone may be the presenting symptoms of an acute hemolytic transfusion reaction. The severity of the reaction is also variable.

Some types of acute transfusion reactions can be accompanied by signs and symptoms that are *not* listed in Table 46–2. Signs and symptoms of acute hemolytic transfusion reactions can include nausea, flushing, dyspnea, oliguria, and generalized bleeding. Also, chest radiographs of patients suffering from transfusion-related acute lung injury reveal bilateral infiltrates that are predominantly perihilar and in the lower lung fields. Finally, the symptoms and signs in Table 46–2 may not necessarily be transfusion-related but rather may be due to myriad non–transfusion-related causes and their appearance happens to coincide with the transfusion.

Table 46–1. Frequencies of Acute Transfusion Reactions

TYPE OF REACTION	ESTIMATED FREQUENCY (PER TRANSFUSED UNIT)
Mild allergic reaction	1/33–1/100
Febrile transfusion reaction	1/100–1/200
Septic reaction	1/2000–1/20,000*
Volume overload	1/100–10,000
Acute hemolytic transfusion reaction (symptomatic)	1/12,000–1/33,000
Nonimmune hemolysis	Unknown†
Anaphylactic reaction	1/18,000–1/170,000
Transfusion-related acute lung injury	1:5,000‡
Cytokine reaction	Unknown

*Platelet units.
†Although the actual incidence of nonimmune hemolysis is not well documented, it appears to be rare.
‡Milder forms may not be rare but are likely to go unrecognized.

Table 46–2. Symptoms and Signs of Acute Transfusion Reactions

TYPE OF REACTION	ANXIETY	CHILLS, RIGORS	DYSPNEA	FLANK PAIN	HIVES	FEVER	TACHYCARDIA	HYPOTENSION
Acute hemolytic transfusion reaction	+++	++	++	+++	–	++	++	+++
Febrile transfusion reaction	+	++	–	–	–	++	+	–
Mild allergic reaction	+	–	–	–	+++	–	–	–
Anaphylactic reaction	++	–	++	–	+	+	++	+++
Septic reaction	+	++	++	–	–	++	++	+++
Nonimmune hemolysis	–	–	–	–	–	–	–	–
Volume overload	+	–	++	–	–	–	+	–
Transfusion-related acute lung injury	+	+++	+++	–	–	+++	+	+++
Cytokine reaction	++	++	+	–	–	++	–	+++

Scoring scale: –, not present; +, mild sign or symptom; ++, moderate sign or symptom; +++, severe sign or symptom.

DIAGNOSTIC EVALUATION

First, before diagnostic evaluation, the transfusion should be stopped as soon as symptoms and signs suspicious of a transfusion reaction are observed. The intravenous line should be kept open for fluid support, if needed, or in case the transfusion is restarted (e.g., if a mild allergic reaction is diagnosed). Using Tables 47–1 and 47–2, one can formulate a differential diagnosis before laboratory results are available. Unless the reaction is clearly limited to a mild allergic reaction, specimens should be sent for laboratory evaluation.

Second, one should make sure that the patient is receiving the correct product. For example, is John Doe, medical record #123, receiving a product labeled for John Doe, medical record #123?

Third, the specimens in Table 46–3 should be sent as soon as possible for laboratory evaluation: post-transfusion blood specimens (one for serum, i.e., not anticoagulated, and one anticoagulated), the transfused product or products, and urine for urinalysis to determine if there is hemoglobinuria.

Fourth, the transfusion service or blood bank should be notified.

Care must be taken when evaluating the signs, symptoms, and laboratory test results for transfusion reactions because they can be variable. In particular, a patient may have an acute hemolytic transfusion reaction without evidence of renal failure, shock, or disseminated intravascular coagulation. Indeed, the initial symptoms of an acute hemolytic transfusion reaction may be limited to fever with or without chills. Likewise, the first sign of a contaminated unit causing a septic transfusion reaction may be fever without hypotension. A variety of bacteria can cause a septic transfusion reaction, but shock from a contaminated unit is most likely due to endotoxin from Gram-negative organisms. A Gram stain of the blood product can often help in quickly determining the type of organism in the product.

MANAGEMENT AND DISCUSSION OF THERAPIES

Complications of transfusion reactions should be managed in a standard manner: (1) stopping the transfusion immediately, (2) providing general supportive intensive care unit (ICU) care, and (3) performing specific interventions as indicated. For example, if circulatory shock develops during a transfusion, the transfusion should be stopped and the shock treated with intravenous fluids and vasopressors. In addition, if anaphylaxis is suspected as the cause of the hypotension, it should be treated with epinephrine (see Chapter 8).

If *bacterial contamination* of the transfusion unit is suspected, broad spectrum antibiotics should be started to cover Gram-positive (including staphylococcal species) and Gram-negative pathogens. In a suspected acute hemolytic transfusion reaction, urine output and renal function should be monitored and measures taken to promote diuresis. Intravenous fluids, diuretics, mannitol, and low-dose dopamine have been advocated, analogous to treatment of acute tubular necrosis.

Treatment for *transfusion-related acute lung injury* includes discontinuing the transfusion and providing supportive care, including ventilatory support if needed. Although recommendations for treatment have included diuretics, oxygen, high-dose corticosteroids, and albumin infusions, there is little scientific evidence for

Table 46–3. Laboratory Findings Associated with Acute Transfusion Reactions

TYPE OF REACTION	DIRECT ANTIGLOBULIN TEST*	VISIBLE HEMOLYSIS*	HEMOGLOBINURIA*	GRAM STAIN OF BLOOD PRODUCT	CULTURE OF BLOOD PRODUCT	BILIRUBIN, LACTIC DEHYDROGENASE
Acute hemolytic transfusion reaction	+	+	+	–	–	Increased
Febrile transfusion reaction	–	–	–	–	–	–
Mild allergic reaction	–	–	–	–	–	–
Anaphylactic reaction	–	–	–	–	–	–
Septic reaction	–	–	–	May be positive	+	–
Nonimmune hemolysis	–	+	+	–	–	–
Volume overload	–	–	–	–	–	May be increased
Transfusion-related acute lung injury	–	–	–	–	–	–
Cytokine reaction	–	–	–	–	–	–

*This assumes that these tests were negative before transfusion. Otherwise, an increase in the strength of the direct antiglobulin test or the amount of hemolysis or hemoglobinuria may be observed.

any of these therapies. Laboratory testing of the patient's blood and the donor unit can help determine the cause of the reaction. Practically, however, the diagnosis is based on clinical suspicion and ruling out other causes of acute respiratory distress syndrome (see Chapter 73).

The symptoms of *cytokine reactions* resolve with supportive therapy, and there are no long-term sequelae. However, cytokine reactions may initially resemble acute hemolytic reactions or anaphylaxis, both of which should be considered and ruled out. These reactions may be prevented by discontinuance of ACE inhibitors and prestorage leukodepletion.

Regarding treatment of *nonimmune hemolysis,* if the patient exhibits only hemoglobinemia and hemoglobinuria, supportive therapy may be sufficient, while intensive management will be necessary for those cases with hypotension, shock, and renal dysfunction.

Patients with *volume overload* should be treated with diuretics as needed. In some cases, it may be possible to have the transfusion service split red blood cell units into two smaller transfusable volumes or to reduce the volume of platelets in order to minimize the total volume transfused.

Minor Transfusion Reactions

Febrile transfusion reactions are treated with antipyretic agents. Acetaminophen is usually sufficient, but in cases of rigors, meperidine (intramuscularly or subcutaneously) may be necessary. The probability of future transfusions resulting in febrile reactions can be decreased by using *leukoreduced products.* Filters are often used to deplete the blood products of leukocytes, but platelets and red blood cells may be leukoreduced at collection and not require any additional filtering. Premedication with antipyretic agents may be appropriate for selected patients receiving multiple transfusions with repeated reactions.

If a patient experiences a mild allergic transfusion reaction, the transfusion should be temporarily discontinued while maintaining intravenous access, and an antihistamine (25 to 50 mg of diphenhydramine hydrochloride intravenously) should be administered. If symptoms improve in 30 minutes, the transfusion can be restarted. If symptoms do not improve, the blood product should be disconnected and sent along with other specimens for evaluation as detailed earlier.

CLINICAL PEARLS AND PITFALLS

Certain types of blood products are predictably associated or not associated with certain types of transfusion reactions (Table 46–4).

SUMMARY AND COMMENTS

Although most transfusion reactions are minor, life-threatening reactions do occur. Common symptoms such as fever and chills may herald mild reactions (e.g., febrile or mild allergic reactions) or, alternatively, may represent the first symptom of a life-threatening reaction, such as acute hemolytic transfusion reaction, transfu-

Table 46–4. Transfusion Products Associated with Various Types of Acute Transfusion Reactions

TYPE OF REACTION	PRODUCTS COMMONLY IMPLICATED	PRODUCTS RARELY IMPLICATED
Acute hemolytic transfusion reaction	RBCs	Platelets, FFP
Febrile transfusion reaction	Platelets, RBCs	FFP
Mild allergic reaction	RBCs, platelets, FFP	—
Anaphylactic reaction	RBCs, platelets, FFP	—
Septic reaction	Platelets (RBCs on occasion)	FFP
Nonimmune hemolysis	RBCs	—
Volume overload	RBCs, FFP	Platelets
Transfusion-related acute lung injury	RBCs, platelets, FFP	—
Cytokine reactions	RBCs, platelets, FFP	—

RBCs, red blood cells; FFP, fresh frozen plasma.

sion-related acute lung injury, or bacterial contamination. Hence, no reaction should be ignored. This chapter's topics have been limited to transfusion reactions that develop during or immediately after the transfusion. Other subacute or chronic adverse reactions to transfusion include transmission of infectious disease, graft versus host disease, post-transfusion purpura, delayed hemolytic transfusion reactions, immunomodulation, and iron overload.

In general, if a reaction occurs during a transfusion, the transfusion should be stopped and the transfusion service notified. Once a potentially significant transfusion reaction has been reported, blood bank protocols designed to minimize the risk of transfusion reactions require that a laboratory work-up be conducted. While the laboratory work-up is proceeding, blood products cannot routinely be released. If a product is urgently needed, direct communication with the transfusion service will facilitate access to potentially life-saving blood products. Every transfusion service has a physician who can be consulted when questions arise concerning transfusion reaction investigation and management.

BIBLIOGRAPHY

Capon SM, Goldfinger D: Acute hemolytic transfusion reaction, a paradigm of the systemic inflammatory response: New insights into pathophysiology and treatment. Transfusion 35:513–20, 1995.
This is a good in-depth review of the pathophysiology and treatment of acute hemolytic transfusion reactions.

DeChristopher PJ, Anderson RR: Risks of transfusion and organ and tissue transplantation—practical concerns that drive practical policies. Am J Clin Pathol 107:S2–S11, 1997.
This contains an overview of frequencies of adverse effects of blood component transfusion.

Hume HA, Popovsky MA, Benson K, et al: Hypotensive reactions: A previously uncharacterized complication of platelet transfusion? Transfusion 36:904–909, 1996.
This discusses the pathophysiology of this newly recognized transfusion reaction.

Jeter EK, Spivey MA: Noninfectious complications of blood transfusion. Hematol Oncol Clin North Am 9:187–204, 1995.
This is a good comprehensive review.

Owen HG, Brecher ME: Atypical reactions associated with use of angiotensin-converting enzyme inhibitor and apheresis. Transfusion 34:891–894, 1994.
This study supports discontinuing ACE inhibitors prior to apheresis to avoid severe reactions.

Sazama K, DeChristopher PJ, Dodd R, et al: Practice parameter for the recognition, management, and prevention of adverse consequences of blood transfusion. Arch Pathol Lab Med 124:60–70, 2000.
Comprehensive practice guidelines approved by the College of American Pathologists that cover both acute and long-term adverse consequences of blood transfusion. It is available online from the web site www.cap.org.

Wagner S: Transfusion-related bacterial sepsis. Curr Opin Hematol 4:464–469, 1997.
This is a comprehensive review of transfusion-related bacterial sepsis.

47

Limb Swelling

Indira Gurubhagavatula
Gregory Tino

Swelling of the limbs is common among critically ill patients. Although it has myriad causes, deep venous thrombosis (DVT) is one of the most important because it may result in a life-threatening pulmonary embolism (PE). This chapter reviews the pathophysiology of limb swelling and presents an algorithm for the evaluation and management of the patient who experiences limb swelling in the intensive care unit (ICU). It focuses particularly on the diagnosis, prevention, and treatment of DVT.

PATHOPHYSIOLOGY

One third of body water is extracellular. This volume is distributed between the interstitial (75%) and the intravascular (25%) spaces by Starling forces, that is, the hydrostatic and colloid osmotic pressures within each compartment. *Edema* is the pathologic increase in the interstitial component of the extracellular fluid volume and results from an imbalance in Starling forces or destruction of capillary wall integrity, or both.

The distribution of edema is an important factor in determining its cause. *Generalized* edema may be insidious in onset with a patient gaining 3 to 5 L in excess fluid before it becomes clinically evident. It may result from hypoalbuminemia; cardiac, renal, or hepatic disease; or positive pressure ventilation that attenuates release of atrial natriuretic factor (Table 47–1). On clinical examination, generalized edema may appear to be confined to the pleural or peritoneal cavity or dependent zones such as the sacrum. *Localized* edema usually results from occlusion of venous or lymphatic channels (see Table 47–1).

In the 19th century, Virchow proposed that the triad of venous stasis, endothelial injury, and hypercoagulability is fundamental for the development of DVT. Stasis from factors such as prolonged bed rest and vasodilatory effects of sepsis may increase the likelihood of leukocyte adhesion to vessel walls and subsequent intimal injury. Other triggers for injury include direct trauma, surgical manipulation, and venous catheter insertion. Injury exposes thrombogenic matrix proteins and activates the extrinsic pathway of coagulation. In addition, hypercoagulability is associated with medical conditions commonly seen in ICUs, such as malignancy and disseminated intravascular coagulation. Transient hypercoagulability may occur during critical illness or after surgery from decreased fibrinolysis, increased catecholamine-induced platelet aggregation, and reduced hepatic clearance of clotting factors. Finally, some patients may have inherited hypercoagulable states.

DIAGNOSTIC EVALUATION OF LIMB SWELLING

A focused history and physical examination are crucial in the initial evaluation of patients with edema. The distribution, acuity of onset, and presence of associated

541

Table 47–1. Causes of Edema in the Intensive Care Unit

	LOCALIZED	GENERALIZED
Venous and Lymphatic Obstruction	Portal vein obstruction Postoperative and iatrogenic (vein removal or ligation, groin dissection, after mastectomy, central venous catheter placement, dressing, cast, tourniquet) Thrombosis, thrombophlebitis Trauma (compartment syndrome, a ruptured Baker cyst, hematoma, fracture)	Cardiovascular causes (congestive heart failure, constrictive pericarditis) Positive pressure ventilation, especially with high positive end-expiratory pressure
Increased Capillary Permeability	Angioneurotic edema Burn injury Infection (cellulitis, abscess, osteomyelitis, gas gangrene)	Sepsis and systemic inflammatory response syndrome (SIRS) Anaphylaxis
Hypoalbuminemia		Cirrhosis Nephrosis Cachexia Catabolic state

symptoms should be determined. In particular, the presence of DVT risk factors (Table 47–2) should be sought. An algorithm for the physical examination, diagnostic testing, and treatment of localized and generalized edema is shown in Figure 47–1.

Physical Examination

Physical examination is an insensitive and nonspecific tool for identifying DVT, with a false-positive rate of about 50% (compared with the "gold standard" of venography). Physical findings may develop late in the course of disease or may be absent altogether. The most useful physical finding is *unilateral edema*. Other findings, with their prevalences, include localized pain (56%), tenderness (55%),

Table 47–2. Risk Factors for Deep Venous Thrombosis

Advanced age Burns Congestive heart failure Direct trauma to vein (hip or knee surgery, central venous catheter insertion, and so on) Hypercoagulable state (acquired, inherited) Malignancy Pregnancy, postpartum state	Premenopausal estrogen use Prior history of DVT Prolonged venous stasis (more than 3 days bed rest, prolonged inactivity, surgery longer than 30 minutes, paralysis) Trauma (fractures of long bone, pelvis, spine)

DVT, deep venous thrombosis.

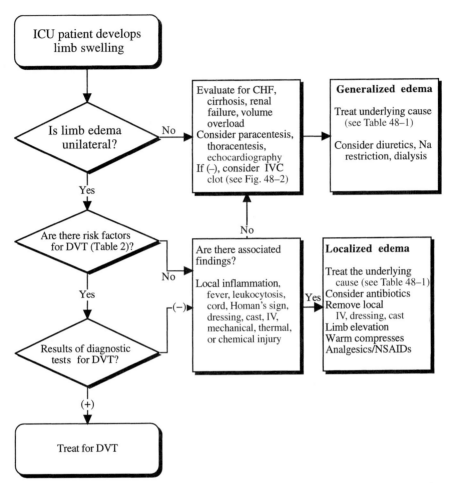

Figure 47–1. Schematic flow diagram for evaluation and treatment of limb swelling. DVT, deep venous thrombosis; CHF, congestive heart failure; IVC, inferior vena cava; IV, intravenous; Na, sodium; NSAIDS, nonsteroidal anti-inflammatory drugs.

warmth (42%), erythema (34%) and palpable cord (6%). Homan's sign (13%) is the development of calf pain on passive dorsiflexion of the foot, but it is not specific for DVT. Low-grade fever or prominent superficial limb veins may be evident. In cases of extensive thrombosis, massive swelling, diminished peripheral pulses, and cyanosis may occur.

The presence of multiple risk factors should raise strong suspicion of DVT even with few physical findings. In contrast, when physical findings occur without DVT risk factors, one should search for conditions other than DVT.

Impedance Plethysmography

Impedance plethysmography (IPG) is a rapid, safe, inexpensive, and well-validated bedside test for DVT. IPG measures venous outflow in the leg before and after occlusion of blood flow by a pneumatic cuff placed around the thigh. The cuff is inflated and then abruptly deflated. Electrical resistance is recorded by means of circumferential calf electrodes. The initial venous volume is plotted against the volume 3 seconds after cuff deflation and is compared with a discriminant line.

IPG has several advantages. Its greatest value is its high sensitivity (96 to 100%) in excluding *proximal* (above the popliteal fossa) lower extremity DVT in *symptomatic* patients. In asymptomatic patients, the sensitivity falls to as low as 50%. Its accuracy is also relatively operator-independent.

IPG, however, has several limitations. One is its high false-positive rate (decreased specificity) in specific clinical settings, which, unfortunately, are common in the ICU (Table 47–3). IPG also cannot detect nonocclusive proximal DVT or isolated calf DVT. Serial tests are required to exclude clot propagation if initial results are negative and clinical suspicion is high. An algorithm for the use of IPG is provided in Figure 47–2.

Ultrasonography, Duplex Scanning, and Color Flow Doppler

Doppler ultrasonography requires directing an ultrasound beam at a vein. Moving blood reflects the beam back at a changed frequency that generates sound. Ultrasonography can evaluate vein patency and venous valve competency in the common femoral, superficial femoral, and popliteal veins. It is 76 to 96% sensitive and 84 to 100% specific for diagnosis of DVT, but results vary according to the experience and expertise of the personnel performing and interpreting the test results. *Duplex scanning* refers to the combination of Doppler ultrasonography with real-time (B-mode) ultrasonography. Using the latter, veins may be visualized directly and assessed for compressibility and the presence of increased intraluminal echogenicity, which represents thrombus. The sensitivity of duplex scanning is 89 to 100% and the specificity is 97 to 100%, again with the potential for different test characteristics locally. *Color flow Doppler ultrasonography* is a newer and more rapid modality than duplex scanning. Blood flowing toward the detector appears red, blood flowing away blue, and stationary structures gray. Absence of flow in a vein despite compression and Valsalva indicates the presence of thrombus. Its

Table 47–3. Conditions Associated with False-Positive Impedance Plethysmographic Results

Increased Central Venous Pressure	**Reduced Local Venous Outflow**
Airway obstruction, e.g., asthma	Extrinsic compression of femoral or
Cardiac tamponade	iliac vein
Congestive heart failure	Severe arterial insufficiency from
Cor pulmonale	Arterial occlusive disease
Intrinsic PEEP (auto-PEEP)	Severe hypotension
Mechanical ventilation	Use of vasoconstrictor
Increased Intra-abdominal Pressure	Unresolved prior DVT
Tense ascites or intra-abdominal hemorrhage	
Near-term pregnancy	

PEEP, positive end-expiratory pressure; DVT, deep venous thrombosis.

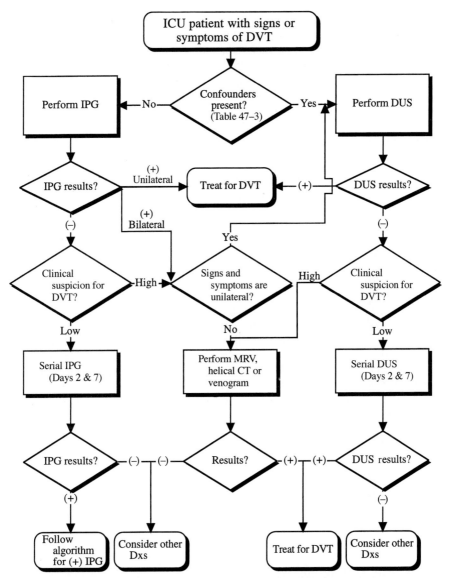

Figure 47–2. Schematic flow diagram of evaluation for deep venous thrombosis (DVT) using impedance plethysmography (IPG). PPV, positive predictive values; DUS, Doppler ultrasonography; MRV,
magnetic resonance venography; Dxs, diagnoses; CT, computed tomography.

reported sensitivity for detecting proximal DVT is 92 to 100% when compared
with venography, and its specificity is 100%.

Ultrasonography and color flow Doppler are noninvasive, widely available and,
unlike IPG, can diagnose conditions other than DVT (such as a Baker's cyst, soft
tissue masses, adenopathy, fluid collections, and pseudoaneurysms). They may also

be used for the diagnosis of upper extremity DVT. However, in contrast to IPG, they require expensive equipment, a skilled operator, and up to 30 to 60 minutes to perform the test. In addition, the interpretation of results is subjective. Ultrasonographic studies may be technically limited by structural and anatomic features, such as the presence of orthopedic devices, central venous or arterial catheters; open wounds; burns; or morbid obesity.

Venography

Venography has been the gold standard for the diagnosis of DVT since the 1980s. However, it requires considerable expertise to perform and interpret. In fact, misinterpretation occurs in as many as 10% of cases. Futhermore, up to 5 to 10% of studies cannot be completed because of technical failures, such as inadequate venous filling. Complications include pain, *induction* of thrombus in 1 to 2% of patients, infection, phlebitis, bleeding, and the risks of radiocontrast administration.

Magnetic Resonance Venography

Among the newer technologies available for the diagnosis of DVT is magnetic resonance venography (MRV), which offers a noninvasive means of direct visualization of veins without radiocontrast injection. From the images obtained, an array of projectional views can be constructed and the entire venous system thus visualized. The presence and the age of intraluminal clot as well as nonthrombotic causes of edema can often be established. Moreover, imaging of iliac veins, heart, and central vessels is also possible. Current limitations of MRV include expense, lack of universal availability, and lack of portability.

PROPHYLAXIS AGAINST DEEP VENOUS THROMBOSIS

Prophylaxis against thromboembolic disease is indicated for all ICU patients who are immobilized and have the potential for prolonged venous stasis (see Table 47–2). Both pharmacologic and mechanical means are at the ICU physician's disposal.

Pharmacologic Prophylaxis

Low-dose heparin, 5000 units given subcutaneously (SQ) every 8 to 12 hours, reduces the incidence of DVT and PE in patients in the ICU and reduces mortality from PE. When combined with antithrombin III, heparin accelerates its action. Heparin also inactivates clotting Factors IX, X, XI, and XII. The most important effects are its inhibition of the conversion of Factor X to Xa and its antithrombin effect. Approximately 50 to 70% of cases of thromboembolism are prevented in postoperative patients treated with low-dose heparin. Although injection or wound hematomas may occur, the risk of major bleeding is not increased even postoperatively.

Adjusted-dose subcutaneous heparin is given to patients who are at somewhat higher risk for thromboembolism, including those undergoing total hip replacement. The dose of SQ heparin is 7500 to 15,000 units every 12 hours and is increased to maintain the activated partial thromboplastin time (PTT) drawn 6 hours after administration at 1.5 to 2 times control. In patients undergoing total hip replacement, this therapy reduces DVT risk from 39 to 13%.

Dextran is as effective as low-dose heparin if given at the time of surgery and on the first postoperative day for some patients but is ineffective in patients undergoing major orthopedic surgery, such as hip replacement or hip fracture repair. Since it may cause serious allergic reactions, its routine use should be discouraged.

Low molecular weight (LMW) heparins, which are obtained by gel filtration of standard heparin, require less frequent (once daily) dosing. The risk of heparin-induced thrombocytopenia may be lower, whereas the risk of bleeding complications is the same or less compared with standard (unfractionated) heparin. However, the PTT cannot be used to adjust dose. Several studies have compared enoxaparin (one of several LMW heparins) with standard heparin, dextran, and placebo for prophylaxis in total hip replacement. The efficacy of enoxaparin was at least equal to that of standard heparin and better than dextran. The rate of fatal PE or the need for postoperative transfusion was lower than that with dextran. More studies are needed that compare various LMW heparins to each other and to determine their cost-effectiveness. Enoxaparin is now being used routinely at some institutions for DVT prophylaxis in patients undergoing hip and knee surgery.

Warfarin is used for DVT prophylaxis in patients at high risk for DVT, such as those undergoing hip repair or replacement. Warfarin is the most commonly used oral anticoagulant and is also available for intravenous use. It inhibits the action of the four vitamin K-dependent factors: II, VII, IX, and X. After initiation of therapy, the prothrombin time (PT) is primarily affected by Factor VII, which which has the shortest half-life of the four—6 hours. Because Factors IX, X, and II have half-lives of 24 to more than 48 hours, the PT must be elevated for at least 48 hours to ensure inhibition of these factors and attainment of an effective antithrombotic state. The measured PT time reflects the dose given 1 to 2 days earlier. Because many drugs interact with warfarin, careful review of medication profiles is mandatory.

Mechanical Prophylaxis

The most popular method of mechanical DVT prophylaxis is the use of lower extremity pneumatic compression devices. When applied externally to the legs, pneumatic compression devices reduce the incidence of DVT from 22.9 to 6.7%. They reduce venous stasis by direct compression of veins in a pulsatile fashion, and they also offer a local and systemic fibrinolytic effect. Thus, if placement of the device on one leg is precluded by the presence of an orthopedic device, wound, or other mechanical considerations, it may still be applied to the other leg or to an arm, or both. Pneumatic compression devices are recommended for DVT prophylaxis when SQ heparin is contraindicated (e.g., because of the risk of intracranial bleeding). They are also being used in conjunction with SQ heparin in patients at high risk for DVT because evidence suggests that using both together is more effective than using either one alone. Compression devices are relatively safe, but they should not be used in patients who already have DVT because that may precipitate embolism.

Several types of *interruptive filters* placed in the inferior vena cava below the renal veins will prevent PE but not DVT (Table 47–4). The Greenfield filter is a conical, six-pronged percutaneously placed device whose tip captures emboli while blood flows around the sides. Recurrent emboli via collaterals may occur as soon as 4 months after filter placement but with an incidence of less than 4%. Patency rates from several studies are 95 to 98% at 10 years. Other percutaneously placed filters are also available.

Inferior vena cava ligation with sutures or clips compares less favorably to inferior vena cava filter placement because it requires general anesthesia and laparotomy and has poorer flow rates and more sequelae of venous stasis than does a filter placement.

TREATMENT OF DEEP VENOUS THROMBOSIS

The most feared complication of DVT is PE. Untreated DVT may also lead to post-thrombophlebitis syndrome, manifested as varicose veins, edema, skin pigmentation, extremity pain, liposclerosis, and sometimes frank ulceration. The two main treatment options for DVT include (1) anticoagulation with heparin followed by warfarin and (2) thrombolytic therapy.

Anticoagulation prevents clot extension, embolization, and early recurrence. It is indicated for patients with proximal DVT (in veins proximal to the popliteal vein) or for those with calf vein DVT that has propagated above the popliteal fossa. Propagation rates of 5.6 to 23% have been described in postoperative patients and of approximately 10% in symptomatic patients. Almost all occurrences of PE associated with calf DVT are due to proximal propagation. Most data support serial IPG or Doppler ultrasonographic studies to follow isolated calf vein DVT over the first week after DVT diagnosis, reserving the use of anticoagulant therapy only after proximal extension has been documented (see Fig. 47–2).

Unless contraindicated, initial treatment should consist of continuous anticoagulation with intravenous heparin. Heparin acts immediately and has a half-life of 60 to 90 minutes. The usual dose is a bolus of 80 units/kg followed by a continuous infusion of 18 units/kg per hour of infusion. Weight-based dosing (see Table 12–4

Table 47–4. Indications for Inferior Vena Cava Filter Placement

....

After pulmonary or cardiac embolectomy
Cardiopulmonary reserve insufficient to tolerate another PE (see Fig. 76–1)
Complication of anticoagulation
Contraindication to anticoagulation
Massive DVT or thrombus at high risk for embolization
Occurrence of PE despite 2 days of full anticoagulation ("failure of anticoagulation")
Prophylaxis in selected orthopedic surgical or trauma patients who have suffered
　　multiple long bone or pelvic fractures.

....

PE, pulmonary embolism; DVT, deep venous thrombosis.

for dosing algorithm) achieves therapeutic effect more quickly than does fixed dosing (i.e., a 5000-unit bolus followed by an infusion of 1000 units per hour) while remaining as safe and efficacious. Higher doses of heparin are needed early in treatment, and lower doses are sufficient later. Therefore, the PTT should be monitored frequently early in anticoagulation and less often once a stable dose is reached. Dose should be adjusted to keep the PTT at 1.5 to 2 times normal (usually 50 to 80 seconds).

Patients who have a large clot burden may require more than 24 hours to achieve therapeutic anticoagulation. Risk of recurrence is decreased if therapeutic PTT is reached within 24 hours. Approximately 5 to 6% of patients treated with heparin experience thrombocytopenia and 5 to 10% experience bleeding, so hemoglobin and platelet count should be monitored. Thrombocytopenia is usually mild but may be severe in patients previously treated with heparin. Heparin-induced thrombocytopenia is occasionally associated with paradoxical arterial thrombosis, the so-called white dot syndrome (see Chapter 45). If severe bleeding or marked thrombocytopenia occurs, heparin should be stopped. In patients requiring large doses of heparin (at least 35,000 units/day) or in those with an elevated PTT resulting from the presence of an antiphospholipid antibody (e.g., a lupus anticoagulant), a heparin assay that measures anti-Factor Xa activity has been shown to be safe and effective for monitoring anticoagulation to avoid unnecessary dose escalation. Its use may also lower bleeding risk when compared with the use of PTT.

Subcutaneous *LMW heparin* appears to be at least as safe and effective as continuous intravenous heparin and more convenient to administer. However, its routine use requires confirmation by additional randomized clinical trials comparing it with conventional heparin.

Oral *warfarin* may be administered along with heparin in stable patients without contraindication to oral anticoagulation to reduce length of stay, hospital costs, and the incidence of heparin-associated thrombocytopenia. Heparin is continued for a minimum of 4 to 5 days and stopped thereafter without taper, once the prothrombin time has been at therapeutic levels for 2 days. The starting dose of warfarin should be 5 to 10 mg per day. It should be titrated to maintain international normalized ratio of 2 to 3, with higher levels in patients with recurrent DVT or PE. An intravenous form of warfarin is now available for use.

If oral anticoagulation is contraindicated, or if the patient demonstrates resistance (e.g., due to malignancy), alternative forms of therapy should be considered, including chronic treatment with adjusted-dose SQ heparin (5000 to 7500 units three times per day) or inferior vena cava filter placement.

Thrombolytic therapy is usually reserved for cases of acute, massive DVT because of the threefold increase in bleeding risk compared with heparin alone and the 1% risk of cerebral hemorrhage. However, lytic therapy may reduce the incidence of post-thrombophlebitic syndrome. Treatment initiated within 5 to 7 days of the onset of symptoms is more likely to dissolve clots successfully than treatment given 1 to 3 weeks after the onset of symptoms. Showering of emboli may occur during therapy, and placement of an inferior vena cava filter before initiation of lytic therapy is important in patients with low cardiopulmonary reserve.

Upper Extremity Deep Venous Thrombosis

Early studies suggested that 1 to 2% of all DVT occurs in the upper extremities, but the prevalence is probably higher now because of the widespread use of subclavian and internal jugular venous catheters in the ICU. The frequency of catheter-associated DVT is 13 to 35%. Clot formation is related to catheter size and composition, duration of placement, number of venipuncture attempts, substance infused, and occurrence of infection. Coating catheters with heparin-benzalkonium has reduced the incidence of catheter-associated clot. Use of aseptic technique, minimization of venipuncture attempts, prompt catheter removal, and ensuring that the tip rests in a high-flow vessel such as the superior vena cava reduces the risk further. Diagnosis requires using ultrasonography, computerized tomography, MRV or venography. Although upper extremity DVT was not routinely treated in the past with anticoagulation, current practice is to initiate timely therapy in order to prevent the 5 to 12% incidence of PE as well as other potential complications, such as septic thrombophlebitis, superior vena cava syndrome, venous gangrene, or chronic limb disability.

BIBLIOGRAPHY

Bergqvist D, Lowe GDO, Berstad A, et al: Prevention of venous thromboembolism after surgery: A review of enoxaparin. Br J Surg 79:495–498, 1992.
This article presents a brief review of low molecular weight heparins in thromboprophylaxis.

Carpenter JP, et al: Magnetic resonance venography for the detection of deep venous thrombosis: Comparison with contrast venography and duplex Doppler ultrasonography. J Vasc Surg 18:734–741, 1993.
This article compares blinded readings of duplex scanning, venography, and magnetic resonance venography among 85 patients and concludes that magnetic resonance venography is an accurate diagnostic technique for imaging DVT.

Goldhaber SZ, Buring JE, Lipnick RJ, et al: Interruption of the inferior vena cava by clip or filter. Am J Med 76:512–516, 1984.
This is a brief review of clips and filters used for caval interruption.

Horattas MC, Wright DJ, Fenton AH, et al: Changing concepts of deep venous thrombosis of the upper extremity—Report of a series and review of the literature. Surgery 104:561–567, 1988.
This is a retrospective review of patients in whom symptomatic axillary or subclavian vein thrombosis developed; pulmonary embolization was seen in 12% of the patients. The article reviews diagnosis and treatment of upper extremity DVT.

Hoyt DB, Swegle JR: Deep venous thrombosis in the surgical intensive care unit. Surg Clin North Am 71:811–830, 1991.
This article presents a thorough review of diagnosis, prophylaxis, and therapy for DVT in critically ill surgical patients.

Huisman MB, Buller HR, ten Cate JW, Vreekan J: Serial impedance plethysmography for suspected deep venous thrombosis in outpatients. The Amsterdam General Practitioner Study. N Engl J Med 314:823–828, 1986.
In 426 patients suspected of having acute DVT, the value of serial IPG is compared with venography. None of the 289 patients with normal IPG results acquired pulmonary embolus during a 6-month follow-up period.

Hull RD, Hirsh J, Carter CJ, et al: Diagnostic efficacy of impedance plethysmography for clinically suspected deep-vein thrombosis. Ann Intern Med 102:21–28, 1985.
A randomized trial of IPG versus IPG plus leg scanning in 634 patients found that IPG alone is an effective way of evaluating symptomatic patients.

Mudge M, Leinster SJ, Hughes LE: A prospective 10-year study of the post-thrombotic syndrome in a surgical population. Ann Roy Coll Surg Engl 70:249–252, 1988.
This article discusses a 10-year prospective study of 564 patients undergoing laparotomy to determine the incidence of post-thrombotic syndrome.

Richlie DG: Noninvasive imaging of the lower extremity for deep venous thrombosis. J Gen Intern Med 8:271–277, 1993.
This is a succinct, thorough review of plethysmography, ultrasound, and color-flow Doppler, with their respective strengths and limitations.

Turpie AGG, Levine MN, Hirsh J, et al: A randomized controlled trial of a low-molecular-weight heparin (enoxaparin) to prevent deep-vein thrombosis in patients undergoing elective hip surgery. N Engl J Med 315:925–929, 1986.
This article presents a study of 100 patients undergoing hip surgery to determine whether LMW heparin is safe and effective in preventing DVT. Comparison with placebo revealed a DVT incidence of 12% in the treated group versus 42% in the placebo group.

Wheeler HB: Diagnosis of deep vein thrombosis: Review of clinical evaluation and impedance plethysmography. Am J Surg 150:7–13, 1985.
This article reviews the value of history, physical examination, and IPG in the diagnosis of DVT.

Wheeler HB, Hirsh J, Wells P, Anderson FA: Diagnostic tests for deep vein thrombosis: Clinical usefulness depends on probability of disease. Arch Intern Med 154:1921–1928, 1994.
This is a review of the important principles in interpretation of diagnostic tests, offering a useful algorithm for the diagnosis of DVT.

48 Ventilator Alarm Situations

Daniel J. Reily
Paul N. Lanken

Contemporary microprocessor-based mechanical ventilators provide a wide selection of ventilatory modes that can customize assisted ventilation to individual patients. These technologically advanced ventilators incorporate a variety of alarms to alert intensive care unit (ICU) clinicians to numerous potentially dangerous situations. Ventilator alarms are designed to inform, but not dictate, the actions necessary to correct the potential hazard. For this reason, it is imperative that ICU practitioners be familiar with the function of the array of these alarms, how to evaluate ventilator alarm situations, and how to successfully manage those situations.

TYPES OF VENTILATOR ALARMS

The type and number of alarms that are functional on a ventilator vary depending on which ventilatory mode is being used. In addition, identical alarms may have different meanings and response times in different modes. Finally, alarms can signify different levels of clinical urgency (Table 48–1).

In face of this complexity, the ability to categorize ventilator alarms is essential. All alarms can be categorized into three types based on whether they indicate (1) a ventilator failure, (2) a patient-ventilator interface problem, or (3) a patient-related event.

Because most modern ventilators function by combining a microprocessor-based electromechanical system with a pneumatic system, *ventilator failure* can result from a malfunction in its electronic or pneumatic systems. Ventilator manufacturers incorporate *preset alarms* to ensure the safety of these systems. In the

Table 48–1. Level of Urgency of Ventilator Alarms

LEVEL*	PRIORITY	TYPE OF EVENT	EXAMPLES
1	Highest	Immediately life-threatening	Electrical power failure Loss of pneumatic power Exhalation valve failure
2	High	Eventually life-threatening if problem persists	High airway pressure Low exhaled volume Inverse inspiratory:expiratory time (I:E) ratio
3	Low	Not life-threatening or a one-time event	Short period of high respiratory rate One-time high airway pressure

*Level is indicated by tone, pitch, or volume of the audio alarm, or by information on the ventilator's visual display, or both.

553

case of a true ventilator failure and not user error, for example, a power cord being disconnected, there is little choice but to recognize the problem quickly and replace the ventilator.

Patient-ventilator interface problems refer to the interaction of the ventilated patient with the ventilator. Thresholds for alarms arising from problems at this interface are usually set by a respiratory care practitioner and relate closely to the ventilator's monitoring capabilities. Significantly, these alarms may alert the ICU clinician to problems in how ventilatory support is being provided to the patient. They can signify a range of situations, for example, from a patient becoming disconnected from the ventilator to the peak inspiratory flow failing to meet a patient's inspiratory demand.

Patient-related event alarms are synonymous with "monitoring alarms." They are designed to detect changes in the patient's underlying physiologic condition. When a simple physiologic monitor alarm, for example, an electrocardiographic monitor, activates, the reason for the alarm arises from a patient-related event and not the functioning of the monitor itself. In contrast, a ventilator with its alarms serves not only as a physiologic monitor but also as a therapeutic intervention whose effects are continuously self-monitored. ICU clinicians often have difficulty in recognizing when a problem arises from the patient or from the ventilator and in distinguishing patient-ventilator interface problems from those solely attributable to the patient (patient-related events).

Each commonly used ventilator alarm is designed to detect a certain acute abnormality, as indicated by its name. Many alarms, however, overlap in the underlying conditions that they detect, as well as in the clinical consequences that they aim to prevent (Table 48–2). For example, if the patient becomes disconnected from the ventilator, multiple alarms activate. Early-response alarms monitor low inspiratory pressure, low exhaled tidal volume and low positive end-expiratory pressure (if positive end-expiratory pressure had been applied before the discon-nection). Later alarms include low expired minute ventilation and apnea. Not only do these ventilator-associated alarms form a redundant safety net, but they also are complemented by nonventilator alarms, such as a pulse oximeter, or electrocar-diographic lead monitoring. Tables 48–3 to 48–7 list conditions in which alarming is used frequently, with their differential diagnoses, categorized according to site of the problem, and matched with appropriate corrections.

VENTILATOR ALARMS: IDENTIFYING THE SITE OF THE PROBLEM

Certain alarms fall into both patient–ventilator interface alarms and patient-event alarms categories. Alarms for airway pressures, respiratory rate, and exhaled volumes can have different meanings in different applications and, for this reason, serve as useful examples to consider in detail.

High and Low Airway Pressure Alarms

Peak airway pressure, also called peak inflation pressure or peak inspiratory pressure (PIP), is the maximal airway pressure needed to deliver a certain tidal

Table 48–2. Common Ventilator Alarms

NAME OF ALARM	DETECTS	DESIGNED TO PREVENT
High inspiratory pressure	Acute increase in peak airway pressure	Barotrauma
Low inspiratory pressure	Large air leak	Delivery of inadequate tidal volume
	Patient disconnection from ventilator circuit	Hypoventilation, hypoxemia
		Patient discomfort
	Insufficient response by the ventilator to the patient's inspiratory demand	Excessive work of breathing
Low PEEP or CPAP pressure	Small leak in the system	Loss of end-expiratory pressure
		Decrease in Pao$_2$
High end-expiratory pressure	Resistance to exhalation	Partial or complete obstruction of expiratory breathing circuit
Low exhaled tidal volume	Air leak	Insufficient ventilatory support
	Decrease in spontaneous tidal volumes	Hypoventilation
Low exhaled minute ventilation	Decrease in mechanical or spontaneous volumes	Insufficient ventilatory support
		Hypoventilation
	Decreased lung compliance*	Respiratory compromise
	Onset of respiratory muscle fatigue*	
High exhaled minute ventilation	Increase in lung compliance*	Hyperventilation
		Dynamic hyperinflation
	Excessive ventilation	Acute respiratory alkalosis
High respiratory rate	Respiratory distress, including anxiety, pain	Respiratory compromise
		Patient discomfort
	Self-cycling ventilator	Hyperventilation
	Onset of respiratory muscle fatigue	Dynamic hyperinflation
		Acute respiratory alkalosis
Inverted inspiratory: expiratory ratio	Self-cycling ventilator	Hyperventilation
	Insufficient expiratory time	Dynamic hyperinflation (air trapping with auto-PEEP)
	Inadvertent inspiratory pause	
Apnea	Respiratory arrest	Hypoventilation with hypercapnia
		Hypoxemia
Low oxygen-air inlet pressure	Disconnection of oxygen or compressed air source	Hypoxemia
	Fall in oxygen or air pressure to less than minimal level	Insufficient pressure to power the ventilator's pneumatic system
Power disconnect	Electrical power failure	Failure of all components of the ventilator that require electrical power to operate
	Ventilator unplugged by mistake	
Low or high Fio$_2$	A variance between the set Fio$_2$ and the analyzed Fio$_2$	Hypoxemia
		Oxygen toxicity
		Misinformed clinical decisions based on incorrect Fio$_2$
Ventilator inoperative	Malfunction in the ventilator serious enough to be unsafe for patient use	All potentially harmful effects of the ventilator on the patient
		Insufficient ventilatory support

*Pertains to pressure control and pressure support modes of ventilation.
PEEP, positive end-expiratory pressure; CPAP, continuous positive airway pressure.

Table 48–3. Ventilator Alarm Conditions: High Peak Airway Pressures Due to High Airway Resistance

PROBLEM	SITE OF EVENT	CORRECTIVE ACTION
Coughing	Patient	Suction; increase sedation
Airway occlusion due to mucous plugs	Patient	Suction; bronchoscopy; give intratracheal N-acetylcysteine
Biting on endotracheal tube	Patient	Suction to confirm obstruction at mouth level; insert a bite block
Bronchospasm	Patient	Treat bronchospasm
Patient asynchrony with ventilator	Patient-ventilator interface	Adjust settings to better meet patient needs; reassure anxious patient
Ventilator circuit obstructed by condensed water	Ventilator	Drain water from circuit

volume to the patient. High PIPs result when airway resistance increases, when lung compliance decreases, or when both occur. If PIP increases without a decrease in compliance, airway resistance must have increased. *High peak pressure alarms* are commonly caused by problems with a patient's airway, such as partial obstruction of an endotracheal tube caused by biting or kinking or increased secretions or bronchospasm (Tables 48–3 and 48–4).

Low airway pressure alarms (Table 48–5) are often associated with air leaks in the ventilator's breathing circuits, for example, around the cuff of an endotracheal tube, or when the patient's inspiratory effort persists during the inspiration cycle (resulting from enhanced respiratory efforts). The negative pressure that the patient

Table 48–4. Ventilator Alarm Conditions: High Peak Airway Pressures Due to Low Respiratory System Compliance

PROBLEM	SITE OF EVENT	CORRECTIVE ACTION
Tension pneumothorax	Patient	Decompress acutely with needle, insert chest tube
"Flash" pulmonary edema	Patient	Treat cardiac cause, e.g., ischemia
Endotracheal tube tip in right main bronchus	Patient-ventilator interface	Confirm with auscultation, reposition ETT and secure
Inverse I:E ratio	Patient-ventilator interface	Shorten inspiration; extend expiration
"Bucking" (resisting positive pressure breath)	Patient-ventilator interface	Sedation, change to more compatible mode; reassure patient
Excessively large tidal volume delivered	Patient-ventilator interface	Decrease tidal volume delivered

I:E, inspiratory:expiratory; ETT, endotracheal tube.

Table 48–5. Ventilator Alarm Conditions: Low Inspiratory Pressure, Low Continuous Positive Airway Pressure, or Low Positive End-Expiratory Pressure

PROBLEM	SITE OF EVENT	CORRECTIVE ACTION
Leak in system	Patient-ventilator interface	Find and correct leak
Faulty exhalation valve	Ventilator	Correct malfunction
Patient disconnection	Patient	Evaluate and reconnect patient
Insufficient peak flow rate	Patient-ventilator interface	Increase flow to meet the inspiratory demand
Ventilator not properly sensing patient's inspiratory effort	Patient-ventilator interface	Adjust ventilator settings to synchronize with patient's efforts

generates during inspiration reduces the peak pressure to less than the threshold set for the low airway pressure alarm.

High and Low Respiratory Rate Alarms

An increase in respiratory rate is one of the first signs that the patient may be experiencing difficulties in breathing. If the ventilator is not providing adequate support, for example, because of a leak in the circuit or a mechanical malfunction, the patient's respiratory rate increases to compensate for insufficient ventilatory support. Patient-related reasons for activation of a *high respiratory rate alarm* include anxiety, pain, an acute neurologic event (resulting in central neurogenic hyperventilation), hypoxemia, hypercapnia, metabolic acidosis, respiratory distress, or respiratory muscle fatigue (Table 48–6).

A *low respiratory rate alarm* activates when a patient becomes apneic or the patient's respiratory drive has been acutely suppressed because of sedation (or other causes of central nervous system depression).

Table 48–6. Ventilator Alarm Conditions: High Respiratory Rate

PROBLEM	SITE OF EVENT	CORRECTIVE ACTION
Hypoxia	Patient-ventilator interface	Increase F_{IO_2}
Anxiety	Patient	Increase sedation
Pain	Patient	Increase analgesic
Respiratory muscle fatigue	Patient-ventilator interface	Increase ventilatory support
Dyspnea	Patient-ventilator interface	Increase ventilatory support, treat symptoms with opioids
Low ventilator sensing threshold	Patient-ventilator interface	Adjust sensitivity
Cardiac pulsations	Patient-ventilator interface	Adjust sensitivity
Central neurogenic hyperventilation	Patient-ventilator interface	Give opioids; paralyze patient as last resort

Table 48–7. Ventilator Alarm Conditions: Low Exhaled Tidal Volume

PROBLEM	SITE OF EVENT	CORRECTIVE ACTION
Leak in circuit	Patient-ventilator interface	Correct leak
Patient disconnected	Patient-ventilator interface	Reconnect patient
Leak through chest tube	Patient	Adjust alarms
Patient's spontaneous tidal volume decreased	Patient	Adjust ventilatory support
Decreased lung compliance (in PS)	Patient	Evaluate patient
Alarm set improperly	Patient-ventilator interface	Adjust alarms
Leak around tracheal cuff	Patient-ventilator interface	Evaluate, reposition and reinflate ETT

PS, pressure support mode of ventilation; ETT, endotracheal tube.

Low Exhaled Volume Alarm

A ventilator's breathing circuit and an endotracheal tube provide the means for the ventilator to deliver a volume of gas to the patient's lungs. It is imperative that this be a sealed system to ensure that the patient actually receives the gas volume generated by the ventilator. If there is a leak in this system, the patient receives a smaller than desired tidal volume; this, in turn, results in activation of the *low exhaled volume alarm*. Unless the patient is spontaneously breathing (as noted earlier in discussing low peak pressure alarms), most low exhaled volume alarms can be attributed to a leak in the circuit or a leak around the endotracheal tube cuff (Table 48–7). As a rule, ventilators are accurate in delivering volumes equal to their set tidal volumes.

A number of patient-related events can trigger a low exhaled volume alarm. This commonly occurs when the patient's spontaneous tidal volumes decrease, often in conjunction with an increase in the patient's respiratory rate, and is referred to as "rapid shallow breathing." This often signifies the onset of respiratory muscle fatigue. When using pressure control or pressure support modes of ventilation, low (or high) changes in exhaled tidal volume (without a leak in the mechanical system) are a good reflection of changes in respiratory system compliance. In response, the ICU clinician should make ventilator changes to prevent hypoventilation, hyperventilation, or overdistention of the lung. One should keep in mind that if a patient has one or more chest tubes in place that have air leaks, the measured exhaled volume will always be less than the delivered tidal volume because of these air leaks.

SETTING AND RESPONDING VENTILATOR ALARMS

Role of Respiratory Care Practitioners in the Intensive Care Unit

Although all health care professionals working in the ICU should be knowledge-able about ventilator alarms, respiratory care practitioners have primary responsibility for ventilator management and for setting all alarms. These individuals (generally identified as Registered Respiratory Therapists [RRT] or Certified Respiratory Therapy Technicians [CRTT]) have had specialized training to deal with ventilators, ventilator quality control, and ventilator-related problems, and they serve as resource persons for ventilator alarms in the ICU. If the ventilator's alarms are set incorrectly, they can lead to false alarms, that is, activating in the absence of a true ventilator mishap or patient event. These false alarms, often called *nuisance alarms,* can compromise patient safety if they lead to failure of ICU staff to respond to true events.

The Alarm Package

Microprocessor-based ventilator alarms can be visual or audible, or both. They also usually signal a message to direct the clinician to the problem. An audio alarm may have been initiated, but by the time the caregiver reaches the bedside the situation may have corrected itself. Most ventilators are equipped with a memory display, which identifies the reason why the alarm originally activated. The alarm package on microprocessor-based ventilators also has a priority level to alert the practitioner to the seriousness of the alarm and, consequently, to the promptness required in responding to the alarm (see Table 48–1).

Built-in Ventilatory Safety Devices

All ventilators have certain safety devices built in to ensure patient safety. Non–microprocessor-based ventilators have only pressure monitoring capabilities. Microprocessor ventilators continuously perform a self-assessment. Although manufacturers have safety features unique to their own products, some are common among most brands in current use. These safety devices are usually designed to protect the patient from any harmful effects caused by ventilator malfunction.

Back-up apnea ventilation is a built-in safety device that serves two main functions: first, it provides as an emergency mode of ventilation when the microprocessor senses a ventilator malfunction and, second, it activates if the ventilated patient becomes apneic for a period longer than the set parameters allow. For some ventilators, the clinician has the option to choose these parameters. For others, the parameters are set by the manufacturer.

The ventilator and the ventilator circuit are a closed system, that is, they are closed to atmospheric pressure. As such, all ventilation and gas sources are provided via the ventilator's pneumatic system. If the ventilator suddenly stops functioning, but the patient is still capable of spontaneous breathing, the patient cannot actually inspire because of the lack of an adequate gas supply. Some ventilators have an inspiratory safety valve that opens the patient's circuit to ambient air if the ventilator suddenly fails.

Most microprocessor-based ventilators require a preuse test before they can be used to ventilate a patient. This assures proper calibration and function beforehand. This test also evaluates the ventilator circuit, making sure all connections are properly sealed and preventing unwanted air leaks. It can even measure the compliance of the circuit, which allows the ventilator to increase its generated tidal volume in order to compensate for the volume needed to expand the tubing during inspiration.

Responding to Ventilator Alarms

When responding to ventilator alarms, one's first priority must be to ensure patient safety. A good rule of thumb is to ventilate the patient manually if one is in doubt

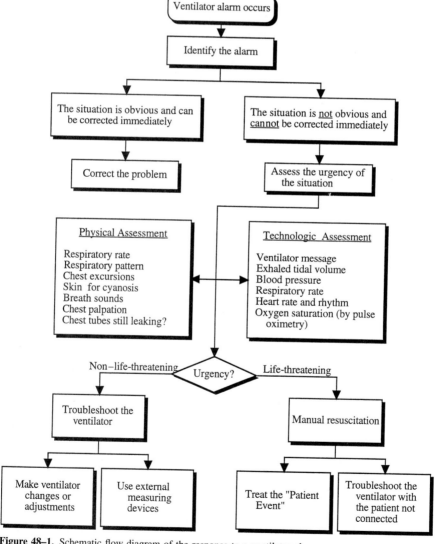

Figure 48–1. Schematic flow diagram of the response to a ventilator alarm.

about the adequacy of the patient's ventilatory support. Likewise, if a potentially dangerous situation cannot be corrected immediately, the patient should be promptly switched from ventilator to a manual resuscitator. After ensuring patient safety, one should take a general stepwise approach when responding to ventilator alarms (Fig. 48–1).

BIBLIOGRAPHY

Kirby RR, Banner MJ, Down JB, et al: Clinical Application of Ventilatory Support. New York: Churchill Livingstone, 1990.
This book presents a practical application to monitoring lung mechanics, including troubleshooting changes in a patient's clinical course.

MacIntyre NR, Day SD: Essentials for ventilator-alarm systems. Respir Care 37:1108–1112, 1992.
The original paper that defined the terminology used in the discussion of ventilator alarm systems.

Pierson DJ, Kacmarek RM: Foundations of Respiratory Care. New York: Churchill Livingstone, 1992.
This is an extensive review of the principles of mechanical ventilation, including a detailed description of the evaluation of the patient ventilator system.

Tobin MJ (ed): Principles and Practice of Mechanical Ventilation. New York: McGraw-Hill, 1994.
This is an excellent, comprehensive analysis of the classification, response requirements, and evaluation of ventilator alarms.

Tobin MJ (ed): Principles and Practice of Intensive Care Monitoring. New York: McGraw-Hill, 1998.
As a companion volume to the preceding reference, it comprehensively reviews aspects of monitoring in the ICU, including ventilator alarms.

49

Acute Coronary Syndromes: Acute Myocardial Infarction and Unstable Angina

Joseph R. McClellan

The anatomic basis for most cases of acute myocardial infarction (MI) and unstable angina is the acute fissuring and rupture of an atherosclerotic plaque in an epicardial coronary artery with formation of superimposed thrombus. Plaques that rupture tend to have a thin fibrous coat over a central collection of foam cells, lipid, and necrotic debris. The vulnerable plaque typically ruptures near its junction with normal endothelium, and this exposes collagen and atheromatous material, which, in turn, leads to thrombosis. The extent of the thrombotic reaction dictates the clinical course and subsequent clinical syndrome. If the injury is severe and deep, the thrombotic reaction may lead to either partial or total occlusion. In addition, a variety of vasoactive mediators are released from the endothelial wall that can cause vasospasm and transient complete occlusion. *Rest angina* frequently results from this type of transient arterial occlusion. If there is a prolonged lack of antegrade blood flow, however, an acute MI occurs.

The triggers of acute plaque rupture are not fully defined. Most likely, acute hemodynamic stress is the trigger, but acute and chronic endothelial inflammation may also play a role. There is a circadian variation in the occurrence of all acute cardiovascular events, including MI, sudden death, and stroke, with their peak frequency in the first 2 hours after awakening. On arising and assuming an upright posture there are a variety of acute circulatory adjustments, including the release of catecholamines, which results in increased cardiovascular tone and hemodynamic stress. In addition, in these hours there is an increase in blood viscosity and platelet aggregation. Beta-blocker therapy eliminates the higher morning incidence of acute cardiovascular events, which suggests that catecholamine release and hemodynamic stress are important causative events.

Left ventricular (LV) dysfunction and cardiogenic shock are the major causes of in-hospital mortality in patients with acute MI. Patients with extensive, transmural infarction may develop severe ventricular dysfunction and hypotension. Reduced blood pressure causes a further reduction in coronary perfusion and leads to progressive deterioration in myocardial function. Cardiogenic shock occurs when more than 40% of the total myocardial mass is damaged (see Chapter 6). Reperfusion with a thrombolytic agent or primary angioplasty reduces the occurrence of cardiogenic shock.

Patients with unstable angina and non–Q wave MI typically have preserved ventricular function, but severe, prolonged ischemia may lead to stunning and reduced contractile function. *Ventricular remodeling* is a term that encompasses all the changes that occur in LV size, shape, and function after an acute MI. Characteristically, the infarcted area of myocardium expands, which may result in progressive LV enlargement and a detrimental effect on both LV function and prognosis. Reducing LV wall stress early in the course of an acute infarct improves

563

LV function and decreases LV size. Because they reduce both preload and afterload, intravenous nitroglycerin and angiotensin-converting enzyme inhibitors are important drug interventions to reduce LV wall stress and infarct size.

Reperfusion therapy with thrombolytic agents or angioplasty, and the presence of collateral circulation, may also have a beneficial effect on infarct size. "The open heart artery hypothesis" holds that a patent infarct-related artery improves outcomes by preventing the transmurality of infarction (which would otherwise result in progressive ventricular dilation) and by providing a conduit for collateral circulation to the rest of the coronary arterial tree. Patients with a patent infarct-related artery also have a reduced frequency of ventricular aneurysm formation and improved myocardial electrical stability.

RISK STRATIFICATION

In unstable angina, the short-term risks of acute MI and in-hospital mortality are approximately 10% and 5%, respectively. These are increased with frequent or prolonged episodes of chest pain, especially if associated with significant ST-segment depression. The importance of the clinical presentation is illustrated by the Duke Angina Score (Table 49–1), which provides important prognostic information. Recurrent silent ischemia during continuous electrocardiographic (ECG) monitoring and large perfusion defects on exercise or pharmacologic stress tests also identify a high-risk group of patients.

In acute MI, the risk of death depends on the extent and severity of infarction and whether significant complications develop. Both clinical (Kilip Class, Table 49–2) and hemodynamic criteria (Table 49–3) are important predictors of outcome. LV function is the most important prognostic indicator. Other clinical predictors of poor outcome include age (especially > 70 years old), anterior location, prior infarction, presence of crackles on chest examination, female gender, and diabetes. A combination of two or more of these factors progressively increases the short-term mortality of acute MI.

More recent studies, using multivariate analyses, suggest that cardiac troponin I or T levels have independent additional prognostic value for patients with

Table 49–1. Duke Angina Score and Prognosis

ANGINA SCORE*	SURVIVAL (%) AT 5 YEARS	INFARCT FREE (%) AT 5 YEARS
0	86	75
6	83	71
12	76	63
21	72	54

*Angina Score = Angina Course Score × [1 + daily frequency] + 6 (if ST segment changes are present) where Angina Course Score = 3 if unstable variant; 2 if progressive with nocturnal; 1 if progressive, no nocturnal; 0 if stable.

From Califf RM, et al. Importance of clinical measures of ischemia in the prognosis of patients with documented coronary artery disease. J Am Coll Cardiol 11:20–26, 1988.

Table 49–2. Kilip Classification for Acute Myocardial Infarction

CLASS	SIGNS/SYMPTOMS	HOSPITAL MORTALITY (%)
I	Normal examination, no congestive heart failure	8
II	Mild congestive heart failure, rales < 50% of lung fields, S3 present	30
III	Pulmonary edema, rales > 50% of lung fields	44
IV	Cardiogenic shock	>80

From Kilip T. Treatment of myocardial infarction in a coronary care unit. Am J Cardiol 70:457, 1967.

unstable angina, non–Q wave acute MI, and Q wave acute MI. These levels can predict risk of subsequent cardiac events as well as predict subsets of patients who will have significant responses to therapeutic interventions.

CLINICAL DIAGNOSIS

Medical History

The wide spectrum of clinical presentations for both unstable angina and acute MI cause difficulties in diagnosis for both patients and physicians. Acute MI is frequently unrecognized or "silent"; for example, in the Framingham Population Study, more than 25% of patients who sustained an MI had the event discovered only during routine follow-up visits. The occurrence of silent infarction is more common in women, the elderly, and in patients who have impaired pain perception (e.g., diabetics). In addition, up to 8% of patients who present to an emergency

Table 49–3. Hemodynamic Subsets in Acute Myocardial Infarction

CLASS	HEMODYNAMICS		MORTALITY (%)	TREATMENT
	Cardiac Output (L/min/m²)	PAWP (mm Hg)		
I	≥2.2	≤18	3	None
II	≥2.2	>18	9	Diuretics, ACEI
III	<2.2	≤18	23	Volume expansion
IV	<2.2	>18	51	Acute PTCA, IABP, inotropes

ACEI, angiotensin-converting enzyme inhibitors; PTCA, percutaneous transluminal coronary angioplasty; IABP, intra-aortic balloon pump; PAWP, pulmonary capillary wedge pressure.

From Forrester JS, et al. Medical therapy of acute myocardial infarction by application of hemodynamic subsets. N Engl J Med 295:1356, 1976.

department with an acute MI are incorrectly diagnosed and sent home. Conversely, an estimated 1 million patients who do not have coronary heart disease are hospitalized unnecessarily to "rule out" an acute MI.

Initiation of potentially lifesaving therapy depends on the prompt, accurate recognition of patients presenting with an acute coronary syndrome. Although the quality of the discomfort is variable, patients with angina usually have a midline component to their pain syndrome. Classically substernal in location, angina may involve only the epigastrium, throat, or jaw. It is usually precipitated by events that increase myocardial oxygen consumption, such as exercise and emotional stress, and lasts between 1 and 15 minutes. The pain is almost never only sharp or pleuritic or fleeting in character (i.e., lasting only seconds). The discomfort may or may not radiate, and rest and nitroglycerin usually relieve it. The diagnosis of acute MI is suggested when chest discomfort that is similar to typical angina but more severe lasts longer than 30 minutes.

Unstable angina encompasses patients who present with new onset or accelerated angina characterized by greater frequency, increased duration, or occurrence with less effort or at rest. Unfortunately, different definitions for this syndrome have been used in reported series, making comparisons among populations quite difficult. Because of this problem, a classification scheme has been proposed that provides uniformity to the characterization of these patients and allows improved comparison (Table 49–4). The multicenter Chest Pain Study evaluated the initial clinical symptoms with a series of simple questions and the ECG and developed an algorithm to help identify patients with MI. For example, patients with pain described as stabbing, reproduced by palpation, or radiating to the back, abdomen, or legs had a low likelihood of acute infarction.

However, patients with acute MI frequently have symptoms other than chest discomfort as their initial manifestation. For example, in the elderly, acute dyspnea, mental confusion, sweating, and syncope are common modes of presentation. Up to one half of diabetic patients who develop an acute MI are not diagnosed on presentation and do not receive appropriate initial therapy. Because diabetics with

Table 49–4. Braunwald's Proposed Classification of Unstable Angina

RELATIONSHIP TO REST PAIN	RELATIONSHIP TO CAUSE	RELATIONSHIP TO ANTIANGINAL THERAPY
I. New onset of severe angina or accelerated angina; no rest pain	A. Secondary: develops in the presence of extracardiac condition	1. Absent or minimal therapy
II. Angina at rest within 1 month but not within past 48 h (subacute)	B. Primary: absence of extracardiac conditions	2. Presence of appropriate therapy
III. Angina at rest within past 48 h (acute)	C. Postinfarction: within 2 weeks of myocardial infarction	3. Maximal tolerated doses, all three categories (beta blockers, calcium antagonists, and nitrates including IV nitrates)

IV, intravenous.
From Braunwald E. Unstable angina. A classification. Circulation 80:410–414, 1989. © American Heart Assoc.

MI have morbidity and mortality at twice the rate of nondiabetics, prompt recognition and treatment is especially important.

There are a variety of noncardiac causes of chest discomfort, each with characteristic clinical features (see Chapter 34). Reflex esophagitis is the most common cause of noncardiac chest pain that can be confused with pain of cardiac origin. Musculoskeletal discomfort, anxiety disorders, and pulmonary and gastrointestinal disorders may also mimic cardiac pain. Careful clinical assessment and follow-up evaluation are needed to accurately define the cause of chest discomfort. Frequently, many patients are admitted to the hospital with a diagnosis of "rule out MI" and are discharged after cardiac enzyme evaluation is negative and a stress test is normal. These patients have a great deal of uncertainty regarding the actual cause of their chest discomfort, and further evaluation and intervention are essential in their postdischarge care.

Physical Examination

Although patients with angina or unstable angina have very few, if any, physical findings that suggest an underlying cardiac abnormality between attacks, during an acute anginal episode multiple findings may be appreciated. These include elevation of jugular venous pressure, a palpable ectopic bulge on palpation of the precordium, an S3 gallop, and the murmur of mitral regurgitation.

The physical examination's features of acute MI vary with the location of the infarction as well as with the extent and severity of ventricular dysfunction. The patient's general appearance usually reflects ongoing discomfort and apprehension. The patient may be profoundly diaphoretic with cool, clammy extremities and a reduction in peripheral perfusion. The initial blood pressure may be low, especially in patients with extensive infarction or with activation of the parasympathetic nervous system, resulting in bradycardia and peripheral vasodilatation. Alternatively, the pain of infarction may lead to intense vasoconstriction and elevation in blood pressure. The heart rate may be increased, normal, or decreased. Patients are usually tachypneic in response to pain and apprehension or as a result of an increase in pulmonary venous pressure or pulmonary edema. Jugular venous pressure is often elevated with inferior MI and right ventricular (RV) infarction. Precordial examination may reveal an ectopic impulse from a bulging akinetic myocardial segment. A fourth heart sound (S4) is almost always audible. Unfortunately, an S4 is a frequently present, nonspecific finding especially in elderly patients with hypertension. A variety of other physical findings, such as an S3 gallop, pericardial rub, or the murmurs of mitral regurgitation or ventricular septal defect, identify these complications.

ECG Findings

The initial ECG in patients with acute coronary syndromes is usually abnormal. Careful analysis and comparison with a previous tracing improves diagnostic accuracy and is vitally important in the initial assessment. A totally normal ECG occurs infrequently (<6%) in patients with an acute MI and portends an excellent short-term prognosis. The typical changes of an acute infarction, initially present in approximately one half of patients, include peaked, tall, symmetric T waves, ST-segment elevation more than 1.0 mm in two contiguous ECG leads, ST-segment/T-wave changes, and the development of pathologic Q waves.

The number of leads with ST-segment elevation also provides an estimate of the infarct size. Development of ST-segment depression in patients with acute MI may be an electrical phenomenon (a so-called reciprocal change, such as may occur in anterior [V_1–V_3] leads after a posterior wall MI) or represent additional, extensive ischemia or infarction. Other imaging modalities are necessary to define the extent of myocardial involvement.

Although the ECG diagnosis of MI with left bundle branch block remains difficult, three useful criteria are (1) ST-segment elevation greater than 1 mm in leads with positive R wave (concordant with the QRS complex), (2) ST-segment depression in leads V_1 to V_3, and (3) ST-segment elevation more than 5 mm in leads with negative R wave (discordant with the QRS complex).

Isolated ST-segment depression in leads V_1 to V_3 may represent a true posterior infarction or inferior ischemia. With RV infarction, there is ST-segment elevation in V_1 and in right-sided leads V_3R to V_6R. These findings are sensitive and specific indicators of RV infarction. Transient ST-segment depression in association with chest pain strongly suggests underlying coronary disease and also increases the likelihood of a subsequent cardiac event (MI or death).

Patients with unstable angina may also have transient ST-segment elevation. In general, patients with ST-segment depression have more multivessel disease, greater impairment in LV function, and decreased survival when compared with patients with transient ST-segment elevations. Isolated ST-segment elevation in aVR reflects global myocardial ischemia. Unstable angina and non–Q wave MI present with similar ECG findings. Non–Q wave MI is more likely when chest pain lasts more than 2 hours and it is confirmed by enzymatic changes. In unstable angina, the typical ECG pattern of critical left anterior descending stenosis, characterized by abnormal ST segments and negative T waves in leads V_1 to V_3, defines a subgroup of patients with extensive ischemia, abnormal wall motion, and high cardiac event rates.

Biochemical Markers of Cell Injury

Myocardial enzymes are released into the plasma with myocardial injury (see Table 34–2, Chapter 34). After the onset of infarction the total creatine kinase (CK) begins to rise in 6 to 12 hours and peaks in 12 to 24 hours. The CK-MB isoenzyme (isoenzyme of creatine kinase with muscle and brain subunits) increases within 6 hours of cell injury and peaks between 10 and 12 hours. The detection of a characteristic rise and fall in CK and the CK-MB isoenzyme confirms the diagnosis of acute MI. CK-MB also has two subforms (MB_1 and MB_2), and separate analysis allows earlier detection of cell injury. The MB_2 isoform is released into the serum before MB_1, and an increase in the ratio of MB_2/MB_1 is an early, reliable marker of myocardial damage.

A variety of other biochemical markers that reflect cell injury are released in both unstable angina and acute MI (Table 34–2, Chapter 34). Cardiac *troponins* are structural proteins found in cardiac muscle that regulate calcium and the interaction with actin and myosin. During cellular injury both troponin T and I are released from damaged cells. Troponin T is detectable in serum 2 to 4 hours after cellular injury and may be present for up to 10 days. In both unstable angina and acute MI, troponins are also important prognostic indicators and identify patients at increased risk of further cardiac events. The serum myoglobin level also increases early during acute infarction and is useful in early diagnosis. The rate of rise of both troponins and myoglobin also increases during successful thrombolysis and is useful in deciding whether therapy has been successful. Overall, these biochemical markers allow rapid assessment of cellular damage and reperfusion in patients with a suspected acute MI and may facilitate early thrombolytic or interventional therapy.

Noninvasive Imaging

Two-dimensional echocardiography can be performed easily, quickly, and repeatedly at the bedside and is a valuable modality in the diagnosis, management, and recognition of complications of acute MI. It can be especially useful when ECG changes are equivocal and the detection of a new wall motion abnormality can confirm the presence of acute ischemia or infarction. Echocardiography, however, cannot distinguish a remote infarction from a new cardiac event. Resting myocardial perfusion imaging with Tc-99m sestaMIBI is a sensitive technique for diagnosis and risk stratification of patients with chest pain. A resting defect confirms the presence of ischemia or infarction, and a normal image obtained during chest pain identifies patients with a very low likelihood of a serious cardiac event during short-term follow-up. The combination of excellent sensitivity and a very low subsequent cardiac event rate in patients with a normal perfusion imaging scan makes this method especially useful in the assessment of patients with acute chest pain. Further studies are necessary to assess the relative values of biochemical markers and acute imaging techniques in identifying patients with chest pain who are at high risk for a cardiac event. Acute imaging with Tc-99m sestaMIBI in patients with MI has also been useful in enhancing understanding of the determinants of infarct size and assessing the effects of reperfusion.

MANAGEMENT

Unstable Angina

Aspirin substantially reduces major complications in patients with unstable angina and is the single most important initial therapy (Fig. 49–1). Numerous random controlled clinical trials have demonstrated that aspirin results in striking reductions (between 20–50%) in both acute MI and death in patients with unstable angina. As soon as possible, patients should chew a 325-mg tablet of aspirin and then continue with daily aspirin therapy. Ticlopidine is an alternative platelet inhibitor to be used in patients not able to take aspirin (e.g., due to allergy).

Platelet glycoprotein (GP) IIb/IIIa inhibitors are a significant advance in the therapy of ischemic heart disease. By blocking the IIb/IIIa receptor, platelet aggregation is inhibited. Clinical trials have demonstrated that these agents markedly reduce death and MI in patients with unstable angina and do not substantially

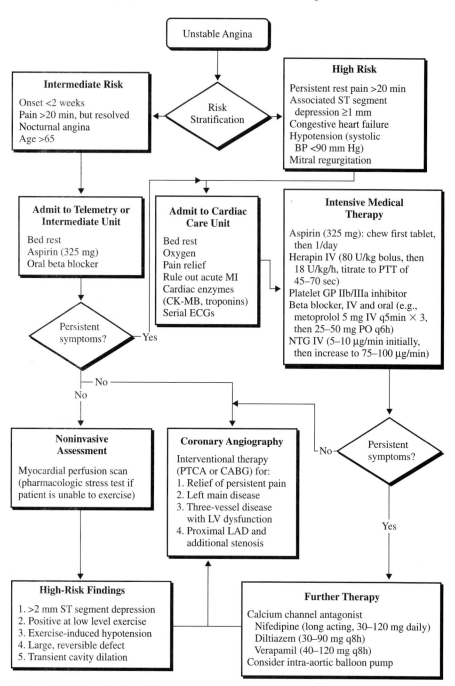

Figure 49–1. Schematic flow diagram for the management of unstable angina. IV, intravenous; MI, myocardial infarction; CK-MB, creatine kinase, MB subunits; ECGs, electrocardiograms; GP, glycoprotein; PO, by mouth; q6h, every 6 hours; PTCA, percutaneous transluminal coronary angioplasty; CABG, coronary artery bypass grafting; LAD, left anterior descending [artery]; LV, left ventricular; PTT, partial thromboplastin time; NTG, nitroglycerin.

increase bleeding complications. Platelet GP IIb/IIIa therapy also reduces ischemic complications in patients who undergo coronary, catheter-based interventions.

Heparin also provides a series of benefits in unstable angina. The frequency and duration of ischemic episodes and the occurrence of refractory angina are reduced with heparin therapy. Heparin also reduces the complications and improves the overall success of coronary angioplasty. In contrast, thrombolytic therapy has *not* been demonstrated to benefit patients with unstable angina.

Beta blockers decrease the determinants of myocardial oxygen demand and result in a modest (about 11%) reduction in the risk of MI, but they have not been demonstrated to reduce overall mortality. *Intravenous nitroglycerin* (NTG) also decreases the frequency and duration of myocardial ischemia but does not reduce the occurrence of cardiac events. Likewise, *calcium channel blockers* are effective in decreasing angina but do not reduce the risk of death or MI. Because short-acting dihydropyridine compounds produce vasodilatation and reflex tachycardia, they may be detrimental to patients with unstable angina and, if used at all, should be given only with a beta blocker.

Acute Myocardial Infarction

General Measures

On arrival, intravenous access is immediately established to be able to treat serious dysrhythmias (Fig. 49–2). Arterial puncture and insertion of deep venous lines, however, should be avoided because these may complicate or prevent the use of thrombolytic therapy. Oxygen is usually administered to prevent hypoxemia, and it frequently provides symptomatic relief.

Patients with acute MI usually recognize that they have a serious, life-threatening event; fear, anxiety, and apprehension are universal accompaniments. One major initial therapeutic goal is to relieve pain and allay anxiety. Pain relief may also result in physiologic improvement by reducing the determinants of myocardial oxygen consumption (lowering blood pressure and heart rate). Although there has been a recent trend to initiate intravenous NTG for pain relief, this does not replace giving analgesics. In most instances, one should give morphine sulfate by bolus (3–5 mg IV), followed by 2 to 3 mg IV every 5 minutes until relief of pain or until 16 to 24 mg has been administered.

Medical Therapy

Aspirin alone reduces mortality by 20 to 25%; and, if there are no strong contraindications, the patient should chew one 325-mg tablet immediately with the same dose continued daily. *Intravenous NTG* has numerous beneficial effects, including coronary vasodilatation, platelet inhibition, and reductions in infarct size and LV wall stress. It may also improve survival. Intravenous NTG infusion is begun at 5–10 μg/min and increased to 1 to 2 μg/kg per minute as long as blood pressure is adequate. Because tolerance to intravenous NTG develops rapidly, NTG is usually given for only the first 24 to 48 hours. *Beta blockers* also reduce mortality, decrease myocardial oxygen consumption, and improve electrical stability. Therapy should be initiated intravenously especially with a large anterior MI and tachycar-

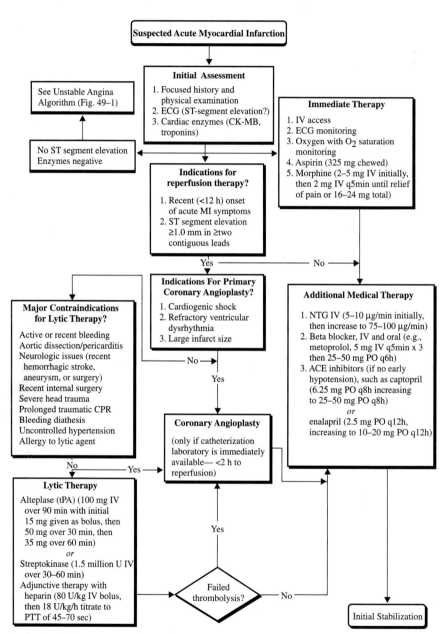

Figure 49–2. Schematic flow diagram for the initial management of acute myocardial infarction. ECG, electrocardiogram; CK-MB, creatine kinase, MB subunits; IV, intravenous; MI, myocardial infarction; q5min, every 5 minutes; ACE, angiotensin-converting enzyme; CPR, cardiopulmonary resuscitation; NTG, nitroglycerin; PTT, partial thromboplastin time; tPA, tissue plasminogen activator.

dia. *Angiotensin-converting enzyme inhibitors* also reduce mortality, decrease LV wall stress, and improve LV remodeling. They may be detrimental, however, if there is significant hypotension. If the blood pressure is adequate, low-dose oral therapy can begin on the first day and subsequently titrated, while carefully following the blood pressure, to normal therapeutic doses. *Heparin* is an antithrombotic agent and an especially important adjunctive therapy in patients who receive tissue plasminogen activator (tPA). Heparin should be continued for 48 to 72 hours with the partial thromboplastin time maintained between 55 and 85 seconds. Heparin is also important in the prevention of systemic emboli in patients with extensive anterior infarctions. These patients should be anticoagulated with heparin during their hospitalization and continued on warfarin for at least 3 more months.

Calcium channel blocking agents have not been demonstrated to reduce the mortality or morbidity of acute MI and have little role in its management. As noted earlier, the short-acting dihydropyridine compounds are likely deleterious and should not be used alone. *Prophylactic lidocaine* reduces the likelihood of ventricular fibrillation, but meta-analysis suggests that its prophylactic use increases overall mortality, so it should not be used in this manner. *Magnesium* has been evaluated in numerous trials, but recent results of a large clinical trial (ISIS-4) did not demonstrate a significant benefit.

New antithrombotic agents including hirudin and bivalirudin (Hirulog) have been evaluated as adjunctive therapy in patients with MI in two large clinical trials (TIMI-9 and GUSTO IIb). Results did not demonstrate substantial benefit or reduced cardiac event rates. *Platelet glycoprotein IIb/IIIa receptor antagonists* are also being evaluated in clinical trials. Initial results suggest benefit, especially in decreasing cardiac events after interventional procedures and as an adjunct to thrombolytic therapy.

Reperfusion Therapy: Thrombolysis and Coronary Angioplasty

Thrombolytic therapy in patients with acute MI and ST-segment elevation results in about a 25% reduction in the likelihood of in-hospital mortality and in improved long-term survival. The absolute mortality benefit substantially increases when collateral circulation is present and when treatment is begun early. There is a 2% per hour reduction in mortality; that is, an expected mortality of 11 to 12% (if treatment is delayed until >6 hours) is reduced to 2% if thrombolytic agents are started within 1 hour of the onset of symptoms. Clearly, "time is muscle."

The goals of reperfusion therapy are to rapidly identify suitable candidates (including the elderly) who do not have exclusion criteria and institute reperfusion therapy as soon as possible (see Fig. 49–2). Patients with contraindications to thrombolytic therapy should be considered for an alternate reperfusion strategy (i.e., primary angioplasty). Because tissue plasminogen activator (tPA) costs approximately 10 times more than streptokinase, substantial controversy has been generated over which thrombolytic agent to use; and more than 100,000 patients have been randomized in clinical trials to answer this question. The studies indicate that both streptokinase and tPA are effective thrombolytic agents. The GUSTO I trial demonstrated a 1% decrease in mortality (from 8% to 7%), that is, a relative decrease of 14%, with tPA as compared with streptokinase, with the most benefit found in patients younger than the age of 75 with anterior infarcts. Benefit of thrombolysis with either agent, however, will be limited unless more attention is placed on streamlining emergency department procedures to ensure the shortest possible interval from arrival to the hospital and initiation of thrombolysis and on educating physicians not to exclude appropriate candidates for their use.

Primary angioplasty is also an effective initial therapeutic strategy for patients with acute MI. When immediately available, this approach provides a survival benefit equal to thrombolysis and also decreases the risk of stroke and other hemorrhagic complications of thrombolytic agents. The major concern, however, is logistical. If the catheterization procedure cannot be performed rapidly, thrombolysis should be immediately instituted. Primary angioplasty is a valuable alternative in patients with a major contraindication to lytic therapy or who present with large anterior infarcts and shock. Rescue angioplasty is also useful in patients who have failed thrombolytic therapy, again especially in those patients with large anterior infarcts. Angioplasty is not recommended in patients who have successful restoration of prompt antegrade blood flow after thrombolytic therapy, even if significant residual stenosis is present. In some large-scale, clinical trials, the strategy of immediate angioplasty after successful thrombolysis resulted in an *increase* in mortality.

COMPLICATIONS OF ACUTE MYOCARDIAL INFARCTION

Cardiogenic Shock

Although the frequency of cardiogenic shock in acute MI has decreased to 7% compared with 15% in the prethrombolytic era, the mortality remains high at 60 to 90% (Table 49–5). Shock usually results from extensive loss of myocardial mass and contractile function but may occur with other mechanical complications of infarction. Clinical and hemodynamic assessment are both valuable in risk stratification and the therapeutic approach to patients with shock (see Table 49–3). Shock may occur because of relative or absolute hypovolemia, especially in patients with increased vagal tone and peripheral venodilation. The approach to the patient in cardiogenic shock is discussed in Chapter 6.

Hemodynamic monitoring is often necessary to optimize volume status, cardiac output, and peripheral oxygen delivery. Intra-aortic balloon pumps (IABPs) provide a beneficial hemodynamic effect by increasing coronary perfusion in diastole as well as augmenting stroke volume by creating reduced afterload during systole. IABPs are also especially useful with persistent, refractory chest pain and myocardial ischemia. Inotropic agents augment cardiac output at the expense of increased myocardial oxygen consumption and may ultimately increase infarct size. Unfortunately invasive monitoring, IABPs, and inotropic drug therapy have not appreciably reduced the mortality of cardiogenic shock. Direct restoration of blood flow with coronary angioplasty, within hours of the onset of shock, reduces mortality and should be considered in every patient with extensive infarction and cardiogenic shock. The development of effective LV assist devices (LVADs) provides an additional approach to patients with refractory shock (see Chapter 86). These devices are currently used primarily as bridges to cardiac transplantation, but trials are underway to evaluate the permanent implantation of LVADs.

Table 49–5. Complications of Acute Myocardial Infarction and Their Management

COMPLICATION	MANAGEMENT
Hypertension	Relieve pain with morphine (see Fig. 49–2)
	IV NTG; ACE inhibitors; beta blockers (see Fig. 49–2)
Hypotension due to hypovolemia	Usually in setting of inferior wall or right ventricular MI
	Rapid IV infusion of crystalloid
	Hemodynamic monitoring (see Table 49–3)
Shock (see also Chapter 16)	Ensure adequate ventilation and oxygenation
	Acute primary PTCA
	Hemodynamic monitoring
	Intra-aortic balloon pump
	Inotropic drugs (dobutamine, 2–10 μg/kg/min; dopamine, 2–5 μg/kg/min)
Bradycardia and atrioventricular block (see also Chapter 30)	Atropine, 0.5–1.0 mg if low heart rate with symptoms or hypotension
	Stand-by external pacer for patients at risk for complete heart block (new LBBB with first-degree block; new bifascicular block, e.g., RBBB and LAH)
	Temporary transvenous pacer for anterior MI with complete heart block and inferior MI with heart block with symptoms or hypoperfusion
Supraventricular tachycardia (see also Chapter 31)	Direct current cardioversion if symptoms or hemodynamic instability
	Adenosine: 6–12 mg IV bolus
	Beta blockers to slow heart rate (esmolol by IV infusion; or metoprolol, 5 mg IV q5 min × 3; or propranolol, 0.5–2 mg IV over 5 min)
	Procainamide, IV 750 mg–1 g load (given at ≤ 50 mg/min), then at 1–2 μg/min
Ventricular tachycardia or fibrillation	Defibrillate immediately
	Lidocaine, 0.5–1 mg/min IV bolus, then 1–4 mg/min infusion
	Beta blockers (metoprolol, 5 mg IV q5min × 3, then 25–50 mg PO q6h)

IV, intravenous; NTG, nitroglycerin; ACE, angiotensin-converting enzyme; MI, myocardial infarction; PTCA, percutaneous transluminal coronary angioplasty; LBBB, left bundle branch block; RBBB, right bundle branch block; LAH, left anterior (fascicular) block; PO, by mouth.

Dysrhythmias and Conduction Disturbances

Ventricular ectopic contractions frequently occur in acute MI and may herald ventricular tachycardia or fibrillation. *Ventricular fibrillation* may also occur without any warning dysrhythmia and requires immediate defibrillation. Lidocaine is usually effective in controlling ventricular tachycardia and preventing further ventricular fibrillation. *Isolated ventricular premature contractions* do not require treatment. Meta-analysis of the numerous prophylactic lidocaine trials suggests that this strategy may actually increase overall mortality. Alternative drug therapies are procainamide and amiodarone. The persistence of significant ventricular dysrhythmias is an ominous prognostic sign and requires additional evaluation and treatment.

Accelerated idioventricular rhythms, usually at rates between 60 and 100, also frequently occur, especially with inferior infarction. In general, this rhythm disturbance is benign, self-limited, and well tolerated and does not usually require treatment.

Sinus tachycardia occurs frequently and is often the result of pain, apprehension, or fever. However, sinus tachycardia may also be a compensatory response to impaired ventricular function and reduced cardiac output. Similarly, *atrial fibrillation* may also occur as a manifestation of LV failure with increased LV diastolic pressure, which causes stretching of the left atrium. It may also occur with atrial ischemia or infarction or in association with pericarditis. When these dysrhythmias develop, they should trigger a re-evaluation of ventricular function and overall management. Tachycardia increases myocardial oxygen consumption and may increase infarct size. Treatment with beta blockers should be done while carefully assessing for evidence of heart failure. Because of its very short duration of action, intravenously administered esmolol is often a good initial agent to control the ventricular rate.

Abnormalities in atrioventricular (AV) conduction occur because of ischemia in the specialized cardiac conduction system. The right coronary artery supplies the AV node approximately 90% of the time, and inferior infarction often results in conduction disturbances localized to the AV node. Commonly with inferior MI, there will be first-degree (prolonged PR interval), Mobitz I (Wenckebach) block, or complete heart block with an adequate "escape" pacemaker from the AV junction. This type of complete heart block usually does not require pacing therapy and resolves in 3 to 7 days. However, patients with inferior MI and heart block have more extensive LV damage, more associated RV infarction, and a threefold increase in mortality as compared with patients with inferior MI and no heart block.

The His bundle and distal conduction system (right and left bundles) are supplied by septal branches from both the left anterior descending and right coronary arteries. Complete heart block with anterior MI usually occurs only with severe, extensive infarction and may be heralded by the development of 2:1 AV block (Mobitz II) or left or right bundle branch block. Transvenous pacing is usually required to stabilize patients with anterior MI and complete heart block, but the mortality remains high because of the extent and severity of ventricular dysfunction. Patients who survive are likely benefited by permanent pacemaker implantation. Stand-by, transcutaneous external (Zoll) pacemakers have reduced the need for "prophylactic" transvenous pacer insertion in patients with anterior MI who develop distal conduction system disease (e.g., new bundle branch block).

Right Ventricular Infarction

Right ventricular infarction is a common but frequently unrecognized complication that can lead to both decreased RV diastolic compliance and systolic dysfunction. The clinical triad of elevated jugular venous pressure, hypotension, and clear lung fields in the setting of acute inferior MI strongly suggests this diagnosis. Other evidence of RV infarction includes Kussmaul's sign, tricuspid regurgitation, a right-sided S3 gallop, exaggerated pulsus paradoxus, and ST-segment elevation in V_1 and the right-sided leads on the ECG. RV infarction substantially increases the risk of death (from 5% in patients without RV involvement to 30% in patients with RV infarction) and the risk of complications, including AV block, cardiogenic shock, and ventricular fibrillation. The primary treatment is vigorous volume expansion to raise the LV filling pressure and restore LV stroke volume. Most patients have improvement in RV function in 2 to 3 days after the acute MI.

Papillary Muscle Dysfunction and Rupture

Severe ischemia or infarction can lead to papillary muscle dysfunction or rupture and varying severity of mitral regurgitation. The posteromedial papillary muscle, in association with inferior infarction, is most commonly affected because it has a single blood supply. The peak occurrence of rupture is on day 2 to 4 after acute MI, and the clinical severity depends on the extent of damage to the papillary muscle apparatus and chordal structures. The most common clinical presentation is the appearance of a new systolic murmur and acute pulmonary edema. The presence of papillary muscle rupture and dysfunction is confirmed by echocardiographic demonstration of abnormalities in the mitral valve apparatus and severe mitral regurgitation. Vasodilatation and IABP insertion may assist with initial stabilization; and, even though the overall operative mortality is approximately 25%, immediate surgery is usually the best therapeutic option.

Ventricular Septal Defect and Cardiac Rupture

Both ventricular septal defect and free wall rupture are more likely in the elderly and in patients with systemic hypertension. Ventricular septal defects may occur with either anterior or inferior infarction and are more likely seen with extensive infarction. The size of the defect and extent of left-to-right shunting determine the clinical features. Patients with septal rupture are usually recognized by the development of shock and a new systolic murmur. Again, bedside echocardiography can document the location, size, and amount of shunt flow. Early surgery provides the best chance for survival.

Acute cardiac rupture can occur without warning and presents as sudden severe hypotension with a relatively unchanged ECG. Free wall rupture is usually a catastrophic event, and only emergent surgery will prevent death. Occasionally, rupture will be subacute with symptoms of pericardial pain, nausea, and persistent vomiting or acute agitation.

Mural Thrombus and Systemic Emboli

The likelihood of mural thrombus formation and early systemic emboli are related to the size and location of the infarct. The *overall* frequency of mural thrombi is 20%, with a 2% risk of systemic emboli, but the risk is even higher if the LV apex is involved. For example, patients with a large anterior MI have a 60% prevalence of thrombus and a 6% risk of emboli. Because the embolic risk is substantially reduced with anticoagulation, patients with anterior and apical infarction should receive heparin during their hospitalization and warfarin for at least 3 months after discharge. Reperfusion therapy resulting in a patent artery also reduces the occurrence of mural thrombosis.

Acute Pericarditis

Acute MI is the most common cause of acute pericarditis and is clinically recognized in approximately 20% of patients with an acute MI. The clinical presentations range from detection of an asymptomatic friction rub to severe discomfort, fever, and associated atrial and ventricular dysrhythmias. Pericardial pain typically is different from the pain due to infarction—it is sharper in quality, pleuritic, and varying in intensity with motion, swallowing, or coughing. Classically, the pain is relieved when sitting and may radiate to the left shoulder. On physical examination, there is a three-component pericardial rub, and the ECG demonstrates PR-segment depression and concave ST-segment elevation in multiple leads (see Chapter 53, Fig. 53–2A). Aspirin (650 mg q4–6 h) and nonsteroidal anti-inflammatory agents are equally effective in relieving symptoms.

BIBLIOGRAPHY

Braunwald E, Maseri A, Armstrong PW, et al: Rationale and clinical evidence for the use of glycoprotein IIb/IIIa inhibitors in acute coronary syndromes. Eur Heart J Suppl D:D22–D30, 1998.
This is a recent consensus statement by a group of international experts on use of platelet glycoprotein IIb/IIIa inhibitors in acute coronary syndromes.

Collins R, Peto R, Baigent C, Sleight P: Aspirin, heparin, and fibrinolytic therapy in suspected acute myocardial infarction. N Engl J Med 336:847–860, 1997.
Recent review and critical interpretation of large-scale clinical trials of use of these agents in suspected acute myocardial infarction with recommendations for routine use of aspirin and fibrinolytic therapy.

De Zwaan C, Frits WHM, Gorgels AGM, et al: Unstable angina. Are we able to recognize high-risk patients? Chest 112:244–250, 1997.
This is a concise and practical review of identification of the patient with unstable angina who is at high risk of death or nonfatal myocardial infarction.

Fibrinolytic Therapy Trialists' Collaborative Group: Indications for fibrinolytic therapy in suspected acute myocardial infarction: Collaborative overview of early mortality and major morbidity results from all randomized trials of more than 1000 patients. Lancet 343:311–322, 1994.
This is a meta-analysis of clinical trials from the early 1990's assessing the efficacy and safety of thrombolytics in acute MI.

Fuster V, Badimon L, Cohen M, et al: Insights into the pathogenesis of acute coronary syndromes. Circulation 77:1213–1220, 1988.
This is a classic description of the pathogenesis of acute coronary syndromes.

Hamm CW, Heeschen C, Goldmann B, et al: Benefit of abciximab in patients with refractory unstable angina in relation to serum troponin T. N Engl J Med 340:1623–1629, 1999.
Elevated troponin T levels identify a high risk group that benefits from abciximab (a glycoprotein IIb/IIIa inhibitor) before and during percutaneous transluminal coronary angioplasty.

Ross AM, Coyne KS, Reiner JS, et al: A randomized trial comparing primary angioplasty with a strategy of short-acting thrombolysis and immediate planned rescue angioplasty in acute myocardial infarction: the PACT trial. J Am Coll Cardiol 34:1954–1962, 1999.
This recent study of 606 patients suggests that reduced dose thrombolytics may have a beneficial effect on outcomes of primary angioplasty and that an approach combining thrombolytics and angioplasty may be better than either single approach.

Ryan TJ, Antmann EM, Brooks NH, et al (1999 Update): ACC/AHA guidelines for the management of patients with acute myocardial infarction: A report of the American College of Cardiology/American Heart Association Task Force on Practice Guidelines. J Am Coll Cardiol 34:890–911, 1999.

This is an updated comprehensive consensus document covering evaluation and management of patients with acute MI. A summary or the full report is available at www.acc.org *(American College of Cardiology) or* www.americanheart.org *(American Heart Association).*

Savonitto S, Ardissino D, Granger CB: Prognostic value of the admission electrocardiogram in acute coronary syndromes. JAMA 281:707–713, 1999.

This retrospective study of patients enrolled in the GUSTO-IIb (Global Use of Strategies To Open Occluded Arteries in Acute Coronary Syndromes) clinical trial found that electrocardiograms upon presentation were highly predictive of death and myocardial infarction in a multivariate analysis.

Sgarbossa EB, Pinski SL, Barbagelata A, et al: Electrocardiographic diagnosis of evolving acute myocardial infarction in the presence of left bundle branch block. GUSTO-1 (Global Utilization of Streptokinase and Tissue Plasminogen Activator for Occluded Coronary Arteries) Investigators. N Engl J Med 334:481–487, 1996.

This presented the derivation and validation of a clinical prediction rule to help identify patients who present with left bundle branch block and possible acute MI in order to give them appropriate treatment without delay.

Shlipak MG, Lyons WL, Go AS, et al: Should the electrocardiogram be used to guide therapy of left bundle-branch block patients with suspected myocardial infarction? JAMA 281:714–719, 1999.

This study reported that the predictive rule developed by Sgarbossa and coworkers in the preceding citation had poor predictive value. See further discussion in the latter's letter to the editor and the author's response (JAMA 282:1224–1225, 1999).

Van de Werf F: Cardiac troponins in acute coronary syndromes. N Engl J Med 335:1388–1389, 1996.

Editorial describing studies supporting the utility of troponins I and T as risk and response stratifying parameters in unstable angina and acute MI.

Zijlstra F, Hoorntje JCA, de Boer M-J, et al: Long-term benefit of primary angioplasty as compared with thrombolytic therapy for acute myocardial infarction. N Engl J Med 341:1413–1419, 1999.

Faxon DP, Heger JW: Primary angioplasty—enduring the test of time. N Engl J Med 341:1461–1465, 1999.

The study by Zijlstra and associates and accompanying editorial by Faxon and Heger revisit an issue that has been studied for the last 20 years and both conclude that, under certain conditions (rapid access to an experienced catheterization laboratory), primary angioplasty is better than thrombolytic therapy and should be the treatment of choice. A more cautionary view is expressed in a letter to the editor by Boersma E, Akkerhuis M, Simoons ML, et al: N Engl J Med 342:890–892, 2000.

50

Thoracic Aortic Aneurysms and Dissections

Bonnie L. Milas
Alberto Pochettino

Because patients with thoracic aortic aneurysms or dissections may be admitted to a cardiac care unit or to a medical or surgical intensive care unit (ICU), clinicians working in any of these units need to be familiar with the diagnosis, evaluation, and management of these conditions.

AORTIC ANEURYSMS

Dilatation of the aortic diameter to more than 50% greater than the mean for normal individuals defines an aortic aneurysm. *True aneurysms* involve all three layers of the aortic wall, whereas *pseudoaneurysms* involve fewer layers. The latter typically result from a rupture contained by surrounding structures—for example, pleura, thrombus, or abscess wall. *Fusiform aneurysms* involve the entire circumference of the aortic wall; *saccular aneurysms* are localized and result from weakness of a small area of aortic wall.

Within the thorax, approximately 60% of aneurysms involve the ascending aorta, 30% are localized to the descending aorta, and only 10%, mostly saccular, are within the aortic arch alone. Thoracoabdominal aneurysms involve variable portions of both the thoracic and abdominal aorta.

Atherosclerosis is commonly associated with aneurysms of the arch and descending thoracic aorta. In contrast, ascending aortic aneurysms are typically associated with collagen-vascular defects, either clearly defined, such as Marfan or Ehlers-Danlos syndrome, or less well defined, such as annuloaortic ectasia. Poststenotic dilatation is an additional cause of ascending aortic aneurysms. This occurs in patients with aortic stenosis or mixed aortic stenosis and regurgitation.

Microscopic findings in ascending aortic pathology most commonly demonstrate fragmentation of elastin fibers within the media. This results in a reduction of the tensile strength of the aortic wall, leading to dilatation. A dilated, thin ascending aorta is prone to an intimal tear, which, in turn, becomes the lead point of an aortic dissection. Other rare causes of thoracic aortic pathology include vasculitis (which most commonly causes occlusive disease), infections and trauma (which mostly give rise to pseudoaneurysms), and tertiary syphilis (which causes medial degeneration of the ascending aorta and arch, resulting in aneurysm formation).

AORTIC DISSECTIONS

Aortic dissection is a condition in which blood escapes from the aortic lumen through a tear in the intima and develops a channel within the aortic media. The adventitia becomes the only layer preventing a free rupture. The false lumen dissects downstream until the media is strong enough to counteract the force that is propagating the channel, a new intimal tear (re-entry point) forms distally to decompress the false channel, or the false channel thromboses due to sluggish flow. An intimal tear is identified either at surgery or by imaging studies in almost all patients with aortic dissections.

Complications

Aortic dissection places the patient at risk for catastrophic complications. Rupture can occur anywhere in the involved aorta. If the proximal ascending aorta ruptures, acute cardiac tamponade may result. The expanding false lumen can also cause stenosis, occlusion, or dissection of the origin of branch vessels, compromising blood flow to the heart, brain, mesentery, liver, spinal cord, or extremities. When the dissection involves the ascending aorta, the aortic commissures can be displaced by the expanding false lumen, causing prolapse of the involved aortic valve leaflets and significant aortic insufficiency.

Classification

Aortic dissections were first classified by DeBakey according to the site of intimal tear and the extent of the false lumen along the aorta. A simpler and more clinically based classification was developed at Stanford (Table 50–1). Type A dissections involve the ascending aorta alone or both the ascending and descending aorta. Type B dissections involve *only* the descending aorta—that is, distal to the left subclavian artery. Patients with type A dissections commonly are hypertensive, with some element of annuloaortic ectasia or collagen-vascular defect, such as Marfan's syndrome; most do not have atherosclerotic disease. In contrast, patients with type B dissections typically have advanced atherosclerotic disease and labile hypertension. They are older and often have serious comorbid conditions related to systemic atherosclerosis.

Treatment

The Stanford group demonstrated better hospital survival in patients with type A dissections treated surgically, whereas medical therapy resulted in better survival rates for patients with type B dissections. As a result, emergent surgical repair is

Table 50–1. Stanford Classification of Thoracic Aortic Dissections

TYPE	DESCRIPTION
Type A	Dissections involving the ascending aorta (may also involve the descending aorta)
Type B	Dissections involving *only* the descending thoracic aorta (distal to left subclavian artery)

the therapy of choice for patients with type A dissections. Medical management is the preferred approach to patients with type B dissections, with surgery having only a limited role.

The goals of surgery in type A aortic dissections are to prevent rupture of the ascending aorta, prevent or correct malperfusion of the coronary arteries or the brachiocephalic vessels, and prevent or treat aortic insufficiency. Because it is not possible to replace the entire dissected aorta, management of the residual dissected aorta is dictated by symptoms. For example, malperfusion syndromes are treated by extra-anatomic bypass. The goal of surgical treatment in type B dissections is to correct malperfusion syndromes and, if needed, to treat acute aortic rupture.

TRAUMATIC AORTIC INJURIES

When penetrating injuries involve the ascending aorta, they are usually fatal. Blunt injuries to the aorta, typically due to deceleration injuries sustained in motor vehicle accidents, can cause disruption of the ascending aorta, which is also usually lethal. Deceleration injuries to the *descending* aorta usually occur just distal to the left subclavian artery at the aortic isthmus. At this point, the aorta is fixed to the posterior chest wall by the intercostal arteries and anteriorly to the pulmonary artery by the ligamentum arteriosum. Sudden deceleration applies stress to the aorta at these points of fixation. If the aorta ruptures, immediate exsanguination and death result. Although containment of the rupture by parietal pleura may permit survival long enough for the patient to get to a hospital (a contained aortic disruption), the patient's ultimate survival depends on prompt diagnosis and surgical repair (see Chapter 97).

DIAGNOSTIC AND CLINICAL CONSIDERATIONS

Most aortic aneurysms are asymptomatic until late in their course. As a consequence, they are usually detected as incidental findings during medical evaluation. When symptoms develop, they usually relate to rapid growth or pressure on surrounding structures (Table 50–2).

The hallmark presentation of *acute aortic dissection* is sharp (or "tearing"), severe pain that is either retrosternal or midscapular (Table 50–3). It typically

Table 50–2. Diagnostic Considerations for Aortic Aneurysms

Asymptomatic (in most cases)
Aortic valvular insufficiency
Chest pain (anginal pain may occur if coronary blood flow is compromised)
Dysphagia
Dyspnea (due to compression of trachea)
Hemoptysis
Hoarseness (due to pressure on left recurrent laryngeal nerve)
Wheezing (due to tracheal compression)

Table 50–3. Diagnostic Considerations for Acute Aortic Dissections

···

TYPE A OR B DISSECTIONS

Diaphoresis
Hypotension
Radiation of pain to back or abdomen
Severe retrosternal or midscapular pain
Syncope

TYPE A DISSECTIONS

Aortic insufficiency murmur
Ischemic electrocardiographic changes
Signs of cardiac tamponade
   Distant heart sounds
   Electrical alternans
   Elevated jugular or central venous pressure
   Hypotension
   Pulsus paradoxus
Hemiplegia or visual changes
Absent upper extremity pulses or blood pressure differential

TYPE B DISSECTIONS*

Abdominal pain, metabolic acidosis, or melena (due to mesenteric ischemia)
Absent lower extremity pulses
Motor or sensory deficit isolated to one limb
Oliguria, anuria, rising BUN and creatinine levels (due to renal ischemia)
Paraplegia (due to anterior spinal cord ischemia)

···

*Also applies to type A dissections extending past the left subclavian artery.
BUN, blood urea nitrogen.

radiates down the patient's back as the dissection propagates and is frequently associated with syncope, diaphoresis, or hypotension.

Traumatic aortic disruption may be difficult to detect. Injured patients often have multisystem trauma and are unable to report retrosternal or intrascapular pain. Therefore, a high index of suspicion must be maintained based on the physical evidence of trauma and the mechanism of injury. Signs associated with a contained aortic disruption include a widened mediastinum seen on chest radiograph, unexplained hypotension, pulse deficits or the presence of a blood pressure differential between upper and lower extremities, and excessive blood loss via chest tube (Table 50–4) (see Chapter 97).

Table 50–4. When to Suspect Traumatic Aortic Rupture

···

       Postdeceleration injury
       Evidence of anterior chest wall injury
       Hypotension
       Increased output of blood flow via chest tube
       Pulse deficit or blood pressure differential in limbs
       Widened mediastinum on chest radiograph

···

Diagnosis

The diagnosis of an aortic pathologic condition is usually confirmed by chest computed tomography (CT), magnetic resonance imaging (MRI), magnetic resonance angiography scan (MRA), or transesophageal echocardiography. Which modality to employ depends on local availability and practice patterns. Although aortography was used extensively in the past, it is now usually reserved for elective delineation of abdominal visceral blood supply or to image stable traumatic aortic disruptions. The coronary anatomy should be defined by cardiac catheterization in the older patient with a previous history of angina or a positive stress test, or if acute electrocardiographic or clinical findings suggest acute myocardial ischemia. Likewise, if clinical circumstances permit, carotid or peripheral vascular studies are warranted in patients with atherosclerotic aortic disease.

Medical Management (Table 50–5)

Patients with acute thoracic aortic pathology are at risk for abrupt hemodynamic decompensation or exsanguination due to leakage or rupture of the aorta. Immediate management priorities include acquisition of intravenous access with two large-bore intravenous catheters and availability of an adequate number of units of blood for rapid transfusion. An arterial catheter should be placed in the extremity demonstrating the highest systolic arterial pressure. Placement of a central venous line or a pulmonary artery catheter in order to assess and monitor hemodynamic status should be considered before aggressive vasodilation. Simultaneous volume resuscitation during vasodilator therapy may be necessary in volume-depleted patients.

There are two critical pharmacologic objectives: (1) meticulous control of blood pressure aiming for a systolic blood pressure of 105 to 115 mm Hg and (2) simultaneous reduction of myocardial ejection velocity so that aortic shear forces

Table 50–5. Medical and Preoperative Management of Thoracic Aortic Disease

Insert two large bore IV catheters
Type and cross for 6 units of red blood cells
Insert arterial catheter in limb with highest blood pressure
Monitor end organ perfusion (see Table 50–6)
Monitor limb pulses
Vasodilator therapy by continuous IV infusion to keep systolic blood pressure within 105- to 115-mm Hg range (e.g., sodium nitroprusside or nicardipine). See Chapter 52 for details of their usage.
Concomitant beta-blocker therapy to keep heart rate at 60–80/min and cardiac index at 2.0–2.5 L/min/m^2 (e.g., IV infusion of esmolol). See Chapter 52 for details.
Preoperative pain management using opioids, but avoid obtundation to allow serial neurologic examinations.
Volume resuscitation
Chest radiograph

IV, intravenous

are decreased. For the former, blood pressure control should be achieved by continuous intravenous infusion of rapidly acting vasodilators, such as nitroprusside or nicardipine (see Chapter 52). To reduce myocardial ejection velocity, one should give a rapidly acting, easily titratable beta-blocker—for example, a continuous intravenous infusion of esmolol (see Chapter 52). The dose of beta-blocker should be titrated aiming for a heart rate between 60 and 80 beats per minute (and, if measured, a cardiac index between 2.0 and 2.5 L/min/m^2). If beta-blocker therapy is strongly contraindicated, one can use verapamil to achieve the same goals.

If vasodilators are used alone, myocardial ejection velocity can increase because of the vasodilator-induced decreased afterload—that is, decreased resistance to left ventricular ejection. Concurrent beta-blockade *must* be instituted with the vasodilator therapy to decrease the risks of dissection propagation or aneurysm rupture. Finally, control of pain with opioids is an important adjunct to vasodilator therapy and beta-blockade.

End-organ function (including mental status, urine output, and the presence of abdominal or extremity pain) should be assessed frequently until definitive repair is made or symptoms are controlled (Table 50–6).

Postoperative Care (Table 50–7)

Control of Blood Pressure and Blood Loss

As a first priority, one must continue to control blood pressure meticulously to avoid disruption of aortic suture lines and to decrease the risk of rupture of the residual dissected aorta.

Postoperative bleeding can result from hypothermia, depletion of coagulation factors, thrombocytopenia, or inadequate surgical hemostasis. The patient with

Table 50–6. Monitoring End-Organ Perfusion

Cardiac

12-lead ECG
Presence and degree of anginal pain
Signs of aortic insufficiency and congestive heart failure
Signs of cardiac tamponade

Neurologic

Level of consciousness
Motor or sensory deficit

Gastrointestinal

Abdominal examination
Liver function studies
Coagulation profile

Renal

BUN and creatinine levels
Hourly urinary output

ECG, electrocardiogram; BUN, blood urea nitrogen.

Table 50–7. Postoperative Management of Thoracic Aortic Surgical Patients

Perform same interventions as preoperative care (Table 50–5) except as noted below.
For patients with potential intraoperative spinal cord ischemia (distal descending thoracic
  aortic repairs), maintain mean blood pressure > 80 mm Hg.
Assess for bleeding and coagulopathy.
Monitor end-organ perfusion (same as Table 50–6) except as noted below.
Complete neurologic examination when patient is responsive.
If patient is unresponsive, check for residual neuromuscular blocker effect by twitch monitor.
  If residual neuromuscular blocker effect is present, reverse neuromuscular blocker.
  If still unresponsive, pharmacologically reverse benzodiazepines and opioids.
  If still unresponsive, obtain neurologic consultation and STAT head CT scan without
    contrast or brain MRI with contrast.
If patient has focal neurologic deficit, obtain neurologic consultation and STAT head CT scan
  without contrast or brain MRI with contrast.
If patient has signs of spinal cord injury, obtain MRI of spinal cord and somatosensory-
  evoked potential tests.
Epidural anesthesia is preferred for post-thoracotomy patients for pain management.
Postoperative spinal drainage to decrease ICP if elevated.

CT, computed tomography; MRI, magnetic resonance imaging; ICP, intracranial pressure; STAT, immediately.

excessive bleeding postoperatively should first be warmed and have any coagulation deficits corrected. If chest tube output of blood exceeds 150 to 200 mL/hour in the postoperative period, surgical re-exploration should be considered.

End-Organ Evaluation

Various techniques used during surgical repair of the thoracic aorta expose the patient to periods of ischemia, which can include complete circulatory arrest under deep hypothermia (18° C). After surgical repair, end-organ performance must be monitored to ensure the adequacy of perfusion to the entire vascular tree. The same clinical and laboratory indicators that were used in the preoperative period should be used postoperatively to determine the adequacy of end-organ perfusion (see Table 50–6).

Certain considerations apply for specific interventions. For example, reconstruction of the distal descending thoracic aorta or the proximal abdominal aorta can cause spinal cord ischemia. In these patients, perfusion of the spinal cord via collateral vessels can be augmented by maintaining their *mean* arterial pressure at greater than 80 mm Hg. Likewise, after aortic root surgery with reimplantation of the coronary arteries, a 12-lead electrocardiogram should be obtained on arrival in the ICU to evaluate for myocardial ischemia. Finally, after descending aortic surgery, a chest radiograph should be obtained to confirm re-expansion of the left lung.

A neurologic examination should be performed as soon as the patient is responsive in the ICU. This should focus on mental status and the patient's ability to move all extremities because both the brain and spinal cord are at risk from interruption of blood flow or embolization of atherosclerotic debris or air. If a cerebrospinal drainage catheter was placed for surgery and an elevated cerebrospinal fluid pressure is noted postoperatively, cerebrospinal fluid drainage is indicated.

Testing for somatosensory evoked potentials can also be used to aid in determining spinal cord integrity.

Intraoperatively administered barbiturates, benzodiazepines, opioids, and neuromuscular blockers can delay the ability to assess neurologic function. A patient who is unresponsive to commands 6 to 12 hours postoperatively following aortic surgery requires further evaluation. A twitch monitor can be used to determine the presence of residual neuromuscular blockade. If there is diminished response by twitch monitor, neuromuscular blockade should be reversed pharmacologically. If there is a strong response by twitch monitor but the patient does not respond to commands, one should give naloxone to reverse opioids and flumazenil to reverse benzodiazepines. If the patient remains unresponsive after performing such reversals or if a responsive patient exhibits a focal neurologic deficit, a formal neurologic consultation and noncontrast head CT scan (to avoid contrast-induced renal injury) or MRI scan of the brain should be obtained. Although a bland infarction would not usually be detectable by CT scan until postoperative day 2 or 3, an intracranial hemorrhage could be visualized immediately postoperatively. An MRI of the spinal cord is indicated after descending aortic surgery to assess spinal cord injury in patients suspected of having this complication.

Pain Management

Pain management is particularly important after descending thoracic aortic surgery because of potentially severe pain from the thoracotomy incision. Epidural analgesia is effective and should be instituted after hemodynamic stability is attained, bleeding has subsided, the coagulation profile and platelet count have normalized, and the absence of neurologic injury has been determined. Under these circumstances, if an epidural catheter had not been placed preoperatively, postoperative placement is indicated. Alternatively, if a spinal drain is in place, it can be used to deliver a single dose of opioid into the intrathecal space before its removal.

BIBLIOGRAPHY

Crawford ES, Coselli JS: Thoracoabdominal aneurysm surgery. Semin Thorac Cardiovasc Surg 3:300–322, 1991.
This excellent article is exhaustive in its scope and has sections on proximal aortic surgery, descending aortic surgery, and trauma, among others

Feliciano DV: Trauma to the aorta and major vessels. Chest Surg Clin North Am 7:305–323, 1997.
This is a review of the issues surrounding trauma to the intra- and extrathoracic aorta.

Kwitka G, Roseberg JN, Nugent M: Thoracic aortic disease. In: JE Kaplan (ed): Cardiac Anesthesia. Philadelphia: WB Saunders, 1993, pp 758–780.
This article presents an evaluation and management of thoracic aortic disease from the anesthesiologist's perspective.

Marini CP, Cunningham JN: Issues surrounding spinal cord protection. Adv Cardiac Surg 4:89–107, 1993.
This is a review of the perioperative risks to and protective strategies for the spinal cord during surgery to the thoracic aorta.

Miller DC, Stinson EB, Oyer PE, et al: Operative treatment of aortic dissections. Experiences with 125 patients over a sixteen-year period. J Thorac Cardiovasc Surg 78:365–382, 1979.
This is a highly influential study that established superiority for surgical therapy for type A dissections and medical therapy for type B dissections.

Stone C, Downing SW, Griepp RB, et al: Diseases of the thoracic aorta. In: LH Edmunds (ed): Cardiac Surgery in the Adult. New York: McGraw Hill 1997, pp 1125–1267.
This is a large review chapter on thoracic aortic disease and its operative and perioperative management.

51 Cardiogenic Pulmonary Edema

David DeNofrio
Evan Loh

Pulmonary edema commonly occurs in patients in the intensive care unit (ICU), and among its many causes, the most frequent and readily reversible is cardiogenic pulmonary edema. This chapter presents the pathophysiology of alveolar fluid accumulation, differential diagnoses associated with cardiogenic pulmonary edema, and its evaluation and management.

Cardiogenic pulmonary edema is defined as excess fluid in the lungs due to increased pulmonary capillary pressure, whereas in *noncardiogenic* pulmonary edema, the excess fluid occurs primarily from a change in the permeability of the alveolar-capillary membrane. In cardiogenic pulmonary edema, the increase in pulmonary *capillary* pressure is caused by increased pulmonary *venous* pressure. The result is an increased net filtration of water across the pulmonary endothelium and its accumulation in the interstitial and alveolar spaces of the lung.

PATHOPHYSIOLOGY

Functional Anatomy of the Alveolar-Capillary Membrane

The alveolar-capillary membrane is composed of alveolar epithelium, interstitial space, and capillary endothelium. Based on the thickness of the interstitial space, the alveolar-capillary membrane can be divided into two distinct areas: (1) a thin side that is highly efficient in gas exchange and (2) a thick side that allows transudate to collect and drain to lymphatics. The thin side promotes gaseous diffusion of oxygen and carbon dioxide across the membrane, whereas the thick side provides the connective tissue support for the pulmonary capillary network and a reservoir for edema fluid.

Ultrastructurally, interstitial edema appears initially as widening of the thick side. This fluid is then removed from the lung by drainage into terminal lymphatic vessels that arise near terminal bronchioles and eventually connect with hilar lymphatics to return the fluid to systemic veins. Normal lymphatic flow from the lungs is estimated to be about 20 mL/hour at rest, but this may increase manyfold in states of pulmonary edema. Excess fluid in the pericapillary interstitial spaces of the lung stimulates juxtacapillary receptors ("J receptors"), which are vagal afferents that stimulate breathing and promote lymphatic drainage of fluid from the lung by "lymphatic pumping." When the capacity of this lymphatic drainage system for removing interstitial fluid from the lungs is exceeded by fluid inflow, fluid accumulates in the lungs as alveolar edema (Fig. 51-1).

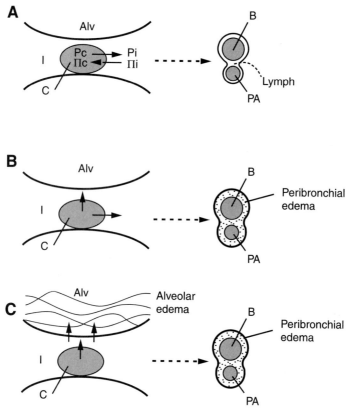

Figure 51–1. Development of cardiogenic pulmonary edema. *A,* Fluid balance between the alveoli and microvessels in the lung is determined by the Starling relationship. Normally, a small amount of lymph drains from the lung via lymphatics. *B,* Increased pulmonary capillary pressure raises microvascular pressure, increasing filtration of protein-poor liquid across the pulmonary endothelium into the interstitial space, resulting in *interstitial edema.* This is located in the alveolar-capillary membrane and in the peribronchial sheath around the airways and pulmonary arteries. *C,* With continued increases in pulmonary capillary pressure, fluid crosses the alveolar-capillary membrane causing *alveolar edema.* Alv, alveolus; B, bronchus; C, capillary; I, interstitial space; Pc, capillary (microvascular) hydrostatic pressure; Pi, interstitial hydrostatic pressure; Πc, capillary oncotic pressure; Πi, interstitial oncotic pressure; PA, pulmonary artery; *dashed arrow,* flow of lymph from alveolar-capillary membrane to bronchovascular interstitial space and terminal lymphatics; *solid arrows,* flow of fluid across capillary endothelium and alveolar epithelium. (Adapted from West JB: Pulmonary Pathophysiology—the Essentials, 5th ed. Philadelphia: Lippincott Williams & Wilkins, 1998.)

The Starling Relationship

Fluid balance between microvasculature and interstitial space in the lung is determined by the Starling equation (Equation 1):

$$Qf = K[(Pc - Pi) - \sigma(\Pi c - \Pi i)] \qquad \text{(Equation 1)}$$

where Qf represents the net flow of water across a semipermeable membrane (which in this case is the pulmonary capillary membrane), K is a filtration coefficient describing the conductance of the membrane for water, Pc is the microvascular hydrostatic pressure, Pi is the interstitial hydrostatic pressure, σ is the reflection coefficient for the protein permeability of the membrane (when $\sigma = 1$, the membrane is impermeable to protein and when $\sigma = 0$, it is freely permeable), and Πc and Πi are the oncotic pressures (osmotic pressures due to proteins) in the capillaries and interstitial space, respectively (see Fig. 51–1).

Increased pulmonary venous pressure raises capillary pressure (Pc). This, in turn, leads to increased net filtration of protein-poor fluid across the pulmonary endothelium into the interstitial space. The fluid is a transudate with low protein concentration, since σ appears to be relatively high normally and the membrane functions like a molecular sieve. When this fluid flows into the interstitium, it results in increased interstitial hydrostatic pressure (Pi) and a dilution of interstitial protein concentration which, in turn, decreases interstitial oncotic pressure (Πi). Both of these latter effects are homeostatic, that is, they tend to reduce the net pressure gradient of the right-hand side of Equation 1, $[(Pc - Pi) - \sigma(\Pi c - \Pi i)]$. Under conditions of very high Pc, however, these homeostatic mechanisms (which also include increased lymphatic pumping described earlier, resulting from stimulation of respiration by J receptors) become overwhelmed and the result is acute cardiogenic pulmonary edema.

Alveolar Fluid Accumulation

In experimental animal models, acute pulmonary edema occurs when the pulmonary capillary pressures exceed plasma colloid osmotic pressure. In humans, this value is 25 to 28 mm Hg. Patients with *chronic* congestive heart failure, however, have an increased lymphatic capacity for fluid removal and higher pulmonary capillary pressures are required for the development of pulmonary edema.

Once alveolar flooding occurs, lung compliance falls because of surfactant inactivation and washout. Gas exchange is also impaired because of ventilation-perfusion mismatch, resulting in hypoxemia. Decreased lung compliance increases the elastic work of breathing, whereas hypoxemia stimulates chemoreceptors. Both of these effects increase respiratory effort and add to the generalized sensation of breathlessness.

DIFFERENTIAL DIAGNOSIS OF ACUTE RISES IN PULMONARY CAPILLARY PRESSURE

Sudden impairment of pulmonary venous outflow that results in increased pulmonary capillary pressure is the central pathophysiologic factor leading to the development of acute cardiogenic pulmonary edema. Common causes include valvular heart disease and impaired left ventricular systolic or diastolic function or both (Table 51–1). The resolution of cardiogenic pulmonary edema depends on the accurate identification and initiation of therapy directed at its cause. If correctly identified, pure cardiogenic pulmonary edema often responds to appropriate therapy within hours.

Table 51–1. Causes Of Acute Cardiogenic Pulmonary Edema

....

Aortic valve	Ventricle
Aortic dissection	Systolic dysfunction
Aortic stenosis/regurgitation	Acute viral myocarditis
Hypertrophic obstructive cardiomyopathy	Chronic valvular heart disease
Mitral valve	Hypertensive heart disease
Atrial myxoma	Myocardial ischemia/infarction
Chordae tendinae rupture	Diastolic dysfunction
Left atrial thrombosis	Left ventricular hypertrophy
Mitral valve stenosis/regurgitation	Myocardial ischemia
Mitral valve thrombosis	Restrictive cardiomyopathy
Papillary muscle ischemia or rupture	
Pericardium	
Constrictive pericarditis	
Tamponade	

....

Left Atrium Causes

Left atrial outflow obstruction can be caused by stenosis of the native or prosthetic mitral valve (i.e., thrombus, endocarditis). Mitral stenosis secondary to rheumatic heart disease is a common cause of chronically elevated pulmonary venous pressures that are tolerated without pulmonary edema. Nevertheless, the latter may still develop when elevated heart rates (i.e., rapid atrial fibrillation) decrease the diastolic time for left ventricular filling.

Acute mitral insufficiency is also a common cause of cardiogenic pulmonary edema, most frequently seen as the result of a ruptured-ischemic papillary muscle in the setting of acute myocardial infarction. Acute mitral insufficiency markedly increases left ventricular end-diastolic and left atrial pressures. The retrograde transmission of these elevated pressures into the pulmonary venous circulation leads to an acute increase in pulmonary capillary pressure with rapid flooding of the alveolar air space. Ruptured chordae tendinae can also occur following an acute myocardial infarction and in patients with chronic mitral insufficiency secondary to myxomatous mitral valve degeneration. The resultant mitral insufficiency from this cause mimics the presentation with a ruptured papillary muscle.

Left Ventricular Dysfunction

Systolic Dysfunction

Impaired left ventricular contractility is the most common cause of cardiogenic pulmonary edema. Left ventricular systolic dysfunction can be secondary to coronary artery disease with acute coronary insufficiency, acute viral myocarditis, hypertension, valvular heart disease, an idiopathic dilated cardiomyopathy, or a combination of these conditions.

A common cause of left ventricular systolic dysfunction prompting admission to an ICU is myocardial infarction. This can occur in patients with myocardial ischemia (stunning) or myocardial cell death in the setting of an acute myocardial infarction (see Chapter 49).

Acute viral myocarditis is a less common but equally devastating cause of systolic dysfunction. This can usually be diagnosed with a history of an antecedent viral prodrome, elevated sedimentation rate and creatine phophokinase level, and diagnostic pathologic findings revealing focal or diffuse lymphocytic infiltrates with evidence of myocyte necrosis on endomyocardial biopsy. The myocyte contractile dysfunction is due to a combination of myocyte death, direct lymphocyte cytotoxicity, and cytokine release (i.e., tumor necrosis factor-alpha). Patients can have marked depression of both right and left ventricular systolic function, accompanied by elevated pulmonary artery wedge pressures.

Whether to treat this subgroup of patients with immunosuppressive therapy is unclear. Recent prospective randomized trials have failed to demonstrate any reduction in mortality or improvement in left ventricular function in patients with acute myocarditis treated with immunosuppressive therapy.

Diastolic Dysfunction

Diastolic dysfunction is defined by impaired left ventricular filling secondary to decreased compliance of the ventricle. The latter results in an elevated left ventricular end-diastolic pressure. Diastolic dysfunction occurs in patients with concentric left ventricular hypertrophy secondary to hypertension, idiopathic left ventricular hypertrophy, myocardial fibrosis, infiltrative processes, impaired myocardial relaxation, and ischemia.

Patients with left ventricular hypertrophy in the setting of acute hypertensive crisis can have impairment of left ventricular emptying leading to increased left ventricular end-diastolic pressure. In this case, decreased left ventricular compliance arises from increased wall stress and subendocardial ischemia. Acute cardiogenic pulmonary edema occurring in patients with hypertrophic obstructive cardiomyopathy or a restrictive or infiltrative cardiomyopathy, for example, amyloid, is often associated with increased heart rates or atrial dysrhythmias or both. These conditions decrease diastolic filling times, leading to increased pressures.

Left Ventricular Volume Overload

In response to chronic (but not acute) volume overload, the left ventricle progressively dilates with compensatory hypertrophy. This change in both ventricular geometry and number of sarcomeres tends to augment stroke volume and normalize left ventricular wall stress, as is evident by inspection of Laplace's law (Equation 2).

$$s = P \times r / (2 \times h) \qquad \text{(Equation 2)}$$

where s = average circumferential wall stress, r = radius at the endocardial surface, P = ventricular intracavitary pressure, and h = wall thickness. An increased wall thickness (h) in the denominator lessens the effects on wall tension (s) by the increased radius (r) in the numerator.

Aortic insufficiency (acute or chronic) may also precipitate pulmonary edema.

Acute aortic insufficiency is usually the result of infective endocarditis or acute aortic dissection. Chronic aortic dissection is most commonly due to hypertension. Retrograde aortic dissections that involve the sinus of Valsalva, however, can also be a presentation of patients with cystic medial necrosis (Marfan syndrome). These so-called type A dissections can also occlude the coronary ostium, resulting in angina or myocardial infarction, or cause hemorrhage into the pericardium, resulting in tamponade physiology (see Chapter 50).

Left Ventricular Outflow Obstruction

The left ventricle's response to outflow obstruction depends on whether the obstruction is acute or chronic. In acute obstruction, the left ventricle responds to the increases in left ventricular systolic pressure and wall stress by ventricular dilatation and decreased stroke volume. The decreased cardiac output is followed by an acute rise in left atrial and pulmonary venous and capillary pressures.

In contrast, in chronic obstruction, the left ventricle responds to the gradual rise in left ventricular afterload with concentric left ventricular hypertrophy in an attempt to normalize wall stress (Equation 2). As the obstruction progresses, left ventricular end-diastolic pressure rises, but the mean left atrial pressure changes little. Finally, with further obstruction, left ventricular systolic function fails with decreased cardiac output and stroke volume and, at this point, the left atrial and pulmonary artery capillary pressures rise with resultant pulmonary edema.

Left ventricular outflow obstruction can be the result of critical aortic stenosis (both supra- and subvalvular stenosis), hypertrophic cardiomyopathy, severe systemic hypertension, or a combination of these conditions. Chronic aortic stenosis is associated with a hypertrophied left ventricular wall, which requires high end-diastolic filling pressures to preserve cardiac output. These not only cause pulmonary edema but also impair diastolic coronary blood flow, resulting in chronic subendocardial ischemia. Critical aortic stenosis is usually defined by an aortic valve area less than or equal to 0.7 cm^2 and a systolic gradient greater than or equal to 50 mm Hg in the face of preserved cardiac output.

Another form of chronic outflow tract obstruction seen in the ICU setting is caused by hypertrophic cardiomyopathy. The pulmonary edema that results from this disorder has a mechanism similar to that of aortic stenosis but with one important difference. The hypertrophy results in flow acceleration below the level of the aortic valve. This is due to dynamic outflow obstruction that worsens acutely with hypovolemia or tachycardia (decreased diastolic filling of the left ventricle). Under these conditions, restoration of euvolemia and therapy for the tachycardia are of paramount importance.

DIAGNOSTIC EVALUATION

Clinical Features

Patients with acute cardiogenic pulmonary edema present with extreme breathlessness, anxiety, diaphoresis, peripheral vasoconstriction and hypoperfusion, and evidence of increased sympathetic nervous system activity, for example, tachycardia. Patients may also complain of a cough, productive for pink frothy liquid (pulmonary edema), and the sensation of air hunger. They are usually sitting bolt upright (orthopnea), breathing rapidly, and using accessory muscles of respiration.

Physical Examination

On initial examination, patients usually exhibit a cool periphery, suggesting a low-flow state with compensatory vasoconstriction. Blood pressure should be symmetric in the extremities. If not, one should suspect aortic dissection with encroachment on the coronary ostia or aortic insufficiency, or both, as the diagnosis. A widening of the aortic pulse pressure with a short diastolic decrescendo murmur at the left sternal border are also clues to aortic dissection. Patients with tamponade and low cardiac output may exhibit a *pulsus paradoxus* and electrical alternans on the electrocardiogram (ECG) (see Chapter 53). Lung examination typically reveals crackles bilaterally, but occasionally asymmetric rales can be observed.

The cardiac examination may have several findings, depending on the cardiac cause of the pulmonary edema. Patients with pulmonary hypertension secondary to acute left heart failure will have an increased P_2 without evidence of elevated right heart pressures (i.e., no jugular venous distention or hepatojugular reflex). Patients with cardiac tamponade may exhibit Kussmaul's sign (increased inspiratory venous pressure). Patients with dilated cardiomyopathies and systolic heart failure will have an enlarged diffuse point of maximal impulse that is laterally displaced and may exhibit an S_3 and S_4 gallop. In these individuals, right-sided heart failure can be assessed by the presence of a right ventricular lift and right-sided S_3. Chronic volume overload is manifested by elevated jugular venous pressure. A systolic heart murmur may reflect valvular aortic stenosis or valvular mitral regurgitation. A systolic murmur with an associated parasternal thrill is suggestive of an acute ventricular septal rupture due to myocardial infarction.

Laboratory Evaluation

An arterial blood gas analysis should be performed in all patients with acute dyspnea and suspected cardiogenic pulmonary edema to help determine the need for assisted ventilation. Mechanical ventilation can significantly decrease the work of breathing, improve the A-a gradient (PAO_2–PaO_2), and relieve the patient's anxiety. These changes will lead to decreased heart rate and sympathetic nervous system activity. Cardiac enzymes should also be analyzed to rule in myocardial infarction as a possible cause if left ventricular systolic dysfunction is suspected. Serum chemistry panels should also be obtained. An elevated blood urea nitrogen:creatinine ratio is usually found in patients with poor cardiac output and can indicate either a "prerenal" state secondary to hypovolemia or poor perfusion due to congestive heart failure. Low serum sodium and elevated total bilirubin levels may be indicative of severe congestive heart failure with hepatic congestion secondary to right-sided volume overload. A low albumin level may indicate a low vascular oncotic pressure as a contributing cause of pulmonary infiltrates and suggests chronic hepatic congestion or malnutrition or both.

Noninvasive Testing

Chest Radiographs

Portable chest radiographs usually, but not always, demonstrate heart enlargement, suggesting that congestive heart failure is secondary to left ventricular dysfunction or pericardial tamponade. A widened mediastinum with an enlarged cardiac silhouette suggests an aortic dissection with retrograde dissection into the pericardium. Finally, pulmonary edema *without* evidence of cardiac enlargement on the chest radiograph is most consistent with acute ischemia-infarction, mitral regurgitation, or ventricular septal defect if it is cardiogenic pulmonary edema or with acute respiratory distress syndrome (ARDS) (see Chapter 73) if it is not.

Cephalization is an early finding that represents increased perfusion of the upper lung fields as a result of increased pulmonary arterial and venous pressures. Perivascular cuffing by edema fluid, prominent interstitial markings, and the appearance of Kerley B lines (lymphatics perpendicular to visceral pleura) are also commonly seen. As the edema worsens, there can be bilateral perihilar infiltrates, opacification, and pleural effusions. Development and resolution of radiographic findings may lag behind the patient's clinical status by several hours.

Electrocardiography

An ECG should be performed in all patients with cardiogenic pulmonary edema to look for electrocardiographic evidence of myocardial ischemia or infarction. Other important findings may be diffuse ST elevation, that is, a pattern consistent with pericarditis, and electrical alternans, suggestive of a pericardial effusion.

Two-Dimensional Echocardiography

An assessment of left ventricular systolic and diastolic function can be rapidly obtained at the bedside by two-dimensional echocardiography. The two-dimensional transthoracic echocardiogram analysis of Doppler flow patterns and velocities can help determine the cause of cardiogenic pulmonary edema. Abnormalities in aortic and mitral valve function as well as outflow obstruction due to hypertrophic cardiomyopathy can be identified and their severity determined by measuring flow velocities across the valves. Pericardial fluid and tamponade physiology can also be easily identified by bedside transthoracic echocardiography.

Transesophageal echocardiography should be employed when there are questions of aortic dissection or prosthetic valvular incompetence. Both magnetic resonance imaging and transesophageal echocardiography have high sensitivity in diagnosing acute aortic dissection. The choice of imaging modality used should be based on the experience and availability with each technique at an individual center (see Chapter 50). Hemodynamically unstable patients, however, preferably should have a transesophageal echocardiogram obtained at the bedside.

Invasive Monitoring

The placement of *intra-arterial catheters* to monitor blood pressure closely and to perform frequent arterial blood gas determinations should be strongly considered in patients admitted to the ICU with pulmonary edema.

Pulmonary artery catheterization is helpful in distinguishing cardiogenic from noncardiogenic pulmonary edema. Elevations in right atrial and right ventricular end-diastolic pressures indicate right-sided heart failure. Although the most common cause of right ventricular failure is left ventricular failure, one should always consider new intracardiac shunts or pre-existing or new pulmonary hypertension, especially if left ventricular function is preserved. Measuring oxygen saturation in the right heart chambers may indicate a step-up suggesting a ventricular septal defect. "V waves" on the pulmonary artery wedge tracing are usually the result of acute mitral regurgitation or left ventricular systolic failure. Elevated pulmonary artery diastolic pressure out of proportion to pulmonary artery wedge pressure in patients with a chest radiograph consistent with pulmonary edema should make one suspicious of other causes of pulmonary hypertension, such as acute respiratory distress syndrome. Finally, measurements of cardiac output and systemic vascular resistance, easily obtainable using the thermodilution technique, can guide both resuscitation and inotropic therapy (see Chapters 5 and 6). Complications from pulmonary artery catheterization include ventricular arrhythmias, right bundle branch block, pulmonary infarction, infection, vascular thrombosis, and pulmonary artery rupture (see Chapter 9).

Left heart catheterization should be considered in patients suspected of having coronary artery disease as the cause for their left ventricular dysfunction. Left heart catheterization can also provide valuable information on the severity of aortic or mitral valvular stenosis (if that is in question after obtaining an echocardiogram). Classic subaortic gradients can also be established accurately in patients with hypertrophic cardiomyopathy.

MANAGEMENT

Supplemental Oxygen and Mechanical Ventilation

Patients should receive supplemental oxygen via nasal prongs or face mask in order to keep the O_2 saturation greater than 90%. If hypoxemic or hypercapnic respiratory failure develops (see Chapter 1), mechanical ventilation should be used to decrease the work of breathing, decrease sympathetic nervous system activity, and improve arterial oxygenation. *Noninvasive positive-pressure ventilation* (see Chapters 27 and 77) has been used successfully in this group of patients, especially if the pulmonary edema resolves over the next 24 hours.

Morphine Sulfate

Morphine sulfate should be administered as an intravenous (IV) bolus at a dose of 2 to 4 mg. Repeat IV boluses of 2 to 4 mg given at 15- to 20-minute intervals to titrate to effect, that is, to control air hunger, dyspnea, and tachypnea. Morphine reduces anxiety, the work of breathing, and the central sympathetic outflow, resulting in arteriolar and venous dilatation. Patients should be watched closely, however, for respiratory depression. If respiratory depression develops, naloxone should be administered at a dose of 0.4 to 0.8 mg IV. In general, morphine should not be administered to patients with chronic obstructive pulmonary disease unless they are receiving assisted ventilation beforehand.

Diuretics

Furosemide is the most commonly used diuretic in patients presenting with cardiogenic pulmonary edema. Although usually given in a dose of 40 mg IV, the dose may be increased as needed based on the patient's response. The maximal amount of intravenous furosemide given at one dose is 200 mg. Furosemide works initially by direct pulmonary venous dilatation, which decreases pulmonary congestion. Peak diuresis usually occurs 30 minutes after administration with a further reduction in pulmonary capillary pressure. If diuretics fail, one may need to resort to acute hemodialysis and ultrafiltration in patients with pulmonary edema and chronic or acute renal failure (see Chapter 16).

Vasodilators

Systemic vasodilators should be used to decrease systemic and pulmonary vascular pressures. Although nitroglycerin can be administered sublingually or topically, buccal and topical absorption may be erratic. Hence, nitroglycerin should be administered as an IV infusion. Intravenous nitroglycerin is administered at a dose of 5 μg/min and titrated upward as needed to improve pulmonary congestion or until the patient's arterial pressure falls to less than 100 mm Hg. In patients presenting with hypertensive emergency, acute aortic regurgitation, or acute mitral regurgitation, nitroprusside therapy should be administered at an initial dose of 40 μg/min IV and titrated upward as needed to improve pulmonary congestion or until systemic arterial pressure falls to less than 100 mm Hg (see Chapter 52).

There is strong evidence that angiotension-converting enzyme inhibitors improve survival in patients with left ventricular dysfunction after an acute myocardial infarction as well as in those with congestive heart failure. However, data are limited in patients with acute cardiogenic pulmonary edema. Its utility in this condition is supported by a placebo-controlled, randomized, double-blind study of intravenous enalaprilat. This demonstrated that early intravenous administration of a 1-mg dose of this agent in patients with acute pulmonary edema improved preload, afterload, and arterial oxygenation while maintaining cardiac output and creatinine clearance.

Inotropic Agents

Patients with systolic left ventricular dysfunction and normal to high filling pressures should be considered for intravenous inotropic support to improve cardiac performance and improve systemic perfusion. This is usually achieved by using a beta-agonist or phosphodiesterase inhibitor or both.

Dobutamine, a synthetic sympathomimetic amine, acts mainly on $beta_1$, $beta_2$, and $alpha_1$ receptors. Its hemodynamic effects include increasing stroke volume, stroke work, and cardiac output, and decreasing systemic vascular resistance due to decreased sympathetic nervous system activity. Dobutamine should be started as an intravenous infusion at 2.5 μg/kg/min, and if tolerated, can be gradually increased to 7 to 15 μg/kg/min.

Milrinone, a phosphodiesterase inhibitor, may increase myocardial inotropy by inhibiting degradation of cyclic adenosine monophosphate. Other effects of milrinone include reducing systemic vascular resistance and improving left ventricular diastolic compliance. All of these lead to an increase in cardiac index and a decrease in left ventricular afterload and filling pressures. Patients should receive an intravenous loading dose of 50 μg/kg over 10 minutes and then a maintenance dose starting at 0.375 to 0.5 μg/kg/min.

Balloon Counterpulsation

Patients with refractory cardiogenic pulmonary edema and cardiogenic shock should be considered for mechanical circulatory support. Indications are usually a cardiac index less than 2.0 L/min/m^2, a systolic arterial pressure less than 90 mm Hg, and a pulmonary artery wedge pressure greater than 18 mm Hg (despite adequate pharmacologic support). Intra-aortic balloon counterpulsation causes both a reduction in afterload and an increase in diastolic blood pressure. The former increases cardiac output, whereas the latter improves diastolic coronary blood flow. This technique is contraindicated in patients with severe peripheral vascular disease (due to the potential for limb ischemia) or with aortic insufficiency (due to worsening of the aortic insufficiency with inflation of the balloon in diastole). It is commonly used as a bridge to more definitive interventions, such as balloon angioplasty or coronary artery bypass surgery (see Chapters 6 and 49).

BIBLIOGRAPHY

American College of Cardiology/American Heart Association Task Force on Practice Guidelines (Committee on Evaluation and Management of Heart Failure): Guidelines for the evaluation and management of heart failure. Circulation 92:2764–2784, 1995.
This contains a section dedicated to the diagnosis and treatment of acute heart failure and acute cardiogenic pulmonary edema.

Annane D, Bellissant E, Pussard E, et al: Placebo-controlled, randomized, double-blind study of intravenous enalaprilat efficacy and safety in acute cardiogenic pulmonary edema. Circulation 94:1316–1324, 1996.
Patients were given a 2-hour intravenous infusion of enalaprilat with a significant decrease in pulmonary artery wedge pressure and mean pulmonary artery pressure without change in cardiac output. Enalaprilat was found to be effective and well tolerated in this small study.

Braunwald B: Heart Disease: A Textbook of Cardiovascular Medicine, 4th ed. Philadelphia: WB Saunders, 1992.
Chapter 20, titled "Pulmonary Edema: Cardiogenic and Noncardiogenic" is a general review on the pathophysiology and current classification of pulmonary edema.

Fishman AP: Pulmonary Disease and Disorders, 3rd ed. New York: McGraw-Hill, 1997.
Chapter 60, titled "Pulmonary Edema" is an in-depth review of Starling's equation and ultrastructural anatomy of the alveolar-capillary membrane.

Grossman W, Baim DS: Cardiac Catheterization, Angiography and Intervention, 4th ed. Philadelphia: Lea & Febiger, 1991.

This textbook outlines the diagnostic techniques of left and right heart catheterization as well as intra-aortic balloon counterpulsation and other forms of cardiopulmonary support.

Hillberg RE, Johnson DC: Noninvasive ventilation. N Engl J Med 337:1746–1752, 1997.

This article reviews the utility of noninvasive ventilation delivered by use of a continuous positive airway pressure (CPAP) mask in improving oxygenation, decreasing respiratory work, and reducing the need for endotracheal intubation in patients with congestive heart failure and pulmonary edema.

52   Hypertensive Crisis

Raymond Townsend

Admission rates to the intensive care unit (ICU) for hypertensive crises have been declining, partly because of better-tolerated and longer-acting antihypertensive drug therapy. Hypertensive crises are likely to occur in patients who have abruptly stopped their antihypertensive medication, recently used sympathomimetic drugs (prescription, nonprescription, or illicit), or who have lost blood pressure control because of the superimposition of a secondary form of hypertension (e.g., renal artery stenosis or pheochromocytoma). This chapter presents an organized approach on how to assess the threat of severely elevated blood pressure and how to choose and use an initial antihypertensive agent.

DEFINITIONS

A *hypertensive crisis* exists when the target organs of hypertension (brain, heart, retina, and kidney) become compromised or damaged in conjunction with elevated blood pressures. These often exceed 200/140 mm Hg. Exceptions occur, such as in the eclampsia of pregnancy (see Chapter 72), in which hypertensive end-organ damage may occur at lower blood pressures (often in the range of 160/110 mm Hg in patients who were normotensive before the onset of their illness). These circumstances, however, are noteworthy exceptions because most hypertensive crises occur in patients with *pre-existing,* often poorly controlled, high blood pressure. It is important to distinguish true *emergencies* in which rapid blood pressure reduction is necessary from *urgent* hypertension in which blood pressure elevations can be treated more slowly and with oral medication alone. It must be emphasized that the diagnosis of a hypertensive crisis does not rest on blood pressure readings alone, but it also requires the concomitant impairment of underlying organ systems. Many clinical situations in which there is a severe elevation of blood pressure warrant the designation of a "crisis" (Table 52–1).

PATHOPHYSIOLOGY AND CLINICAL CHARACTERISTICS

Autoregulation

Blood pressure represents a balance between the cardiac output and the peripheral vascular resistance. In crisis situations, the problem is due to a marked increase in vascular resistance. Organ systems, in addition to responding to neural and humoral factors affecting blood flow, possess an intrinsic ability to control perfusion, that is, *autoregulation.* The goal of autoregulation is to preserve blood flow over a wide range of blood pressure. This phenomenon has been most apparent clinically in the cerebral circulation (Fig. 52–1). Chronic, poorly controlled hypertension shifts the lower and upper ends of the autoregulation curve rightward so that, although hypertensive patients tolerate higher blood pressures, the cerebral circula-

603

Table 52–1. Hypertensive Crises*

Cardiovascular Presentations

Aortic dissection
Left ventricular failure
Myocardial infarction
Postoperative vascular or coronary artery bypass surgery
Unstable angina

Neurologic Presentations

Hypertensive encephalopathy
Intracranial hemorrhage
Subarachnoid hemorrhage
Thrombotic stroke

Miscellaneous Presentations

Preeclampsia or eclampsia of pregnancy
Renovascular hypertension
States of severe catecholamine excess
    Clonidine withdrawal
    Illicit drug use (LSD, cocaine, phencyclidine)
    Phenylpropanolamine use
    Pheochromocytoma
    Tyramine, MAO inhibitor drug interaction

*A hypertensive crisis is the occurrence of severe hypertension with one or more of the clinical conditions listed in this table.

LSD, lysergic acid diethylamide; MAO, monoamine oxidase.

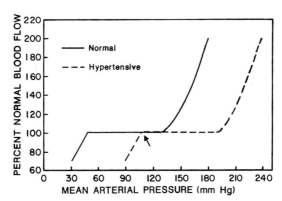

Figure 52–1. Schematic representation of autoregulation of cerebral circulation for normals *(solid line)* and for chronic hypertensives *(dashed line)*. Autoregulation is illustrated by the horizontal segments of each curve in which the blood flow is held constant over a range of increasing mean arterial pressure. Note that the range over which blood pressure is autoregulated is shifted to the right in chronically hypertensive patients. In these patients, decreased cerebral perfusion may result if mean arterial pressure is lowered below the takeoff of the lower "arm" of their perfusion-pressure graph *(arrow)*. (Modified from Strandgaard S, Oleson J, Skinhoj E, et al: Autoregulation of brain circulation in severe arterial hypertension. Br Med J 1:507–510, 1973.)

tion does not adapt acutely to lower blood pressures that are easily tolerated in normotensive individuals. As a result, when neurologic symptoms result from hypertensive crisis, it is important to lower blood pressure only by 20 to 25% less than presenting levels to avoid precipitating further neurologic deterioration.

Vasospasm

Blood vessels intrinsically constrict in response to increased pressure, that is, they exhibit *vasospasm.* This may be superseded by a striking decrease in vascular resistance in hypertensive crises, causing a "breakthrough" vasodilatation (the rightward end of the autoregulation curve in Fig. 52–1) and giving vessels a "sausage-like" appearance of spasm alternating with dilatation. Vasospasm contributes to organ dysfunction by reducing blood flow. The associated vasodilatation is linked with the formation of edema, thrombus, and fibrinoid necrosis. One clinical correlate of this vascular damage is the appearance of hemorrhages, cotton-wool spots, and exudates in the retina.

Volume Depletion

Patients presenting with a hypertensive crisis are often volume-depleted because of the pressure-related natriuresis. This relative hypovolemia activates the renin-angiotensin and the sympathetic nervous systems, both of which potentiate the blood pressure elevation in a vicious cycle. It is important to assess volume status carefully before perfunctorily administering diuretics in a hypertensive crisis.

Electrocardiographic Changes

In the course of rapid blood pressure reduction one may note new electrocardiographic changes, even in the absence of known prior coronary artery disease. These changes consist of T-wave flattening or inversion and occur irrespective of the antihypertensive agent used. Although such changes may represent true ischemia, they are often attributed to a decrease in ventricular chamber size associated with rapid blood pressure reduction.

DIAGNOSTIC EVALUATION

History and Physical Examination

The evaluation of a patient presenting in a potential hypertensive crisis should be carried out quickly so that therapy can be administered promptly. Certain features in the history and physical examination can help identify hypertensive patients requiring immediate attention from those with elevated blood pressure but who are not in imminent risk of end-organ damage (Tables 52–2 and 52–3).

The history data in Table 52–2 can help differentiate hypertensive encephalopathy (which worsens over several days) from an acute intracranial hemorrhage or

Table 52–2. Focused History in Severe Hypertension

Was antihypertensive therapy recently interrupted?
Were neurologic symptoms present?
Were they sudden (minutes to hours) or gradual (over days)?
Is there
   A severe headache?
   A visual disturbance?
   Nausea or vomiting?
Is severe dyspnea present?
Is the patient pregnant?
Does the patient have worsening angina?
Any recent vascular surgery (including CABG)?
Has the patient taken sympathomimetic agents, including cold remedies,
   MAO inhibitors, other antidepressants, or cocaine?

CABG, coronary artery bypass grafting; MAO, monoamine oxidase.

thrombosis (which typically has a much more acute onset). In addition, the history may also identify clues as to why the patient has a hypertensive emergency. The physical examination can identify objective findings of organ compromise, contributing more evidence in favor of lowering blood pressure rapidly.

Laboratory Studies

Additional studies that should be ordered on admission include evaluation of renal function (serum creatinine, blood urea nitrogen, electrolytes, and a urinalysis), chest radiograph, myocardial isoenzyme determination (creatine phosphokinase, troponin I [see Table 34–2, Chapter 34]), and plasma and urine catecholamine determinations (only when pheochromocytoma is seriously suspected). A complete blood count and peripheral smear should be performed to look for microangiopathic changes in red blood cells indicating fibrinoid necrosis in the circulation. One must not wait, however, to obtain the results of these tests before initiating therapy.

Table 52–3. Focused Physical Examination in Severe Hypertension

Are pressures equal in both arms?
Are femoral pulses present?
Is grade III or IV retinopathy present?
Is the patient oriented to person, place, and time?
Are pupils equal?
Is the neck stiff?
Are rales or an S_3 heart sound present?
Are abdominal bruits present?
Are there neurologic deficits?

GENERAL APPROACH TO MANAGEMENT

How Fast to Reduce Blood Pressure

After evaluation in a monitored setting (electrocardiogram and continuous or frequent intermittent blood pressure monitoring), the initial steps in reducing blood pressure pharmacologically depend on the organ system with greatest impairment at presentation. Therapy can be initiated in many emergency departments. The "safest" level to which blood pressure can be reduced is rarely known in an individual, but empirically a 25% reduction in blood pressure is usually well tolerated.

An arterial catheter for pressure monitoring should be inserted when nitroprusside is given as a continuous intravenous (IV) infusion. Arterial catheterization is also indicated when frequent blood gas analyses are needed or if blood pressure reduction will be difficult because of lability. Importantly, patients with prior angina or known coronary artery disease or those with a history of transient ischemic attacks or carotid bruits on examination may experience symptoms related to these conditions as their blood pressure is reduced, particularly if such reduction is carried out quickly.

How fast to reduce the blood pressure depends on the clinical presentation. For neurologic presentations of hypertensive crises, a gradual reduction of blood pressure over an hour or more is indicated. For cardiovascular presentations, blood pressure should be reduced in a matter of minutes.

Neurologic Presentations

In patients with neurologic presentations, it is important to avoid the use of antihypertensive drugs that may impair mental status (clonidine, methyldopa, reserpine). Employ short-acting agents and be prepared to reduce IV drug therapy, allowing blood pressure to rise if the patient's neurologic condition deteriorates as blood pressure is reduced. Searching for secondary forms of hypertension (particularly renovascular disease) should be postponed (but not forgotten) until the patient's clinical situation has clearly stabilized and the renal function has remained at or returned to baseline. In patients with intracranial hemorrhage or a new stroke, there is debate about whether and how much to lower blood pressure. The prognosis in these circumstances is poor despite therapeutic interventions.

Occasionally, blood pressure falls spontaneously when these patients reach a health care setting. As a consequence, the following guidelines can be used:

1. Treat diastolic blood pressure (BP) greater than 140 mm Hg with nitroprusside immediately.
2. Wait 20 minutes for systolic BP greater than 230 mm Hg or diastolic BP in 121 to 140 mm Hg range and then give intravenous labetalol (miniboluses, see Table 52–5).
3. Wait at least 1 hour to start oral therapy for systolic BP of 180 to 230 mm Hg or diastolic BP in 105 to 120 mm Hg range.
4. Do not treat blood pressures of less than 180/105 mm Hg.

Cardiovascular Presentations

In patients with left ventricular failure and hypertension, intravenous nitroglycerin and nitroprusside are both effective therapies, but nitroprusside usually reduces systemic blood pressure more rapidly and with better control. In patients with severe hypertension accompanying unstable angina (with or without myocardial infarction), intravenous nitroglycerin is considered the preferred agent. In this clinical setting, the "steal" phenomenon (shunting of blood away from ischemic areas by normally responsive resistance vessels, thereby worsening ischemia) has been associated with nitroprusside.

SPECIFIC PHARMACOLOGIC AGENTS (Table 52–4)

Diazoxide

Diazoxide is chemically related to the sulfonamide-derived diuretics of the thiazide class. When initially introduced, it was given as a 300-mg bolus and it often produced sustained blood pressure reductions that persisted for many hours. However, some patients experienced severe hypotension requiring pressor support, whereas others had worsening of angina or acute myocardial infarction. Other drawbacks to the use of diazoxide include hyperglycemia, fluid retention (requiring diuretics), and tachycardia (often requiring use of a beta-blocker). Currently, diazoxide is given as either a 1 mg/kg bolus or 50 to 150 mg IV bolus, repeated as needed for blood pressure control. In addition, since diazoxide *increases* shear

Table 52–4. Choice of Initial Agent in Hypertensive Crises

SETTING	FIRST CHOICE	SECOND CHOICE	AGENTS TO AVOID
Aortic dissection	Nitroprusside plus beta-blocker	Trimethaphan plus beta-blocker	Diazoxide, hydralazine
Catecholamine excess	Labetalol	Phentolamine (for suspected pheochromocytoma)	
Hypertensive encephalopathy	Nitroprusside	Labetalol	Methyldopa, reserpine, clonidine
Intracranial hemorrhage with diastolic blood pressure:			
>140 mm Hg	Nitroprusside	Labetalol, diazoxide	
121–140 mm Hg	Labetalol	Nitroglycerin	
Left ventricular failure	Nitroprusside	Nitroglycerin	Labetalol
After vascular surgery	Nicardipine	Nitroprusside, nitroglycerin	
Preeclampsia or eclampsia	Hydralazine	Labetalol	Nitroprusside, trimethaphan
Unstable angina with or without myocardial infarction	Nitroglycerin	Labetalol	Diazoxide, hydralazine

force (the change in pressure compared with the change in time [dP/dT] for the pulse wave), it should *not* be used in aortic dissection. Finally, because diazoxide increases heart rate and worsens angina, it should be avoided in unstable angina patients with or without myocardial infarction.

Enalaprilat

Although effective in reducing severely elevated blood pressure, IV enalaprilat has less efficacy than other available agents.

Hydralazine

Intravenous hydralazine works quickly and effectively in hypertensive crises. Drawbacks include worsening of coronary ischemia, usually due to a marked increase in heart rate. Thus, hydralazine is best avoided in unstable angina, myocardial infarction, or aortic dissection. Hydralazine is still the drug of choice in eclampsia (see Chapter 72).

Labetalol

Intravenous labetalol has been used both as repeated small boluses and continuous intravenous infusion to treat hypertensive crisis. Labetalol has mixed beta-blocking and alpha-blocking activity. Unlike most drugs used in hypertensive crises, the heart rate usually slows rather than increases when labetalol is used. Labetalol is contraindicated in patients in whom beta-blockade will worsen underlying conditions (see Table 52–4). IV labetalol infusion can be performed safely without an arterial line.

Nicardipine

Nicardipine is one of a few IV dihydropyridine calcium channel antagonists currently in use to treat hypertension. Nicardipine is more water soluble than are compounds such as nifedipine, facilitating its intravenous administration. Nicardipine does not usually produce sudden falls in blood pressure. The IV injection site for nicardipine should be rotated at least once a day because phlebitis occurs frequently (~40% of patients) after 24 hours of infusion. As with labetalol, an arterial line is not usually necessary when the only indication is for monitoring the antihypertensive effect of nicardipine.

Nitroglycerin

The use of intravenous nitroglycerin for hypertensive crisis has found increasing popularity in the management of unstable angina, myocardial infarction, left ventricular failure, and the postoperative hypertension accompanying coronary artery bypass grafting. At low doses, its venodilatory effects predominate. Both arterial and venous dilatation occur at increased doses.

The side effects of nitroglycerin infusion are partly related to the use of propylene glycol or ethanol as solvents. These can lead to ethanol intoxication, gout, acidosis, hyperosmolality, and coma. Patients with renal impairment are at greatest risk from propylene glycol. Nitroglycerin less commonly releases nitrite (NO_2^-), which serially oxidizes hemoglobin to produce methemoglobinemia, ultimately reducing oxygen transport.

Nitroprusside

Nitroprusside of sodium was found to possess antihypertensive effects in 1929. However, initial concerns over the deterioration of the compound on exposure to light and the liberation of cyanide molecules from the native chemical structure hampered its development until approval by the Food and Drug Administration in 1974.

Nitroprusside Metabolism

The principal steps of nitroprusside metabolism follow:

1. Cyanide ions (CN^-) are liberated from nitroprusside by red blood cell or endothelial sulfhydryl groups.
2. Cyanide ions are rapidly metabolized by rhodanase enzymes and sulfur-containing cofactors such as thiosulfate to thiocyanate (SCN^-) ions in the liver.
3. Thiocyanate ions are returned to the circulation and excreted by the kidney.
4. Hepatic disease, a lack of sulfhydryl groups, or renal disease can impair the metabolism of nitroprusside.

Cyanide Toxicity

Cyanide toxicity is uncommon but should be suspected when a loss of antihypertensive efficacy (tachyphylaxis), metabolic acidosis, air hunger, confusion, headache, giddiness, or an arterial blood gas determination showing normal PaO_2 but decreased oxyhemoglobin saturation is seen. Cyanide toxicity is usually not seen at infusion rates of nitroprusside less than 2 μg/kg per minute. It is treated by infusing sodium nitrite (which induces methemoglobinemia and binds cyanide), followed by sodium thiosulfate (which facilitates the metabolism of cyanide to thiocyanate). Eli Lilly markets a Cyanide Antidote Kit, which facilitates treating nitroprusside-related cyanide toxicity.

Thiocyanate Toxicity

Thiocyanate toxicity has also been reported, occurring most frequently in undialyzed patients with impaired renal function or in patients receiving high infusion rates. The manifestations of thiocyanate toxicity include tinnitus, blurred vision, delirium, anorexia, and seizures. In patients receiving nitroprusside for more than 24 hours, it is prudent to monitor serum thiocyanate levels. Thiocyanate levels less than 10 mg/dL (1.7 mmol/L) are well tolerated. Thiocyanate is removed by hemodialysis.

Other Cautions

1. Avoid concurrent administration of clonidine or methyldopa because fatalities from abrupt hypotension and myocardial infarction have occurred when these drugs were given concurrently with nitroprusside.
2. Discontinue infusion if the intravenous line becomes discolored (blue, green, or dark red).
3. Use nitroprusside with increased caution in elderly patients who are more sensitive to the drug.
4. Be aware that clinical hypothyroidism may worsen because thiocyanate inhibits the uptake and binding of iodine.

Dosing

New labeling and use suggested by the Food and Drug Administration recommends a starting dose of 0.3 μg/kg per minute because of the occurrence of cyanide toxicity at the previous starting dose. Adding 10 mL of 10% sodium thiosulfate to each 100 mg (dissolved in solution) of nitroprusside reduces the risk of thiocyanate toxicity (if prolonged use of nitroprusside is anticipated) but does not cause a loss of antihypertensive efficacy.

Trimethaphan

At the time of this writing, commercial production of trimethaphan (Arfonad) has been suspended, although it may reappear if produced generically. Trimethaphan was used predominantly in aortic dissection and occasionally to manage hypertension in neurosurgical patients. Trimethaphan can cause meconium ileus in newborns and should be avoided in eclampsia.

Fenoldopam

Fenoldopam has recently been approved for short-term (up to 48 hours) management of severe hypertension. It appears to be a dopamine agonist (for the D_1 receptor) and acts as a vasodilator. Fenoldopam acts quickly and, when titrated, reaches a new balance in about 15 minutes. It is administered without a bolus dose and appears to cause less tachycardia (the most common adverse effect noted with its use) when the starting dose is between 0.03 and 0.1 μg/kg per minute. There is no rebound effect if the dosage is reduced or interrupted. There could, however, be an adverse interaction with beta-blockers in that excessive hypotension is theoretically possible if the rise in heart rate with fenoldopam infusion is blocked. There are no known contraindications to its use in severe hypertension.

A change to an oral agent can be initiated any time after stabilization of blood pressure on fenoldopam.

INITIAL THERAPY

Each hypertensive crisis requires its own evaluation (Tables 52–5 and 52–6). The choice of initial agent should be guided by the relative merits of one drug over another in a specific hypertensive crisis and by the familiarity the critical care specialist has with each agent.

Hypertensive encephalopathy and other acute neurologic situations respond well and reliably to nitroprusside, although labetalol and nicardipine are also effective. Likewise, *left ventricular failure* in isolation responds well and reliably to nitroprusside. However, the presence of *unstable angina* with or without *myocardial infarction* would favor the use of IV nitroglycerin because nitroprusside may adversely affect the coronary circulation in these instances. *Dissecting aneurysms* have traditionally been managed with trimethaphan and an intravenous beta-blocker (the latter reduces aortic shear pressures), although nitroprusside and an intravenous beta-blocker are equally useful. In *preeclamptic* patients, labetalol has been used successfully, although hydralazine and methyldopa are also still used. In postoperative patients, nitroglycerin or nitroprusside is useful in patients who have undergone *coronary bypass* procedures, and nicardipine is useful in patients who have undergone *other vascular surgery.*

Once the patient's condition has stabilized and any nausea or vomiting or other gastrointestinal complications (such as postoperative ileus) have subsided, oral therapy should be instituted and the intravenous agent titrated downward.

Table 52–5. Dosing of Selected Antihypertensive Agents

DRUG	INITIAL DOSE	MAXIMAL DOSE	ONSET OF ACTION	DURATION
Diazoxide	1 mg/kg bolus over 5 min	600 mg	<2 min	6–12 h
Enalaprilat	1.25 mg every 6 h	5 mg every 6 h	15 min	6 h
Fenoldopam	0.1 μg/kg/min	1.6 μg/kg/min	15 min	1 h
Hydralazine	10 mg	60 mg every 6 h	<5 min	3–8 h
Labetalol				
bolus	20 mg over 2 min	Total of 300 mg	<5 min	1–4 h but variable
continuous	0.5–2.0 mg/min	300 mg	—	—
Nicardipine	5 mg/h	15 mg/h	<60 min	<1 h
Nitroglycerin	5 μg/min	100 μg/min	<5 min	<5 min
Nitroprusside	0.3 μg/kg/min	10 μg/kg/min	<1 min	<2 min
Trimethaphan	1 mg/min	4 mg/min	<5 min	<10 min

IV, intravenous.

Table 52–6. Side Effects, Costs, and Contraindications of Selected
Antihypertensive Agents

DRUG	MAIN SIDE EFFECT	OTHER SIDE EFFECTS	RELATIVE COST*	CONTRAINDICATIONS
Diazoxide	Profound hypotension	↑ Heart rate, ↑ glucose, N/V, flushing, sodium retention	$$	Thiazide allergy
Enalaprilat	Hypotension	Angioedema, ↑ creatinine in bilateral renal artery stenosis	$$$	Angioedema
Fenoldopam	↑ Heart rate	Headache, flushing, N/V, hypotension	$$	Severe volume depletion
Hydralazine	↑ Heart rate	Headache, flushing, N/V	$	Angina, acute myocardial infarction, mitral stenosis
Labetalol (bolus or continuous)	Nausea	Fatigue, dizziness, scalp tingling	$$	Asthma, COPD, overt cardiac failure, more than first-degree heart block, severe bradycardia
Nicardipine	Headache	↑ Heart rate, phlebitis	$$$$	Severe aortic stenosis
Nitroglycerin	Headache	↑ or ↓ in heart rate, flushing, N/V, methemoglobinemia	$	Constrictive pericardial disease
Nitroprusside	Cyanide or thiocyanate toxicity	↑ Heart rate, N/V	$	Unstable angina
Trimethaphan	Orthostatic hypotension	Bowel atony, loss of visual accommodation	$$	Severe volume depletion

*Acquisition cost of drug for 24 h at maximal dosage (approximate range: $10/day for nitroprusside versus
>$200/day for nicardipine).
N/V, nausea/vomiting; COPD, chronic obstructive pulmonary disease.

BIBLIOGRAPHY

Brott T, Reed RL: Intensive care for acute stroke in the community hospital setting. The first 24 hours.
Stroke 20:694–697, 1989.
*Practical guidelines are provided for the management of hypertension in stroke, an area that
remains controversial.*

Cressman MD, Vidt DG, Gifford RW, Jr, et al: Intravenous labetalol in the management of severe
hypertension and hypertensive emergencies. Am Heart J 107:980–985, 1984.
*This article provides an excellent evaluation of intravenous labetalol, presenting a balanced view
of effectiveness and tolerability.*

Curry SC, Arnold-Capell P: Toxic effects of drugs used in the ICU. Nitroprusside, nitroglycerin, and
angiotensin-converting enzyme inhibitors. Crit Care Clin 7:555–581, 1991.
*This is a "must-have" review. All practitioners of ICU medicine should strongly consider having
this issue on their reference shelves.*

Gifford RW Jr: Effect of reducing elevated blood pressure on cerebral circulation. Hypertension 5(Suppl III):17–20, 1983.
This article explains the basis for safely reducing blood pressure 25% from initial values at presentation in hypertensive crisis.

Gretler DD, Elliott WJ, Moscucci M, et al: Electrocardiographic changes during acute treatment of hypertensive emergencies with sodium nitroprusside or fenoldopam. Arch Intern Med 152:2445–2448, 1992.
Electrocardiographic (T-wave) changes occur commonly during blood pressure reduction in hypertensive crises irrespective of the agent used.

Mabie WC: Management of acute severe hypertension and encephalopathy. Clin Obstet Gynecol 42:519–531, 1999.
This is a recent review of treatment of hypertensive crisis in pregnancy (with 73 references).

Mann T, Cohn PF, Holman LB, et al: Effect of nitroprusside on regional myocardial blood flow in coronary artery disease. Results in 25 patients and comparison with nitroglycerin. Circulation 57:732–738, 1978.
This article demonstrates greater dilatory effect of nitroprusside on the "resistance" level of the coronary circulation as opposed to the more salutary effects of nitroglycerin on the "conductance" vessels.

Nightingale SL: From the Food and Drug Administration. JAMA 265:847, 1991.
This article describes new nitroprusside labeling for legal purposes because many reviews of hypertensive emergencies recommend the higher 0.5 g/kg per minute starting dosage.

Post JB 4th, Frishman WH: Fenoldopam: a new dopamine agonist for the treatment of hypertensive urgencies and emergencies. J Clin Pharmacol 38:2–13, 1998.
This is a review of fenoldopam to treat hypertensive crisis (with 65 references).

Strandgaard S, Oleson J, Skinhoj E, Lassen NA: Autoregulation of brain circulation in severe arterial hypertension. Br Med J 1:507–510, 1973.
This is a classic physiologic study of cerebral autoregulation.

53 Pericardial Tamponade

Steven A. Malosky
Victor A. Ferrari

Pericardial tamponade occurs when fluid accumulation within the pericardial space raises intrapericardial pressure, causing impaired diastolic filling of the heart. Initially, this impairment in cardiac filling is manifested only as tachycardia and elevated central venous pressures because compensatory mechanisms maintain cardiac output. As the effusion enlarges and intrapericardial pressure continues to rise, however, cardiac output and systolic blood pressure eventually fall and may be followed by shock and death if not treated promptly. In describing the syndrome of pericardial tamponade, it is difficult to improve on the seminal description provided by Richard Lower, a 17th century Cornish physiologist. He wrote ". . . Just as the Heart labors when affected by disease within, so it does when oppressed from without by disease of its covering. So it happens that when that same covering of the Heart is filled with an effusion, and the walls are compressed with water on every side, so that they cannot dilate to receive the blood; then truly the pulse diminishes until at length it is suppressed by even more water, when syncope, and death itself follows."

ANATOMY OF THE PERICARDIUM

The heart and great vessels are surrounded by and tethered to the pericardium. The pericardium has two layers consisting of a serous membrane and a fibrous sac. The serous membrane lines the outside of the heart and proximal great vessels (visceral pericardium or epicardium) as well as the inside of the fibrous sac (parietal pericardium). The potential space between the visceral and parietal pericardium is the pericardial space. The pericardial sac is attached anteriorly to the sternum, posteriorly to the vertebral column, and inferiorly to the diaphragm. It is drained by an extensive lymphatic system by which interstitial fluid, pericardial fluid, and lymph are routed from the pericardial space to the venous system via lymphatic channels in the right pleural space and the thoracic duct.

The pericardial space normally contains between 20 and 60 mL of colorless fluid that is an ultrafiltrate of serum, containing 1.7 to 3.5 g/dL of protein and electrolytes in concentrations similar to serum. Pressure within the pericardial space is influenced by both intracardiac pressure and surrounding intrapleural pressures. Normally, mean intrapericardial space pressure is close to zero, with fluctuations from -5 cm H_2O to $+5$ cm H_2O during respiration.

FUNCTION OF THE PERICARDIUM

The function of the pericardium remains a puzzle. A number of investigators have suggested various roles, including prevention of excessive dilatation of the heart, prevention of adhesions to surrounding chest structures, and maintenance of the heart in a stable geometric position within the chest. It is clear that the pericardium prevents distention of the heart under artificial fluid loading conditions in animals, although the relevance of this to humans is questionable. One important role may be to maintain a stable diastolic coupling between the left and right ventricles during a range of hemodynamic states. Notably, congenital absence of the pericardium has no adverse effect on survival or exertional capacity.

CAUSES OF PERICARDIAL EFFUSION

Fluid accumulation within the pericardial space is a prerequisite for the development of cardiac tamponade (with the rare exceptions of massive pleural effusions and pneumopericardium that can produce tamponade physiology without pericardial fluid). Because the pericardium is relatively indistensible, in the acute setting as little as 100 to 200 mL of rapidly accumulating fluid (such as after trauma or iatrogenic injury during an invasive procedure) can cause tamponade. In the chronic setting, pericardial effusions may contain up to 2 L of fluid without causing tamponade because the pericardium can be stretched to accommodate the slowly increasing volume of fluid. Fluid can accumulate within the pericardium as a result of infection or inflammation of the pericardium (serositis, pericarditis) or from neoplastic disorders (Table 53–1). Purulent pericarditis results from bacterial infection of the pericardium and is characterized by a syndrome of fever, chest pain, and a pattern suggesting pericarditis on the electrocardiogram. Blood or thrombus in the pericardium after trauma or thoracic surgery may also result in tamponade, even though it is generally loculated. Patients with chronic pericardial disease and a thickened and poorly compliant pericardium can also develop tamponade from small loculated effusions.

DIAGNOSIS

Tamponade should be suspected in any critically ill patient in whom unexplained hypotension or shock develops. A change in mental status or the onset of oliguria may be early signs of systemic hypoperfusion. Enlargement of the cardiac silhouette on chest radiography should also alert the clinician to the possibility of a pericardial effusion.

Patients may be admitted to the ICU because of tamponade due to a pericardial effusion from many different causes (see Table 53–1). In addition, they are at risk for the development of tamponade from iatrogenic causes while in the ICU, for example, hemopericardium due to central venous catheter perforation of the superior vena cava or right atrium or puncture of the right atrium or ventricle by a pacemaker wire.

Symptoms

Symptoms tend to play a minor role in the diagnosis of tamponade, especially in the ICU setting. Before the onset of tamponade, the diagnosis of pericardial effusion may be difficult. Chest discomfort is a noteworthy complaint (depending

Table 53–1. Differential Diagnosis of Pericardial Effusion

INFECTIOUS	NEOPLASTIC	CONNECTIVE TISSUE DISEASE
Viral	Metastatic spread	Systemic lupus erythematosus
Coxsackie virus	Contiguous spread	Rheumatoid arthritis
Influenza	Pericardial tumor	Sjögren's syndrome
Echovirus		Scleroderma
HIV-related		Whipple's disease
Bacterial		Reiter's syndrome
Tuberculous		Ankylosing spondylitis
Fungal		

CARDIAC DAMAGE	OTHER SYSTEMIC DISEASES	MISCELLANEOUS
Post myocardial infarction (MI)	Uremia, chronic renal	Puncture of superior vena cava
Dressler's syndrome	failure	or right atrium by central
(postpericardiotomy	Amyloidosis	venous catheter
syndrome)	Hemochromatosis	Puncture of right atrium or
Trauma (blunt-penetrating)	Myxedema	ventricle during right heart
Myocardial rupture (post MI)		catheterization
After thoracic-cardiac surgery		Aortic dissection
		Air (pneumopericardium)

DRUG-INDUCED
Procainamide
Hydralazine
Minoxidil
Quinidine

HIV, human immunodeficiency virus.

on the presence of pericarditis) and is often described as sharp in quality and constant or prolonged in duration. If pericarditis is present, the chest pain may be relieved by the patient leaning forward or changing position. With large chronic effusions, extracardiac mechanical compression of the esophagus or the recurrent laryngeal or phrenic nerves may result in dysphagia, hoarseness, cough, or singultus. Once tamponade-induced falls in cardiac output or blood pressure occur, patients who remain conscious generally appear anxious or confused (due to cerebral hypoperfusion) and may complain of dyspnea.

Physical Examination

Early in tamponade, the vital signs generally reveal tachycardia without hypotension and a slightly increased respiratory rate (Table 53–2). Paradoxical pulse (pulsus paradoxicus) usually develops later, but this can also occur from obstructive airway disease alone. Paradoxical pulse refers to a decline in systolic blood

Table 53–2. Pathophysiology of Tamponade

	INTRAPERICARDIAL PRESSURE		HEMODYNAMIC PARAMETERS		
PHASE	Absolute	Relative	Heart Rate	Cardiac Index	Systemic Blood Pressure
I. Early signs	4–8 mm Hg	< RA		WNL	WNL
II. Pretamponade	10 mm Hg (jugular venous distention is present)	= RA ($\uparrow$) = RVEDP ($\uparrow$) but < PAWP and < LVEDP	$\uparrow$	Slightly $\downarrow$	Paradoxical pulse is present
III. Frank tamponade	15–30 mm Hg	= RA ($\uparrow\uparrow$) = RVEDP ($\uparrow\uparrow$) = PAEDP ($\uparrow\uparrow$) = PAWP ($\uparrow\uparrow$) = LVEDP ($\uparrow\uparrow$)	$\uparrow\uparrow$	$\downarrow\downarrow$	$\downarrow\downarrow$

RA, right atrial pressure; RVEDP, right ventricular end-diastolic pressure; PAEDP, pulmonary artery end-diastolic pressure; PAWP, pulmonary artery wedge pressure; LVEDP, left ventricular end-diastolic pressure; WNL, within normal limits; $\uparrow$, increased; $\uparrow\uparrow$, marked increase; $\downarrow$, decreased; $\downarrow\downarrow$, marked decrease.

pressure of greater than 10 to 15 mm Hg on inspiration. It is thought to be caused by impaired left ventricular filling due to compression of the left ventricle between the rapidly filling right ventricle (distended with systemic venous return during inspiration) and the incompressible pericardial fluid.

Jugular venous distention is a nearly constant finding (but sometimes absent in loculated posterior effusions after cardiac surgery), but the neck veins may be difficult to visualize in obese patients. Although it may be subtle, changes in the jugular venous pulse contour should be sought, looking for a prominent x descent and attenuation (or absence) of the y descent, reflecting impairment of early diastolic filling (Fig. 53–1). The heart sounds may be muffled but can usually be heard unless the effusion is massive. The point of maximal cardiac impulse is typically nonpalpable, but a pericardial friction rub is often heard or palpable. The extremities are frequently cool with mottled skin and weak pulses.

Electrocardiography

A large pericardial effusion may cause low voltage on the electrocardiogram, defined as less than 5 mV absolute voltage for the QRS complex in the limb leads (I, II, III, aVF, aVL, and aVR) (Fig. 53–2*B*). In the individual patient, however, it is usually more helpful to compare his or her current electrocardiogram amplitude to prior tracings, if available.

Pericarditis frequently produces characteristic, although sometimes subtle, electrocardiographic findings (Fig. 53–2*A*). *PR segment depression* is sometimes present and is best seen in leads II, aVF, and V_3 through V_6. In contrast, lead aVR usually shows PR elevation, that is, electrocardiographic changes opposite those

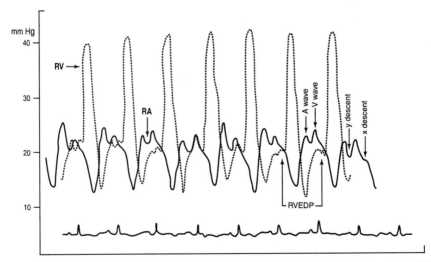

Figure 53–1. Simultaneous right atrial (RA) pressure tracing *(solid line)* and right ventricular (RV) pressure tracing *(broken line)* in a patient with tamponade. Note (1) increased RA pressure, (2) equalization of RA pressure with RV end-diastolic pressure (RVEDP), and (3) attenuated y descent with a pronounced x descent of the RA pressure tracing.

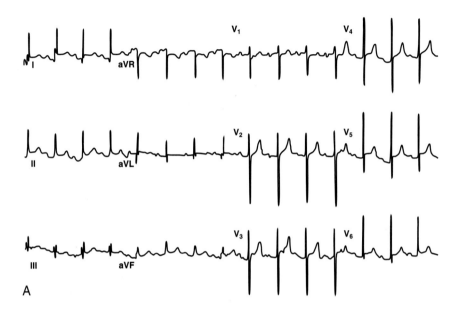

A

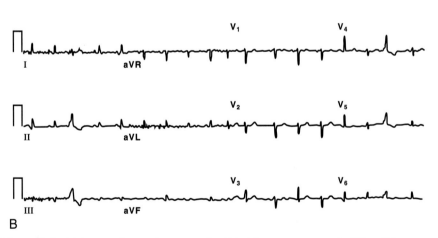

B

Figure 53–2. *A,* Electrocardiogram in acute pericarditis. Note concave upward, diffuse ST segment elevation and PR depression (except in aVR, which shows the opposite changes). The upright T waves denote the acute phase of pericarditis. *B,* Electrocardiogram in large pericardial effusion. Note the low-amplitude QRS voltage in the limb leads (<5 mV) and the alternation in QRS axis, particularly in lead V_3 (so-called electrical alternans).

seen in the other leads. *Diffuse ST segment elevation* is concave upward and may mimic an acute myocardial infarction. This can usually be distinguished from infarction by its diffuse distribution and upward concavity. Reciprocal ST depression is generally seen in lead aVR. *T wave inversion* may or may not be seen but is usually present late in the course of pericarditis.

A less common finding in the setting of pericardial effusion is "electrical alternans," in which the amplitude of the QRS complex alternates from beat to beat or in a periodic manner (Fig. 53–2B). This reflects rhythmic changes in the QRS axis and occurs most commonly with a large pericardial effusion. Electrical alternans can also be seen with severe heart failure, limiting its specificity.

Chest Radiography

Although the cardiac silhouette is enlarged in the presence of a large pericardial effusion, the absence of an enlarged cardiac silhouette does not exclude the diagnosis of tamponade. This is because the volume of pericardial fluid causing tamponade may be small if it accumulates rapidly or after chest surgery. The presence of a large pleural effusion should be noted because it alone may cause tamponade physiology. A widened mediastinum may reflect an aortic dissection, which can rupture into the pericardial space with ensuing tamponade. A nodule in the lung field or a missing breast because of prior mastectomy may suggest the source of a metastatic neoplastic effusion. Similarly, a severe pneumonia may be the source of an infected pericardial effusion. One final point is to take note of the position of any central venous catheters or transvenous pacemaker wires because migration of a tip through the superior vena cava, right atrium, or right ventricle may cause a hemopericardium.

Echocardiography

The echocardiogram is the most important study to obtain in evaluating tamponade; without it, the diagnosis remains in question. Emergency echocardiograms can be obtained relatively quickly in most hospitals and, except in cardiac arrest, needle drainage of a presumed pericardial effusion should never be attempted without an echocardiogram to demonstrate the size and location of the effusion (which also aids in selecting the preferred therapeutic approach). The most obvious finding on echocardiography is the presence of a pericardial effusion (Fig. 53–3). The effusion may not be particularly large, nor does it have to be circumferential (after cardiac surgery, a thrombus or effusion located posteriorly or overlying the right atrium can produce tamponade).

Additional findings on the echocardiogram that distinguish a simple pericardial effusion from actual tamponade physiology include diastolic collapse of the right atrium, right ventricle (see Fig. 53–3) or left atrium, or a combination of the three; abnormally wide variation in Doppler flow velocity across the atrioventricular valves with respiration; and absence of (normal) inspiratory decrease in diameter of the inferior vena cava.

Clinical situations in which some of the usual echocardiographic findings of tamponade (diastolic collapse of the right-sided heart chambers) may be masked

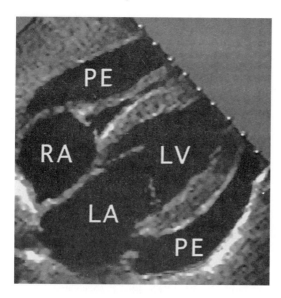

Figure 53–3. Two-dimensional echocardiographic view of three chambers of the heart showing right atrium (RA), left atrium (LA), left ventricle (LV), and a large circumferential pericardial effusion (PE) located anterior to the RA and posterior to the LA and LV. Note the collapsed right ventricle immediately to the right of the RA.

are acute or chronic pulmonary hypertension, right ventricular (RV) failure or infarction (with increased RVEDP), and after cardiac surgery (due to tethering of the right side of the heart anteriorly after sternotomy).

Pulmonary Artery (Swan-Ganz) Catheterization

Many critically ill patients have pulmonary artery catheters in place, which can be helpful in establishing a diagnosis of tamponade. As a practical point, one should make sure that the pressure tracings obtained from the pulmonary artery catheter are accurate by reconfirming the zero level of the transducer and then examining the tracing carefully in case it is overly damped or flattened. If it is, one should aspirate and flush the catheter and transducer with saline to eliminate bubbles.

The hallmark of pericardial tamponade is elevation and equalization of the diastolic filling pressures of both ventricles, that is, right and left ventricular end diastolic pressures (RVEDP and LVEDP). Since the LVEDP cannot be measured directly with a pulmonary artery catheter, the pulmonary artery wedge pressure (PAWP) is used (technically, the PAWP is a surrogate of left atrial pressure, not LVEDP, but in the absence of mitral valve disease, the mean left atrial pressure approximates the LVEDP). Thus, the classic finding in support of a diagnosis of tamponade is an elevated right atrial pressure (>7 to 8 mm Hg) with mean right atrial pressure = RVEDP = PAWP (Fig. 53–4; see Table 53–2). Reduced cardiac output is a late finding, as is reduced mixed venous oxygen saturation (<65%). In addition to the elevation and equalization of filling pressures, the morphologic characteristics of the right atrial pressure tracing often supports the diagnosis of tamponade. In tamponade (see Fig. 53–1), the x descent is steep and the y descent is attenuated, reflecting reduced passive diastolic filling of the right ventricle with dependence of ventricular filling on atrial systole. These characteristic changes in

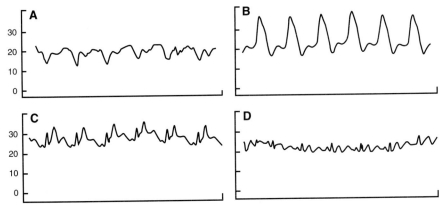

Figure 53–4. Representative hemodynamic tracings obtained by use of a Swan-Ganz catheter in a patient with cardiac tamponade. *A,* Right atrial (RA) pressure. *B,* Right ventricular (RV) pressure. *C,* Pulmonary artery (PA) pressure. *D,* Pulmonary artery wedge pressure (PAWP). Note that there is equalization of the mean RA, RV, and PA end-diastolic pressures, and the mean PAWP.

the right atrial pressure tracing may not be evident when using a flotation pulmonary artery catheter because of damping due to the small bore of the right atrial lumen.

Adjunctive Imaging Studies

If metastatic disease is suspected, computed tomography or magnetic resonance imaging of the chest and lungs may be useful in evaluating lung masses or bony lesions or detecting mediastinal lymphadenopathy. Occasionally, tumors may present with invasion of the pericardium or cardiac chambers, and either of these imaging techniques can document their presence and extent.

Differential Diagnosis of Tamponade

Several common disorders can mimic tamponade in the ICU setting, including right ventricular infarction (see Chapters 6 and 49), major pulmonary embolism (see Chapter 76), tension pneumothorax (see Chapter 32) and severe auto–positive end-expiratory pressure (auto-PEEP) (see Chapter 2). All may present with dyspnea, tachycardia, jugular venous distention, and hypotension or shock (Table 53–3).

THERAPY

Once the diagnosis of pericardial tamponade has been established, one must decide the type of drainage procedure to use. Medical therapy alone is ineffective in treating tamponade. Intravenous fluid administration can help to maintain preload

Table 53–3. Causes Mimicking Pericardial Tamponade

CAUSE	HYPOTENSION AND TACHYCARDIA	HYPOXEMIA	JUGULAR VEINS	ELECTROCARDIOGRAPHIC CHANGES	ECHOCARDIOGRAPHIC FINDINGS
Pericardial tamponade	Prominent	Not prominent	Elevated	Low voltage and ST changes (see Fig. 53–2)	Pericardial effusion (see Fig. 53–3)
RV infarction	Prominent	Not prominent	Elevated	RV infarction pattern	Dilated RV with regional wall motion abnormalities
Major pulmonary embolus	Prominent	Prominent	Elevated	RV strain pattern	Dilated and hypokinetic RV; hyperdynamic LA and LV
Tension pneumothorax	Prominent	May be prominent	Elevated	Low voltage and RV strain	Shifted heart and mediastinum
Severe auto-PEEP (in ventilated patients)	Prominent	May be prominent	Elevated	Low voltage due to hyperinflated lung	Poor technical quality (due to lung disease); underfilled LA and LV

RV, right ventricle; LA, left atrium; LV, left ventricle; PEEP, positive end-expiratory pressure.

but is only a temporizing measure. The basic options are percutaneous needle or catheter drainage (performed by an interventional cardiologist) versus open or thoracoscopic drainage such as a pericardial window (performed by a cardiothoracic surgeon). Decisions about which type of approach to use are often based on convention and local expertise rather than on data from controlled clinical trials. Recurrent or persistent effusions after percutaneous drainage generally require a surgical solution.

Percutaneous Approach (Pericardiocentesis)

Pericardiocentesis can be a relatively high-risk procedure if not carried out under controlled conditions. It should be performed in the catheterization laboratory whenever feasible. Pericardiocentesis should be attempted only when echocardiography has documented the presence of 1 cm or more (depth) of anterior-circumferential freely flowing pericardial fluid. Pericardial effusions that are posterior or loculated, or due to a thrombus, cannot be drained percutaneously. Effusions that have recurred after a recent pericardiocentesis should generally be drained surgically.

A pericardiocentesis needle (18-gauge, 5 to 7 cm in length) is inserted one fingerbreadth below the xiphoid process and directed toward the mid-left clavicle at an approximately 30- to 45-degree angle from the patient's chest wall (the patient is positioned in a semiupright sitting position).

When the cause of the effusion is unknown, pericardial fluid should be sent for cytologic examination, Gram staining and routine bacterial culture, fungal culture, total protein determination, lactate dehydrogenase measurement, and smear and culture for acid-fast bacilli. In addition, the following laboratory studies should be obtained: blood urea nitrogen and serum creatinine, thyroid function tests, blood cultures (when appropriate), antinuclear antibody and rheumatoid factor, purified protein derivative (PPD) skin test and anergy panel, sputum for acid-fast bacilli smear and culture, and human immunodeficiency virus serologic tests (in an otherwise unexplained effusion). In addition, if there is justification for trying to identify a specific viral-type cause, for example, coxsackievirus, echovirus or *Mycoplasma,* serologic tests for these agents can be sent under appropriate clinical circumstances.

Complications include laceration of the right atrium, right ventricle, or coronary artery (with ensuing precipitation of worsened tamponade); ventricular arrhythmias and fibrillation; laceration of the stomach, lung, or colon; pneumothorax; a major vagal reaction; and death (a 3% mortality rate).

Surgical Drainage

Surgical drainage is generally reserved for recurrent symptomatic effusions (or those judged likely to recur) as well as for effusions with adhesions or loculations such that they cannot be approached percutaneously. In the subxiphoid approach, a small incision is made below the xiphoid and the dissection is carried down to the pericardium, which is then grasped and incised. A chest tube draining to gravity is then placed within the pericardial space. This technique has relatively low risk and can be performed under local anesthesia if necessary.

For loculated effusions, a left lateral thoracotomy needs to be performed under general anesthesia. Partial pericardial resection (a pericardial "window") is then performed, allowing pericardial fluid to drain into the left pleural space, which itself is drained by a chest tube. Infected pericardial effusions are generally drained via a median sternotomy with partial pericardial resection and drainage via a mediastinal chest tube.

A new approach to drainage of pericardial effusion is the thoracoscopic technique, which in the appropriate patient and setting can further minimize risk and discomfort while effectively draining the effusion as well as resecting part of the pericardium.

BIBLIOGRAPHY

Fowler NO: Cardiac tamponade—a clinical or an echocardiographic diagnosis? Circulation 87:1738–1741, 1993.
  This is an editorial by one of the experts in pericardial disease, discussing the role of echocardiography in redefining some aspects of pericardial disease.

Holt JP: The normal pericardium. Am J Cardiol 26:455–465, 1970.
  For those interested, this is a more detailed description of normal pericardial physiology.

Kern MJ, Aguirre FL: Hemodynamic rounds—interpretation of cardiac pathophysiology from pressure waveform analysis: Pericardial compressive hemodynamics, Part I. Catheter Cardiovasc Diagn 25:336–342, 1992.
  This article provides a concise explanation of atrial pressure waveform analysis in the diagnosis of pericardial disease.

Reddy PS, Curtiss EI, Uretsky BF: Spectrum of hemodynamic changes in cardiac tamponade. Am J Cardiol 66:1487–1491, 1990.
  This is a lucid, clinically oriented study and discussion of the hemodynamics of tamponade.

Soler-Soler J, Permanyer-Miralda G, Sagrista-Sauleda J: A systematic diagnostic approach to primary acute pericardial disease—the Barcelona experience. Cardiol Clin 8:609–620, 1990.
  This article presents a clinically oriented discussion of the diagnostic evaluation of acute pericarditis and effusion.

Zayas R, Anguita M, Torres F, et al: Incidence of specific etiology and role of methods to specific etiologic diagnosis of primary acute pericarditis. Am J Cardiol 75:378–382, 1995.
  This study examines the sensitivity and specificity of commonly performed diagnostic tests in pericarditis and pericardial effusion.

54

Hypothermia and Hyperthermia

C. Crawford Mechem

Hypothermia and hyperthermia are potentially fatal emergencies caused by environmental exposure, underlying disease processes, or drugs. Although therapy is often initiated in the prehospital setting or emergency department, multiple organ system involvement often necessitates intensive care unit (ICU) management.

HYPOTHERMIA

Hypothermia is defined as a core temperature less than 35° C (95° F). It is categorized as *mild* if core temperature is 32 to 35° C (89.6 to 95° F), *moderate* at 28 to 32° C (82.4 to 89.6° F), or *severe* at less than 28° C (82.4° F).

Pathophysiology

Body temperature reflects the balance between heat production and heat loss. The four physiologic mechanisms of heat loss are evaporation, convection, radiation, and conduction. Conduction is enhanced by exposure to water, which increases thermal conductivity 20- to 30-fold. In response to cold stress, the hypothalamus attempts to stimulate heat production through shivering and increasing thyroid, catecholamine, and adrenal activity. Vasoconstriction simultaneously minimizes heat loss in hypothermic patients.

Clinical Manifestations

As the hypothermic patient's compensatory mechanisms are overwhelmed, temperature-dependent physiologic changes occur. Patients with *mild hypothermia* demonstrate tachypnea, tachycardia, ataxia, dysarthria, impaired judgment, shivering, and diuresis. *Moderate hypothermia* is characterized by decreased pulse and cardiac output, hypoventilation, central nervous system depression, hyporeflexia, decreased renal blood flow, and loss of shivering. Atrial fibrillation and other arrhythmias may be seen. The electrocardiogram may manifest an Osborn or J wave (Fig. 54–1); this secondary wave follows the S wave, most prominently in leads aVL, aVF, and V_{1-6}. In *severe hypothermia*, coma, hypotension, bradycardia, ventricular arrhythmias, asystole, pulmonary edema, oliguria, and areflexia occur. The differential diagnosis for hypothermia and predisposing factors are shown in Table 54–1.

Because many standard thermometers read only to 34.4° C, the diagnosis of hypothermia depends on the use of a lower-reading glass or electronic thermometer to determine core temperature. After making the diagnosis, laboratory evaluation should be undertaken to identify potential complications. Characteristic findings are presented in Table 54–2.

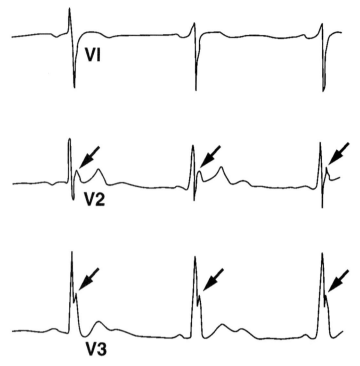

Figure 54–1. Precordial electrocardiographic leads illustrating the Osborn or "J" wave *(arrow)* in a hypothermic patient. (Courtesy of Behzad B. Pavri, M.D.)

Management

The management of hypothermia starts by stabilizing the airway, breathing, and circulation. It also includes preventing further heat loss, initiating rewarming, and treating complications (Fig. 54–2). Early endotracheal intubation facilitates clearing of secretions produced by cold-induced bronchorrhea in patients with altered mental status or a decreased gag reflex. Blood pressure may be supported by crystalloid infusions. Dopamine administration should be considered in cases refractory to volume resuscitation. Core temperature should be monitored closely during therapy to prevent iatrogenic worsening of hypothermia or overshoot hyperthermia.

Rewarming techniques are divided into passive external rewarming, active external rewarming, and active internal rewarming. *Passive external rewarming* is the method of choice for *mild* hypothermia. After wet clothing is removed, blankets or other types of insulation are applied, allowing the patient's intrinsic heat production to generate passive warming. This process requires sufficient physiologic reserve to generate heat by shivering or increasing metabolic rate.

Active rewarming techniques provide heat to the patient directly. These include warm blankets, heating pads, radiant heat, or warm baths directly to the patient's skin. These methods are indicated for moderate to severe hypothermia or for

Table 54–1. Differential Diagnosis for Hypothermia

Central nervous system disorders
   Head trauma
   Stroke
   Wernicke's encephalopathy
Drugs
   Ethanol
   Phenothiazines
   Sedative hypnotics
Environmental exposure (prehospital, operating room)
   Endocrine and metabolic disorders
   Hypoadrenalism
   Hypoglycemia
   Hypopituitarism
   Hypothalamic disease
   Hypothyroidism
   Malnutrition
   Hemorrhage with massive transfusion
Medical or surgical acute disorders
   Pancreatitis
   Sepsis
   Stroke
   Uremia
   Iatrogenic (overshoot in cooling heat stroke victims)
   Diffuse exfoliative dermatitis

Table 54–2. Laboratory, Electrocardiographic, and Radiographic Findings in Hypothermia

TESTS	FINDINGS
Arterial blood gas determination	Metabolic acidosis, respiratory alkalosis, or both
Amylase determination	Increase due to hypothermia-induced pancreatitis
Chest radiograph	Aspiration pneumonia, vascular congestion, pulmonary edema
Electrocardiogram	Prolongation of PR, QRS, QT intervals; ST segment elevations; T-wave inversions; Osborn J wave; atrial fibrillation or sinus bradycardia
Electrolytes	No consistent abnormality
Glucose	Increase, decrease, or no change
Hemoglobin, hematocrit	Increase due to hemoconcentration
PT, PTT	Increase due to inhibition of coagulation cascade
Platelet count	Decrease due to splenic sequestration
WBC count	No consistent abnormality

PT, prothrombin time; PTT, partial thromboplastin time; WBC, white blood cell.

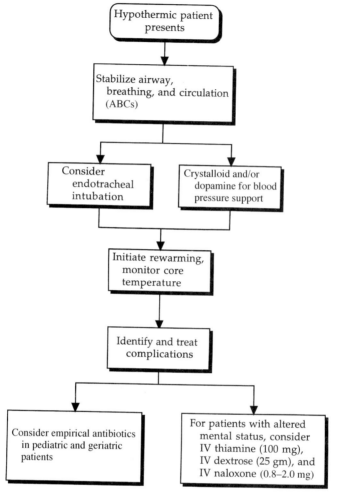

Figure 54–2. Schematic flow diagram outlining management of the hypothermic patient.

patients with mild hypothermia who lack physiologic reserve, are unstable, or fail to respond to passive external rewarming. A risk of active external rewarming is *core-temperature afterdrop*. This complication occurs when the extremities and trunk are warmed simultaneously. As extremities are rewarmed, cold blood that had pooled in the vasoconstricted extremities of the hypothermic patient flows into the core circulation, causing a drop in core temperature. This can be avoided by rewarming the trunk before the extremities by active internal warming.

Active internal rewarming is the most aggressive therapeutic strategy and may be used alone or combined with active external rewarming in moderate or severe hypothermia. Effective techniques include pleural and peritoneal irrigation with warm saline, continuous arteriovenous or conventional hemodialysis, and cardiopulmonary bypass. Giving humidified, inspired gas; warm intravenous fluids; and bladder or gastrointestinal irrigation with warm saline are adjunctive.

The hypothermic heart is sensitive to movement; rough handling, especially of the severely hypothermic patient, may precipitate *arrhythmias*. Although atrial fibrillation or flutter often resolves spontaneously with rewarming, management of ventricular arrhythmias may be problematic. Animal studies suggest that bretylium (5 to 10 mg/kg intravenously) is the drug of choice for ventricular fibrillation and may be an effective *prophylactic* agent against ventricular arrhythmias in patients with core temperatures less than 28° C. Ventricular arrhythmias and asystole may be refractory to conventional therapy until the patient has been rewarmed. Hypothermic patients in cardiac arrest should receive defibrillation and pharmacologic therapy as indicated. However, if unsuccessful, cardiopulmonary resuscitation and aggressive rewarming must be initiated promptly. Further efforts at resuscitation should be attempted once the core temperature is 30 to 32° C and should be continued until the temperature is 32 to 35° C.

HYPERTHERMIA

Hyperthermia may be defined as an elevation of body temperature to greater than the normal diurnal range of 36 to 37.5° C resulting from failure of thermoregulation. The causes of severe hyperthermia (core temperature >40° C [104° F]) in ICU patients are heat stroke, neuroleptic malignant syndrome (NMS), and, rarely, malignant hyperthermia.

Heat stroke is defined as body temperature greater than 40.5° C (104.9° F) with associated dysfunction of the central nervous system in the setting of an excessive environmental heat load. There are two types of heat stroke: *exertional* and *classic*. *Exertional heat stroke* generally occurs in young, otherwise healthy individuals who engage in heavy exercise during periods of high ambient temperature and humidity. *Classic heat stroke* affects individuals with underlying chronic medical conditions that either impair thermoregulation or prevent them from leaving the hot environment.

NMS is an idiosyncratic reaction to neuroleptic antipsychotic agents. It is characterized by hyperthermia, altered mental status, autonomic dysfunction, and muscle rigidity. NMS may mimic sepsis syndrome, including hypotension and anion gap metabolic acidosis.

Malignant hyperthermia is a rare, autosomal dominant disorder precipitated by exposure to anesthetic agents, most commonly succinylcholine and halothane. Malignant hyperthermia presents with severe hyperthermia and muscle rigidity.

Pathophysiology

The body's heat load results from its metabolic processes plus heat absorbed from the environment. In response to rising ambient temperature, the anterior hypothalamus stimulates efferent fibers of the autonomic nervous system to produce sweating and cutaneous vasodilation. Evaporation is the principal mechanism of heat loss in a hot environment but becomes ineffective when the relative humidity is greater than 75%. Convection, conduction, and radiation play lesser roles.

In heat stroke, the body is unable to dissipate the excess heat load, and a dangerous increase in core temperature results. When the temperature is greater than 42° C (107° F), oxidative phosphorylation becomes uncoupled and enzymes cease to function. Hepatocytes, vascular endothelium, and neural tissue are most sensitive to these effects, but all organ systems may be adversely affected.

NMS is believed to result from dopamine receptor blockade in the central nervous system or withdrawal of dopaminergic agonists. The frequency of NMS is directly related to the antidopaminergic potency of the neuroleptic agent. Although haloperidol appears to be the most common cause, all neuroleptic agents may cause this disorder, even when used to treat nausea. Hyperthermia results from increased muscle activity and altered hypothalamic thermoregulation.

Malignant hyperthermia results from the uncontrolled efflux of calcium from the sarcoplasmic reticulum and the associated increase in muscle activity.

The differential diagnosis for hyperthermia is extensive and includes infectious, endocrine, central nervous system, and toxic causes (Table 54–3). The diagnosis of heat stroke, NMS, or malignant hyperthermia is based on a careful history and physical examination of a patient with severe hyperthermia. The context in which symptoms develop usually suggests the cause. Rectal or core temperature should be determined in all patients. Severely hyperthermic patients may manifest sinus tachycardia, tachypnea, and hypotension or normal blood pressure with a widened pulse pressure.

Physical findings in heat stroke include cutaneous vasodilation, rales due to noncardiogenic pulmonary edema, excessive bleeding due to disseminated intravascular coagulation, and evidence of central nervous system dysfunction such as altered mental status and seizures. The skin may be moist or dry, depending on underlying medical conditions, hydration status, and the speed with which the heat stroke developed. NMS may present with diaphoresis, autonomic instability, muscle rigidity, fluctuating mental status, choreoathetosis, and tremors. Malignant hyperthermia is characterized by core temperatures up to 45° C (113° F) and muscle rigidity. The onset of malignant hyperthermia is usually within 1 hour of general anesthesia administration but may be delayed as long as 11 hours.

No laboratory finding is pathognomonic. However, such studies can be used to

Table 54–3. Differential Diagnosis of Hyperthermia

Environmental exposure	Hypothalamic stroke
Sepsis	Status epilepticus
Encephalitis	Cerebral hemorrhage
Brain abscess	Neuroleptic malignant syndrome (NMS)
Meningitis	Alcohol, sedative-hypnotic withdrawal
Tetanus	Salicylate, lithium toxicity
Typhoid fever	Sympathomimetic toxicity
Thyroid storm	Anticholinergic toxicity
Pheochromocytoma	Dystonic reaction
Catatonia	Serotonin syndrome
	Malignant hyperthermia

exclude other diagnoses and screen for possible complications. Baseline studies should include a complete blood count and prothrombin and partial thromboplastin times because of the risk of disseminated intravascular coagulation, as well as electrolyte, blood urea nitrogen, and creatinine determinations; urinalysis; and measurement of creatine phosphokinase levels because of the possibility of rhabdomyolysis. Liver function tests should be performed in the setting of heat stroke. Toxicologic screening may be indicated if a medication effect is suspected. A chest radiograph may demonstrate pulmonary edema, whereas an electrocardiogram may reveal evidence of heat-related myocardial damage. A head computed tomographic scan and lumbar puncture should be considered to assess central nervous system causes.

Management of heat stroke, NMS, and malignant hyperthermia requires rapid cooling while stabilizing respiration and circulation and treating complications (Fig. 54–3). Continuous core temperature monitoring with a rectal or esophageal probe is mandatory, and cooling measures should be stopped once a temperature of 39 to 39.5° C has been achieved to reduce the risk of iatrogenic hypothermia. In cases of suspected NMS or malignant hyperthermia, the potential offending agents must be stopped immediately.

Several cooling techniques exist and are the most effective for victims of heat

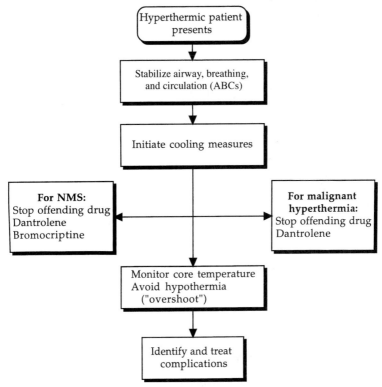

Figure 54–3. Schematic flow diagram outlining management of the hyperthermic patient. NMS, neuroleptic malignant syndrome.

stroke. Evaporative cooling is the modality of choice because it is effective, noninvasive, and easily performed. The naked patient is sprayed with a mist of lukewarm water while air is circulated with large fans. Resultant shivering may be suppressed with intravenous benzodiazepines or with chlorpromazine (25 to 50 mg intravenously unless NMS is suspected). Immersing the patient in ice water results in rapid cooling but makes monitoring and access difficult. Applying ice packs to the axillae, neck, and groin is effective but poorly tolerated in the awake patient. Cold peritoneal lavage is rapid but contraindicated in pregnant patients or those with previous abdominal surgery. Cold humidified oxygen, cold gastric lavage, cooling blankets, and cold intravenous fluids are adjunctive.

In NMS and malignant hyperthermia, cooling techniques are secondary to pharmacologic treatments. Drug therapy in NMS includes the dopamine agonist, bromocriptine, 2.5 to 7.5 mg orally every 8 hours, and dantrolene, 0.8 to 3 mg/kg intravenously every 6 hours (up to 10 mg/kg/24 h). Dantrolene is a nonspecific skeletal muscle relaxant that blocks the release of calcium from the sarcoplasmic reticulum. Although the efficacy of these agents has not been demonstrated in controlled trials, the results of several case reports support their use. Nitroprusside used to treat hypertension in NMS has been demonstrated to facilitate cooling by means of cutaneous vasodilation.

For malignant hyperthermia, the mainstay of pharmacologic management is dantrolene administration, 2.5 mg/kg intravenously every 8 hours. After an initial response, it may be continued at a dose of 1.2 mg/kg orally four times a day for 3 days.

CLINICAL PEARLS AND PITFALLS

1. Hypothermia and hyperthermia may be missed unless a true core temperature is obtained.
2. Initiation of therapy is often necessary before the cause is determined.
3. Early administration of parenteral antibiotics should be considered if occult sepsis is a possibility.
4. In severely hyperthermic patients, rapid cooling is best achieved by evaporation of lukewarm mist with fans. Cooling should be discontinued at a temperature of 39.5° C.
5. Heat stroke victims should not be assumed to be hypovolemic.
6. Bretylium is the drug of choice for prophylaxis or treatment of ventricular arrhythmias in severe hypothermia.
7. Resuscitation of the hypothermic patient in cardiac arrest should be continued until the core temperature reaches at least 32° C.

BIBLIOGRAPHY

Carbone JR: The neuroleptic malignant and serotonin syndromes. Emerg Med Clin North Am 18:317–325, 2000.
   This is a recent review that compares neuroleptic malignant syndrome (NMS) with serotonin syndrome (SS) (with 55 references).
Chan TC, Evans SD, Clark RF: Drug-induced hyperthermia. Crit Care Clin 4:785–808, 1997.
   This is a comprehensive review of malignant hyperthermia, neuroleptic malignant syndrome, and hyperthermic effects of sympathomimetic and anticholinergic poisonings (with 110 references).

Danzl DF, Pozos RS: Accidental hypothermia. N Engl J Med 331:1756–1760, 1994.
This review emphasizes the treatment of hypothermia.

Desforges JF: Hyperthermia. N Engl J Med 329:483–487, 1993.
This is a detailed review describing the pathophysiology and management of hyperthermia.

Harchelroad F: Acute thermoregulatory disorders. Clin Geriatr Med 9:621–639, 1993.
This article reviews hyperthermia and hypothermia in the geriatric population.

Jolly BT, Ghezzi KT: Accidental hypothermia. Emerg Med Clin North Am 10:311–327, 1992.
This is a detailed review of the diagnosis and management of hypothermia.

Lazar H: The treatment of hypothermia. N Engl J Med 337:1545–1547, 1997.
This editorial reviews current methods and accompanies Walpoth and colleagues' reference further on.

Orts A, Alcarez C, Delaney KA, et al: Bretylium tosylate and electrically induced cardiac arrhythmias during hypothermia in dogs. Am J Emerg Med 10:311–316, 1992.
This article presents the animal research leading to the use of bretylium in hypothermic patients.

Schneider SM: Neuroleptic malignant syndrome: Controversies in treatment. Am J Emerg Med 329:483–487, 1993.
This article is a good overview of the presentation and management of NMS.

Seraj MA, Channa AB, Al Harthi SS, et al: Are heat stroke patients fluid depleted? Importance of monitoring central venous pressure as a simple guideline for fluid therapy. Resuscitation 21:33–39, 1991.
This article discusses fluid status determination in heat stroke victims in Saudi Arabia.

Tek D, Olshaker JS: Heat illness. Emerg Med Clin North Am 10:299–310, 1992.
This is an overview of heat stroke and other heat-related illnesses.

Walpoth BH, Walpoth-Aslan BN, Heinrich P, et al: Outcome of survivors of accidental deep hypothermia and circulatory arrest treated with extracorporeal blood warming. N Engl J Med 337:1500–1505, 1997.
This report convincingly demonstrates the superiority of extracorporeal rewarming to treat severe hypothermia with or without cardiac arrest in previously healthy young patients.

55

Smoke and Carbon Monoxide Inhalation

Christopher D. O'Brien
Scott Manaker

Inhalation injury from smoke and toxic products of combustion is associated with 50 to 80% of the 6000 fatalities resulting from fires in the United States each year. From the late 1980s to the late 1990s, mortality rates for surface burn injuries have declined. The majority of victims died of smoke-related pulmonary injury and carbon monoxide (CO) poisoning. In addition, more than 3800 individuals die yearly from intentional and accidental exposures to other sources of CO. Indeed, CO remains the leading cause of death from poisoning in the United States, with most of its victims at the extremes of age or socioeconomically disadvantaged. This chapter focuses on the causes, pathophysiology, and management of inhalation injuries with emphasis on CO poisoning.

INHALATION INJURY

Respiratory injuries related to smoke inhalation result from thermal effects, toxic products of combustion, or asphyxia (respiratory or cellular). Exposure to super-heated gases may produce mucosal injury of the upper or lower airway, depending on the victim's level of consciousness and the water content of the smoke. Because of its high specific heat, steam is particularly injurious to the lower airway. Smoke inhalation may result in chemical injury by deposition of acid or alkaline combustion products in the upper and lower airway. These toxic combustion products adsorb to the particulate fraction (soot and liquid droplets), deposit on respiratory mucosa, and lead to both local corrosion and systemic toxicities from their subsequent absorption. The extent and location of the injury depends on particle size, minute ventilation, duration of exposure, and toxicant water solubility. Small particles (<0.06 micron) are deposited primarily in the lung parenchyma (potentially bypassing the upper airway), whereas larger particles (2 to 5 microns) are distributed throughout the respiratory tract. The increasing prevalence of synthetic compounds in the environment has produced a burgeoning list of combustion products that may complicate an inhalation injury (Table 55–1).

Most smoke inhalation deaths result from asphyxia. Fires consume oxygen, which may lower the ambient oxygen concentration to less than 10% in poorly ventilated areas. However, the two major asphyxiants, CO and hydrogen cyanide, are responsible for more than 80% of smoke inhalation–related fatalities. When oxygen is consumed in a closed-space (low oxygen) fire, pyrolysis (incomplete combustion) predominates and CO levels may rapidly exceed 0.1%, sufficient to lead to death within minutes. In this setting, up to 27% of smoke-inhalation victims may also demonstrate significantly elevated blood cyanide levels. In some cases, the synergistic effects of other toxic products of combustion, such as hydrogen sulfide, may also play a role in asphyxiation.

Table 55–1. Toxic Products of Combustion

CHEMICAL	SOURCES	INJURY PRODUCED
Aldehydes	Plastic from furniture	Upper airway injury and CNS depression
Acrolein	Acrylics from windows, wood finishes, or wall coverings	Diffuse airway and alveolar injury
Ammonia	Phenolics and nylon	Upper airway injury
Anhydrides	Chemical, paint, plastics	Airway injury, asthma; pulmonary hemorrhage with high-dose exposure
Carbon dioxide	Closed space fires (as high as 10% CO_2)	Respiratory acidosis, CNS depression
Cyanide	Carpets, upholstery, nylon polyurethane products from isocyanates	Acidosis, shock, asthma, airway injury, hypersensitivity pneumonitis
Hydrogen chloride	Fabrics, polyvinyl chloride	Mucosal burns and edema, dysrhythmias, shock
Hydrogen fluoride	Polytetrafluoroethylene (Teflon) from pipes or kitchen utensils	Upper airway injury
Nitrogen dioxide	Nitrocellulose	Alveolar injury

Modified from Sheppard D: Noxious gases: Pathogenetic mechanism. In: Baum G, Wolinsky E (eds): Textbook of Pulmonary Diseases, 4th ed. Boston, Little, Brown, 1989, pp 840–841.

CNS, central nervous system.

CARBON MONOXIDE POISONING

CO is a colorless, odorless, tasteless, nonirritant gas that is normally present at ambient concentrations of less than 0.001%. CO avidly combines with hemoglobin to form carboxyhemoglobin (CO-Hgb). The concentration of CO-Hgb can be measured by co-oximetry and expressed as a percentage of total hemoglobin. Patients presenting with acute CO poisoning demonstrate a range of neurologic, cardiovascular, and systemic symptoms that roughly correlate to the CO-Hgb level. However, the CO-Hgb level predicts the degree of initial CO exposure *poorly* and does not reflect the CO levels in the tissues.

At low CO-Hgb levels (<10%), patients are usually asymptomatic. However, individuals with pre-existing cardiopulmonary disease, such as coronary artery disease or chronic obstructive pulmonary disease, may suffer exacerbations of their condition. Patients with CO-Hgb levels greater than 20 to 25% may experience headache, nausea, confusion, and dizziness. Coma and seizures secondary to cerebral edema occur at CO-Hgb levels greater than 50%. Myocardial ischemia and ventricular arrythmias may occur at CO-Hgb levels greater than 20%, with death likely at levels greater than 60% (Table 55–2). Overall mortality from acute CO intoxication ranges from 0 to 31%, depending on the severity of exposure and subsequent treatment. Significant morbidity persists in up to 40% of CO poisoning victims.

A syndrome of delayed neurologic sequelae can occur 3 to 40 days after apparent recovery from acute CO exposure. Victims of this insidious phenomenon demonstrate variable degrees of aphasia, apraxia, apathy, disorientation, hallucina-

Table 55–2. Carboxyhemoglobin Concentration and Clinical Effects

CARBOXYHEMOGLOBIN % CONCENTRATION	SEVERITY	EXPECTED SYMPTOMS
5–10	Mild	Psychomotor impairment
10–20		Headache, dyspnea
20–30		Nausea, lethargy, mild weakness
30–40	Moderate	Vomiting, syncope, severe weakness
50	Severe	Loss of consciousness, seizures, dysrhythmias
60	Potentially lethal	Coma
70	Lethal	Death

Modified from Ruddy RM: Smoke inhalation injury. Pediatr Clin North Am 41:317–336, 1994.

tions, bradykinesia, cogwheel rigidity, gait disturbances, incontinence, personality changes, and mood changes that may be permanent. Without treatment, up to 40% of CO-poisoned patients may suffer some manifestation of these delayed neurologic sequelae.

Although smoke inhalation is the most commonly recognized source of CO poisoning, many other environmental sources of CO may yield both acute and chronic CO toxicity. Exhaust from internal combustion engines, and other devices that may involve incomplete combustion, can produce CO accumulation in closed or poorly ventilated areas. Unlike victims of acute CO poisoning, patients suffering from chronic CO intoxication may experience only nonspecific, low-grade symptoms, making accurate diagnosis notoriously difficult. The actual incidence of non–fire-related CO poisoning is not well defined. However, since more than a third of these cases may go undiagnosed, chronic CO intoxication has been labeled an occult epidemic.

PATHOPHYSIOLOGY OF CARBON MONOXIDE POISONING

CO blocks oxygen transport from the alveolus to the tissues by preferentially binding to hemoglobin with 230-fold greater affinity than oxygen. The amount of CO uptake depends on the minute ventilation, the relative concentrations of CO and oxygen, and the duration of exposure. The binding of a single CO molecule to hemoglobin produces a conformational change, which makes hemoglobin more oxygen avid and results in a leftward shift of the oxyhemoglobin dissociation curve (see Appendix A, Fig. 1). Although dissolved blood oxygen tension (Pa_{O_2}) remains unchanged, not only do oxygen content of arterial blood (Ca_{O_2}) and oxygen delivery (Do_2) to tissues decrease but so does the ability of hemoglobin to offload O_2 at the capillary level. As the blood oxygen content falls, an increased minute ventilation and a respiratory alkalosis ensue, causing further uptake of CO and an additional leftward shift of the oxyhemoglobin dissociation curve (see Appendix A, Fig. 1). Although direct co-oximetry detects CO-Hgb, pulse oximetry does not. This results in the so-called oximetry gap.

Approximately 10 to 15% of CO binds to extravascular proteins, including myoglobin, cytochrome C oxidase, guanylate cyclase, and nitric oxide synthase. The dissociation of CO from myoglobin and cytochrome oxidase is significantly slower than that from hemoglobin. Therefore, persistent derangements of oxidative metabolism and myocardial and skeletal muscle function may occur despite normal CO-Hgb levels. The delay in CO dissociation from these proteins has been postulated to explain the acute and delayed toxicity seen in CO poisoning. Furthermore, fetal hemoglobin has a significantly greater affinity for CO than does hemoglobin A, explaining the occurrence of fetal demise in gravid women successfully treated for CO poisoning.

The half-life of CO-Hgb when a patient is breathing ambient oxygen (21%) at sea level is approximately 320 minutes. If one breaths 100% oxygen, this is reduced to 60 minutes. Breathing 100% oxygen under 2.5 to 3.0 atmospheres of pressure reduces the half-life of CO-Hgb to only 23 minutes. In addition, 100% oxygen at 2.5 to 3.0 atmospheres increases the dissolved plasma oxygen to 6 mL/ dL, which is sufficient to supply basal oxygen requirements to the tissues in the absence of functional hemoglobin. This acceleration of CO excretion and augmentation of oxygen delivery underlies the use of normobaric and hyperbaric oxygen therapy in acute CO poisoning in which initial mortality appears to result from hypoxia-related ventricular dysrhythmias and cardiovascular collapse. In contrast, CO-induced delayed neurologic sequelae do not appear to be caused by hypoxia alone. Rather, it is hypothesized that the characteristic perivascular neural injury of CO poisoning is due to the derivation of oxygen free radicals and the production of oxidative injury. Although seemingly counterintuitive, hyperbaric oxygen therapy may prevent formation of oxygen species responsible for brain lipid peroxidation and thus limit the extent and frequency of delayed neurologic sequelae.

DIAGNOSIS AND EVALUATION

Smoke inhalation should be considered in any victim rescued from an accident or fire scene, whether or not surface burns are present. Smoke inhalation is an important diagnostic consideration when altered mental status exists, as many victims may not manifest overt signs of surface injury despite severe inhalation damage or asphyxiant exposure. The initial patient evaluation follows the algorithms of Advanced Trauma Life Support Program (see Chapter 93), as associated trauma is common and may worsen precipitously if not identified.

Early recognition of CO poisoning and airway compromise, the two major inhalation injuries, is crucial. The classic predictive signs and symptoms of inhalation injury (hoarseness, stridor, cervical and oropharyngeal burns, singed facial hair, carbonaceous sputum) are notoriously insensitive in predicting either CO poisoning or airway injury. Since arterial oxygen tension or pulse oximetry may be normal despite severe CO poisoning, early measurement of arterial or venous CO-Hgb by co-oximetry is mandatory in all potential victims. Similarly, early laryngoscopic or fiberoptic examination of the upper airway may confirm inhalation injury (pharyngeal or laryngeal soot, airway edema, erythema, and mucosal blistering) and facilitate management decisions.

Smoke inhalation victims may manifest both thermal and chemical injury. Therefore, their initial clinical presentation is highly variable and may underestimate the severity of illness. Abnormal breath sounds (crackles or rhonchi) suggest lower airway or parenchymal injury but may be delayed for 24 hours after injury. Similarly, initial chest radiographs may be unremarkable despite significant hypoxemia. In patients with significant upper airway injury on initial evaluation, fiberoptic bronchoscopy examines the subglottic airway for evidence of severe injury. Initially, abnormal lower airway findings include mucosal edema, erythema, blistering, hemorrhage, ulceration, soot deposition, and airway narrowing. Subsequently, crusts, mucous plugs, and bronchial casts may form from sloughed epithelium. Increasingly available portable spirometry facilitates identification of patients most at risk for airway compromise: up to 30% of inhalation-injury patients manifest an upper airway obstruction on their flow-volume loops. Ultimately, the early diagnosis of airway injury identifies patients at increased risk for mortality and enables physicians to anticipate both early and late sequelae, including atelectasis, bacterial pneumonia, and acute respiratory distress syndrome.

All suspected victims of CO poisoning should undergo an assiduous examination for other potential toxins and comorbid conditions, particularly patients with an altered mental status or victims of intentional poisoning. A complete blood count, serum chemistry panels, a blood gas determinaton with a CO level measured by co-oximetry, and a toxicology screen should be obtained. In any smoke inhalation victim, the presence of a metabolic acidosis or venous Po_2 greater than 40 mm Hg raises the possibility of concomitant hydrogen cyanide exposure. However, an anion gap metabolic acidosis is consistent with lactic acidosis due to CO poisoning alone when oxygen delivery is sufficiently compromised. The possibility of concomitant toxin or volatile ingestion causing the acidosis should be ruled out. Serial creatine kinase and lactate dehydrogenase levels should be obtained, and the patient should undergo electrocardiographic monitoring if the initial electrocardiogram is abnormal (sinus tachycardia, ST interval changes). All victims of CO poisoning should undergo early psychometric testing and serial neurologic examinations to identify any deficit. Patients manifesting any neurologic findings (or those in whom there is a history of such a deficit at the scene) should be treated with hyperbaric oxygen. Later in the course of CO poisoning, neuroimaging studies (computed tomography, magnetic resonance imaging) may reveal characteristic abnormalities of CO toxicity, including bilateral necrosis of the globus pallidus, cerebral cortex, hippocampus, and substantia nigra.

Although diagnosing CO poisoning is straightforward in victims of smoke inhalation or attempted suicide, the identification of chronic or acute CO toxicity from other sources is challenging. The most sensitive indicator of CO poisoning is a history of possible CO exposure from the use of kerosene heaters, wood stoves, or indoor grills; overly insulated or airtight homes, where backdrafting occurs through furnace exhaust chimneys; being enclosed in vehicles with faulty exhaust systems, including boats and pick-up trucks with caps; the use of methylene chloride–containing solvents with CO produced through hepatic metabolism; or other exposures to products of incomplete combustion. The physical findings, signs, and symptoms of acute and chronic poisoning may mimic exacerbation of a variety of conditions, including myocardial ischemia, chronic obstructive pulmonary disease, acute stroke, seizure, migraine headache, depression, or nonspecific viral illness. The sign of cherry red skin or mucous membranes, or both, is specific, although present in less than 10% of patients with acute CO poisoning. Pulse oximetry does not detect CO-Hgb and should never be employed for diagnosis or screening. Despite the universal employment of co-oximetry, the CO-Hgb level is extremely unreliable in predicting the severity and prognosis of most CO exposures. It is a poor screening test, particularly if obtained long after the exposure ends. Indeed, the best screening test for possible CO toxicity remains the history and the clinician's inclusion of this entity in the differential diagnosis.

MANAGEMENT

Initial management of the smoke inhalation victim follows the guidelines for trauma resuscitation: early establishment of a stable airway and management of life-threatening concurrent injuries. Control of the airway through orotracheal or nasotracheal intubation is always indicated when the primary or secondary survey suggests potential airway compromise. Signs and symptoms such as stridor, hoarseness, full-thickness burns of the face or neck, mucous membrane burns, severe central nervous system depression, or laryngoscopic evidence of laryngeal edema mandate early intubation. All patients should be treated with 100% oxygen by tight-fitting face mask or via endotracheal tube until CO poisoning has been excluded. Similarly, therapy for concomitant cyanide poisoning (see Table 57–1, Chapter 57) should be considered for patients at risk: entrapped victims with severe CO poisoning; patients exposed to fires involving nylon, polyurethane, melamine, wool, or silk; or individuals with unexplained persistent acidosis or a reduced arteriovenous difference in oxygen content.

Supportive therapy includes humidification of the upper respiratory tract to alleviate mucous membrane dryness and discomfort while minimizing inspissation of secretions. Bronchodilator therapy with beta agonists may relieve bronchospasm related to inhalation injury. However, anticholinergic agents should be avoided because of their potential drying effects. Corticosteroid administration in patients with airway edema from inhalation injury has been associated with increased mortality in limited controlled studies and therefore is not recommended. The use of corticosteroid therapy for bronchospasm from smoke inhalation is less well defined and has been used empirically in patients with symptoms refractory to other therapy. Despite the high incidence of infection associated with surface burn and inhalation injuries, prophylactic systemic antibiotics are not indicated because they promote early emergence of resistant organisms.

The therapy guidelines for all CO poisoning victims are similar regardless of the CO exposure source (Fig. 55–1). All patients suspected of CO exposure should receive 100% supplemental oxygen by tight-fitting mask or by endotracheal intubation if severely obtunded. Once initiated, normobaric oxygen therapy (NBO) should be continued until CO-Hgb levels are less than 5% and no signs of cardiovascular, neurologic, or other initial symptoms exist (6 to 12 hours). Cardiac monitoring is essential, as ventricular arrhythmias cause most early deaths in CO-poisoned victims. Most CO-exposed patients warrant admission to the hospital or extended observation in the emergency ward. An asymptomatic patient with a CO-Hgb less than 10% and no initial neurologic or hemodynamic instability (including transient loss of consciousness) may be safely discharged.

All patients evaluated for significant CO poisoning should be considered for early referral to the nearest hyperbaric oxygen (HBO) therapy facility. The decision to initiate HBO in a CO poisoning victim should follow the algorithm in Figure

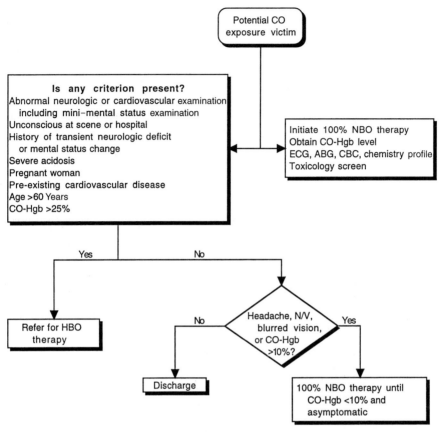

Figure 55–1. Schematic flow diagram to treat carbon monoxide (CO) poisoning. ABG, arterial blood gas; ECG, electrocardiogram; CBC, complete blood count; CO-Hgb = carboxyhemoglobin; HBO, hyperbaric oxygen; NBO, normobaric oxygen; N/V, nausea and vomiting. (See Fig. 25–1, Chapter 25 for mini-mental status examination. (Modified from Thom SR: Smoke inhalation. Emerg Med Clin North Am 7:371–387, 1989.)

55–1. Most studies support the contention that HBO hastens resolution of symptoms in patients with acute severe CO intoxication (depressed mental status or frank coma, myocardial ischemia, severe acidosis, or persistent neurologic deficits). Furthermore, HBO therapy reduces the risks for delayed, CO-induced, permanent neurologic sequelae. This reduction has been observed consistently in multiple, large-scale observational studies. Thus, emergent referral of severely poisoned CO patients to a hyperbaric center is warranted.

In moderate CO poisoning (transient loss of consciousness, neuropsychologic abnormalities), few data indicate HBO confers a mortality benefit when compared with NBO. However, a recent, prospective, randomized trial in patients with mild to moderate CO poisoning indicated a reduction in the incidence of delayed neurologic sequelae when treated with early HBO (two treatments initiated within 6 hours of exposure). Some experts suggest that subgroups of patients with higher morbidity and mortality risk from moderate CO poisoning should also be considered for HBO even in the absence of persistent or transient mental status or neurologic abnormalities. This includes patients with pre-existing cardiovascular disease, patients older than 60 years of age, pregnant women (with increased mortality risk to the fetus), and patients with prolonged CO exposure ("soaking") or CO-Hgb levels greater than 25 to 30%. Patients with mild CO intoxication, defined as having constitutional symptoms but no loss of consciousness and no cognitive deficits on neuropsychologic screening, should be treated with NBO therapy and monitored closely, but they do not require referral to a hyperbaric facility.

BIBLIOGRAPHY

Hardy KR, Thom SR: Pathophysiology and treatment of carbon monoxide poisoning. Clin Toxicol 32:613–629, 1994.
This is an excellent review of epidemiologic data, pathophysiology, and outcome studies involving CO poisoning. A comprehensive description of clinical presentations, management strategies, and the delayed neurologic sequelae syndrome is included.

Mozingo DW, Barillo DJ, Pruitt BA: Acute resuscitation and transfer management of burned and electrically injured patients. Trauma Q 11:94–113, 1994.
This article presents a comprehensive review of burn injury management with an excellent section detailing the presentation and management of smoke inhalation.

Ruddy RM: Smoke inhalation injury. Pediatr Clin North Am 41:317–336, 1994.
This is a detailed review of smoke inhalation causes, presentation, management, and complications in adult and pediatric patients.

Thom SR, Taber RL, Mendiguren II, et al: Delayed neuropsychologic sequelae after carbon monoxide poisoning: Prevention by treatment with hyperbaric oxygen. Ann Emerg Med 25:474–480, 1995.
This article presents a randomized, prospective (but nonblinded) clinical trial evaluating HBO therapy in moderate and mild CO poisoning. A good overview of delayed neurologic sequelae is included.

Tibbles PM, Edelsberg JS: Hyperbaric-oxygen therapy. N Engl J Med 334:1642–1648, 1996.
This is an excellent review of the theory behind HBO and its clinical applications.

Tibbles PM, Perotta PL: Treatment of carbon monoxide poisoning: A critical review of human outcome studies comparing normobaric oxygen with hyperbaric oxygen. Ann Emerg Med 24:269–276, 1994.
This article presents an excellent overview of outcome studies performed up to 1994. A well-documented set of treatment recommendations is outlined based on the available literature.

56

Burns

Daniel O. Hensell
Frederick DeClement

Burns are common clinical problems with which clinicians in the intensive care unit (ICU) should be familiar. Small burns can be treated and autografted on an outpatient basis by a burn specialist. Massive burn injuries are best treated in a regional burn unit. Critical care specialists are often involved with a burn injury when the burn is a secondary diagnosis, that is, when the patient's primary problem is medical (smoke inhalation, lightning) or surgical (trauma). A burned patient with trauma may be kept in an ICU for treatment and stabilization of the trauma before transfer to a burn center for the more prolonged burn care and rehabilitation.

EXTENT OF BURN

Since the pathophysiology of the burn injury correlates well with the area of skin involved, the percentage of the body's surface area that is burned must be estimated. Detailed diagrams, such as that of Berkow, can be used to determine the percent of total body surface area (BSA) affected. A more practical method to use is the Rule of Nines: the head-neck and each upper extremity contributes 9% BSA, the front or back of the trunk and each lower extremity contributes 18% BSA, and the perineum contributes 1% BSA. Perhaps an even simpler and more rapid method of estimating percent of BSA burned is using the palmar surface of the patient's hand. The palmar surface including the surface of the digits approximates 1% BSA (although in actuality it is only 0.85%). Similarly, the palmar surface of the hand minus the palmar area of digits can be considered 0.5% BSA. In calculating the percent of BSA of injury, first-degree burns are excluded. Although the area involved would normally be calculated at admission, later re-evaluation is necessary because some burns may become evident later after removal of soot and dirt. In addition, some areas of normally pigmented collapsed bullae of partial-thickness injury could later be debrided with dressing changes.

While evaluating the more apparent burn wounds, other less apparent but critical problems, for example, the classic ABCs of airway, breathing, and circulation plus trauma survey, must not be overlooked. For example, at the time of initial examination the patient may be hypotensive, have vasoconstriction, and be wet and partially clad. Care must be taken to avoid hypothermia in these circumstances. Although cardiovascular monitoring is performed routinely, continuous core temperature monitoring is necessary, especially when wounds are redressed or when patients are bathing or waiting in an operating room.

CATEGORIZATION OF BURNS

Depth Of Burn

The depth of burns is reflected by the standard terminology of first-, second-, and third-degree burns (Table 56–1).

Table 56–1. First-, Second-, and Third-Degree Burns

DEGREE	DEPTH OF INJURY	APPEARANCE	EXAMPLE	COMMENT
First	Only superficial epidermal layer	Red; no bullae	Sunburn	Commonly caused by flash-type energy source
Second	Superficial partial thickness	Bullae present or previously present; moist reddened surface beneath prior bullae	Scald by hot water	Expect to heal in 14 days Healed skin is dull and pink
Second (deep)	Deep partial thickness	White appearance beneath the bullae	Hot tar or grease	Caused by adherent energy source Many need 30 days to heal Often excised and autografted
Third	Full thickness	No bullae Dry leathery texture White or gray ischemia Occasionally translucent eschar	Sustained exposure to flames	Requires excision and autograft closure

Unusual Types of Burns

Chemical burns are usually due to acid or alkali. All should be treated initially by intense lavage for more than 30 minutes using saline or tap water. Efforts at neutralization of the chemical agent are not useful. The resulting neutralization reaction will be exothermic and perhaps cause additional thermal tissue damage.

Hydrofluoric acid contact is an exception. First aid of burns resulting from hydrofluoric acid requires magnesium or calcium gel (using a water-soluble lubricant as a base), with delayed care requiring subcutaneous injection of 10% calcium gluconate at 0.5 mL/cm^2. Multiple injections require digital blocks or even light general anesthesia. Areas of hydrofluoric acid injury may exhibit pain and no redness or minor redness with delayed pain. Exposure around the fingernails can be treated by calcium injections beneath the edges, with the rare requirement for drilling holes in the nails if later collections develop.

High-voltage electrical injuries are more insidious than other burns in that the burned area is difficult to evaluate. Significant injury can occur beneath normal skin and cause difficulty with estimation of burn size and fluid requirements. Although a common electrical injury involves a flash burn from a nearby short circuit, the more serious high-voltage contact injuries involve an entry and exit wound. These sites have especially severe damage and very thick eschar. Extremity muscle injury may require an alkaline diuresis and low-dose dopamine for treatment of rhabdomyolysis and myoglobinuria (to maintain a urine output greater than 100 mL/h).

Such wounds of extremities also have a high risk for the development of a *compartment syndrome*. Under these circumstances, compartment pressures should be monitored using a central venous pressure–type manometer or pressure transducer with a needle and infused saline (see Chapter 95). Compartment pressures are considered elevated when they (expressed in centimeters of water) equal, exceed, or are within 20 mm Hg of the diastolic pressure (in millimeters of mercury). More commonly, areas of an extremity surrounding the entry or exit wounds are firm and tight, and the diagnosis of elevated compartment pressure can be made by inspection. If this occurs, a fasciotomy is required on admission.

Typically, high-voltage burns are re-explored every third day for débridement and evaluation of tissue salvage. These injuries are characterized by delayed tissue necrosis as well as delayed appearance of peripheral neuropathies and early onset of cataracts.

Lightning injury is different from high-voltage injury. The chief concerns are cardiac arrhythmias, severe autonomic dysfunction, and small skin burns that characteristically follow areas of metal contact, such as coins or zippers.

Frostbite injuries should be treated as burns. After careful rewarming, involved areas should be treated with great care to avoid any tissue trauma or shearing forces. Any débridement should be carried out several weeks after injury because areas of blackened bullae may spontaneously slough to reveal pink, healed skin beneath.

BURN MANAGEMENT

Fluid Resuscitation

The initial care of a major burn injury requires fluid resuscitation to counter hypotension secondary to the capillary permeability of the burn. The most common resuscitation formula involves lactated Ringer's (LR) with no glucose using the Parkland formula: 4 mL LR $\times$ % burn $\times$ body weight (kg) = volume (mL) per 24 hours (Fig. 56–1). The volume of resuscitation is calculated from the time of injury and *not* the time the patient first receives medical care. Often a "catch up" of fluids is required. If myoglobinuria appears, the infusion rate should be increased. Concomitant smoke inhalation may require an increase in the Parkland formula from 4 mL LR to 5 mL LR. In the elderly, the value of 3 mL LR may be substituted. Half the calculated fluid is given in the first 8 hours and the remaining half over the ensuing 16 hours.

This formula provides an approximation only so that hourly urine output must be closely observed. If oliguria (<30 mL/h) occurs, increasing the infusion rate or adding colloid or low-dose dopamine should be chosen over giving diuretics or vasopressors. By the second 24 hours, the patient has usually sustained maximal edema. In an effort to return the third-spaced fluid, a colloid in the form of salt-poor albumin (SPA) is usually administered. This is calculated as 0.1 mL SPA $\times$ % burn $\times$ body weight (kg) = volume (mL) of 25% SPA given over an 8-hour period, that is, from hour 24 to hour 32. At 24 hours, glucose may be added to the fluids with a change from LR to D5 1/2 normal saline or D5 1/4 normal saline, guided by serum electrolyte determinations. By the second 24 hours, fluids should be decreased, but in slow increments because a rapid decrease will cause return of hypotension and oliguria.

By the third day after injury, the extravasated fluid will begin mobilizing, as indicated by diuresis, with return to preburn weight by the fifth day after the burn

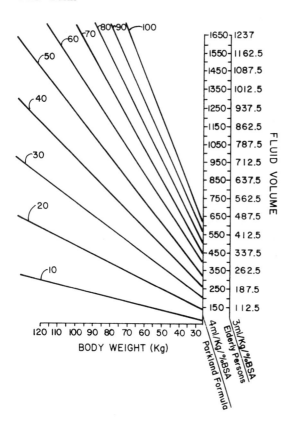

Figure 56–1. Nomogram for estimating volume of lactated Ringer's to be given *per hour* over the first 8 hours (starting at the time of the burn; see text). To use the nomogram, start at the point representing the patient's weight (kg) on the horizontal axis, move vertically to intersect the diagonal line (corresponding to the patient's percent burn), and then move horizontally to intersect the vertical axis to get the hourly fluid volume over first 8 hours. (See text for further details.) (Adapted from Brooker AF, Pezeshki C: Tissue pressure to evaluate compartmental syndrome. J Trauma 19:689–691, 1979.)

episode. Thereafter, some increased fluids still must be administered to account for evaporative loss from the burn wound, using the formula (25 + % burn) × BSA (m²) = mL/h.

Pain Management

It is not unusual that burn patients require high analgesic doses. The analgesic of choice is morphine. An initial loading dose can be as high as 8 mg as an intravenous bolus and thereafter titrated by continuous infusion according to the patient's response and hemodynamics. It is often necessary to add anxiolytics, especially for patients with a history of alcohol abuse.

Hematologic and Electrolyte Issues

Blood test results on admission would be expected to show hemoconcentration, with the hemoglobin and hematocrit dropping during resuscitation. After the diuresis phase, the hemoglobin commonly drops further even in the absence of surgery or trauma. The white blood cell count also is greatly elevated at admission and similarly drops to as low as 2000/μL within several days of injury. It then recovers spontaneously to a mildly elevated level. The drop in white blood cell count is felt to be due to margination and does not signify any pathologic condition or effects of topical therapy. Similarly, the platelet count drops to a lesser degree on approximately the third to fifth day with gradual recovery. Magnesium and calcium concentrations tend to remain stable from the LR resuscitation, although they gradually drop later, with the decrease in total calcium concentration parallel to the fall in serum albumin. In view of the anemia following the burn episode and the likelihood of upcoming surgery, recombinant erythropoietin (Epogen or Procrit) (4000 units subcutaneously three times weekly) can be administered in the early phase. Even with this, most burn patients require multiple red blood cell transfusions.

Escharotomy

The evaluator of the burn on admission should be alert to any circumferential third-degree burns because they will require escharotomy. On extremities where the burn depth is less clear, these burns can be watched closely by following distal pulses by Doppler ultrasonography. If a full-thickness wound is present over a hemithorax or the entire chest, respiratory compromise may occur. Escharotomies are performed with Bovie electrocautery in a secluded area (e.g., an operating room) that will allow aspiration of the smoke plume. They should be performed with the patient under light general anesthesia with the incisions made down to the subcutaneous fatty tissue level. Extremities, including joints, should have longitudinal incisions along the medial and lateral aspects. The anterior chest wall should have bilateral anterior axillary incisions that connect transversely across the infraclavicular line and in a chevron fashion following the subcostal margins. Areas over the sternum should not be incised because of the risk of osteomyelitis. As the fluid resuscitation is carried out, a significant amount of the administered fluid will extravasate so that appropriately performed escharotomy wounds will readily spread when incised. Hand burns may require escharotomy on the digits if both palmar and dorsal aspects are of full-thickness depth. These incisions should be carried out longitudinally, dorsal to the flexion crease, which indicates the underlying neurovascular bundle, and lateral to the midline digital extensor tendon mechanism.

At times, a deep partial-thickness burn in a circumferential pattern or on the anterior chest may benefit from chemical escharotomy. Using an enzyme agent (Collagenase or Travase), one can place longitudinal stripes on the medial and lateral aspects of extremities and around the chest, repeated once or twice at 8-hour intervals. Use is limited to narrow stripes because the agents are painful and may cause bleeding.

Wound Care

Local care of burn wounds involves washing and dressing changes daily. The most common local agent used is silver sulfadiazine (SSD) (Silvadene, Thermazine). This agent should be used daily unless there is a sulfa allergy. A contact allergic reaction to SSD appears as a dermatitic redness and rash around the wound. Any intact bullae of a partial-thickness injury and remnants of collapsed bullae should be left in place as biologic dressings. Often, serous wound discharge and SSD combine to form a yellow material that may be misinterpreted as purulence. Also, the silver content of the SSD precipitates and may cause harmless black staining of the wound edges or dressings. Electrical burns, because of their very thick eschar, may be better treated with mafenide (Sulfamylon) application every 8 hours and no dressings because only this agent will penetrate the thick eschar.

Nutrition

Burn injuries lead to greater metabolic demands than does other trauma. Thus, the nutritional therapy of burn care must be aggressive. In burns of greater than 20% BSA, a nasogastric tube should be placed on admission because ileus is common. Efforts should be made to begin enteral feeding on the day of admission, and gastric residual fluid should be measured to determine if enteral feedings should continue. All tubes, for example, nasogastric and endotracheal, in burn patients are best affixed with umbilical tape and not adhesive tape. To increase the gastrointestinal motility, metoclopramide (Reglan) and cisapride (Propulsid) are often administered. Enteral feeding is the preferred means, with the nasogastric tube replaced by a smaller soft nasoenteral feeding tube after several days or even later by a gastrostomy or jejunostomy tube. Continuous feeding amounts should be accelerated as rapidly as possible to a maximal caloric need, calculated using the Harris-Benedict formulas (Table 56–2) or as recommended by a nutritional consultation. Since gastric bleeding due to stress ulcers in a burn patient is well described (Curling ulcer), patients should also be given sucralfate (Carafate) by nasogastric tube or H_2 histamine receptor blockers intravenously (in a dose sufficient to keep gastric pH greater than 4. Generally, use of parenteral lipids as fat supplements in burn patients should be minimized because they may compromise the hepatic reticuloendothelial system. Multiple vitamins are given daily. Often lactobacillus (Lactenex) and nystatin are given enterally in an empirical attempt to minimize intestinal pathogen translocation. The enteric feeding formula should have a significant fiber content and be combined with a program of regular laxative or enema use. Attention to nutritional care must be aggressive with extra attention to small details. As an example, prior to surgery, patients should be kept in a fasting state only after 4:00 AM instead of after midnight.

Burns of Special Areas

Burns of special areas require special care. Burns around the face and head may do well with no dressings and triple antibiotic application daily, with ophthalmologic evaluation if indicated. Burned ears can be treated with mafenide and no dressings because this agent may decrease the incidence of chondritis and avoids the risk of pressure necrosis. If ears are wrapped, care must be taken to place padding behind them to avoid pressure. All burned extremities should be kept elevated, with hand burns benefiting by an early occupational therapy consultation. Digits should be kept in a straight position and wrapped individually. Burns of the back and buttock

Table 56–2. Estimates for Daily Caloric and Protein Needs

For Caloric Needs (total Kcal) for Weight Maintenance (Harris-Benedict Formulas)

For Males:
[65.5 + 13.7 × weight (kg) + 5 × height (cm) − 6.7 × age (yr)] × Activity Factor*
 × Injury Factor†
For Females:
[665.1 + 9.6 × weight (kg) + 1.8 × height (cm) − (4.7 × age (yr)] × Activity Factor*
 × Injury Factor†

For Protein Needs

Protein = 2–2.5 gm/kg or a ratio of Kcal:nitrogen (g) of 100:1

*ACTIVITY FACTOR		†INJURY FACTOR	
Confined to bed	1.2	Surgery	1.1–1.2
Ambulatory	1.3	Infection	1.2–1.6
Fever	1.13 for each ° C	Trauma	1.4–1.8
	greater than 37° C	Sepsis	1.4–1.8
		Ventilator	1.3
		Skin breakdown	1.3–1.5
		Radiation therapy or chemotherapy	1.6
		Burn injury	
		<20%	1.2–1.4
		20–25%	1.6
		25–30%	1.7
		30–35%	1.8
		35–40%	1.9
		40–45%	2.0
		>45%	2.1

Data from Long CL, Schaffel N, Geiger JW, et al: Metabolic response to injury and illness: Estimation of energy and protein needs from indirect calorimetry and nitrogen balance. JPEN 3:452–457, 1979; Gottschlich MM, Matarese L, Shonts E (eds): Nutrition Support Core Curriculum. Silver Spring, MD: American Society for Parenteral and Enteral Nutrition (ASPEN) Publishers, 1992; and Williamson J: Actual burn nutrition care practices: A national survey (Part II). J Burn Care Rehab 10:185–941, 1989.

will benefit by use of pressure-reducing mattresses and beds. The risk of pulmonary embolism is always present, requiring pneumatic stockings or subcutaneous heparin use or both. This risk becomes greater when the lower extremities have wounds or donor sites for skin grafting that cause pain with motion.

Complications

By far the most common complication of burns is infection. The highest risk of bacterial invasion from skin flora in the eschar occurs approximately 5 to 7 days after the burn episode. The initial organism is usually *Staphylococcus* progressing to methicillin-resistant *Staphylococcus* and later to *Pseudomonas* colonization of the wounds. No prophylactic antibiotics are administered for the burn injury except in patients with valvular heart disease or vascular implants, for example, a pacemaker. Signs of systemic sepsis include change of mental status and ileus, with infection of the burn wound usually appearing as a cellulitis indicated by widening of the reddened margin and often increased edema around the area. Surveillance cultures may be obtained by initial surface swabbing of the wound on admission and later culture of eschar pieces obtained at each burn excision procedure. A history of the patient's injury may give a clue to some unusual pathogen that may cause early sepsis, for example, rolling in a puddle or dirt. Tetanus prophylaxis must be addressed. Because of their immunosuppressive effects, steroids should never be used in a burn injury.

Bacteremia is extremely common. Pulmonary artery lines should be avoided if possible, and central venous line use should be minimized. Unfortunately, sites for peripheral lines in patients with burned extremities are limited. However, lines may be placed through burns without hesitation. The alternative is to change the central line sites (not over a guide wire) conscientiously at regular intervals. Similarly, the constant risk of bacteremia affects other procedures, for example, choosing external fixation of orthopedic injury versus internal fixation. The best prophylaxis for infection is early excision with removal of the pathogen-bearing eschar as soon as is feasible, even as early as the first day after the burn episode. Edema around the area of injury does not affect graft take or procedures. When the amount of autograft is inadequate, cadaver allograft can be used.

Ethics of Burn Care

The ethics of burn care have been advanced by the availability of information from multiple burn units relating survival rates to age and burn size. Previously, providing palliative care alone was recommended on admission only in cases of obviously fatal burns. With this more recent prognostic data, the decision to limit care in other burn patients whose prognoses are poor can be based on more accurate information. Under these circumstances, burned patients who previously would have endured a long course of suffering before dying may be limited to supportive care alone when their particular percent BSA burn and age would make survival highly unlikely or unprecedented.

BIBLIOGRAPHY

Brooker AF, Pezeshki C: Tissue pressure to evaluate compartmental syndrome. J Trauma 19:689–691, 1979.
  This presents a description of various methods for measuring compartment pressure and their clinical significance from an orthopedic trauma viewpoint.

Harris J, Benedict F: A biometric study of basal metabolism in man. Publ No. 279, Carnegie Institute of Washington. Philadelphia: JB Lippincott, 1919.
  This article was cited in the American Dietetic Association Manual of Clinical Dietetics, Chicago, 1988. It contains a description of the application of the Harris-Benedict formula as it applies to burns.

Nguyen TT: Current treatment of severely burned patients. Ann Surg 223:14–25, 1996.
  This is an overview of burn care with brief analysis of the development of current methods. Common resuscitation protocols are compared, with discussion of wound closure and scar management.

Robson MC, Burns BF, Smith DJ Jr: Acute management of the burned patient. Plast Reconstr Surg 89:1155–1168, 1992.
  This article reviews burn care with emphasis on wound management.

Saffle JR, Davis B, Williams P: Recent outcomes in the treatment of burn injury in the United States: A report from the American Burn Association Patient Registry. J Burn Care Rehab 16:219–231, 1995.
This article presents current U.S. survival data in relation to age and percent of burn.

Sheridan RL, Petras L, Basha G, et al: Planimetry study of the percent of body surface represented by the hand and palm: Sizing irregular burns is more accurately done with the palm. J Burn Care Rehab 16:605–606, 1995.
This is an analysis of the palmar template for body surface area determination that offers more precision than the "rough estimate" of the 1940s.

57

Drug Overdoses and Toxic Ingestions

Jeanmarie Perrone
Fred Henretig

Most patients admitted to the intensive care unit (ICU) for a drug overdose survive and recover fully. Successful management of patients after a serious ingestion depends on emergency department (ED) personnel initiating the critical interventions of airway management and gastrointestinal decontamination, which are continued in the ICU.

Not all "drug overdoses" are intentional. Toxic ingestions may be accidental or result from ingestion of products stored inappropriately, for example, lye stored in a soda bottle. Iatrogenic dosing errors and excess self-medication of drugs with narrow therapeutic:toxic ratios (salicylates, theophylline, lithium) also occur. Occasionally, chronic medications precipitate acute toxicity due to a drug interaction or a change in drug metabolism. Although initial management of poisonings mainly emphasizes the route and manner in which the toxicity occurred, disposition of patients following ICU care depends on whether the overdose was intentional or not.

Although coma in many patients admitted to the ICU is attributed to a drug ingestion, patients with unclear histories should undergo evaluation for other causes of altered mental status. Intracranial pathologic conditions should be excluded by computed tomographic (CT) scans of the head, and lumbar puncture should be generally performed in febrile patients (see Chapter 64).

MECHANISMS OF INJURY

Direct Drug Effects

Nearly all drugs or chemicals produce harmful biologic effects if taken in excessive amounts. Pathologic effects may occur at the site of exposure due to cytotoxic chemical reactions, for example, caustic acid or alkali ingestions, that result in damage to all exposed cells. Systemic toxicity is due to selective effects of the toxin or a metabolite on specific targets, such as binding to specific receptors (therapeutic drugs), disruption of metabolic pathways, (cyanide, salicylates, iron), cellular production of toxic metabolites (acetaminophen in liver, methanol in retina, ethylene glycol in kidney), and enzymatic inhibition (Na^+/K^+-ATPase by digitalis; anticholinesterase by organophosphates). Some toxins produce effects by several mechanisms, for example, isoniazid causes hepatotoxicity via a cytochrome P-450 pathway metabolite and neurotoxicity via inhibition of pyridoxal $5'$-phosphate.

Complications

Aspiration occurs in poisoned patients as a complication of vomiting, orogastric lavage, endotracheal intubation, or loss of airway reflexes due to obtundation. Early assessment and definitive airway management are critical in preventing aspiration. Noncardiogenic pulmonary edema and the acute respiratory distress syndrome (ARDS) may complicate recovery following life-threatening ingestions. Rhabdomyolysis can occur in patients after prolonged periods of immobilization due to obtundation, protracted agitation or seizures, or cocaine or amphetamine use. Under these circumstances, aggressive rehydration and maintenance of urine output are important. Acute renal failure may occur directly, for example, from ethylene glycol or *Cortinarius* mushroom ingestions, or secondarily, for example, from drug-induced hypotension. Acute hepatic failure most commonly occurs after acetaminophen poisoning but may occur as part of the syndrome of multiple organ system failure.

MANAGEMENT

Diagnostic Approach

One should always begin with an assessment of the airway, breathing, and circulatory status (ABCs) and reassess these vital signs frequently (Fig. 57–1). Empty pill bottles or discussions with family members regarding medicines available in the home are helpful in focusing the diagnostic work-up. Physical examination should screen for manifestations of common toxic syndromes ("toxidromes"), for example, anticholinergic, opioid, or salicylate toxicity. An electrocardiogram screens for conduction defects associated with cyclic antidepressants, calcium channel antagonists, beta-blockers, or digoxin. Toxicology screening should be performed if the results will be available in a sufficiently short time frame to be clinically relevant.

Therapeutic Approach

After initial stabilization of the ABCs, certain therapies should be considered in all poisoned patients. Suspected hypoglycemia should be treated with an intravenous (IV) bolus of concentrated dextrose solution (50 mL of 50% dextrose). Patients with the triad of signs suggesting opioid toxicity (respiratory depression, pinpoint pupils, and coma) should be treated with the opioid antagonist naloxone (Table 57–1). IV fluid therapy is important in many patients with overdoses to compensate for volume losses associated with vomiting. IV benzodiazepine sedation is indicated for agitated or uncooperative patients because it may prevent rhabdomyolysis, hyperthermia, and injuries to the patient or staff.

One of the most critical interventions in a poisoned patient is gastrointestinal decontamination. Syrup of ipecac, however, has *no* role in the ED or ICU management of the poisoned patient. Orogastric lavage via a large-bore tube (Ewald tube) may be critical in patients ingesting agents not bound by activated charcoal,

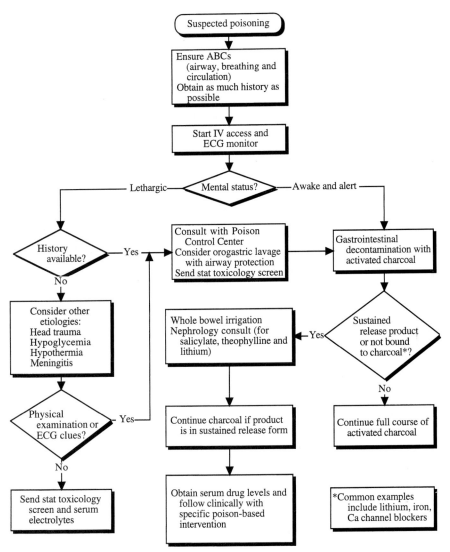

Figure 57–1. Schematic flow diagram of diagnostic and therapeutic approach to patients in whom drug overdose or poisoning is suspected.

such as iron or lithium. In addition, seriously poisoned patients may benefit from the extra 10 to 40% drug removal that can be achieved with orogastric lavage. It should be considered in any patient manifesting signs of toxicity following a potentially life-threatening ingestion, but it should be performed only after the patient's airway is judged to be protected, often necessitating endotracheal intubation.

Oral activated charcoal can diminish absorption of many drugs and can enhance drug excretion for some agents via gastrointestinal dialysis (the diffusion of high

Table 57–1. Antidotes and Adjuncts in the Therapy of Selected Poisonings

TOXIN	ANTIDOTE	DOSING FOR ADULTS AND COMMENTS
Anticholinergic agents	Physostigmine	1–2 mg IV over 5 min. Use with caution for severe delirium (may cause seizures, asystole, cholinergic crisis).
Benzodiazepines	Flumazenil	0.2 mg IV over 30 sec. Repeat at 1-min intervals as needed (second dose 0.3 mg, then 0.5 mg) until total of 3 mg. Not indicated if cocaine or tricyclic antidepressants have been ingested concurrently, or if chronic use of benzodiazepines is present or suspected.
Beta-blockers	Glucagon	5–10 mg IV. Titrate repeat doses. May use infusion of 2–10 mg/h
Calcium channel blockers	Calcium gluconate	1 g (10 mL of 10% solution) IV over 5 min with electrocardiographic monitoring. Repeat as needed, check serum calcium after third dose.
	Glucagon	Same dosing as for beta-blockers (less experience, but some promising case reports).
Cyanide	Sodium nitrite	300 mg IV over 2–4 min.
	Sodium thiosulfate	12.5 g IV over 10 min. Thiosulfate alone may be preferable in smoke inhalation victims or CNS toxicity related to prolonged nitroprusside infusion.
Digoxin	Antidigoxin antibodies (Digibind)	Vials (No.) = ingested dose (mg)/0.6, or (digoxin level [ng/mL] $\times$ 5.6 $\times$ weight [kg])/600 or 10–20 for a life-threatening arrhythmia.
Iron	Deferoxamine	Maximal rate of 15 mg/kg/h IV for severe cases. Caution; hypotension with high rates; duration should not exceed 24 h without consultation with poison control center.
Isoniazid	Pyridoxine	Attempt to match gram for gram of isoniazid ingested, if known. Use 5 g if unknown. May repeat once in severe cases.
Methanol, ethylene glycol	Ethanol	Loading dose 10 mL of 10% solution/kg. Maintenance 1.0–1.5 mL/kg (double during dialysis). Aim for ethanol level of 100 mg/dL.
	4-methylpyrazole (fomepizole)	Initial loading dose of 15 mg/kg IV over 30 min with further dosing per poison control center.
Opioids	Naloxone	1–2 mg IV. Repeat as needed up to 8–10 mg. Infusion: two thirds of reversal dose/h, titrate to effect.
Organophosphate insecticides	Atropine	2 mg IV. Repeat as needed until excessive pulmonary secretions are controlled.
	Pralidoxime	1–2 g IV, repeat at 1 h if significant weakness is present, then q6h for 24–48 h in severe cases. Consider infusion of 2.5% solution at 500 mg/h in very severe cases. End point is persistent relief of nicotinic and cholinergic signs.
Tricyclic antidepressants	Sodium bicarbonate	1–2 mEq/kg IV. Titrate to arterial pH of 7.5 or electrocardiographic alterations (see text).

Modified from Kulig K, Bar-Or D, Cantrill SV, et al: Management of acutely poisoned patients without gastric emptying. Ann Emerg Med 14:562–567, 1985.

plasma drug levels back into the gut lumen to be bound to activated charcoal and excreted) or interruption of enterohepatic circulation of active metabolites. Sustained release preparations (e.g., calcium channel blockers) and drugs not bound to activated charcoal (e.g., lithium, iron) may be cleared from the gut using whole bowel irrigation. Bowel irrigation is performed with polyethylene glycol–electrolyte lavage solutions (e.g., GoLYTELY, CoLYTE) administered via nasogastric tube at a rate of 1 to 2 L/h in adults.

The regional poison control center should be consulted to obtain general management and toxin-specific therapeutic advice, since many common toxins have specific therapies or antidotes (see Table 57–1).

COMMON TOXIC INGESTIONS

Acetaminophen

Acetaminophen is one of the most commonly ingested medications. Few hospitalized patients become seriously ill from acetaminophen overdose because of early diagnosis and antidote treatment with *N*-acetylcysteine (NAC). Life-threatening hepatotoxicity, however, occurs in the few who present late after their ingestions or in whom clinicians fail to recognize acetaminophen when it is coingested with other drugs.

Patients with a history of acetaminophen ingestion should have a 4-hour (after the estimated time of ingestion) acetaminophen level obtained and interpreted using the Rumack-Matthew nomogram (Fig. 57–2). Nausea, vomiting, and occasional right upper quadrant abdominal pain are associated with toxic hepatitis from ingestions a day or two earlier. Patients with jaundice or coagulopathy or those reporting a large acetaminophen dose 1 to 3 days previously should be presumed to have hepatotoxicity. When presentations are delayed more than 24 hours after ingestion, acetaminophen levels may be low or zero, but significant elevations in transaminases and prothrombin time reflect severe acetaminophen poisoning.

Therapeutic doses of acetaminophen are metabolized in the liver by glucuronidation (60%), sulfation (30%), or by the P-450 cytochrome oxidase system (4%). The last pathway results in a toxic intermediate, *N*-acetyl-*p*-benzoquinoneamine (NAPQI). NAPQI is then normally reduced by glutathione, which prevents toxicity. With increasing dose or overdose, more acetaminophen metabolism is shunted into the P-450 system, depleting glutathione. As a result, NAPQI accumulates and induces centrilobular necrosis of the liver. The antidote NAC replenishes the glutathione and prevents hepatic necrosis.

Patients with toxic acetaminophen levels require a loading dose of NAC (140 mg/kg) and subsequent dosing every four hours (70 mg/kg) for an additional 17 doses. Although most effective within the first 8 hours after overdose, NAC therapy has been shown to be clearly beneficial up to 24 hours after overdose. Some studies suggest that NAC therapy initiated even 24 hours after ingestion in patients with fulminant hepatic failure also decreases morbidity and mortality. If the patient was treated with activated charcoal in the 1 to 2 hours prior to receiving the first dose of NAC, one should consider giving a repeat loading dose of NAC (since the charcoal can also bind the NAC).

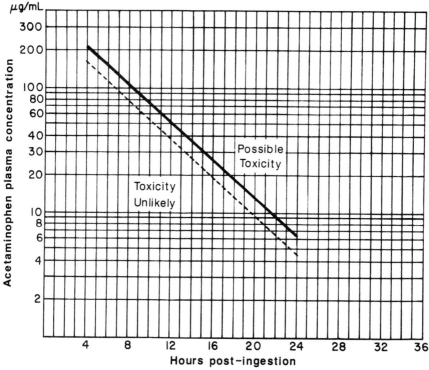

Figure 57–2. The Rumack-Matthew nomogram *(solid line)* estimates the likelihood of hepatotoxicity in acute acetaminophen overdose. *N*-acetyl cysteine (NAC) therapy is recommended if the acetaminophen plasma level at 4 hours (or later) after ingestion plots above the broken line. For example, patients with levels greater than or equal to approximately 150 μg/mL at 4 hours or greater than or equal to approximately 35 μg/mL at 12 hours after ingestion should be treated with NAC (see text). The broken line allows a 25% variability below the solid line to take into account inaccuracies in estimated time of ingestion or measurement of plasma level. (Adapted from Rumack BH, Matthew H: Pediatrics 55:871–876, 1975.)

Calcium Channel and Beta-Adrenergic Receptor Antagonists

Accidental or intentional ingestions of small quantities of the potent calcium channel or beta-adrenergic receptor antagonists can result in significant toxicity and many fatalities. Patients often present with bradycardia and hypotension with obtundation, seizures, or coma. This poisoning must be considered in any young person with unexplained bradycardia, but it may be misdiagnosed as a complicated myocardial infarction or conduction defect in older patients. Sustained release preparations may produce toxicity for days, and sudden decompensation may occur at any time.

Because beta-blockers decrease intracellular cyclic adenosine monophosphate, a specific therapeutic role has been suggested for the hormone glucagon. Glucagon increases myocardial cyclic adenosine monophosphate via a non–beta-adrenergic receptor–mediated mechanism. Calcium channel antagonists block the slow inward calcium channels and cause conduction defects, negative inotropic and chronotropic effects, and peripheral vasodilation. Intravenous calcium competitively antagonizes these effects, and glucagon may also act as a positive inotropic and chronotropic agent that can overcome the calcium channel blocker effects (see Table 57–1).

Following acute management and stabilization, gastrointestinal decontamination must address the problem posed by many sustained release preparations of these agents and their potential for prolonged toxicity. Appropriate management includes orogastric lavage, activated charcoal administration, and whole bowel irrigation.

Therapy for bradycardia begins with atropine (0.5–1.0 mg IV bolus), followed by 10% calcium chloride or calcium gluconate. Calcium therapy may be repeated to a total dose up to several grams if there is a clinical response. If the response to calcium is inadequate, glucagon should be given (3 to 10 mg IV bolus followed by a 2- to 5-mg/h IV infusion). Epinephrine infusions may be necessary if hypotension is refractory. In isolated cases with massive ingestion and poor response to pharmacologic therapy, placement of a transvenous pacer or an intra-aortic balloon pump, or both, has been successful.

Digitalis

Although the mortality rate of digitalis poisoning has dramatically improved with the use of digoxin-specific antibody fragments (Digibind), both acute and chronic digitalis poisoning continue to occur. Acute digitalis poisoning presents with emesis and the development of myriad tachy- or bradydysrhythmias. Potassium elevations greater than 5.0 mEq/L indicate significant toxicity and reflect digitalis-induced inhibition of the Na^+/K^+-ATPase pump. In chronic poisoning, gastrointestinal symptoms are less prominent, and making the diagnosis requires a high level of suspicion in any patient with dysrhythmias and a history of digoxin use.

Following acute stabilization of a patient with potential digitalis toxicity, oral activated charcoal should be administered. Immediate serum potassium and digoxin levels should be obtained and electrocardiographic monitoring should be initiated. Bradycardia, conduction defects, ventricular ectopy, and atrial tachycardia or fibrillation (with arteriovenous nodal block preventing rapid ventricular response to atrial tachycardias) may be seen with digoxin poisoning (see Chapters 30 and 31). Any dysrhythmia is an indication for Digibind therapy. Other indications include a serum potassium elevation of greater than or equal to 5 mEq/L. In the setting of an unknown overdose with bradycardia when the differential diagnosis includes calcium channel blockers, beta-blockers, and digoxin, treatment with Digibind should occur before giving calcium because calcium can potentially exacerbate digoxin poisoning.

Psychotropic Medications

Cyclic Antidepressants and Phenothiazines

Cyclic antidepressants continue to be the leading cause of death by overdose. All overdose patients should be screened by electrocardiography for possible tricyclic ingestion. Prolongation of QRS duration (>100 msec) is more highly associated with serious toxicity than are serum levels, which are not readily available. For example, patients with QRS duration greater than 100 msec have a 35% incidence of seizures and those with a QRS greater than 160 msec have a 50% incidence of ventricular dysrhythmias. A positive R wave in lead aVR and an S wave in leads I and aVL are also associated with toxicity.

Patients with either tricyclic antidepressant or phenothiazine ingestions may present with lethargy and the anticholinergic signs of tachycardia, dry mouth, dilatated pupils, decreased bowel sounds, and urinary retention. Seizures or dysrhythmias or both most often signify serious cyclic antidepressant ingestion, but two phenothiazines, thioridazine (Mellaril) and mesoridazine (Serentil), also exhibit cardiotoxicity. Patients with recent ingestions (within the prior 30 to 90 minutes) may be asymptomatic initially but rapidly deteriorate in the first hour in the emergency department. Orogastric lavage and activated charcoal should be initiated early. Obtundation often mandates endotracheal intubation. If the QRS is greater than 100 msec, one should initiate alkalinization of the serum to pH 7.45 to 7.55 with sodium bicarbonate (IV bolus followed by infusion). Alkalinization decreases drug binding to the myocardium, expands the plasma volume, and overcomes the sodium channel blocking type IA cardiotoxic effects induced by the cyclic antidepressant. One should manage seizures with a benzodiazepine or barbiturate, since a resultant lactic acidosis exacerbates the cardiotoxicity. If hypotension persists despite sodium bicarbonate and other fluid therapy, a direct vasoconstrictor such as norepinephrine will be more effective than indirectly acting vasopressors.

Lithium

Lithium toxicity differs from other psychotropic drug toxicity. Lithium ingestions provoke considerable vomiting and diarrhea. As dehydration ensues, renal lithium excretion decreases because lithium, a cation, is reabsorbed with sodium in the proximal tubule. Vigorous volume expansion with normal saline enhances lithium excretion in the kidney. Since lithium does not bind to activated charcoal used in gastrointestinal decontamination, orogastric lavage should be considered for recent ingestions, followed by whole bowel irrigation to limit distal gastrointestinal absorption. A lithium level, serum electrolytes, and renal function should be checked immediately.

The principal toxicity of lithium is to the central nervous system (CNS) with distinct acute and chronic toxicities. Acute ingestions manifest elevated serum levels, reflecting rapid absorption yet slow distribution to intracellular compartments and the CNS. Therefore, patients may be asymptomatic despite high serum levels. At this time, lithium is most accessible to dialysis. Any patient with lithium levels greater than 4.0 mEq/L should undergo hemodialysis, since renal elimination is insufficient to prevent significant neural accumulation of lithium. Any patient with serious neurologic symptoms (altered mental status, seizures, or coma) from lithium should also undergo hemodialysis. Unfortunately, not all patients with elevated levels and neurologic signs recover fully, even with hemodialysis.

Salicylates

Salicylates are commonly found in many over-the-counter analgesics and combination cold preparations. Rheumatology patients often take high-dose aspirin daily and may develop chronic salicylism as its therapeutic index diminishes.

Acute salicylate toxicity often manifests with vomiting and auditory disturbances (tinnitus, hearing loss). Hyperpnea or tachypnea may contribute to the classic mixed acid-base disturbance of a primary respiratory alkalosis and a metabolic acidosis. Severe hyperthermia or sweating may occur. Agitation or confusion may occur and progress to seizures with higher salicylate levels. A serum salicylate level should be obtained early and followed serially to determine the extent and course of the ingestion.

Gastrointestinal decontamination of salicylate poisoning may include orogastric lavage, but most patients can be effectively treated with multiple doses of activated charcoal. Urinary alkalinization should be performed in any symptomatic patient until the salicylate level is less than 30 to 40 mg/dL. Adding three ampules of sodium bicarbonate (44 mEq/ampule) to 1 L of 5% dextrose in water (D5W) infused IV at a rate of 200 to 300 mL/h alkalinizes the urine. Since salicylate poisoning is commonly accompanied by fluid losses (vomiting, sweating, tachypnea), the saline load is usually well tolerated. However, cerebral edema and salicylate-induced noncardiogenic pulmonary edema may complicate alkalinization therapy, especially in elderly patients.

In general, levels greater than 100 mg/dL mandate hemodialysis. Rapidly rising levels, severe acid-base disturbances, neurologic complications, or volume overload precluding alkalinization may also require hemodialysis. Early consultation with a nephrologist is advisable in any significant salicylate poisoning.

Sedative-Hypnotics

Barbiturates

Widely available as sedative-hypnotic and anticonvulsant agents, barbiturates act at the gamma-aminobutyrate–chloride channel receptor, resulting in synaptic inhibition. In excess, they cause global CNS depression and hypotension by decreasing sympathetic tone; massive overdose also directly depresses myocardial contractility. Based on lipid solubility, ultrashort-, short-, intermediate-, and long-acting barbiturates have correspondingly rapid CNS penetration. Doses exceeding the hypnotic dose by 5- to 10-fold result in significant toxicity, although tolerance develops in chronic users.

Clinical effects include dose-related CNS depression with mild symptoms of lethargy, ataxia, and nystagmus. The patient with a massive overdose presents with deep coma and typically miotic pupils. Apnea, hypothermia, bradycardia, and hypotension are also common. Some patients with reversible barbiturate toxicity exhibit no evidence of brainstem function and appear clinically brain dead. Laboratory investigation reveals elevated barbiturate levels (coma usually occurs with >20 μg/mL for short-acting barbiturates and >60 μg/mL for phenobarbital). Barbiturate habituation is common, and these patients may manifest a severe delirium tremens–like withdrawal syndrome.

The treatment of barbiturate overdose is largely supportive, with ventilatory assistance and cardiovascular support to reverse hypotension (intravenous volume and vasopressor infusion as necessary). Enhanced elimination with alkaline diuresis (useful only for phenobarbital) and repeated gastric administration of activated charcoal has not improved clinical outcome. Saline loading to enhance diuresis may predispose to pulmonary edema, and charcoal administration has been associated with complications due to gastrointestinal obstruction and tracheal aspiration in nonintubated patients. Hemoperfusion has been advocated for patients expected to have prolonged coma (serum levels >100 μg/mL for phenobarbital or >50 μg/mL for other barbiturates).

Benzodiazepines

Like barbiturates, benzodiazepines also function via the gamma-aminobutyrate receptor and produce dose-dependent CNS depression. Unlike barbiturates, however, first-generation benzodiazepines (diazepam, chlordiazepoxide) have rarely been associated with significant respiratory or cardiovascular depression. In recent years, newer short-acting agents have occasionally been linked to cardiorespiratory compromise. All benzodiazepines may produce life-threatening CNS and respiratory depression when ingested along with large amounts of ethanol or other sedative-hypnotic agents. As with barbiturates, benzodiazepine dependence is also common, and withdrawal may present as a severe delirium tremens–like syndrome.

Laboratory testing by qualitative immunoassay is widely available. Many rapid screens use oxazepam as the immunoreagent, and therefore some of the newer benzodiazepines that are not metabolized to oxazepam go undetected. Management of benzodiazepine toxicity is supportive, with no proven benefit for enhanced elimination. The role of a specific antagonist, flumazenil, in overdose management is controversial. Since its effect is brief (1 to 2 hours) and its use may precipitate seizures (in a benzodiazepine-dependent patient or with concomitant cocaine or tricyclic antidepressant ingestion), it is usually not recommended in patients admitted to the ICU.

Serotonergic Agents

Serotonin syndrome (SS) is a complication of serotonergic agents, which are drugs that increase the central nervous system serotonin neurotransmission. Although SS may occur after an overdose of such an agent, more often SS occurs relatively soon after an increase in dose of a primary serotonergic agent or the addition of a second agent. Serotonergic drugs are legion, including selective serotonin reuptake inhibitors, such as fluoxetine, cyclic antidepressants, monamine oxidase (MAO) inhibitors, amphetamines such as "Ecstasy" (3,4-methylenedioxymethamphetamine or MDMA), and opioids such as meperidine, tramadol and dextromethorphan.

SS is a challenge to diagnose since it has no confirmatory laboratory tests and its signs and symptoms vary in diversity and severity. Common clinical manifestations include one or more of the following: (1) abnormal mental status, such as confusion, agitation, or unresponsiveness; (2) autonomic nervous system dysfunction, such as hyperthermia, diaphoresis, and hypertension; (3) neuromuscular dysfunction, such as myoclonus, hyperreflexia, and muscle rigidity (especially of the lower extremities). SS can result in multiple organ system failure, but generally it has a good prognosis. Treatment remains supportive and all serotonergic agents should be discontinued. Use of specific antidotes awaits results of controlled clinical trials.

Theophylline

Although theophylline was once a relatively common ingestant, its decreased use in the management of obstructive airway disease has diminished its availability for toxic ingestion. Acute theophylline toxicity is manifested by prominent vomiting and tachycardia. Early management includes an antiemetic, such as metoclopramide (10-mg increments up to 1 mg/kg), to prevent emesis and to allow administration of oral activated charcoal. In cases of continued intractable vomiting, one of the more expensive antiemetics (ondansetron, granisetron) should be given.

A regimen of multiple doses of activated charcoal should be given at 1 to 2 g/kg initially followed by 0.5 g/kg every hour until toxicity resolves. Theophylline has high affinity for activated charcoal, and the resultant gastrointestinal dialysis is nearly as effective as hemodialysis. Overdose of sustained-release theophylline preparations should be managed with the addition of whole bowel irrigation.

Serious morbidity and fatalities in theophylline poisoning usually result from seizures or dysrhythmias. Rarely, profound hypotension occurs from excessive beta$_2$-adrenergic receptor–mediated peripheral vasodilation. Seizures should be managed with benzodiazepines followed, if needed, by phenobarbital. Diltiazem is preferred over adenosine for supraventricular tachycardia because the latter is antagonized by theophylline. Beta-blockers may be indicated to antagonize beta$_2$-mediated hypotension in patients without a history of asthma or chronic obstructive pulmonary disease. More aggressive treatment of elevated theophylline levels depends on the patient's clinical status and the absolute level. Seizures, dysrhythmias, or acute theophylline ingestions resulting in levels greater than or equal to 100 mg/dL should be treated with hemodialysis or, preferably, hemoperfusion. As with salicylism, chronic theophylline toxicity can result in more serious manifestations at lower serum drug levels.

BIBLIOGRAPHY

Ashbourne JF, Olson KR, Khayam-Bashi H: Value of rapid screening for acetaminophen in all patients with intentional drug overdose. Ann Emerg Med 18:1035–1038, 1989.
This study examined acetaminophen levels in all patients presenting with any overdose and convincingly demonstrated the need to obtain serum acetaminophen levels in any patient who presents after intentional ingestion of any drug.

Boehnert M, Lovejoy FH: Value of the QRS duration versus the serum drug level in predicting seizures and ventricular arrhythmias after an acute overdose of tricyclic antidepressants. N Engl J Med 313:474–479, 1985.
This prospective study demonstrated that the QRS duration is the best predictor of serious toxicity in tricyclic antidepressant toxicity.

Carbone JR: The neuroleptic malignant and serotonin syndromes. Emerg Med Clin North Am 18:317–325, 2000.
This is a recent review that compares neuroleptic malignant syndrome (NMS) with serotonin syndrome (SS) (with 55 references).

Harrison P, Keays R, Bray G, et al: Improved outcome of paracetamol-induced fulminant hepatic failure by late administration of acetylcysteine. Lancet 1:1572–1573, 1990.
This is a retrospective analysis of outcome from NAC therapy initiated 10 hours or more after ingestion, demonstrating decreased morbidity and mortality in 100 patients with fulminant hepatic failure.

Henretig F: Sedative-hypnotic poisoning. In: Harwood-Nuss A (ed): The Clinical Practice of Emergency Medicine, 2nd ed. Philadelphia: JB Lippincott, 1996.
A review of ingestions of nonbarbiturate, nonbenzodiazepine sedative-hypnotics.

Kulig K: Initial management of ingestions of toxic substances. N Engl J Med 326:1677–1681, 1992.
This is a good overview of general treatment principles.

Kulig K, Bar-Or D, Cantrill SV, et al: Management of acutely poisoned patients without gastric emptying. Ann Emerg Med 14:562–567, 1985.
This is a description of a prospective randomized study of 592 poisoned patients who were randomized to receive either gastric emptying (syrup of ipecac or orogastric lavage) followed by activated charcoal or activated charcoal alone. Clinical outcomes were compared.

Mills KC: Serotonin syndrome. A clinical update. Crit Care Clin 4:763–783, 1997.
This is a comprehensive review of the serotonin syndrome, including serotonin physiology and psychopharmacology, pathophysiology, clinical features, and therapy of serotonin syndrome (with 113 references).

Mofenson HC, Greensher J: The unknown poison. Pediatrics 55:336, 1974.
This article originated the concept of the "toxidrome" approach to evaluation of the poisoned patient.

Perrone J, Hoffman RS, Goldfrank LR: Special considerations in gastrointestinal decontamination. Emerg Clin North Am 12:285–299, 1994.
This article presents a review of trends in gastrointestinal decontamination of the poisoned patient.

Shannon M: Predictors of major toxicity after theophylline overdose. Ann Intern Med 119:1161–1167, 1993.
This prospective study examined risk factors for major toxicity following theophylline overdose and found that the theophylline level was the best predictor in acute ingestions and underlying age was the best predictor in chronic ingestions.

Smilkstein MJ, Knapp GL, Kulig KW, et al: Efficacy of oral N-acetylcysteine in the treatment of acetaminophen overdose: Analysis of a national multicenter study (1976–1985). N Engl J Med 319:1557–1562, 1988.
This is a summary analysis of the efficacy of oral NAC in the treatment of acetaminophen poisoning in 2540 patients over a 10-year period.

58

Acute Pancreatitis

Douglas O. Faigel
David C. Metz

Acute inflammation of the pancreas has multiple causes and may manifest as mild disease or result in multiple organ system failure, sepsis, and death. The typical presentation of acute pancreatitis is abdominal pain in association with elevated blood levels of pancreatic enzymes. It may occur as an initial or recurrent attack. The pathogenesis is felt to be pancreatic autodigestion caused by intraparenchymal activation and release of proteolytic enzymes from zymogen granules. The resultant destruction and inflammation can result in a variety of local complications for which a clinically based system of classification has been developed (Table 58–1).

ETIOLOGY

More than 90% of cases of acute pancreatitis are due to ethanol abuse or cholelithiasis or are idiopathic. A wide variety of other agents, including medications and toxins, accounts for the remaining 10% (Tables 58–2 and 58–3). Biliary microlithiasis (which is bile containing small crystals of cholesterol monohydrate, calcium bilirubinate, or calcium carbonate) is also now recognized as an important cause of acute and recurrent pancreatitis. It may account for up to 30% of what was previously thought to be idiopathic pancreatitis.

CLINICAL PRESENTATION

The hallmark of acute pancreatitis is abdominal pain associated with elevated blood levels of pancreatic enzymes. The pain generally comes on suddenly and rises to a peak within a few hours. It is steady and typically midepigastric and bores through to the back. The patient prefers to remain still in bed and may assume a hunched-over or semifetal position in an attempt to release tension on the retroperitoneum; exaggerating the lumbar lordosis exacerbates the pain. Nausea and vomiting are present in more than 80% of patients. The presence of bluish discolorations of the flanks (the Grey Turner sign) or periumbilical area (Cullen sign) is rare and is not seen at presentation. These signs may develop several days into the illness because of dissection of peripancreatic bleeding into the subcutaneous tissues. Bowel sounds are diminished or, if a paralytic ileus is present, absent. An abdominal radiograph may reveal a *sentinel loop*: a paralyzed air-filled segment of proximal small bowel in close proximity to the inflamed pancreas. The abdomen is typically soft but with exquisite tenderness to deep palpation. Peritoneal signs may be present in complicated cases. Subcutaneous fat necrosis may be present and resembles erythema nodosum or panniculitis. Altered mental status may be due to shock or complications of alcoholism (e.g., delirium tremens, the Wernicke-Korsakoff syndrome).

The serum amylase level rises in acute pancreatitis within 2 to 12 hours of the onset of symptoms and remains elevated for 3 to 5 days. Persistently raised levels suggest the possibility of local complications. The lipase level may remain elevated

Table 58–1. Classification System for Acute Pancreatitis

TERM	DEFINITION	COMMENTS
Severe acute pancreatitis	Acute pancreatitis associated with organ failure or certain local complications (necrosis, abscess, or pseudocyst) or both. Most often it is the clinical expression of the development of *pancreatic necrosis.*	It is characterized by 3 or more Ranson criteria (see Table 58–2) or 8 or more points in the APACHE II system.* *Mild* acute pancreatitis has only interstitial edema and, as a rule, runs an uncomplicated course.
Acute fluid collections	These collections, localized in or near the pancreas, occur early in the course of acute pancreatitis and always lack a defined wall.	They are common, occurring in 30–50% of patients with severe pancreatitis, and most regress spontaneously. Those not regressing are an early stage in the development of acute pseudocysts and pancreatic abscesses.
Pancreatic necrosis	Diffuse or focal area(s) of nonviable pancreatic parenchyma, typically associated with peripancreatic fat necrosis. Pancreatic necrosis may be sterile or become infected (which triples the risk of death).	Dynamic contrast enhanced computed tomography shows a well-marginated zone of nonenhancing pancreatic parenchyma >3 cm or involving more than 30% of the pancreas.
Acute pseudocysts	Collections of pancreatic fluid, enclosed by a defined wall of fibrous or granulation tissue, arising from acute pancreatitis. They are usually rich in pancreatic enzymes and most often sterile.	They may be palpable but most often are discovered by imaging studies, which show a well-defined wall. Their formation requires 4 or more weeks from the onset of acute pancreatitis.
Pancreatic abscesses	Circumscribed intra-abdominal collections of pus, in or near the pancreas, but containing little or no pancreatic necrosis. Do *not* use this term to describe *infected pancreatic necrosis* (the mortality of which is double that of a pancreatic abscess).	These occur 4 or more weeks after the onset of acute pancreatitis and likely arise as a result of limited necrosis with subsequent liquefaction and infection.
Pancreatic ascites	The presence of free fluid with pancreatic enzymes inside the peritoneal cavity.	Pancreatic ascites may be sterile or infected.
Infected pseudocyst	Variably used to describe infected pancreatic necrosis or pancreatic abscesses.	Use of this ambiguous term should be avoided.
Hemorrhagic pancreatitis	This term should be used only when hemorrhage in the gland is directly visualized.	Incorrectly used as a synonym for *pancreatic necrosis,* which may not be hemorrhagic.
Pancreatic phlegmon	Originally this referred to a palpable mass of sterile edematous tissues, but later used to describe pancreatic necrosis with infection.	Use of this ambiguous term should be avoided.

Modified from Bradley EL III: A clinically based classification system for acute pancreatitis. Arch Surg 128:586–590, 1993.

*Knaus WA, Draper EA, Wagner DP, et al: APACHE II: severity of disease classification system. Crit Care Med 13:818–829, 1985.

longer than the amylase level. Elevation of both enzymes to levels greater than 10 times the upper limit of normal is highly specific but only 80 to 90% sensitive for acute pancreatitis. For example, patients with underlying chronic pancreatitis may not be able to generate such high serum enzyme levels because of prior loss of pancreatic parenchyma.

DIFFERENTIAL DIAGNOSIS

There are multiple causes for an elevated amylase level that are not due to acute pancreatitis (Table 58–4). Several deserve special comment. Perforated peptic ulcer may present with pain and elevated pancreatic enzymes resulting from spillage

Table 58–2. Selected Causes of Acute Pancreatitis

Major causes (~90% of cases)
  Ethanol abuse
  Gallstones, including microlithiasis
  Idiopathic
Other causes (~10% of cases)
  Medications and toxins (see Table 58–2)
  Metabolic conditions
    Hyperlipidemia
    Hypercalcemia
    End-stage renal failure
    Hypothermia
  Infections
    Viral (mumps, coxsackie virus, hepatitis A or B, echovirus, adenovirus, cytomegalovirus,
      varicella, Epstein-Barr virus, human immunodeficiency virus)
    Bacterial *(Mycoplasma pneumoniae, Salmonella, Campylobacter jejuni, Mycobacterium,*
      Legionella, Leptospira)
    Intraductal parasites *(Ascaris, Clonorchis)*
  Trauma
    Blunt
    Postoperative (especially after intra-abdominal surgery or cardiopulmonary bypass)
    Endoscopic retrograde cholangiopancreatography (ERCP)

Table 58–3. Medications and Toxins Associated with Acute Pancreatitis

CATEGORY	DEFINITE ASSOCIATION	PROBABLE ASSOCIATION
Antihypertensive agents		ACE inhibitors
		Methyldopa
Anti-inflammatory and		Acetaminophen
analgesic agents		Corticosteroids
		Mesalamine
		NSAIDs
		Salicylates
Antimicrobial agents	Didanosine (ddI)	Erythromycin
	Pentamidine	Metronidazole
	Sulfonamides	Nitrofurantoin
	Tetracyclines	
Chemotherapeutic	6-MP, azathioprine	
agents	L-Asparaginase	
Diuretics	Furosemide	Chlorthalidone
	Hydrochlorothiazide	Ethacrynic acid
Toxins	Ethanol	
	Methanol	
Others	Estrogens (via hyperlipidemia)	
	Intravenous lipid infusions	
	Valproic acid	

6-MP, 6-mercaptopurine; NSAIDs, nonsteroidal anti-inflammatory drugs; ACE, angiotensin-converting enzyme.

Table 58–4. Selected Non-Pancreatitis Causes of Hyperamylasemia

Intra-abdominal emergencies	Salivary adenitis
Perforated viscus (stomach, duodenum, jejunum)	Poor renal clearance
Mesenteric infarction	Renal insufficiency
Biliary obstruction	Macroamylasemia
Acute cholecystitis	Miscellaneous
Ruptured ectopic pregnancy	Metabolic, diabetic ketoacidosis
Salpingitis	Acute and chronic liver disease

into the peritoneal cavity. Abrupt onset of pain, peritoneal signs, and free air on radiography differentiates this entity from pancreatitis. Acute cholecystitis may sometimes be associated with mild hyperamylasemia. The pain of cholecystitis is typically right-sided, and ultrasonography or computed tomography can suggest the diagnosis. A stone in the bile duct (choledocholithiasis) may cause cholangitis with biliary colic, elevated liver-associated enzymes, and jaundice with or without concomitant pancreatitis. Bowel ischemia or infarction due to mesenteric vascular occlusion, volvulus, and hernia are important considerations because of the need for prompt surgical treatment. Salpingitis and ruptured ectopic pregnancy may cause abdominal pain and elevated amylase levels and may occasionally be confused with acute pancreatitis.

PROGNOSIS

Dynamic computed tomographic scanning during bolus intravenous injection of contrast may both provide a diagnosis (by demonstrating inflammation and ruling out other entities) and help with prognosis (by assessing the degree of inflammation and necrosis). Nonenhancing areas within the gland correlate with the presence of necrosis. Fluid collections and evidence of inflammation around the pancreas are well seen.

The degree of severity of disease as evident on the computed tomographic scan correlates well with clinical course and outcome. For example, patients with only interstitial edema of the pancreas on computed tomography (CT) usually have a mild clinical course with low risk of local or systemic complications, and recovery is the rule. In contrast, patients with evidence of pancreatic necrosis usually have severe pancreatitis with a high risk of local and systemic complications (Table 58–5) and about a 25% risk of death.

Severity of disease and prognosis can also be gauged by clinical scoring systems. Ranson and coworkers introduced the first such system in 1974, often referred to as Ranson's Criteria (Table 58–6), based on findings on admission to the hospital and at 48 hours after admission. This system has proven to be useful to define those with severe acute pancreatitis (see Table 58–1) and their mortality risks.

MANAGEMENT

Patients with severe acute pancreatitis require admission to the intensive care unit (ICU) for management by a multidisciplinary team, including an intensivist, a gastroenterologist, and a surgeon. Initial management requires supportive care with adequate fluid and electrolyte replacement and careful monitoring for organ failure

Table 58–5. Local and Systemic Complications of Acute Pancreatitis

SYSTEM	COMPLICATION
Cardiovascular	Hypotension and circulatory shock
	Rupture of pseudoaneurysm
	Splenic rupture or hematoma
Central nervous system	Psychosis
Gastrointestinal	Bowel obstruction (mechanical versus paralytic)
	Gastrointestinal hemorrhage
	Ulceration
	Gastric varices
Hematologic	Coagulopathy (disseminated intravascular coagulation)
	Retinopathy
Metabolic	Hyperglycemia
	Hypocalcemia
Renal	Acute renal failure
	Right-sided hydronephrosis
Respiratory	Acute respiratory distress syndrome

and other systemic complications. Potential offending medications (see Table 58–3) should be discontinued, and reintroduction should be avoided because rechallenge can lead to fulminant disease. Patients should receive nothing by mouth. Nasogastric suction should be instituted for persistent vomiting, ileus, or obstruction but does not alter ultimate outcome. Total parenteral nutrition should be considered if a prolonged (>5 days) nothing-by-mouth status is anticipated. Adequate opioid analgesia is required. There is no benefit of one opioid over another, but high doses of meperidine (previously felt to be the agent of choice) may result in seizures, particularly in patients with renal failure, and should be avoided.

Primary and prophylactic medical and surgical therapies have been largely unsuccessful, with the exception of gallstone pancreatitis. Therapies designed to put the pancreas at rest by inhibiting pancreatic secretion with nasogastric suction, histamine H_2-receptor blockers, atropine, glucagon, somatostatin, or fluorouracil have *not* been shown to change the course of the disease. Prophylactic antibiotic

Table 58–6. Ranson's Criteria for Severity and Prognosis in Acute Pancreatitis*

CRITERIA ON ADMISSION	CRITERIA WITHIN 48 HOURS OF ADMISSION
Age >55 years	Decrease in hematocrit >10% (absolute)
WBC >16,000/μL	BUN increase >5 mg/dL [1.79 mmol/L]
Glucose >200 mg/dL [11.1 mmol/L]	Calcium <8 mg/dL [2.0 mmol/L]
LDH >350 IU/L	Pao$_2$ <60 mm Hg
AST >250 U/L	Base deficit >4 mEq/L [4 mmol/L]
	Fluid sequestration >6 L

*Predicted mortality for patients with non-gallstone pancreatitis: <3 criteria, 0% mortality; 3–5 criteria, 10–20% mortality; 6 or more criteria, >50% mortality.

AST, aspartate aminotransferase; BUN, blood urea nitrogen; LDH, lactic dehydrogenase; WBC, white blood cell count.

From Ranson JHC, Rifkind KM, Roses DF, et al: Prognostic signs and the role of operative management in acute pancreatitis. Surg Gynecol Obstet 139:69–81, 1974.

therapy with ampicillin is not beneficial, but broad spectrum antibiotic coverage, such as with imipenem, has been shown to decrease infectious complications. Luiten and coworkers have recently shown that colonization of the gut with Gram-negative bacteria (other than *Escherichia coli*) to be a risk factor for development of infected pancreatic necrosis and increased mortality. These investigators previously showed a decrease in morbidity and mortality in patients with severe pancreatitis by treatment with intravenous cefotaxime and selective decontamination of the digestive tract (SDD). Because concern remains that such prophylactic antibiotic regimens may eventually result in infections by resistant organisms, this approach needs further confirmation before it can be endorsed as a general recommendation. Early surgical therapies such as peritoneal lavage and pancreatic resection likewise do not appear to be of benefit. Surgical treatment of pancreatitis caused by gallstones is not beneficial and when performed in the early acute phase may have a mortality rate as high as 48%. Endoscopic retrograde cholangiopancreatography (ERCP) with sphincterotomy and stone extraction is indicated when there is evidence of biliary obstruction due to a stone (e.g., increasing jaundice) or of acute cholangitis. In patients with biliary pancreatitis but without signs of obstruction or cholangitis, ERCP and sphincterotomy have not been shown to be beneficial.

Supportive treatment is aimed largely at the systemic and local complications that may occur (see Table 58–5). Shock is due to massive third spacing of fluid and peripheral vasodilatation. *Cardiovascular collapse* may be an early cause of death in patients with severe pancreatitis and requires aggressive volume replacement and vasopressors. *Hypoxemia* is common and may occur in a majority of patients during the first 2 days. It is generally asymptomatic with a normal chest radiograph and resolves as the pancreatitis improves. However, up to 20% of patients with severe pancreatitis develop the acute respiratory distress syndrome (see Chapter 73) requiring mechanical ventilation. Development of *acute respiratory distress syndrome* portends a greater than 50% mortality. *Pleural effusions* are usually left-sided and exudative, with high amylase levels; they resolve as the pancreatitis improves. Persistent and large effusions may indicate a pancreaticopleural fistula. *Coagulopathy* is generally due to disseminated intravascular coagulation, for which there is no specific treatment, but factor replacement may be required if bleeding is present or invasive procedures are planned. *Acute renal failure* is generally due to acute tubular necrosis from renal hypoperfusion; if the condition requires dialysis, a greater than 50% mortality is predicted. *Hyperglycemia* may occur transiently in 50% of patients and, if severe, requires insulin therapy. *Hypocalcemia* is multifactorial because of saponification of calcium salts in areas of fat necrosis, hypoalbuminemia, hypomagnesemia, and abnormalities of glucagon, calcitonin, and parathyroid hormone secretion or responsiveness. Treatment of hypocalcemia should be guided by the ionized calcium level. Sudden *blindness,* which occurs rarely but may be permanent, arises from Purtscher's angiopathic retinopathy (discrete flame-shaped hemorrhages with cotton-wool spots). Idiopathic pancreatic *encephalopathy* with confusion, delirium, and coma may be due to effects of brain hypoperfusion and metabolic abnormalities. It must be differentiated from other causes of altered mental status, including the sequelae of alcoholism.

The most common gastrointestinal complication is *paralytic ileus.* Treatment is nasogastric decompression and observation. Occasionally, mechanical obstruction may occur resulting from involvement of the bowel by the inflammatory process.

This, too, can be managed conservatively, although if persistent, surgical resection of the affected loop may be required. *Gastrointestinal hemorrhage* may occur from stress ulcerations, bleeding from gastric varices, or a ruptured pseudoaneurysm. *Stress ulcerations* can be managed endoscopically and with histamine H_2-receptor antagonists. *Gastric varices* develop as a consequence of splenic vein thrombosis, which may complicate either acute or chronic pancreatitis. The diagnosis is confirmed by angiography, and splenectomy is curative. Erosion of major peripancreatic arteries, usually in association with a pseudocyst, may result in *pseudoaneurysm formation*. Bleeding from a ruptured pseudoaneurysm reaches the gastrointestinal tract via the pancreatic duct or directly via the rupture of the pseudocyst into the bowel lumen. Intra- or *retroperitoneal hemorrhage* can also occur. Treatment of this unusual condition is by angiographic embolization or surgery. Extension of pancreatic inflammation may cause splenic rupture or right-sided hydronephrosis.

Local pancreatic complications include the development of *fluid collections, pseudocysts,* and *localized infection* (see Table 58–1). They occur primarily in patients with necrotizing pancreatitis. Sterile fluid collections can be managed expectantly because most will resolve. Ten to 15% of patients will acquire pseudocysts, and two thirds of these will resolve spontaneously, generally within 6 weeks. Complications of pseudocysts include pain, bleeding, infection, bowel obstruction, and rupture. Surgical treatment is indicated for pseudocysts that are greater than 6 cm and have persisted for more than 6 weeks, are enlarging on serial examinations, or have led to a complication. Pancreatic abscesses and infected pancreatic necrosis are treated with surgical drainage and systemic antibiotics. In patients with acute pancreatitis who improve with supportive treatment, no further therapy is needed. However, if there is no clinical improvement, or if there is further deterioration, severe sterile or infected necrosis must be considered in the absence of obvious local or systemic complications. In both sterile and infected necrosis, there may be fever and leukocytosis ($>20,000/\mu L$). Although there is no consensus as to the role of surgery for severe sterile necrosis, most experts agree that extensive surgical débridement is indicated for infected necrosis. However, differentiating sterile from infected necrosis may be challenging. Intrapancreatic air on CT indicates the presence of gas-forming organisms and is an indication for surgery. CT-guided aspiration for Gram stain and culture has been advocated as being both highly sensitive and specific for infection, with Gram stain by itself being 98% sensitive. Percutaneous drainage of the infected area with pigtail catheters is generally not effective because of the thick consistency of the necrotic debris, but it may help stabilize patients until more definitive débridement can be performed.

SUMMARY

Acute pancreatitis remains a serious cause of morbidity and mortality. Initial assessment is aimed at determining the cause and differentiating mild from severe disease based on prognostic signs and CT findings. Patients with severe pancreatitis require admission to the ICU, aggressive fluid resuscitation, treatment of systemic complications, and ERCP if signs of biliary obstruction or acute cholangitis are present. In patients with necrotizing pancreatitis who do not improve or deteriorate while on medical therapy, the presence of infected necrosis should be considered, and CT-guided aspiration should be contemplated. Patients with infected necrosis should undergo surgical débridement. Those with sterile necrosis who do not improve despite prolonged medical therapy may benefit from late surgical débridement.

BIBLIOGRAPHY

Balthazar EJ, Freeney PC, van Sonnenberg E: Imaging and intervention in acute pancreatitis. Radiology 193:297–306, 1994.
This article presents an excellent review of radiologic tests, especially computed tomographic scanning of acute pancreatitis and its complications.

Bradley EL: A clinically based classification system for acute pancreatitis. Arch Surg 128:586–90, 1993.
This article presents the currently accepted terminology for acute pancreatitis as proposed by the International Symposium on Acute Pancreatitis, Atlanta, GA, 1992.

Fan ST, Lai ECS, Mok FPT, et al: Early treatment of acute pancreatitis by endoscopic papillotomy. N Engl J Med 328:228–232, 1993.
This randomized prospective study found that early ERCP and papillotomy decreased morbidity from biliary sepsis in patients with acute pancreatitis and biliary obstruction.

Folsch UR, Nitsche R, Ludtke R, Hilgers RA, et al: Early ERCP and papillotomy compared with conservative treatment for acute biliary pancreatitis. N Engl J Med 336:237–242, 1997.
This random controlled clinical trial showed ERCP and papillotomy not to be beneficial in the absence of biliary obstruction or acute cholangitis.

Forsmark CE, Grendell JH: Complications of pancreatitis. Semin Gastrointest Dis 2:165–176, 1991.
This is an excellent review of local and systemic complications of acute and chronic pancreatitis.

Gerzof SG, Banks PA, Robbins AH, et al: Early diagnosis of pancreatic infection by computed tomography-guided aspiration. Gastroenterology 93:1315–1320, 1987.
This was a prospective study of the utility of CT-guided aspiration to detect infected necrosis in acute pancreatitis.

Lee SP, Nicholls JF, Park HZ: Biliary sludge as a cause of acute pancreatitis. N Engl J Med 325:589–593, 1992.
This was a prospective study establishing biliary microlithiasis as a cause of acute and recurrent pancreatitis and demonstrating the benefit of cholecystectomy or papillotomy in decreasing the chance of recurrence.

Luiten EJT, Hop WD, Lange JF, et al: Controlled clinical trial of selective decontamination for the treatment of severe acute pancreatitis. Ann Surg 222:57–65, 1995.
This randomized clinical study of 102 patients with severe pancreatitis found that selective decontamination of the digestive tract reduced Gram-negative pancreatic infections and mortality.

Luiten EJT, Hop WD, Endtz HP, et al: Prognostic importance of gram-negative intestinal colonization preceding pancreatic infection in severe acute pancreatitis. Results of a controlled clinical trial of selective decontamination. Int Care Medicine 24:438–445, 1998.
This study reported that Gram-negative colonization of the gut (except for E. coli) is a risk factor for subsequent pancreatic infection, usually occurring within 1 week.

Pederzoli P, Bassi C, Vesentini S, Campedelli A: A randomized multicenter trial of antibiotic prohylaxis of septic complications in acute necrotizing pancreatitis with imipenem. Surg Gynecol Obstet 176:480–483, 1993.
This was a randomized study showing significantly fewer infectious complications (but no change in overall mortality) in patients who received prophylactic imipenem.

Steinberg W, Tenor S: Acute pancreatitis. N Engl J Med 330:1198–1210, 1994.
This article presents an excellent comprehensive review of the pathophysiology, diagnosis, and management of acute pancreatitis with an extensive reference list.

Wilmink T, Frick TW: Drug-induced pancreatitis. Drug Safety 14:406–423, 1996.
This is a comprehensive review of drugs that have definite, probable, possible, and doubtful associations with acute pancreatitis. It has 327 references.

59 Acute Liver Failure

Michael R. Lucey

Acute liver injury is a broad term, referring to any acute onset of markedly abnormal liver chemistry profiles in a previously healthy person. The serum transaminase levels are elevated more than five times the upper limit of the normal range and are often increased by 20-fold or more. Acute liver injury can arise from any of the insults listed as causes of fulminant hepatic failure (Table 59–1).

The most important indicator that acute liver injury is progressive and may be life-threatening is the development of acute hepatic encephalopathy. This condition is the key element in the definition of the most serious forms of acute liver injury: fulminant hepatic failure (FHF) and submassive hepatic necrosis (SHN). *FHF* is defined as the development of acute hepatic encephalopathy within 8 weeks of the onset of symptomatic hepatocellular disease in a previously healthy person. *SHN* is defined as the development of acute hepatic encephalopathy within 9 to 24 weeks of the onset of symptomatic hepatocellular disease in a previously healthy person. FHF and SHN are always accompanied by severe coagulopathy.

FHF and SHN are clinical syndromes caused by acute necrosis of a large proportion of hepatocytes. It is estimated that 2000 cases occur in the United States annually and that 80% of these patients die. Outcome is determined by the course of encephalopathy, which is measured on a four-point scale (Table 59–2). Cerebral edema, leading to increased intracranial pressure, is a common feature of severe FHF and may cause permanent cerebral injury and death.

DIFFERENTIAL DIAGNOSIS

The causes of FHF are shown in Table 59–1. Chronic liver disease may present with an acute onset and mimic FHF. Wilson's disease is an example of this type of presentation, so it is usually included in the list of causes of FHF. A history of

Table 59–1. Causes of Acute Liver Failure

CATEGORY	EXAMPLES
Drugs	Acetaminophen, halothane, phenytoin
Miscellaneous	Acute fatty liver of pregnancy, Reye's syndrome, Wilson's disease, malignant infiltration
Toxins	*Amanita phalloides,* carbon tetrachloride
Vascular	Budd-Chiari syndrome, cocaine, heat stroke, ischemia ("shock liver"), veno-occlusive syndrome
Viral hepatitis	Hepatitis A, B, D, E, C*, G*, CMV, HSV, EBV, varicella
Idiopathic	

*Uncertain cause of acute liver failure.
CMV, cytomegalovirus; HSV, herpes simplex virus; EBV, Epstein-Barr virus.

Table 59–2. Grading Scale for Hepatic Encephalopathy

GRADE	SYMPTOMS	SIGNS	ELECTROENCEPHALOGRAPHIC FINDINGS
I	Subtle change in mental status, difficulty in computation, emotional lability	No asterixis	Normal or symmetric slowing, triphasic waves
II	Drowsy, unequivocal loss of computation, memory loss	Asterixis	Abnormal symmetric slowing, triphasic waves
III	Sleepy but arousable, can answer simple questions only	Asterixis (if able to comply)	Abnormal symmetric slowing, triphasic waves
IVa	Coma, no response to commands, responds to pain	Unable to comply for asterixis testing, Babinski reflex is present	Abnormal slow delta waves (2–3/ min)
IVb	Coma, no response to commands or pain	Same as in IVa	Same as in IVa

heavy alcohol use also suggests chronic injury, even though alcoholics are at particular risk of acetaminophen-induced FHF. A characteristic clinical scenario leading to acute liver failure including FHF arises when an alcohol abuser stops drinking and takes acetaminophen to soothe abdominal pain or headache. Indeed, the "misadventure" of combining alcohol and acetaminophen is probably the most common cause of severe acute liver failure in the United States at present.

PREDICTING OUTCOME IN FULMINANT HEPATIC FAILURE AND SUBMASSIVE HEPATIC NECROSIS

Prognostic Criteria From Kings College Hospital

Studies from the liver unit at Kings College Hospital in London have established prognostic criteria for determining the prognosis of FHF (Table 59–3). In general, the clinical course of encephalopathy is the most informative datum in a particular patient: the deeper the coma, the worse the outcome. For example, FHF patients who have grade III or grade IV encephalopathy have a higher mortality than do patients whose encephalopathy never progresses beyond grade II.

Etiology

Hepatitis A virus– and hepatitis B virus–induced FHF have a better outcome than does idiopathic FHF. FHF due to phenytoin or halothane has a poor prognosis. In contrast, the majority of patients with acetaminophen-induced FHF who have grade III coma recover spontaneously.

Table 59–3. Prognostic Criteria Predicting Need for Liver Transplantation

Acetaminophen toxicity

pH <7.3 (irrespective of grade of encephalopathy) *or* prothrombin time >100 sec* and serum creatinine level >3.4 mg/dL (300 μmol/L) in patients with grade III or grade IV encephalopathy

All other causes

Prothrombin time >50 sec* (irrespective of encephalopathy) *or* any three of the following variables (irrespective of grade of encephalopathy):
Age >40 yr
Liver failure due to drug idiosyncrasy or idiopathic hepatitis previously called NANB
Duration of jaundice prior to encephalopathy >7 days
Prothrombin time >25 sec*
Serum bilirubin >17.5 mg/dL (300 μmol/L)

Modified from O'Grady JG, Alexander GJM, Hayllar KM, William R: Early indicators of prognosis in fulminant hepatic failure. Gastroenterology 97:439–445, 1989.
*Prothrombin times should be doubled for patients in the United Kingdom because of differences in methodology.
NANB, non-A, non-B.

Clinical Presentation and Comorbidities

Poor prognostic factors include age greater than 40 years as well as delayed onset of encephalopathy after the onset of jaundice. The latter indicates lack of spontaneous recovery; for this reason, SHN has a particularly poor outcome. Renal failure and acidosis (particularly in acetaminophen-induced FHF) also indicate a poor prognosis.

MANAGEMENT

All patients with FHF should be transferred to an intensive care unit (ICU) at a liver transplant center. Early transfer of patients with *any* degree of encephalopathy is crucial. Patients with acute hepatic injury that has not yet manifested encephalopathy may be managed in their local hospitals, but their physicians should alert a transplant center so that expeditious transfer can be arranged. Management should be directed toward the issues discussed in the following sections.

Diagnosis

One should run a battery of serologic tests for infections: anti–hepatitis B core antigen antibody of IgM class, hepatitis B surface antigen, anti–hepatitis A virus antibody of IgM class, and antibodies to cytomegalovirus, Epstein-Barr virus, herpes simplex virus, and varicella. The last four conditions are rare causes of FHF in immunocompetent patients. FHF caused by herpes simplex virus appears to have a predilection for pregnant women.

Serum ceruloplasmin levels should be determined and eyes should be examined by slit-lamp microscope for Kayser-Fleischer rings to assess for Wilson's disease. A family history of liver symptoms or neurologic failure in early life, a history of gradual intellectual deterioration or psychiatric symptoms in the patient before the onset of liver failure, or an unusually low serum alkaline phosphatase level (<80 IU/dL) may be clues to the presence of Wilson's disease.

One should also look for toxic insults such as the ingestion of wild mushrooms (amanita) or drugs (see Table 59–1). Finally, the physician should consider whether the patient represents the acute presentation of previously unrecognized chronic liver disease, as discussed earlier.

Specific Therapy

Patients with FHF who have ingested acetaminophen should receive a full course of *N*-acetylcysteine (NAC). This course is irrespective of whether the ingestion was part of a suicide attempt or simply for pain relief. Treatment with NAC should be instituted even if 24 to 36 hours have elapsed since the ingestion of acetaminophen (see Chapter 57). In Europe, NAC can be administered intravenously, whereas in the United States, NAC is available only as an enteral preparation. The standard NAC oral regimen consists of a loading dose of 140 mg/kg, followed by a maintenance dose of 70 mg/kg every 4 hours for a total of 18 doses. NAC should be administered via a nasogastric tube when patients are unable to take it by mouth. Although there are considerable data to support a role for circulating benzodiazepines in the development of acute (and chronic) hepatic encephalopathy, flumazenil has no role in the treatment of FHF (unless within a defined research protocol).

Avoidance of Renal Failure

Aminoglycosides, radiographic dye, and other potentially nephrotoxic agents should be used cautiously. Some practitioners advocate early use of continuous arteriovenous hemofiltration and dialysis or continuous venovenous hemofiltration and dialysis for better management of fluid balance (see Chapter 16).

Metabolic Fluxes

FHF, especially when caused by acetaminophen or one of the microvesicular fat deposition disorders (acute fatty liver of pregnancy), is often complicated by *hypoglycemia.* This may cause coma, which can be confused with cerebral edema. Correcting hypoglycemia in FHF often requires large amounts of dextrose. Hypokalemia and acidosis may also complicate FHF.

Hematologic Stability

Coagulopathy should be corrected by fresh frozen plasma before invasive procedures, such as placement of central venous catheters or an intracranial pressure (ICP) monitor, or whenever there is evidence of serious hemorrhage (intracranial hemorrhage, gastrointestinal bleeding). In most circumstances, it is not appropriate to give fresh frozen plasma simply to correct a prolonged prothrombin time. Furthermore, the uncorrected prothrombin time is a useful parameter to monitor recovery or deterioration of hepatic synthetic function.

Hypotension

Hypotension is common in FHF, despite high cardiac output, and is associated with low systemic vascular resistance. Hypotension may exacerbate low cerebral perfusion pressure (CPP) due to a raised ICP (see Chapter 42).

Assisted Ventilation

Mechanical ventilation via an endotracheal tube should be undertaken in patients with grade IV encephalopathy, or in patients with *any* evidence of hypoxia or respiratory distress because noncardiogenic pulmonary edema is a complication of FHF. Mechanical ventilation can also maintain a desired level of hypocapnia as an adjunct to controlling an elevated ICP (see Chapter 42).

Control of Infection

Repeated cultures of blood, urine, and ascites are advisable because patients with FHF are at increased risk of infection. This is particularly important because infection-induced sepsis may prevent liver transplantation, and the syndrome of high cardiac output and hypotension, associated with acute liver failure, mimics bacterial sepsis.

Management of Encephalopathy

Lactulose is given to all patients with acute hepatic encephalopathy. Its benefit is maximal when the patient is passing three to four soft stools per 24 hours. This is usually achieved by giving 30 mL every hour until a stool is passed and then giving 30 mL three times a day. Not only is there is no extra benefit to giving greater amounts of lactulose, it may be harmful by causing diarrhea, contracting intravascular volume (potentially precipitating renal failure), and depleting potassium. Patients with acute liver injury but without acute encephalopathy should be fed a balanced diet containing at least 80 g of protein per day. Patients with FHF can tolerate 60 g of protein per day, which should be administered orally, enterally, or parenterally, depending on the clinical circumstances. No convincing controlled clinical trials support withholding protein completely or administering specially formulated oral or parenteral amino acid feedings.

Cerebral Edema

Cerebral edema is the single most dangerous early complication of FHF. Patients may have rapid and extreme changes in CPP, especially precipitated by positional changes and movement. At their most severe, acute elevations in ICP may present with seizures, changes in pupillary responses, and decerebrate or decorticate posturing.

The treatment of raised ICP in FHF is intravenous mannitol. Only mannitol has been shown to be of therapeutic benefit in the syndrome of elevated ICP in FHF. Dexamethazone or other corticosteroids are of no value. The utility of barbiturate coma and ventilator-driven hypocapnia in reversing elevations in ICP associated with FHF are unknown but are often tried on an empirical basis. One should also treat for possible hypoglycemia as a cause of new neurologic signs (until this complication is ruled out).

Because ICP is subject to rapid changes, ICP monitoring is often used in the management of severely ill patients with FHF (see Chapter 42). Monitoring ICP serves two purposes: first, it facilitates attempts to reduce ICP and restore CPP whenever ICP rises and second, it enables the caregivers to recognize persistently elevated ICP and reduced CPP, which may cause irreversible brain injury before the patient undergoes liver transplantation. Unfortunately, the specific thresholds that infallibly predict irreversible brain injury are uncertain.

ICP monitoring is not advised before the patient is transferred to a liver transplant center. Rather, early transfer before development of grade III or IV coma is recommended. A protocol for placement of an epidural ICP catheter is shown in Table 59–4. The final decision should be made on a case-by-case basis in consultation with a neurosurgeon. In general, treatment should begin when CPP falls to less than 60 mm Hg (Table 59–5).

ICP monitoring should be discontinued when (1) a liver transplant has been successfully completed and the coagulopathy and neurologic examination are improving, (2) the patient ceases to be eligible for liver transplantation, or (3) brainstem function is absent with CPP less than 30 mm Hg or ICP greater than 60 mm Hg for more than 6 hours.

Liver Transplantation

Liver transplantation is a lifesaving procedure for patients with FHF or SHN who are not responding to medical management. Notwithstanding the aforementioned prognostic factors, the most important indicators that the patient needs liver transplantation are the level of encephalopathy and a trend of worsening encepha-

Table 59–4. Criteria for Placement of an Epidural Catheter
to Monitor Intracranial Pressure

All eligibility criteria for liver transplantation are met
Family member is available to give informed consent
Head computed tomographic scan within 24 h shows no evidence of intracranial bleeding
Mean arterial blood pressure >70 mm Hg
Prothrombin time ≤25* sec, platelets >100,000/μL after aggressive replenishment
Patient receiving mechanical ventilation
Stage IV coma, but with some brainstem function on neurologic examination

*Prothrombin times should be doubled for patients in the United Kingdom because of differences in methodology.

Table 59–5. Treatment of Low Cerebral Perfusion Pressure

....

Manipulate the height of the head

Vasopressor support to maintain mean arterial blood pressure at ≥60 mm Hg above ICP (but not more than systolic arterial pressure of 180 mm Hg or a mean pressure of 120 mm Hg)

Osmotic diuresis with 20% mannitol to maintain serum osmolality at 300–310 mOsm/L (but not >320 mOsm/L)

Hyperventilation by mechanical ventilation to maintain $Paco_2$ at 25–30 mm Hg

If serum sodium is <146 mEq/L and renal and cardiac parameters permit, give an intravenous bolus (50 mL) of 3% saline

Corticosteroids should not be used

Intracranial hemorrhages should not be evacuated

....

ICP, intracranial pressure.

lopathy. Unfortunately, because acute hepatic encephalopathy can vary between grade II and III in a matter of minutes, this judgment remains difficult.

For this reason, some authorities have used coagulation factor levels, particularly the Factor V level of less than 20% of normal, as an indicator of when to perform transplantation. Even if a patient with FHF is placed on the transplant list, obtaining a suitable donor organ quickly can be problematic. For example, it is not unusual for a patient listed in the highest priority status in North America to wait 72 hours or longer. During this time, further deterioration, especially worsening cerebral edema, may make transplantation impossible. Although the outcome of liver transplantation in FHF is somewhat worse than liver transplantation for other causes, 1-year survival rates of 50 to 60% are commonplace.

BIBLIOGRAPHY

Basile AS, Hughes RD, Harrison PM, et al: Elevated brain concentrations of 1-4-benzodiazepines in fulminant hepatic failure. N Engl J Med 325:473–478, 1991.
Postmortem study shows the elevated benzodiazepine concentrations in brains of some persons dying from FHF.

Bernstein D, Tripodi J: Fulminant hepatic failure. Crit Care Clin 14:181–197, 1998.
This is a review of clinical features and management of FHF written for intensivists (with 85 references).

Blei AT, Olafsson S, Webster S, Levy R: Complications of intracranial pressure monitoring in fulminant hepatic failure. Lancet 341:157–158, 1993.
Survey of complications that result from placement of ICP monitors.

Canalese J, Gimson AES, Davis C, et al: Controlled trial of dexamethazone and mannitol for the cerebral edema of fulminant hepatic failure. Gut 23:625–269, 1982.
Controlled trial showing benefit of mannitol infusions to treat cerebral edema associated with FHF.

Castells A, Salmeron JM, Navasa M, et al: Liver transplantation for acute liver failure: Analysis of applicability. Gastroenterology 105:532–538, 1993.
Descriptive study of liver transplantation in FHF.

Harrison PM, Keays R, Bray GP, et al: Improved outcome of paracetamol-induced fulminant hepatic failure by late administration of acetylcysteine. Lancet 335:1572–1583, 1990.
Important study indicates that NAC should be administered up to 24 hours after ingestion of acetaminophen in patients with toxic liver injury.

Lee WM: Acute liver failure. N Engl J Med 329:1862–1872, 1993.
Good review of acute liver failure and FHF.

Lidofsky SD, Bass NM, Prager MC, et al: Intracranial pressure monitoring and liver transplantation for fulminant hepatic failure. Hepatology 16:1–7, 1992.
Descriptive study of the use of ICP monitoring in FHF.

Mutiner D: Fulminant and subfulminant hepatic failure. In: Neuberger J, Lucey MR (eds): Liver Transplantation: Practice and Management. London, UK: BMJ Books, 1994, pp 72–85.
Good general review.

OGrady JG, Alexander GJM, Hayllar KM, William R: Early indicators of prognosis in fulminant hepatic failure. Gastroenterology 97:439–445, 1989.
Important analysis of prognoses from a large center.

Schrodt FV, Rochling FA, Casey DL, Lee WN: Acetaminophen toxicity in an urban county hospital. N Engl J Med 337:1112–1117, 1997.
Informative retrospective review of acetaminophen toxicity cases in nontransplant center.

Smilkstein MJ, Knapp GL, Kulig KW, Rumack BH: Efficacy of oral *N*-acteylcysteine in the treatment of acetaminophen overdose. N Engl J Med 319:1557–1562, 1988.
Large review shows the efficacy of NAC in acetaminophen overdose.

60

Lower Gastrointestinal Bleeding and Colitis

Roberta J. Hunter
Michael L. Kochman

LOWER GASTROINTESTINAL BLEEDING

When lower gastrointestinal (GI) bleeding occurs acutely in a patient in the intensive care unit (ICU), it may be a primary event or may be due to local trauma or another acute medical condition. Prompt diagnosis of the cause of the bleeding should be combined with definitive therapy to improve the patient's hemodynamic status and outcome. This chapter provides an overview to assist the ICU clinician in recognizing and treating the most common of the multitude of causes for lower GI bleeding.

Lower GI bleeding is defined as intestinal bleeding that occurs from a source distal to the ligament of Treitz. One's clinical impression as to the source of GI bleeding may be misleading. For example, when all cases of suspected acute lower GI bleeding are thoroughly investigated, 15 to 20% are found to be bleeding from the small intestine proximal to the ligament of Treitz or from other upper gastrointestinal sources.

Approximately 80% of all patients with acute lower GI bleeding will stop bleeding spontaneously, but a quarter of these individuals will have recurrent bleeding during the same hospitalization. Mortality, estimated to be between 10 and 15%, is increased for the group with recurrent or persistent bleeding. No bleeding source can be identified in 8 to 12% of suspected cases of lower GI bleeding, even after extensive diagnostic testing.

History and Causes

Initial assessment of patients with gastrointestinal bleeding, including lower GI bleeding, should begin with measurement of blood pressure (Fig. 60–1). One should simultaneously start appropriate resuscitative measures for restoring intravascular volume. Concomitantly with these measures, one should obtain a directed history and do a focused physical examination relevant to lower GI bleeding.

The causes of acute lower GI bleeding are diverse (Table 60–1). In patients less than 50 years of age, hemorrhoids are the most common cause, whereas in patients older than 50 years of age, diverticulosis and angiodysplasia (arteriovenous malformations) are most frequent. Whether or not bleeding is associated with pain may be helpful in suggesting the likely diagnosis. Rectal pain may indicate an anal fissure or hemorrhoidal source. Abdominal pain may indicate inflammatory bowel disease, ischemia, or infectious colitis. Painless lower GI bleeding, especially in an elderly patient, should increase one's suspicion of a diverticulum or angiodysplasia as the cause. Pain that worsens after eating occurs with mesenteric ischemia, whereas pain that worsens with passing of stool suggests an anal fissure.

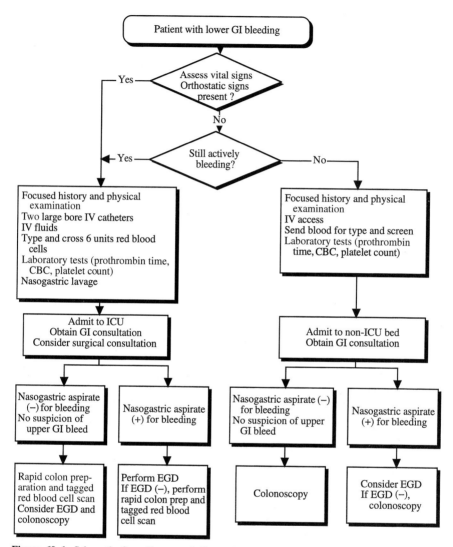

Figure 60–1. Schematic flow diagram of diagnostic evaluation and initial management, including triage, for a patient who presents with a history or signs suggesting lower gastrointestinal bleeding (see text). GI, gastrointestinal; IV, intravenous; CBC, complete blood count; EGD, esophagogastroduodenoscopy.

The characteristics of the patient's stool in acute lower GI bleeding confirm the diagnosis of GI bleeding and give clues about its origin. Although *hematochezia*, the passage of reddish stools, is classically indicative of a lower gastrointestinal source, up to 20% of patients with an upper GI source may also exhibit this finding. Hematochezia, in combination with orthostatic hypotension, should always increase concern about the possibility of the upper GI tract as a source of bleeding. Frank bright red blood per rectum is usually from a perianal source. Blood on the

Table 60–1. Potential Sources for Presumed Lower Gastrointestinal Bleeding

Massive upper gastrointestinal bleeding
Small intestine sources distal to the ligament of Treitz
   Arteriovenous malformation
   Diverticula
   Inflammatory bowel disease
   Meckel's diverticulum
   Neoplasm
   Vasculoenteric fistula (postsurgical)
Large intestine sources
   Arteriovenous malformation
   Colitis (infectious or radiation-induced)
   Colonic varices (idiopathic or due to portal hypertension)
   Diverticulosis
   Endometriosis
   Hemorrhoids
   Inflammatory bowel disease
   Intussusception with mucosal compromise
   Ischemia
   Neoplasm
   Solitary rectal ulcer
   Vasculitis

outside of a well-formed stool likely represents an anal canal lesion such as hemorrhoids, fissures, or polyps. Many causes of acute lower GI bleeding may produce maroon stools. Melena may originate from a lower GI source, such as the distal small bowel or proximal colon. A history of change in stool habits or stool caliber suggests neoplastic causes. If the patient has bloody diarrhea, one should consider inflammatory bowel disease or infectious colitis. A history of an endoscopic procedure with biopsy or polypectomy within 14 days should raise the possibility of bleeding from that site.

Physical Examination

Physical examination may be helpful in determining the cause of lower GI bleeding. Complaints of pain out of proportion to the physical findings should raise one's suspicion for ischemia of the small bowel or colon, or both. In combination with a history of atrial fibrillation, recent myocardial infarction, or in a patient on pressors or with systemic hypotension, such disproportionate abdominal pain suggests inadequate perfusion of the mesenteric arteries. A pulsatile mass suggests an aortic aneurysm or the formation of a vasculoenteric fistula. Stigmata of chronic liver disease may indicate the existence of varices anywhere along the gastrointestinal tract, including the small intestine, colon, and rectum. Rectal examination should be performed, as a rectal mass may be palpated or fissures may be seen. The patient's stool should always be tested for occult blood to ensure that its abnormal appearance is actually due to hemoglobin and is not secondary to ingested bismuth, beets, or oral iron supplementation.

Management

Patients with gastrointestinal hemorrhage, including lower GI bleeding, should be admitted to the ICU *if* they meet appropriate clinical criteria of severity or concomitant disease (Table 60–2). Specific management of a patient with lower GI bleeding is dictated by the specifics and the acuity of the situation. The surgical service should be consulted if the patient has massive bleeding (requiring more than 6 units of blood) or develops signs of an acute surgical abdomen.

Investigations of the Colon

In general, *colonoscopy* should be the first test performed in the evaluation of suspected lower GI bleeding if bleeding has ceased. It has the advantage of being potentially both diagnostic and therapeutic. However, it requires an oral cleansing of the colon to allow complete mucosal examination. This is not a major disadvantage if patients spontaneously stop bleeding (as occurs in 80% of all patients with lower GI bleeding). After adequate oral cleansing of the bowel, the diagnostic accuracy of emergency colonoscopy is high (70 to 92%).

Alternatively, *anoscopy* or *sigmoidoscopy* or both, may be performed in selected patients during the bleeding episode or after cessation of bleeding. However, this should be followed later by double-contrast barium enema for a complete evaluation of the colon. This second option has been advocated as the more cost-effective approach in patients less than 50 years of age.

Satisfactory bowel cleansing is generally difficult to achieve in patients who continue to bleed actively. Nonetheless, colonoscopy as a first test may still be effective even in the presence of active lower GI bleeding if the colon receives special preparation. For this purpose, a balanced electrolyte solution is administered orally or via a nasogastric tube at the rate of 240 mL every 15 minutes. This provides reasonably satisfactory cleansing of the bowel in 4 to 6 hours. Once the rectal effluent becomes clear of stool and blood, colonoscopy is performed. Under these circumstances, it has been reported to yield more specific diagnoses and

Table 60–2. Criteria for Admission to the Intensive Care Unit with Acute Lower Gastrointestinal Bleeding

Patients should be admitted to the ICU if they have any of the following:
Orthostatic signs*
Evidence of active hemorrhage
Hemoglobin <10 g/dL or ≥3 g/dL drop from previous baseline
History of previous GI bleeding episode
History of dysfunction of any of the following organ systems:
   Cardiac
   Pulmonary
   Hepatic
   Renal

* Orthostatic signs are seen when a change in position from supine to erect causes two or more of the following: (1) pulse increase of 20 beats per minute, (2) systolic blood pressure drop ≥20 mm Hg, and (3) diastolic blood pressure drop ≥10 mm Hg.
ICU, intensive care unit; GI, gastrointestinal.

opportunities for therapy when compared with other interventions, such as angiography and surgery. The only absolute contraindications to colonoscopy in the acute setting are persistent circulatory shock and a perforated viscus.

If the patient continues to bleed but is otherwise hemodynamically stable, a technetium-99m–labeled *red cell scintigraphy scan* may help localize the site of hemorrhage. Its advantages include the ability to detect bleeding rates as low as 0.05 to 0.1 mL/min and to detect intermittent or recurrent bleeding. Its major disadvantages include variable sensitivity and erroneous localization of the site of bleeding in up to 25% of cases. In addition, it does not provide the potential for therapeutic intervention. This test is most helpful in assessing if patients are bleeding vigorously enough to permit visualization by selective angiography.

Angiography also has the potential for being both a diagnostic and therapeutic intervention. However, bleeding rates of 0.5 to 1.0 mL/min are required for angiographic localization. Angiography does not require a bowel preparation and if it reveals the site of bleeding, it allows for more selective surgical resection. Angiography may be therapeutic if intra-arterial vasopressin is used. Instillation of vasopressin should be considered a temporizing maneuver only because rebleeding may occur in up to 50% of cases if no definitive therapy is undertaken. A significant disadvantage of angiography is that the patient must be actively bleeding at rates greater than the threshold of detection at the time of the study. It also carries a 10% complication rate. Complications include arterial thrombosis and embolization and renal failure from radiocontrast exposure.

Small Bowel Investigations

If a bleeding site cannot be found in the colon, investigation of the small bowel is warranted. In the stable patient, enteroclysis (a contrast enema of the small bowel) or small bowel enteroscopy may be performed. The diagnostic yield for enteroclysis is reported to be as high as 20% in patients with prior negative upper GI and colon evaluations. The yield on enteroscopy may be higher when performed intraoperatively. A suture may then be placed where the abnormality is identified, facilitating surgical resection or oversewing of the site. A radionuclide scan to detect a bleeding Meckel's diverticulum may be performed in selected patients at high risk for this disorder, such as teenagers and young adults.

Surgical Interventions

Surgical therapy for lower GI bleeding should be recommended for patients in whom exsanguination is occurring because of uncontrolled hemorrhage but only after they have had a negative upper GI evaluation. Subtotal colectomy may be the simplest procedure if a bleeding site cannot be localized. For patients with diffuse diverticulosis and an uncontrolled hemorrhage, the operative mortality is about 10%. Surgery may also be considered in patients with recurrent bleeding despite colonoscopic or angiographic intervention, or both, and in patients with diffuse colonic disease, such as diffuse angiodysplasia or chronic ischemia.

COLITIS

The discussion of colitis will be limited to the forms of colitis likely to be seen in the ICU, for example, infectious colitis and ischemic colitis. Patients with inflammatory bowel diseases rarely require acute admission to the ICU, and their management will not be considered in this chapter.

Clostridium difficile Colitis

Etiology and Pathogenesis

Clostridium difficile is a common pathogen in hospitalized patients. In this setting, *C. difficile* spores are readily available for transmission, leading to nosocomial outbreaks because they can survive on surfaces for months. They may be cultured from a variety of surfaces, including floors, toilets, scales, room furniture, and mops. *C. difficile* is a Gram-positive, spore-forming anaerobic bacillus that produces two toxins. Toxin A, an enterotoxin, is the main pathogenic factor. It causes opening of tight cellular junctions in bowel epithelium and results in increased epithelial permeability. Toxin B, a cytotoxin, leads to changes in cell shape, for example, rounding of the cell. This forms the basis of the cytolytic cell culture assay commonly used to diagnose the presence of *C. difficile* toxin.

The normal human colon is resistant to colonization by *C. difficile* by virtue of its normal endogenous bacteria. However, use of antibiotics can lead to an environment in which *C. difficile* may predominate. Antibiotics commonly associated with this complication include ampicillin, amoxicillin, clindamycin, cephalosporins, and aminoglycosides.

Clinical Features

Typical clinical features of *C. difficile* infection include watery diarrhea and crampy lower abdominal pain. The patient may have received antibiotics for several days during the 4 to 6 weeks before the onset of symptoms. Laboratory evaluation may show an elevated white blood cell count, electrolyte abnormalities consistent with diarrhea-induced volume depletion, and white blood cells in the stool. Flexible sigmoidoscopy performed at the bedside without prior bowel preparation may reveal pseudomembranes. However, the absence of these membranes does not exclude the diagnosis because up to one third of infected patients may have disease only in the right colon.

Severe or fulminant *C. difficile* infection may be heralded by increasing abdominal pain, dehydration, and worsening abdominal distention as the colon dilates and becomes atonic. Diarrhea may then disappear. The white cell count may rise into the tens of thousands. Serial abdominal examinations and radiographs are indicated under these circumstances. Severe localized abdominal pain with signs of peritonitis may represent the development of a perforation. If this or severe sepsis develops, a subtotal colectomy may be necessary.

Treatment

Metronidazole or vancomycin is used for the treatment of *C. difficile* colitis. If possible, other antibiotics should be discontinued. As a rule, antidiarrheal agents should be avoided. Oral metronidazole (500 mg q8h) or oral vancomycin (125 mg q6h) for 7 to 10 days usually suffices for most cases with metronidazole being less expensive. In severe infection, metronidazole may be given intravenously (500 mg q8h), or vancomycin may be given via a nasogastric tube (125 mg q6h) for 10 days. Response to therapy with resolution of diarrhea can be expected in the first 72 hours for more than 95% of patients. However, 10 to 20% of patients will have a relapse after discontinuation of the therapy. Follow-up toxin assays, however, are required only in symptomatic individuals.

Typhlitis

Typhlitis is an infection within the bowel wall in the cecum, typically occurring in immunocompromised patients who have received chemotherapy or glucocortico-steroids. The exact cause is uncertain. No single organism has been identified as pathogenic. Gram-positive rods and cocci, Gram-negative bacilli, enterococci, and *Candida* have been shown to be present by culture.

The diagnosis may be difficult to make because its symptoms resemble side effects of the primary chemotherapy. These symptoms include fever, nausea, vomiting, and abdominal pain. The abdomen may be tender and the cecum palpable as a boggy mass in the right lower quadrant. Abdominal radiographs may reveal a right-sided soft tissue density or an ileus with complete or partial obstruction. Although barium enema may demonstrate nodular mucosa, it is not the test of choice because it carries a risk of perforation. The preferred test is the abdominal computed tomographic scan, which may show cecal wall thickening, a right lower quadrant soft tissue mass, or cecal pneumatosis. Ultrasonography may also be helpful and reveal a target or halo sign of a solid mass with echogenic center.

Overall survival from typhlitis is only 40 to 50%. Initial treatment is supportive with complete bowel rest, intravenous hydration, broad spectrum antibiotic admin-istration, and consideration of the addition of antifungal agents if the patient fails to improve within 72 hours. The abdominal examination must be followed closely to monitor for the development of peritoneal signs. The surgical service should be made aware of the patient if such signs develop or if the patient continues to deteriorate despite intensive therapy. The decision to take the patient to the operating room must take into consideration the patient's overall prognosis from any underlying neoplastic disease as well as the fact that some studies have found no improvement in outcome despite surgical intervention. The surgical procedure of choice is a right hemicolectomy with removal of all necrotic debris.

Ischemic Colitis

Ischemic colitis falls into occlusive and nonocclusive categories (Table 60–3). Abdominal pain is typically a presenting symptom in 75 to 98% of patients with

Table 60–3. Causes of Ischemic Colitis

OCCLUSIVE CAUSES	NONOCCLUSIVE CAUSES
Abdominal aortic aneurysm	Cardiac dysfunction
Abdominal surgery	Ergotamine
Embolism	Hypovolemia
Thrombosis	Intravenous pressors
Tumor compression	Local hemodynamic disturbances
Vasculitis	Systemic hypotension
	Vasopressin infusion

ischemic colitis of any form. In these patients, the abdominal examination may demonstrate distention, and blood may be present in the stool.

Seventy-five percent of mesenteric infarctions occur secondary to mesenteric arterial embolus. The typical patient is elderly and has atrial fibrillation without other vascular disease. Abrupt onset of abdominal pain out of proportion to the physical examination findings, spontaneous gastrointestinal emptying with bloody diarrhea, and an appropriate cardiac history should raise a high level of suspicion for mesenteric infarction. Plain radiographs may show a thickened bowel wall. Angiography is the definitive test, with the most common lesion demonstrated being occlusion of the superior mesenteric artery. Treatment is embolectomy with re-establishment of blood flow and resection of any nonviable bowel.

Mesenteric arterial and venous thrombosis may present in a manner similar to that of an arterial embolus. These conditions may have a more insidious onset over time. In arterial thrombosis, anticoagulation may be helpful, but surgical therapy is often needed. Anticoagulation may be used in venous thrombosis if the thrombosis is incomplete. Surgical intervention is required for complete thrombosis and bowel infarction.

Nonocclusive causes of ischemic colitis have clinical features that may develop gradually in the setting of other systemic diseases. Abdominal pain, distention, and gastrointestinal bleeding may be the first manifestation of this entity in a patient in the ICU. Diagnosis is suspected from the correct clinical context and may be confirmed with angiography. Treatment includes supportive care, including nasogastric decompression, optimizing treatment of underlying hemodynamics, and antibiotics to cover enteric organisms. An infusion of papaverine may be used in selected patients if vasospasm is demonstrated on angiography.

BIBLIOGRAPHY

DeMarkles MP, Murphy JR: Acute lower gastrointestinal bleeding. Med Clin North Am 77:1085–1100, 1993.
    This article emphasizes the cause and evaluation of moderate to severe acute lower gastrointestinal bleeding.

Dusold R, Burke K, Carpentier W, Dyck WP: The accuracy of technetium-99m–labeled red cell scintigraphy in localizing gastrointestinal bleeding. Am J Gastroenterol 89:345–348, 1994.

This article reviews the role for technetium-labeled red blood cell scans in the management of lower gastrointestinal bleeding.

Evers ML, Nelson DA: Managing the triage of GI hemorrhage as a function of stability. N J Med 92:159–162, 1995.
This article presents a triage tool to assist in the identification of patients with GI hemorrhage. Criteria include orthostasis; current, active GI hemorrhage; hemoglobin less than 10 g/dL or a 3 g/dL drop from a known baseline; and history of underlying organ system dysfunction.

Fekety R, Kim KH, Brown D, et al: Epidemiology of antibiotic-associated colitis: Isolation of *Clostridium difficile* from the hospital environment. Am J Med 70:906, 1981.
This epidemiologic review of C. difficile stresses the importance of enteric isolation precautions, careful hand washing, and the cleansing of potentially contaminated surfaces and objects in the hospital environment to decrease the nosocomial spread of this infection.

Hiruki T, Fernandes B, Ramsay J, Rother I: Acute typhlitis in an immunocompromised host: Report of an unusual case and review of the literature. Dig Dis Sci 37:1292–1296, 1992.
Typhlitis is reviewed in detail, and its potential pathogenetic role in the development of septicemia in immunocompromised hosts is discussed.

Jensen DM, Machicado GA, Jutabha R, et al: Urgent colonoscopy for the diagnosis and treatment of severe diverticular hemorrhage. N Engl J Med 342:78–82, 2000.
Among 121 patients presenting with severe hematochezia and diverticulosis, there were 10 patients with definite diverticular bleeding, all of whom responded well to local colonoscopic treatment. See also Letters to Editor about this article in N Engl J Med 342:1608–1611, 2000.

Jensen DM: Current management of severe lower gastrointestinal bleeding. Gastrointest Endosc 41:171–173, 1995.
This is a review of the management of lower gastrointestinal bleeding.

Makela JT, Kiviniemi H, Laitinen S, Kairaluoma MI: Diagnosis and treatment of acute lower gastrointestinal bleeding. Scand J Gastroenterol 28:1062–1066, 1993.
In this series, the cause of bleeding was detected in 76% (203 of 266) of the cases during initial investigation, and the cause remained unclear after subsequent examinations in 17% of the cases.

Miller LS, Barbarevech C, Friedman LS: Less frequent causes of lower gastrointestinal bleeding. Gastroenterol Clin North Am 23:21–52, 1994.
The less frequently encountered causes of gastrointestinal bleeding—including solitary rectal ulcer syndrome, colonic varices, mesenteric vascular insufficiency, and others—are reviewed.

Parkes BM, Obeid FN, Sorensen VJ, et al: The management of massive lower gastrointestinal bleeding. Am Surg 59:676–678, 1993.
The results of this study suggest that segmental resection should be performed only when the bleeding site is identified angiographically. Subtotal colectomy should be reserved for massive bleeding with negative angiographic findings and life-threatening clinical events.

Pothoulakis C, LaMont JT: *Clostridium difficile* colitis and diarrhea. Gastroenterol Clin North Am 22:623–637, 1993.
This thorough review covers the epidemiology, diagnosis, therapy, and clinical outcomes associated with C. difficile.

Richter JM, Christensen MR, Kaplan LM, Nishioka NS: Effectiveness of current technology in the diagnosis and management of lower gastrointestinal hemorrhage. Gastrointest Endosc 41:93–98, 1995.
In this series, colonoscopy yielded a diagnosis in 90% of patients, provided the opportunity for successful therapy in 9 of 13 patients (69%), and shortened hospital stay. Diagnostic yield, therapeutic opportunity, and cost-effectiveness are maximized with early investigation.

61 Upper Gastrointestinal Bleeding

Brian R. Stotland
Gregory G. Ginsberg

Upper gastrointestinal (GI) bleeding is defined as bleeding from a source proximal to the ligament of Treitz (Table 61–1). It is considered *severe* when it results in shock or orthostatic hypotension or, a decrease in hemoglobin (Hgb) by 3 to 4 g/dL or if the patient needs a transfusion of at least 2 units of packed red blood cells. Severe upper GI bleeding generally necessitates admission to an intensive care unit (ICU) (Table 61–2). Although upper GI bleeding occurs more commonly in men, the overall mortality rate of 5 to 10% is similar for both sexes.

ASSESSMENT

When a patient presents with GI bleeding, regardless of the source, the initial management should focus on two main aspects: (1) volume resuscitation with appropriate intravenous fluids and blood products and (2) identification of the source of bleeding to allow selective therapy. The rapid initial assessment should include determination of vital signs and postural blood pressure changes, a focused history and physical examination, and gastric lavage.

Focused History

In addition to the presenting symptoms, one should inquire about a history of prior GI bleeding, peptic ulcer disease, bleeding diathesis, renal or liver disease, alcohol

Table 61–1. Causes of Upper Gastrointestinal Bleeding and Their Frequency

CAUSE	FREQUENCY
Erosive gastritis	29.6%
Duodenal ulcer	22.8%
Gastric ulcer	21.9%
Varices (esophageal, gastric)	15.4%
Esophagitis	12.8%
Erosive duodenitis	9.1%
Mallory-Weiss tear	8.0%
Neoplasm	3.7%
Esophageal ulcer	2.2%
Stomach ulcer	1.9%
Osler-Weber-Rendu syndrome	0.5%
Other	7.3%

From Silverstein FE, Gilbert DA, Tedesco JF, et al: The national ASGE survey on upper gastrointestinal bleeding. I. Study design and baseline data. Gastrointest Endosc 27:73–79, 1981.

Table 61–2. Indications for Admission to the Intensive Care Unit
for Upper Gastrointestinal Bleeding

....

Active bleeding
Hemodynamically unstable
Known or suspected portal hypertension
Significant comorbid disease
Coagulopathy (e.g., prothrombin time elevated with INR >2)
Possible sentinel bleed (previous abdominal aortic graft)

....

INR, international normalized ratio.

abuse, use of nonsteroidal anti-inflammatory drugs (NSAIDs), or chronic anticoagulation. It is important to assess the possibility of cirrhosis or other causes of portal hypertension because management of variceal bleeding is distinct. The source of bleeding may be suggested by the history. Retching or vomiting immediately before the onset of bleeding suggests a Mallory-Weiss tear. A prior history of abdominal aortic aneurysm repair should prompt consideration of an aortoenteric fistula. Recent instrumentation of the pancreas, liver, or biliary tract should raise the suspicion of hemobilia or hemosuccus pancreaticus. A history of chronic epistaxis and skin telangiectasias indicates the possibility of hereditary hemorrhagic telangiectasia (Osler-Weber-Rendu syndrome).

If the patient has a clear history of vomiting bright red blood or "coffee grounds" (representing the presence of blood in the stomach long enough to be acidified by gastric acid to turn brown in color), the diagnosis of upper GI bleeding is straightforward. However, occasionally bleeding from the posterior pharynx or the lung may be confused with upper GI bleeding. A history of *melena* is nonspecific. Melena results from bacterial degradation of red blood cell heme. It commonly arises when the bleeding source is from the upper GI tract but may also be observed if the bleeding is from a small bowel source or a slow bleed from the right colon.

Focused Physical Examination and Laboratory Evaluation

The physical examination should start with the patient's hemodynamic status. Aside from directing immediate resuscitation, initial vital signs have prognostic importance, that is, 50% of patients presenting with shock have rebleeding episodes. An orthostatic pulse rise of more than 20 beats per minute implies at least 500 mL of blood loss. An accompanying fall in diastolic pressure of 10 mm Hg or more implies at least 1000 mL of blood loss. The initial examination should also include a survey for stigmata of chronic liver disease, such as spider angiomas, gynecomastia, palmar erythema, ascites, and splenomegaly. Findings suggestive of underlying malignancy or cutaneous lesions associated with diseases that can cause GI bleeding, such as hereditary hemorrhagic telangiectasia, may also be detected.

Initial laboratory evaluation should include a complete blood count with a platelet count, coagulation studies (prothrombin time [PT], and partial thromboplastin time [PTT]), and determination of serum electrolytes, creatinine, blood urea nitrogen (BUN), bilirubin, and liver-associated enzyme levels. The initial blood draw should include a sample to be sent for STAT typing and cross-matching.

Intestinal metabolism of blood raises serum BUN so that a BUN:creatinine ratio greater than 20 (when both BUN and creatinine are expressed in mg/dL) supports the diagnosis of upper GI bleeding. However, this is a nonspecific finding and can be seen in hypovolemia alone.

Gastric Lavage

Even when the patient has an obvious history of upper GI bleeding, gastric lavage is indicated to clear the stomach in anticipation of endoscopy in order to decrease the risk of aspiration for the patient and to improve visualization for the endoscopist. In this regard, a large-bore tube (e.g., an Ewald tube) may be needed because it is less likely to be occluded by blood clots. There is no therapeutic advantage to the use of iced saline (versus room temperature tapwater or saline) for the lavage fluid. If there is no evidence of recent bleeding in the initial gastric aspirate, that is, no red blood or coffee grounds, the nasogastric tube may be removed.

There is a 30% mortality rate when *both* the gastric aspirate and stool contain red blood. However, up to 16% of those actively bleeding from the upper GI tract may have clear gastric fluid on lavage. This may be due to intermittent bleeding or bleeding beyond the gastric pylorus without blood refluxing into the stomach. Identification of bile in the gastric aspirate is notoriously *inaccurate* and should not be used as proof of lack of an upper GI bleeding source.

APPROACH TO MANAGEMENT

Generic Care

Initial management is individualized based on the patient's hemodynamics, the rate of bleeding, and accompanying medical problems. General recommendations for the patient in the ICU starts with assuring ample intravenous access (Table 61–3). For hypotensive patients who are undergoing exsanguination, large-bore (8 Fr) catheters, so-called trauma lines (which must be used with corresponding wide-bore tubing and special three-way stopcocks) should be used. Alternatively, 8 Fr catheter introducer sheaths, which are routinely used for insertion of pulmonary artery catheters, can also be used (but without small-bore stopcocks). Normal saline or Ringer lactate solution should be given initially to keep the heart rate at less than 100 beats per minute and the systolic blood pressure higher than 100 mm Hg, if possible. Once available, it is preferable to replace lost blood volume with transfused packed red blood cells. This is particularly true for patients with cirrhosis who tend to redistribute crystalloids to the extravascular space and acquire massive total body fluid overload. Deciding when to transfuse is dependent on the patient's hemodynamic stability, underlying conditions, and comorbidities and the risk of further bleeding. Early consultation with a gastroenterologist and a general surgeon is recommended for patients in the ICU with upper GI bleeding.

During the first few hours after a bleeding episode, the plasma volume and Hgb concentration decrease proportionately so that the Hgb concentration is often

Table 61–3. Initial Management in the Intensive Care Unit

Secure two wide-bore intravenous (IV) access lines (at least two 16 [or less, preferably 18] gauge peripheral IV lines or one 16- or 18-gauge peripheral IV line and one central venous catheter)
Give volume replacement, initially with crystalloid
Monitor central venous pressure if patient has underlying cardiac, renal disease, or shock
Send hemoglobin (Hgb) and hematocrit, platelet count, coagulation studies (PT, PTT) STAT; follow Hgb frequently
Type and cross-match or type and screen for at least 6 units of packed red blood cells
Give unmatched O negative blood via "trauma lines" and wide-bore tubing in patients in shock with exsanguinating hemorrhage
Insert Foley catheter to monitor urinary output
Obtain abdominal radiograph
Consult gastroenterologist and general surgeon early

PT, prothrombin time; PTT, partial thromboplastin time.

normal despite significant bleeding. Later, when the plasma volume is overexpanded from crystalloid therapy, the Hgb may *underestimate* the quantity of red blood cells present. The goals of transfusion of blood products can be summarized as follows: (1) packed red blood cells are given to improve oxygen delivery and provide a buffer in case further bleeding should occur, (2) fresh frozen plasma is administered to correct defects in coagulation, and (3) platelets are given to treat thrombocytopenia or platelet dysfunction. For example, keeping the Hgb greater than or equal to 10 g/dL is a commonly used end point for most patients with upper gastrointestinal bleeding.

Standard ICU monitoring should include continuous electrocardiographic and systemic blood pressure monitoring (by means of an arterial catheter) or, alternatively, electrocardiographic and intermittent but frequent systemic blood pressure measurements by automated cuff. Patients with a history of congestive heart failure or significant heart disease should be candidates for central venous pressure or pulmonary arterial pressure monitoring. Patients with respiratory insufficiency or altered mental status, that is, those with increased risk for aspiration, should undergo tracheal intubation. Similarly, patients with active hematemesis should be kept in the left lateral decubitus position (to decrease risk of aspiration), and tracheal intubation should be considered for airway protection. The importance of frequent repeated clinical assessments of the patient's condition by ICU staff cannot be overemphasized.

Endoscopic and Angiographic Interventions

Once the patient is stabilized (and rarely in the unstable patient who is undergoing exsanguination), urgent endoscopy should be considered. This procedure is indicated in resuscitated patients with active hemorrhage, in those requiring transfusion of blood products, or in those with evidence of hypovolemia, known or suspected portal hypertension, or suspected aortoenteric fistula. Patients who rebleed after initial stabilization should also undergo urgent endoscopy. Endoscopy can be deferred for up to 24 hours in patients with self-limited bleeding and no hemodynamic instability. Esophagogastroduodenoscopy (EGD) correctly identifies the source of bleeding in most cases. It is also valuable in providing prognostic

Table 61–4. Endoscopic Findings in Peptic Ulcers and Their Risk of Rebleeding

ENDOSCOPIC FINDING	RISK OF REBLEEDING
Arterial (pulsatile) bleeding	85%
Nonbleeding visible vessel	40–50%
Adherent clot	20–30%
Oozing without visible vessel	<20%
Flat blood spot at ulcer base	<10%
Clean base	<5%

From Silverstein FE, Gilbert DA, Tedesco JF, et al: The national ASGE survey on upper gastrointestinal bleeding. I. Study design and baseline data. Gastrointest Endosc 27:73–79, 1981.

information and initiating the proper therapy. The accuracy in identifying the bleeding source is highest within the first 12 to 18 hours of hospital admission (approximately 90%) and falls by 30% or more after 24 hours. Accurate identification of endoscopic features can predict the risk of rebleeding (Table 61–4). Since radiologic contrast studies offer no therapeutic benefit, and contrast agents may interfere with subsequent endoscopy, they have no role in the initial evaluation of upper GI bleeding.

In preparation for upper endoscopy, the patient should have electrocardiographic and hemodynamic monitoring, ideally with automated noninvasive intermittent blood pressure monitoring, as well as respiratory monitoring by continuous pulse oximetry. Equipment for endotracheal intubation should be readily available. A trained endoscopy nurse or ICU nurse must monitor the patient's vital signs and clinical condition during the endoscopy procedure and be ready to provide oropharyngeal suctioning. Conscious sedation using an opioid and a benzodiazepine are usually administered with supplemental oxygen. Reversal agents (naloxone and flumazenil) should be readily available.

EGD with endoscopic therapy has been demonstrated to decrease morbidity in acute upper GI bleeding. Meta-analyses of trials of endoscopic therapy for bleeding from peptic ulcers estimate that the odds ratio for further bleeding is 0.23 to 0.38, that is, the risk patients have for continued bleeding after endoscopy is 23 to 38% of the risk that patients without EGD have. EGD also reduces the risk of the need for surgery. The odds ratio for overall mortality in patients undergoing endoscopic therapy is 0.55 to 0.62 compared with pharmacologic therapy alone.

When endoscopic diagnosis or therapy is unsuccessful because of obscured visibility or persistent bleeding, angiography may be considered an alternative to emergency surgery. Angiography may effectively localize the source of bleeding, and vascular embolization may be effective in patients in whom endoscopic therapy failed or who are poor surgical candidates.

EVALUATION AND MANAGEMENT OF DIFFERENT CATEGORIES OF UPPER GASTROINTESTINAL BLEEDING

Gastric and Duodenal Peptic Ulcers

Ulcer disease occurs in approximately 10% of the population, and bleeding develops in about 15% of patients with ulcers. The two main causes of ulcers are the use of NSAIDs and infection with *Helicobacter pylori*. Once identified, a gastric or duodenal peptic ulcer may have one of several features that suggest recent or active hemorrhage and that predict the risk of rebleeding (see Table 61–4). Gastric ulcers as a group have a higher overall rebleeding rate than do duodenal ulcers. Endoscopic therapeutic intervention is beneficial only in the presence of high-risk features, that is, arterial bleeding or a visible vessel. If one finds an adherent clot, one should gently wash it. If it washes off easily and reveals active bleeding or a visible vessel, intervention is indicated. Since 80% of all upper GI bleeds will stop spontaneously, only lesions predisposed to rebleeding should be treated endoscopically.

Endoscopic interventions of proven benefit in bleeding peptic ulcers include treatment by contact devices (contact electrocautery or heater probes), injection therapy, and laser photocoagulation. Prospective trials of contact devices used with forceful coaptation of the vessel wall have shown them to decrease rebleeding, shorten hospital stay, decrease transfusion requirements, and lower hospital costs. It is best performed with a 10 Fr probe, a low wattage setting, and a long duration of pulses (10 to 30 seconds). Injection therapy has been used alone or in combination with contact devices for ulcer bleeding. When used alone and regardless of the choice of injectant, injection therapy achieves results comparable to contact devices. Endoscopic laser therapy has also been shown to be efficacious in upper GI bleeding. However, it is often impractical because of its expense and lack of portability. Ultimately, which modality to use depends on the anatomic characteristics of the lesion, the equipment available, and the experience of the endoscopist.

In general, these procedures are considered safe and effective in the proper subset of patients. However, complications from all types of endoscopic therapy occur and include ulceration, induced or worsened bleeding (20%) and perforation (1%). Precipitated bleeding usually can be controlled endoscopically, whereas perforation is more likely to occur during a second round of endoscopy.

It is generally recommended that H_2-receptor antagonists be used in patients with bleeding peptic ulcers, but none of these agents has been shown to be effective in stopping active bleeding or in decreasing early rebleeding. Their use aims to enhance healing and decrease late rebleeding from peptic ulcers. Continuous intravenous infusion of H_2-receptor antagonists more effectively suppresses gastric acid than does bolus therapy. Although proton pump inhibitors, for example, omeprazole, are more efficient in suppressing acid than are H_2-receptor antagonists, they are not yet available for intravenous use in the United States.

Patients who rebleed after endoscopic therapy usually do so within 48 hours of the initial procedure. Hypovolemic shock on presentation predicts a high risk of recurrent bleeding. In long-term follow-up, the rate of recurrent hemorrhage after endoscopic hemostasis for peptic ulcer disease is approximately 33%. This rate may be reduced by eradication of *H. pylori* when present, avoidance of NSAIDs, and long-term gastric acid suppression as the clinical situation dictates.

Most patients with rebleeding should undergo a repeat attempt at endoscopic therapy. This also serves to clarify the source of bleeding if surgery is needed. Even if cessation of bleeding is not achieved, bleeding may be temporarily slowed to achieve greater patient stability while arranging for surgery. The timing of surgery needs to be individualized and should be influenced by the requirement for transfusion, hemodynamic stability, patient's age, and comorbid illnesses.

Rebleeding does not absolutely necessitate surgery. However, rebleeding from a large posterior duodenal ulcer is more likely to require surgery because of the potential risk of penetration into the gastroduodenal artery. Emergency operations for bleeding peptic ulcers have a 10 to 20% risk of mortality.

Stress Ulcer and Gastritis

Bleeding from stress ulcers or severe gastritis occurs commonly in critically ill patients admitted to the ICU for other diagnoses. Certain conditions are associated with an increased risk of stress ulcerations and bleeding (Table 61–5). Their cause is likely multifactorial and includes hypersecretion of acid, altered mucosal defense, and drug-induced injury. Patients at high risk for the development of a stress ulcer in the ICU should be treated prophylactically (see also Chapter 10). When compared with placebo, there is less clinically important bleeding when H_2-receptor antagonists are administered (odds ratio 0.44; 95% confidence interval 0.22 to 0.88). However, patients receiving H_2-receptor antagonists may have an increased risk for nosocomial pneumonia (odds ratio 1.25; 95% confidence interval 0.78 to 2.00). This may be due to an increase in gastric bacterial colonization in the achlorhydric stomach. Patients treated prophylactically with sucralfate have rates of clinically important bleeding similar to those seen with H_2-receptor antagonist therapy (odds ratio 1.28; 95% confidence interval 0.27 to 6.11) and possibly less nosocomial pneumonia (odds ratio 0.78; 95% confidence interval 0.60 to 1.01). Despite this, patients in the ICU who receive H_2-receptor antagonists or sucralfate have similar rates of overall mortality (probably reflecting the underlying disease and severity of illness). Although less effective than therapy with H_2-receptor antagonists or sucralfate, liquid antacids may also be used for prophylaxis. They are less expensive, but they require that the dose be titrated to keep gastric pH greater than 3.5. Hemorrhagic gastritis and ulceration may still occur despite all types of prophylaxis. If upper GI bleeding develops while a patient is in the ICU, it should be managed similarly to a patient presenting de novo.

Esophageal Varices

Increased portal vein resistance, usually resulting from liver disease, results in increased flow in portosystemic venous shunts. This may induce the formation of varices in the esophagus and, less commonly, in the stomach. Rarely varices can

Table 61–5. Risk Factors for the Development of Stress
Gastritis in Patients in the Intensive Care Unit

Mechanical ventilation for ≥48 h	Trauma
Coagulopathy	Renal failure
Increased intracranial pressure (Cushing's ulcer)	Liver failure
Burns (Curling's ulcer)	Multiple organ system failure
Sepsis syndrome	

form more distally in the GI tract. Gastric fundal varices may also arise from splenic vein thrombosis (such as occurs as a rare complication of acute pancreatitis). All varices are susceptible to spontaneous rupture and can result in massive hemorrhage. Although bleeding from esophageal or gastric varices accounts for only 15% of all upper GI bleeding, it accounts for 30% of severe upper GI hemorrhage. It also carries a 15 to 40% mortality rate. On average, when compared with other causes of GI bleeding, variceal bleeding is associated with higher rebleeding rates, transfusion requirements, length of hospitalization, and mortality risk. If no portal pressure lowering procedure is performed, those who survive their first bleeding episode have a 70% risk of a second episode.

Many therapeutic modalities are available for bleeding esophageal varices. They include endoscopic, mechanical, pharmacologic, radiologic, and surgical therapies.

Endoscopy

At endoscopy, up to 50% of patients with known portal hypertension who present with upper GI bleeding are found to be bleeding from nonvariceal sources. Thus, endoscopy is critical to define the bleeding source and to direct therapy. If actively bleeding esophageal varices or signs of recent esophageal variceal hemorrhage are identified, endoscopic therapy (sclerotherapy or variceal ligation) should be carried out immediately. This therapy is successful in up to 90% of cases but has rebleeding rates of 3 to 66%, depending on technique and follow-up regimen.

Sclerotherapy is proved to help control active bleeding, to decrease the rebleeding rate, and to reduce early mortality. These benefits are independent of site of injection (intra- vs. intervariceal) and choice of sclerosant (2% sodium tetradecyl sulfate, 5% sodium morrhuate, or 5% ethanolamine oleate). Potential complications associated with sclerotherapy include esophageal ulceration, altered esophageal motility, esophageal stricture, perforation, pleural effusion, procedure-related bacteremia, and respiratory infection due to aspiration. Sclerotherapy is associated with a 10 to 30% complication rate and a 0.5 to 2% procedure-related mortality rate.

Endoscopic variceal ligation involves the application of tight rubber bands directly onto the varix to strangulate and eventually induce its sloughing. Three prospective comparative trials have demonstrated that ligation is superior to sclerotherapy. A meta-analysis indicated that when compared with sclerotherapy, ligation significantly reduced rebleeding (odds ratio 0.52) and mortality (odds ratio 0.67) with fewer side effects. Side effects related to variceal ligation primarily relate to the insertion of special overtubes to allow repeated passes of the endoscope. The use of an overtube has become unnecessary with the development of banding cylinders that can carry multiple bands at a time.

Tamponading Tubes

In patients in whom endoscopic therapy fails and who require stabilization while awaiting radiologic or surgical therapy, temporary use of a Sengstaken-Blakemore or Minnesota tube is recommended. Both tubes have gastric and esophageal balloons that can tamponade the gastroesophageal junction and, if necessary, the esophageal varices themselves. They stop the bleeding in up to 80% of patients.

However, this success is short-lived and should be viewed only as a temporizing measure to allow stabilization until more definitive treatment can be carried out. The tubes have a 10 to 30% rate of major complications, including aspiration, esophageal necrosis, and perforation and tracheal compression.

Experience with the proper use of either type of tube is essential to minimize complications. Before trying to insert a tamponading tube, the patient should undergo tracheal intubation for airway protection. Once properly positioned (preferably with the proper position confirmed radiographically), the gastric balloon is inflated and traction is applied. Tamponade of the gastroesophageal junction is often sufficient to arrest bleeding. If bleeding continues, the esophageal balloon is inflated. It is preferable to leave the balloon or balloons inflated for less than 24 hours at a time to prevent pressure necrosis to the esophageal and gastric mucosa. Although the Minnesota tube has an esophageal aspiration port, the Sengstaken-Blakemore tube does not. If the latter is going to be inserted, a nasogastric tube connected to suction should be attached proximal to its esophageal balloon before insertion.

Pharmacologic Therapy

Pharmacologic therapy plays a significant adjunctive role in the management of variceal bleeding. Arginine vasopressin infusion can reduce portal blood flow and pressure. Although it has been shown to help control hemorrhage in 52% of patients (compared with 18% with placebo), it has not been proved to reduce mortality. The usual dose is 0.4 to 0.6 units/minute. Potential side effects include cardiac, peripheral vascular, and GI ischemia. The addition of nitroglycerin (preferably given intravenously) has been shown to improve variceal hemostasis and to reduce ischemic side effects. Clinical trials have shown a nonstatistically significant trend toward improved outcome with the combination of vasopressin and nitrates when compared with placebo.

Somatostatin and its synthetic analog octreotide also reduce splanchnic blood flow and portal pressure but do not induce changes in systemic blood pressure or cardiac ischemia. Recent clinical trials have shown that octreotide significantly reduces requirements for transfusion as well as rebleeding rates and may decrease early mortality (trend not statistically significant in most trials) when used in conjunction with either sclerotherapy or ligation. In addition, octreotide alone may be as effective as sclerotherapy alone in controlling active hemorrhage. The drug is given in a continuous intravenous infusion at 25 to 50 μg/hour for 2 to 5 days, often with an initial bolus of 25 to 50 μg. Since somatostatin and octreotide do not have the side effect profile of vasopressin, they do not require the concomitant use of nitrates. However, they cost several times more than vasopressin.

Propanolol, a nonselective beta-blocker, has been proven to provide prophylaxis against variceal hemorrhage, but it has no role in the acute management of variceal bleeds.

Shunt Procedures

Patients with bleeding varices due to portal hypertension who do not respond to pharmacologic and endoscopic treatment should be considered for a shunt procedure. A transjugular intrahepatic portosystemic shunt (TIPS) functions in a manner similar to a surgically created portosystemic shunt. It can rapidly lower portal pressure and achieve immediate control of variceal bleeding. However, there is a 10% procedure-related complication rate and a 1 to 2% associated mortality rate. In addition, 10 to 30% of patients will experience a new onset or worsening of hepatic encephalopathy after TIPS. Finally, approximately 50% of TIPS stenose after 6 to 12 months, requiring revision by balloon dilation.

Variceal bleeding that cannot be successfully controlled with medical and endoscopic therapy is an accepted indication for TIPS. It can often serve as a lifesaving bridge to liver transplantation. However, TIPS placement is contraindicated in patients with elevated total bilirubin or creatinine levels or with hepatic encephalopathy refractory to medical treatment.

If TIPS is not available, patients with refractory variceal bleeding should be considered for a surgical shunt. The distal splenorenal shunt is probably the preferred surgical shunt, but ultimately the type of shunt selected depends on the severity of liver disease, presence of ascites, degree of encephalopathy, and experience of the surgeon. An alternative surgical procedure, esophageal transection, may be lifesaving when performed by an experienced surgeon in the patient in whom acute exsanguination is occurring.

Gastric and small and large bowel varices may also bleed on occasion. Such bleeding is generally less responsive to the standard therapeutic measures mentioned previously than is esophageal variceal bleeding. In addition, sclerotherapy for gastric varices has been associated with an increased complication rate. When there is significant hemorrhage from varices distal to the esophagus, early consideration should be given to a decompressive shunt procedure.

Other Causes of Upper Gastrointestinal Bleeding

There are a host of other causes of upper GI bleeding (see Table 61–1). Erosive gastritis and duodenitis are epithelial lesions that do not involve large blood vessels, yet they may still cause significant blood loss. Common causes include NSAID use, alcohol consumption, and physiologic stress. Specific therapy includes avoidance of the offending agent, acid suppression (preferably with the use of omeprazole) and general supportive measures.

Mallory-Weiss lesions are linear tears of the mucosa located at the gastroesophageal junction, usually caused by retching. Although more than 90% of bleeding from Mallory-Weiss tears stops spontaneously, persistent bleeding may be treated with endoscopic therapy.

Vascular anomalies may occur anywhere along the GI tract. Angiodysplasia, arteriovenous malformations, Dieulafoy's lesions, and gastric antral vascular ectasia are reported causes of upper GI bleeding. All are usually amenable to endoscopic therapy. Aortoenteric fistulas develop in the third part of the duodenum after abdominal aortic aneurysm repair in 0.5 to 2.4% of patients. Their management is surgical, but endoscopy is useful to rule out other causes of bleeding.

Hemobilia presents with the triad of jaundice, GI bleeding, and right upper quadrant pain in 40% of patients. The most common cause is iatrogenic, such as after liver biopsy or percutaneous transhepatic cholangiography. The diagnosis is made by endoscopy (witnessing blood emerging from the major papilla) or angiography. Angiographic or surgical treatment is recommended.

BIBLIOGRAPHY

American Society for Gastrointestinal Endoscopy Standards of Practice Committee: The role of endoscopy in the management of non-variceal acute upper gastrointestinal bleeding: Guidelines for clinical application. Gastrointest Endosc 38:760–764, 1992.
This is an evidence- and consensus-based review and guideline for the application of endoscopic therapies for acute nonvariceal upper GI bleeding.

Avgerinos A, Armonis A: Balloon tamponade and efficacy in variceal hemorrhage. Scand J Gastroenterol 207(Suppl):11–16, 1994.
This is a good review of data and experiences with esophageal balloon tamponade for the management of esophageal variceal bleeding.

Beson I, Ingrand P, Person B, et al: Sclerotherapy with or without octreotide for acute variceal bleeding. N Engl J Med 333:555–560, 1995.
This article showed the superiority of octreotide plus sclerotherapy versus sclerotherapy alone in reducing rebleeding.

Bornman PC, Theodorou NA, Shuttleworth RD, et al: The importance of hypovolemic shock and endoscopic signs in predicting recurrent hemorrhage from peptic ulceration: A prospective evaluation. BMJ 291:245, 1985.
This article identifies clinical and endoscopic features that predict patients at higher risk for rebleeding.

Cook DJ, Fuller HD, Guyatt GH, et al: Risk factors for gastrointestinal bleeding in critically ill patients. Canadian Critical Care Trials Group. N Engl J Med 330:377–382, 1994.
This study identifies independent risk factors associated with increased risk of GI bleeding in patients in the ICU.

Cook DJ, Guia HJH, Salena BJ, Laine LA: Endoscopic therapy for acute non-variceal upper gastrointestinal hemorrhage: A meta-analysis. Gastroenterology 102:138–148, 1992.
Results of pooled data comparing modalities show them to be equally effective.

Cook DJ, Guyatt G, Marshall J, et al: A comparison of sucralfate and ranitidine for the prevention of upper gastrointestinal bleeding in patients requiring mechanical ventilation. N Engl J Med 338:791–797, 1998.
Large multicenter blind, placebo-controlled trial found that critically ill patients treated with ranitidine (50 mg every 8 h) had a significantly lower rate of clinically important GI bleeding compared with those treated with sucralfate. There were, however, no significant differences in rates of ventilator-associated pneumonia, length of stay in ICU or ICU mortality.

Cook DJ, Reeve BK, Guyatt GH, et al: Stress ulcer prophylaxis in critically ill patients. Resolving discordant meta-analyses. JAMA 275:308–314, 1996.
Pooled data analysis resolves discrepancies in prior systematic reviews and demonstrates H_2-receptor antagonist therapy to be effective in decreasing the risk of bleeding from stress gastritis.

Katz PO, Salas L: Less frequent causes of upper gastrointestinal bleeding. Gastroenterol Clin North Am 22:879, 1993.
Less common sources of upper GI bleeding and their management is reviewed.

Laine L, Cook D: Endoscopic ligation compared with sclerotherapy for treatment of esophageal variceal bleeding. A meta-analysis. Ann Intern Med 123:280–287, 1995.
Variceal band ligation is equal in efficacy to sclerotherapy and is associated with fewer side effects and requires fewer sessions to achieve obliteration.

McCormick PA, Dick R, Burroughs AK: Review article: The transjugular intrahepatic portosystemic shunt (TIPS) in the treatment of portal hypertension. Aliment Pharmacol Ther 8:273–282, 1994.
This article describes the TIPS procedure and reviews its indications and applications.

Navarro VJ, Garcia-Tsa G: Variceal hemorrhage. Crit Care Clin 11:391–414, 1995.
This is a good review of the evaluation and management of variceal hemorrhage.

62 Hemolytic Anemia

Marc J. Kahn

The term *hemolysis* was first used in 1901 by William Hunter in his treatise, *Pernicious Aenemia,* when he described that certain anemias could come not only from decreased production of red blood cells but also from their destruction. This chapter focuses on the variety of mechanisms and causes that destroy red blood cells.

CLINICAL CLUES TO HEMOLYSIS

It is important to identify the clinical clues that indicate red blood cell destruction is taking place. Simply speaking, *hemolysis* can be defined as a decrease in the number of circulating erythrocytes without evidence of frank blood loss. In general, this should be accompanied by evidence that bone marrow is compensating for this reduction in erythrocytes. The most obvious example of a marrow response, an elevation in the reticulocyte count, should generally be observed whenever hemolysis is occurring. Other laboratory findings consistent with a diagnosis of hemolysis are elevations in unconjugated bilirubin and lactate dehydrogenase levels, hemoglobinemia, hemoglobinuria, and a reduction in the serum haptoglobin concentration. These results are consistent with, but not diagnostic of, the presence of hemolysis because these tests have low sensitivity and specificity. As with other hematologic disorders, review of the peripheral blood smear is essential for the correct diagnosis of a hemolytic anemia; certain peripheral smear findings can indicate specific pathophysiologic processes (Fig. 62–1).

The hemolytic anemias can be divided into two major groups: those that are inherited and those that are acquired (Table 62–1).

INHERITED HEMOLYTIC ANEMIAS

Inherited hemolytic anemias, which may be contributing factors in illnesses leading to stays in the ICU, will be mentioned only briefly because they seldom are the sole or primary cause for admission to an ICU. The inherited hemolytic anemias can be related to disorders of the erythrocyte membrane, enzymes, globin chain production, and globin chain structure.

Red Blood Cell Membrane Disorders

Disorders of the erythrocyte membrane are thought to cause hemolysis by shortened red blood cell survival and splenic destruction. These disorders include hereditary spherocytosis, hereditary elliptocytosis, hereditary pyropoikilocytosis, and hereditary stomatocytosis. These disorders are due to mutations in erythrocyte membrane support proteins such as ankyrin, spectrin, protein 4.1, and others. They

705

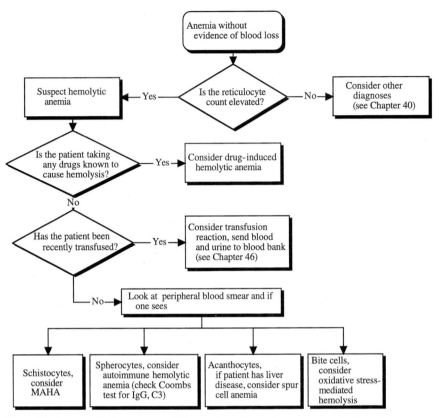

Figure 62–1. Schematic flow diagram of diagnostic work-up of suspected acquired hemolytic anemia. MAHA, microangiopathic hemolytic anemia.

are characterized by lifelong red blood cell destruction and varied levels of anemia. Some of these disorders are associated with splenic dysfunction and they may predispose patients to bacteremias (as asplenia does).

Red Blood Cell Enzyme Disorders

Disorders of erythrocyte enzymes can lead to hemolytic episodes. Such enzyme defects include deficiencies of pyruvate kinase (also called *nonspherocytic hemolytic anemia*), which usually presents in children with unexplained anemia. One enzyme defect that has clinical importance in adults is glucose-6-phosphate dehydrogenase deficiency (G6PD). G6PD is an enzyme that generates nicotinamide-adenine dinucleotide phosphate, which, in turn, is used by erythrocytes and other cells as an antioxidant.

G6PD deficiency has its highest prevalence among Kurdish Jews, with an estimated prevalence of more than 60%. As the gene coding for G6PD is on the X chromosome, affected individuals tend to be males. These individuals, as a rule,

Table 62–1. Differential Diagnosis of Hemolytic Anemia

Inherited Hemolytic Anemias

Membrane defects (spherocytosis, elliptocytosis, pyropoikilocytosis, stomatocytosis)
Enzyme defects (Embden-Meyerhof pathway defects, hexose monophosphate shunt defects,
  nucleotide enzyme defects)
Thalassemias
Hemoglobinopathies

Acquired Hemolytic Anemias

Immune hemolysis
  Autoimmune
    Paroxysmal cold hemoglobinuria
    Warm antibody hemolytic anemia
    Cold agglutinin disease
  Alloimmune
  Drug-induced
Microangiopathic hemolytic anemia (MAHA)
Infection-related hemolysis
Spur cell anemia

do not have significant hemolysis unless subjected to oxidant stress, which is usually caused by drugs or fever. Others can have variations in the protein composition of the enzyme itself via point mutations in the encoding gene and also be subject to episodic hemolysis. Such is the case for African Americans with G6PD deficiency. This leads to varying sensitivities to certain drugs or foods. Although the typical drugs that cause hemolysis in patients with G6PD deficiency include primaquine, doxorubicin, and phenazopyridine, many more medications should be avoided in persons deficient in G6PD (Table 62–2).

Diagnosis is made by review of the peripheral smear that may show red blood cell fragmentation or Heinz bodies (inclusions of denatured hemoglobin seen in smears stained with methylene blue). Laboratory analysis of G6PD levels and phenotype should be performed at times other than during or immediately after hemolytic episodes because the cells that remain after a hemolytic episode tend to be those with higher levels of G6PD. Proper treatment of this disorder is avoidance of exposure to these compounds. Once hemolysis occurs, it tends to be self-limited and the care remains supportive.

Table 62–2. Medications to be Avoided in Persons with
         Glucose-6-Phosphate Dehydrogenase Deficiency

Acetanilid	Nitrofurantoin	Sulfamethoxazole
Dapsone	Phenazopyridine	Sulfanilamide
Methylene blue	Primaquine	Sulfapyridine
Nalidixic acid	Sulfacetamide	Toluidine Blue
Niridazole		

Globin Chain Production and Structure Disorders

Disorders of globin chain production and structure include the thalassemias and hemoglobinopathies, such as hemoglobin S and hemoglobin C. These mutations cause unstable hemoglobins, which shorten red blood cell survival. These conditions can exacerbate or cause other medical conditions but rarely prompt ICU stays by themselves.

ACQUIRED HEMOLYTIC ANEMIAS

Acquired hemolytic anemias can be severe and, by themselves, result in the patient's ICU admission (Table 62–3).

Autoimmune Hemolytic Anemias

Autoimmune hemolytic anemias (AHAs) result from the destruction of red blood cells when antibodies recognize antigens on their surfaces. There are three types of autoimmune hemolytic anemias: (1) paroxysmal cold hemoglobinuria, (2) warm antibody autoimmune hemolytic anemia, and (3) cold agglutinin disease.

Paroxysmal Cold Hemoglobinuria

Paroxysmal cold hemoglobinuria is exceedingly rare and is characterized by both recurrent episodes of massive hemolysis after exposure to cold and the presence of the Donath-Landsteiner antibody (an antibody to the P antigen on red blood cells). This IgG antibody binds to the erythrocyte in the cold and causes complement-mediated hemolysis on warming. It is classically associated with congenital or tertiary syphilis. Therapy has been supportive, with complete remission on treatment of the infection. With the advent of effective therapy for syphilis in modern times, paroxysmal cold hemoglobinuria is more often seen in children after a viral infection. It is usually a single episode without recurrences. Clinical

Table 62–3. Treatment of Acquired Hemolytic Anemias

Disorder	Treatment
Paroxysmal cold hemoglobinuria	Usually self-limited; can treat underlying disease
Warm antibody	Prednisone; may also need danazol, IgG, or splenectomy
Cold agglutinin disease	Keep patient warm; prednisone not helpful
Drug-induced	Remove offending agent
Acute hemolytic reaction	Immediately stop transfusion; support blood pressure, control bleeding, and maintain urine output
Microangiopathic hemolytic anemia	Treat underlying condition; avoid giving platelets
Infectious causes	Treat underlying infection
Spur cell anemia	Supportive care

features include aching pains in the back and legs, abdominal pain, fevers, and chills followed by hemoglobinuria and occasional jaundice. This condition is usually self-limited and does not require specific therapy.

Warm Antibody Autoimmune Hemolytic Anemia

Common autoimmune hemolytic anemias are divided into warm antibody–induced hemolytic anemia and cold antibody–induced hemolytic anemia (also called *cold agglutinin disease*). The temperature classification is derived from the temperature at which red blood cell destruction occurs—37° C in the case of warm hemolytic anemia and temperatures less than normal body temperature in the case of cold agglutinin disease.

Warm antibody–induced hemolytic anemia occurs when antibodies of the IgG class bind to Rh-type or other antigens on the erythrocyte surface at body temperature. Hemolysis is usually the result of splenic destruction of erythrocytes. Macrophages, in the Billroth cords of the spleen, recognize the Fc portion of the antibody bound to the erythrocyte via their Fc receptors. Antibody-coated cells may also be recognized by the Kupffer cells in the liver, but this is less common. On recognition and binding by macrophages, partial phagocytosis results in the red blood cells becoming spherical. They are subsequently ingested by these cells. Complement-mediated erythrocyte destruction is rare in warm antibody-induced hemolytic anemia.

Warm hemolytic anemia can be primary, that is, occurring without underlying disease, or secondary, such as that due to lymphoproliferative disorders (typically chronic lymphocytic leukemia or lymphoma). This condition is also associated with connective tissue disorders, such as systemic lupus erythematosus, other neoplasms, such as ovarian carcinoma, chronic inflammatory diseases, such as ulcerative colitis, and ingestion of drugs, such as alpha-methyldopa.

The presenting complaints of individuals with warm antibody autoimmune hemolytic anemia (AHA) are usually secondary to anemia, that is, decreased exercise tolerance, shortness of breath, or rarely exacerbation of angina. Occasionally, patients present with jaundice, fever, or hepatosplenomegaly.

Review of the peripheral smear is essential in making a diagnosis of warm antibody AHA. Because of partial ingestion of erythrocytes by splenic macrophages, the cells assume a spherocytic shape to maximize their volume for a given surface area. Spherocytes on the peripheral smear are therefore the hallmark of warm antibody AHA. The peripheral smear may also show polychromasia and an elevated reticulocyte count. Diagnosis of warm antibody AHA also requires a positive direct Coombs test to demonstrate the presence of immunoglobulin or complement, or both, on the surface of the patient's erythrocytes. These patients also may have free antibody in their plasma, which would also result in a positive indirect Coombs' test finding.

Transfusing patients with warm antibody AHA is problematic for two reasons. First, it is often difficult to crossmatch these individuals because of the presence of a panreactive antibody in their plasma. Second, the transfused cells have a short half-life because of the hemolytic process. Therefore, transfusion should be avoided in all but the most serious conditions in which immediate increase in the oxygen carrying capacity of the blood is needed. Even then, the least incompatible blood should be transfused slowly and care taken to follow the hematocrit because the transfused blood is not likely to sustain the hematocrit for long.

Treatment of warm antibody AHA involves preventing macrophage recognition and destruction of the antibody-coated cells. The traditional treatment is glucocorticoid administration. These agents appear to work by decreasing macrophage recognition of antibody-coated cells as well as decreasing production of the autoantibody. Patients are treated with oral prednisone at a dose of 60 to 100 mg daily. Alternatively, the equivalent daily dose of intravenous methylprednisolone may be used. High-dose glucocorticoid therapy is continued for 10 to 14 days at which point the prednisone is tapered to a dose of 30 mg daily. Prednisone is then slowly tapered over several months. Approximately two thirds of patients with warm antibody AHA respond to prednisone and 20% have a complete remission.

Other therapeutic modalities include splenectomy, which removes the site of erythrocyte destruction. However, splenectomy is effective in only about two thirds of patients. Alternatively, immunosuppressive agents, such as cyclophosphamide or azathioprine, the nonvirilizing androgen danazol, intravenous immunoglobulin G (IgG), and the purine analog 2-chlorodeoxyadenosine have been used with varied success. The overall prognosis for warm antibody AHA is variable, with frequent relapses common.

Cold Agglutinin Disease

Cold agglutinin disease is characterized by the presence of monoclonal antibodies of the IgM class that react with erythrocytes at temperatures less than body temperature, usually between 28 and 31° C. The target antigen on the erythrocyte is usually an oligosaccharide of the I/i system which is a precursor to the ABH and Lewis blood group antigens. As IgM can readily fix complement, a patient's red blood cells become coated with complement. This results in cell injury by direct lysis and hepatic macrophage and splenic macrophage opsinization. Usually, the progression of the complement cascade is halted at the formation of C3b because of protective proteins on the red blood cell surface.

Cold agglutinin disease may be a primary disorder but is more often associated with infections, such as *Mycoplasma* pneumonia or mononucleosis, or with pre-existing B-cell neoplasms.

The clinical presentation of patients with cold agglutinin disease is usually a chronic hemolytic anemia without jaundice. The peripheral smear may show spherocytosis that is much less pronounced than in the case of warm antibody AHA. In addition, autoagglutination may be seen on the peripheral smear, particularly if the blood is cooled. This disorder can be confirmed by the presence of complement (C3b) on the red blood cell surface. Because IgM readily dissociates from the erythrocyte, it usually is not detected on the cell surface.

The treatment of patients with cold agglutinin disease is supportive. Patients must be kept warm, particularly their extremities. Glucocorticoids, danazol, immunoglobulin, and splenectomy are, as a rule, not beneficial. In severe anemia, red blood cell transfusions can be given but must be warmed before use. Likewise, intravenous fluids must be warmed before infusion to prevent antibody from attaching to erythrocyte membranes. Although the primary form of the disease is usually chronic with a benign course, the postinfectious forms are generally self-limited.

DRUG-INDUCED HEMOLYTIC ANEMIA

Since the first description of drug-induced hemolytic anemia by Sedormid in 1949, the list of drugs associated with hemolytic anemia has grown steadily. They can cause hemolytic anemia by several well-described mechanisms. The first mechanism is via a hapten process. *Penicillin* is the prototype of this process. Penicillin, when given in high doses, can become bound to the red blood cell membrane. IgG antibodies are then produced to this complex, causing red blood cell destruction by splenic macrophages. In the case of *quinidine*, red blood cells are destroyed when drug-antidrug complexes become bound to the red blood cell membrane. This has also been called an *innocent bystander reaction. Alpha-methyldopa* is able to induce the formation of antibodies, usually IgG, against red blood cell antigens.

The clinical presentation of drug-induced hemolytic anemia is similar to autoimmune hemolytic anemias. Hemolysis tends to be mild, and the only treatment needed in most circumstances is discontinuation of the offending drug.

ACUTE HEMOLYTIC TRANSFUSION REACTIONS

The major source of mortality from blood transfusion involves the transfusion of allogeneic incompatible blood (see also Chapter 46). The overwhelming majority of these mishaps are due to clerical error in which properly crossmatched blood is given to the wrong patient. After the infusion of alloincompatible blood, the patient usually experiences fever, low back pain, chest pain, hypotension, nausea, and vomiting. Shock may soon follow and lead to multiorgan failure; hemoglobinuria can also contribute to the development of acute renal failure. A consumptive coagulopathy develops in up to one third of patients.

The hemolytic process is due to intravascular destruction with complement as well as to hepatic and splenic clearance of the incompatible erythrocytes. Laboratory findings include the presence of hemoglobinemia (which can be detected at the bedside by pink staining of the patient's plasma when held up to a light) and hemoglobinuria. Demonstration that the blood recipient's plasma agglutinates the transfused red blood cells is also evidence for a major transfusion reaction.

The management of such individuals is the immediate cessation of the transfused blood product. That product as well as samples of patient's blood and urine should be sent to the transfusion service (blood bank) for analysis. Bleeding is a major complication of an acute hemolytic reaction and is usually caused by a consumptive coagulopathy. Some authors suggest that heparin may be helpful in this instance. When used, heparin is usually given at several hundred units an hour at a constant infusion without a bolus. It is also important to maintain the fibrinogen level at greater than 100 mg/dL in patients with acute hemolytic reactions. This is best accomplished with cryoprecipitate. To protect the kidneys from the toxic insult, the systolic blood pressure should be maintained at greater than 100 mm Hg by the use of fluids, blood products, and vasopressors, if necessary. Although the use of mannitol is controversial, maintaining a urine output of at least 100 mL/hour for the first 24 hours is important to preserve renal function. This can be carried out by giving loop diuretics (e.g., furosemide) or mannitol and intravenous hydration.

MICROANGIOPATHIC HEMOLYTIC ANEMIA

Microangiopathic hemolytic anemia (MAHA) occurs when circulating erythrocytes are sheared by fibrin strands deposited in the microcirculation. This results in fragmentation of red blood cells. As fibrin is usually deposited by thrombotic processes, patients with MAHA are frequently thrombocytopenic. MAHA is felt to be primary in the case of thrombotic thrombocytopenic purpura (TTP) and hemolytic uremic syndrome. In these conditions (see Chapter 63), MAHA is accompanied by fever and microthrombosis of small vessels in the kidney or central nervous system, or both. Other conditions that predispose to MAHA include malignant hypertension, eclampsia, organ rejection, cancer, collagen vascular disorders, congenital arteriovenous malformations, and drugs such as cyclosporine A and mitomycin C.

The clinical features of MAHA relate to the underlying disease causing the process. Common findings include anemia, thrombocytopenia, renal dysfunction, fever, and central nervous system abnormalities. The peripheral smear is diagnostic of this condition. Classic features include the presence of fragmented red blood cells (schistocytes), decreased platelets, and nucleated red blood cells. High levels of lactate dehydrogenase occur and can be used to follow the course of the disease.

Treatment of MAHA is usually directed toward treating the underlying disorder. In the case of TTP or hemolytic uremic syndrome, plasmapheresis has greatly altered the natural history, causing resolution in more than 80% of patients. Plasmapheresis should be prompt, immediately following diagnosis. Although red blood cells can be used to treat the underlying anemia in cases of MAHA, they should be washed to prevent the accidental infusion of platelets or platelet particles. Platelet transfusions should be avoided in the case of TTP because their use may cause sudden death; this is likely due to acute microthrombosis in vital organs.

OTHER HEMOLYTIC CONDITIONS

A variety of infectious organisms can cause hemolytic episodes through a variety of mechanisms. First, organisms can invade the erythrocyte directly, as is the case with *malaria, babesiosis,* and *bartonellosis.* Alternatively, the organism can elaborate a hemolytic toxin such as *Clostridium perfringens.* In both circumstances, treatment is supportive, with therapy directed against the infecting organism.

Patients with advanced liver disease caused by alcohol and cirrhosis can rarely acquire a rapidly progressive hemolytic anemia characterized by acanthocytes (spur cells) on the peripheral smear. This condition is usually accompanied by jaundice and splenomegaly. It is usually progressive, with death occurring in weeks to months.

BIBLIOGRAPHY

Berkowitz FE: Hemolysis and infection: Categories and mechanisms of their interrelationship. Rev Infect Dis 13:1151–1162, 1991.
This article presents a thorough review of the subject. It includes a discussion of drug-induced hemolysis.

Beutler E: Glucose-6-phosphate dehydrogenase deficiency. N Engl J Med 324:169–174, 1991.
This article presents a classic description of this disorder with emphasis on molecular pathophysiology. It is easy to read and well referenced.

Castro O, Branbilla DJ, Thorington B, et al: The acute chest syndrome in sickle cell disease: Incidence and risk factors. Blood 84:643–649, 1994.
This prospective cohort study of over 3700 patients with sickle cell disease reviews the incidence, risk factors, and mortality of acute chest syndrome in this population.

Centers for Disease Control and Prevention. Hemolysis associated with 25% human albumin diluted with sterile water—United States, 1994-1998. MMWR Morb Mortal Wkly Rep 48:157–159, 1999.
This describes 10 cases of this unusual form of acute hemolysis due to administration of a hypotonic solution.

Palek J, Lux SE: Red cell membranes skeletodefects in hereditary and acquired hemolytic anemias. Semin Hematol 20:189–224, 1983.
This is a nice review of structural defects in erythrocytes that lead to hemolysis.

Rosse WF: Autoimmune hemolytic anemia. Hosp Pract 20:105–119, 1985.
This is an older reference, but it is still elegant in its simplicity. It was written by an accomplished author in the field.

Vichinsky EP, Neumayr LD, Earles AN, et al: Causes and outcomes of the acute chest syndrome in sickle cell disease. N Engl J Med 342:1855–1865, 2000.
This large, multicenter study of 671 episodes of acute chest syndrome found that it is commonly precipitated by fat embolism and infection, especially community acquired pneumonia. The overall mortality was 3%.

63

Idiopathic and Thrombotic Thrombocytopenias

David G. Morrison
Marc J. Kahn

Moderate to severe thrombocytopenia is a major feature of several disorders that often lead to admission to the intensive care unit (ICU). Immune (idiopathic) thrombocytopenic purpura (ITP) and thrombotic thrombocytopenic purpura (TTP) are two such conditions. Early and accurate diagnosis and rapid application of appropriate therapy are keys to the successful management of patients with these disorders. Accurate diagnosis requires differentiating the thrombocytopenia of ITP and TTP from each other as well as from other thrombocytopenic conditions. The diagnostic work-up should begin with a carefully focused history and physical examination, followed by an examination of the peripheral blood smear (Fig. 63–1). Blood products should *not* be given to a nonbleeding patient with thrombo-

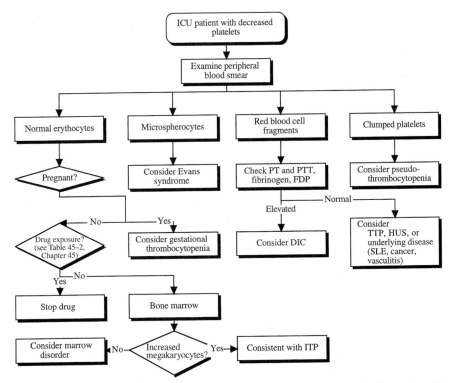

Figure 63–1. Schematic diagram to evaluate ICU patient with thrombocytopenia. PT, prothrombin time; PTT, partial thromboplastin time; FDP, fibrin degradation products; DIC, disseminated intravascular coagulation; TTP, thrombocytic thrombocytopenic purpura; HUS, hemolytic uremic syndrome; SLE, systemic lupus erythematosus; ITP, idiopathic thrombocytopenic purpura.

Table 63–1. Safeguards for Patients in the Intensive Care Unit
With Thrombocytopenia From Any Cause

No antiplatelet drugs that interfere with platelet function (aspirin, NSAIDs, high doses of penicillin, or semisynthetic penicillins)
No intramuscular injections
All blood draws need direct pressure and pressure dressings
After removing central venous catheters or arterial lines, one must exert direct pressure over the site for a minimum of 10 min followed by a pressure dressing
Flush lines with normal saline and avoid heparin unless absolutely necessary
Avoid indwelling bladder catheters, rectal tubes, nasotracheal and nasogastric tubes
Evaluate for other coagulopathies and obtain hematologic consultation if the need for anticoagulation is anticipated

NSAIDs, nonsteroidal anti-inflammatory drugs.

cytopenia until the smear is inspected, particularly to rule out the presence of TTP. Moreover, during the initial evaluation, patients should be safeguarded from iatrogenic bleeding complications due to a low platelet count (Table 63–1).

IMMUNE THROMBOCYTOPENIC PURPURA

Mechanism and Diagnosis

Autoantibodies directed against the patient's platelets cause ITP. These antibodies are usually directed against the platelet glycoproteins Ib/IX or IIb/IIIa, and their binding results in platelets being destroyed in the spleen. Destruction occurs by splenic macrophage Fc-receptor recognition of antibody-coated platelets. Patients with ITP usually have mucosal bleeding, severe anemia, or incidental thrombocytopenia on routine blood counts. Fortunately, severe bleeding such as intracranial hemorrhage is rare in ITP.

ITP is characterized by a decrease in the number of platelets seen in the peripheral smear. Occasionally, large platelets can be found. Erythrocytes and leukocytes should appear normal. Bone marrow examination may show an increased number of megakaryocytes, indicating an appropriate response to the increased platelet destruction. Platelet antibody testing is usually unhelpful because of low sensitivity and specificity.

ITP remains a diagnosis of exclusion after other causes of thrombocytopenia are ruled out. Table 63–2 lists the differential diagnoses of thrombocytopenia without microangiopathy. Evan's syndrome is also an antibody-mediated disease, with antibodies directed against both platelets and erythrocytes. The destruction of erythrocytes occurs with the same mechanism as does the destruction of platelets.

ITP has been associated with other conditions in up to 20% of cases. In this setting, it is often called secondary ITP. Causes of secondary ITP include collagen vascular diseases, lymphoproliferative disorders, infections, and other autoimmune syndromes. Thrombocytopenia is also a common manifestation of human immunodeficiency virus (HIV) disease, presumably caused by increased platelet destruction on an immune basis. The clinical features of HIV-associated ITP are similar to

Table 63–2. Differential Diagnosis of Thrombocytopenia Without Microangiopathy*

ITP	Alcohol
Evan's syndrome	Drug-induced thrombocytopenia
Incidental gestational thrombocytopenia	Systemic lupus erythematosus
Bone marrow failure	

* Microangiopathy denotes the presence of schistocytes (fragmented red blood cells) on peripheral smear. ITP, immune thrombocytopenic purpura.

those of idiopathic ITP. However, ITP associated with HIV infection in patients with hemophilia is of particular concern because these patients are at much higher risk for catastrophic bleeding than are patients with primary ITP.

Treatment

Treatment of ITP depends on the platelet count and clinical presentation. Spontaneous bleeding in ITP is rare with platelet counts greater than 50,000/μL. This number of platelets is also sufficient for most surgical procedures. Although rare, spontaneous bleeding has been reported in ITP patients with platelet counts in the 30 to 50,000/μL range. Since as many as 5% of adults and 40% of children with ITP have spontaneous remissions, it is safe to observe patients with ITP and platelet counts greater than 30,000/μL if they are not actively bleeding.

Actively bleeding patients with ITP require urgent management. Platelet transfusions are usually ineffective because of shortened platelet survival despite platelet counts increasing transiently in some patients. Pretreatment with intravenous immunoglobulin (IVIG) at a dose of 0.4 to 1.0 g/kg may increase the life span of the transfused platelets and cause an increase in the platelet count several days later by modulating the immune response. This therapeutic modality is expensive, costing between $5000 and $10,000 per treatment course. Antifibrinolytic agents such as epsilon-aminocaproic acid can effectively reduce hemorrhage, but the use of these agents is complicated by an increased incidence of thrombosis.

Glucocorticoids have become the mainstay of treatment for ITP that is symptomatic or when the platelet count falls to less than 30,000/μL. The typical daily dose of prednisone is 1 mg/kg. This inexpensive treatment elevates platelet counts in about two thirds of treated patients. Most patients exhibit a decline in platelet count when the prednisone dose is tapered and therefore require additional therapy. Splenectomy can produce sustained increases in platelet counts in more than two thirds of patients with ITP. Pneumococcal vaccine should be given 2 weeks before splenectomy to reduce the severity of complications due to postsplenectomy pneumococcal bacteremias. Some patients have a relapse of ITP months or even years after splenectomy. This is attributable to the presence of an accessory spleen. Such spleens occurs in up to 20% of patients and are easily detected by radionuclide scanning. After the removal of accessory spleens, ITP resolves in many such patients.

ITP may become refractory to conventional therapy in some patients. Modalities of therapy for refractory ITP include the use of immunosuppressive agents, such as azathioprine, cyclophosphamide, or vinca alkaloids. Alternatively, danazol, an androgenic steroid, can be useful for sustaining partial remissions or a decrease the glucocorticoid dose. Small case series report that combination chemotherapy and high-dose dexamethasone is efficacious in the management of chronic refractory ITP. Lastly, immunoadsorption of plasma through a staphylococcal protein A column has been used successfully in small numbers of patients with refractory ITP.

IMMUNE THROMBOCYTOPENIC PURPURA IN PATIENTS WITH HUMAN IMMUNODEFICIENCY VIRUS OR IN PREGNANCY

Pregnancy and HIV infection are two special circumstances associated with ITP. Although HIV-positive patients are clinically similar to other patients with ITP, they manifest dramatic elevations in platelet counts when they receive zidovudine therapy. Presumably, the antiretroviral agents inhibit virally mediated ITP.

Pregnancy can lead to thrombocytopenia from a variety of causes, including thrombocytopenia of pregnancy, ITP, and preeclampsia and eclampsia. The management of ITP early in pregnancy is similar to the management of ITP in nonpregnant patients except that splenectomy is contraindicated. The critical management decision in ITP during pregnancy focuses on delivery of the fetus. Although rare, infants born to women with ITP may be thrombocytopenic. As a precaution, many obstetricians recommend prednisone therapy for the mother beginning several weeks before delivery. Fetal scalp vein platelet count determinations have been suggested as one means to assess the fetal platelet count. Because thrombocytopenia is rare in the infant and because cesarean section poses a risk to the thrombocytopenic mother, some authors conclude that conventional delivery should be undertaken with immediate and frequent monitoring of the newborn's platelet count.

THROMBOTIC THROMBOCYTOPENIC PURPURA AND RELATED DISORDERS

Mechanism and Diagnosis

TTP, hemolytic uremic syndrome (HUS), and HELLP (microangiopathic *h*emolysis, *e*levated *l*iver function tests, *l*ow *p*latelet *c*ounts) syndrome represent a clinical spectrum of the same pathogenic event occurring in different patient subgroups. The primary event is likely a disorder of the interaction of high molecular weight von Willebrand's factor and blood vessel walls, which produces activation of circulating platelets. Regardless of its exact mechanism, the primary aberration is a thrombotic microangiopathy. Table 63–3 lists the differential diagnosis for thrombocytopenia with microangiopathy.

Patients with TTP typically present with the relatively abrupt onset of several or all of the following *classic pentad* of cardinal signs and symptoms: (1) fever, (2) mucosal bleeding due to thrombocytopenia, (3) altered central nervous system

Table 63–3. Differential Diagnosis of Thrombocytopenia With Microangiopathy

TTP (thrombotic thrombocytopenic purpura)	Septic abortion
HUS (hemolytic uremic syndrome)	Systemic vasculitis
Disseminated intravascular coagulation	Carcinoma
HELLP (hemolytic anemia, elevated liver function tests, low platelet counts)	Solid organ rejection
Malignant hypertension	Mitomycin C, cisplatin, cyclosporine A
Preeclampsia, eclampsia	Cholesterol emboli syndrome

function (which may manifest itself only as a headache), (4) renal dysfunction or hematuria, and (5) hemolytic anemia due to a microangiopathic process (this is also called *microangiopathic hemolytic anemia* [MAHA]). The diagnosis of TTP does not require all five findings, but all patients diagnosed with TTP must manifest microangiopathy. This condition occurs when erythrocytes are fragmented by strands of fibrin deposited in the microvasculature. HUS is similar to TTP, but neurologic dysfunction is absent or mild, whereas renal dysfunction is more pronounced. HELLP syndrome occurs in pregnant or peripartum patients and is probably part of the spectrum of preeclampsia. TTP and related disorders are true emergencies and must be managed as such.

Definitive diagnosis is made by inspection of the peripheral blood smear. Patients with TTP and related disorders have schistocytes (fragmented blood cells) on their smears. In addition, the platelet count is markedly diminished, and nucleated red blood cells can also be found. The reticulocyte count is usually elevated unless the bone marrow has been infarcted. Lactate dehydrogenase (LDH) levels are elevated because of intravascular destruction of red blood cells, with release of their stores of intracellular LDH. As such, serial LDH levels are useful markers of disease activity.

Treatment

Platelet transfusions must **not** be given to patients with TTP. They should be avoided for all but life-threatening bleeding. The problem with platelet transfusions is that they have been associated with sudden death due to microthrombosis in vital organs, such as the heart and brain. Primary therapy of TTP remains plasma exchange via apheresis therapy. Initially, patients should have a daily exchange of 1 to 2 plasma volumes. Removed plasma is usually replaced with fresh frozen plasma. This avoids the coagulopathy resulting from removal of clotting factors by the apheresis therapy. However, replacement with plasma deficient in high molecular weight von Willebrand multimers (cryosupernatant) may produce higher response rates. The optimal number and total duration of plasma exchanges for the treatment of TTP remain unclear. Plasma exchange usually continues daily until the patient improves clinically and the platelet count improves. When the platelet count and LDH levels normalize, the plasma exchange is gradually tapered. Each plasma exchange costs about $1000, and the overall response rate is about 80%.

Glucocorticoids are administered to all patients with TTP at a dose equivalent to prednisone of 1 mg/kg per day. Although randomized trials have not established the true benefit of daily steroid administration, the response rate of TTP to prednisone alone is about 10%, and there may a potential additive effect with plasma exchange therapy. The adjunctive use of antiplatelet agents such as aspirin, dipyridamole, or sulfinpyrazone should be avoided because they may increase the risk of bleeding.

Before establishment of plasma exchange as the primary treatment modality for TTP, splenectomy and glucocorticoid administraton were often used as combination therapy. Despite increased complications from thrombocytopenia, experienced surgeons can usually perform splenectomies in patients with TTP safely, with a response rate as high as 50%. Early splenectomy is associated with a better response rate than splenectomy that is performed late in the course of TTP, but this difference may only reflect selection bias.

Other agents, including vincristine (2 mg weekly), azathioprine, cyclophosphamide, and IVIG have been used anecdotally in the treatment of TTP with varied success. Most patients with TTP survive, but the mortality rate is still significant at about 20%. Relapses commonly occur in survivors. These are treated similarly to initial bouts of TTP.

Associated Disorders

HUS is more prevalent than TTP in young children. In many cases, HUS is preceded by bloody diarrhea from verotoxin-producing bacteria such as *Escherichia coli* 0157:H7 or *Shigella dysenteriae* 1. Patients with HUS become anuric and may have seizures. Most patients recover with supportive measures only, although plasma exchange has also been used with apparent success.

Other conditions such as cancer have been associated with TTP-like illnesses. The malignancy is usually widely metastatic, and treatment of the underlying malignancy usually results in resolution of TTP. Chemotherapeutic drugs, such as mitomycin C or, less commonly, cisplatin, have also been associated with TTP. Staphylococcal protein A column apheresis has led to resolution in some patients with chemotherapy-induced TTP.

Diverse drugs such as cyclosporine A, FK506 (tacrolimus [Prograf]), quinine, cocaine, and ticlopidine (Ticlid) have been associated with TTP. Treatment consists of removal of the offending drug and consideration of plasma exchange.

SUMMARY

A careful history and physical examination and the review of the peripheral blood smear will usually allow the diagnosis of ITP or TTP. However, most patients with thrombocytopenia in the ICU will have low platelet counts due to other causes, such as sepsis, liver disease with hypersplenism, heparin or other drugs, and disseminated intravascular coagulation (see Chapter 45). A high index of suspicion and hematologic consultation will permit the ICU clinician to differentiate these more common causes of thrombocytopenia from the less common disorders of ITP and TTP, leading to their successful diagnosis and treatment.

BIBLIOGRAPHY

Bennett CL, Connors JM, Carwile JM, et al: Thrombotic thrombocytopenic purpura associated with clopidogrel. N Engl J Med 342:1773–1777, 2000.
This is the first reported case series of 11 patients who developed TTP during or soon after treatment with clopidogrel, which at the time had largely replaced ticlopidine in clinical practice because of the latter's association with TTP and other adverse effects.

Berchtold P, McMillan R: Therapy of chronic idiopathic thrombocytopenic purpura in adults. Blood 74:2309–2317, 1989.
This article presents a thorough review of the therapeutic modalities available for the treatment of chronic ITP.

Burrows RF, Kelton JG: Thrombocytopenia at delivery: A prospective survey of 6715 deliveries. Am J Obstet Gynecol 162:731–734, 1990.
This article distinguishes between gestational thrombocytopenia and ITP. Gestational thrombocytopenia is not associated with excess fetal complications.

Crowther MA, Heddle N, Hayward CPM, et al: Splenectomy done during hematologic remission to prevent relapse in patients with thrombotic thrombocytopenic purpura. Ann Intern Med 125:294–296, 1996.
This article presents a case series providing evidence for splenectomy in preventing the relapse of TTP.

Jacobs P, Wood L, Novitzky N: Intravenous gammaglobulin has no advantages over oral corticosteroids as primary therapy for adults with immune thrombocytopenia: A prospective randomized trial. Am J Med 97:55–59, 1994.
This is a small but important study. IVIG is clearly effective for ITP, but only as a component of a more comprehensive treatment algorithm. Steroid therapy may require 7 to 10 days for full efficacy before resorting to expensive IVIG therapy. However, IVIG should be administered before splenectomy.

Law C, Marcaccio M, Tam P, et al: High-dose intravenous immune globulin and the response to splenectomy inpatients with idiopathic thrombocytopenic purpura. N Engl J Med 336:1494–1498, 1997.
Retrospective cohort study showing that a favorable response to IVIG correlated with a good to excellent response to splenectomy; likewise, a poor response to IVIG portended a poor response to splenectomy.

Moschowitz E: An acute pleiochromic anemia with hyaline thrombosis of the terminal arterioles and capillaries: An undescribed disease. Arch Intern Med 36:89–93, 1925.
This initial clinical description still forms the basis for the diagnostic criteria for TTP and hence the "pentad of Moschowitz."

Rock GA, Shumack KH, Buskard NA, et al: Comparison of plasma exchange with plasma infusion in the treatment of thrombotic thrombocytopenic purpura. Canadian Apheresis Group. N Engl J Med 325:393–397, 1991.
Although both are efficacious, plasma exchange is more effective than plasma infusion in the initial treatment of TTP.

Wong CS, Jelacic S, Habeeb RL, et al: The risk of the hemolytic uremic syndrome after antibiotic treatment of *Escherichia coli* O157:H7 infections. N Engl J Med 342:1930–1936, 2000.
This prospective cohort study found that antibiotic treatment of children with E. coli O157:H7 infection actually increased the risk of the hemolytic uremic syndrome.

64

Acute Central Nervous System Infections

Stephen Gluckman

Acute infections of the central nervous system (CNS) are generally categorized as meningitis or encephalitis. Although it may be difficult to differentiate between them at presentation, the difference in their diagnostic considerations and therapeutic approaches is important. *Encephalitis* refers primarily to a brain parenchymal infection characterized by a clinical presentation of cerebral dysfunction, for example, obtundation, confusion, or focal abnormalities, or a combination of these conditions. Encephalitis is most commonly caused by viruses. In *meningitis*, initial abnormalities usually include fever, headache, and meningeal signs. If cerebral dysfunction does occur with meningitis, it is the secondary result of cerebral edema, increased intracerebral pressure, or alterations in cerebral blood flow, or a combination of these factors. Although most cases of meningitis are due to viruses or bacteria, some may be due to noninfectious agents. This chapter focuses on acute syndromes of meningitis and encephalitis with an onset of hours to a few days.

EPIDEMIOLOGY AND ETIOLOGY

Viral Central Nervous System Infections

Aseptic meningitis refers to meningitis in which no common bacterial pathogen can be identified. Although most patients with aseptic meningitis are not ill enough to be admitted to an intensive care unit (ICU), occasionally the cause of the CNS disease is in doubt or patients are unusually ill. In the past, the specific cause of cases of aseptic meningitis (and encephalitis) were often undetermined. However, more recent diagnostic techniques, particularly the use of the polymerase chain reaction (PCR), have resulted in the identification of a pathogen in 55 to 70% of cases.

Many CNS viral pathogens are more closely associated with either a meningitis or an encephalitis. However, infection with any virus can produce either syndrome. In addition, measles, mumps, varicella-zoster, rubella, and influenza have been associated with *postinfectious encephalitis*.

Bacterial Central Nervous System Infections

Uncomplicated adult *bacterial meningitis* in the United States is primarily due to *Streptococcus pneumoniae* and *Neisseria meningitidis*. However, many factors influence the likelihood of infection with other organisms (Table 64–1). Splenectomy, immunoglobulin deficiency, pneumococcal pneumonia, alcoholism, chronic liver or renal disease, diabetes mellitus, and cerebrospinal fluid leaks all predispose the patient to infection with *S. pneumoniae*. Meningitis due to *Hemophilus influen-*

723

Table 64–1. Predisposing Factors to Specific Bacterial Meningitis Pathogens

PREDISPOSING FACTOR	PATHOGENS
Age	
Young adult	*Neisseria meningitidis*
Adult (any age)	*Streptococcus pneumoniae*
Older adult	*Listeria monocytogenes*
Impaired host defense	
Granulocytopenia	Aerobic Gram-negative bacilli, *Staphylococcus aureus*
Defect in cell-mediated immunity	*L. monocytogenes*
Terminal complement deficiency	*N. meningitidis*
Postsplenectomy	*S. pneumoniae*
Open head trauma, postneurosurgery	Aerobic Gram-negative bacilli, *S. aureus, S. epidermidis*
Cerebrospinal fluid shunt	*S. epidermidis*
Basilar skull fracture	*S. pneumoniae*

zae is uncommon in adults, except in those with sinusitis, otitis media, epiglottitis, immunoglobulin deficiencies, and alcoholism. *Listeria monocytogenes* should be considered in persons with a defect in cell-mediated immunity (e.g., solid organ transplant, human immunodeficiency virus (HIV) infection, chronic corticosteroid use, Hodgkin's disease), as well as in alcoholics, the elderly, and persons with iron overload, chronic liver or renal disease, and diabetes.

PATHOGENESIS

Acute meningitis and encephalitis are primarily caused by relatively few pathogens with unique abilities to invade the cerebrospinal fluid (CSF). As a rule, viral and bacterial CNS pathogens gain entry into the CSF via a hematogenous route. Some viruses may also gain access by retrograde spread along nerves. Bacteria occasionally invade the CNS from a contiguous focus or by direct inoculation during or after trauma or neurosurgery.

In bacterial meningitis, once these agents gain access to the CSF fluid, there are few host defenses available to control their rapid multiplication. CSF is devoid of phagocytic cells or effective humoral immunity via immunoglobulins or complement. The pathogens induce an inflammatory response that is mediated by a number of cytokines within the CSF, particularly interleukins 1 and 6 and tumor necrosis factor. These cytokines induce phagocytes to adhere to endothelium and enter the CSF. The resultant inflammation and microvascular injury produces brain edema, increased intracerebral pressure, decreased tissue perfusion, and direct tissue injury. Better understanding of this pathogenesis has led to new considerations for therapeutic intervention with drugs that can modulate the inflammatory response.

Viral encephalitis can be either primary or postinfectious. Primary infection is characterized by direct viral invasion of the CNS, which can be demonstrated by light or electron microscopy. The virus can often be cultured from brain tissue or identified by immunofluorescent staining. In postinfectious encephalitis, the virus cannot be detected in tissue nor recovered in culture. Although the neurons are not involved, perivascular inflammation and demyelination are prominent.

CLINICAL PRESENTATION AND COMPLICATIONS

Most patients with *acute viral meningitis* present with fever, headache, and nuchal rigidity. The headache is typically severe and either frontal or diffuse. Photophobia is also common. Meningismus limits head flexion but not rotation. In contrast, both flexion and rotation are limited in patients with cervical arthritis, Parkinson's disease, and neuroleptic malignant syndrome. Additional symptoms include nausea, vomiting, diarrhea, and myalgias. Patients with viral meningitis are usually uncomfortable but do not appear toxemic. Although most patients have a nonspecific presentation, associated clinical clues to the cause might include an enteroviral exanthem, mumps parotitis, or herpes genitalis. The duration of viral meningitis is generally less than a week, and it usually resolves without sequelae.

Acute bacterial meningitis also presents with fever, headache, and findings of meningeal irritation. In addition, an altered sensorium with a nonfocal neurologic examination is common. It can range from mild confusion to complete unresponsiveness. If these symptoms occur, focal neurologic findings include cranial nerve palsies, hemiparesis, and aphasia. They are often associated with complications such as subdural empyema, cortical vein thrombosis, sagittal or cavernous sinus thrombosis, or hydrocephalus. Focal or generalized seizures may also occur. Because papilledema is *not* a feature of uncomplicated meningitis, this finding suggests the presence of a complication or an alternative diagnosis.

In certain groups of patients, the presentation of bacterial meningitis is more likely to be atypical. Meningitis in the elderly may be subtle with only a change in mental status. In patients who have sustained head trauma, the findings of an associated meningitis may be attributed to the injury. In neutropenic patients, the inflammatory response in the CSF may be attenuated. For these reasons, bacterial meningitis must be considered in any patient with an altered mental status, especially if febrile.

The general physical examination may occasionally give clues to the cause of the bacterial meningitis. A localized source of infection, such as pneumonia or sinusitis, may be found. Characteristic cutaneous findings of meningococcemia, that is, petechiae or purpura, suggest that organism, but these findings can also be seen with other pathogens. Other possible clues include the presence of a CSF shunt, a dural sinus, or CSF rhinorrhea.

The clinical distinction between viral meningitis and encephalitis is based on the state of brain function. Patients with meningitis may be uncomfortable, lethargic, or distracted by headache, but their cerebral function remains normal. Abnormalities in brain function in encephalitis, however, are common and include altered mental status, motor or sensory deficits, and speech or movement disorders. Seizures and postictal states can be seen with meningitis alone and should not be construed as definitive evidence of encephalitis. Encephalitis with herpes simplex virus type 1 (HSV-1) has a particular affinity for the medial temporal and inferior frontal lobes of the brain. Because of this, symptoms such as bizarre behavior, speech disorders, and gustatory or olfactory hallucinations are characteristic of infection with this organism. Accompanying herpes labialis is seen in less than 10% of cases. Furthermore, the appearance of herpetic skin lesions can be a nonspecific complication of many febrile illnesses. Therefore, the presence or absence of mucocutaneous herpes infection is *not* of diagnostic importance in evaluating patients for HSV-1 encephalitis.

GENERAL DIAGNOSTIC APPROACH

Examination of the CSF obtained by lumbar puncture is the key initial test in the evaluation of a patient for CNS infection. The CSF findings will confirm or rule out the presence of CNS inflammation. Although the specific pattern of results generally allow the clinician to distinguish a bacterial from a nonbacterial process, the CSF findings with aseptic meningitis and encephalitis are indistinguishable.

In most patients, the presentation of an acute meningitis is sufficiently distinct from the presentation of a CNS mass lesion that imaging before a lumbar puncture is unnecessary and might potentially delay therapy (Fig. 64–1). Findings that should prompt either computed tomography or magnetic resonance imaging of the brain before lumbar puncture are papilledema, any sign of brainstem compression,

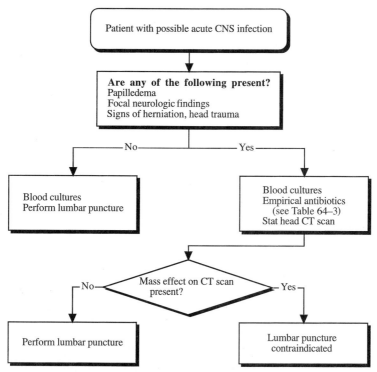

Figure 64–1. Schematic flow diagram outlining steps in the initial evaluation of a patient suspected of having an acute central nervous system infection (see text for details). CT, computed tomography.

or focal neurologic findings (other than occurring in a postictal state), and evidence of head trauma. If meningitis is a consideration and findings suggest the possibility of increased intracranial pressure, *antibiotic therapy should not be delayed while obtaining CNS imaging studies before lumbar puncture.* The CSF should routinely be sent for cell count and differential, glucose and protein determinations, Gram stain, and bacterial culture. In addition, several milliliters of CSF should be saved in a refrigerator pending the results of these initial tests in case further testing is needed. Generally the results of the initial tests reflect whether or not the process is bacterial (Fig. 64–2). If bacterial meningitis is not diagnosed, this reserved fluid can be tested for other pathogens.

The CSF findings in patients with viral and bacterial CNS infections are shown in Table 64–2. In *viral meningitis* or *encephalitis,* the predominant cell is the lymphocyte, although early in the course granulocytes (neutrophils) may be in the majority. In equivocal situations, a repeat CSF examination 8 hours after the first will show a shift from granulocytes to lymphocytes in most cases. The CSF

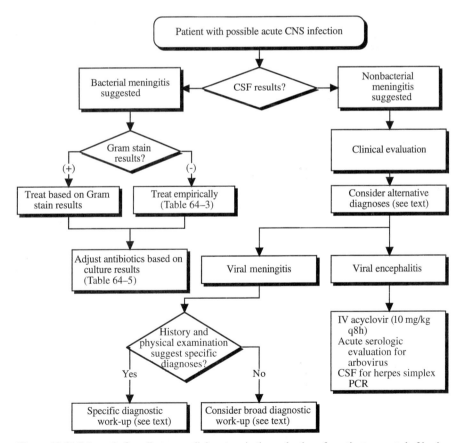

Figure 64–2. Schematic flow diagram outlining steps in the evaluation of a patient suspected of having an acute central nervous system infection based on the initial results of cerebrospinal fluid (CSF analysis) (see Table 63–2 and text for details). PCR, polymerase chain reaction.

Table 64–2. Typical Cerebrospinal Fluid Findings in Viral and Bacterial Meningitis

	VIRAL	BACTERIAL
WBCs (cells/μL)	<1000	>1000
% Granulocytes	<50*	>90
Glucose	Normal†	Decreased
Protein	Elevated	Elevated
Gram stain	Negative	Positive in 80–90% of cases

* Early in viral meningitis there may be a predominance of granulocytes.
† See text for discussion of normal and decreased values.
WBCs, white blood cells.

glucose level is usually normal, but a mild decrease can be seen with HSV, mumps, some enteroviruses, and lymphocytic choriomeningitis. The presence of red blood cells in the appropriate setting suggests HSV-1 encephalitis.

In *bacterial meningitis,* the white blood cell count is expected to be greater than 1000 cells/μL, but lower values are occasionally seen. CSF with less than 10 white blood cells/μL has a 99% negative predictive value for bacterial meningitis. In most cases greater than 90% of these cells are granulocytes. A lymphocyte predominance may be seen in when the total count is low. This is most commonly due to *L. monocytogenes.* A decreased CSF glucose concentration is expected but is not specific for bacterial meningitis. It can also be seen in carcinomatous meningitis, tuberculous meningitis, some viral meningitides, or when the serum glucose is low. A decreased CSF glucose level in bacterial meningitis is due to both anaerobic glycolysis and a decrease in its active transport. CSF glucose values of less than 10 mg/dL are highly specific for bacterial meningitis but are uncommon. CSF glucose levels are less than 40 mg/dL in 60% of cases and a ratio of CSF:serum glucose is less than 0.3 in 70% of instances. Since values for cell count, percent granulocytes, and glucose can individually overlap with aseptic meningitis, it is important to look at the entire pattern when evaluating the CSF results. CSF glucose levels of less than 34 mg/dL, a CSF:serum glucose ratio of less than 0.3, a CSF protein concentration greater than 220 mg/dL, CSF white blood cell count greater than 2000/μL, or a CSF granulocyte count greater than 1180/μL were found to be independent predictors of bacterial rather than viral meningitis with a specificity of 99%. Because CSF bacterial antigen tests are no more sensitive than is the CSF Gram stain, the routine use of these tests in adults is generally not indicated. They are potentially useful, however, in a patient who has been started on antibiotics before the initial lumbar puncture.

APPROACH TO THE PATIENT WITH A NONBACTERIAL CENTRAL NERVOUS SYSTEM INFECTION

The general approach to a nonbacterial CNS infection is outlined in Figure 64–1. With the exception of HSV-1, HIV, and possibly varicella, there are no specific drugs for viral CNS infections. Because of these limited therapeutic implications, the approach to a patient with clinical and CSF features of viral meningitis or encephalitis should limited to:

1. **Empirical treatment for HSV-1 with acyclovir if there is evidence of encephalitis**
   Early treatment is clearly associated with a better outcome. The dose is 10 mg/kg intravenously every 8 hours in patients with normal renal function. The duration is 10 to 14 days.

2. **Careful consideration for another, potentially treatable cause (e.g., non-steroidal anti-inflammatory drug–associated sterile meningitis, CNS vasculitis)**

3. **Observation for clues of specific viruses**
   A focal encephalitis, especially with localization to the temporal lobes by electroencephalography, computed tomography, or magnetic resonance imaging suggests HSV-1. Other enteroviral illnesses beginning at home (as suggested by illnesses with pleurodynia, pancreatitis, parotitis, febrile exanthem) suggest an enteroviral meningitis. Parotitis suggests mumps or enteroviral infection. Measles and varicella are associated with characteristic rashes. Recent high risk exposure suggests possible acute HIV infection.

4. **The pursuit of a viral cause other than HSV should be individualized, depending on the clinical information as indicated in the following sections**
   Although there is no specific treatment for most viruses, patients and their families often benefit from an explanation of an illness as severe as meningitis or encephalitis.
   a. When HSV-1 is a consideration, request a CSF polymerase chain reaction for HSV. This is the most rapid and specific test available and has replaced other modalities. Brain biopsy can establish the diagnosis, but there are occasionally false-negative results. CSF culture has a low sensitivity. Measurement of serum HSV antibodies alone is not helpful.
   b. Culture the CSF for enteroviruses, HSV-2 and mumps. Culture the throat for enteroviruses and mumps. Culture the stool for enteroviruses.
   c. Obtain routine serologic studies for HIV, although the serologic results are often negative at the time of presentation with acute HIV infection. Seroconversion occurs several weeks later with recovery. In contrast, PCR for HIV is positive in high titer during acute disease.
   d. Obtain an "acute" serologic profile for the arboviruses (including West Nile virus in affected regions) to be paired with a "convalescent" blood study 2 to 3 weeks later. Mumps can be diagnosed on a single specimen.

APPROACH TO THE PATIENT WITH A BACTERIAL CENTRAL NERVOUS SYSTEM PROCESS

When CSF examination suggests a bacterial process, empirical antibiotics are indicated until the culture results are known. The initial choice should be guided by the findings on the CSF Gram stain and any specific clinical features that might alter the microbiologic picture (Tables 64–3 and 64–4; see also Table 64–1).

Table 64–3. Initial Empirical Therapy of Presumed Bacterial Meningitis

CLINICAL	ANTIBIOTIC
Adult <50 yr with no predisposing factors	Ceftriaxone or cefotaxime plus vancomycin*
Adult >50 yr	Same as above plus ampicillin
Decreased cell-mediated immunity†	Same as above plus ampicillin
After head trauma or neurosurgery	Ceftazidime plus vancomycin
Granulocytopenia	Ceftazidime plus vancomycin
Cerebrospinal fluid shunt infection	Ceftriaxone or cefotaxime plus vancomycin

*Vancomycin is now added to the initial regimen by many physicians because of the increasing prevalence of resistant *Streptococcus pneumoniae*.

† Examples include patients receiving steroids chronically, with lymphoma, HIV disease, or solid organ transplant.

Once a specific bacterial cause of meningitis has been identified by culture, the antimicrobial regimen can be modified (Table 64–5). *Pseudomonas aeruginosa* should be treated with ceftazidime (or an antipseudomonal penicillin) plus an aminoglycoside. If there is no response to systemic therapy, consideration should be given to intrathecal or intraventricular aminoglycoside dosing. Some clinicians add an aminoglycoside to the regimen in patients with proven *Listeria* meningitis because of in vitro synergy (although improved in vivo efficacy has not been demonstrated). *Staphylococcus epidermidis*, the predominant pathogen in CSF shunt infections, should be treated with vancomycin. Rifampin has been added in patients who do not improve. Although some persistent shunt infections have been

Table 64–4. Recommended Doses of Antibiotics for Bacterial Meningitis in Adults with Normal Renal and Hepatic Function

ANTIBIOTIC	DOSE (TOTAL/DAY)	DOSING INTERVAL (HOURS)
Amikacin	15 mg/kg	8
Ampicillin	12 g	4
Cefotaxime	12 g	4
Ceftazidime	6 g	8
Ceftriaxone	4 g	12
Chloramphenicol	4–6 g	6
Ciprofloxacin	800 mg	12
Gentamicin	5 mg/kg	8†
Nafcillin	12 g	4
Oxacillin	12 g	4
Ofloxacin	800 mg	12
Penicillin G	20–24 million units	4
Rifampin	600 mg	24
Tobramycin	5 mg/kg	8†
Trimethoprim-sulfamethoxazole	20 gm/kg*	12
Vancomycin	2 g	12†

* Dosage based on the trimethoprim component.

† Adjust dose by serum level.

Table 64-5. Specific Antimicrobial Therapy for Bacterial Meningitis

ORGANISM	STANDARD THERAPY	ALTERNATIVE THERAPIES
Streptococcus pneumoniae		
Sensitive to penicillin (mean inhibitory concentration [MIC] <0.1 µg/mL)	Penicillin G	Third-generation cephalosporin,* chloramphenicol, cefuroxime
S. pneumoniae		
Resistant to penicillin (MIC = 0.1–1.0 µg/mL)	Third-generation cephalosporin	Vancomycin
(MIC >2.0 µg/mL)	Vancomycin	
Nesseria meningitidis	Penicillin G	Third-generation cephalosporin, cefuroxime, chloramphenicol
Hemophilus influenzae		
beta-lactamase (−)	Ampicillin	Third-generation cephalosporin, chloramphenicol, cefuroxime
beta-lactamase (+)	Third-generation cephalosporin	Chloramphenicol, fluoroquinolone†
Enterobacteriaceae	Third-generation cephalosporin	Piperacillin, chloramphenicol, trimethoprim-sulfamethoxazole
L. monocytogenes	Ampicillin§	Trimethoprim-sulfamethoxazole
Pseudomonas aeruginosa	Ceftazidime‡	Piperacillin,‡ fluoroquinolone,† imipenem‡
Staphyloccus aureus		
methicillin-sensitive	Nafcillin or oxacillin	Vancomycin
methicillin-resistant	Vancomycin	Trimethoprim-sulfamethoxazole
S. epidermidis	Vancomycin§	

* Ceftriaxone, cefotaxime, ceftazidime.
† Levofloxacin, ofloxacin, ciprofloxacin, and others.
‡ The addition of an aminoglycoside should be considered (see text).
§ The addition of rifampin should be considered (see text).

cured when vancomycin has been injected directly into the shunt, in general, the shunt must be removed under these circumstances.

In a patient with a history of allergy to penicillin, chloramphenicol should be substituted. If indicated, attempts to desensitize the patient to specific antibiotics can be made later.

Although the duration of antimicrobial therapy for bacterial meningitis has not been scientifically determined, 10 to 14 days is standard for pneumococcus, meningococcus, and hemophilus. Gram-negative meningitis and meningitis due to *L. monocytogenes* is usually treated for 3 weeks.

ADJUNCTIVE THERAPY

1. If there are signs of increased intracranial pressure (ICP), treatment to lower it should be started and monitoring ICP invasively should be considered in severe cases (see Chapter 42).
2. Fever increases brain metabolic activity. This, in turn, increases cerebral blood flow, which may have detrimental effects by raising ICP. Antipyretic agents should be used to keep the temperature less than 38° C.
3. The inappropriate secretion of antidiuretic hormone commonly complicates intracerebral infections. One should be follow serum electrolyte levels attentively and adjust intravenous fluid management appropriately to avoid hyponatremia (see Chapter 81) because this will exacerbate brain edema.
4. Recurrent seizures can produce neuronal damage and should be controlled. Prophylactic antiseizure therapy, however, is not indicated.
5. Adjunctive corticosteroids should be considered. The rapid bactericidal activity of many of the antibiotics causes lysis of bacteria, which provokes the release of proinflammatory mediators. Because these mediators have the potential to increase inflammation and brain injury, blunting the inflammatory response has a sound rationale.

    Adjunctive dexamethasone has been shown to be beneficial in the treatment of bacterial meningitis in children. Pediatric controlled trials show a decrease in the number of days of hospitalization, a decrease in the frequency of hearing loss, and no steroid-related side effects. Despite the absence of similar studies for adults with meningitis, on the basis of the extensive animal data and the proven benefit in children, it has been suggested that dexamethasone be considered for use in adults with bacterial meningitis. This decision should be individualized. Two groups of patients, in particular, should be considered for adjunctive dexamethasone treatment. The first are patients with the highest bacterial loads, for example, bacteria visible on Gram stain. They are most likely to have a bacteriolysis-related severe inflammatory response. The second group are patients with elevated ICP. If used, the recommended dose of intravenous dexamethasone is 0.15 mg/kg every 6 hours for 4 days.

BIBLIOGRAPHY

Centers for Disease Control and Prevention: Outbreak of West Nile-like viral encephalitis—New York, 1999. MMWR Morb Mortal Wkly Rep 48:845–849, 1999.

West Nile virus, not previously known to be present in North America, was later identified as the cause of this report of a cluster of encephalitis cases in New York City in August 1999. This virus should be tested for serologically in patients with encephalitis who live in or near affected areas (see CDC website, www.cdc.gov, *for up-to-date information regarding affected regions).*

Connolly KJ, Hammer SM: The acute aseptic meningitis syndrome. Infect Dis Clin North Am 4:599–622, 1990.
This article presents a discussion of the major viral and nonviral causes of this syndrome and the approach to a patient.

Durand ML, Calderwood SB, Weber DJ, et al: Acute bacterial meningitis in adults. N Engl J Med 328:21–28, 1993.
This is a descriptive series of 27 years of bacterial meningitis at the Massachusetts General Hospital.

Lyons MK, Meyer FB: Cerebrospinal fluid physiology and the management of increased intracranial pressure. Mayo Clin Proc 65:684–707, 1990.
This article reviews cerebrospinal fluid composition, formation, absorption, the blood-brain barrier, and the management of increased intracranial pressure.

Quagliarello VJ, Scheld WM: Bacterial meningitis: Pathogenesis, pathophysiology, and progress. N Engl J Med 327:864–872, 1992.
This is primarily a review of the inflammatory mediators of meningitis and their therapeutic implications.

Quagliarello VJ, Scheld WM: Drug therapy: Treatment of bacterial meningitis. N Engl J Med 336:708–716, 1997.
This is an updated review of current therapy for bacterial meningitis that addresses limitations of data supporting the use of dexamethasone as adjunctive therapy in adults.

Roos KL, Scheld WM: The management of fulminant meningitis in the intensive care unit. Infect Dis Clin North Am 3:137–154, 1898.
This is a good review of bacterial meningitis that includes the adjunctive therapy of meningitis.

Rotbart HA: Enteroviral infections of the central nervous system. Clin Infect Dis 20:971–981, 1995.
This article reviews the epidemiologic, clinical, and diagnostic aspects of enteroviral CNS infections and comments on future therapy.

Tsai TS: Arboviral infections in the United States. Infect Dis Clin North Am 5:73–102, 1991.
This article presents an extensive review of all clinical aspects of arboviral CNS infections.

Tunkel AR, Wispelwey B, Scheld WM: Bacterial meningitis: Recent advances in pathophysiology and treatment. Ann Intern Med 112:610–623, 1990.
This article presents a complete review of pathophysiology and treatment of bacterial meningitis. This covers some of the issues about corticosteroid adjunctive therapy.

Whitley RJ: Viral encephalitis. N Engl J Med 323:242–250, 1990.
This is a brief review of the clinical manifestations of the major viral encephalitides.

Whitley RJ, Lakeman F: Herpes simplex virus infections of the central nervous system: Therapeutic and diagnostic considerations. Clin Infect Dis 20:414–420, 1995.
The pathogenesis, diagnosis, and treatment of HSV-1 infections of the CNS are discussed.

65

Community Acquired Pneumonia

Ebbing Lautenbach
Patrick J. Brennan

Pneumonia is defined as inflammation and consolidation of lung tissue resulting from an infectious agent. Pneumonia is the sixth leading cause of death in the United States and is the most common infectious disease resulting in mortality. Although new antimicrobial agents have been developed to treat community acquired pneumonia, the incidence of this disease resulting from resistant pathogens continues to rise. Finally, increased populations at high risk, particularly those with acquired immunodeficiency disease or those receiving immunosuppressive therapy, have contributed to the increasing importance of opportunistic pathogens as causes of community acquired pneumonia.

CLINICAL DIAGNOSIS AND CAUSES

Although the majority of patients with community acquired pneumonia present with the classic signs and symptoms of fever, cough, and sputum production, the signs and symptoms are neither sensitive nor specific. For example, the elderly with community acquired pneumonia often show none of these traditional indicators of infection. Instead, the most reliable sign of pneumonia in this group is an increased respiratory rate.

Atypical Versus Typical Pneumonia

Some clinicians have suggested that *typical* and *atypical* community acquired pneumonia can be distinguished based on clinical presentation. Community acquired pneumonia due to "atypical" organisms (*Mycoplasma pneumoniae, Chlamydia pneumoniae, Legionella* species and viruses) was believed to be characterized by a prior viral-like syndrome (myalgias, arthralgias, and sore throat), nonproductive cough, absence of pleurisy and rigors, lower fever, and absence of consolidation on auscultation compared with community acquired pneumonia due to "typical" organisms (*Streptococcus pneumoniae, Hemophilus influenzae, Staphylococcus aureus,* and Gram-negative bacteria). When studied systematically, however, these characteristics were found to be no more common in atypical than in typical pneumonias. In addition, the time course of pneumonia, often believed to be more subacute in atypical community acquired pneumonia, was found to be the same as in typical community acquired pneumonia. Finally, there were no consistent distinctions when comparing laboratory data and chest radiographs of patients with typical and atypical pneumonias. Clinical demographics may give clues to the cause, but definitive diagnosis depends on laboratory and microbiologic testing to identify a specific pathogen.

735

Pathogens

Although its rate of isolation has decreased over the past several decades, *S. pneumoniae* remains the most frequently identified cause of community acquired pneumonia. Despite new diagnostic techniques, the cause of community acquired pneumonia remains unknown in up to 45% of cases. In a review of 15 studies of community acquired pneumonia conducted between 1960 and 1985, the five most common pathogens identified (in order of frequency)) were *S. pneumoniae, H. influenzae, viruses, M. pneumoniae, and Staphylococcus aureus.* More recent studies have shown that organisms, such as *Legionella* species, aerobic Gram-negative rods, and *C. pneumoniae* have become common causes of community acquired pneumonia.

Because the initial treatment of community acquired pneumonia is often empirical, knowledge of the most likely pathogens is vital. The causative organism may often be suspected based on the patient's risk factors or comorbid illnesses (Table 65–1). *S. pneumoniae,* however, remains the most common cause in **all** groups

Table 65–1. Most Likely Pathogens for Community Acquired Pneumonia

Young adults (age <30)	*Streptococcus pneumoniae*
	Mycoplasma pneumoniae
	Chlamydia pneumoniae
Heavy cigarette smokers	*S. pneumoniae*
	Haemophilus influenzae
	Moraxella catarrhalis
HIV-positive patients (CD4$^+$ lymphocytes <200/μL)	*Pneumocystis carinii*
	S. pneumoniae
	H. influenzae
	Mycobacterium tuberculosis
	Fungi
Nursing home residents	*S. pneumoniae*
	Gram-negative bacilli (especially, *Klebsiella pneumoniae*)
	Influenza A or B
	Staphylococcus aureus
	Anaerobes
	M. tuberculosis
Patients with a recent flu-like illness	*S. pneumoniae*
	S. aureus
	H. influenzae
Neutropenic patients	*S. pneumoniae*
	Gram-negative bacilli (especially, *Pseudomonas aeruginosa*)
Alcohol abusers	*S. pneumoniae*
	K. pneumoniae
	S. aureus
	Anaerobes
Solid organ transplant recipients (>3 mo after transplant)	*S. pneumoniae*
	H. influenzae
	Legionella species
	P. carinii
	Cytomegalovirus

except in those with human immunodeficiency virus (HIV). In the latter group, *Pneumocystis carinii* is the most prevalent cause of community acquired pneumonia. Severe recurrent pneumonias with *S. pneumoniae* or *H. influenzae* should suggest an underlying immunocompromised state, for example, HIV infection or multiple myeloma. *Legionella* infections by species other than *Legionella pneumophila* may also be more common in the immunosuppressed patient and, if such infections occur, one should assess the patient's immune status.

DIAGNOSTIC EVALUATION

Chest Radiograph

When community acquired pneumonia has a typical clinical presentation, an infiltrate on chest radiograph generally confirms the diagnosis. The chest radiograph may be normal, however, if taken in the first 24 hours of a bacterial pneumonia or in the setting of severe neutropenia. Likewise, 10 to 30% of patients with *P. carinii* pneumonia may have normal chest radiographs at presentation.

Gram Stain and Culture of Sputum

Although its usefulness has been widely debated, a Gram stain and culture of expectorated sputum may be valuable in establishing the cause of community acquired pneumonia and guiding initial therapy. Although only 60 to 70% of patients with community acquired pneumonia can produce sputum on admission to hospital, performing these tests on a sputum sample is noninvasive and relatively inexpensive. In patients eventually diagnosed with pneumonia due to *S. pneumoniae,* 62 to 89% demonstrate lancet-shaped Gram-positive diplococci on initial Gram stain (a diagnostic test sensitivity of 62 to 89%). Alternatively, finding many polymorphonuclear neutrophils and no organisms on Gram stain suggests infection with *M. pneumoniae, C. pneumoniae,* or *Legionella* species.

Sputum cultures *must* be interpreted in light of the findings of the corresponding sputum Gram stain. Isolation of a predominant organism by culture is more clinically compelling when compatible with the findings on Gram stain. Isolation of a predominant organism that is not part of the normal respiratory flora may be useful in modifying antibiotics. Because of difficulty in isolation, cultures for *M. pneumoniae, C. pneumoniae, Legionella* species, and respiratory viruses are not routinely performed.

The clinical value of a sputum Gram stain and culture depends largely on the quality of the sputum specimen. Having greater than 25 polymorphonuclear neutrophils and less than 10 squamous epithelial cells per low power field can be used as criteria to assess whether the sputum is an adequate sample from the lower respiratory tract. Prior antibiotic therapy decreases the usefulness of sputum cultures because the chance of isolating an organism from sputum decreases by up to 50% after just one to two doses of antibiotic. Bronchoscopy may be valuable in diagnosing community acquired pneumonia but is usually reserved for patients who do not respond to initial empirical antibiotics, patients who are critically ill, or patients in whom resistant organisms are suspected. In one study, an etiologic diagnosis was obtained in 79% of patients with community acquired pneumonia when fiberoptic bronchoscopy and protected specimen brush cultures were used.

Blood Cultures and Thoracentesis Results

Although positive blood culture results are considered to be definitive (i.e., highly specific) in establishing the cause of community acquired pneumonia such results occur in only about 10% of patients with community acquired pneumonia (i.e., low sensitivity). Of these, 60 to 70% of cultures grow *S. pneumoniae.* The low prevalence of positive blood cultures may, in part, be the result of the prior administration of antibiotics.

Pleural effusions are found in 10 to 50% of reported patients with community acquired pneumonia. A diagnostic thoracentesis should be performed if the effusion is large, the clinical presentation usual, or the patient fails to respond to initial therapy. Pleural effusions with a pH greater than 7.3, glucose levels greater than 60 mg/dL, and lactate dehydrogenase levels less than 1000 IU/dL usually resolve with antibiotic therapy alone. If the fluid is grossly purulent, has a pH less than 7.0 or glucose level less than 60 mg/dL, or has organisms seen on Gram stain, the patient, in general, should undergo chest tube drainage. Of note, one should not send specimens with thick pus to the laboratory for measurement of pH—not only are they likely to plug up the arterial blood gas analyzers but also the information about the pH is unnecessary in view of the gross appearance indicating an empyema.

Other Diagnostic Tests

Measuring acute and convalescent serologic titers for various atypical respiratory pathogens has no practical role in the management of community acquired pneumonia because the results are not available to guide therapy. As such, they should not be ordered in the routine patient with community acquired pneumonia.

The presence of a *urine antigen* for *Legionella* is highly sensitive to document infection with *L. pneumophila* (serogroup 1), which causes 70 to 90% of cases of *Legionella* pneumonia. It does not, however, rule out infection by other serogroups of *L. pneumophila* or other *Legionella* species (both of which combined cause 10 to 30% of community acquired pneumonia due to *Legionella*). Although other tests are available for diagnosing community acquired pneumonia due to *Legionella,* such as cultures of sputum or tracheal aspirate, direct fluorescent antibody testing, and acute anti-*Legionella* serum titer, none are as sensitive as the urine antigen test. The sensitivity of cultures also declines after the start of anti-*Legionella* antibiotic administration.

A rapid screen for a variety of respiratory viruses—performed on nasopharyngeal washings or swab or, less preferably (due to dilution), on bronchoalveolar lavage fluid—can be useful as a test with high sensitivity in confirming a viral cause within 24 hours.

RISK FACTORS FOR MORTALITY AND COMPLICATIONS

A meta-analysis of 127 study cohorts that included 33,148 patients with community acquired pneumonia examined risk factors for mortality (Table 65–2). Although overall mortality was 13.7%, it was 36.5% in patients who were admitted to the intensive care unit (ICU). Another meta-analysis of 41 studies established the frequency of common complications of community acquired pneumonia (Table 65–3).

TREATMENT

Antibiotic Selection

Severely ill patients with community acquired pneumonia are as a rule admitted to the ICU or an intermediate care unit. Since one cannot often determine the cause of community acquired pneumonia on admission, initial treatment must be

Table 65–2. Risk Factors* For Mortality in Community Acquired Pneumonia
....

Age	>65 yr
Symptoms, signs	Dyspnea
	Temperature <37° C
	Respiratory rate >20 breaths per min
	Systolic blood pressure <100 mm Hg
	Altered mental status
Comorbid illnesses	Alcohol abuse
	Coronary artery disease
	Congestive heart failure
	Diabetes mellitus
	Immunosuppression
	Neoplastic disease
Laboratory data	White cell count <10,000/μL
	BUN >7.1 mmol/L
	Bacteremia
Chest radiograph	>1 lobe involvement
	Bilateral pleural effusions
Pathogens	
Bacterial	*Pseudomonas aeruginosa*
	Klebsiella pneumoniae
	Escherichia coli
	Staphylococcus aureus
	Mixed bacterial species
Viral	Influenza A
	Parainfluenza
	Respiratory syncytial virus

....

*Patients infected with human immunodeficiency virus (HIV) were excluded from analysis; HIV infection is a risk factor for mortality as CD4+ lymphocyte counts fall (see Chapter 17).

BUN, blood urea nitrogen.

Adapted from Fine MJ, Smith MA, Carson CA, et al: Prognosis and outcomes of patients with community-acquired pneumonia. JAMA 275:134–141, 1996, and Hasley PB, Albaum MN, Li Y-H, et al: Do pulmonary radiographic findings at presentation predict mortality in patients with community-acquired pneumonia? Arch Intern Med 156:2206–2212, 1996.

Table 65–3. Frequency of Complications of Community Acquired Pneumonia

Hepatic abnormalities*	12.3%
Pleural effusion	10.6%
Renal failure	10.4%
Congestive heart failure	8.6%
Respiratory failure	7.8%
Shock	7.7%
Lung abscess	6.3%
Pneumothorax	5.7%
Empyema	5.2%

*Jaundice, liver function test abnormalities, or hepatic failure.

Adapted from Fine MJ, Smith MA, Carson CA, et al: Prognosis and outcomes of patients with community-acquired pneumonia. JAMA 275:134–141, 1996.

empirical (Tables 65–4 and 65–5). If the causative pathogen is identified during the course of therapy, treatment should be converted to the most appropriate, least expensive antibiotic. It should be noted that overall, 4 to 5% of *S. pneumoniae* strains in the United States have intermediate or high resistance to penicillin, with some areas reporting resistance rates as high as 25%. Other parts of the world have noted greater than 50% of *S. pneumoniae* to be resistant to penicillin. In addition, these isolates are also frequently resistant to other commonly used

Table 65–4. Empirical Antibiotics For Community Acquired Pneumonia in Severely Ill* Patients Who Are **Not** Immunosuppressed

CLASS OF ANTIBIOTIC	ANTIMICROBIAL ACTIVITY	EXAMPLE (DOSAGE)
Macrolide antibiotic	*Legionella,* mycoplasma, and *Chlamydia* species	Erythromycin (1g IV q6h)
	plus	
Third-generation cephalosporin (without antipseudomonal activity)	*Streptococcus pneumoniae, Haemophilus influenzae, Klebsiella pneumoniae* and other aerobic Gram-negative bacilli (not *Pseudomonas aeruginosa*)	Ceftriaxone (1–2 g IV q24h)
	or, as a single agent,	
Fluoroquinolone	*S. pneumoniae, H. influenzae, K. pneumoniae,* and other aerobic Gram-negative bacilli (including many *P. aeruginosa*), *Legionella,* mycoplasma, *Chlamydia* species	Levofloxacin (500 mg IV once a day)

*Severely ill patients are defined as having one or more of the following: respiratory rate >30 breaths per min; PaO_2/FIO_2 <250; mechanical ventilation; >1 lobe involvement; blood pressure <90/60 mm Hg; vasopressors >4 h; or acute renal failure.

Data from American Thoracic Society: Guidelines for the initial management of adults with community-acquired pneumonia: Diagnosis, assessment of severity, and initial antimicrobial therapy. Am Rev Respir Dis 148:1418–1426, 1993; Bartlett JG, Breinan RF, Mandell LA; File TM: Community-acquired pneumonia in adults: Guidelines for management. Clin Infect Dis 26:811–838, 1998.

Table 65–5. Empirical Antibiotics for Community Acquired Pneumonia in Severely Ill* Patients Who **Are** Immunosuppressed (But Not HIV +)†

CLASS OF ANTIBIOTIC	ANTIMICROBIAL ACTIVITY	EXAMPLE (DOSAGE)
Macrolide antibiotic or fluoroquinolone (see Table 65–4)	*Legionella,* mycoplasma, and *Chlamydia* species	Erythromycin (1 g IV q6h) or Levofloxacin (500 mg IV once a day)
	plus, either	
Third-generation cephalosporin with antipseudomonal activity	*Streptococcus pneumoniae, Haemophilus influenzae, Klebsiella pneumoniae,* and other aerobic Gram-negative bacilli, including *Pseudomonas aeruginosa*	Ceftazidime (1–2 g IV q8h) Cefepime (1–2 g IV q12h)
	or	
Third-generation cephalosporin (without antipseudomonal activity)	*S. pneumoniae, H. influenzae, K. pneumoniae*	Ceftriaxone (1–2 g IV q24h)
	combined with	
Another antipseudomonal agent (check local sensitivities before prescribing specific agent)	*P. aeruginosa*	Imipenem/cilastatin (500 mg IV q6h) Levofloxacin (500 mg IV q24h)

*Severely ill as defined in Table 65–4.

†*In addition* to the above regimen, in general, patients who are or suspected to be human immunodeficiency virus–positive, should receive co-trimoxazole (unless contraindicated) for *Pneumocystis carinii* (see Chapter 17)

Data from American Thoracic Society: Guidelines for the initial management of adults with community-acquired pneumonia: Diagnosis, assessment of severity, and initial antimicrobial therapy. Am Rev Respir Dis 148:1418–1426, 1993 *and* Bartlett JG, Breiman RF, Mandell LA, File TM: Community-acquired pneumonia in adults: Guidelines for management. Clin Infect Dis 26:811–838, 1998.

antibiotics, such as erythromycin, floxins (fluoroquinolones), tetracycline, and trimethoprim-sulfamethoxazole. One should **always** consider the current local resistance patterns when making empirical treatment decisions.

Duration of Therapy

Although the duration of treatment remains somewhat arbitrary, 10 days is usually recommended for common bacterial pneumonias, 10 to 14 days for those due to *M. pneumoniae* and *C. pneumoniae,* and 14 to 21 days for *Legionella* pneumonias (although comparative studies of different duration of treatment for *Legionella* are lacking). Changing from intravenous to oral therapy is generally carried out when the patient has been afebrile (less than 38° C) for 24 hours, with a respiratory rate less than 24 breaths per minute, oxygen saturation on room air greater than 95%, and chest radiograph stable or improving.

CLINICAL COURSE

Resolution

After the initiation of therapy for community acquired pneumonia, fever usually resolves in 2 to 4 days (more rapidly with *S. pneumoniae*). White cell elevation resolves after about 4 days. Abnormal clinical findings, however, may persist beyond 7 days in 20 to 40% of patients with *M. pneumoniae* and *C. pneumoniae* (with cough sometimes lasting up to 3 to 4 weeks). Resolution of chest radiographic findings generally lags behind clinical improvement. In patients younger than 50 years of age who are otherwise healthy, the radiograph clears completely by 4 weeks in only 60%. In older patients and those with bacteremia, chronic obstructive pulmonary disease, alcohol abuse, or other chronic illness, the radiograph clears by 4 weeks in only about 25% and may require 12 or more weeks for full resolution in these patients.

Nonresolution or Recurrence of Community Acquired Pneumonia

Failure of a community acquired pneumonia to resolve occurs in 13 to 26% of patients. This may be due to the nature of the infecting pathogen, the regimen selected for empirical therapy, anatomic factors affecting clearance of infection, or other noninfectious processes that may mimic community acquired pneumonia (Table 65–6). In a cohort of patients with nonresolving pneumonia, fiberoptic bronchoscopy was diagnostic in 86% of patients in whom a final diagnosis was made. Of those in whom no specific diagnosis was made, all had clear radiographs at 6 months.

When bronchoscopy is unrevealing, computed tomography of the chest might provide additional useful information. For example, it may more clearly define the

Table 65–6. Selected Causes of Apparent Empirical Antibiotic Failure

Anatomic factor	Endobronchial obstruction
Antibiotic-related factors	Altered drug metabolism
	Continued fever due to antibiotic (drug fever)
	Inadequate dosing
	Inadequate spectrum
	Poor absorption or penetration
Infectious factors	Empyema or lung abscess
	Resistant organism
	Unsuspected infection elsewhere
	Unusual organism*
Noninfectious factors	Acute respiratory distress syndrome
	Congestive heart failure
	Malignancy
	Pulmonary hemorrhage
	Recurrent aspiration

*Pneumocystis carinii, Mycoplasma tuberculosis, fungal, viral.

nature of a pulmonary infiltrate and can also be used to evaluate the presence of a loculated empyema, interstitial disease, cavitation, or adenopathy. Rarely, open lung biopsy may be required for definitive diagnosis.

Recurrent pneumonia is defined as the occurrence of two or more episodes of pneumonia separated by at least a 1-month period of radiographic and symptomatic resolution. This is most commonly associated with bronchiectasis, chronic obstructive pulmonary disease, and congestive heart failure, but bronchial obstruction and chronic aspiration must also be considered.

Bibliography

American Thoracic Society: Guidelines for the initial management of adults with community-acquired pneumonia: Diagnosis, assessment of severity, and initial antimicrobial therapy. Am Rev Respir Dis 148:1418–1426, 1993.
This article offers consensus-based guidelines for treatment of community acquired pneumonia.

Applebaum PC: Antimicrobial resistance in *Streptococcus pneumoniae:* An overview. Clin Infect Dis 15:77–83, 1992.
This article provides a summary of this increasingly important problem.

Bartlett JG, Mundy LM: Community-acquired pneumonia. N Engl J Med 333:1618–1624, 1995.
This article presents a concise review of the evaluation and treatment of community acquired pneumonia.

Bartlett JG, Breiman RF, Mandell LA, File TM: Community-acquired pneumonia in adults: Guidelines for management. Clin Infect Dis 26:811–838, 1998.
These new guidelines from the Infectious Disease Society of America (IDSA) endorses the use of fluoroquinolones in empirical therapy.

Chen DK, McGeer A, de Azavedo JC, et al: Decreased susceptibility of *Streptococcus pneumoniae* to fluoroquinolones in Canada. N Engl J Med 341:233–239, 1999.
This reported increasing resistance of S. pneumoniae to fluoroquinolones (from 0% in 1993 to 2.9% in 1997 and 1998 in adults) as fluoroquinolone use increased, probably as a result of selective pressure. This emphasizes the need for the practitioner to be aware of current local patterns of resistance when choosing empirical therapy for community acquired pneumonia.

Fang GD, Fine M, Orloff J, et al: New and emerging etiologies for community-acquired pneumonia with implications for therapy. Medicine 69:307–316, 1990.
Legionella *species and* Chlamydia pneumoniae *were the third and fourth most common causes of community acquired pneumonia in this Pittsburgh study of 359 patients.*

Feinsilver SH, Fein AM, Niederman MS, et al: Utility of fiberoptic bronchoscopy in nonresolving pneumonia. Chest 98:1322–1326, 1990.
This presents an analysis of situations in which bronchoscopy is likely to provide the correct diagnosis.

Fine MJ, Smith MA, Carson CA, et al: Prognosis and outcomes of patients with community-acquired pneumonia. JAMA 275:134–141, 1996.
This meta-analysis of 127 study cohorts reported outcomes in community acquired pneumonia.

Hasley PB, Albaum MN, Li Y-H, et al: Do pulmonary radiographic findings at presentation predict mortality in patients with community-acquired pneumonia? Arch Intern Med 156:2206–2212, 1996.
Multivariate analysis of a prospective cohort of 1906 ambulatory and hospitalized patients with community acquired pneumonia found that the presence of bilateral pleural effusions (but not having two or more lobes involved) was an independent predictor for increased 30-day mortality rate (relative risk = 2.8 with 95% confidence intervals of 1.4–5.8).

Mundy LM, Auwaerter PG, Oldach D, et al: Community-acquired pneumonia: Impact of immune status. Am J Respir Crit Care Med 152:1309–1315, 1995.
This article presents a 1-year study of the causes of community acquired pneumonia in 385 patients—221 were immunosuppressed.

Ortqvist A, Kalin M, Lejdeborn L, Lundberg B: Diagnostic fiberoptic bronchoscopy and protected brush culture in patients with community-acquired pneumonia. Chest 97:576–582, 1990.
Bronchoscopy identified the cause of community acquired pneumonia in 79% of patients.

Rein MF, Gwaltney JM, O'Brien WM, et al: Accuracy of Gram's stain in identifying pneumococci in sputum. JAMA 239:2671–2673, 1978.
This article presents an analysis of the utility of this test in diagnosing the cause of community acquired pneumonia.

66

Necrotizing Fasciitis and Related Soft Tissue Infections

Joseph H. Gorman, III
Robert C. Gorman
Jon B. Morris

Necrotizing fasciitis of an extremity was first described as "hospital gangrene" in 1871 by Joseph Jones, a Confederate Army surgeon. A review of more than 2600 cases of necrotizing fasciitis during the Civil War revealed a mortality of 46%. Despite modern advances in antibiotics and surgical therapy, the current mortality rate of this rapidly progressive disease remains virtually unchanged.

Two major factors contribute to the continued poor outcome of patients with serious soft tissue infections. The first and most important is *diagnostic delay.* Many studies have shown that prognosis and outcome depend on the time to diagnosis. Because of the benign and subtle way this deadly disease often presents, its diagnosis is delayed. Also contributing to this delay is the confusion created by the plethora of names of soft tissue infections, depending on the anatomic location and the causative organisms.

The second major cause of the high mortality in patients afflicted with necrotizing fasciitis is the high frequency of pre-existing systemic disease. Many of these patients are elderly and have diabetes mellitus, hypertension, peripheral vascular disease, malnutrition, alcoholism, or drug abuse.

SOFT TISSUE INFECTIONS

Layers of Soft Tissue

The "soft tissue" can be divided into four layers: (1) the skin, (2) subcutaneous tissue or superficial fascia, (3) deep fascia, and (4) muscle.

The *skin* is a two-layer membrane consisting of the epidermis and dermis. These layers are tightly fused above the subcutaneous tissue. When intact, the skin presents an almost impenetrable barrier to microorganisms. The blood supply of the skin runs horizontally at the junction of the dermis and subcutaneous tissue (Fig. 66–1).

The subcutaneous tissue or *superficial fascia* consists of fat and loose connective tissue between the dermis and the deep fascia. Most soft tissue infections occur at this level. The subcutaneous tissue is only loosely fixed to the deep fascia. This junction between superficial fascia and deep fascia is a potential space, called the *fascial cleft.* Infection can spread rapidly in this plane, impeded only where the superficial fascia is adherent to bone.

The *deep fascia* is a layer of strong connective tissue that overlies and separates major muscle groups. Where present, the deep fascia effectively deters the spread

745

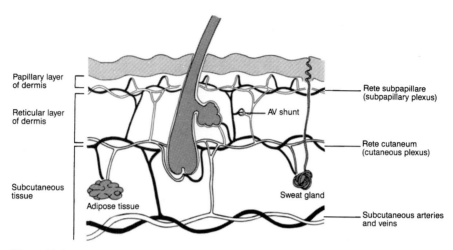

Figure 66–1. The dermal vasculature consists of superficial and deep plexuses that are connected by numerous communicating vessels. This rich blood supply is responsible for the skin being spared until relatively late in cases of necrotizing fasciitis, despite the infection-induced thromboses occurring in the vessels of the subcutaneous tissue. (From Ham's Histology, 9th ed. Philadelphia: J. B. Lippincott, 1987, p. 467.)

of infection from the superficial fascia into the muscle. Where absent, for example, in the face and scalp, superficial infections can quickly spread into deeper tissues.

Skeletal muscle is the deepest layer of soft tissue and is made up of long multinucleated cells enclosed in the sarcolema. Multiple cells are held together by a fibrous epimysium in which nerves and blood vessels run. The blood supply is extensive, with each muscle fiber receiving blood from several capillary beds. The richness of this blood supply is, in part, responsible for muscle's high resistance to infection.

Dividing the soft tissue into these four anatomic layers is helpful both descriptively and therapeutically. Infectious processes that affect the two most superficial layers are usually self-limited or can be treated effectively with nonsurgical therapy, that is, local hygiene and antibiotics. Infections of the deep fascia and muscle, which can spread rapidly and produce large areas of tissue destruction and severe sepsis, virtually always require surgical therapy.

Pathogenesis

Although soft tissue infections can originate from defects in systemic defenses, they more commonly develop as a result of *local damage* to the usually impenetrable corneal layer of the epidermis, which allows microorganisms to invade. This epidermal damage can be caused by trauma as subtle as that associated with tape removal, hair plucking, or occlusive dressings that retain water and macerate the skin. Although damage to the skin is, in most cases, necessary for soft tissue infection, it is by no means sufficient. Other factors such as the size of the bacterial inoculum, local host defense, and traumatic damage to surrounding tissues influence whether an infection results.

Normal tissue can be extremely resistant to infection. One study reported that injection of 2×10^9 *Staphylococcus aureus* was required to produce infections consistently in normal guinea pig soft tissues. Traumatized and underperfused tissue, however, needed a much smaller inoculation. All serious soft tissue infections require some combination of skin breakdown, microorganism inoculation, and tissue devitalization or compromised local defense (either by trauma or by systemic disease).

CLINICAL MANIFESTATIONS AND DIFFERENTIAL DIAGNOSIS

Skin Infections

Most infections confined to the skin are caused by streptococcal and staphylococcal infections. Examples of these types of infection, nonspecifically called pyodermas, include impetigo, ecthyma, and erysipelas (Table 66–1).

Impetigo consists of two forms, a bullous form caused by *S. aureus* and an epidemic form caused by group A *Streptococcus pyogenes*. Impetigo begins as a small red papule, progresses to a vesicle, and eventually ruptures, leaving its hallmark ulcer with a yellow crust. Untreated, the ulcer may last for months, but cellulitis and lymphangitis are rare. Glomerulonephritis is a feared complication of the streptococcal variant, and epidemic nephritis has been described after

Table 66–1. Soft Tissue Layers and Infections

LAYER INVOLVED	INFECTION	CAUSATIVE BACTERIA AND COMMENTS
Skin	Impetigo	*Staphylococcus* (bullous form) Group A *Streptococcus pyogenes* (epidemic form)
Skin	Ecthyma	Deeper form of impetigo
Skin	Erysipelas	*S. pyogenes*; has distinct violaceous border
Skin	Pyoderma	*Pseudomonas aeruginosa*; typically in immunocompromised hosts; "pyoderma gangrenosa" is a blue-red ulcer surrounding a necrotic base
Skin	Embolic ulcers	*P. aeruginosa* and *S. aureus*
Superficial fascia (Subcutaneous tissue)	Cellulitis	*S. pyogenes*, usually without preceding trauma; Gram-negative bacilli and anaerobes occur with cellulitis due to bowel perforations or animal/human bites (see text)
Fascial cleft and deep fascia	Necrotizing fasciitis	Clostridial species; mixed aerobes-anaerobes; *Vibrio* species, *S. pyogenes*
Muscle	Myonecrosis	Clostridial species and other mixed aerobes-anaerobes can produce subcutaneous gas; group A beta-hemolytic *S. pyogenes* (so-called flesh-eating bacteria) causes necrotizing fasciitis with myonecrosis
	Abscess	*S. aureus*; associated with less pain or systemic toxicity; usually occurs after trauma

outbreaks of impetigo. Prompt treatment with penicillin reduces the risk of nephritis.

Ecthyma is essentially a deeper form of impetigo. It also begins as a vesicle but produces a large "punched out" ulcer with a violaceous border and a thick eschar. Although superficial pseudomonal pyoderma in the immunocompromised patient can present with lesions that are similar to both impetigo and ecthyma, these lesions can usually be differentiated by their blue-green exudate and fruity odor. Embolic pustular lesions in patients with systemic *Pseudomonas aeruginosa* and *S. aureus* also present with ulcers similar to impetigo. These ulcers can usually be differentiated from impetigo, however, by their more purulent appearance and the clinical setting.

Erysipelas is a painful and indurated lesion with a sharply circumscribed border, commonly associated with a fever and leukocytosis. This type of infection is always confined to the skin, but if left untreated can progress to cellulitis or even necrotizing fasciitis. *S. pyogenes* is almost always the cause.

Superficial Fascial Infections

Infections of the superficial fascia without necrosis or suppuration are commonly referred to as *cellulitis*. Localized tenderness, heat, erythema, and swelling usually accompany systemic symptoms, such as malaise, fever, and chills. Obvious signs of skin trauma may be absent. Cellulitis can be differentiated from a more superficial erysipelas type of infection by the absence of a distinct indurated border. Clinically, the difference means little because the therapy for both is intravenous antibiotics. The most common inciting organism is *S. pyogenes,* and the infection is usually secondary to minor skin trauma.

Mixed Gram-negative cellulitis is characteristically seen as a result of a disruption in bowel mucosa or infected bite wounds. When the bowel is the source of infection, organisms include *Escherichia coli, Klebsiella, Enterobacter, Serratia,* and *Bacteroides* species. Human bites are often accompanied by *Eikenella corrodens* infection, whereas dog and cat bites may be complicated by *Pasteurella multocida* infections. Both these latter Gram-negative bacilli are sensitive to penicillin.

Fascial Cleft and Deep Fascial Infections

Once infecting organisms reach the potential space between the subcutaneous tissue and the deep fascia, the fascial cleft, they are free to spread horizontally along this potential space. In doing so, they produce a rapidly progressive and destructive infective process. Once the infection of this space is established, the disease follows two different courses, usually depending on the infecting organism and immune status of the host.

First, it can present as a rapidly progressive fulminant infection, with the skin developing large bullae containing black fluid and bacteria. Without therapy, these lesions progress to full-thickness burn-like eschars and lead to progressive shock and death.

Second, it may present more subtly with little superficial evidence of the underlying progressive spread of tissue destruction. With this presentation, the only clinical signs may be a faint line of erythema at the leading edge of the infection and a thin "dishwater" drainage. Pain may be out of proportion to the physical findings, or anesthesia may be present because of destruction of subcutaneous nerves. The limited skin findings in the second type of presentation are likely due to sparing of the superficial subcutaneous vascular plexus that runs horizontally at the interface between the dermis and subcutaneous tissue (see Fig. 66–1).

In both types of presentation, the deep fascia itself and the underlying muscle are not affected, but the majority of the subcutaneous tissue from the deep fascia "outward" is destroyed by a relentless devitalization created by infectious vascular thrombosis. Although most cases of necrotizing fasciitis require a mixture of synergistic bacteria to produce disease, *S. pyogenes* and *Clostridia* and *Vibrio* species can produce a fulminant course on their own. Crepitus secondary to gas production may extend widely beyond the areas of obvious infection. Gas production, however, is not pathognomonic for clostridial infections; other mixed synergistic aerobic and anaerobic infections may also produce gas but to a lesser extent.

Fournier's disease, first reported in 1883, is a necrotizing fasciitis of the scrotum and surrounding perineum, penis, and abdominal wall. The most common causes are local trauma, periurethral extravasation of infected urine, or perirectal abscess. Since the subcutaneous tissue is sparse, the scrotal skin is directly applied to the fascia and fasciitis in this area tends to spread rapidly and involve the skin early in the course. Because of this, diagnosis is usually made quickly and, as a result, the prognosis is somewhat better than that for necrotizing fasciitis in other locations.

Muscle Infections

Deep pyogenic muscle infections can be difficult to diagnose initially because they are often obscured by overlying normal skin and subcutaneous fat. These infections range in severity from a relatively benign staphylococcal abscess to life-threatening clostridial or *S. pyogenes* myonecrosis. Staphylococcal and clostridial infections are usually caused by trauma. Clostridial infections are more explosive at onset with a shorter incubation time (<24 hours), excruciating pain, extensive gas production, a sweet but foul odor, and rapidly progressive systemic toxicity. Staphylococcal abscesses are more indolent (incubation over 3 to 4 days), pain and gas production are much less pronounced, there is a more sour than sweet odor, and systemic toxicity is much more limited. *S. pyogenes* myonecrosis is virtually always accompanied by necrotizing fasciitis and severe systemic toxicity.

DIAGNOSIS AND MANAGEMENT

Approach to Diagnosis

The depth of a soft tissue infection correlates well with the severity of disease. Infections confined to the skin and subcutaneous tissues can almost always be treated successfully with either enteral or parenteral antibiotics. Most often these infections are caused by staphylococcal and streptococcal species that can be treated with penicillins or first-generation cephalosporins (see Chapter 14). What must be kept in mind is that all soft tissue infections represent a spectrum of disease, that is, even simple superficial infections, if treated inadequately, can progress to deeper, more life-threatening infections. In addition, the presentation of deep severe infections can at first be benign and thus deceiving. In fact, some instances of erysipelas are more impressive clinically than is early necrotizing fasciitis.

When necrotizing fasciitis presents with fulminating sepsis, large black bullae, and frankly necrotic skin, the diagnosis and clinical decision are straightforward. The patient should be hemodynamically stabilized and taken emergently to the operating suite for wide debridement of all infected tissue. The more difficult case is the patient in whom necrotizing fasciitis presents with only mild erythema, watery discharge, and tenderness (Fig. 66–2). Survival in this group of patients can be seriously affected by diagnostic delay.

In a retrospective study, 29 patients with operative findings indicating necrotizing fasciitis were divided into two groups. The first group received definitive surgical therapy within 24 hours of hospital admission, whereas surgical therapy in the second group was delayed for longer than 24 hours. Mortality in the early surgery group was 6% versus 25% in the late surgery group. The authors found that overreliance on negative diagnostic test results (fine needle aspiration and negative plain films), equivocal physical findings, and admission to a nonsurgical service were associated with a delayed correct diagnosis.

Although tests like fine needle aspiration and plain radiographs (looking for gas) are helpful when positive, negative studies cannot rule out deep necrotizing infections. Magnetic resonance imaging (MRI) and CT may increase sensitivity. CT is much more sensitive for gas than plain radiographs, but not all necrotizing infections produce gas. MRI may offer a diagnostic advantage by its capacity to delineate fascial planes well. One study correlating surgical findings with preoperative MRI examinations determined that T2-weighted images could reliably differentiate between infectious cellulitis and necrotizing fasciitis. It was found that cellulitis produced a dome-shaped *heterogeneous* area of high intensity with high-intensity streaking in the hypodermis. Necrotizing fasciitis was found to produce a well-defined *homogeneous* dome-shaped area of high intensity deep in the hypodermis. Although the use of MRI scanning holds promise, controlled outcome studies of its usefulness are lacking. Since it is relatively untested in a controlled manner, overreliance on it in certain clinical settings could be dangerous if surgery is delayed.

Treatment

A patient with significant risk factors for necrotizing fasciitis—such as diabetes mellitus, advanced age, peripheral vascular disease, malnutrition, immunosuppression, alcoholism, or drug abuse—with even equivocal clinical findings should promptly receive parenteral antibiotics and be observed closely (see Fig. 66–2). If symptoms do not improve in 12 hours, or if they worsen, surgical exploration is indicated. Parenteral antibiotics should be given that are effective against known or suspected pathogenic bacteria (see Table 66–1). For example, for Fournier's

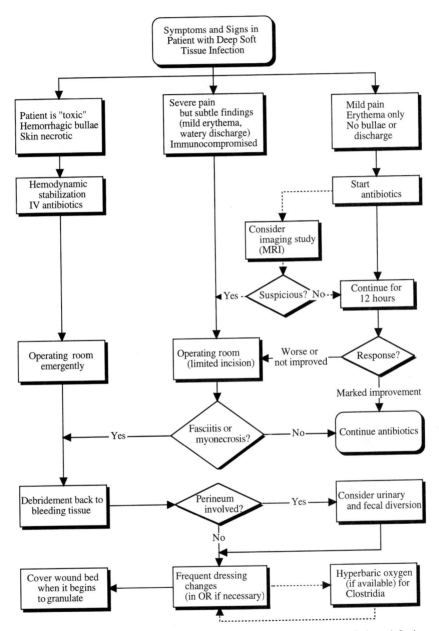

Figure 66–2. Diagnostic and therapeutic algorithm for management of deep soft tissue infections.

disease, appropriate coverage includes agents active against *Staphylococcus, Streptococcus,* enterococci, anaerobes, and Gram-negative aerobic bacilli. In addition, some clinicians advocate coverage of *S. pyogenes* necrotizing fasciitis with both penicillin (for bacteria in the growth phase) and clindamycin (for bacteria in the stationary phase).

Initial exploration consists of making several small incisions in the area in question. If necrotizing fasciitis is present, a clamp or probe passes with little resistance along the fascia. When this finding is present, the area of devitalized tissue should be widely debrided down to unaffected fascia. Although all devitalized tissue should be removed, as much of the overlying perfused skin should be preserved as possible. Because this infection usually spreads from the fascial cleft outward, the superficial horizontally running dermal blood supply is often maintained until late in the course. Some authors recommend guiding the extent of the excision by sending intraoperative frozen sections, but determination of coagulation necrosis by this method can be difficult and may lead to underestimation of the infection. It is usually safer to resect the devascularized subcutaneous tissue back to the point where bleeding begins.

In addition to sharp dissection, hydrotherapy with a pulse irrigator may help remove dead tissue while preserving as much viable, perfused tissue as possible. If the perineum is extensively affected, colonic diversion and superpubic bladder drainage to divert the fecal and urine streams should be strongly considered. The wound should be packed loosely with dry or damp gauze. For severe cases, dressing changes should take place daily in the operating room for wound inspection and further debridement. When the wound is completely clean and granulation tissue begins to form, dressing changes can take place in the ICU with sedation.

The benefit of adding hyperbaric oxygen (HBO) therapy to antibiotics and radical surgical debridement for treatment of necrotizing fasciitis is controversial. One study reported a decrease in mortality for necrotizing fasciitis from 66 to 23% and a decrease in the average number of debridements per patient from 3.3 to 1.2 when HBO was added to the treatment regimen. More recently, a second group reported that HBO had no effect on morbidity and mortality. Retrospective studies support both sides. Although HBO therapy may add slightly to the overall effectiveness of treatment, it is no replacement for aggressive surgical excision therapy.

In contrast to its controversial general adjunctive role, the use of HBO in the treatment of clostridial myonecrosis is more solidly established. One experimental study found that when HBO therapy was added to antibiotics and surgery, the survival rates for clostridial myonecrosis in a dog model of disease increased from 70 to 95%. When administered at 3 Atm for 90 minutes/day in addition to surgery and antibiotics, HBO has been found to identify the demarcation between viable and devitalized tissue more clearly. This allows surgeons to be more conservative during follow-up debridements.

SUMMARY

Soft tissue infections represent a wide spectrum of disease ranging from benign superficial infections to deep, rapidly progressive and life-threatening ones. Infections of the skin and subcutaneous tissue are usually easily treated with antibiotics alone, whereas infections of the fascial cleft and muscle almost always require surgical debridement in addition to antibiotics.

Symptoms and clinical presentation of both superficial and deep infections can be benign at first. A high index of suspicion must be maintained in susceptible patients who present with equivocal physical findings. Although imaging tests such as MRI and CT may be helpful in making a diagnosis, negative radiologic studies are no substitute for early surgical exploration in suspicious cases.

BIBLIOGRAPHY

Centers for Disease Control and Prevention: Nosocomial Group A Streptococcal infections associated with asymptomatic health-care workers—Maryland and California, 1997. MMWR 48:163–166, 1999.
This reports an unusual cluster of nosocomial Group A Streptoccal infections manifesting as wound or postpartum infections with toxic shock syndrome, which can be acquired from asymptomatic carriers.

Francis KR, Lamaute HR, Davis JM, Pizzi WF: Implications of risk factors in necrotizing fasciitis. Am Surg 59:304–308, 1993.
This article presents a study of the risk factors associated with the development of necrotizing fasciitis.

Green RJ, Dafoe DC, Raffin TA: Necrotizing fasciitis. Chest 110:219–229, 1996.
This is a concise review of etiology, microbiology, diagnosis, and treatment (with 105 references).

Lille ST, Sato TT, Engrav LH, et al: Necrotizing soft tissue infections: Obstacles in diagnosis. J Am Coll Surg 182:7–11, 1996.
This is a 10-year retrospective analysis of the risk factors associated with increased mortality in necrotizing fasciitis.

Riseman JA, Zamboni WA, Curtis LM: Hyperbaric oxygen therapy for necrotizing fasciitis reduces mortality and the need for debridement. Surgery 108:847, 1990.
This article discusses how hyperbaric therapy in conjunction with antibiotics and debridement reduces morbidity and mortality.

Roettinger W, Edgerton MT, Kurtz LD: Role of inoculation as a determinant of infection in soft tissue wounds. Am J Surg 126:354, 1973.
This is an analysis of the importance of the location of the initial infection site.

Sheridan RL, Shank ES: Hyperbaric oxygen treatment: A brief overview of a controversial topic. J Trauma 47:426–435, 1999.
This is a comprehensive review of hyperbaric oxygen therapy, including its use as an adjunct to treat necrotizing fasciitis.

Shupak A, Shoshani O, Goldenberg I, et al: Necrotizing fasciitis: An indication for hyperbaric oxygen therapy? Surgery 118:873–878, 1995.
This article presents a retrospective study of hyperbaric therapy suggesting that it does not appreciably alter outcome in necrotizing fasciitis.

Stamenkovic I, Lew PD: Early recognition of potentially fatal necrotizing fasciitis. The use of frozen section biopsy. N Engl J Med 310:1689–1693, 1984.
This article discusses how the rapid performance of frozen section for diagnosis can speed definitive therapy.

Tibbles PM, Edelsberg JS: Hyperbaric oxygen therapy. N Engl J Med 334:1642, 1996.
This is a review of hyperbaric therapy, its mechanisms, and indications for use.

67

Acute Neuromuscular Weakness

Shawn J. Bird
James W. Teener

The development of acute neuromuscular weakness is one of the more common neurologic syndromes requiring admission to the intensive care unit (ICU). Because ventilatory performance depends on skeletal muscle activity, hypercapnic respiratory failure often complicates acute neuromuscular disease. In addition, weakness of expiratory, pharyngeal, and laryngeal muscles causes difficulty in swallowing and coughing, both of which increase the risk of aspiration.

GENERAL APPROACH TO ACUTE NEUROMUSCULAR WEAKNESS

Monitoring for Respiratory Compromise

The same general approach to respiratory failure applies to all neuromuscular disorders. The vital capacity (VC) is the respiratory parameter to monitor because it reflects the mechanical function of the lungs and respiratory muscles. In addition, it can easily be performed at the bedside at frequent intervals to demonstrate the patient's trend. Measurement of negative inspiratory force (NIF) may give similarly useful information. Although oxygenation should also be monitored (by use of a pulse oximeter), abnormalities of arterial blood gases are an *insensitive* measure of respiratory muscle weakness because they are often a late abnormality. How frequently should the VC be measured is dependent on the disease and the rate of progression of weakness, for example, every 2 hours may be necessary in a myasthenic crisis.

Intubation and Assisted Ventilation

With close monitoring, endotracheal intubation should be performed as an elective procedure before precipitous respiratory collapse (and not in response to this complication). Intubation is warranted in patients with a VC less than or equal to 15 mL/kg or in those with a VC trending to 15 mL/kg plus clinical signs of respiratory fatigue, such as increasing respiratory rate, tachycardia, use of accessory muscles of respiration, and paradoxical motion of the diaphragm ("respiratory paradox"). Oropharyngeal weakness, inability to handle secretions, and risk of aspiration or airway obstruction also may necessitate intubation (Table 67–1). Facial weakness (and inability to get a good air seal) may make measurements of VC less reliable and, in these circumstances, the clinical signs and symptoms of respiratory fatigue are especially helpful. As long as the patient does not need an artificial airway to clear secretions or prevent airway occlusion, noninvasive

Table 67–1. Guidelines for Starting Assisted Ventilation* for Patients with Acute Neuromuscular Weakness

....

Ventilatory Ability (Vital Capacity [VC])*

VC <15 mL/kg body weight *or*
VC falling steadily toward 15 mL/kg with signs of respiratory distress or paradoxical respirations

Airway Integrity

Inability to clear oral secretions *or*
Intermittent aspiration *or*
Obstruction of airway in certain positions

Oxygenation

Same as with other medical conditions

....

*Consider use of noninvasive ventilation in patients who do not need an artificial airway to clear secretions.

ventilation may serve as a useful temporizing modality to provide assisted ventilation, particularly if the respiratory muscle weakness can be reversed quickly (see Chapters 2 and 77).

Differential Diagnosis

Acute neuromuscular weakness may occur in patients with known disorders, such as myasthenia gravis (MG). Patients with a pre-existing neuromuscular disorder, such as amyotrophic lateral sclerosis, may also present with acute weakness in the setting of another illness (such as infection). Frequently, however, the cause of the weakness is unknown. This necessitates a diagnostic work-up because pharmacologic and other interventions vary according to specific causes. In the differential diagnosis of acute neuromuscular weakness, certain clues from the history and examination can help to identify its cause (Table 67–2).

Electrophysiologic studies (nerve conduction studies and needle electromyography, which are collectively called electromyography [EMG]) are usually required to fully investigate these disorders. This is particularly true in individuals with an abnormal mental status (common in the ICU setting) who may not be able to cooperate with a motor and sensory examination. The electromyogram allows full investigation of the presence and nature of peripheral motor and sensory involvement. It can distinguish among disorders of nerve, muscle, and neuromuscular junction (Table 67–3) and provides prognostic information by quantifying the extent of nerve or muscle injury. Of the few indications for performing a nerve biopsy, suspected vasculitis is the most common. Muscle biopsy should likewise be reserved for when a specific cause is likely to be identified.

GUILLAIN-BARRÉ SYNDROME

Guillain-Barré syndrome (GBS) is the most common cause of acute flaccid quadriparesis in the United States. This disorder is an acute, inflammatory demyelinating polyneuropathy that is primarily characterized by progressive limb weakness and areflexia. In two thirds of those affected, it occurs 2 to 4 weeks after a viral-like

Table 67–2. Differential Diagnosis of Acute Neuromuscular Weakness

CAUSE BY LOCALIZATION	SUGGESTIVE CLINICAL FEATURES	IMPORTANT DIAGNOSTIC TESTS
Spinal Cord	Sensory level; early urinary symptoms; spares cranial muscles	See Appendix F for sensory dermatomes
Acute epidural compression (disc, abscess, tumor)	Local neck or radicular pain; history of trauma or tumor	MRI or myelogram
Other causes (transverse myelitis, cord hemorrhage)	History of trauma (hemorrhage)	MRI or myelogram; LP
Anterior Horn Cell (Motor Neuron)	Weakness without sensory or reflex loss	
Poliomyelitis or enterovirus-related polio syndrome	Antecedent systemic viral illness	LP
Paralytic rabies	History of animal bite	Viral cultures of CSF, saliva
Multiple Radiculopathies		
Carcinomatous or lymphomatous meningitis	History of carcinoma or lymphoma*	LP with cytologic studies
Lyme polyradiculoneuropathy	History of ECM; prodromal headache	LP; serum and CSF Lyme titer
Peripheral Neuropathy	Weakness with sensory and reflex loss	
Guillain-Barré syndrome†	Early loss of reflexes; facial weakness	LP; EMG
Acute intermittent porphyria‡	Associated gastrointestinal or psychiatric illness	Urine porphyrins
Massive intoxication (arsenic or thallium)‡	Illness with nausea, vomiting, and hypotension 2 to 3 wk prior	Serum arsenic or thallium
Critical illness polyneuropathy	Develops after period of critical illness	EMG
Neuromuscular Junction	Weakness without sensory or reflex loss	
Myasthenia gravis	Dysphagia, dysarthria, ptosis, diplopia	EMG, RNS; AChR antibodies
Botulism	Pupillary unreactivity	EMG, RNS
Hypermagnesemia	History of renal failure	Serum magnesium
Organophosphate toxicity	History of exposure	EMG, RNS
Persistent neuromuscular blockade	History of neuromuscular blocking agent	EMG, RNS
Myopathy	Weakness without sensory or reflex loss	
Hypokalemic myopathy	History of $\downarrow K^+$, diuretic use, or RTA	Serum K^+
Acute quadriplegic myopathy	History of use of steroids or NMBAs	EMG

*Neurologic disorder often the presenting feature.
†Demyelinating neuropathy.
‡Axonal neuropathy.
LP, lumbar puncture; EMG, nerve conduction studies and needle electromyography; RNS, repetitive nerve stimulation studies; ECM, erythema chronica migrans; NMBAs, neuromuscular blocking agents; RTA, renal tubular acidosis; MRI, magnetic resonance imaging; CSF, cerebrospinal fluid; AChR, acetylcholine receptor.

Table 67–3. Summary of Electrophysiologic Abnormalities

	DEMYELINATING NEUROPATHY (GUILLAIN-BARRÉ SYNDROME)	AXONAL NEUROPATHY	MYASTHENIA GRAVIS*	MYOPATHY
Nerve conduction studies				
Motor amplitudes	↓ †	↓	Normal	Normal– ↓
Sensory amplitudes	↓ †	↓	Normal	Normal
Repetitive stimulation studies	Normal	Normal	Decrement	Normal
Needle EMG studies				
MUP morphology	Normal– ↑	Normal– ↑	Normal– ↓	↓
MUP recruitment	↓	↓	Normal– ↑	↑

*This could also include other disorders of neuromuscular transmission (e.g., botulism).
†Specific features of demyelination (conduction block, marked conduction velocity slowing).
Decrement, reduction in motor response with successive stimuli at 2 to 3 Hz; EMG, electromyography; MUP, motor unit potential, recorded with needle electrode, referring to morphology, amplitude and duration; MUP recruitment, firing at a given muscle contractile force.

respiratory or gastrointestinal illness. Less commonly, it follows identifiable acute infections, including *Mycoplasma, Campylobacter jejuni,* and viruses (cytomegalovirus [CMV], Epstein-Barr virus [EBV], herpes simplex virus [HSV], and human immunodeficiency virus [HIV]). GBS also rarely follows surgery or certain immunizations. Recognition of this disorder is important because early detection of respiratory failure may limit complications and early therapy may limit nerve fiber loss and the extent of ultimate disability.

Clinical Presentation

The typical individual with GBS presents initially with distal limb numbness or tingling paresthesias, followed by ascending weakness of the limbs. Weakness usually predominates over any sensory findings on examination, although sensory symptoms such as paresthesia and pain are common. In addition to limb weakness, which often begins in the legs and then ascends to the arms, facial weakness is present in 40% of cases. Less commonly, bulbar involvement, manifested by dysarthria and dysphagia, and ocular involvement, with limitation of extraocular movements, are present. Respiratory motoneuron involvement occurs, and mechanical ventilation is required in 30% of cases. Deep tendon reflexes are almost always lost, particularly in weak limbs. Bladder involvement is rare, although urinary retention is sometimes seen. In certain individuals, the weakness may begin in the arms and descend into the legs, or respiratory and bulbar involvement may occur early.

The pace of progression can vary dramatically, from rapid (complete quadriparesis and intubation over 24 to 48 hours) to slow (progression over 3 or 4 weeks). In addition, respiratory decline may not always parallel the degree of limb weakness and must be followed carefully. Clinical recovery depends on the severity of the disorder, the degree of axonal loss, and early medical therapy. Predictors of *poor outcome* are patients older than 60 years of age, those with rapidly progressive disease (time to maximal deficit <7 days), and those with markedly reduced distal motor amplitudes on EMG studies. The mortality was 1 to 5% in several large series. Mortality is most often due to secondary complications, such as pulmonary embolism, sepsis, and other systemic disorders.

Pathogenetic Mechanism

The pathogenesis of GBS involves an autoimmune attack on the myelin of peripheral and cranial nerves. Clinical and experimental evidence support both humoral and cellular mechanisms in its pathogenesis. The dysfunction in nerve conduction is caused by segmental demyelination. This produces a relatively rapid and reversible block of conduction without loss of integrity of the underlying axon or nerve fiber. Varying degrees of axonal damage occur as a result of a "bystander effect" from the adjacent attack on myelin. How much axonal loss occurs is *the* critical factor that determines long-term disability.

Disorders that can mimic GBS should always be considered. The most important one is *acute cervical spinal cord compression.* Nearly half of patients with acute cervical myelopathy present with reduced reflexes and tone, as part of a spinal injury syndrome (see Chapter 98). The expected features of spasticity and hyperreflexia develop later. Epidural spinal cord compression due to tumor, abscess, or hematoma is important to recognize because it may be treatable by emergency decompression. One must suspect this entity on clinical grounds. Important clues to this diagnosis include absence of facial weakness in the setting of profound limb weakness, a level of sensory loss on the trunk (see sensory dermatomes in Appendix F), and prominent urinary incontinence. When in doubt, spinal cord imaging is necessary. Other acute causes of severe neuropathy are uncommon (see Table 67–2).

GBS is a clinical diagnosis, and often laboratory abnormalities become helpful only after the early critical period. Diagnosis is made by recognition of an acutely developing quadriparesis with sensory symptoms and hyporeflexia. Investigation of possible alternative diagnoses or initiation of therapy should not be delayed while waiting for diagnostic confirmation by laboratory studies. Only a few select laboratory tests are helpful in confirming the diagnosis, identifying possible associated illnesses, and assisting with prognosis.

Laboratory studies that may support the diagnosis are the cerebrospinal fluid (CSF) examination and electrophysiologic tests (EMG). The CSF protein is elevated infrequently in the first 48 hours, but most patients with GBS demonstrate this abnormality 7 to 10 days into their illness. There are usually only a few cells in the spinal fluid. If there are more cells present (particularly >50 white blood cells/μL), GBS associated with HIV seropositivity or, less commonly, carcinomatous meningitis or Lyme disease should be considered. Nerve conduction studies play the primary role in identifying specific features of demyelination that are characteristic of GBS (see Table 67–3). As with CSF analysis, however, these specific features of demyelination are often not seen within the first several days of the illness but appear in most patients after 1 week.

If the possibility of acute axonal neuropathy secondary to vasculitis is a consideration, biopsy of nerve or muscle, or both, may be indicated. Otherwise, biopsy is rarely helpful in the setting of GBS. Other laboratory abnormalities may include an occasional mild elevation in sedimentation rate or lymphopenia from a preceding viral or mycoplasmal infection. Stool cultures for *C. jejuni* may identify this associated infection in patients with a preceding diarrheal illness. Many of these patients have severe or abrupt onset of disease. Rarely Lyme disease may present with an acute neuropathy, but this is more typically a polyradiculopathy rather than classic GBS. Most importantly, HIV infection may be associated with development of GBS. All patients with a CSF pleocytosis or with risk factors for HIV (and perhaps all those with GBS) should have serum tested for HIV seropositivity. GBS occurs in HIV-seropositive patients without acquired immunodeficiency syndrome. The prognosis or treatment of GBS in the setting of HIV does not differ from that without HIV infection.

Therapy

Treatment includes the medical management of both the respiratory failure and other complications of paralysis and specific immunotherapeutic intervention. The latter includes plasma exchange (PE) (also called apheresis) or intravenous immunoglobulin (IVIG). Currently most patients with GBS undergo a course of PE or IVIG. PE has been established as effective in GBS in three large randomized controlled trials. In a North American GBS-PE trial, severely affected patients treated with PE, on average, were able to walk unassisted 3 months earlier and required mechanical ventilation half as long as those who were not treated with PE. PE should be started as soon as possible in those unable to walk unassisted or those with respiratory involvement because irreversible nerve loss may occur with delays. Early relapse is seen following PE in 10% of patients and is clustered in the month after first treatment. If this occurs, further improvement will be seen after additional PE treatments.

Therapy with IVIG is an alternative to PE. Three randomized, placebo-controlled trials demonstrated its comparable efficacy to PE. Whether the potential benefit of a combination of these two therapies warrants the added risks and cost is uncertain at this time (Table 67–4). Early relapse after IVIG administration may also be seen. Other immunosuppressive agents, including corticosteroids, have not been demonstrated to be efficacious and are not recommended.

Autonomic abnormalities are common in patients with GBS in the ICU setting. Sinus tachycardia and hypertension, the most commonly encountered forms of dysautonomia, usually require no treatment. Hypertension ($>220/120$ mm Hg) may need treatment. This should be carried out with caution, however, because hypertension in this setting is mostly paroxysmal, and treatment may result in periods of marked *hypotension.* Orthostatic hypotension usually responds to intravascular volume expansion. Electrocardiographic changes with ST-T segment and T-wave abnormalities may be seen and an occasional patient experiences heart block requiring pacemaker placement. Most of these changes, however, are temporary and require no treatment.

Neuropathic pain is a common problem early in the course of GBS. Such pain is often deep and achy and involves the truncal musculature, extending into the limbs. It probably reflects inflammatory disease in the nerve roots. This pain can

Table 67–4. Plasma Exchange and Intravenous Immunoglobulin in
Guillain-Barré Syndrome and Myasthenia Gravis

	PLASMA EXCHANGE	INTRAVENOUS IMMUNOGLOBULIN
Major limitations	Inadequate venous access Hemodynamically unstable patient Availability* Temporary effect in MG	Contraindicated in IgA deficiency Renal failure Severe CHF Temporary effect in MG National shortage of IVIG
Common complications	Hypotension Catheter-related (sepsis, clot, hemorrhage at the site, pneumothorax during insertion) Transient coagulopathy (due to loss of clotting factors)	Headache, chills, fever, hypertension or hypotension during the infusion Fluid overload
Standard treatment	PE of 250 mL/kg total plasma volume over 4–6 exchanges	IVIG 400 mg/kg/day for 5 days
Cost of total course†	$4400–9000	$5600–$10,000

*Should be available in all tertiary centers.
†Treatment costs only, exclusive of hospitalization.
MG, myasthenia gravis; CHF, congestive heart failure; IVIG, intravenous immunoglobulin; PE, plasma exchange.

be severe and occasionally is the overwhelming symptom at presentation. It should be treated aggressively because it often resolves over days to weeks. Later in the course of disease, patients may experience neuropathic pain of a different sort related to the underlying nerve injury. This pain is usually burning, dysesthetic pain akin to that seen in patients with diabetic neuropathy and may be treated effectively with tricyclic antidepressants.

MYASTHENIA GRAVIS

MG is an autoimmune disease in which antibodies directed against skeletal muscle acetylcholine receptors (AChR) interfere with neuromuscular transmission and produce weakness. MG should be suspected in any patient who has weakness without sensory abnormalities (see Table 67–2). Patients typically describe weakness that fluctuates and often worsens with repetitive activity. Ocular and bulbar muscles are most commonly involved, but any pattern of weakness may be seen.

Myasthenic Crisis

Neuromuscular respiratory failure caused by MG is called a *myasthenic crisis*. It may be precipitated in patients with stable myasthenia by a variety of factors including infection, surgery, medications, or tapering of immunosuppression. A number of medications can increase weakness in MG and should be avoided or used with great caution in myasthenic patients (Table 67–5).

Table 67–5. Drugs to Be Avoided or Used with Caution in Myasthenia Gravis

Antibiotics	**Psychotropic**
Aminoglycosides	Lithium
Lincomycin	Chlorpromazine
Clindamycin	**Rheumatologic Agents**
Polymyxin B	
Colistin	D-Penicillamine
Colistimethate	Chloroquine
Bacitracin	**Other**
Antimalarials	Sodium lactate
Chloroquine	Magnesium sulfate
Quinine	Neuromuscular blocking agents
Cardiovascular Agents	Ophthalmic beta-blockers
Quinidine	**Problematic at High Doses**
Procainamide	Opioids
Bretylium	Muscle relaxants
Verapamil	Respiratory depressants
Beta-blockers	CNS depressants
Lidocaine	Corticosteroids

CNS, central nervous system.

Patients in myasthenic crisis typically experience increasing generalized weakness, although occasionally they present with respiratory insufficiency out of proportion to their limb weakness. Severe bulbar weakness that produces dysphagia and aspiration often complicates the respiratory failure. The recognition of a crisis is relatively straightforward in a known myasthenic patient.

Diagnosis

A number of measures can be employed to confirm the diagnosis of MG (Table 67–6). In approximately 80% of patients with generalized myasthenia, elevated

Table 67–6. Suggested Laboratory Tests in Suspected Myasthenia Gravis

DIAGNOSTIC STUDIES*	OTHER HELPFUL STUDIES
Edrophonium (Tensilon) test (90%)†	Chest computed tomography for thymoma
AChR antibody titer (85%)	Thyroid function studies
EMG, RNS (80%)	Autoimmune screen (if clinical suspicion)
Single fiber EMG (>90%)‡	Screen for conditions that may complicate steroid therapy§

*Parenthesis indicates approximate sensitivity of test in generalized MG.
†Requires ptosis or other observable muscle weakness.
‡Useful if other diagnostic studies are negative.
§Examples include tuberculosis, diabetes, peptic ulcer disease, hypertension, and renal disease.
AChR, acetylcholine receptor; EMG, nerve conduction studies and needle electromyography; RNS, repetitive nerve stimulation studies.

levels of antibody directed against the acetylcholine receptor can be measured. Pharmacologic and electrophysiologic testing may confirm the diagnosis. Edrophonium (Tensilon) is a short-acting acetylcholinesterase inhibitor that is administered intravenously. It should rapidly improve ocular misalignment, ptosis, or other weakness if it is due to myasthenia. In patients with ocular abnormalities, the test has a sensitivity of approximately 90%. Atropine should be available to treat the rare complications of hypotension and bradycardia.

The classic finding on EMG testing of myasthenic patients is a decrement in compound muscle action potential amplitude with recurrent stimulation (see Table 67–3). A decrement greater than 10 to 15% is seen in approximately 85% of patients who have moderately severe generalized MG. Single-fiber EMG is a more sensitive technique for examining neuromuscular transmission. Ninety percent of patients with even mild myasthenia have abnormal single-fiber EMG studies.

Myasthenia may be associated with other autoimmune disorders, particularly autoimmune thyroid disease. Systemic lupus erythematosus, rheumatoid arthritis, pernicious anemia, ulcerative colitis, pemphigus, Sjögren's syndrome, and autoimmune ovarian failure have also been reported to coexist with MG. Ten percent of patients with MG have thymoma. Most cases are benign, but occasionally malignant thymoma is identified. All patients with a new diagnosis of MG should undergo computed tomography of the chest.

Therapy

The treatment options for the patient who is experiencing increasing weakness because of MG are dependent on the severity and pace of deterioration. Initially, patients are treated with increasing doses of acetylcholinesterase inhibitors, such as pyridostigmine. At high doses, complications due to muscarinic cholinergic side effects are frequently encountered, and glycopyrrolate or other atropine-like drugs are needed to treat the diarrhea and excessive secretions. A potential complication of high-dose acetylcholinesterase inhibitor therapy is *cholinergic crisis.* This rare phenomenon of increasing weakness is typically encountered in patients receiving acetylcholinesterase inhibitors intravenously or intramuscularly rather than orally. If a cholinergic crisis is suspected, acetylcholinesterase inhibitors should be discontinued.

When weakness becomes severe and respiratory failure threatens, treatment with acetylcholinesterase inhibitors alone is not sufficient. Treatment modalities for myasthenic crisis include corticosteroids, PE, and IVIG (see Table 67–4). PE is considered the therapy of choice for myasthenic crisis. Since improvement with corticosteroids usually occurs after a several week delay, they are used as an adjunct to PE. Corticosteroids, however, can exacerbate weakness in the first 2 weeks of their administration, which mandates careful observation of respiratory function.

One particular danger in myasthenic crisis is that generalized weakness can often mask the usual signs of respiratory distress, such as accessory muscle use. Also, weak respiratory muscles may fatigue, causing precipitous respiratory failure. A patient at risk for respiratory failure should have VC monitored every 2 to 4 hours. Elective intubation or noninvasive ventilation should be considered as the VC approaches 15 mg/kg body weight (see Table 67–1). Once a patient is receiving assisted ventilation, dosages of acetylcholine esterase inhibitors can be reduced to exclude cholinergic crisis as a cause of the increasing weakness and to reduce respiratory tract secretions. While intubated, the patient should have the NIF and VC measured daily. As the NIF nears -20 cm H_2O and VC rises to 10 to 15 mL/kg, weaning can start. Another sign of recovery is when intubated patients can lift their head off the bed. Patients who have experienced myasthenic crisis typically have relatively severe disease and require long-term immunosuppressive therapy.

NEUROMUSCULAR COMPLICATIONS OF CRITICAL ILLNESS

Critical illness polyneuropathy, persistent neuromuscular blockade, and acute quadriplegic myopathy are three distinct syndromes that may develop in critically ill patients as a consequence of the illness or its treatment (Table 67–7). Nerve and muscle dysfunction are common in ICU patients and may result in difficulty weaning from mechanical ventilation and a prolonged ICU stay.

Critical Illness Polyneuropathy

Critical illness polyneuropathy (CIP) is a sensory-motor axonal nerve disorder that may develop in the setting of the systemic inflammatory response syndrome (SIRS) and usually its severe form, sepsis (see Chapter 8, Table 8–1). The pathophysiology of CIP is uncertain, since evidence to support drugs, toxins, nutritional deficiencies, autoimmune disorders, or specific infectious agents as causative is lacking.

On clinical examination, those with CIP have limb weakness, atrophy, and reduced reflexes. Sensory loss can be demonstrated in patients able to cooperate

Table 67–7. Critical Illness Polyneuropathy and Acute Quadriplegic Myopathy

	CRITICAL ILLNESS POLYNEUROPATHY	ACUTE QUADRIPLEGIC MYOPATHY
Risk factors	Sepsis or SIRS	NMBAs or steroids, or both
Clinical findings	Sensory and motor deficits	Purely motor
Creatine phosphokinase	Normal	Normal to slightly ↑
Pathology of biopsied tissue	Nerve—axonal loss	Nerve—normal
	Muscle—denervation	Muscle—patchy myosin loss; minimal necrosis
Clinical course	Slow recovery	Often rapid recovery
Nerve conduction studies	↓ Sensory and motor potential amplitudes	Normal sensory potentials
		↓ ↓ Motor potential amplitudes
Spontaneous activity	Yes; often prominent	None or sparse
MUP morphology	Normal to long-large	↓ Amplitude and ↓ duration
MUP recruitment	Increased recruitment ratio (neurogenic)	Early full (myopathic)
Muscle excitability	Normal	Absent or ↓ ↓

SIRS, systemic inflammatory response syndrome; NMBAs, neuromuscular blocking agents; MUP, motor unit potential.

with the examination. Failure to wean from the ventilator, a feature common to other neuromuscular disorders in this setting, may be the first recognized manifestation. The severity of the neuropathy correlates with the total time of critical illness. Those who survive the critical illness with mild to moderate neuropathy recover peripheral nerve function fully over months. Those with severe neuropathy, requiring axonal regeneration for recovery, have either no recovery or a significant persistent deficit.

EMG studies typically demonstrate reduced motor and sensory response amplitudes, without evidence of demyelination (see Table 67–3). Phrenic nerve conduction studies are notable for reduced or absent responses bilaterally. Needle EMG examination of the chest wall muscles or the diaphragm may also demonstrate denervation and can confirm the presumed neuromuscular cause of the failure to wean from the respirator.

Persistent Neuromuscular Blockade

The effects of *neuromuscular blocking agents* (NMBAs) used in the ICU can persist in individual patients, creating unexpected weakness and inability to wean from mechanical ventilation. Metabolic derangements, particularly renal failure, can slow the clearance of certain neuromuscular blocking agents and their active metabolites, producing prolonged paralysis (see Chapter 4, Table 4–7). This effect is easily detected with nerve conduction studies with repetitive stimulation. Prolonged blockade may last for days and should be considered in any patient who remains weak after discontinuation of NMBA. Weakness should not persist beyond 2 weeks after stopping the blocking agent, however, and typically lasts for only a few days. There is no specific treatment.

Acute Quadriplegic Myopathy

Neuromuscular blocking agents and corticosteroids have been strongly linked to the development of a myopathy in the setting of critical illness, that is, acute quadriplegic myopathy (AQM). This myopathy, however, may also occur with the same risk factors as CIP, particularly sepsis (see Table 67–7). In addition to AQM, other names of this syndrome include *acute myopathy with myosin-deficient fibers* and *critical illness myopathy*. The typical clinical picture of AQM is that of a patient who is intubated and has been treated with corticosteroids and NMBAs. As the medical crisis resolves, it becomes apparent that the patient is quadriplegic or quadriparetic. Some patients have only mild weakness, but many are severely affected, and weaning from the ventilator is often delayed because of the myopathy. Sensation is spared and reflexes are decreased in parallel with the decrease in strength. After patients recover from the acute illness, there is usually improvement in strength within 1 to 3 months.

Serum creatine phosphokinase levels are most often normal or minimally elevated. Nerve conduction studies in AQM reveal diminished motor nerve amplitudes in the setting of normal sensory response amplitudes. Needle EMG often reveals myopathic features (see Table 67–3). Muscle biopsy may reveal loss of myosin adenosine triphosphatase staining, and electron microscopy confirms loss of myosin thick filament. It has recently been shown that muscle is electrically inexcitable in AQM. Clinical recovery of patients parallels recovery of muscle membrane excitability, indicating that weakness in AQM is primarily the result of muscle membrane inexcitability, although myosin loss may also contribute.

BIBLIOGRAPHY

Dalakas MC: Intravenous immune globulin therapy for neurologic diseases. Ann Intern Med 126:721–730, 1997.
This is an excellent review of the mechanism, side effects, and uses of IVIG in GBS, myasthenia, and other neurologic disorders.

Drachman DB: Myasthenia gravis. N Engl J Med 330:1797–1810, 1994.
This is an excellent review of the basic science as well as the clinical aspects of MG.

Guillain-Barré Study Group: Plasmapheresis and acute Guillain-Barré syndrome. Neurology 35:1096–1104, 1985.
This article presents a randomized controlled trial of PE versus conventional treatment in 245 patients with GBS that firmly established PE as efficacious.

Hughes RA: Management of acute neuromuscular paralysis. J R Coll Physicians Lond 32:254–259, 1998.
This is an excellent review of the differential diagnosis and management of weakness and neuromuscular respiratory failure.

Hund E: Myopathy in critically ill patients. Crit Care Med 27:2544–2547, 1999.
This is a recent, concise review of the topic, with emphasis on the types of myopathic changes seen on muscle biopsies (with 69 references).

Hund EF, Borel CO, Cornblath DR, et al: Intensive management and treatment of severe Guillain-Barré syndrome. Crit Care Med 21:433–446, 1993.
This review summarizes the presentation, complications, and therapeutic approaches to the severely weak GBS patient.

Lacomis D, Petrella JT, Giuliani MJ: Causes of neuromuscular weakness in the intensive care unit: A study of ninety-two patients. Muscle Nerve 21:610–617, 1998.
This is a retrospective review that found 42% of patients had acute myopathy and 13% acquired CIP.

Ng NKP, Howard RS, Fish DR, et al: Management and outcome of severe Guillain-Barré syndrome. Q J Med 88:243–250, 1995.
This study details the ICU experience with 79 patients with GBS, with data on status on admission, specifics of treatment, and the nature and incidence of significant complications.

Plasma Exchange–Sandoglobulin Guillain-Barré Trial Group: Randomized trial of plasma exchange, intravenous immunoglobulin, and combined treatments in Guillain-Barré syndrome. Lancet 349:225–230, 1997.
This trial involving 383 patients established that IVIG and PE are both effective in GBS.

Rich MM, Teener JW, Raps EC, et al: Muscle is electrically inexcitable in acute quadriplegic myopathy. Neurology 46:731–736, 1996.
This article demonstrates the unique physiology of patients with AQM.

Stangel M, Hartung H-P, Marx P, et al: Side effects of high-dose intravenous immunoglobulins. Clin Neuropharmacol 20:385–391, 1997.
This is a review of the adverse effects of intravenous immunoglobulins and how one can minimize these risks (with 43 references).

Van der Meche FGA, Schmitz PIM, and the Dutch Guillain-Barré Study Group: A randomized trial comparing intravenous immunoglobulin and plasma exchange in Guillain-Barré syndrome. N Engl J Med 326:1123–1129, 1992.
This article discusses a trial of 147 patients who received either PE or IVIG in which both groups did as well.

68

Brain Death and Management of Potential Organ Donors

Joseph B. Schellenberg
Paul N. Lanken

Patients who sustain brain injury from various causes may have irreversible damage to their central nervous system. When the injury is sufficiently severe to damage the cortex and brainstem with disruption of normal responsive and homeostatic mechanisms, the patient may meet the criteria for "brain death" (death by neurologic criteria). All states in the United States accept brain death as legally valid, and most have statutes modeled after The Uniform Determination of Death Act. The latter states "An individual who has sustained either (1) irreversible cessation of circulatory and respiratory functions, or (2) irreversible cessation of all functions of the entire brain, including the brain stem, is dead. A determination of death must be made in accordance with accepted medical standards." This chapter discusses those accepted medical standards and how to test for them.

Making a timely and accurate diagnosis of brain death is an essential skill of intensivists. It is important for several reasons: (1) caring for the family's needs, (2) allocating limited intensive care unit (ICU) resources fairly and wisely, and (3) providing opportunities for organ donation. In general, it requires a review of the patient's medical history, two neurologic examinations, and the use of a confirmatory diagnostic test (Fig. 68–1).

As a rule, hospitals have incorporated these elements into their policies and protocols concerning brain death. One should always refer to the institutional policy when diagnosing brain death because it should be written to take into account the applicable laws and local practices.

DETERMINATION OF BRAIN DEATH (Fig. 68–1)

Medical History

The initial evaluation of the potentially brain dead patient should focus on the patient's history. There should be an identifiable cause for the patient's condition, such as head trauma, cerebrovascular accident, or prolonged hypoxemia-ischemia as in cardiopulmonary arrest. Next, the clinician must exclude reversible causes of coma, for example, underlying toxic or metabolic causes. Any treatable metabolic causes in the absence of an intrinsic cerebral pathologic condition must be corrected before continuing the evaluation. These include gross physiologic disturbances, such as hypothermia, hypoxemia, or hypotension; metabolic derangements, such as acidosis, hypo- or hyperglycemia, renal or hepatic encephalopathy; and serious electrolyte disorders, such as hypo- or hypernatremia and hypo- or hypercalcemia.

Four Steps for Determining Brain Death in Adults

Step 1. Confirm Compatible History

Confirm plausible mechanism of injury (trauma, stroke, prolonged hypoxic–ischemic event)

Step 2. Rule Out Complicating Conditions

Rule out hypothermia (core temperature must be > 32° C)
Rule out circulatory shock
Rule out persistent effects of neuromuscular blocking agent (if patient received such an agent)
Rule out other reversible causes of coma or apparent coma (e.g., drug intoxication, metabolic causes, or locked-in syndrome)

Step 3. Perform Two Neurologic Examinations Showing No Brain Function

No response to painful stimuli
No movement except spinal reflexes
No pupillary reflexes
No corneal reflexes
No oculocephalic reflex
No oculovestibular reflex
No gag reflex
No ventilatory response to hypercapnia
 (see Apnea Test, Table 68–1)

Step 4. Perform a Confirmatory Test

Electroencephalogram (EEG) showing isoelectric tracing
Four-vessel cerebral angiogram showing absence of flow
Radionuclide perfusion brain scan showing absence of flow

Figure 68–1. Recommended steps in making a brain death determination (see text for details). Intervals between two neurologic examinations should be at least 24 hours in cases of hypoxic-ischemic brain injury and at least 12 hours in other types of brain injury; the second examination can be omitted if the four-vessel cerebral angiogram or perfusion brain scan confirms no flow to the brain. Consistent with policies of many hospitals, a confirmatory test, usually an electroencephalogram, is recommended for *all* patients undergoing brain death determination.

Drug overdose or toxic exposure should always be ruled out in patients presenting to the ICU in coma and who otherwise appear brain dead. In most cases, if a patient has received sedatives or analgesics before the evaluation for brain death, adequate time (usually four times the excretion half-life of the substance, but one must take into account hepatic or renal dysfunction when present) for elimination of the substance must occur. If plasma levels of the potentially confounding drug correlate well with its degree of drug-induced central nervous system depression, one can measure plasma concentration of the involved substance to determine if the level of the drug is clinically significant in causing the patient's coma.

Particular attention must be given to patients in whom neuromuscular blocking agents were used because some may have prolonged neuromuscular blockade due to their underlying disease processes, altered renal or hepatic elimination, or coadministration of potentiating drugs (see Chapter 4). A peripheral nerve stimulator should be used in all patients undergoing evaluation for brain death who received neuromuscular blocking agents. A sustained muscle contraction in response to a 5 second tetanic stimulus may be more informative than the usual train-of-four response in determining the integrity of the neuromuscular response.

Physical Examination in Brain Death Determination

The examination of the potentially brain dead patient focuses particular attention on the absence of brainstem reflexes. Because of the critical role of these examinations in brain death determinations, many hospitals mandate consultation with a neurologist to perform these examinations when patients are not already on a neurologic or neurosurgical service.

Pupillary reflexes should be assessed in a dimmed room with the patient's eyes initially closed. One eye is then opened and a bright light applied. The pupil should be observed for 30 seconds and then the test should be repeated in the opposite eye. A normal response is brisk constriction of the pupil. In brain death, the pupils must be nonreactive ("fixed") but not necessarily dilated.

The *corneal reflex* can be assessed by lightly brushing the cornea with a sterile cotton swab or gauze. A normal response is a blink to the stimulus. In brain death, there should be no response. Excessive abrasion of the cornea should be avoided if the patient is a potential cornea donor.

The *oculocephalic reflex* (doll's eye reflex) assesses vestibular and proprioceptor responses. In an intact reflex, as the patient's head is rotated laterally from one side to the other, the patient's eyes move in the opposite direction. In a brain dead patient, the eyes remain fixed with the lateral turn. This maneuver should not, however, be performed in patients with potentially unstable cervical fractures.

Like the oculocephalic reflex, the *oculovestibular reflex* (cold caloric reflex) assesses vestibular and midbrain function. Since it generally provides a stronger stimulus of the two reflexes, it is preferred in determinations of brain death. The external auditory canals should first be inspected to ensure that the tympanic membranes are intact and unobstructed. The head should be midline and elevated at 30 degrees to allow for maximal stimulation of the horizontal semilunar canal. A soft catheter is inserted into the canal and the ear is slowly (20 seconds or more) irrigated with at least 50 mL of iced water. The eyes are observed for approximately 1 minute. If the reflex is intact, both eyes deviate toward the irrigated ear. In a brain dead patient, the eyes do not move at all. Any other response is not consistent with brain death.

The *apnea test* is used to confirm brain death clinically only when the aforementioned preconditions have been met and when all other brainstem reflexes are absent. Since it requires an intact phrenic nerve and functioning diaphragm, it should not be performed if patients have a high cervical fracture or neuromuscular disease impairing diaphragmatic function. Maintaining adequate oxygenation during the test and documenting a rise in $Paco_2$ to a level that would stimulate respiration in an intact patient is critical to performing a successful apnea test (Table 68–1).

Table 68–1. Steps in Performing the Apnea Test

1. Preoxygenate patient with 100% oxygen for at least 15 min.
2. Confirm that arterial pH $\leq$7.44 and $Paco_2$ = 36–45 mm Hg at the start of the test.
3. Disconnect patient from the ventilator and give supplemental oxygen to keep Sao_2 at 98%. (This can be done by T-piece or, preferably, by delivering oxygen at 2–6 L/min via a 14 Fr suction catheter [with its suction port taped closed] inserted into the endotracheal tube until it is 1–2 cm above the tip of the endotracheal tube.)
4. Observe patient for spontaneous respiratory efforts for 10 min.
5. After 10 min, obtain an arterial blood gas sample and place patient back on mechanical ventilation ($Paco_2$ can be expected to rise 2–4 mm Hg/min in the absence of ventilation).
6. $Paco_2$ at the end of the observation period should be at least 60 mm Hg. If not, repeat the test with a longer observation period.
7. For patients who lack a normal response to elevated $Paco_2$ (chronic obstructive pulmonary disease with baseline hypercapnia or obesity hypoventilation syndrome), follow the hospital policy dealing with such circumstances or perform a confirmatory test without attempting the apnea test.

Note: The apnea test should be performed only after the absence of other brainstem reflexes has been documented on both the first and second neurologic examinations because it may aggravate hemodynamic instability.

Confirmatory Testing in Brain Death

Certain techniques have been established as confirmatory tests for brain death. Under certain conditions, they may also expedite the diagnosis of brain death in potential organ donors.

Electroencephalography in brain death is characterized by an isoelectric recording referred to as electrocerebral inactivity or electrocerebral silence. An isoelectric recording can also occur in patients who have received toxic levels of central nervous system depressants and subsequently fully recover. This emphasizes the importance of eliminating the possibility of potentially confounding conditions (see Fig. 68–1) before establishing the diagnosis of brain death. The recording must be made in accordance with the appropriate specifications and be performed under the supervision of a neurologist familiar with these protocols. Precautions should taken if local ICU environments prove to have enough electrical interference to prevent a true isoelectric recording from being obtained.

Cerebral evoked responses, including brainstem auditory evoked responses recorded after auditory click and somatosensory evoked responses recorded after median nerve stimulation, assess whether certain brainstem pathways are intact. These tests show promise as adjunctive tests in predicting poor outcome in comatose patients after hypoxic-ischemic injuries (see Chapter 69), but their usefulness as a confirmatory test for brain death remains to be established.

Not surprisingly, the absence of cerebral blood flow strongly correlates with clinical brain death and pathologic evidence of brain necrosis. Brain blood flow can be assessed by a number of imaging methods, but only angiography and radionuclide scanning have been established as confirmatory tests to determine brain death.

Failure to visualize the intracranial vessels after intravenous injection of radiocontrast is considered to be the gold standard confirmatory test for the diagnosis of brain death. Unfortunately, the cost of the study, the risk of transporting the patient to the radiology department, and the potential nephrotoxicity of the contrast limit its routine use. Radionuclide imaging with technetium (Tc^{99m}) or iodine (I-123)-based agents is safe, accurate, and can be performed at the bedside of the critically ill patient. Because its resolution is less than conventional angiography, it really can only assess for the presence or absence of cerebral cortical flow and not brainstem flow. Under most conditions, however, when used in conjunction with the findings of the clinical examination (see Fig. 68–1), absence of nuclide uptake within the brain is accepted as diagnostic for brain death.

Cautions When Making Brain Death Determinations

When making the diagnosis of brain death, it is important to avoid confounders of the neurologic examination. For example, fixed pupils can occur from anticholinergic drugs (mydriasis), opioids (meiosis), or pre-existing medical conditions, such as prostheses. The oculocephalic and oculovestibular reflexes can be suppressed from neuromuscular blocking agents, ototoxic drugs, or drugs that damage vestibular functioning. Apnea and lack of motor activity can occur because of neuromuscular blocking agents, sedatives, or neuromuscular disease. An isoelectric electroencephalogram can result from an overdose of sedative drugs as well as hypoxia, hypothermia, and profound metabolic encephalopathy.

Finally, since death is a legal as well as medical event, as noted earlier, one must know how the laws of one's particular jurisdiction influence making brain death determinations. Although uncommon, one may encounter local statutes that conflict with what is presented in this chapter because not all states or countries treat brain death uniformly.

COMMUNICATION WITH THE FAMILY

Although the procedure to determine brain death has become well established in most ICUs in the United States, two major problems persist. One has to do with coping successfully with the challenges of medical management of the brain dead patient, which is addressed later in this chapter. The other has to do with dealing with the family's lack of understanding about brain death as communicated to them by the ICU team.

How the concept of brain death and its implications for organ transplantation is communicated to the patient's family leaves a great deal of room for improvement. For example, one recent survey of families of brain dead patients found that 52% of nondonor families (those who refused organ donation) still believed that *a brain dead patient could recover*. Indeed, 39% of donor families and 47% of nondonor families said that they *never* received an explanation about brain death from a physician or other health care professional. It should not be difficult to understand why a family that does not comprehend that being brain dead means being really dead would refuse to donate that patient's organs.

MANAGEMENT OF THE POTENTIAL ORGAN DONOR

Goals of Aggressive Therapy

The goal of aggressive intervention is to maintain organs suitable for transplantation in the brain dead patient while waiting for permission for transplantation and until transfer of the patient's care to the transplantation team in the operating suite.

Despite increased interest in using ICU patients as non–heart beating cadaveric donors after their life support is withdrawn, the greatest supply of organs for donation come from brain dead donors with an intact circulation. Recent experience has shown that aggressive management of the potential organ donor during and after determination of brain death can increase the total number of successful donors and the number of organs procured per donor. The importance of this cannot be overemphasized because the gap between the number of patients awaiting transplants and the number of available organs continues to widen.

Without aggressive support, studies have shown that cardiac arrest occurs in 20% of potential organ donors within 6 hours of making the determination of brain death and in 50% of potential organ donors within 24 hours of brain death. Although a complete description of organ procurement procedures is beyond the scope of this chapter, knowledge of the anticipated physiologic disorders in the brain dead patient and an organized approach to their treatment is essential to all intensivists (Table 68–2).

In many ICUs, clinically savvy members of the regional organ procurement organization can assist the ICU team in the medical management of the brain dead patient, such as providing written protocols to guide this therapy.

Loss of Homeostatic Mechanisms

As described previously, loss of homeostatic mechanisms is the hallmark of brain death. For this reason hypothermia is common in these patients and must be treated aggressively with active rewarming. Rewarming techniques include the use of external warming devices, warmed saline gastric lavage, and warming ventilator gases to 40 to 41° C (see also Chapter 54).

Table 68–2. Physiologic Complications of Brain Death

DISORDERED SYSTEM	MANIFESTATIONS
Central homeostasis	Hypothermia
Cardiopulmonary	"Autonomic storm" with hypertension and tachycardia
	Subsequent hypotension with loss of vascular tone
	Bradycardia or tachycardia
	Pulmonary edema
Endocrine	Central diabetes insipidus
	Hypothyroidism
	Adrenal insufficiency
Hematologic	Disseminated intravascular coagulopathy

Cardiovascular Changes

Cardiovascular changes in brain death include an initial sympathetic "storm" with associated hypertension and tachycardia followed by profound hypotension requiring intensive therapy. Before cessation of brain stem function, as intracerebral pressure rises the medulla oblongata becomes ischemic. This results in unopposed sympathetic activity, which causes significant hypertension and tachycardia. This is frequently brief and often does not require intervention with antihypertensive agents.

Soon after brain death, hypotension frequently occurs from several factors. Absolute hypovolemia can be present because of traumatic fluid loss, third spacing, diabetes insipidus (DI), or the use of diuretics for the treatment of cerebral edema. Neurogenic shock characterized by a loss of vascular tone and venous pooling can also occur from a loss of central vasomotor control. Initial therapy should be volume replacement with isotonic crystalloid. Blood products may be used if the hemoglobin is less than 10 g/dL or if there is a coexisting coagulopathy warranting therapy. In patients who do not respond to volume loading, pressor agents should added. The choice of which pressor agent to use is somewhat arbitrary, but dopamine, norepinephrine, and epinephrine are commonly used. In patients who have pulmonary edema, cardiac dysfunction, persistent hypotension, or high positive end-expiratory pressure requirements, insertion of a pulmonary artery catheter to guide therapy should be considered.

Endocrine and Fluid-Electrolyte Changes

Central DI occurs commonly after brain death because of a lack of central secretion by the pituitary gland. It is defined by hypernatremia, hyperosmolar plasma, and hypotonic polyuria (>4 mL/kg/h). If untreated, DI can result in hypovolemia and such severe electrolyte abnormalities that the patient's organs are deemed unacceptable for transplantation.

Therapy for DI involves replacement of water losses and arginine vasopressin. The water replacement should be based on the calculated free-water deficit (see Chapter 81), but a good starting point is to infuse replacement sodium-free fluid at the rate of the urinary output from the previous hour. If dextrose-containing solutions are used, care must be taken to avoid hyperglycemia. Arginine vasopressin should be given with urine outputs greater than 200 mL/h. Administered as an aqueous intravenous infusion, it should be titrated to decrease urine output to 100 to 200 mL/h. This is usually in the range of 0.5 to 1.0 units/h. Patients who require prolonged therapy are candidates for desmopressin, a synthetic vasopressin analog with less pressor effect.

Electrolyte abnormalities should be monitored and treated when present. Although circulating thyroid hormone (thyroxine) and cortisol levels have been shown to decrease after brain death, replacement therapy is not routinely recommended. Glucocorticoid replacement should, however, be considered in cases of refractory hypotension.

INVOLVING THE REGIONAL ORGAN PROCUREMENT ORGANIZATION

According to many state laws, obtaining consent for transplantation from family members, screening potential organ donors, and deciding on organ allocation are the responsibility of representatives of regional organ procurement organizations. In addition, the appropriate organ procurement organization should be made aware of all potential organ donors undergoing brain death determinations to maximize timely and coordinated interactions among all relevant parties.

BIBLIOGRAPHY

A definition of irreversible coma. Report of the Ad Hoc Committee of the Harvard Medical School to examine the definition of brain death. JAMA 205:337–340, 1968.
This landmark consensus article brought the concept of brain death into the medical mainstream.

Ali MJ: Essentials of organ donor problems and their management. Anesth Clin North Am 12:655–671, 1994.
This is a good review of the physiologic changes after brain death and a practical approach to the management of the clinical problems that the changes create (with 70 references).

Hunt S, Baldwin J, Baumgartner W, et al: Cardiovascular management of a potential heart donor: A statement from the transplantation committee of the American College of Cardiology. Crit Care Med 24:1599–1601, 1996.
A concise approach to maintaining cardiac function and hemodynamic stability in the brain dead organ donor.

Monsein L: The imaging of brain death. Anaesth Intensive Care 23:44–50, 1995.
This article reviews the confirmatory radiographic studies available for the diagnosis of brain death.

Pallis C: Reappraising death. BMJ 285:1409–1412, 1982.
This is the first of a series of nine articles critiquing the concept of brain death and how it is determined clinically in the United States and United Kingdom.

Power B, Van Heerden P: The physiological changes associated with brain death—current concepts and implications for treatment of the brain dead organ donor. Anaesth Intensive Care 23:26–36, 1995.
This article provides an organ systems–based review of the physiology of brain death.

President's Commission for the Study of Ethical Problems in Medicine and Biomedical and Behavioral Research. Guidelines for the determination of death. JAMA 246:2184–2186, 1981.
This is a summary statement by the medical consultants to the Commission that forms the basis for many hospital policies on determination of death by neurologic criteria.

President's Commission for the Study of Ethical Problems in Medicine and Biomedical and Behavioral Research. Defining Death. Complete report on the medical, legal and ethical issues in the determination of death. Washington, DC: U.S. Government Printing Office, July 1981.
This is a landmark consensus document endorsing the concept of brain death and its legalization.

Schafer JA, Caronna JJ: Duration of apnea needed to confirm brain death. Neurology 28:661–666, 1978.
By measuring $Paco_2$ at intervals of apnea in 10 patients undergoing brain death determinations, the authors found that the threshold for $Paco_2$ may approach 60 mm Hg and that 10 minutes or more of apnea may be necessary to reach that $Paco_2$ level.

Youngner S, Landefeld S, Coulton C, et al: "Brain death" and organ retrieval: A cross-sectional survey of knowledge and concepts among health professionals. JAMA 261:2205–2210, 1989.
A study showing that many health care providers involved in the care of critically ill patients did not have a consistent concept of brain death.

69

Prognosis After Cardiopulmonary Arrest

Darren B. Taichman
Paul N. Lanken

Cardiopulmonary resuscitation (CPR), combined with Advanced Cardiac Life Support (ACLS) (see Appendix E), has resulted in the survival of many victims of cardiopulmonary arrest. Although the overall survival rate at discharge for patients with in-hospital cardiac arrest is low (about 10 to 15%), some of these patients may survive in states that they might have regarded as worse than death before their arrest. Neurologic impairment is common after CPR, with many patients having severe and permanent loss of neurologic function. Indeed, up to 40% of those who survive the initial 24 hours after cardiac arrest are comatose for 3 days or longer. A minority of these patients may have advance directives to stop life support if survival in a state of profound neurologic impairment is likely. More commonly, however, no oral or written advance directive was made by the patient to guide this decision. In such cases, both health care providers and family members face difficult medical and ethical decisions.

These decisions would be easier to make if one had a reliable means to identify patients early after arrest who were likely to recover fully as well as those who were likely to die, remain in a persistent vegetative state, or otherwise survive with severe neurologic impairment. Knowing the likelihood of each of these outcomes could guide intensivists and families in making decisions in accord with the patient's previously expressed preferences or life values. Forgoing life support under circumstances in which the patient's neurologic prognosis looks bleak may prevent unwanted therapies and interventions and reduce the emotional suffering of families. For these reasons, making prognoses for neurologic recovery in comatose patients after a hypoxic-ischemic injury, such as cardiopulmonary arrest, is an essential skill for all intensivists.

This chapter focuses on only one cause of coma: coma after nontraumatic hypoxic-ischemic injury, such as that resulting from cardiopulmonary arrest and CPR. However, because prognosis of coma differs with different causes of the coma, one must not use the prognostic information in this chapter to judge prognosis in other types of coma. For example, coma due to traumatic causes (see Chapter 96) differs importantly in treatment and prognosis when compared with nontraumatic coma. Likewise, causes of nontraumatic coma—for example, stroke or metabolic-toxic disorders—other than hypoxia-ischemia can have markedly different prognoses.

COMA AFTER HYPOXIC-ISCHEMIC INJURY

Coma is defined as an absence of consciousness and indicates severe dysfunction of both cerebral hemispheres or the upper brainstem, or both. A comatose patient does not open the eyes regardless of the stimulus, make comprehensible sounds or

775

Table 69–1. Clinical Signs Used for Prognosis After Hypoxic-Ischemic Injury

NEUROLOGIC TEST	RESPONSES IN RANK ORDER*
Pupillary light reflex	Present
	Absent
Oculocephalic or oculovestibular response	Normal
	Limited
	Absent
Eye opening	Spontaneous
	To noise
	To pain
	None
Spontaneous eye movements	Orienting
	Roving conjugate
	Roving dysconjugate
	Other movement
	None
Motor response (best limb)	Obeying
	Localizing
	Withdrawal
	Flexor (decorticate)
	Extensor (decerebrate)
	None
Verbal response	Oriented
	Confused
	Inappropriate
	Incomprehensible
	None

*Responses are ranked hierarchically with best response at the top of the list for each test.

Data from Levy DE, Caronna JJ, Singer BH, et al: Predicting outcome from hypoxic-ischemic coma. JAMA 253:1420–1426, 1985.

words, obey commands, or move or localize extremities appropriately to painful stimuli. Abnormal levels of consciousness or motor function, or both, are common initially after CPR, and patients demonstrate varying degrees of recovery at differing rates. Coma persisting beyond the first day after CPR is generally an ominous sign.

The site of dysfunction may be assessed by serially monitoring a few, reliable clinical signs that are readily apparent on physical examination (Table 69–1). Abnormal speech, environmental recognition, and response to commands usually reflect disordered forebrain function. One can assess the integrity of the brainstem, in part, through examination of the eyes. Other than voluntary gaze, the brainstem controls important ocular activities, such as corneal and pupillary responses, eye opening, and conjugate movements. Damage to the brainstem may also cause the absence of motor responses to pain. Abnormal limb posturing may also indicate brainstem injury but may alternatively represent deep forebrain injury without necessarily indicating brainstem involvement.

Like coma, the *vegetative state* is another abnormal and diminished level of consciousness and also involves an absence of evident cognitive awareness. In distinction to coma, however, the vegetative state is accompanied by periods of eyes-open wakefulness, occurring at times in sleep-wake–like cycles.

Finally, in distinction to altered consciousness, "brain death" (death by neurologic criteria) implies not only the absence of evident cognitive awareness but also of irreversible loss of function of the entire brain (see Chapter 68).

PROGNOSTIC APPROACH TO THE COMATOSE PATIENT AFTER CARDIOPULMONARY RESUSCITATION

Prior Studies of Prognosis

Several important studies have assessed prognostic factors in the comatose patient after CPR. Most have been retrospective analyses of a cohort of patients. The outcomes measured have usually been overall patient survival and neurologic recovery. Although there were some differences between investigations, recovery and level of neurologic function were generally defined similarly (Table 69–2). The results of two of these studies form the basis of the approach to assessing prognosis described in this chapter.

These studies identified several neurologic tests and responses that can help in determining the likelihood of a patient recovering from coma. Given the potential implications of any prognostic system on patient care and outcome, preference has been given to the use of physical findings with the least interobserver variability (see Table 69–1). For example, the presence or absence of pupillary light reflexes (a finding known to have minimal interobserver variation) is used, whereas deep tendon reflexes are not.

Serial Markers of Neurologic Recovery

The basic assessment of prognosis in a comatose patient focuses on the presence or absence of a few ocular and limb motor findings performed serially over several days to monitor changes (Tables 69–3 and 69–4). Serial examinations are important because no single system can predict each individual's outcome with perfect

Table 69–2. Levels of Neurologic Recovery

LEVEL	DESCRIPTION
No recovery	Coma until death
Vegetative state	Eyes-open wakefulness without evidence of cognitive awareness
Severe disability	Conscious but dependent on others for performing ADLs
Moderate disability	Conscious but unable to resume the prior level of activity (but not dependent on others for ADLs)
Good recovery	Resumes prior level of activity and function

ADLs, activities of daily living (to move from bed to chair, to walk, to change one's clothes, and to feed, bathe, and toilet oneself).

Data from Levy DE, Caronna JJ, Singer BH, et al: Predicting outcome from hypoxic-ischemic coma. JAMA 253:1420–1426, 1985.

Table 69–3. Best Predictors of Poor Outcomes After Hypoxic-Ischemic Injury

TIME SINCE ONSET OF COMA	PHYSICAL FINDINGS PRESENT	PERCENT IN COMA OR VEGETATIVE STATE AT 1 YEAR (95% CI)*	PERCENT WITH SEVERE DISABILITY AT 1 YEAR (95% CI)	PERCENT WITH MODERATE DISABILITY OR GOOD RECOVERY (95% CI)
Initial examination (6–12 hr)	Absent pupillary light reflex	94 (84–99)	6 (1–16)	0 (0–7)
1 day	Motor responses no better than flexor AND spontaneous eye movements were neither orienting nor roving conjugate	95 (88–98)	4 (84–98)	1 (0–6)
3 days	Motor response no better than flexor	93 (84–98)	7 (2–16)	0 (0–5)
1 wk	Motor response not obeying commands AND initial spontaneous eye movements were neither orienting nor roving conjugate AND eye opening at 3 days was not spontaneous†	100 (87–100)	0 (0–13)	0 (0–13)
2 wk	Oculocephalic response not normal AND motor response was not obeying commands at 3 days AND eye opening has not improved at least 2 grades†	100 (80–100)	0 (0–20)	0 (0–20)

*95% confidence limits. See Table 69–2 for definitions of outcomes.
†Note that prognosis at the indicated interval is based, in part, on findings at an earlier time point.
Data from Levy DE, Caronna JJ, Singer BH, et al: Predicting outcome from hypoxic-ischemic coma. JAMA 253:1420–1426, 1985.

accuracy. In addition, certain findings lack significant prognostic information at early time points but become meaningful later. For example, the presence of flexor or extensor motor posturing in the first day after cardiac arrest is not predictive of future course, whereas such posturing persisting beyond 3 days after CPR reliably predicts an inability to achieve independent functioning in the future.

Between 1973 and 1977, Levy and colleagues (Levy et al., 1985) studied neurologic criteria for prognosis in more than 200 comatose patients after nontrau-

Table 69–4. Best Predictors of Good Outcomes After Hypoxic-Ischemic Injury

TIME SINCE ONSET OF COMA	PHYSICAL FINDINGS PRESENT	PERCENT IN COMA OR VEGETATIVE STATE AT 1 YEAR (95% CI)*	PERCENT WITH SEVERE DISABILITY AT 1 YEAR (95% CI)	PERCENT WITH MODERATE DISABILITY OR GOOD RECOVERY (95% CI)
Initial examination (6–12 h)	Pupillary light reflex present AND motor response extensor or better AND spontaneous eye movements roving conjugate or orienting	41 (22–61)	19 (6–38)	41 (22–61)
1 day	Motor response withdrawal or better AND eye opening improved at least 2 grades†	7 (1–22)	3 (0–17)	63 (44–80)
3 days	Motor response withdrawal or better AND spontaneous eye movements normal	8 (1–25)	15 (4–35)	77 (56–91)
1 wk	Motor response obeying commands	6 (1–21)	22 (9–40)	72 (53–86)
2 wk	Oculocephalic response normal	4 (0–20)	15 (4–35)	81 (61–93)

*95% confidence limits. See Table 69–2 for definitions of outcomes.
†Note that prognosis at the indicated interval is based, in part, on findings at an earlier time point.
Data from Levy DE, Caronna JJ, Singer BH, et al: Predicting outcome from hypoxic-ischemic coma. JAMA 253:1420–1426, 1985.

matic coma (71% of these cases were directly attributable to cardiac arrest). They analyzed their results by recursive partitioning to develop a set of prognostic algorithms to be applied at the following five time points after hypoxic-ischemic injury: initial examination (within 6 to 12 hours), 1 day, 3 days, 7 days, and 14 days. The algorithms were developed taking into account the status of each response at these five time points in order to arrive at a predicted likelihood of best functional status within 1 year. The resulting stratification of patients according to their physical findings and predicted 1-year best neurologic recovery are summarized in Tables 69–3 and 69–4. Only the best predictors of a poor outcome or of a good outcome are presented because these are likely to be the most influential in guiding decisions regarding levels of life support.

The worsening of prognosis with the persistence of abnormal neurologic findings evident in Tables 69–3 and 69–4 illustrates a conclusion reached in these and essentially all studies on the subject: the longer a patient takes to recover, the less likely a good recovery is. Patients destined to do well usually show early progress.

Table 69–5. Risk Factors for Mortality After Hypoxic-Ischemic Injury

....

As measured at the third day of coma:
Abnormal brainstem function (any of the following: absent pupillary response, absent corneal
   response, or absent or dysconjugate roving eye movements)
No withdrawal response to pain
No verbal response
Creatinine level ≥1.5 mg/dL (≥132.6 μmol/L)
Age >70 yr
Note: The presence of four risk factors on day 3 of coma predicts 96% mortality at 2 mo.

....

From Hamel MB, Goldman L, Teno J, et al: Identification of comatose patients at high risk for death or severe
disability. JAMA 273:1842–1848, 1995.

It is worth noting that the presence of certain findings was associated with a
relatively good chance of recovery. The presence of any of the following at 1 day
after the onset of coma was associated with at least a 50% chance of ultimately
regaining some degree of independent function: (1) confused, inappropriate speech
or better (see Table 69–1); (2) orienting spontaneous eye movements; (3) normal
oculocephalic or oculovestibular responses; and (4) ability to follow commands.

Adjunctive Tests to the Serial Marker Approach

Hamel and colleagues (1995) studied more than 200 nontraumatic comatose
patients (31% cases due to cardiac arrest) and similarly found the lack of motor
response and presence of abnormal ocular findings predictive of a poor outcome
(Table 69–5). In addition, they evaluated the value of coexistent medical conditions
in predicting outcome. In summary, the presence of four out of five readily
identifiable risk factors (Table 69–5) on the third day of coma predicted less than
a 5% chance of survival at 2 months. Importantly, this study subsequently validated
these predictive rules in 349 additional patients.

Nonpredictive Factors

Factors *not* found to be predictive of patient outcome include the patient's functional status before the neurologic insult, sex, the cause of the coma, location of
the precipitating event (e.g., in or outside the hospital), or the presence of post-
anoxic seizures. Likewise, the utility of the Glasgow Coma Scale as a predictor of
outcome in these patients has been disappointing.

Caveats

An incorrect conclusion of good or poor prognosis based on these or other
algorithms could have dire consequences if incorporated into decisions regarding
further care. Therefore, it is vital to keep in mind several important limitations to
the use of the prognostic algorithms presented earlier. First, no system is perfect

and cannot accurately predict outcome for all patients. Any system's ability to predict outcome is limited by differences between the original study population and other patients in whom the system is subsequently applied. Coma, for example, is only one of many possible sequelae of systemic hypoxia and ischemia, and individual patients will likely differ with respect to comorbidities. Advances in available therapies to prevent ischemia-reperfusion injuries during CPR may also influence outcomes in the future. Finally, all studies are subject to statistical realities and the inability to eliminate error completely.

With regard to the study by Levy and colleagues (1985), although this is a landmark study, its conclusions have not been validated by application to another large prospective cohort of patients after CPR. Independent validation, however, is now virtually impossible because of changes in ICU practice (increased rates of withdrawing life support in ICUs since the 1970s when the study was performed) that preclude the use of the same outcome (best neurologic status within 1 year). Another problem is that the study's prediction rules will tend to "contaminate" the study of other cohorts of similar patients because, as the definitive work in this area, its predictive rules have been widely adapted to clinical practice.

Furthermore, because none of these studies included "younger" populations (indeed, the age range evaluated is often not stated), none of these predictive rules can be confidently applied to children or even young adults.

In addition, when assessing for neurologic impairment, one must take care to rule out the confounding effects of pre-existing neurologic deficits, the influence of drugs (e.g., anticholinergic agents on pupillary reactions, depressants on corneal reflexes, or paralytic agents on motor function) or ongoing medical conditions (e.g., hypotension or metabolic derangements).

Finally, the *lack* of the findings indicating a poor prognosis should not be interpreted as necessarily predicting a good outcome. Although the predictive value of certain motor responses, loss of ocular reflexes, or other signs (see Table 69-3) for a poor outcome is substantial, the converse is unproved. For example, a good recovery is not predicted because the pupillary reflex alone is intact initially. One must be cautious not to misinterpret these guidelines and erroneously conclude that a good neurologic recovery is likely or certain.

Despite these important caveats and limitations, following the approach described previously can make a reasonable assessment of prognosis in comatose patients. Specifically, some individuals with only a slight chance of full neurologic recovery can be identified reliably and this information can be used with reasonable confidence in guiding discussions of further care. Ultimately, the decision to continue or refrain from further life support must be made by a process that is based on medical knowledge combined with respect for the patient's preferences or life values (see Chapter 22 for more discussion about this decision-making process).

FUTURE DIRECTIONS

The utility of measuring sensory evoked potentials in assessing neurologic prognosis has been undergoing evaluation. By this method, the presence or absence of cortical function is tested by stimulating a peripheral nerve (e.g., the median) while checking if the cerebral cortex has an electrical response to the stimulus as measured by surface electrodes. Specific evoked potentials (termed *peaks*) indicate the integrity of specific neurologic pathways. In a prospective cohort of 441 patients with nontraumatic coma (nearly half due to ischemia-hypoxia) studied by Madl et al. (1996), a certain sensory evoked potential ("N20" peak) was bilaterally absent in 86 patients. All these patients died within 100 days, with none regaining consciousness before death. The use of benzodiazepine (midazolam) or opioid (fentanyl) sedatives did not affect the sensory evoked potential measurements in this study.

In an earlier study of 66 unconscious patients after cardiac arrest, these same authors demonstrated that the absence or delay of another evoked potential (N70) was similarly associated with 100% mortality (Madl et al., 1993). Although these results are promising, they require prospective validation in other centers before their widespread use can be recommended.

BIBLIOGRAPHY

Attia J, Cook DJ: Prognosis in anoxic and traumatic coma. Crit Care Clin 14:497–511, 1998.
Systematic review of published studies of patients in coma due to anoxia and to trauma (with 32 references).

Bedell SE, Delbanco TL, Cook EF, Epstein FH: Survival after cardiopulmonary resuscitation in the hospital. N Engl J Med 309:569–576, 1983.
This analysis of 294 consecutive patients after cardiopulmonary arrest while hospitalized identified prearrest medical conditions (e.g., pneumonia) and characteristics of the arrest itself (e.g., resuscitation for longer than 30 minutes) associated with higher mortality. The attitudes of patients after resuscitation were also presented.

Berek K, Aichner F: Prognosis of cerebral hypoxia after cardiac arrest. Curr Opin Crit Care 5:211–215, 1999.
Recent concise review of predictors of outcomes after cardiac arrest; not limited to comatose survivors (with 43 references).

Edgren E, Hedstrand U, Kelsey S, et al: Assessment of neurological prognosis in comatose survivors of cardiac arrest. Lancet 343:1055–1059, 1994.
This article describes a prospective cohort of 262 patients, demonstrating the poor prognoses associated with the persistent absence of withdrawal to pain after 3 days. It also demonstrates the unreliability of assessments made within the first few hours.

Hamel MB, Goldman L, Teno J, et al: Identification of comatose patients at high risk for death or severe disability. JAMA 273:1842–1848, 1995.
This article describes a large prospective cohort study of 596 patients in nontraumatic coma, identifying risk factors for poor prognosis. This important study found that the patient's medical comorbidities plus neurologic deficits predicted prognosis.

Levy DE, Caronna JJ, Singer BH, et al: Predicting outcome from hypoxic-ischemic coma. JAMA 253:1420–1426, 1985.
This was a landmark study of 210 comatose patients, identifying physical findings predictive of prognosis. Numerous flow diagrams using a recursive partitioning algorithm categorize patients according to likely prognosis when evaluated at serial times after injury.

Madl C, Grimm G, Kramer L, et al: Early prediction of individual outcome after cardiopulmonary resuscitation. Lancet 341:855–858, 1993.
Evaluation of sensory evoked potentials in a study involving predicting the outcome of unconscious patients after cardiac arrest. Includes a brief review and explanation of the method for the nonneurophysiologist.

Madl C, Kramer L, Yeganehfar W, et al: Detection of nontraumatic comatose patients with no benefit of intensive care treatment by recording of sensory evoked potentials. Arch Neurol 53:512–516, 1996.
This article describes a prospective cohort study of 441 patients to determine the utility of sensory evoked potentials in assessing prognosis.

70   Status Epilepticus

Andrew Siderowf
Mark M. Stecker

Status epilepticus (SE) is defined as persistent seizure activity lasting 30 minutes or more or two or more seizures over the same time period without a return to normal consciousness between episodes. However, for practical purposes, most hospitalized patients in SE are treated long before they meet these formal criteria, especially if they become medically unstable.

CLINICAL CATEGORIES

Generalized convulsive status epilepticus (GCSE) is the most common form of SE seen in the intensive care unit (ICU) and has the highest morbidity and mortality (Table 70–1). It is characterized by tonic stiffening of the trunk and extremities, followed by rhythmic jerking movements. After the seizure, there is typically transient confusion and generalized hypotonia. Early in the course of SE, these different elements are distinct. As SE persists, the difference between these phases diminishes and seizure activity becomes less evident. *Complex partial status epilepticus* is manifested primarily by impaired consciousness. Automatisms (repetitive "automatic" movements), apparent psychosis, eye deviation or eyelid fluttering, and tonic-clonic movements may occur. In *simple partial status epilepticus*, seizures do not impair consciousness but typically involve episodic motor or sensory changes. Simple partial seizures often consist of rhythmic jerking localized to one extremity. In *absence status epilepticus*, consciousness is impaired, with only minimal motor signs. The electroencephalogram (EEG) in patients with this type of SE shows generalized spike and wave activity. In *nonepileptic status* (or *psychogenic status*), the patient displays behaviors superficially similar to epileptic seizures but has no epileptic activity on EEG.

PATHOPHYSIOLOGY AND COMPLICATIONS

On the cellular level, loss of inhibition by GABAergic interneurons on neurons with intrinsic pacemaker capability probably plays a central role in epileptogenesis, leading to synchronous, repetitive firing of large populations of neurons. Loss of inhibition may also play a key role in the failure of seizure termination that differentiates SE from ordinary seizures. Neuronal damage that occurs in SE is likely mediated in part by excitatory neurotransmitters, such as aspartate and glutamate. Excessive release of these excitatory amino acids causes elevations of intracellular calcium, production of reactive oxygen species, and ultimately neuronal death. Changes in the cellular microenvironment, including hypoxia, acidosis, elevated extracellular potassium levels, and breakdown of the blood-brain barrier, also contribute to neuronal death.

Status epilepticus leads to widespread systemic effects. Heart rate and blood

783

Table 70–1. Classification, Description, and Complications of Status Epilepticus

TYPE OF SEIZURE	COMMON CAUSES	CLINICAL BEHAVIOR	MAJOR COMPLICATIONS	ESTIMATED TIME TO COMPLICATIONS

Generalized convulsive seizure SE (GCSE)	Anticonvulsant withdrawal
	Chronic epilepsy
	Drugs
	  Cocaine
	  Cyclosporine
	  Ethanol
	  Imipenem
	  Isoniazid
	  Lithium
	  Lidocaine
	  Penicillin
	  Quinolones
	  TCAs
	  Theophylline
	Infectious
	  Encephalitis
	  Meningitis
	Metabolic
	  Hepatic failure
	  Hyponatremia
	  Renal failure
	Structural
	  Anoxia
	  Head injury
	  Hemorrhage, AVM
	  Stroke
	  Tumor
		Repetitive, generalized body movements
		Usually demonstrates clear evolution with initial tonic contractions followed by clonic contractions. The rate and amplitude of the clonic contractions varies over time.
		Usually stereotyped
		Patient is *always* unresponsive
		After partial treatment, prolonged convulsive status or in the setting of severe brain injury only, "subclinical" manifestations may persist
		Low-amplitude focal twitching with unresponsiveness
		Frequent variations in the level of consciousness
		Intermittent nystagmoid eye deviations
			Systemic
			Anoxia (rare if <10 min)
			Aspiration
			Hyperpyrexia
			Hypoglycemia
			Hypotension or hypertension
			Metabolic acidosis
			Rhabdomyolysis
			Neurologic
			Brain injury (most common with SE lasting >6 h)
			Postictal state (including Todd's paralysis)
				Systemic:
				15–40 min
				Neurologic:
				1–6 h or more for permanent side effects
				Duration of postictal state will increase rapidly with the duration of SE.

Complex partial seizure	As above	As above, but may also experience automatisms, head turning, arm and leg posturing	As above	As above. Time to significant systemic complications is substantially greater.
Simple partial SE	As above, plus hyperglycemia in HHNK	Focal twitching in an extremity or other body part (examine eyes, tongue, abdomen, and feet); Stereotyped intermittent sensory disturbances	Systemic — Injuries to an extremity with rhabdomyolysis; Neurologic	As above. Time to systemic injury is much longer in this group than in the two previous groups.
Absence SE	Genetic epilepsy; Juvenile myoclonic epilepsy; Progressive myoclonic epilepsy; Spike-Wave stupor; Lithium intoxication	Altered responsiveness but may be intermittently alert enough to follow commands; Observe for intermittent twitching in eyes or other body parts	As above	Similar to above
Nonepileptic seizures	Psychiatric (although there may be an organic basis)	Pleomorphic; May resemble generalized complex SE, complex partial SE, or absence status at times; Look for preserved consciousness in the face of bilateral movements	Although the risk of systemic complications is much lower than in the other forms of SE, there is certainly risk for aspiration or injury; Iatrogenic effects of antiseizure drugs	

AVM, arteriovenous malformation; HHNK, hyperglycemic hyperosmolar nonketotic coma (see Chapter 79); SE, status epilepticus; TCAs, tricyclic antidepressants.

pressure rise initially and hypotension develops later. Hyperpyrexia results from tonic muscle contraction and failure of central regulatory mechanisms. More than one third of patients have respiratory acidosis before mechanical ventilation, and another third have lactic acidosis. Electrolyte disturbances, including hyperglycemia, hypoglycemia, hyperkalemia, and hyperphosphatemia, may occur. Aspiration pneumonia and renal failure due to rhabdomyolysis also occur commonly.

Mortality from GCSE ranges from 2 to 25%, but it is difficult to separate mortality due to SE from that due to underlying causes. Prognosis is especially poor in patients with anoxic brain injury, in whom mortality is 70 to 80%, and in patients with multiple organ system failure, in whom mortality reaches 90%. The best prognosis is in SE due to alcohol or anticonvulsant withdrawal. SE lasting more than 24 hours has been associated with a sixfold increase in mortality compared with patients in whom SE persists less than 4 hours. Patients with refractory SE who require barbiturate coma have mortality as high as 77%. Permanent cognitive impairment may result from GCSE and prolonged complex partial SE. Simple partial and absence SE are associated with a lower degree of morbidity and mortality than generalized tonic-clonic and complex partial SE.

DIFFERENTIAL DIAGNOSIS AND ETIOLOGY

Status epilepticus should be considered in all patients with altered mental status in the ICU. One's clinical suspicion should be especially high in the presence of any abnormal movements. Complex partial SE, absence SE, and partially treated GCSE can all present with subtle motor findings. Furthermore, sedatives or neuromuscular blocking agents may mask typical signs. For these reasons, *all* patients in the ICU with unexplained impairments in consciousness should routinely have an EEG. Conversely, other conditions can produce abnormal movements that may be mistaken for seizures. *Myoclonus* can occur in the setting of toxic-metabolic encephalopathy. Myoclonic jerks are typically less rhythmic than the movements associated with seizures. They are more responsive to position or stimulus and do not evolve over time like seizures. Occasionally, *tremor* due to Parkinson's disease, drug intoxication, or withdrawal may be mistaken for seizure activity. *Psychogenic seizures* may be clinically indistinguishable from epileptic seizures, but the EEG is normal during such events.

Common causes of SE include alcohol abuse, anticonvulsant withdrawal, metabolic abnormalities (e.g., hyponatremia, hypocalcemia, severe hepatic failure), intractable epilepsy, central nervous system infections, vascular lesions, trauma, and tumors. Idiopathic SE accounts for up to one third of cases. Drugs commonly used in the ICU such as cyclosporine, theophylline, imipenem, high-dose penicillin, and lidocaine may cause seizures.

DIAGNOSTIC EVALUATION

The diagnostic evaluation in SE is directed toward recognizing the type of seizure and identifying any underlying cause (Tables 70–2 and 70–3). Historical factors of particular interest include prior seizures or anticonvulsant use, alcoholism or other drug use, head injury, or recent febrile illness. Level of consciousness should

Table 70–2. Diagnostic Approach to the Patient with Suspected Status Epilepticus

Neurologic Examination

Assess level of consciousness
Observe any spontaneous movements—are they
    Rhythmic (seizure) or arrhythmic (myoclonus)
    Provokable by stimulation or position (myoclonus)
    Focal or generalized
    Correlated (seizure) or uncorrelated (myoclonus) in different areas
    Tonic-clonic (seizure)
    Demonstrating clear evolution over time (seizure)
Focal abnormalities (e.g., hemiparesis, forced eye deviation)
Papilledema
Nuchal rigidity

Laboratory Tests

Complete blood count, serum electrolyte determination, liver function tests,
    fingerstick glucose determination, magnesium and calcium levels
Medication levels (e.g., phenytoin, theophylline)
Toxicology screen
Electroencephalography, computed tomographic scanning (see Table 70–3)
Lumbar puncture*

* Lumbar puncture should be performed if there is any significant suspicion of meningitis and only after clinical convulsions have terminated. If the neurologic examination is focal, a computed tomographic scan of the head should be performed first.

be assessed. Any abnormal movements of any part of the body, especially the eyes, should be noted. When there is suspicion of infection, lumbar puncture should be performed but it should be postponed until an intracranial mass lesion has been excluded. Most patients with SE should undergo an imaging study of the brain. Almost all patients can be safely transported for a noncontrast computed tomographic scan of the head. This is sufficient to exclude hemorrhage, large tumors, and impending herniation. A magnetic resonance imaging scan of the brain is more sensitive in detecting structural causes of SE. It should be performed once the patient is stabilized if the computed tomographic scan was not diagnostic.

Electroencephalography has a central role in the evaluation and management of SE, especially when there are only subtle motor signs. Patients with convulsive SE whose clinical seizures stop but who fail to awaken after initial therapy often require an EEG to rule out further seizures, that is, subclinical SE. In refractory SE, there is often little clinical evidence of ongoing seizure activity and the EEG is necessary to guide treatment.

MANAGEMENT AND DISCUSSION OF THERAPIES

Although SE should be treated promptly, as a rule there is time for assessment, initiation of diagnostic evaluation, and review of a plan of action before the first anticonvulsant agent is given. A methodical approach will achieve timely seizure control and avoid iatrogenic complications. GCSE, complex partial SE, and non-convulsive generalized SE are treated similarly. Patients with focal SE are at less

Table 70–3. Degree of Urgency for Electroencephalography, Head Computed Tomographic Scan, and Therapy in Status Epilepticus

CLINICAL SCENARIO	CLINICAL SUSPICION OF STATUS EPILEPTICUS	TIMING OF ELECTROENCEPHALOGRAPHY	TIMING OF COMPUTED TOMOGRAPHIC SCAN	URGENCY OF TREATMENT
Unresponsive; tonic-clonic movements; nonfocal neurologic examination	Very high	Urgent (<1 h) unless there is prompt response to treatment	When stable	Urgent (do first)
Unresponsive; spontaneous movements suggestive of seizure; focal examination or papilledema	High	Urgent (1 h) after CT scan	Urgent	Urgent (do first)
Unresponsive; spontaneous movements suspicious but nondiagnostic for SE; nonfocal examination	Moderate (if no other causes are evident such as head injury, toxic-metabolic encephalopathy)	Urgent (do first)	After EEG (unless suspicion of acute structural lesion is high)	Pending EEG
Unresponsive; spontaneous movements not highly suggestive of seizure; focal examination or papilledema	Moderate	Urgent (1–2 h) if CT scan is normal and clinical history does not suggest cause other than SE	Urgent (do first)	Based on results of CT scan, EEG
Unresponsive; spontaneous movements suggest myoclonus; nonfocal examination	Low	Elective (within 8–10 h)	Depends on clinical situation	Elective

EEG, electroencephalography; SE, status epilepticus; CT, computed tomography.

risk for significant brain injury and they need not be treated as aggressively unless the seizures lead to self-injury or aspiration.

The first priority is to ensure an adequate airway, breathing, and circulation (the classic "ABCs" of resuscitation). Initially, the patient should be placed on his or her side to minimize the risk of aspiration. Objects placed in the patient's mouth can break teeth or lead to aspiration of the inserted object. Supplemental oxygen should be given. The patient need not automatically be intubated at this point, but patients who require high-dose barbiturates will ultimately need intubation. Blood pressure, if low, should be supported, whereas hypertension should be managed cautiously because treatment of SE will generally cause blood pressure to fall. Glucose and thiamine should be given if there is a question of hypoglycemia and two reliable intravenous access sites should be secured.

The basic pharmacologic approach to SE (Fig. 70–1) includes three phases: (1) initial treatment with a benzodiazepine, (2) therapy with phenytoin, and (3) therapy with barbiturates or alternatives for refractory seizures. Other options are available, but it is generally best to use a familiar drug regimen rather than the newest alternative (Table 70–4). Diazepam and lorazepam are both acceptable in the initial treatment of SE, but lorazepam is preferred because of its longer duration of action (diazepam, which has a longer pharmacokinetic half-life, has a shorter duration of activity due to rapid redistribution to non–central nervous system locations). Respiratory depression is the major side effect of benzodiazepines, especially when combined with barbiturates. In patients at high risk for respiratory depression, smaller doses of benzodiazepines and larger doses of phenytoin may be given initially.

Phenytoin controls a high percentage (60 to 80%) of seizures not effectively terminated by benzodiazepines, and it provides a longer duration of anticonvulsant action than does lorazepam. For most adults, the loading dose of 20 mg/kg is sufficient to produce blood levels of only 10 to 15 mg/L. If an initial dose of phenytoin is not effective, a second loading dose of 10 mg/kg can be given to obtain a blood level of about 25 mg/L. Phenytoin must be given at a rate of 50 mg/min or slower with appropriate cardiac monitoring to avoid complications of arrhythmia and hypotension. If hypotension occurs, the infusion may continue at a slower rate.

Fosphenytoin, a phenytoin precursor (with a 15-min conversion half-life to phenytoin), is also approved to treat SE. Unlike phenytoin, it does not use propylene glycol as a diluent and it has a pH of 9 (vs. 12 for phenytoin). The glycol and extreme pH are thought to contribute to the adverse affects of phenytoin. As a result, fosphenytoin, which uses the same loading doses as phenytoin to treat SE, can be given at a faster rate (100 to 150 mg/min) compared with phenytoin (maximal of 50 mg/min) and can achieve therapeutic plasma phenytoin levels faster (see Table 70–4). Its availability in hospitals, however, is currently limited by its cost since it is much more expensive than phenytoin.

Seizures that are refractory to benzodiazepines and adequate doses of phenytoin can be treated with barbiturates. Patients receiving high doses of benzodiazepines and barbiturates should be tracheally intubated for respiratory support if they have not been already. High-dose barbiturates often cause hypotension, and dopamine should be readily available when infusions are initiated. Other systemic side effects include hypothermia, profound sedation, abolition of brainstem reflexes, and paralytic ileus. Prolonged barbiturate coma carries a significant risk of mortality and may be reasonably withheld from terminally ill patients. It is appropriate to consider palliative therapy, depending on the preferences of the patient's family.

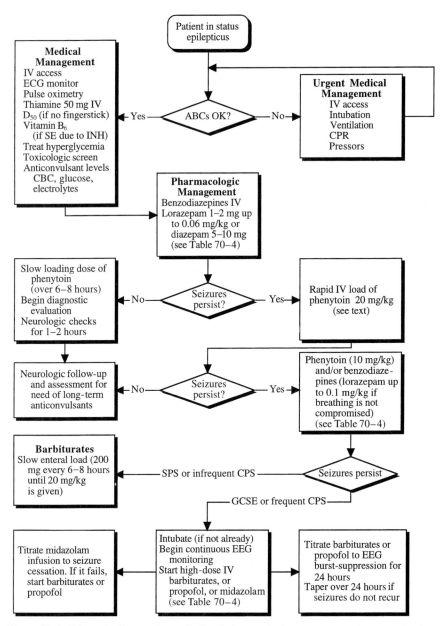

Figure 70–1. Schematic diagram for medical and pharmacologic management of status epilepticus. ABCs, airway, breathing, circulation; CBC, complete blood count; CPR, cardiopulmonary resuscitation; CPS, complex partial seizures; D_{50}, 50 g dextrose; ECG, electrocardiogram; EEG, electroencephalogram; GCSE, generalized convulsive status epilepticus; INH, isoniazid; IV, intravenous; SPS, simple partial seizures.

Anesthetic doses of *pentobarbital* may be required for treatment of refractory SE. Pentobarbital is preferred to phenobarbital because of its shorter serum half-life. A usual loading dose of pentobarbital is 10 mg/kg, although substantially higher doses may be needed, followed by a continuous infusion at a rate of 0.5 to 4 mg/kg/h. The infusion is titrated to maintain the EEG in a 3:1 burst-suppression pattern (isoelectric periods that are three times longer than bursts of electrical activity). After electrical seizures subside, pentobarbital should be tapered over 12 to 24 hours. If seizures recur, a small bolus is given to return the EEG to the same burst-suppression pattern and the infusion is continued for another 48 to 60 hours. If seizures recur after this period, the prognosis is poor, and reinstituting therapy is likely to be of little benefit.

Several alternatives to barbiturates for treatment of refractory SE have become available. These agents offer some advantages over traditional therapy but are not as well proven and are more expensive. Continuous midazolam infusion produces less hypotension than barbiturates and may be safer in critically ill patients. The short-acting anesthetic agent, propofol, has been used successfully to treat SE. Its rapid offset of action may reduce the prolonged sedation caused by high-dose barbiturate therapy. Inhalational anesthetic agents such as isoflurane can be used to titrate the EEG to the appropriate degree of burst suppression. However, their use is limited to the operating room, and they are associated with a high risk of recurrence once they are tapered. Various studies have used other agents such as lidocaine, chloral hydrate, and paraldehyde for SE, but none of these has been thoroughly studied.

Many patients in the ICU have renal or hepatic failure, or both, which make pharmacotherapy of SE additionally challenging. In general, however, the initial management of SE does not change materially in spite of failure of clearance mechanisms. It is important to obtain frequent serum levels of anticonvulsants in this group of patients.

CLINICAL PEARLS AND PITFALLS

Pearls

1. Use familiar medications rather than the newest drug for treating SE.
2. Bilateral motor activity with preserved consciousness is rare in epilepsy.
3. Rhabdomyolysis is rare in seizures lasting less than 7 minutes.
4. Fever may make seizures much harder to control.
5. Have two intravenous access sites so that phenytoin is not administered through the same tubing as other anticonvulsants.

Pitfalls

1. Motor signs may become subtle during prolonged seizures.
2. Neuromuscular blockade conceals clinical manifestations of SE.
3. Rapid phenytoin infusion can cause hypotension and arrhythmias.
4. Barbiturates commonly cause hypotension.
5. A 1 g loading dose of phenytoin is insufficient to control SE in most adults.

Table 70–4. Medications Used in Treating Status Epilepticus

MEDICATION (TRADE NAME)	MAJOR SIDE EFFECTS	TIME TO ONSET	DURATION OF EFFECT	ADMINISTRATION	SERUM LEVELS	STRENGTH OF EVIDENCE	HOSPITAL COST*
Diazepam (Valium)	Sedation Respiratory failure Hypotension (usually mild)	10–15 sec	15 min	Effective dose range: 0.1–0.3 mg/kg IV Rate of administration: 0.06 mg/kg/min IV	300 ng/mL	High	$0.50
Fosphenytoin (Cerebyx)	Same as phenytoin Pruritus	10–20 min	Same as phenytoin	Effective load: 20 mg/kg IV Rate of administration: 100–150 mg/min (less if BP falls) May repeat 10 mg/kg IV if seizures persist	Same as phenytoin	High	Load: $100 to $200
Lorazepam (Ativan)	Sedation Respiratory failure Hypotension (usually mild)	2–3 min	6 h	Effective dose range: 0.02–0.2 mg/kg IV Rate of administration: 0.02 mg/kg/min IV (watch for delayed effects)	30 ng/mL	High	$16.00
Midazolam (Versed)	Sedation Respiratory failure Hypotension (mild)	0.5–2.0 min	1–3 h	Effective load: 0.2 mg/kg IV Maintenance: 0.75–10 µg/kg/min IV	Not applicable	Moderate	Load: $14.00 Maintenance: $5.00/h

Drug	Adverse effects	Onset	Half-life	Dosing	Therapeutic level	Availability	Cost
Phenytoin (Dilantin)	Hypotension Arrhythmia Asystole (rare) Heart block (rare)	15–30 min	22 h	Effective load: 20 mg/kg IV Rate of administration: 50 mg/min (less if BP falls) May repeat 10 mg/kg IV if seizures persist	18–25 µg/mL	High	Load: $2.25
Phenobarbital (Luminal)	Hypotension (severe) Sedation Respiratory Failure	20–30 min	87–100 h (half-life)	Effective load: 20 mg/kg IV Rate of administration: 50 mg/min IV (Slower rates are used if patient has significant cardiac or respiratory problems)	20–50 µg/mL	High	Load: $20.00
Pentobarbital (Nembutal)	Hypotension (severe) Sedation Respiratory failure	20–30 min	11–50 h	Effective load: 10 mg/kg IV Maintenance: 0.5–4 mg/kg/h	10–50 µg/mL	High	Load: $10.00 Maintenance: $5.00/h
Propofol (Diprivan)	Hypotension Sedation Recurrent seizures with rapid discontinuation Respiratory depression Risk of infections	30–60 sec	5 min (redistribution half-life)	Effective load: 2 mg/kg IV (over 10 min) Maintenance: 1–12 mg/kg/h IV (Do *not* taper faster than 5% of maximum rate per h)	2.5 µg/mL	Limited	Load: $50.00 Maintenance: $30.00/h

* All cost estimates are based on a 60-kg patient receiving maximal doses and only represent the relative hospital acquisition costs.
BP, blood pressure; IV, intravenous.

6. The duration of the anticonvulsant effect from a single dose of a benzodiazepine is short, so one should also treat with longer-acting anticonvulsants.

BIBLIOGRAPHY

Alldredge BK, Lowenstein DH: Status epilepticus: new concepts. Curr Opin Neurol 12:183–190, 1999.
This is a recent, comprehensive review by experts in the field (with 53 references).
Lothman E: The biochemical basis and pathophysiology of status epilepticus. Neurology 40(Suppl 2):13–23, 1990.
This article provides a good description of the basic pathophysiology underlying status epilepticus.
Lowenstein DH, Alldredge BK: Status epilepticus at an urban public hospital in the 1980's. Neurology 43:483–488, 1993.
This article describes the factors relating to outcome in patients with status epilepticus.
Simon RP: Physiologic consequences of status epilepticus. Epilepsia 26(Suppl 1):S58–S66, 1986.
This article provides a description of the systemic effects of status epilepticus.
Treiman DM, Meyers PD, Walton NY, et al: A comparison of four treatments for generalized convulsive status epilepticus. N Engl J Med 339:792–798, 1998.
This prospective randomized study found that lorazepam was successful as the initial drug in about two thirds of patients with overt generalized convulsive SE and more efficacious than phenytoin alone.
Walker MC, Smith SJM, Shorvon SD: The intensive care treatment of convulsive status epilepticus in the UK. Anaesthesia 50:130–135, 1995.
Treatment of status epilepticus in the UK is described and a description of many treatments rarely used in the United States is included.
Working Group on Status Epilepticus: Treatment of convulsive status epilepticus. JAMA 270:854–859, 1993.
This article describes the "standard" approach to status epilepticus with reasons for each step in the protocol.
Yaffe K, Lowenstein DH: Prognostic factors of pentobarbital therapy for refractory generalized status epilepticus. Neurology 43:895–900, 1993.
This article provides a description of the use and outcome of high-dose barbiturate therapy for refractory status epilepticus.

71

Stroke

Jin-Moo Lee
Eric C. Raps

Stroke is the third leading cause of death in the United States, claiming 150,000 lives annually. Although in some series, the 30-day mortality for stroke exceeds 20%, it is more often debilitating than fatal. In the United States, stroke causes moderate to severe morbidity in more than 350,000 individuals each year. Depending on size, type, and location, an acute stroke may be considered a medical emergency requiring intensive care unit (ICU) monitoring and care for life-threatening complications. New therapies can reduce neurologic deficits provided that they are given within a brief window of time after onset. Therefore, time is of the essence when treating a patient with acute stroke.

DEFINITIONS AND CLASSIFICATION OF STROKES

Stroke is a broadly defined term referring to the abrupt onset of persistent (>24 hours) neurologic symptoms caused by inadequate blood flow to a particular area of brain or by hemorrhage into or around the brain, which compresses brain tissue and secondarily compromises perfusion. In contrast, a *transient ischemic attack* (TIA) is a focal neurologic deficit that resolves within 24 hours, with the vast majority resolving within 2 hours. If there is not prompt resolution and the deficit persists, a cerebral infarction or stroke has occurred.

Classification

Strokes can be classified into two major categories: (1) *ischemic strokes*, composing approximately 80% of all strokes and (2) *hemorrhagic strokes*, composing the remaining 20% (Table 71–1). The three causes responsible for ischemic strokes are *embolism, thrombosis*, and *hypoperfusion*. Hemorrhagic strokes are subclassi-

Table 71–1. Classification of Strokes

ISCHEMIC	HEMORRHAGIC
Embolic	Intracerebral hemorrhage
Cardiac embolus	Hypertensive
Artery-to-artery embolus (internal carotid artery as origin)	Amyloid angiopathy
Thrombotic	Subarachnoid hemorrhage
Large vessel	Aneurysm
Small vessel (or lacunar infarct)	Arteriovenous malformation
Hypoperfusion	

fied based on the compartment into which the bleeding occurs: *subarachnoid* and *intracerebral hemorrhage*.

Distinguishing between ischemia and primary intracerebral hemorrhage is important when evaluating a patient with an acute stroke. Patients with hemorrhagic strokes typically present with symptoms developing over minutes to hours. Headache, vomiting, and seizures are more commonly seen in patients with intracerebral hemorrhage. Signs of obtundation or coma early in the course of a stroke strongly suggest an intracerebral hemorrhage due to mass effect on the reticular activating system. Evaluation by computed tomography (CT) or magnetic resonance imaging (MRI) is critical to the early diagnosis of hemorrhagic stroke.

Differential Diagnosis

Although arriving at the diagnosis of stroke is usually not clinically challenging, abrupt onset of a neurologic deficit may be caused by other conditions. *Migraine headaches* can be associated with transient focal neurologic symptoms preceding or during the early phase of the headache. Rarely, these deficits may persist and result in frank infarction. *Focal seizures* may manifest with deficits such as aphasia or sensory symptoms that can mimic a stroke. In addition, postictal neurologic deficits (*Todd's paralysis*) may persist for greater than 24 hours after a seizure.

PATHOPHYSIOLOGIC MECHANISMS

Ischemic Strokes

Ischemic strokes can arise from one of four different mechanisms: (1) embolism, (2) small vessel occlusion, (3) thrombosis, or (4) hypoperfusion (see Table 71–1). *Emboli* are the cause of up to 40% of all ischemic strokes and originate from more proximal sites. Artery-to-artery embolism (usually from atherosclerotic plaques in the internal carotid artery) and cardiac embolism account for the majority of embolic strokes. Atrial fibrillation increases the risk of cardioembolic stroke 5-fold, and the presence of associated valvular heart disease raises the risk 17-fold.

Hyaline-lipid deposition (*lipohyalinosis*) in the walls of small cerebral arteries is associated with chronic hypertension and results in *small vessel occlusions*. Known as lacunar infarcts, these typically involve small penetrating arteries, including the lenticulostriates or basilar penetrators in the subcortical and brainstem regions. Although typically less than 1 cm in diameter, lacunar infarcts may cause substantial deficits when they occur in critical areas such as the internal capsule, thalamus, or basis pontis.

Thrombosis is also a common cause of stroke. A thrombus may form in the setting of a ruptured atherosclerotic plaque or from an underlying hypercoagulable state.

Hypoperfusion of the brain—for example, arising from brief episodes of cardiac arrest or hypotension—may result in multiple areas of brain ischemia. Especially vulnerable are the so-called watershed territories involving areas of brain at the border zone of two different vascular supplies. Watershed infarcts can be bilateral and typically involve areas bordering the territories of the middle cerebral and anterior cerebral artery.

Hemorrhagic Strokes

Clinical manifestations of intracerebral hemorrhage (ICH) and subarachnoid hemorrhage (SAH) sometimes overlap, but the pathophysiology, etiology, and prognosis of the two conditions differ remarkably. *Hypertension* is the most common risk factor associated with ICH. The proximate cause of the bleeding is a ruptured Charcot-Bouchard microaneurysm formed at sites of vascular branching, where mechanical stress is maximal. Chronic hypertension, lipohyalinosis, and fibrinoid necrosis all contribute to weakening of the walls of arterioles and the formation of these microaneurysms. They typically occur along the lenticulostriate arteries, thalamoperforating arteries, and paramedian branches of the basilar artery, which correspond to common sites of bleeding in deep subcortical structures (putamen, thalamus, pons, and cerebellum).

The second most common cause of ICH is *amyloid angiopathy*, an infiltrative disorder of intracranial vessels that is unrelated to systemic amyloidosis. Amyloid angiopathy is often seen in elderly patients who may have an associated dementia. Other rare causes of ICH include *vasculitis* (systemic lupus erythematosus, polyarteritis nodosa, primary central nervous system vasculitis), bleeding diatheses (caused by anticoagulant therapy, thrombolysis, severe thrombocytopenia, disseminated intravascular coagulation), and cerebral neoplasms (especially glioblastoma and metastatic tumors).

Nontraumatic SAH usually results from rupture of intracranial *aneurysms* or bleeding from *vascular malformations*. Saccular or berry aneurysms arise from a congenital defect in the medial muscular layer of the intracerebral arteries. Aneurysms are located commonly at the junction of the anterior cerebral and anterior communicating arteries, at the junction of the posterior communicating and internal carotid arteries, at the middle cerebral artery trifurcation, and at the top of the basilar artery.

Neuronal Injury

The occlusion of a cerebral artery produces a central core of nonviable brain tissue that is surrounded by a zone of viable tissue, known as the *penumbra*. Blood supply to this region is substantially reduced but is not as poor as in the infarcted territory. Neuronal death in the penumbra occurs as a consequence of "excitotoxicity," that is, the dysregulated release of excitatory neurotransmitters (especially glutamate) leading to damage of their target neurons. The excitotoxic activation of these neurons, via glutamate receptors, leads to a cascade of events, including calcium influx, protease and DNAse activation, and free radical generation as well as programmed cell death (apoptosis). If blood supply is restored or the excitotoxic cascade is blocked within a temporal window, the penumbral area may be salvaged. This therapeutic window is targeted by new techniques in the emergent care of patients with acute strokes.

Complications of Strokes

Although up to 30% of ischemic strokes result in *hemorrhagic transformation*, only a fraction of these patients show signs of neurologic deterioration. Hemorrhagic transformation is more likely to occur in strokes of large volume that show mass effect. Hematoma evacuation must be considered when hemorrhagic transformation occurs in infarcts involving the posterior fossa, as marked neurologic deterioration may result from compression of the brainstem. *Cerebral edema* is another life-threatening complication of large ischemic strokes. Maximal swelling usually occurs 24 to 72 hours after a stroke and leads to clinical deterioration if it produces substantial mass effect (see Chapter 42).

One third of all patients with SAH have *acute hydrocephalus*, caused by the obstruction of cerebrospinal fluid (CSF) flow through the ventricular system. These patients typically exhibit drowsiness and, if severe, coma with posturing. The diagnosis can be confirmed by CT and requires prompt intervention with external ventricular drainage. Delayed hydrocephalus, due to blockage in absorption of CSF by the parasagittal arachnoid villi, occurs in a small fraction of patients and may require permanent ventricular shunting.

Recurrence of bleeding after SAH is a major cause of morbidity and mortality, affecting 25 to 40% of patients in the first 3 to 4 days after their initial bleeding event. Two thirds of these recurrent hemorrhages are fatal. Surgical obliteration of the aneurysm is the treatment of choice, but optimal timing of the procedure is in dispute (see further on).

Vasospasm is another complication of SAH, generally occurring between the 4th and 10th day after the initial event. Focal neurologic symptoms or confusion are manifestations of vasospasm, which, if persistent, may result in infarction. Calcium channel blockers, particularly nimodipine, may prevent vasospastic infarction but may require concomitant hydration and volume expansion to ameliorate hypotension.

DIAGNOSTIC APPROACH

After a clinical diagnosis of acute stroke has been made, it is imperative to distinguish hemorrhagic from ischemic stroke as rapidly as possible and to start appropriate therapy to maximize neurologic recovery (Figs. 71–1 and 71–2). A CT scan is usually the first neuroimaging study to be performed because it is readily available and highly sensitive to acute bleeds. In the absence of evidence for hemorrhage, an ischemic infarct is presumed. Within the first 12 hours after their onset, ischemic infarcts are commonly undetectable by CT.

Ischemic Stroke

The size and location of an ischemic infarct may help elucidate the mechanism that caused the stroke (see Fig. 71–1). In the acute setting, one must rely on the neurologic examination to localize the infarcted area (Table 71–2). One important

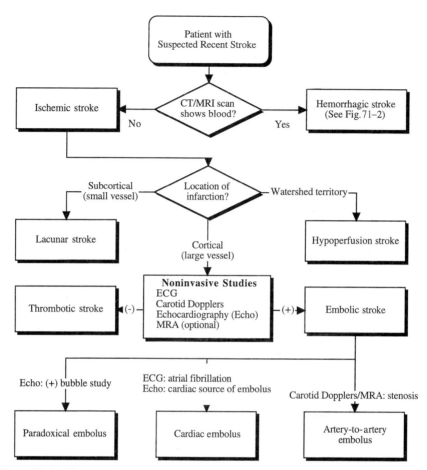

Figure 71–1. Schematic diagram for diagnostic evaluation of nonhemorrhagic stroke. Patients who present within 3 hours of onset of the first symptom of stroke and have no intracranial hemorrhage by computed tomography (CT) should be evaluated for thrombolytic therapy with alteplase (see text). MRI, magnetic resonance imaging; ECG, electrocardiography; MRA, magnetic resonance angiography.

distinction to make is between cortical and subcortical infarcts because these two locations imply different stroke mechanisms and potential complications. A stroke involving the cortex implicates the occlusion of a large artery and suggests an embolic event. In contrast, a subcortical stroke usually involves small vessels and implies lipohyalinosis as the mechanism. A repeat scan more than 24 hours after onset is often helpful. MRI is superior to CT in identifying small infarcts and infarcts located in the posterior fossa. Virtually all patients with ischemic strokes should undergo a noninvasive neurovascular assessment with carotid ultrasonography to evaluate the presence of hemodynamically significant extracranial stenoses in the large arteries. In certain instances, magnetic resonance angiography or transcranial Doppler may be used to assess intracranial disease. Regardless, cere-

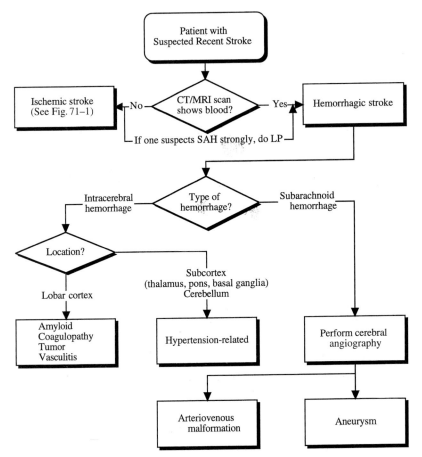

Figure 71–2. Schematic diagram for diagnostic evaluation of hemorrhagic stroke. CT, computed tomography; MRI, magnetic resonance imaging; SAH, subarachnoid hemorrhage; LP, lumbar puncture.

Table 71–2. Clinical Signs Suggesting Stroke Localization

CORTICAL LOCATION	SUBCORTICAL LOCATION	BRAINSTEM LOCATION
Aphasia	Pure motor hemiparesis involving face, arm, leg	Cranial nerve deficits
Neglect of contralateral side		Bilateral weakness or sensory deficit
Hemianopsia (field cut)		Ataxia
Forced eye deviation	Pure hemisensory deficit involving face, arm, leg	Vertigo, nystagmus
Hemiparesis or hemisensory deficit or both, involving face, arm, or leg only		Diplopia, skew deviation
		Crossed signs (i.e., ipsilateral facial nerve deficit, with contralateral hemiparesis)
		Obtundation, loss of consciousness

bral angiography remains the "gold standard" for assessing extracranial and intracranial artery stenosis, ulceration, and other arteriopathies. Angiography, however, is not indicated for all stroke patients because it poses risks by its invasive nature. Indications for cerebral angiography include stroke in a young person, suspicion of vasculitis, venous strokes, and patients with extracranial carotid stenosis who are being considered for carotid endarterectomy.

All patients with cerebral ischemia should have a routine electrocardiogram to assess the possibility of cardiac arrhythmias prone to emboli, for example, atrial fibrillation. If such an arrhythmia is suspected or a cardioembolic source is possible, Holter monitoring should be performed and an echocardiogram obtained. Strong indications of a cardiac or proximal aortic source of emboli should prompt transesophageal echocardiography even in the presence of an unrevealing transthoracic echocardiogram. A contrast ("bubble") study should be performed to assess the possibility of a right-to-left shunt via a patent foramen ovale or atrial septal defect resulting in a "paradoxical embolus."

Further work-up of rare causes of stroke may be warranted in the appropriate clinical setting. For example, a stroke in a young person (<45 years) should prompt a complete evaluation for hypercoagulable states (e.g., measuring levels of protein C, protein S, antithrombin III, and antiphospholipid antibody) as well as for vasculitis (measuring antinuclear antibody, erythrocyte sedimentation rate, and possibly obtaining a cerebral angiogram). Sleep apnea has also been identified recently as a potential stroke risk factor but through an unclear mechanism.

Hemorrhagic Stroke

The diagnosis of ICH can be made by CT, which provides information about the size, location, degree of mass effect, and amount of edema (see Fig. 71–2). Blood appears hyperdense acutely on CT and is frequently surrounded by areas of low density, reflecting edema or areas of infarction. Angiography should be considered in young patients with lobar hemorrhage and in nonhypertensive patients to exclude arteriovenous malformation, aneurysm, or arteritis. Although CT is preferable to MRI in the acute phase, a follow-up MRI scan may be warranted in patients without an underlying cause to rule out a neoplastic process.

The diagnosis of SAH is usually clear: most patients present with the acute onset of the "worst headache of my life" frequently in association with vomiting and a stiff neck. CT demonstrates subarachnoid blood in the majority of cases; 10 to 15% of SAHs, however, are undetected by CT. Therefore, if the suspicion of SAH is high, a lumbar puncture must be performed to exclude this diagnosis. Characteristically, patients with SAH have either xanthochromic (yellow-colored) CSF or persistently elevated red blood cell levels in all tubes of collected CSF. Cerebral angiography is the mainstay for diagnosing the underlying cause of SAH and should be performed as soon as possible. As many as 20% of patients with SAH have multiple aneurysms, necessitating four-vessel angiograms in all patients. If the arteriogram does not reveal an aneurysm, it should probably be repeated in 1 to 2 weeks, as vasospasm can interfere with the visualization of these lesions. A transcranial Doppler study may be helpful in identifying the vasospastic complications of SAH.

ACUTE MANAGEMENT

Ischemic Stroke

Recent developments have revolutionized treatment of acute ischemic stroke. Salvaging the ischemic penumbra by reperfusion or neuroprotection is the goal, but it must be achieved within a narrow therapeutic time window. In a recent double-blinded randomized controlled trial, alteplase, also called tissue plasminogen activator (tPA), was shown to significantly improve outcome when given to patients *within 3 hours* of onset of acute ischemic stroke (and no evidence of intracranial hemorrhage on CT). tPA was given intravenously at a dose of 0.9 mg/kg (maximal dose = 90 mg) with 10% of the dose given as a bolus (given over 1 minute) and the remainder given over 1 hour as a continuous infusion. Antithrombotic and antiplatelet drugs were withheld for the first 24 hours. Patients treated with tPA had significant improvement in neurologic outcome at 3 months using four different measures of neurologic deficit or disability. The benefits were independent of the type of ischemic stroke. Although symptomatic hemorrhagic transformation within 36 hours occurred at a much higher rate in the tPA group (6.5% versus 0.6%), no difference in overall 3-month mortality was observed (17% in the tPA group versus 21% in the placebo group). In contrast, trials involving streptokinase showed significantly *increased* mortality in treated groups.

A host of experimental drugs, known as *neuroprotective agents,* aimed at preventing the destructive cascade triggered in the ischemic penumbra are under investigation. Although results from several earlier trials have been negative, optimism remains that efficacy of these types of agents will eventually be demonstrated. These neuroprotective drugs include glutamate receptor antagonists, leukocyte adhesion inhibitors, free radical scavengers, and potassium channel openers.

Supportive measures should be directed at preventing progression of stroke by maintaining cerebral perfusion. After stroke, cerebral blood flow autoregulation is impaired in the area of the infarct and, therefore, low mean arterial blood pressures may lead to stroke extension. The head of the patient's bed should remain flat. It is recommended that *mean* arterial pressure be maintained at 100 to 120 mm Hg. If the mean arterial pressure exceeds 130 mm Hg, treatment with rapidly metabolized agents such as intravenous labetalol should be used. In the acute phase, normal saline should be the intravenous fluid of choice. Experimental evidence suggests that elevated blood glucose may increase infarct size. Hypotonic solutions should be avoided, as they may exacerbate cerebral edema. Prophylaxis for deep venous thrombosis should be instituted.

The use of anticoagulants after acute ischemic stroke is perhaps one of the most controversial topics in neurology. However, accumulating evidence from recent studies suggests that the risk of hemorrhagic transformation with anticoagulant use may outweigh the benefit of recurrent stroke prevention in the first two weeks following stroke, even in the subgroup of patients thought to be at highest risk for recurrent emboli (patients with atrial fibrillation). Aspirin, on the other hand, appears to have a modest but real benefit for recurrent stroke prevention in the acute setting. This benefit is associated with a relatively low rate of hemorrhagic conversion as well as decreased mortality.

Although the focus of this chapter has been acute management, secondary prevention of stroke recurrence also should be discussed. In patients who have a negative embolic work-up or who are not anticoagulation candidates, antiplatelet therapy should be initiated. Aspirin has been shown to reduce the risk of recurrent stroke; however, the precise dose is controversial and ranges between 81 mg/day to 325 mg four times a day. Ticlopidine (250 mg bid) is a more effective antiplatelet agent for secondary stroke prevention but has the troubling side effect of neutropenia. Clopidogrel (75 mg/day), structurally related to ticlopidine, is at least as effective as aspirin without the side effect profile of ticlopidine. Finally, aspirin (25 mg bid) in combination with extended release dipyridamole (200 mg bid) has been shown to be more effective than aspirin (25 mg bid) alone.

Hemorrhagic Stroke

General supportive measures in ICH are directed toward minimizing cerebral edema. Controlled studies have failed to show benefit from steroids in cerebral hemorrhage. Intravenous fluids should be restricted to minimal daily replacement, and hypotonic solutions should be avoided. When necessary, mannitol may be administered and intubation with hyperventilation instituted to reduce cerebral edema (see Chapter 42). Studies involving blood pressure management are lacking, but there is general agreement that systolic blood pressure greater than 190 mm Hg or diastolic blood pressure greater than 110 mm Hg should be avoided. Rapidly metabolized antihypertensive agents such as labetalol or esmolol should be used (see Chapter 52). Surgical intervention in ICH is controversial. In selected cases, clot removal may be beneficial, although no convincing study shows better outcomes in surgically treated patients. Cerebellar hemorrhage is an urgent indication for surgical intervention in order to prevent secondary brainstem compression. Hematoma evacuation should be undertaken while the patient is alert and before the development of pyramidal signs.

The initial management of patients with SAH is directed toward prevention of rebleeding, preparation for surgery, and monitoring for potential complications (see Fig. 42–3, Chapter 42). The patient should be placed in a quiet room with minimal stressful stimulation. Sedation with diazepam is occasionally instituted to prevent excitement and elevation of blood pressure. Hypertension, which may cause repeated rupture, and hypotension, which exacerbates vasospasm, should be avoided. Phenytoin is generally used to avoid complications resulting from seizures. Corticosteroids are also usually employed to reduce meningeal irritation and possible postoperative swelling. Intravascular fluid expansion should be accomplished with normal saline. The best timing for surgery is in dispute, but early surgery (within 3 days of rupture) is becoming the treatment of choice. This decreases the risk of rebleeding and allows aggressive volume expansion for the prevention of vasospasm. Surgery is contraindicated in patients in coma or with severe deficits because of high mortality and low potential for recovery. Vigilance for the complications of SAH should be maintained: (1) prompt decompression for acute hydrocephalus and (2) nimodipine for vasospasm with pressors and volume expansion if hypotension occurs.

BIBLIOGRAPHY

Adams HP Jr, Brott TG, Furlan AJ, et al: Guidelines for thrombolytic therapy for acute stroke: A supplement to the guidelines for the management of patients with acute ischemic stroke. A statement for healthcare professionals from a special writing group of the stroke council, American Heart Association. Circulation 94:1167–1174, 1996.
This is a comprehensive consensus document that includes reviews of medical and surgical therapies with recommendations for current practice in treating ischemic stroke.

Albers GW, Easton JD, Sacco RL, et al: Antithrombotic and thrombolytic therapy for ischemic stroke. Chest 114:683S–698S, 1998.
This is an excellent review article on the use of thrombolytic and antithrombotic drugs for ischemic stroke.

Albers GW, Hart RG, Lutsep HL, et al: Supplement to the guidelines for the management of transient ischemic attacks: A statement from the ad hoc committee on guidelines for the management of transient ischemic attacks, stroke council, American Heart Association. Stroke 30:2502–2511, 1999.
This is an American Heart Association consensus document describing background and recommendations for medical and surgical therapy for transient ischemic attacks.

Barnett HJM, Mohr JP, Stein BM, et al (eds): Stroke: Pathophysiology, Diagnosis and Management. New York: Churchill Livingstone, 1998.
This is a referential textbook on stroke.

Broderick JP, Adams HP Jr, Barsan W, et al: Guidelines for the management of spontaneous intracerebral hemorrhage. A statement for healthcare professionals from a special writing group of the stroke council, American Heart Association. Stroke 30:905–915, 1999.
This is a comprehensive consensus document that includes reviews of diagnosis and management of spontaneous intracerebral hemorrhage, including blood pressure targets.

Caplan LR: Diagnosis and treatment of ischemic stroke. JAMA 266:2413–2418, 1991.
This is a review of the classification and diagnostic work-up of ischemic stroke.

Fisher M (ed): Clinical Atlas of Cerebrovascular Disorder. London: Mosby–Year Book, 1994.
This is an excellent, easy-to-read graphic text of stroke.

Furlan A, Higashida R, Wechsler L, et al: Intra-arterial prourokinase for acute ischemic stroke. The PROACT II study: A randomized controlled trial. JAMA 282:2003–2011, 1999.
This Phase III study of 180 patients with angiographically documented proximal middle cerebral artery occlusion within 6 hours of onset of symptoms showed that intra-arterial infusion of a local thrombolytic agent plus intravenous heparin (vs. intravenous heparin in the control group) resulted in less neurologic disability at 90 days and better rates of recanalization (66 vs. 18% in controls) but with similar mortality rates (25 vs. 27% in controls) and higher rates of intracranial hemorrhage within 24 hours (10 vs. 2% in controls). This agent remains investigational and is undergoing further Phase III clinical trials.

Grotta JC: Current medical and surgical therapy for cerebrovascular disease. N Engl J Med 317:1505–1516, 1987.
This is an excellent compilation of the original literature for strategies in the treatment of stroke.

International Stroke Trial Collaborative Group: The International Stroke Trial (IOST): A randomized trial of aspirin, subcutaneous heparin, both or neither among 19,435 patients with acute ischaemic stroke. Lancet 349:1569–1581, 1997.
This very large controlled clinical trial showed no benefit from heparin and only a modest benefit from aspirin.

The NINDS rt-PA Stroke Study Group: Tissue plasminogen activator for acute ischemic stroke. N Engl J Med 333:1581–1587, 1995.
This is a double-blinded, randomized, controlled study of the use of tPA in acute stroke.

Wechsler LR, Ropper AH: Management of stroke in the intensive care unit. Semin Neurol 6:324–331, 1986.
This is a good discussion of management issues likely to be encountered in an ICU setting.

72 Obstetric and Postobstetric Complications

Samuel Parry
Mark A. Morgan

In Chapter 21, maternal physiologic adaptations to pregnancy were described and guidelines were provided for the care of pregnant patients who are admitted to the intensive care unit (ICU) for nonobstetric indications. This chapter presents the management of pregnant patients in the ICU admitted for *obstetric indications,* including obstetric hemorrhage, preeclampsia or eclampsia, acute fatty liver of pregnancy (AFLP), amniotic fluid embolism, and tocolysis-induced pulmonary edema.

OBSTETRIC HEMORRHAGE

Antepartum Hemorrhage

In any pregnant patient who presents with third trimester vaginal bleeding, ultrasonography should be performed before pelvic examination to exclude the diagnosis of placenta previa and to detect a fetal heart rate.

Differential Diagnosis

There are multiple causes of antepartum hemorrhage (Table 72–1). Abruptio placenta (separation of the placenta from the uterine wall) and placenta previa (placenta implanted over the uterine cervix) may be associated with substantial maternal blood loss in part because of the inability of fibrinized spiral uterine arteries to vasoconstrict. The dissection of blood between the fetal membranes and the maternal decidua often initiates uterine contractions. These contractions may exacerbate the bleeding and precipitate repeated bleeding episodes.

Fetal anemia may be associated with bleeding from placental villous vessels. Primary fetal bleeding is associated with a velamentous cord insertion in which the umbilical cord inserts at a distance from the placenta such that fetal vessels must traverse the placental membranes. A vasa previa occurs when unprotected fetal vessels traverse the uterine cervix. Velamentous cord insertion and vasa previa are rare causes of third trimester vaginal bleeding.

Laboratory Evaluation

Laboratory evaluation includes a complete blood count, prothrombin time and partial thromboplastin time, fibrinogen and fibrin degradation (split) product levels, and a Kleihauer-Betke (KB) stain. A KB stain is an acid elution test that is used to detect fetal hemoglobin in the maternal blood and to calculate the volume of

Table 72–1. Selected Causes of Third Trimester Vaginal Bleeding

CAUSE	RISK FACTORS	COMMENTS
Abruptio placenta	Hypertension Cocaine use Trauma	Usually associated with abdominal tenderness and uterine contractions 20% of cases have concealed hemorrhage (no vaginal bleeding) Rarely visualized by ultrasonography
Placenta previa	Prior cesarean section	Usually no abdominal tenderness, but uterine contractions are common Ultrasonography confirms diagnosis
Uterine rupture	Prior (classic) cesarean section	Acute, persistent, intense abdominal pain
Fetal bleeding	Velamentous umbilical cord insertion Vasa previa	Smear of vaginal bleeding demonstrates nucleated red blood cells, i.e., of fetal origin Apt alkali test shows differential resistance of fetal and maternal oxyhemoglobin to sodium hydroxide

fetomaternal hemorrhage. In an unsensitized Rh-negative mother with antepartum bleeding, Rh immune globulin (Rhogam) should be given to prevent maternal production of anti-D antibodies. A standard vial (300 mg) of Rhogam provides prophylaxis for a 30-mL fetomaternal hemorrhage. Larger fetomaternal hemorrhages, as calculated by KB stain, require additional Rhogam (10 mg/mL fetal whole blood). If the fetomaternal hemorrhage is calculated to exceed 50 mL, the risk for severe fetal anemia is great, and early delivery must be considered.

Maternal coagulation studies are of critical importance in patients with obstetric hemorrhage because of the risk of disseminated intravascular coagulation (DIC) (Table 72–2). In these patients, the coagulation cascade is activated by the release of large amounts of tissue phospholipids or endotoxin, or both, which produce maternal endothelial damage. Obstetric patients diagnosed with DIC should be aggressively supported with fresh frozen plasma or cryoprecipitate and platelets. However, the DIC resolves only when the underlying cause of DIC is resolved.

Table 72–2. Obstetric Conditions Associated with
Disseminated Intravascular Coagulation

Amniotic fluid embolism
Fetal death syndrome
Gestational trophoblastic neoplasia
Obstetric hemorrhage
Preeclampsia, HELLP syndrome, AFLP
Septic abortion

AFLP, acute fatty liver of pregnancy; HELLP, hemolysis, elevated liver enzymes, and low platelets.

Management

A patient with antepartum obstetric hemorrhage requires continuous fetal heart rate monitoring. "Nonreassuring" fetal heart rate patterns may necessitate emergency delivery. Large-bore intravenous access should be established, and aggressive volume replacement with crystalloids or blood components, or both, should be initiated. In the setting of antepartum obstetric hemorrhage, tocolysis may be considered if the mother and fetus are stable and there is evidence for preterm labor in association with cervical dilatation. Because beta-sympathomimetic tocolytics (terbutaline, ritodrine) produce maternal tachycardia and peripheral vasodilatation, both may mask signs of continued bleeding. Thus, magnesium sulfate is probably the tocolytic agent of choice. Delivery options are decided based on maternal and fetal clinical conditions, gestational age, and fetal lung maturity.

Postpartum Hemorrhage

Postpartum hemorrhage may be broadly classified into uterine or nonuterine bleeding. Uterine bleeding, responsible for 90% of cases of postpartum hemorrhage, is generally more severe than nonuterine causes. Because the uterus receives 20% of the maternal cardiac output at term (about 600 mL/minute), rapid control of postpartum uterine bleeding is critical.

Clinical History and Risk Factors

Uterine atony is defined as the failure of prompt myometrial contraction after the third stage of labor. It is associated with multiparity, uterine overdistention (multifetal gestation), protracted labor, and infection. Unfortunately, uterine atony is often idiopathic and cannot be anticipated. *Retained placenta* is frequently associated with uterine atony and difficult delivery of the placenta. Retained placenta usually presents as delayed (>24 hours) postpartum hemorrhage often in association with endomyometritis. *Placenta accreta*, a type of abnormal placentation in which the placenta invades through the maternal decidua and attaches directly to the myometrium, is strongly associated with prior cesarean section and placenta previa. *Uterine rupture* occurs most frequently with vaginal delivery after a previous cesarean section, although the risk for scar dehiscence is less than 1% if the previous incision was confined to the lower uterine segment. Under these conditions, the overall maternal morbidity for a trial of labor has been demonstrated to be less than that of repeat cesarean section.

Nonuterine causes of postpartum hemorrhage include lower genital tract lacerations, which should be suspected after a difficult operative vaginal delivery, hematomas (which may be subclassified as vulvar or pelvic), and coagulopathies. Vulvar hematomas often present as early perineal pain, whereas pelvic hematomas (defined as occurring above the levator ani muscles) usually occur after cesarean delivery.

Physical Examination and Laboratory Findings

The physical examination and laboratory findings typically allow the physician to identify the cause of postpartum hemorrhage rapidly. Physical examination must include an abdominal and pelvic examination, with visualization of the entire vagina and cervix and palpation of the uterine cavity. Pelvic ultrasonography and a complete blood count and coagulation profile may assist in diagnostic and therapeutic decisions. The diagnosis of *uterine atony* is confirmed when brisk vaginal bleeding is encountered after delivery in association with a boggy, flaccid uterus. *Retained placenta* presents similarly (although often many hours later) and ultrasonography may be used to visualize retained products of conception within the uterine cavity. Since the retained placenta is a nidus for infection, the patient may have an elevated temperature and a tender uterine fundus. *Placenta accreta* is readily identified by manual exploration of the uterine cavity and finding placenta remaining adherent to the uterine wall. Pelvic examination including manual exploration of the uterine cavity and visualization of the entire lower genital tract allows the physician to identify *uterine scar dehiscence, lower genital tract lacerations,* and *vulvar hematomas* readily. *Pelvic hematomas* may be concealed but can generally be visualized by ultrasonography when suspected in a postpartum patient with a decreasing hemoglobin and hematocrit.

Management

Although postpartum hemorrhage is generally managed medically, if medical techniques fail or a laceration is identified, surgical procedures are indicated (Table 72–3). Central hemodynamic monitoring is indicated if massive volume replacement is needed. Since physiologic intravascular mobilization of extracellular fluid occurs after delivery, fluid replacement therapy places such a patient at increased risk for pulmonary edema.

POSTPARTUM PREECLAMPSIA

The cause of preeclampsia is yet to be elucidated, but the disease appears to be related to abnormal placentation. This leads to release of unknown endogenous factors, resulting in generalized maternal vasospasm and endothelial cell damage. Diminished blood flow to the uterus and maternal end organs precipitates the various complications associated with severe preeclampsia. Although the cure for preeclampsia is delivery of the fetus and placenta, residual disease frequently persists and may even progress for more than 24 to 48 hours into the postpartum period.

Clinical Diagnosis

The diagnosis of preeclampsia is based simply on the presence of sustained maternal hypertension (defined as systolic blood pressure greater than or equal to 140 mm Hg or diastolic blood pressure greater than or equal to 90 mm Hg) in the second half of pregnancy in a previously normotensive woman in association with proteinuria and nondependent edema. Postpartum complications considered to be due to preeclampsia are listed in Table 72–4.

Table 72–3. Management of Postpartum Hemorrhage

Nonsurgical Approaches

Bimanual uterine compression (facilitated by an empty bladder)

Intravenous oxytocin (20 units in 1000 mL of crystalloid at a brisk infusion rate)

Intramuscular or intramyometrial 15-methyl prostaglandin $F_{2\alpha}$ (0.25 mg), repeat every
   10–15 min

Intramuscular methylergonovine (Methergine) 0.2 mg (may produce transient but extreme blood
   pressure elevations and is contraindicated in hypertensive patients)

Uterine packing performed only after confirming the absence of lower genital tract laceration, uterine
   rupture and uterine inversion. The entire uterus and vagina must be packed. Prophylactic
   antibiotics and continuous oxytocin are recommended. The packing may be removed after
   24–36 h

Angiographic embolization of bleeding vessels

Surgical Approaches

Postpartum dilation and curettage (for retained placenta)

Surgical ligation of pelvic vessels (uterine and hypogastric arteries) to decrease arterial pulse
   pressures (vessels later recanalize and have no effect on subsequent fertility)

Postpartum hysterectomy

Laboratory Abnormalities

Abnormal laboratory test results reflect the clinical manifestations of diminished blood flow to end organs and endothelial cell damage. Decreased renal plasma flow and glomerular capillary endothelial damage result in decreased creatinine clearance, increased serum creatinine levels, increased blood urea nitrogen levls, and oliguria (<50 mL/hour). Intravascular volume depletion secondary to generalized vasospasm causes hemoconcentration. Endothelial cell damage stimulates the coagulation cascade with consumption of platelets and coagulation factors. Hepatocellular necrosis due to decreased hepatic perfusion results in elevated bilirubin and liver enzyme levels.

The HELLP (hemolysis, elevated liver enzymes, and low platelets) syndrome complicates up to 10% of pregnancies with severe preeclampsia. HELLP syndrome was originally defined as including all these factors, but any one of them may represent severe disease. The criteria for the HELLP syndrome include a total

Table 72–4. Postpartum Complications Associated with Severe Preeclampsia

Central nervous system manifestations other than seizures
   (subarachnoid hemorrhage and cerebral infarct)
Disseminated intravascular coagulation
Eclampsia (generalized seizures)
HELLP syndrome
Hepatic infarct and rupture
Oliguria and acute renal failure
Pulmonary edema
Refractory hypertension

HELLP, hemolysis, elevated liver enzymes, low platelets.

greater than or equal to 1.2 mg/dL, lactate dehydrogenase levels) IU/L, an abnormal peripheral smear containing schistocytes and artate aminotransferase (AST) levels greater than 72 IU/L, and platelet counts less than 150,000/μL. Maternal morbidity and mortality correlate with the fall in platelet counts. Those with platelet count less than 50,000/μL are the most severely affected.

Patients with HELLP syndrome often present with malaise, nausea, headache, and right upper quadrant pain. HELLP syndrome must be differentiated from other conditions causing liver disease in pregnancy (Table 72–5). The differential diagnosis of hemolysis and thrombocytopenia includes (1) thrombotic thrombocytopenic purpura (TTP), which presents with a more severe microangiopathic hemolytic anemia, central nervous system, renal manifestations, and fever (see Chapter 63); (2) hemolytic uremic syndrome, which has more severe renal failure; and (3) idiopathic thrombocytopenic purpura (ITP), which is not associated with hypertension, elevated liver enzyme levels, or proteinuria (see Chapter 63).

Management

Therapy of postpartum preeclampsia has three basic goals: seizure prophylaxis, control of hypertension, and supportive therapy for its various complications. Magnesium sulfate has been shown to be the most effective drug for prevention (and treatment) of eclamptic seizures. Standard administration of magnesium sulfate is a 4 to 6 g intravenous loading dose in 50 to 100 mL of 0.9% (normal) saline over 20 minutes, followed by a maintenance dose of 2 g/hour for 24 hours after delivery. The therapeutic range of magnesium for preventing eclamptic seizures is 4 to 7 mEq/L. Plasma magnesium levels should be monitored closely, particularly in patients who have renal dysfunction. An initial magnesium level should be measured 1 hour after the loading dose is completed. Clinical evaluation must include frequent monitoring of mental status, deep tendon reflexes, respiratory effort, and urine output. Patellar reflexes usually are lost at levels of 8 to 10 mEq/L, and respiratory arrest may occur at 13 mEq/L. Calcium gluconate (1 g, available as 10 mL of 10% solution) must be readily accessible for intravenous administration to reverse symptomatic magnesium toxicity (obtundation, apnea).

Antihypertensive agents are typically administered when blood pressure exceeds 180 mm Hg systolic or 110 mm Hg diastolic. Hydralazine has been widely used intravenously as a 5 to 10 mg bolus, which may be repeated every 20 minutes as necessary. Alternatively, labetalol may be given as a 10 mg intravenous bolus, with increasing boluses (20 mg, 40 mg, 80 mg) repeated every 10 minutes to a total dose of 300 mg. After desired blood pressures are attained, an intravenous labetalol drip may be instituted at 1 to 2 mg/minute and then titrated. Occasionally, refractory high blood pressure may require the administration of potent vasodilators, such as sodium nitroprusside, usually with central hemodynamic monitoring.

Several disorders other than refractory hypertension are indications for central hemodynamic monitoring in the postpartum preeclamptic patient: general anesthesia in an unstable patient, pulmonary edema, and oliguria. Because central venous pressure correlates poorly with pulmonary artery wedge pressure in preeclamptic patients, use of a pulmonary artery catheter is preferred (Table 72–5).

Table 72–5. Mechanisms of Oliguria in Patients with Severe Preeclampsia with Associated Hemodynamic Findings

MECHANISMS	PULMONARY ARTERY WEDGE PRESSURE	SYSTEMIC VASCULAR RESISTANCE	CARDIAC OUTPUT	TREATMENT
Intravascular volume depletion (most common)	↓	↑	WNL	IV infusion of crystalloids
Selective renal arteriospasm	WNL to ↑	WNL	WNL	Hydralazine Renal dose dopamine (<5 μg/kg/min)
Depressed left ventricular function	↑	↑	↓	Furosemide Fluid restriction Afterload reduction (see Chapter 6)

Modified from Clark SL, Greenspoon JS, Aldahl D, et al: Severe preeclampsia with persistent oliguria: Management of hemodynamic subsets. Am J Obstet Gynecol 154:490, 1986.
IV, intravenous; WNL, within normal limits.

IVER OF PREGNANCY

AFLP is rare (1 in 10,000 to 100,000 pregnancies). Its cause is unknown. Although approximately 50% of AFLP cases are associated with preeclampsia, these two disease processes have distinct patterns of liver pathology. The histologic and clinical features that differentiate AFLP from other liver diseases in pregnancy are outlined in Table 72–6.

Clinical Manifestations

The clinical manifestations of AFLP include generalized malaise and central nervous system complaints ranging from headache to obtundation and coma. Patients often report nausea and vomiting, right upper quadrant pain, and gastrointestinal bleeding. Examination may reveal jaundice and right upper quadrant tenderness but no hepatomegaly.

Laboratory Abnormalities

Laboratory tests may reveal moderately elevated liver function test results, hypoglycemia (secondary to impaired glycogen synthesis), and a consumptive coagulopathy due to consumption of clotting factors (which is worsened by their decreased hepatic synthesis). Patients may experience hepatorenal failure with oliguria and increased blood urea nitrogen and creatinine levels. Metabolic acidosis may be seen if multiple organ system failure develops.

Treatment

Therapy is supportive, with an emphasis on correcting metabolic derangements, maintaining oxygenation, and restoring renal and mental function. Intravenous fluid therapy should maintain serum glucose at greater than 60 mg/dL. Restricting protein intake and giving lactulose by mouth or nasogastric tube aim to prevent elevations of plasma ammonia. Stress ulcer prophylaxis should be initiated to reduce the risk of gastrointestinal hemorrhage. Coagulation abnormalities may be improved by administering clotting factors, and renal failure may require temporary hemodialysis. These patients are at high risk for nosocomial infection.

Several management options have been attempted to treat patients who are deteriorating despite traditional supportive measures. These strategies include plasmapheresis and liver transplantation. Before 1980, the reported survival rate for AFLP was only 25%; since then, however, improved ICU supportive care has increased survival rates to more than 90%.

AMNIOTIC FLUID EMBOLISM

Amniotic fluid embolism occurs in 1 in 30,000 pregnancies, most commonly during labor. Occasionally it happens early, for example, during a first trimester

Table 72-6. Differential Diagnosis of Liver Disease in Pregnancy

CONDITION	ASPARTATE AMINOTRANSFERASE LEVELS (IU/L)	TOTAL BILIRUBIN (mg/dL)	LIVER HISTOLOGIC FEATURES	OTHER FEATURES
AFLP	<500	<5	Fatty infiltration	Hypoglycemia
				Renal failure
Acute hepatitis B	>1000–2000	>5	Hepatocellular necrosis	Perinatal transmission
HELLP syndrome	>500	<5	Hepatocellular necrosis	Hypertension
				Thrombocytopenia
				Hemolysis with schistocytes
Intrahepatic cholestasis	<300	<5 (mostly direct)	Dilatated bile canaliculi	Pruritus

AFLP, acute fatty liver of pregnancy; HELLP, hemolysis, elevated liver enzymes, low platelets.

dilation and curettage, or late, for example, 48 hours postpartum. Amniotic fluid embolism has been associated with protracted labor. A release of amniotic fluid into the maternal (pulmonary) vasculature appears to be its cause, but it is not clear whether the volume of infusate or the presence of biologically active substances in the amniotic fluid is more important. Fetal squamous cells have been detected in the pulmonary vasculature of pregnant mothers who had a pulmonary artery catheter for reasons other than amniotic fluid embolism. This indicates that amniotic fluid in the maternal pulmonary vasculature is not pathognomonic for amniotic fluid embolism. It also suggests that noxious substances in the amniotic fluid (i.e., arachidonic acid metabolites) may primarily be responsible for the endothelial cell damage and cardiopulmonary changes associated with amniotic fluid embolism syndrome.

Clinical Presentation

Patients with amniotic fluid embolism most commonly present with acute respiratory distress, cyanosis, and cardiovascular collapse. The patient usually has mental status changes that ultimately may lead to coma. Clinical bleeding associated with DIC is seen in 40 to 50% of patients. The cause of DIC is unknown, but trophoblasts are known to have thromboplastin-like effects.

Acute pulmonary hypertension is transient (<1 hour) and often resolves before hemodynamic monitoring and ICU admission. A hemodynamic picture consistent with left ventricular failure (elevated pulmonary artery wedge pressure and low cardiac output) is commonly encountered. Left ventricular failure may result from myocardial hypoxia (due to decreased coronary artery flow) or direct myocardial injury from noxious substances. Pulmonary capillary endothelial injury may also result in acute respiratory distress syndrome.

Treatment

Therapy is supportive and includes maintenance of oxygenation, cardiac output, and blood pressure. The coagulopathy may not resolve quickly, and replacement of clotting factors may be used to maintain adequate clotting function until the patient improves clinically.

TOCOLYSIS-INDUCED PULMONARY EDEMA

Beta-sympathomimetic agents are widely used in the management of preterm labor. Ritodrine and terbutaline are relatively beta$_2$-selective agents that diminish the frequency of extreme maternal sinus tachycardia. When these agents are appropriately administered with free water and with accurate monitoring of the patient's fluid intake and output, the incidence of tocolysis-induced pulmonary edema is less than 1%.

Etiology

The mechanism of tocolysis-induced pulmonary edema has not been completely elucidated. Several mechanisms have been proposed based on the known pharmacologic effects of parenteral beta-sympathomimetics. Their renal effects result in sodium and water retention secondary to enhanced distal tubular sodium reabsorption and increased secretion of vasopressin, respectively. Sodium and water retention, in conjunction with the large amounts of intravenous fluids often administered to these patients, increases the intravascular hydrostatic pressure, driving fluid into the pulmonary interstitium. Additionally, endothelial damage secondary to toxins released by subclinical intrauterine infection (often associated with preterm labor) may cause increased permeability of pulmonary capillaries. These factors contribute to a clinical picture of pulmonary edema resulting from a combination of volume overload and increased permeability.

Clinical Presentation

Beta-tocolysis–induced pulmonary edema often presents with a rapidly progressive shortness of breath in association with chest discomfort and tachypnea. Physical examination reveals bilateral rales, and a chest radiograph demonstrates pulmonary edema. Arterial blood gas analysis typically shows hypoxemia. The possibility of concurrent infection (chorioamnionitis, urinary or respiratory tract) must be carefully investigated.

Management

Therapy for beta-tocolysis–induced pulmonary edema includes oxygen, morphine, or fentanyl administration to relieve dyspnea and decrease venous return; aggressive diuresis with furosemide; and discontinuation of the beta-agonist tocolytic agent. Other tocolytic agents, such as magnesium sulfate or indomethacin, may be considered if intrauterine infection is not present. Caution must be exercised when administering magnesium sulfate, because it can cause respiratory depression at toxic levels, and indomethacin, because it can diminish renal function. The maximal intravenous fluid volume should not exceed 2500 mL/day. Central hemodynamic monitoring is seldom required. However, if the patient fails to improve after diuresis, such monitoring may be needed, and other diagnoses, including pulmonary embolism and peripartum cardiomyopathy, must be considered.

BIBLIOGRAPHY

Clark SL, Cotton DB: Clinical indications for pulmonary artery catheterization in the patient with severe preeclampsia. Am J Obstet Gynecol 158:453–458, 1988.
 The author reports the clinical scenarios in which invasive hemodynamic monitoring is indicated in patients with severe preeclampsia. The most common indication is oliguria, often occurring in conjunction with pulmonary edema.

Clark SL, Greenspoon JS, Aldahl D, et al: Severe preeclampsia with persistent oliguria: Management of hemodynamic subsets. Am J Obstet Gynecol 154:490–494, 1986.
The hemodynamics profiles of nine patients with severe preeclampsia and oliguria are reviewed. Three subsets of patients are identified, including those with intravascular volume depletion, selective renal arteriospasm, and depressed left ventricular function.

Clark SL, Pavlova Z, Greenspoon J, et al: Squamous cells in the maternal pulmonary circulation. Am J Obstet Gynecol 154:104–106, 1986.
Sixteen pregnant women underwent pulmonary artery catheterization for various indications other than amniotic fluid embolism. The detection of fetal squamous cells in the pulmonary arterial circulation of these patients demonstrates that this finding is not pathognomonic for amniotic fluid embolism.

Cotton DB, Gonik B, Dorman K, et al: Cardiovascular alterations in severe pregnancy-induced hypertension: Relationship of central venous pressure to pulmonary capillary wedge pressure. Am J Obstet Gynecol 151:762–764, 1985.
This report demonstrates that central venous pressures do not correlate with pulmonary artery wedge pressures in patients with preeclampsia.

Hatjis CG, Swain M: Systemic tocolysis for premature labor is associated with an increased incidence of pulmonary edema in the presence of maternal infection. Am J Obstet Gynecol 159:723–728, 1988.
This report describes the risk factors for beta-tocolysis–induced pulmonary edema, including sodium and water retention, a narrowed hydrostatic-colloid oncotic pressure gradient, and pulmonary capillary endothelial cell damage secondary to infection.

Hypertension in pregnancy. ACOG Tech Bull 219, 1996.
This technical bulletin provides standards of care for hypertension in pregnancy. It includes a comprehensive bibliography of original papers describing chronic hypertension in pregnancy and pregnancy-induced hypertension.

Lucas MJ, Leveno KJ, Cunningham FG: A comparison of magnesium sulfate with phenytoin for the prevention of eclampsia. N Engl J Med 333:201–205, 1995.
This was a large (more than 1000 preeclamptic women in each group), randomized, controlled trial that demonstrated the superiority of magnesium sulfate versus phenytoin in preventing eclamptic seizures.

Martin JM, Blake PG, Lowry SL, et al: Pregnancy complicated by preeclampsia-eclampsia with the syndrome of hemolysis, elevated liver enzymes, and low platelet count: How rapid is postpartum recovery? Obstet Gynecol 76:737–741, 1990.
This report provides clinical guidelines describing the natural course of HELLP syndrome, which often worsens in the immediate postpartum period.

Roberts WE: Emergent obstetric management of postpartum hemorrhage. Obstet Gynecol Clin North Am 22:283–302, 1995.
This paper provides a comprehensive review of the various causes and therapeutic strategies for postpartum vaginal bleeding.

The Eclampsia Trial Collaborative Group. Which anticonvulsant for women with eclampsia? Evidence from the Collaborative Eclampsia Trial. Lancet 345:1455–1463, 1995.
This was a large, multicenter, randomized controlled trial that demonstrated a decreased risk for recurrent seizures in eclamptic women treated with magnesium sulfate versus diazepam or phenytoin.

73

Acute Respiratory Distress Syndrome

Paul N. Lanken

Acute respiratory distress syndrome (ARDS) is common in the intensive care unit (ICU) setting, with an estimated 50,000 to 100,000 cases per year in the United States. ARDS is the term used to describe the severe form of acute lung injury. Acute lung injury and ARDS are acute respiratory disorders that meet three clinical criteria: (1) poor oxygenation, (2) chest radiographic infiltrates, and (3) absence of congestive heart failure (CHF) (Table 73–1).

Synonyms for ARDS include noncardiogenic pulmonary edema, shock lung, permeability pulmonary edema, and pulmonary capillary leak syndrome. The latter two terms arise from the concept that pulmonary edema in patients with ARDS is due primarily to increased permeability of the alveolar-capillary membrane at normal or modestly elevated pulmonary capillary pressures. In contrast, pulmonary edema in left-sided CHF results from excessive filtration of plasma across the alveolar-capillary membrane as a result of high pulmonary capillary pressure (see Chapter 51).

PATHOGENESIS AND ASSOCIATED CAUSES

Acute respiratory distress syndrome results from injury to the alveolar-capillary membrane that is caused by exogenous agents or by endogenous inflammatory mediators. This injury results in leakage of plasma into the lung's interstitial and alveolar spaces, with the end result being alveolar flooding and respiratory failure. It is a *final common pathway* in response to various causes (Table 73–2). For most of these predisposing conditions, only a minority of patients at risk actually go on to have full-blown ARDS. Although it is unclear why ARDS develops in some at-risk patients, the risk of ARDS increases several-fold if the patient has multiple predisposing conditions. To date, no intervention has been effective in preventing ARDS.

Table 73–1. Criteria for Acute Lung Injury (ALI) and
Acute Respiratory Distress Syndrome (ARDS)

PARAMETER	CRITERIA FOR ALI	CRITERIA FOR ARDS
Hypoxemia	$Pao_2/Fio_2 \leq 300$	$Pao_2/Fio_2 \leq 200$
Chest radiograph	Bilateral infiltrates consistent with pulmonary edema (these may be patchy, interstitial, or alveolar in nature)	
Noncardiac cause	Absence of clinical evidence of left atrial hypertension or, if measured, pulmonary artery wedge pressure ≤ 18 mm Hg	

From Bernard GR, Artigas A, Brigham KL, et al: The American-European Consensus Conference on ARDS. Am J Respir Crit Care Med 149:818–824, 1994.

Table 73–2. Common Causes of Acute Lung Injury
and Acute Respiratory Distress Syndrome

....

Direct Causes of Lung Injury

Aspiration pneumonia
Diffuse pneumonias (viral, pneumocystis, atypical pneumonias, *Legionella*) (see Chapter 65)
Smoke and toxic gas inhalation (see Chapter 55)
Trauma to thorax with lung contusion (see Chapter 97)

Indirect Causes of Lung Injury

Acute pancreatitis (see Chapter 58)
Fulminant hepatic failure (see Chapter 59)
Massive blood transfusion with transfusion-related lung injury (see Chapter 46)
Multiple fractures with fat emboli syndrome
Postcardiopulmonary bypass (see Chapter 86)
Severe sepsis and septic shock (see Chapter 8)

....

CLINICAL CONSIDERATIONS

Clinical Features

Patients with ARDS typically present with acute respiratory distress at the same time as, or shortly after, one or more of the associated causes (see Table 73–2). The physical examination is notable for signs of respiratory distress, rapid shallow respirations with or without scattered inspiratory crackles. They often have orthopnea but no other signs of CHF. Chest radiographs show characteristic diffuse bilateral infiltrates without cardiac enlargement. Initially, the infiltrates may be interstitial and then progress to widespread alveolar densities.

Arterial blood gas results in very early ARDS are most notable for hypoxemia, but often, there is *hypocapnia* with a primary respiratory alkalosis. PaO_2 typically remains low, despite supplemental oxygen. A high respiratory rate and an increased work of breathing rapidly lead to respiratory muscle fatigue, *hypercapnia*, and need for intubation and mechanical ventilation. Because some patients with ARDS may have associated life-threatening conditions, such as hemorrhagic or septic shock, their ARDS may become evident only after initial stabilization and volume resuscitation.

Differential Diagnosis

The differential diagnosis is relatively short and includes cardiogenic pulmonary edema and a few acute conditions with large right-to-left shunts that cause severe hypoxemia. Examples of the latter include severe atelectasis (especially if hypoxic pulmonary vasoconstriction is blunted by vasodilators), opening of a patent foramen ovale as a result of acute pulmonary hypertension arising from a major acute pulmonary embolus, and diffuse pulmonary hemorrhage.

Evidence in favor of CHF includes a cardiac history, an enlarged heart on chest radiograph, and a third heart sound. Rapid improvement after diuresis strongly suggests CHF. As noted in Table 73–1, pulmonary artery wedge pressures (PAWP) of less than or equal to 18 mm Hg support the diagnosis of ARDS. However, similar wedge pressures may be present at the time of measurement in some patients with CHF. Examples include those who undergo diuresis in the interval between the occurrence of pulmonary edema and PAWP determination and those who have "flash pulmonary edema," in which transient ischemia-induced left ventricular dysfunction or papillary muscle dysfunction resolves before PAWP measurement.

PATHOPHYSIOLOGY OF ARDS

Hypoxemia

In early-phase ARDS, the most life-threatening problem is severe hypoxemia. This arises predominantly from a large right-to-left intrapulmonary shunt through numerous fluid-filled alveoli. Its magnitude can be estimated as follows: a 5% shunt is present for every 100 mm Hg decrease in Pao_2 below 700 mm Hg while the patient is breathing 100% oxygen. For example, if Pao_2 on 100% oxygen is 200 mm Hg, then the shunt is approximately 25%. (This estimate is accurate only for Pao_2 values above 150 mm Hg.) Patients with ARDS who need mechanical ventilation usually have shunts in the range of 20 to 50% (normal subjects have right-to-left shunts of 5% or less). Increased right-to-left shunt is the cause of the difficulty in reversing hypoxemia with supplemental oxygen, even with oxygen concentrations of 100%. Because of this, one goal of ARDS management is to decrease the shunt fraction by reopening (recruiting) alveoli with no ventilation.

Low Compliance

Decreased lung compliance in ARDS is due to widespread interstitial and alveolar edema and atelectatic alveoli (microatelectasis). Decreased surfactant activity leads to collapse of alveoli at end-expiration and increased hysteresis between inspiratory and expiratory pressure-volume curves. The low lung compliance results in low respiratory system compliance. For example, a ventilator-delivered tidal volume of 1000 mL produces an end-inspiratory pressure (plateau pressure) of 10 cm H_2O in a patient with a normal compliance of 100 mL/cm H_2O (this assumes that no positive end-expiratory pressure [PEEP] is present) (see Fig. 2–3, Chapter 2). In contrast, the same tidal volume results in a plateau pressure of 50 cm H_2O in a patient with ARDS whose respiratory system compliance is only 20 mL/cm H_2O (again assuming no PEEP). If PEEP *is* present, then the plateau pressure would be even higher.

Loss of alveolar surfactant activity contributes to the low lung compliance in ARDS. At least three different mechanisms decrease alveolar surfactant activity: (1) edema fluid washes surfactant out of alveolar spaces, (2) injury occurring to alveolar type II pneumocytes compromises surfactant production and secretion, and (3) contact with plasma proteins inactivates surfactant. Although loss of surfactant activity contributes to the physiologic abnormalities and respiratory failure in this phase of ARDS, its relative importance remains unclear, and clinical trials testing replacement surfactant therapy have been inconclusive.

Fully Flooded
Alveolus

Partially Flooded
and Collapsed
Alveolus

Fully Collapsed
Alveolus

Normal Alveolus

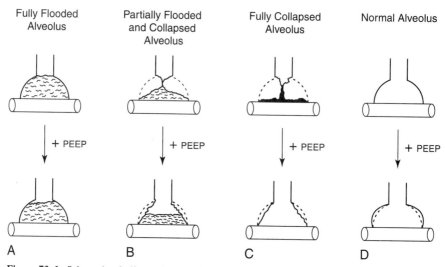

A   B   C   D

Figure 73–1. Schematic of effects of positive end-expiratory pressure (PEEP) on recruitable and non-recruitable regions of lungs with ARDS. Alveoli B and C represent the recruitable lung units. Completely fluid-filled alveolus *(A)* are non-recruitable since PEEP can not open such alveoli. Likewise, completely normal alveoli *(D)* are also considered to be non-recruitable since the PEEP-induced increase in their resting volume represents alveolar *overdistention.* (From Lanken PN: Adult respiratory distress syndrome: Clinical management. In: Carlson RW, Geheb MA [Eds]: The Principles and Practice of Medical Intensive Care. Philadelphia: WB Saunders 1991.)

Although the chest radiograph shows the infiltrates as diffusely uniform, computed tomographic (CT) scans of the lungs of ARDS patients indicate a more patchy distribution of fluid and atelectasis. There are three categories of alveoli: (1) completely filled and nonrecruitable alveoli, (2) atelectatic and recruitable alveoli, and (3) open alveoli (Fig. 73–1). Some have regarded the recruitable and open alveoli as a "baby lung," because they constitute a small fraction of the total lung. Lung protective strategies, such as low tidal volume ventilation, as described later, are based in part on the concept that in ARDS, one is really ventilating a lung for which traditionally sized tidal volumes (10 to 12 mL/kg) are too large, resulting in alveolar overdistention and lung injury.

Increased Minute Ventilation

Patients with ARDS have increased minute ventilation. This results from marked increases in alveolar deadspace, arising from microscopic level changes in ventilation-perfusion (V/Q) ratios that increase the number of alveoli with V/Q greater than 1. Overall dead space to tidal volume ratios are commonly in the 0.7 to 0.8 range (compared with a normal dead space to total ventilation (VD/VT) ratio of 0.3). As a result, the minute ventilation must be increased two to three times in order to keep the $Paco_2$ in the normal range (see Appendix B, Fig. 1). During mechanical ventilation this requires high inspiratory flow rates to maintain an inspiratory-to-expiratory ratio of less than 1. Although high respiratory rates are needed to keep Pa_{CO_2} in the normal range, many clinicians, especially if they are using low tidal volume ventilation, allow Pa_{CO_2} to rise (permissive hypercapnia).

MECHANISMS OF LUNG INJURY

Acute Exudative Phase in Early ARDS

Early-phase ARDS presents as failure of the lungs alone (single-organ failure) or as failure of the lungs with failure of other organs at the same time as part of the syndrome of multiorgan system failure (MOSF). At the beginning of the exudative phase, no morphologic changes may be seen histologically or ultrastructurally other than edema in the interstitium. After gross alveolar edema forms, a pattern of diffuse alveolar damage is present. On histologic examination, protein-rich edema with inflammatory cells fills the alveoli. Hyaline membranes, made up of fibrin strands, form a pseudoepithelium over denuded alveolar basement membranes. The edema may be severe, with lungs from patients with ARDS each weighing more than 1000 g each, a figure that is several times normal.

Overdistention of alveoli resulting from high pressures ("volutrauma" or ventilator-induced lung injury [VILI]) produced by positive pressure mechanical ventilation and PEEP also contributes to the acute exudative phase by augmenting the original injury. Evidence from animal and in vitro lung experiments indicates that subjecting normal lungs to high distending pressures results in the production and release of proinflammatory cytokines and the histologic appearance of diffuse alveolar damage. In addition, ventilation of lungs at physiologically appropriate sized tidal volumes but without any end-expiratory distending pressure, that is, PEEP, can cause release of the same cytokines and lung injury. Based on these reports, it has been hypothesized that traditional volume ventilation with tidal volumes of 10 to 12 mL/kg is an important mechanism that enhances the initial lung injury of ARDS. In addition, systemic release of these proinflammatory mediators from the lung may result in injury to remote organs and subsequent development of MOSF.

When ARDS presents with MOSF syndrome, injury to the lungs and other organs is presumed to be mediated through activation of same endogenous inflammatory mediators and cytokines as the predisposing condition. Neutrophils are hypothesized to be an important mediator of lung injury. They are first sequestered in pulmonary capillaries by endotoxin-mediated complement activation or by cytokine release. After attachment to endothelium and migration into the interstitial and alveolar spaces, they damage endothelial and epithelial cells by producing reactive oxidant species and releasing proteolytic enzymes. Damage to intercellular junctions and cell-substrate connections increases alveolar permeability. In addition, direct injury to endothelium and epithelium by cytokines, such as tumor necrosis factor-alpha, augments the deleterious effects of the neutrophils.

Fibroproliferative Pattern in Late-Phase ARDS

In patients with ARDS who survive the acute exudative phase, alveolar and interstitial remodeling begins after the lung injury is widespread and well established. This may be as early as 1 week after onset. Type II pneumocytes proliferate after loss of the type I cells and eventually differentiate into new type I pneumocytes to reconstitute the alveolar epithelium. In response to mediators released by the inflammatory process in ARDS and toxic concentrations of oxygen, fibroblasts proliferate, migrate, and produce collagen, resulting in alveolar and interstitial fibrosis.

Oxygen toxicity undoubtedly contributes to the pathologic changes in most cases of late-phase ARDS, but its exact role remains uncertain for many reasons. Patients with ARDS are virtually always exposed to a high oxygen concentration, which is by itself a cause of ARDS. The level of FIO_2 that is nontoxic for patients with injured lungs remains unknown. These fibroproliferative changes may be marked and may cause death either from progressive hypoxemic respiratory failure or from nosocomial pneumonia and sepsis, to which patients with late-phase ARDS on ventilators seem to be exquisitely vulnerable.

CLINICAL MANAGEMENT: SPECIFIC THERAPY

Specific therapy for ARDS is directed against the cause of the ARDS, such as an antibiotic against an infection causing diffuse pneumonia, or against one or more steps in its pathogenetic mechanism, such as an agent that blocks a crucial step in lung inflammation or fibrosis. In contrast, *supportive therapy* includes everything else that is done for ARDS patients to preserve their life and restore them to health (Table 73–3).

Specific therapy for early-phase ARDS is limited except in cases involving treatable infections or diffuse pulmonary hemorrhage (see Chapter 75). A controlled clinical trial indicated that a limited course of high-dose corticosteroids does not improve mortality in patients early after the onset of ARDS. In contrast, a much lower daily dose of corticosteroids has become accepted therapy for patients with pneumocystis pneumonia caused by human immunodeficiency virus.

Table 73–3. Therapies for Early-Phase Acute Respiratory Distress Syndrome (ARDS)

Specific Therapies

Antimicrobials in ARDS due to specific treatable infectious causes
Treatment of primary condition causing diffuse alveolar hemorrhage (see Chapter 75)
Corticosteroids in pneumocystis pneumonia and some diffuse alveolar hemorrhage syndromes (see Chapter 75)

Supportive Therapies

Mechanical ventilation with PEEP
Low tidal volume ventilation strategy (see Table 73–4)
Pressure-control ventilation with or without inverse inspiratory-to-expiratory ratio
Prone positioning
Nitric oxide inhalation
Extraordinary methods of gas exchange
    Extracorporeal membrane oxygenation
    Extracorporeal CO_2 removal
    Lowering pulmonary capillary hydrostatic pressure by fluid removal and restriction

Other anti-inflammatory agents have shown promise in animal studies or in preliminary human studies, but confirmation of their efficacy by large, multicenter, controlled clinical trials is lacking.

Some intensivists treat late-phase ARDS with a several-week course of high-dose corticosteroids based on the rationale that persistent inflammation in the lung occurs in many patients with late-phase ARDS and that corticosteroids should be able to suppress this. In addition, many patients with late-phase ARDS have high levels of circulating proinflammatory cytokines, which may be important in perpetuating the fibroproliferative process, and these also can be suppressed by corticosteroids. Although one small, controlled clinical trial and case series from several ICUs suggest that steroids are effective for patients with late-phase ARDS, many intensivists are uncertain of their efficacy or safety. To address this uncertainty, a multicenter, randomized, controlled clinical trial of steroids in late-phase ARDS is ongoing.

CLINICAL MANAGEMENT: SUPPORTIVE THERAPY

Mechanical Ventilation

Almost all patients with ARDS need endotracheal intubation and mechanical ventilation for their survival. The goal of mechanical ventilation is to maintain adequate arterial oxygenation in a patient (usually with a target PaO_2 of 55 to 70 mm Hg) breathing nontoxic oxygen concentrations (usually assumed to be in the 50 to 60% range).

Because ARDS patients have stiff lungs and high VD/VT ratios, they have been commonly treated with high peak inflation pressures and minute ventilations of 25 to 35 L/min to keep their $PaCO_2$ normal. Mechanical ventilators with high flow and pressure capabilities are the standard of practice. Heavy sedation and pharmacologic paralysis, if necessary, are routinely used to decrease peak inspiratory pressures, work of breathing, oxygen consumption, and CO_2 production. In severe cases, the target PaO_2 may be adjusted downward into the 45 to 50 mm Hg range, or even lower, in order to avoid prolonged exposure to potentially toxic oxygen concentrations.

Positive End-Expiratory Pressure

Mechanism of Action

Positive end-expiratory pressure improves arterial oxygenation and decreases right-to-left shunt in most patients with ARDS. PEEP increases the end-expiratory position of the lungs (functional residual capacity) by re-inflating completely atelectatic alveoli and expanding alveoli that are partially atelectatic or open (Fig. 73–2; see also Fig. 73–1). By decreasing the number of alveoli with V/Q ratios of zero or nearly zero, PEEP decreases the shunt fraction and, hence, improves oxygenation. In addition, through its lung recruitment effects, PEEP often improves respiratory system compliance and may make it possible to deliver the same tidal volume at a lower peak airway pressure (Fig. 73–2).

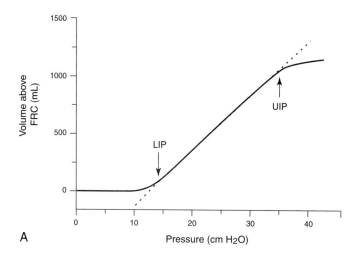

A

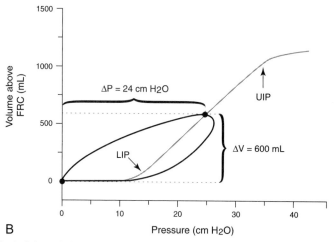

B

Figure 73–2. *A,* Schematic inspiratory static pressure-volume (P-V) curve of the respiratory system (lung and chest wall combined) in ARDS with a lower inflection point (LIP) at ~14 cm H_2O and an upper inflection point (UIP) at ~35 cm H_2O. The abscissa is recoil pressure of the respiratory system and the ordinate is lung volume above functional residual capacity (FRC). *B,* Same static P-V as in *A,* plus a dynamic P-V curve of 600 mL tidal volume starting at PEEP = 0, which is below the LIP. This tidal volume results in a plateau pressure of 24 cm H_2O, which is below the UIP. Static compliance (Cstat = $\Delta V/\Delta P$ = 600 mL/24 cm H_2O) is 25 mL/cm H_2O.

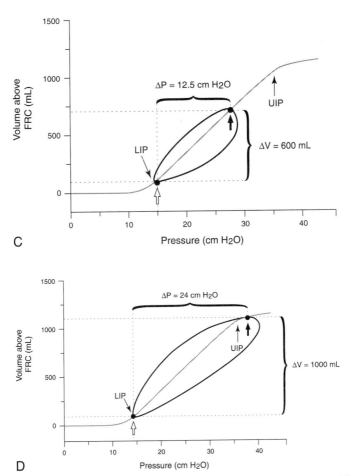

Figure 73–2 *Continued. C,* PEEP of 15 cm H$_2$O has moved the starting point for the 600 mL tidal volume up the static P-V curve to a new FRC *(open arrow),* which is just above the LIP. The tidal volume results in a plateau pressure of 27.5 cm H$_2$O *(closed arrow),* which is still well *below* the UIP. Cstat (ΔV/ΔP = 600 mL/12.5 cm H$_2$O) is increased to 48 mL/cm H$_2$O, compared to *B. D,* Dynamic P-V curve of a 1000 mL tidal volume, starting at 14 cm H$_2$O PEEP, results in a plateau pressure of 38 cm H$_2$O *(closed arrow).* Note the decrease in Cstat (ΔV/ΔP = 1000 mL/24 cm H$_2$O = 41.7 mL/ cm H$_2$O) compared to Cstat derived from the tidal volume of 600 mL in *C.* The 1000 mL tidal volume's plateau pressure exceeds the UIP, which implies alveolar overdistention and is believed to put the lung at risk for ventilator-induced lung injury (see text).

Empiric Method for Setting PEEP

Positive end-expiratory pressure should generally be applied in increments of 2 to 3 cm H_2O and titrated to effect, depending on its indications. For example, when PEEP is used to reverse life-threatening degrees of hypoxemia despite mechanical ventilation with 100% oxygen, PEEP is initiated at 5 or 10 cm H_2O. It is increased rapidly by steps of 3 to 5 cm H_2O until the target Pao_2 is reached or PEEP levels reach 20 or 25 cm H_2O. In this approach, the degree of PEEP-induced lung recruitment is reflected by improvement in Pao_2.

Although increasing PEEP raises the Pao_2 in most cases of ARDS, high PEEP may reduce cardiac output by decreasing venous return to the thorax ("central tourniquet effect"). This reduction in cardiac output can usually be reversed by infusions of inotropic agents or by intravascular volume expansion, although the latter may create more lung edema.

In general, once the target Pao_2 has been achieved by PEEP, Fio_2 is lowered to nontoxic concentrations. Once this is achieved, PEEP is gradually decreased as tolerated. PEEP is lowered stepwise, by use of small decrements, because the abrupt removal of PEEP may result in a precipitous fall in Pao_2, which can take hours to fully recover. For the same reason, routine suctioning of the patient's airways should be minimized, and when suctioning is needed, a closed system should be used. Likewise, because PEEP is critical for oxygenation, it should not be removed in order to measure PAWP.

Best PEEP Determinations

Some have suggested that "best PEEP" for a particular patient be determined by multiplying the Cao_2, oxygen content of arterial blood (see Table 7–3, Chapter 7), at several levels of PEEP by the cardiac index at those levels. One then selects best PEEP as the level that yields maximal oxygen delivery. This approach was based on the hypothesis that increasing cardiac output was a primary goal in treatment of patients with ARDS. Others have advocated that best PEEP should be at the point of maximal compliance of the respiratory system. However, no outcome studies demonstrate the efficacy of either of these recommendations.

More recently, others have advocated that one should set the PEEP at a level determined by measurements of lung recruitment. This is achieved by first measuring the patient's static pressure-volume (P-V) curve with a super syringe. Then, one identifies the lower inflection point (see Fig. 73–2) and sets PEEP at a level just above it. This method may be difficult to do, however, if P-V curves do not show clear, reproducible lower inflection points. In addition, one may need to paralyze the patient to obtain the P-V curve. Finally, P-V curves may change daily, so repeated determinations are recommended. The combination of sufficient PEEP to exceed the lower inflection point and ventilation with a tidal volume small enough so as not to exceed the upper inflection point of the P-V curve (see Fig. 73–2) has been referred to as the "open lung" strategy or the lung protective ventilatory strategy. Controlled clinical trials using this strategy or a low tidal volume ventilation strategy (without measuring lower inflection points) have reported improved survival (described later in more detail).

Rather than relying on the older definition of best PEEP as maximal oxygen delivery or measuring P-V curves, most ICU clinicians adjust PEEP empirically, similar to the approach noted earlier.

Variations in Mechanical Ventilation with PEEP

Low Tidal Volume Ventilation

Based on the evidence that high alveolar distending pressures can cause lung injury, a multicenter clinical trial involving 24 ICUs (by the ARDS Network) tested the efficacy and safety of a low tidal volume ventilation strategy in acute lung injury and ARDS. This strategy used the assist/control mode with a tidal volume of 6 mL/kg predicted body weight (PBW) (Table 73–4). If the plateau pressure (Pplat) at this tidal volume was less than 30 cm H_2O, the patient continued to receive the 6 mL/kg PBW tidal volume. If the Pplat exceeded 30 cm H_2O, however, the tidal volume was lowered stepwise until the Pplat dropped below 30 cm H_2O or the tidal volume reached a minimum of 4 mL/kg PBW (whichever occurred first). Respiratory rates were increased up to 35 breaths/min to treat associated respiratory acidosis. PEEP and FIO_2 were set according to a uniform protocol derived from the clinical practices used in the participating ICUs.

This low tidal volume ventilation strategy was compared in a randomized, controlled clinical trial with a traditional tidal volume ventilation strategy. The latter ventilated patients also in the assist/control mode but at 12 mL/kg PBW. If Pplat at this tidal volume was less than 50 cm H_2O, no change in tidal volume was made. If Pplat exceeded 50 cm H_2O, however, the tidal volume was reduced until Pplat fell below 50 cm H_2O or until the tidal volume reached 4 mL/kg PBW (whichever occurred first).

This study tested the hypothesis that low alveolar pressures would result in better survival for patients with acute lung injury and ARDS. Ventilating at low tidal volumes hypothetically should decrease the degree of alveolar overdistention and associated alveolar injury. Because of the efficacy of the low tidal volume strategy group, this clinical trial ended prematurely in February 1999 after 861 patients were enrolled. This group showed a statistically significant decrease in hospital mortality compared with the traditional tidal volume group. The mortality fell from 39.8% to 31.0%, representing a 22% relative decrease. This study's protocol is summarized in Table 73–4.

Another controlled clinical trial (by Amato et al.), involving two institutions and a smaller number of patients (53), also tested a low tidal volume ventilation strategy. In this lung protective strategy, however, small tidal volumes were combined with PEEP levels that were set above the lower inflection points derived by static P-V curves (see Fig. 73–2) and with additional lung recruitment maneuvers after suctioning or disconnection from the ventilator. This trial also showed a statistically significant reduction in mortality in the lung protection group.

Because the relationship and the mechanism between mechanical forces and alveolar injury are complex, large multicenter, controlled clinical trials are needed to determine whether the lung protective strategy (which used higher PEEP levels than the strategy used in the ARDS Network) has better outcomes than the ARDS Network low tidal volume ventilation strategy.

Table 73–4. NIH NHLBI ARDS Network Low Tidal Volume Ventilation Protocol Summary

Part I. Ventilator Setup and Adjustment

1. Calculate predicted body weight (PBW).*
2. Use assist/control mode and set initial tidal volume (V_T) to 8 mL/kg PBW (if baseline V_T >8 mL/kg).
3. Reduce V_T by 1 mL/kg at intervals ≤2 h until V_T = 6 mL/kg PBW.
4. Set initial rate to approximate baseline $\dot{V}_E$ (but not >35 bpm).
5. Adjust V_T and RR to achieve pH and plateau pressure (Pplat) goals below.
6. Set inspiratory flow rate above patient demand (usually >80 L/min); adjust flow rate to achieve goal of I:E ratio of 1:1.0–1.3.

Part II. Oxygenation Goal: Pao$_2$ = 55–80 mm Hg or Sao$_2$ = 88–95%

1. Use these incremental FIO_2-PEEP combinations to achieve oxygenation goal:

FIO_2	0.3	0.4	0.4	0.5	0.5	0.6	0.7	0.7
PEEP	5	5	8	8	10	10	10	12
FIO_2	0.7	0.8	0.9	0.9	0.9	1.0	1.0	1.0
PEEP	14	14	14	16	18	20	22	24

Part III. Plateau Pressure (Pplat) Goal: ≤30 cm H$_2$O

1. Check Pplat (use 0.5-sec inspiratory pause), Sao$_2$, total RR, V_T, and ABG (if available) at least q 4 h and after each change in PEEP or V_T.
2. If Pplat >30 cm H$_2$O, decrease V_T by 1-mL/kg steps (to a minimum of 4 mL/kg PBW).
3. If Pplat <25 cm H$_2$O and V_T <6 mL/kg PBW, increase V_T by 1 mL/kg until Pplat >25 cm H$_2$O or V_T = 6 mL/kg PBW.
4. If Pplat <30 cm H$_2$O and breath stacking occurs, one may increase V_T in 1-mL/kg PBW increments (to a maximum of 8 mL/kg PBW).

Part IV. pH Goal: 7.30–7.45

Acidosis Management: pH <7.30
1. If pH = 7.15–7.30, increase RR until pH >7.30 or Paco$_2$ <25 mm Hg (maximum RR = 35); if RR = 35 and Paco$_2$ <25 mm Hg, may give NaHCO$_3$.
2. If pH <7.15 and NaHCO$_3$ considered or infused, V_T may be increased in 1-mL/kg PBW steps until pH >7.15 (Pplat goal may be exceeded).

Alkalosis Management: pH >7.45
Decrease RR if possible

From The Acute Respiratory Distress Syndrome Network: Ventilation with lower tidal volumes as compared with traditional tidal volumes for acute lung injury and the acute respiratory distress syndrome. N Engl J Med 342:1301–1308, 2000. (Complete protocol is available *at www.ardsnet.org*).
*Male PBW = 50 + 2.3 (height [inches] −60); female PBW = 45.5 + 2.3 (height [inches] −60)
ABG, arterial blood gas; ARDS, acute respiratory distress syndrome; bpm, breaths per minute; I:E, inspiratory-to-expiratory; NHLBI, National Heart, Lung, and Blood Institute; NIH, National Institutes of Health; PBW, predicted body weight; PEEP, positive end-expiratory pressure; RR, respiratory rate on ventilator; Sao$_2$, oxygen saturation by pulse oximetry; V_T, tidal volume; $\dot{V}_E$, minute ventilation.

Pressure Control and Inverse Ratio Ventilation

Pressure control (PC) ventilation is another method of limiting alveolar pressure and is often used as a "salvage" mode in the face of deteriorating oxygenation in severe ARDS (Fig. 73–3). The flow pattern in PC ventilation is complex and requires a microprocessor-driven mechanical ventilator. PC is often used in conjunction with inverse ratio ventilation (IRV), in which the "inverse ratio" refers to an inspiratory time to expiratory time (I:E) ratio that is less than 1. Conventional I:E ratios, 1:3 to 1:1, provide time for passive expiration to facilitate blood return

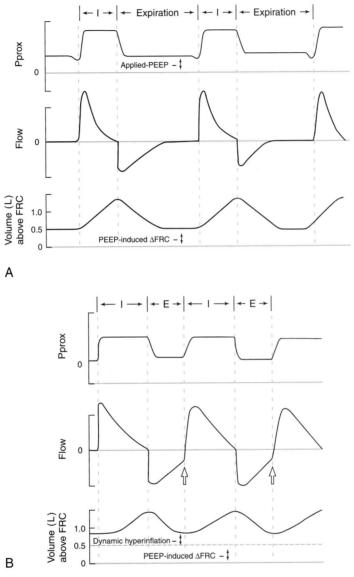

Figure 73–3. Schematic pressure, flow, and volume waveforms during pressure control ventilation (PCV) with applied PEEP. *A,* The inspiratory-to-expiratory (I:E) time is about 1:2. The pressure waveform resembles pressure support mode with the patient triggering each breath (see Fig. 2–5, Chapter 2) but with a marked decelerating flow pattern. The applied PEEP increases the functional residual capacity (FRC) by about 500 mL (PEEP-induced ΔFRC). *B,* In pressure-controlled inverse ratio ventilation (PC-IRV), the I:E time is "reversed," with I>E. Because of this, the next breath starts before expiratory flow has returned to zero *(open arrows),* resulting in auto-PEEP and dynamic hyperinflation of about 300 mL. The latter is in addition to the increased FRC due to the applied PEEP (PEEP-induced ΔFRC). The patient is not initiating any breaths. E, expiration; I, inspiration; PEEP, positive end-expiratory pressure; Pprox, pressure at the proximal end of the endotracheal tube.

to the heart. In pressure control inverted-ratio ventilation (PC-IRV), inspiration is deliberately prolonged so that it exceeds expiration by 50 to 400%. This method "stacks" tidal volumes because there is insufficient time for complete exhalation of the preceding breath. Dynamic hyperinflation (increased functional residual capacity) results and is reflected by the presence of auto-PEEP, an elevated end-expiratory alveolar pressure caused by elastic recoil of incompletely emptied alveoli. PC-IRV increases mean airway pressure compared with conventional mechanical ventilation utilizing the same tidal volume and pressure limit. The associated increase in Pao_2 is probably due to its effects on mean airway pressure and end-expiratory pressure.

The complications of PC-IRV are the same as those of conventional modes. There is the potential for more hemodynamic compromise as a result of higher mean airway pressures and for more barotrauma as a result of high alveolar pressure caused by unrecognized dynamic hyperinflation and auto-PEEP. In addition, IRV almost always necessitates heavy sedation and often paralysis of the patient. Controlled clinical trials are lacking that support the superiority of PC-IRV to conventional modes of mechanical ventilation in efficacy or safety in therapy of ARDS.

Prone Positioning

Some reports have described improvements in oxygenation with the use of prone positioning. The rationale behind this method is based on the computed tomographic findings in ARDS that show localization of lung water in the dependent parts of the lung. It was hypothesized that turning a patient from supine to prone would result in less right-to-left shunt through the fluid-filled alveoli because the prone position gas-filled alveoli would now be in the dependent parts of the lung. Most reports find that the technique results in improved Pao_2 in a majority of patients with ARDS. However, the improvement in oxygenation is temporary, but it may respond repeatedly to further turning. Complications of this method include loss of airway during the turning and pressure ulcers on the chin and face if the prone position is continued for prolonged periods of time.

Nitric Oxide by Inhalation

Like prone positioning, inhaled nitric oxide (NO) has been reported to improve oxygenation on a temporary basis. Because NO leads to relaxation of smooth muscle, it is hypothesized that inhaled NO functions as a selective vasodilator that affects only those alveoli that are ventilated. By this action, it selectively increases blood flow to these ventilated alveoli by lowering arteriolar resistance. It has no effect on nonventilated alveoli, because it is given by inhalation and does not reach them. In addition, it has no systemic effects, because its effects dissipate quickly after combining with hemoglobin.

A controlled clinical trial comparing NO inhalation versus conventional mechanical ventilation in 177 patients with ARDS indicated that NO inhalation improved Pao_2 in about 60% of enrolled patients but that its effects seemed to be transient. Furthermore, no improvements in mortality or length of time on the ventilator were observed in the NO treated group.

In the United States, some ICUs use NO for selected patients with severe ARDS as part of their salvage therapy package. Although NO seems to have little toxicity when it is properly administered, tolerance to the inhaled NO develops so that severe hypoxemia can result if the supply of NO were to stop abruptly. Another drawback of NO is its high cost (up to $4000/day).

Extracorporeal Methods of Gas Exchange

Although limited by local availability and cost, extracorporeal methods to provide oxygenation or carbon dioxide removal have been used in certain centers to treat selected patients with severe ARDS (see Table 73–3). If extracorporeal membrane oxygenation (ECMO) is to be used, it should commence within the first week of ARDS; otherwise, the lung damage appears to be irreversible. Although two controlled clinical trials of patients with severe ARDS have not demonstrated superiority over ventilator-based therapy in terms of survival, some centers in the United States and Europe advocate its use for highly selected patients.

Hemodynamic and Fluid and Diuretic Therapy

Because of increased permeability, the pulmonary edema in ARDS may worsen markedly with increases in pulmonary capillary pressure. Diuretics and fluid restriction are commonly used to lower this pressure. In patients with ARDS and MOSF, however, decreasing intravascular volume is usually limited by problems in maintaining blood pressure, cardiac output, and organ perfusion. Inotropic agents like dopamine are often added to compensate for decreased left-ventricular preload, to maintain renal function, and to keep pulmonary capillary pressure low. Although ARDS patients with a more positive fluid balance have been reported to have worse outcomes, the more positive fluid balance might have been a marker, rather than a cause, of those with worse prognoses. Optimal fluid management in ARDS, especially in MOSF, remains controversial.

Although monitoring of intravascular volume by measuring pulmonary artery wedge pressures has been commonly used in the treatment of ARDS patients, the use of the pulmonary arterial catheter has been reported to be a risk factor for increased mortality in several groups of ICU patients. Whether this association, like the positive fluid balance, merely reflects a selection bias, in other words, whether clinicians are more likely to use pulmonary arterial catheters in patients with MOSF who are sicker and who do not respond to initial hemodynamic therapy, or whether it represents a real risk to patients remains unanswered. In the meantime, one should insert a pulmonary arterial catheter only to answer a specific question or to guide fluid or hemodynamic therapy. Importantly, one should remove it when it is no longer clearly essential for the treatment of the patient. Continued use after 4 days is a strong indication for change in the access site because of increased risk of catheter-associated infections.

General ICU Supportive Care

The survival of patients with ARDS appears to have improved dramatically over the past decade, with mortality rates falling from 40 to 60% in the 1980s to 30 to 40% in the 1990s. In the absence of a "magic bullet" to treat ARDS, this encouraging trend suggests that improvements in general ICU supportive care may have resulted in the better outcomes. Patients with ARDS require comprehensive supportive care. This includes intensive nursing and respiratory care; heavy sedation, commonly with paralysis (see Chapter 4); prophylaxis against stress-related gastric erosions and deep venous thromboses (see Chapter 10); early detection and management of life-threatening barotrauma (see Chapter 32); replacement therapy for renal and other organ failure (see Chapter 16); aggressive nutritional therapy (see Chapter 13); and prevention, early diagnosis, and treatment of nosocomial infections (see Chapters 11 and 14).

LONG-TERM PROGNOSIS

Most patients with ARDS who are weaned from mechanical ventilation have a good prognosis for continued recovery of lung function. Although most patients have no clinically significant residual lung damage after 1 year, many have prolonged physical deficits and emotional distress as a result of effects of their critical illness, prolonged ICU hospitalization, and comorbid conditions.

BIBLIOGRAPHY

Acute Respiratory Distress Syndrome Network: Ventilation with lower tidal volumes as compared with traditional tidal volumes for acute lung injury and the acute respiratory distress syndrome. N Engl J Med 342:1301–1308, 2000.
This multicenter randomized, controlled clinical trial of 861 patients with acute lung injury and acute respiratory distress syndrome showed that a low tidal volume ventilation strategy (summarized in Table 73–4) significantly decreased mortality (from 39.8% to 31.0%, P = 0.007).

Amato MBP, Barbas CSV, Medeiros DM, et al: Effects of a protective-ventilation strategy on mortality in the acute respiratory distress syndrome. N Engl J Med 338:347–354, 1998.
Important report of a controlled clinical trial from two institutions showed a statistically significant decrease in mortality by use of a lung protective strategy of ventilation.

Ashbaugh DG, Bigelow DB, Petty TL, Levine BE: Acute respiratory distress in adults. Lancet 2:319–323, 1967.
Classic original description of ARDS and use of PEEP in its management.

Bernard GR, Artigas A, Brigham KL, et al: The American-European Consensus Conference on ARDS. Am Rev Respir Dis 149:818–824, 1994.
This report presented the currently utilized criteria for defining acute lung injury and ARDS.

Chatte G, Sab J-M, Dubois J-M, et al: Prone position in mechanically ventilated patients with severe acute respiratory failure. Am J Respir Crit Care Med 155:473–478, 1997.
Recent series of 32 ARDS patients, 78% of whom had improved oxygenation after prone positioning.

Davidson TA, Caldwell ES, Curtis JR, et al: Reduced quality of life in survivors of acute respiratory distress syndrome compared with critically ill control patients. JAMA 281:354–360, 1999.
This case control study found that survivors of ARDS had clinically significant reductions in health-related quality of life that seemed to be caused by their ARDS and its sequelae (compared with matched controls of patients with trauma or sepsis without ARDS).

Dellinger RF, Zimmerman JL, Taylor R, et al: Effects of inhaled nitric oxide in patients with acute respiratory distress syndrome: Results of a randomized phase II trial. Crit Care Med 26:15–23, 1998.
Large, randomized, controlled clinical trial that found temporary improvement in oxygenation in about 60% of enrolled patients with ARDS but no improvement in survival or days on ventilator.

Elliot CG, Rasmusson BY, Crapo RO, et al: Prediction of pulmonary function abnormalities after acute respiratory distress syndrome (ARDS). Am Rev Respir Dis 135:634–638, 1987.
Most patients with ARDS recover full functional capacity, and some have residual defects in diffusion capacity.

Gattinoni L, Pesenti A, Bombino M, et al: Relationships between lung computed tomographic density, gas exchange and PEEP in acute respiratory failure. Anesthesiology 69:824–832, 1988.
Classic article describing heterogeneous distribution of fluid in the lung in ARDS and effects of PEEP.

Humphrey HJ, Hall J, Sznajder JI, et al: Improved survival following pulmonary capillary wedge pressure reduction in patients with ARDS. Chest 97:1176, 1990.
An observational study indicating an association between lower pulmonary capillary wedge pressures and improved survival.

Kolobow R, Moretti MP, Gumagalli R, et al: Severe impairment in lung function induced by high peak airway pressure during mechanical ventilation: An experimental study. Am Rev Respir Dis 135:312–315, 1987.
This demonstrated that high alveolar pressures can cause an ARDS-like disorder in animals. Results like this raised the question of whether the same effect occurs in humans.

Milberg JA, Davis DR, Steinberg KP, et al: Improved survival of patients with acute respiratory distress syndrome (ARDS): 1983–1993. JAMA 273:306–309, 1995.
Harborview Hospital in Seattle reported improved survival over 10 years, reaching 64% in 1993, most notably in those with ARDS caused by sepsis and in those younger than 60 years.

Meduri GU, Headley AS, Golden E, et al: Effect of prolonged methylprednisolone therapy in unresolving acute respiratory distress syndrome: A randomized controlled trial. JAMA 280:159–165, 1998.
Promising results of high-dose steroid therapy in late-phase ARDS in a small controlled trial from a single institution.

Ware LB, Matthay MA: The acute respiratory distress syndrome. N Engl J Med 342:1334–1349, 2000.
This is a recent, outstanding and comprehensive review that includes a description and discussion of clinical trials of ventilatory strategies and pharmacologic interventions (with 146 references).

74

Acute Respiratory Failure Due to Asthma and Chronic Obstructive Pulmonary Disease

Melissa D. Cohen
Reynold A. Panettieri, Jr

Acute life-threatening exacerbations of asthma and chronic obstructive pulmonary disease (COPD) occur frequently and they commonly result in admission to the intensive care unit (ICU). The importance of these disorders and their impact on public health is reflected by several compelling epidemiologic observations. Both asthma and COPD are highly prevalent and result in substantial morbidity and mortality. For example, COPD is the fourth leading preventable cause of death because cigarette smoking remains its most common cause.

One of the most alarming observations is the increasing mortality from asthma especially in young African Americans. Reasons proposed for this include (1) a broader definition of asthma to include patients originally thought to have COPD; (2) increased environmental pollutants and allergens; (3) "steroid phobia," that is, reluctance to use oral glucocorticoids by both patients and physicians; (4) overuse of beta-agonist metered dose inhalers (MDIs); (5) inaccurate assessment of the severity of airflow obstruction by both patients and physicians; (6) poor access to medical care by high-risk groups; and (7) improper use of medications or nonadherence to medical regimens.

PATHOPHYSIOLOGY

Asthma is a disease of airway inflammation and hyperreactivity that can trigger bronchospasm within minutes after exposure to a variety of precipitating factors. These factors include allergens, cold air, exercise, and emotional stress. Rapid onset of bronchospasm characterizes the early phase of an asthma attack. The late phase of an asthma attack ("flare") occurs within 2 to 8 hours and may persist for 1 to 2 days. This phase is marked by significant bronchial wall inflammation, mucosal edema, and tenacious secretions that can cause mucus plugs and worsen airway lumen narrowing. The traditional hallmark of asthma is the reversibility of the bronchospasm with bronchodilator therapy. Over time, however, chronic stimulation and inflammation of the airways can cause airway smooth muscle hypertrophy and hyperplasia, resulting in only partially reversible or completely irreversible airflow obstruction.

Complete or partial irreversibility of airflow obstruction predominates in COPD. However, symptomatic relief can often be gained with bronchodilator therapy. This suggests a component of bronchial hyperreactivity and bronchospasm superimposed on the underlying damaged pulmonary architecture. COPD includes

835

chronic bronchitis, emphysema, and chronic diffuse bronchiectasis. Chronic bronchitis is defined as excessive sputum production (>30 mL/day) on most days for at least 3 months of the year for more than 2 successive years. Emphysema is characterized by enlargement of the distal airspaces resulting from destruction of alveoli and loss of lung elasticity. Chronic diffuse bronchiectasis refers to widespread, persistently dilated bronchi associated with bouts of infection. The most common precipitating factors of acute respiratory failure in COPD (a COPD flare) include viral and bacterial respiratory infections, congestive heart failure, nonadherence to medical therapy, and iatrogenic oversedation.

ACUTE ASTHMA FLARES

Clinical Signs and Symptoms

Patients with severe acute exacerbations of asthma (also referred to as *status asthmaticus*) typically present with symptoms of dyspnea, wheezing, and cough. However, it is important to consider other causes in the differential diagnosis of these symptoms, including "cardiac asthma" (secondary to congestive heart failure), upper airway obstruction, pneumonia, "laryngeal asthma" (vocal cord dysfunction syndrome), and anaphylaxis. Because some of these entities may have a component of airway hyperreactivity, it is difficult to distinguish among them solely on the basis of improvement after bronchodilator therapy.

A good clinical assessment of the patient in respiratory distress is necessary for accurate diagnosis and for determining the severity of the attack. However, therapy must begin simultaneously while diagnostic information is being collected. Clinical indicators of severe airflow obstruction include an inability to speak full sentences, orthopnea, diaphoresis, pulsus paradoxus greater than 10 mm Hg, mental status depression (a sign of carbon dioxide narcosis or hypoxemia, or both), central cyanosis, marked accessory muscle use, and evidence of diaphragmatic fatigue such as paradoxical abdominal movement (inward instead of outward movement of the abdominal wall during inspiration while in a supine position). Auscultatory findings may be misleading because wheezing alone does not accurately predict the severity of airway obstruction. Some patients may present with significant wheezing that resolves rapidly after bronchodilator therapy. Conversely, diminished or lack of wheezing may also be a sign of worsening air movement in the setting of progressive airway obstruction. However, distant breath sounds with no wheezing may also be heard in some patients with severe but stable airway obstruction. Having access to a patient's baseline clinical examination is often helpful in assessing the patient's degree of acuity.

If stridor is appreciated, the differential diagnosis of upper airway obstruction includes acute epiglottitis, laryngeal asthma (vocal cord dysfunction syndrome), laryngeal edema due to anaphylaxis, or obstruction from a foreign body or malignancy. Laryngeal asthma (vocal cord dysfunction syndrome) is diagnosed by inspection of the vocal cords during the episode of breathlessness and stridor. Paradoxical closure of the vocal cords during expiration and inspiration is observed in patients with this syndrome. Not only can patients with vocal cord dysfunction syndrome mimic those with true severe asthma flares but the majority of patients with this disorder have coexistent asthma. This makes their evaluation particularly challenging.

Objective Measures of Airflow Obstruction

Since clinical assessment of the degree of airway obstruction has poor sensitivity and specificity in many patients, a peak expiratory flow rate (PEFR) or the forced expiratory volume in 1 second (FEV_1) or both should be measured in all asthmatic patients who can tolerate these measurements. They provide objective measurements of the severity of airflow obstruction. However, if severe airway obstruction or overt respiratory failure is clinically obvious, these measurements should be deferred. Although a PEFR of less than 150 L/minute or a FEV_1 of less than 1 L confirms severe obstruction, a comparison with the patient's measurements of pulmonary function at baseline (if available) is even more helpful. In order to assess the degree of responsiveness to therapy and to monitor the patient's clinical course, it is important to perform these measurements before and after bronchodilator treatments and serially during the acute illness.

Hypoxemia

Hypoxemia is frequently seen during an acute asthma attack because airway narrowing results in ventilation/perfusion ($\dot{V}/\dot{Q}$) mismatching resulting in alveoli with $\dot{V}/\dot{Q}$ less than 1. Mucus plugging of bronchi can also lead to shunting of blood through nonventilated alveoli. Monitoring oxygenation by pulse oximetry alone is usually satisfactory. However, when severe airflow obstruction is suspected or documented, arterial blood gas (ABG) analysis is indicated to assess the patient's ventilatory status. The most common ABG finding during an acute asthma attack is an acute respiratory alkalosis (partial pressure of carbon dioxide in arterial blood [$Paco_2$] in the 30 to 34 mm Hg range) plus mild to moderate hypoxemia. A normal $Paco_2$ occurring in the face of severe airflow obstruction (the so-called "crossover point") necessitates close observation (see Table 1–2). This seemingly normal $Paco_2$ may in reality be an ominous sign of respiratory muscle fatigue and impending hypercapnic respiratory failure. Chest radiographs have limited usefulness in the evaluation of an adult asthma patient unless there is concern for other processes, such as pneumonia or pneumothorax.

ACUTE CHRONIC OBSTRUCTIVE PULMONARY DISEASE FLARES

The evaluation of patients with acute COPD flares requires a slightly different approach from those with acute asthma attacks. In contrast to their utility in asthma flares, spirometric measurements and oxygenation correlate poorly with the degree of severity of an acute COPD exacerbation. Therefore, it is imperative to follow ABG measurements.

However, one should bear in mind that a patient with COPD often has an abnormal ABG determination at baseline. Typical findings at *baseline* in a patient with severe COPD are a mild to moderate degree of hypoxemia plus respiratory acidosis (see Table 1–2). The latter is well compensated by renal bicarbonate retention. It is helpful to compare the results of an ABG determination during an acute flare with those obtained when the patient was in a stable baseline condition. A significant change in $PaCO_2$ from baseline or an absolute degree of acidosis, for example, pH less than 7.25, confirms the diagnosis of an acute COPD flare (Table 74–1).

A chest radiograph is warranted in the evaluation of a patient with a COPD flare to rule out common precipitating causes, such as pneumonia or congestive heart failure. These patients often present with an increase in chronic sputum production. A Gram stain and culture of sputum (or other lower respiratory tract secretions, such as tracheal aspirate) should be performed to direct antibiotic therapy.

MEDICAL MANAGEMENT OF PATIENTS WITH SEVERE AIRFLOW OBSTRUCTION

Overview

The key management issues are similar in both severe acute asthma and COPD flares and include treating reversible bronchospasm and airway inflammation, correcting hypoxemia and respiratory acidosis, managing secretions, removing or treating precipitating factors, and avoiding iatrogenic complications, for example, barotrauma and hemodynamic instability (see Table 74–2). However, because of differences in the underlying pathophysiologic mechanisms, therapeutic tactics may differ for each disorder.

Bronchodilators

There is a large armamentarium of bronchodilating agents as well as various routes of administration used to treat acute bronchospasm (Table 74–2). In adults with acute severe asthma, beta$_2$-selective adrenergic agonists, such as albuterol, have proved to be the bronchodilators of choice over nonspecific beta-agonists, such as epinephrine and isoproterenol. In the acute setting, albuterol is administered by

Table 74–1. Interpretation of Carbon Dioxide Retention in Arterial Blood Gas Analysis

Acute respiratory acidosis	For every 10 mm Hg increase in $PaCO_2$, bicarbonate will increase by 1 mEq/L (± 0.3 mEq/L)* and pH will decrease by 0.08 units
Chronic respiratory acidosis	For every 10 mm Hg increase in $PaCO_2$, bicarbonate will increase by 0.4 mEq/L (± 0.4 mEq/L)* and pH will decrease by 0.03 units

*95% confidence intervals.

Table 74–2. Initial Management of Severe Bronchospasm

Timing

Therapy must be initiated before completion of the physical examination and data collection

Beta-Agonist Therapy

Albuterol 2.5–5.0 mg diluted in 3 mL saline administered via nebulizer
Nebulized treatments should be administered every 20 min
Maximal benefit is usually seen after three treatments

Steroid Therapy

Corticosteroid therapy is begun simultaneously with bronchodilator therapy
Methylprednisolone 125 mg IV × one dose followed by 0.5–1.0 mg/kg IV q6h

Oxygen Therapy

Correct hypoxemia (keep SaO_2 >92%) by administering supplemental oxygen
Use nasal prongs for asthma patient
Patients with COPD who are at risk for carbon dioxide retention require "controlled" oxygen therapy
  and serial arterial blood gas determinations

Assisted Ventilation

If there is worsening hypercapnia, respiratory acidosis, hypoxemia, or signs of respiratory muscle
  fatigue, e.g., respiratory paradox (see text)
Begin noninvasive ventilation in patients with COPD who are awake, alert, and hemodynamically
  stable
Otherwise, proceed with endotracheal intubation (via oral route) and mechanical ventilation

IV, intravenously; COPD, chronic obstructive pulmonary disease.

nebulization because, as a rule, patients in acute respiratory distress cannot coordinate their breathing well enough to use MDIs. Studies have shown no advantage to parenteral administration over inhalational therapy of beta-agonists in patients with acute asthma. Furthermore, parenteral dosing of these agents in adult patients has frequent and serious toxic side effects. They include tachycardia, palpitations, nausea, vomiting, hypokalemia, lactic acidosis, and myocardial ischemia and necrosis. These toxicities have also been observed when high doses of albuterol (>10–15 mg/hour) are given by inhalation.

Current literature shows that in hospitalized patients *not in the ICU,* there is no difference in efficacy between MDI and nebulizer therapy in terms of the bronchodilating response despite a considerable difference in cost to the hospital. However, patients in the ICU are often too dyspneic and anxious to use MDIs properly. Therefore, aggressive bronchodilator therapy via nebulizer treatments should be used initially in all patients in the ICU.

Anticholinergic agents, such as ipratropium bromide (a synthetic analog of atropine without systemic side effects), block muscarinic receptors in the airway, causing bronchial smooth muscle relaxation and decreased submucosal gland secretions. Studies have shown these agents to be less potent than inhaled beta-agonists as single agents in the setting of asthma. Although combining nebulized ipratropium with beta$_2$-agonist treatment may, theoretically, improve bronchodilatation, one study in which ipratropium was given by MDI along with nebulized beta$_2$-agonist therapy failed to demonstrate additional bronchodilatation. Whether recently available nebulized ipratropium will be additive remains to be shown.

Similarly, for patients with COPD flares, the optimal inhaled bronchodilator regimen remains controversial. Most studies demonstrate that there is no clear advantage of beta$_2$-agonists over ipratropium in terms of bronchodilator response. Although some studies favor the use of ipratropium as monotherapy in patients with COPD, and despite the fact that there is little evidence showing beneficial effects from their combined therapy, beta$_2$-agonists and ipratropium are commonly used together in alternating fashion in the acute setting.

Theophylline is a traditional bronchodilating agent that has lost favor in the treatment of acute bronchospasm over recent years for several reasons. First, controlled, randomized trials have shown it has no beneficial effect over standard beta$_2$-agonist and corticosteroid therapy when used either as a single agent or in combination with beta$_2$-agonists and corticosteroids. Second, theophylline's original proposed role as a phosphodiesterase inhibitor, resulting in an increase in cyclic adenosine monophosphate and bronchial smooth muscle relaxation, has been questioned. (Its other proposed mechanisms of action include increasing diaphragmatic contractility and improving mucociliary clearance and anti-inflammatory effects). Third, it has significant toxicities that can occur at or slightly more than traditional therapeutic serum levels.

Given its relatively high risk:benefit ratio, theophylline should not be considered a first-line drug in the treatment of acute bronchospasm. However, it may be continued in the acute setting in patients who take it chronically. If given, theophylline should be dosed carefully (Table 74–3). Its levels must be monitored closely and should be maintained between 8 and 10 mg/dL rather than the higher traditional therapeutic range of 10 to 20 mg/dL. The patient should be observed closely for symptoms and signs of toxicity, which include nausea, vomiting, cardiac arrhythmias, and seizures.

Table 74–3. Theophylline Dosing in Adults with Acute Bronchospasm

DOSING	INTRAVENOUS AMINOPHYLLINE*
Loading dose (over 20 min)†	
History of theophylline use:	
None	6 mg/kg ideal body weight‡ (IBW)
Oral theophylline use	0–3 mg/kg IBW
Maintenance dose§	
Patient category:	
Nonsmoker	0.5 mg/kg IBW/h
Smoker	0.3 mg IBW/kg/h
Critically ill	0.5 mg IBW/kg/h
Congestive heart failure	0.2 mg IBW/kg/h
Severe pneumonia	0.2 mg IBW/kg/h

*Dosing expressed in aminophylline equivalents (theophylline dose = 0.8 × aminophylline dose).

†If possible, serum theophylline levels should be obtained before administration, especially if there is a history of theophylline use.

‡Ideal body weight for adults can be estimated from formulas in Table 12–1.

§Theophylline levels should be measured 12–24 hr after loading and more frequently if symptoms or signs of theophylline toxicity are evident. Target level = 8–10 mg/dL.

From Panettieri RA, Kelley MA: Airflow obstruction caused by bronchospasm. In: Parillo JE, ed. Current Therapy in Critical Care Medicine, 2nd ed. St Louis: Mosby–Year Book, 1991, pp 180–185.

Corticosteroids

Corticosteroid therapy is critically important in the treatment of acute broncho-spasm. Its beneficial effects have been documented in both flares of asthma and COPD in controlled clinical trials. It is essential to begin treatment as soon as possible because the onset of clinical effect takes approximately 6 to 12 hours. Possible mechanisms of action include decreasing inflammation, microvascular permeability, and mucus production and perhaps upregulating $beta_2$-adrenergic receptors in the airway. Current data do not provide evidence for any advantage to using high doses (methylprednisolone 1.5 to 2.0 mg/kg every 6 hours) over lower doses (methylprednisolone 0.5 to 1.0 mg/kg every 6 hours) or administering steroids via the parenteral route versus the oral route. However, in the severely dyspneic patient, intravenous administration is preferred. A methylprednisolone load of 125 mg intravenously, followed by 0.5 to 1.0 mg/kg intravenously every 6 hours is a recommended initial treatment. After there is evidence of clinical improvement, the patient may be switched to an oral steroid, for example, predni-sone, which should be tapered over a minimum of 2 to 3 weeks.

Oxygen Therapy

The hypoxemia associated with an acute asthma attack can usually be corrected with low-flow supplemental oxygen administered via nasal cannula. Oxygen ther-apy is important but is more complicated when treating a patient with a COPD flare. Many patients with COPD become increasingly hypercapnic when their hypoxemia is corrected. Removal of the hypoxic drive to breathe has been one proposed theory to explain this phenomenon. However, more recent studies suggest that the cause may be multifactorial, including oxygen-induced worsening of $\dot{V}/\dot{Q}$ mismatching. Oxygen may increase the fraction of alveoli with $\dot{V}/\dot{Q}$ greater than 1, resulting in increased physiologic deadspace and an increased deadspace:tidal volume ratio. Therefore, it is essential to administer "controlled" oxygen therapy. This can be achieved with the use of a Venturi mask, which, by entraining air, delivers the desired fixed percentage of oxygen (24 to 50%, depending on the entrainment setting). In contrast, nasal prongs deliver oxygen at a certain flow rate, for example, 2 L/minute, and not a concentration. Therefore, the exact concentration of oxygen that the patient inhales with nasal prongs varies according to changes in the patient's minute ventilation. Oxygen should be administered at the lowest concentration in order to maintain a PaO_2 at or slightly greater than 60 mm Hg (or oxygen saturtion in arterial blood [SaO_2] at or slightly greater than 88%). In a patient with COPD, a blood specimen for ABG measurement should be drawn 15 to 30 minutes after every change in fraction of inspired O_2 (FIO_2) to monitor for worsening hypercapnia.

Antibiotics

Despite the lack of supporting data, most patients with a COPD exacerbation lacking an obvious cause are treated empirically with antibiotics. Commonly used agents include trimethoprim-sulfamethoxazole (160 mg/800 mg intravenously or orally every 12 hours), erythromycin (250 to 500 mg intravenously or orally every 6 hours), or ceftriaxone (1 g intravenously every 24 hours). Specific organisms often targeted are *Streptococcus pneumoniae, Haemophilus influenzae, Legionella pneumophila, Chlamydia trachomatis,* and *Mycoplasma pneumoniae.*

Other Interventions

Although little data are available to support its efficacy, maintaining adequate hydration is often recommended based on the idea that it decreases the viscosity of airway secretions and prevents bronchial mucous plugging. Chest physical therapy with postural drainage can aid in the mobilization of thick secretions to decrease mucus plugging and improve oxygenation. Aerosolized *N*-acetylcysteine, a mucolytic agent, has not been shown to be effective in the management of persistent airway secretions and may actually precipitate further bronchospasm.

Aerosolized recombinant human DNase is a potent viscolytic agent that acts by breaking down DNA released by neutrophils in the airway. This therapy is currently being used for treatment of patients with cystic fibrosis. However, no formal studies have been carried out in patients with COPD. Therefore, recombinant human DNase is not recommended for routine COPD management. However, its use may be considered in exceptional cases when accumulation of infected viscous airway secretions persists despite aggressive standard therapy.

The current literature does not recommend the use of magnesium sulfate for the treatment of acute bronchospasm because it adds little benefit to standard therapy with beta-agonists and corticosteroids.

MECHANICAL VENTILATION OF PATIENTS WITH SEVERE AIRFLOW OBSTRUCTION

Asthma Flares

Most patients with an acute, severe asthma attack and acute respiratory acidosis have a good clinical response to aggressive medical therapy and do not require mechanical ventilation. Therefore, as a rule, the decision to intubate an asthmatic patient should be postponed until after initiation of an adequate trial of aggressive bronchodilator and corticosteroid therapy. However, emergent intubation is indicated in all asthmatic patients presenting with cardiac or respiratory arrest, significant mental status depression, or clinical deterioration despite aggressive therapy, as evidenced by worsening hypercapnia, acidosis (pH <7.25), or hypoxemia on serial ABG determinations. Since asthmatic patients often have nasal polyps, it is best to intubate these individuals via the oral route. This also allows the use of a large endotracheal tube ($\geq$8.0 mm), which facilitates suctioning and minimizes airflow resistance due to the artificial airway.

Chronic Obstructive Pulmonary Disease Flares

If intubated, many patients with acute COPD flares may become a "challenge to wean" type of patient (see Chapter 23) because of the baseline pulmonary disease. One option for these patients is to try noninvasive ventilation via a continuous positive airway pressure mask connected to a pressure-cycled assisted ventilation machine or a standard ventilator (see Chapter 77, Table 77–5). Recent studies have shown that in selected patients with acute COPD respiratory failure, the use of noninvasive ventilation can reduce the need for endotracheal intubation, the length of the hospital stay, and the hospital mortality rate. However, this method of ventilation should not be attempted in an obtunded or hemodynamically unstable patient.

The utility of noninvasive ventilation for asthmatic patients remains to be determined, but it may be modest because of limitations in providing high peak airway pressures and patient acceptance of a tightly fitting full or partial face mask while in respiratory distress.

The goal of mechanical ventilation in patients with COPD flares is to gradually correct the acute hypercapnia back to the baseline $PaCO_2$ and not to a normal range. In the short term, overcorrection of PCO_2 will result in acute alkalosis and, in the long term, difficulty in weaning because of suppression of respiratory drive related to an alkalemic pH.

Dynamic Hyperinflation

Patients with severe obstructive airway disease pose a unique challenge during positive pressure ventilation because of the universal occurrence of dynamic hyperinflation (DHI). When these patients are mechanically ventilated, their severe airway obstruction results in prolonged expiratory time. This, in turn, prevents the lungs from completely emptying before the next ventilator breath arrives, a phenomenon known as breath stacking. This causes an incremental increase in lung volume at end-expiration. Because of this phenomenon, alveolar pressure as measured by the plateau pressure at end-inspiration also increases with each subsequent cycled breath. This breath stacking continues until a new steady state is reached at a greater than baseline functional residual capacity (FRC). This intrinsic positive end-expiratory pressure (PEEP) associated with the larger FRC has been referred to as *intrinsic PEEP* or *auto-PEEP*.

The presence of DHI and auto-PEEP can usually be demonstrated at the bedside by occluding the expiratory port of the ventilator just before the *end of* expiration. The magnitude of auto-PEEP can be roughly estimated by observing a rise in airway pressure (see Fig. 2–6). In some ventilators, a built-in shutter valve at end-expiration can be used for the same purpose. If the ventilator has a "flow versus time" display, the presence of DHI and auto-PEEP is indicated by simply observing that the patient's expiratory flow does not return to zero before the start of the next breath (see Fig. 2–7).

Increases in intrathoracic and pleural pressures can decrease venous return to the heart, with resulting decreased cardiac output and systemic hypotension, especially in patients with decreased intravascular volume. One can easily diagnose hypotension due to auto-PEEP because it responds rapidly to disconnecting the patient from the ventilator and slow "bagging" (giving three to four breaths per minute by means of a manual resuscitation bag). These maneuvers should allow sufficient expiratory time for the overinflated lungs to decompress.

Although DHI and auto-PEEP are universally present in any mechanically ventilated patient with severe airway obstruction, auto-PEEP may or may not cause overt clinical problems. If auto-PEEP is clinically problematic, one can decrease it by employing a variety of maneuvers designed to increase expiratory time and to lower the patient's mean intrathoracic pressure (see Chapter 2).

The development of DHI and auto-PEEP also increases the risk of barotrauma. Although no easily measurable index is available to define a threshold for this risk, end-inspiratory lung volume greater than FRC by more than 20 mL/kg has been found to be associated with a higher risk of barotrauma as well as hypotension. High airway resistance in severe obstructive airway disease results in high peak pressures and a large gradient between peak and alveolar pressures. Because some studies suggest that it is the plateau pressure rather than the peak pressure that increases the risk of barotrauma, current recommendations are to maintain plateau pressure at less than 30 cm H_2O.

Recent literature indicates that the absolute level of minute ventilation ($\dot{V}_E$), rather than tidal volume or respiratory rate alone, determines DHI and associated auto-PEEP. Thus, decreasing $\dot{V}_E$ may be more beneficial in lowering DHI than increasing inspiratory flow rate. If plateau pressures continue to rise (>30 cm H_2O), the patient should be managed by "controlled hypoventilation" with "permissive hypercapnia." A moderate respiratory acidosis occurs but is usually well tolerated. However, if arterial pH falls to less than 7.20 to 7.25, some authors recommend treating with a bicarbonate infusion rather than increasing $\dot{V}_E$. Other authors do neither but continue close monitoring for adverse effects of the acidosis.

To achieve this degree of control of $\dot{V}_E$ resulting in permissive hypercapnia requires that the patient not "trigger" the ventilator. This can be accomplished in most patients by heavy sedation alone using a continuous infusion of benzodiazepines, such as lorazepam or propofol (see Chapter 4) However, in some cases, complete pharmacologic muscle paralysis may be necessary to suppress inspiratory efforts and decrease DHI and airway pressure. However, neuromuscular blocking agents must be used with extreme caution and for a minimal duration. Recent studies suggest that the combination of high-dose corticosteroids and a neuromuscular blocking agent given for more than 24 hours increases the risk of a debilitating myopathy and prolonged, even permanent, weakness (see Chapters 4 and 67). This entity has been reported with all nondepolarizing neuromuscular blocking agents, including pancuronium, vecuronium, and atracurium.

Extraordinary Therapies

Unconventional therapies have been attempted in mechanically ventilated patients with severe airflow obstruction who deteriorate despite all conventional treatments. These methods include bronchoscopy to remove mucus plugs, general anesthesia to reduce airway resistance due to bronchospasm, a helium-oxygen (Heliox) mixture to breathe (this provides a less dense gas to overcome frictional resistance when gas flow is turbulent), and partial cardiopulmonary bypass with extracorporeal membrane oxygenation and carbon dioxide removal. There are currently no controlled studies to document the efficacy of these treatments. In addition, many institutions lack the facilities and expertise to perform some of them.

BIBLIOGRAPHY

Albert RK, Martin TR, Lewis SW: Controlled clinical trial of methylprednisolone in patients with chronic bronchitis and acute respiratory insufficiency. Ann Intern Med 92:753–758, 1980.
This classic article presented a double-blind, randomized, placebo-controlled study showing that methylprednisolone improved airflow more than placebo when added to standard therapy in patients with chronic bronchitis and acute respiratory insufficiency.

Brochard L, Mancebo J, Wysocki M: Noninvasive ventilation for acute exacerbations of chronic obstructive pulmonary disease. N Engl J Med 333:817–822, 1995.
Noninvasive ventilation can decrease the need for intubation, length of hospital stay, and in-hospital mortality in selected patients with acute exacerbations of COPD.

Corbridge TC, Hall JB: The assessment and management of adults with status asthmaticus. Am J Respir Crit Care Med 151:L1296–1316, 1995.
State of the art, comprehensive review discusses clinical assessment, pharmacologic management, and mechanical ventilation.

Curtis JR, Hudson LD: Emergent assessment and management of acute respiratory failure in COPD. Clin Chest Med 15:481–500, 1994.
This article presents an extensive review of the management of patients wih COPD and acute respiratory failure.

Douglass JA, Tuxen DV, Horne M: Myopathy in severe asthma. Am Rev Respir Dis 146:517–519, 1992.
A high incidence of a rise in creatine kinase enzyme levels and myopathy was seen in a group of mechanically ventilated patients with severe asthma. The cause may have been related to the use of corticosteroids and vecuronium.

Jantz MA, Sahn SA: Corticosteroids in acute respiratory failure. Am J Respir Crit Care Med 160:1079–1100, 1999.
This is a comprehensive, "state of the art" article that describes and evaluates the evidence for use of corticosteroids in status asthmaticus as well as in other diseases causing respiratory failure (with 326 references).

Kuhl DA, Agiri OA, Mauro LS: Beta-agonists in the treatment of acute exacerbation of chronic obstructive pulmonary disease. Ann Pharmacother 28:1379–1388, 1994.
Beta-agonists given by MDI or nebulizer are equally effective in the acute (non-ICU) setting.

Leatherman J: Life-threatening asthma. Clin Chest Med 15:453–479, 1994.
This article presents an extensive review of the management of severe asthma.

Mountain RD, Sahn SA: Clinical features and outcome in patients with acute asthma presenting with hypercapnia. Am Rev Respir Dis 138:535–539, 1988.
This article discusses a study in which only 5 of 61 (8%) asthmatic patients presenting with hypercapnia required mechanical ventilation. With appropriate medical therapy, most patients with hypercapnia from acute asthma have rapid reversibility, and mechanical ventilation can usually be avoided.

Newman KB, Mason UG, Schmaling KB: Clinical features of vocal cord dysfunction. Am J Respir Crit Care Med 152:1382–1386, 1995.
This is a comprehensive review of the syndrome of vocal cord dysfunction (previously called laryngeal asthma). This syndrome often masquerades as asthma and coexists with asthma. Its hallmark is paradoxical adduction of the vocal cords during the respiratory cycle.

Niewoehner DE, Erbland ML, Deupree RH, et al: Effect of systemic glucocorticoids on exacerbations of chronic obstructive pulmonary disease. N Engl J Med 340:1941–1947, 1999.
Randomized, placebo controlled clinical trial of effectiveness and safety of systemic corticosteroids in patients hospitalized for COPD flares. The steroid treated group had faster improvements in pulmonary function and a slightly shorter length of hospital stay but had more hyperglycemia needing treatment and more readmissions for serious infections.

Pepe PE, Marini JJ: Occult positive end-expiratory pressure in mechanically ventilated patients with airflow obstruction—the auto-PEEP effect. Am Rev Respir Dis 126:166–170, 1982.
This article presents a review of detecting and managing auto-PEEP, along with representative case reports.

Tuxen DV, Lane L: The effects of ventilatory pattern on hyperinflation, airway pressures, and circulation in mechanical ventilation of patients with severe airflow obstruction. Am Rev Respir Dis 136:872–879, 1987.
A study of nine patients with severe airflow obstruction requiring mechanical ventilation showed that small tidal volume and long expiratory time are critical factors in reducing pulmonary hyperinflation, circulatory depression, and the potential for barotrauma.

75

Massive Hemoptysis and Diffuse Pulmonary Hemorrhage

Gerald L. Weinhouse

Patients with massive hemoptysis are distinct from patients with diffuse alveolar hemorrhage. Although the initial management may be similar, the differential diagnosis and definitive treatment for each entity differ markedly.

Massive hemoptysis is variably defined as expectoration of greater than 100 to 1000 mL of blood over a 24-hour period. Many studies use greater than 600 mL/24 hours as their criterion, so much of the medical literature is based on this threshold. Patients with lethal massive hemoptysis die of acute airway obstruction and asphyxia and not from exsanguination. Principles of management are predicated on the "ABCs" (airway, breathing, and circulation) of cardiopulmonary life support, with airway control being of paramount importance.

Diffuse alveolar hemorrhage comprises this clinical triad: (1) extravasation of blood in the terminal airspaces, (2) anemia, and (3) infiltrates on chest radiographs that are indistinguishable from those of pulmonary edema. Hemoptysis may not occur, but bronchoalveolar lavage will yield erythrocytes and hemosiderin-laden macrophages. Patients with lethal diffuse alveolar hemorrhage die of profound hypoxemia and not from exsanguination or airway obstruction

This chapter reviews the causes, diagnostic options, and management approaches to both categories of life-threatening pulmonary hemorrhage.

DIFFERENTIAL DIAGNOSIS OF MASSIVE HEMOPTYSIS
(Table 75–1)

Pseudohemoptysis

Extrapulmonary sites of bleeding may mimic hemoptysis. In particular, *epistaxis* and *hematemesis* should be excluded to avoid inappropriate diagnostic and therapeutic measures and wasting valuable time. Nasopharyngeal examination and gastric lavage can quickly rule out pseudohemoptysis.

Infectious Causes

Historically, *tuberculosis* was the most common cause of massive hemoptysis. Tuberculosis causes hemoptysis by (1) infectious cavities eroding adjacent small blood vessels, (2) rupture of a branch of the pulmonary artery (Rasmussen's aneurysm) within a cavity, (3) erosion of a bronchial wall by a calcified hilar lymph node (broncholith), (4) formation of a mycetoma within an old (inactive) tuberculous cavity, or (5) chronic inflammation from residual bronchiectasis.

Table 75–1. Differential Diagnosis of Massive Hemoptysis

....

Pseudohemoptysis
Infection-related
  Tuberculosis
  Bronchiectasis, e.g., cystic fibrosis
  Mycetoma, e.g., aspergilloma
  Lung abscess
  Necrotizing pneumonia
Neoplasm
  Primary squamous cell carcinoma of the lung, e.g., cavitary squamous cell carcinoma
  Bronchial carcinoid tumors
Iatrogenic
  Rupture of pulmonary artery by Swan-Ganz catheter
  Tracheal–innominate artery fistula due to cuff of tracheostomy tube
Chronic left atrial hypertension, e.g., mitral stenosis

....

Bronchiectasis, such as in cystic fibrosis, frequently results in life-threatening hemoptysis. The infection and chronic inflammation associated with bronchiectasis ultimately lead to proliferation and enlargement of bronchial arteries and veins and systemic-pulmonary vascular anastamoses. Continued infection and inflammation may lead to hemoptysis from rupture of these abnormal vessels.

Patients with *mycetomas* (intrapulmonary fungus balls) are at increased risk for massive hemoptysis. *Aspergillus fumigatus* is the most common offending organism, but other *Aspergillus* and *Mucormycetes* species may also form fungus balls. The wall of the cavity containing the fungus ball becomes hypervascularized with branches of the systemic (bronchial) circulation. Although the precise mechanism of vascular disruption is controversial, it may be mechanical or toxin-mediated. Although seemingly counterintuitive, nonmycetomatous *invasive* fungal infections of the lung are *uncommonly* associated with massive hemoptysis (but may produce scant hemoptysis).

Lung abscesses (due to polymicrobial and anaerobic bacteria) or *necrotizing pneumonias* (such as those caused by *Staphylococcus, Klebsiella,* or *Legionella*) commonly cause mild to moderate hemoptysis but uncommonly cause massive bleeding. Direct necrosis of the walls of blood vessels probably produces the hemorrhage.

Neoplastic Causes

Virtually any tumor can cause hemoptysis, although endobronchial or cavitary lesions bleed most commonly. Squamous cell carcinomas and bronchial carcinoid adenomas are the most frequent cell types associated with massive hemoptysis. Bleeding is usually attributable to necrosis and inflammation rather than direct tumor invasion of blood vessels.

Iatrogenic Causes

Numerous procedures may be complicated by hemoptysis. In the intensive care unit (ICU), pulmonary artery flotation catheters (Swan-Ganz catheters) may cause pulmonary artery rupture. Overinflation of the catheter's balloon relative to the size of the vessel, or advancement of the catheter with the balloon deflated, are two common mistakes that may cause this highly lethal complication (mortality >50%). Because patients with pulmonary hypertension and coagulopathy are at increased risk for this complication, some ICUs prohibit routine "wedging" of Swan-Ganz catheters in these patients.

Although some bleeding is common, bronchoscopy with transbronchial biopsy rarely causes severe hemoptysis. If it occurs, severe bleeding is usually associated with platelet or other coagulation abnormalities or with direct laceration of small arteries by the biopsy forceps.

A tracheal–innominate artery fistula may occur as a consequence of a long-standing aortic graft or tracheostomy. Placement of a tracheostomy tube below the usual site (which is between the second and fourth tracheal rings) may cause an erosion that leads to a communication between the innominate artery and the trachea. A *sentinel bleed* (scant amounts of fresh tracheal bleeding) in a patient with a tracheostomy (except immediately after its insertion) should raise suspicion of a tracheal–innominate artery fistula.

Trauma

Although rare, massive hemoptysis may be associated with either blunt or penetrating chest trauma (see Chapter 97). Blunt trauma can rupture a major bronchus or cause rib fractures that lacerate the lung. Penetrating trauma may lacerate a large pulmonary blood vessel directly.

Cardiovascular Causes

Any cardiovascular lesion producing *pulmonary venous hypertension* may lead to hemoptysis. When pulmonary venous pressures exceed the right atrial pressure, as occurs in congestive heart failure or mitral stenosis (particularly during exertion), flow becomes retrograde into the bronchial veins, creating submucosal bronchial varices. An upper respiratory infection, cough, or sudden increase in pressure in the pulmonary vascular bed may lead to their rupture and hemoptysis. Episodes of hemoptysis associated with pulmonary venous hypertension may be severe but are generally self-limited.

Vascular malformations often originate from the pulmonary circulation. They often drain into submucosal bronchial veins, which then become varicose. Hemoptysis may be due to variceal rupture, but fortunately massive bleeding is rare.

DIFFERENTIAL DIAGNOSIS OF DIFFUSE ALVEOLAR HEMORRHAGE (Table 75–2)

Goodpasture's Syndrome

Glomerulonephritis associated with antiglomerular basement membrane antibody (anti-GBM ab) may present with pulmonary hemorrhage in classic Goodpasture's

Table 75–2. Differential Diagnosis of Diffuse Pulmonary Hemorrhage

After bone marrow transplantation	Idiopathic pulmonary hemosiderosis
Antiphospholipid antibody syndrome	IgA, immunoglobulin A
Behçet's syndrome	IgA nephropathy
Drugs (phenytoin, penicillamine)	Microscopic polyangiitis
Essential mixed cryoglobulinemia	Systemic lupus erythematosus
Goodpasture's syndrome	Wegener's granulomatosis
Henoch-Schönlein purpura	

syndrome. However, the pulmonary manifestations may precede the renal disease by months. Diffuse autoimmune vascular injury produces pulmonary bleeding. Renal biopsy, not open lung biopsy, is the preferred diagnostic approach. In Goodpasture's syndrome, renal biopsy should reveal the characteristic linear, immunofluorescent staining pattern of glomeruli, whereas a lung biopsy may show only nonspecific staining.

Systemic Lupus Erythematosus

Although pulmonary involvement by systemic lupus erythematosus (SLE) is relatively common, diffuse alveolar hemorrhage is uncommon. However, when present, it may precede other signs and symptoms of SLE. Therefore, the diagnosis of SLE should be considered in any patient with diffuse alveolar hemorrhage. An immune complex vasculitis that preferentially affects the pulmonary vascular bed is postulated to be the pathogenic mechanism of hemorrhage.

Bone Marrow Transplantation

Alveolar hemorrhage is more common after autologous bone marrow transplantation than after allogeneic transplantation. Risk factors include age greater than 40 years, total body irradiation, transplantation for solid tumors, high fever, and renal insufficiency. Its pathogenesis remains unknown. However, because it seems to respond to systemic corticosteroid therapy, it is suspected to be immunologically mediated.

Wegener's Granulomatosis

The triad of sinusitis, glomerulonephritis, and lower respiratory tract disease should prompt immediate concern for Wegener's granulomatosis. However, the clinical appearance of the disease sometimes is limited to the respiratory tract (limited form of Wegener's granulomatosis). Life-threatening alveolar hemorrhage as a result of a necrotizing vasculitis may be its presenting sign.

Idiopathic Pulmonary Hemosiderosis

Idiopathic pulmonary hemosiderosis presents in the second or third decade of life, usually in men. It is characterized by recurrent or acute life-threatening hemoptysis. The diagnosis is made by exclusion of other causes.

DIAGNOSTIC APPROACH (Fig. 75–1)

General Diagnostic Studies

One should not overlook the value of a good history and physical examination in the patient with hemoptysis (even though it may be impossible to obtain at the time of initial presentation). The history or physical examination may yield important clues to the cause and the bleeding source earlier than diagnostic laboratory tests.

Initial screening tests should include a complete blood count, including a platelet count, prothrombin time, partial thromboplastin time, blood urea nitrogen, and creatinine determinations, and urinalysis. A chest radiograph is essential for diagnosis and to aid in localizing the bleeding source. An admission electrocardiogram may reveal occult cardiac disease and can provide a baseline in the event that hemodynamic compromise with cardiac injury ensues. Finally, sputum should be sent for Gram stain and routine culture (plus an acid-fast smear and culture if there is suspicion of active tuberculosis on chest radiography).

Special Studies

Bronchoscopy is the initial procedure of choice. It may provide information about both the diagnosis and the location of the bleeding. Early bronchoscopy improves the likelihood of localizing the bleeding site. However, whether to perform flexible or rigid bronchoscopy remains controversial. Flexible bronchoscopy has a greater range of vision and can reach more distally. However, a large volume of blood and clot in the airway will overwhelm its suctioning capability. Rigid bronchoscopy provides superior suctioning and airway control, but it requires general anesthesia, has limited range, and may be more time-consuming to initiate. Fiberoptic bronchoscopy can also be performed via a rigid bronchoscope. Using these two procedures in concert allows one to achieve maximal visualization while providing good suctioning capacity and airway control.

Angiography may serve as an important diagnostic approach if bronchoscopy fails to localize the source of bleeding. Most cases of massive hemoptysis originate from the systemic (bronchial) circulation. However, in lung abscess, tuberculous (Rasmussen's) aneurysm, arteriovenous malformation, or pulmonary artery rupture, the bleeding is from the pulmonary circulation. Angiographic signs suggestive of bleeding include hypervascularity (most common), vascular hypertrophy or tortuosity, bronchopulmonary shunt, aneurysm, capillary stasis, thrombosis, and occasionally extravasation of contrast media.

The *computed tomographic scan* of the lung is considered to be less sensitive than angiography. It infrequently adds information to that obtained by chest

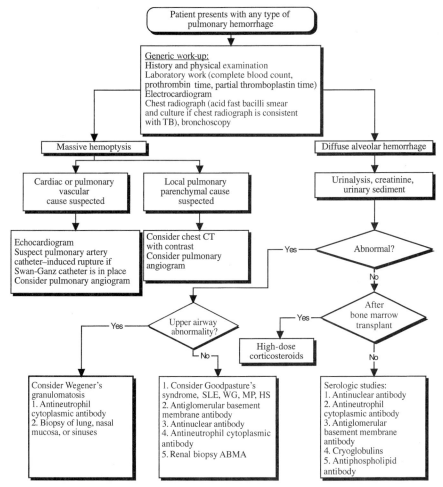

Figure 75–1. Schematic diagram of diagnostic approach to pulmonary hemorrhage. ABMA, antibasement membrane antibody; CT, computed tomography; HS, Henoch-Schönlein purpura; MP, microscopic polyangiitis; SLE, systemic lupus erythematosus; TB, tuberculosis; WG, Wegener's granulomatosis.

radiography and bronchoscopy, particularly since large amounts of blood in the lung may obscure underlying pathology.

To localize the source of hemoptysis by *nuclear medicine* studies (technetium 99m–sulfur colloid isotope-labeled red blood cells), bleeding must be active and brisk at the time of the study. Delays required to label the erythrocytes and low sensitivity limit its utility.

Serologic studies are an important diagnostic tool in diffuse alveolar hemorrhage. However, their results often are not available for several days. Hence, they do not contribute to the acute management of the patient. *Antinuclear antibody* and *anti–double-stranded DNA* support the diagnosis of SLE. However, a small percentage of patients with SLE are seronegative. Suspicion of a pulmonary-renal syndrome mandates measuring titers of both *anti-GBM ab* and *antineutrophil cytoplasmic antibody (ANCA)*. A high titer of anti-GBM ab supports the diagnosis of Goodpasture's syndrome. ANCA titers are reported as either cytoplasmic (C-ANCA) or perinuclear (P-ANCA). A high C-ANCA titer with a positive enzyme-linked immunosorbent assay (ELISA) for antibody to proteinase 3 (PR3) is highly specific and sensitive for Wegener's granulomatosis. A high P-ANCA titer with a positive ELISA for antibody to myeloperoxidase (MPO) is associated with several small-vessel vasculitides, including microscopic angiitis (which can cause diffuse alveolar hemorrhage) as well as Churg-Strauss syndrome and, rarely, some drug reactions. Many other disorders, including infections, can result in positive C-ANCA or P-ANCA, emphasizing the need to test for antibody to PR3 or MPO by ELISA.

THERAPEUTIC APPROACH TO MASSIVE HEMOPTYSIS

Control of the Airway

If bleeding is localized and unilateral, the patient should be placed in the lateral decubitus position with the suspected bleeding side down. This position employs gravity to prevent spillage of blood into the *un*involved lung.

Intubation may be avoided in patients who can maintain oxygenation and ventilation and who can clear the airway by coughing. Because of the importance of an effective cough to clear blood from airways in these circumstances, the use of cough suppressive medication is questionable. In the face of deteriorating oxygenation or ventilation, the patient should be intubated. Because it is often difficult to intubate the patient with massive hemoptysis, the most experienced person available should do it. A large-bore endotracheal tube (ETT) facilitates airway control and allows easy passage of a bronchoscope. An ETT diameter of 8 mm is minimal, and 9 mm is preferable.

In clearly unilateral bleeding, selective intubation of the uninvolved lung will provide ventilation and protection from spill over from the bleeding lung. For bleeding from the right lung, the ETT should be passed into the left mainstem bronchus (over a bronchoscope whose tip is in the left main bronchus) and the cuff carefully inflated. Alternatively, to deal with a bleeding source in the right lung, the ETT can be placed in the usual position above the carina and, by means of a bronchoscope, a Fogarty balloon catheter can be passed into the right mainstem bronchus and inflated to protect the left lung. If bleeding is from the left lung, selective intubation of the relatively short right mainstem bronchus may be the only feasible alternative under dire circumstances despite obstruction of the right upper lobe bronchus by the cuff of the ETT.

Placement of a double-lumen ETT theoretically would allow ventilation of both lungs while preventing aspiration of blood from one lung to the other. Unfortunately, under emergency conditions of massive hemoptysis, these tubes are difficult to place, have a small internal diameter for each individual lumen (needing special narrow-diameter suction catheters, which are not in ready supply in the ICU), and often dislodge or migrate from their requisite precise placement unless the patient is paralyzed.

Control of Bleeding

After establishing control of the airway, hemostasis should be addressed. For the most part, the site of bleeding, available technology, available personnel, and clinical urgency dictate how to accomplish this goal.

Surgery

Selection of patients for surgical management of massive hemoptysis is controversial. Surgery is indicated as definitive therapy for patients with a well-localized process, adequate pulmonary function, and significant risk for recurrent bleeding from the same site. Surgery is also indicated for patients in whom the bleeding is localized and other modalities of therapy have failed.

Arterial Embolization

Bronchial and pulmonary arterial embolization are alternatives to surgery. For patients with poor pulmonary reserve, diffuse disease, or other conditions that make them poor surgical candidates, therapeutic embolization provides a less invasive and potentially lung-sparing solution. This procedure has been especially useful for patients with certain inflammatory diseases, such as bronchiectasis and cystic fibrosis. In these disorders, widely dilated bronchial arteries make the angiographic procedures technically easier, whereas multifocal and recurrent bleeding make surgery less attractive.

If the site of bleeding is identified by arteriography, embolization may be performed immediately. Bronchial arterial embolization is associated with more significant risks than is pulmonary embolization. For example, if arteriography reveals that the anterior spinal artery originates from a bleeding bronchial artery, the procedure may have to be aborted because of the risk of spinal cord injury. In addition, misplacement or reflux of the embolic material into the aorta can cause systemic arterial embolization. However, the procedure is highly effective at stabilizing patients, with acute success reported in 84 to 100% of patients and prolonged success (1 to 60 months) in 70 to 88% of patients.

Endobronchial and Bronchoscopic Techniques

When bleeding is localized to one lung segment, direct tamponade may be possible with a balloon catheter directed toward the site via bronchoscopy. Typically the balloon remains inflated for 24 to 48 hours and may be removed after several hours of observation after deflation. However, long-term management requires definitive, usually surgical, therapy. Although generally safe, balloon tamponade theoretically risks mucosal ischemia or bronchial rupture from balloon overinflation. Furthermore, placing it may be technically difficult and, even if placed in the correct location, it may get displaced by lung expansion during deep inspirations or by coughing.

Thrombin (5 to 10 mL of a solution containing 1000 units/mL) given alone or after fibrinogen (2%, 5 to 10 mL) may seal the bronchus of a bleeding segment. Unfortunately, briskly flowing blood may wash away the fibrin "glue" before a stable clot forms, or residual blood may produce a thrombus in the suction channel of the bronchoscope preventing intrabronchial instillation of clotting factors.

Other bronchoscopic techniques, such as laser coagulation, injection of sclerosing agents, and electrocautery, have been employed successfully when the bleeding site is proximal and visible.

APPROACH FOR SUSPECTED TRACHEAL–INNOMINATE ARTERY FISTULA

If massive hemoptysis occurs in any patient with a tracheostomy tube, one must consider the presence of a tracheal–innominate artery fistula. Immediate consultation with a cardiothoracic surgeon or otorhinolarynologist is indicated. One may attempt to temporize until the patient receives definitive therapy in the operating room by one of several approaches. One can hyperinflate the tube's cuff to try to tamponade the site of the arterial leak. Alternatively, one can remove the tracheal tube and attempt to apply digital compression by inserting a gloved finger into the tracheal stoma and pressing anteriorly against the sternum.

TREATMENT OF DIFFUSE ALVEOLAR HEMORRHAGE

Control of bleeding in patients with diffuse alveolar hemorrhage or poorly localized disease is approached by treating the underlying disease. Because many patients will not have an immediately available diagnosis, initial intervention in these patients will commonly be given empirically to treat the most likely causes, such as Goodpasture's syndrome, SLE, and Wegener's granulomatosis. A full discussion of treatment is beyond the scope of this chapter (see the relevant listings in the Bibliography). However, initial therapy for these entities generally includes "pulse" steroids (methylprednisolone sodium succinate 1g/day) for 3 or more days with cyclophosphamide therapy (2–5 mg/kg/day) plus plasmapheresis for Goodpasture's syndrome (and, in some centers, for SLE).

BIBLIOGRAPHY

Cahill BC, Ingbar DH: Massive hemoptysis. Clin Chest Med 15:147–168, 1994.
  This article is an outstanding, thorough review of the topic.
Green RJ, Ruoss SJ, Kraft SA, et al: Pulmonary capillaritis and alveolar hemorrhage: update on diagnosis and management. Chest 110:1305–1316, 1996.
  This is a highly recommended, comprehensive review of the differential diagnosis of pulmonary capillaritis and alveolar hemorrhage and their management (with 69 references).
Homer RJ: Antineutrophil cytoplasmic antibodies as markers for systemic autoimmune disease. Clin Chest Med 19:627–639, 1998.
  This is an excellent, comprehensive review of cytoplasmic ANCA (C-ANCA) and perinuclear ANCA (P-ANCA) tests and their specificity and sensitivity in various diseases (with 107 references).
Jantz MA, Sahn SA: Corticosteroids in acute respiratory failure. Am J Respir Crit Care Med 160:1079–1100, 1999.
  This is a comprehensive "State of the Art" article that describes and evaluates the evidence for use of corticosteroids in alveolar hemorrhage syndromes (with 326 references).
Jennette JC, Falk R: Small-vessel vasculitis. N Engl J Med 337:1512–1523, 1997.
  This is an outstanding review of vasculitides with particular emphasis on those involving small vessels; all of which may cause diffuse alveolar hemorrhage (with 99 references).
Murin S, Wiedemann HP, Matthay RA: Pulmonary manifestations of systemic lupus erythematosus. Clin Chest Med 19:641–665, 1998.
  This comprehensive review of pulmonary complications of systemic lupus erythematosus includes a section on alveolar hemorrhage and its management (with 209 references).

Myers EN, Carrau MRL: Early complications of tracheotomy. Clin Chest Med 12:589–595, 1991.
This article addresses the treatment of tracheoarterial fistula after tracheostomy.

Nicolls MR, Terada LS, Tuder RM, et al: Diffuse alveolar hemorrhage with underlying pulmonary capillaritis in the retinoic acid syndrome. Am J Resp Crit Care Med 158:1302–1305, 1998.
This is a case report and discussion of diffuse alveolar hemorrhage occurring in a patient with acute promyelocytic leukemia treated with all-trans-retinoic acid.

Prakash UBS, Freitag L: Hemoptysis and bronchoscopy-induced hemorrhage. In: Prakash UBS (ed): Bronchoscopy. New York: Raven Press, 1994, p 227.
This chapter discusses the various modalities of bronchoscopic intervention.

Robbins RA, Linder J, Marlin GS, et al: Diffuse alveolar hemorrhage in autologous bone marrow transplant recipients. Am J Med 87:511–518, 1989.
The risks of this complication in recipients of autologous bone marrow transplantation are reviewed.

Savige J, Gillis D, Benson E, et al: International consensus statement on testing and reporting of antineutrophil cytoplasmic antibodies (ANCA). Am J Clin Pathol 111:507–513, 1999.
This is an international, expert-based consensus statement that warns against diagnosing Wegener's granulomatosis on basis of immunofluorescence (ANCA) results alone and advocates that all positive ANCA be tested by ELISA specific for proteinase 3 (PR3) and myeloperoxidase (MPO).

Waterer GW, Latham B, Gabbay E: Pulmonary capillaritis associated with the antiphospholipid antibody syndrome and rapid response to plasmapheresis. Respirology 4:405–408, 1999.
This is case report of alveolar hemorrhage associated with antiphospholipid antibody syndrome, which was treated with methylprednosolone, cyclophosphamide, and plasmapheresis.

76   Major Pulmonary Embolism

Yevgeniy Gincherman
Harold I. Palevsky

Patients with major pulmonary embolism represent a small but important subset of all patients with venous thromboembolic disease. These individuals experience greatly increased morbidity and mortality, resulting in substantial human and financial costs. Variability in the natural presentation and progression of major pulmonary emboli makes timely detection and treatment difficult. Traditional approaches to the treatment of less extensive pulmonary emboli and deep venous thrombi often prove inadequate for patients with major pulmonary embolism. This chapter discusses the specific indications and use of aggressive and invasive therapy such as local and systemic thrombolytic agents, interventional catheter manipulation techniques, and surgical embolectomy.

DEFINITION, CLINICAL PRESENTATION, AND DETECTION OF MAJOR PULMONARY EMBOLISM

A pulmonary embolus is defined as major if *substantial* hemodynamic or respiratory compromise is present or if a *substantial* percentage of the pulmonary vascular bed is occluded. *Substantial hemodynamic compromise* is the inability to maintain adequate peripheral tissue perfusion as a result of cardiac pump failure. It is often associated with the need for vasopressor agents. *Substantial respiratory compromise* is the inability to maintain arterial oxygenation or adequate ventilation.

Most authors require occlusion of at least 40 to 50% of the pulmonary vascular bed for a pulmonary embolus to be considered major. However, in patients with pre-existing compromise of cardiopulmonary reserve, lesser degrees of occlusion of the pulmonary vasculature can manifest the same degree of cardiopulmonary compromise as does a major pulmonary embolus. Under these circumstances, the compromised circulation reflects both vascular occlusion and the effects of vasoactive mediators. Pulmonary arterial pressure is often elevated with major pulmonary emboli. Mean pulmonary artery pressure usually exceeds 30 mm Hg but may exceed 40 mm Hg in the acute setting. However, 50 mm Hg appears to be the maximal mean pressure that a previously normal right ventricle can generate without failing acutely.

The Miller angiographic severity index is often used to evaluate major pulmonary emboli. In Miller's classification, the right pulmonary artery has nine major segmental branches, and the left pulmonary artery has seven such branches. A filling defect in any of these branches scores 1 point, up to a maximum of 16 points. In addition, each lung is divided into three zones (upper, middle, and lower). Flow in each zone is scored as absent (3 points), severely reduced (2 points), mildly reduced (1 point), or normal (0 points), up to a theoretical maximum of 18 points for both lungs. A score of 20 or more out of the combined maximal score of 34 points has been proposed as an indicator of severely compromised pulmonary vasculature and of the presence of major pulmonary emboli.

Symptoms and signs associated with major pulmonary emboli, as with nonmajor ones, are often nonspecific. For example, presentation may be a syncopal event. Dyspnea, especially with exertion, is frequent, but pleuritic chest pain is not. Pleuritic pain, as a rule, is inversely related to clot size because the smaller clots can travel more distally and cause pleurisy. Tachycardia is common after the acute event and is often accompanied by sharp, small-volume arterial pulses with narrowed pulse pressures. Right ventricular failure may be manifested by jugular venous distention, gallop rhythms, and electrocardiographic signs of acute right ventricle strain. Some patients experience substernal chest pain similar to that seen in myocardial infarction, but their electrocardiographic findings are usually nonspecific.

Clinical and hemodynamic parameters can be further evaluated with the use of transthoracic echocardiography. This noninvasive technique may aid in prompt detection of major pulmonary emboli and guide subsequent treatment. It can easily be used at the bedside in emergency settings, even with unstable patients. Although the left main pulmonary artery is often obscured because of the location of the air-filled left mainstem bronchus, Doppler techniques can be used to estimate pulmonary artery systolic pressure. Many authors contend that chronic pulmonary hypertension is often difficult to distinguish from acute pulmonary hypertension because of major pulmonary embolus. However, if one finds the presence of right ventricular hypertrophy, it makes an acute process, such as pulmonary embolism, less likely to be the sole disorder.

In contrast to transthoracic echocardiography, which rarely allows direct visualization of intraluminal thrombotic material, transesophageal echocardiography can detect emboli in the main pulmonary artery, at its bifurcation, and in the right main pulmonary artery. Transesophageal echocardiography is useful in the evaluation of both acute and chronic pulmonary emboli. In an acute setting, it can provide evidence of the presence of the occlusion of major pulmonary artery branches, obviating the use of more invasive diagnostic methods and permitting prompt progression to therapeutic intervention. Flow artifact in the pulmonary artery, however, may mimic thrombotic material. To summarize, echocardiographic manifestations of acute major pulmonary embolism include right ventricular dilatation with or without right atrial dilatation, abnormal displacement of the intraventricular septum into the left ventricular cavity during systole (due to high right ventricular system pressure), pulmonary artery dilatation, and increased pulmonary arterial pressure (as documented by Doppler techniques).

THERAPY FOR MAJOR PULMONARY EMBOLISM

Over the last 25 years, therapy of major pulmonary embolism has made substantial progress. At present, medical treatments include both peripheral and intrapulmonary administration of standard doses of thrombolytic agents. In addition, intrapulmonary infusion of lower doses of thrombolytic agents can be used to accelerate clot lysis and resolution while trying to reduce the risk of hemorrhage. Since being proposed in the early 1900s, techniques of surgical embolectomy and cardiopulmonary bypass techniques have improved, resulting in less morbidity and mortality. In addition, techniques of transvenous catheter embolectomy and thrombus manipulation have been developed, providing alternatives to the classic surgical approach. A synthesis of recommendations for management of major pulmonary embolism is presented in Figures 76–1 and 76–2.

A recent study of more than 1000 patients with deep venous thrombosis treated with regimens of heparin plus oral anticoagulants found that 2.33% of all patients died of pulmonary embolism despite receiving what is considered standard therapy. Other investigators have reported rates of fatal pulmonary embolism as high as 10% in patients receiving similar therapy. Thus, standard therapy with anticoagulation alone is inadequate in the acute treatment of major pulmonary embolus.

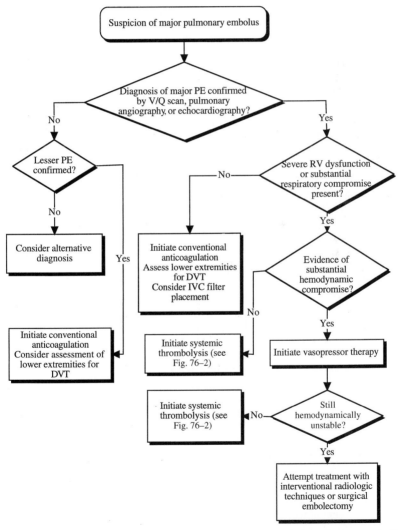

Figure 76–1. Schematic flow diagram for approach to treatment of major pulmonary emboli. PE, pulmonary embolus; V/Q, ventilation/perfusion; RV, right ventricular; DVT, deep venous thrombosis; IVC, inferior vena cava.

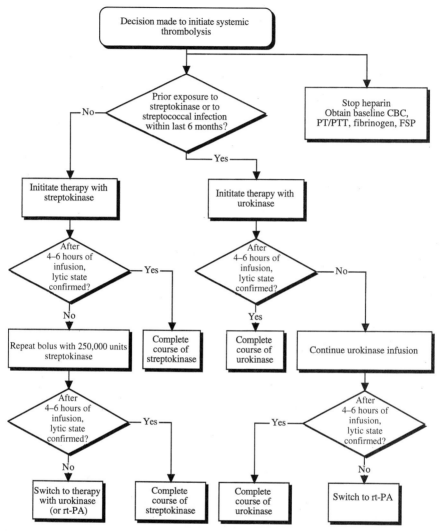

Figure 76–2. Schematic flow diagram for thrombolytic therapy of major pulmonary emboli; systemic lytic state is confirmed when fibrinogen falls and fibrin split products increase markedly. CBC, complete blood count; PT/PTT, prothrombin time/partial thromboplastin time; FSP, fibrin split products; rt-PA, recombinant tissue-plasminogen activator (alteplase).

Intravenous Administration of Thrombolytic Therapy

In the United States, the Food and Drug Administration (FDA) has approved three thrombolytic agents for the treatment of acute pulmonary embolism: streptokinase, urokinase, and recombinant tissue-plasminogen activator (rt-PA), alteplase (Table 76–1). All these agents generate a systemic lytic state and reduce plasma levels of fibrinogen, plasminogen, and alpha$_2$-antiplasmin. Standard dosing protocols for

Table 76–1. Thrombolytic Therapy for Major Pulmonary Embolism

AGENT	LOADING DOSE	HOURLY DOSE	RECOMMENDED DURATION	COST*
Streptokinase	250,000 IU over 30 min	100,000 IU/h	24 h	$400
Urokinase	4400 IU/kg over 10 min	4400 IU/kg/h	12 h	$4000
Alteplase (recombinant tissue-type plasminogen activator)	None	50 mg/h	2 h	$2000

*Cost equals approximate hospital acquisition cost for recommended course of drug (1998).

these agents in the treatment of pulmonary embolism do not include the concurrent use of antithrombotic medications such as aspirin and heparin. Because of this, on completion of the course of thrombolytic therapy, standard anticoagulation must be instituted. Continuous intravenous heparin should be started (without a bolus) after the lytic agent has been stopped and the partial thromboplastin time is less than three times control levels.

Optimal regimens for dosing and duration of thrombolytic treatment have not yet been established. For continuous infusion therapy, setting the duration of treatment for all patients by a single standard protocol suffers because it fails to recognize variations among patients. Others have advocated that once thrombolytic therapy is initiated, it should be continued until either all clot amenable to thrombolysis has been dissolved or a complication of therapy has been identified. For rt-PA, in particular, it is not clear that the FDA-approved short duration of therapy (2 hours) for acute pulmonary emboli is sufficient to lyse the large clot burden found in major pulmonary emboli. One possible approach to determining the duration of drug administration is to follow the level of fibrin degradation products (fibrin split products) and to continue the thrombolytic treatment until they normalize (suggesting cessation of significant clot lysis). Another approach to the duration of thrombolytic therapy uses sequential imaging of the clots, and therapy is maintained as long as continued dissolution of the thrombus is documented. Noninvasive studies, including perfusion lung scanning, magnetic resonance imaging and magnetic resonance angiography (MRI/MRA), and antifibrin and antiplatelet antibody imaging, are preferable to repeated invasive studies.

Combining the observation that increased diffusion of thrombolytic agents into the thrombus takes place when circulating drug levels are high with the relatively long duration of their pharmacologic effects has led to the development of *bolus* dosing protocols for the treatment of major pulmonary emboli. Both animal studies and initial clinical trials with both urokinase and rt-PA suggest that intermittent bolus therapy may be more efficacious with possibly less sustained bleeding risk than the standard continuous infusion regimen. The researchers in the Bolus Alteplase Embolism Group compared reduced-dose bolus rt-PA and conventional infusion in pulmonary embolism thrombolysis. Patients received either 0.6 mg/kg over 15 minutes (maximum of 50 mg) or the standard FDA-approved continuous infusion of 100 mg over 2 hours. Sixty patients were treated with bolus rt-PA and 27 received the standard infusion. Although similar changes in the outcome parameters and similar rates of bleeding complications were documented in both groups, bolus rt-PA administration resulted in less reduction of fibrinogen levels than did the standard infusion. However, larger studies comparing the two regimens that show better outcomes or fewer complications, or both, are needed before adopting the nonstandard approach.

Intrapulmonary Infusion of Thrombolytic Agents

In the 1970s and early 1980s, multiple attempts were made to devise methods of administering thrombolytic agents directly into the pulmonary artery. The theoretical advantage of this approach is twofold. First, local administration of a thrombolytic agent was expected to result in more effective lysis of the clot. Second, it was hypothesized that local administration would produce fewer systemic side effects, most notably less major bleeding. At first, investigators attempted intrapulmonary administration of thrombolytic agents at doses used for peripheral infusion. Contrary to expectations, most researchers found that local infusion of the standard full dose of thrombolytic agents was no more effective than systemic therapy, and rates of major hemorrhage were similar.

After trials of intrapulmonary infusion of standard-dose thrombolytic agents, a number of groups attempted to infuse *low-dose* thrombolytic agents directly into the pulmonary arterial tree with or without concomitant heparin. The UKEP study group compared the efficacy of low- and high-dose intrapulmonary urokinase infusion in 67 and 62 patients, respectively. Two doses of urokinase were used: 2000 IU/kg/hour in conjunction with heparin for 24 hours versus 4400 IU/kg/hour of urokinase alone for 12 hours. Low-dose urokinase combined with heparin was as effective in clot lysis as the standard higher dose as documented by pulmonary angiograms (performed 30 to 48 hours after initiation of therapy). However, similar rates of major bleeding were observed in the two groups. In addition, various bolus infusion regimens have been given as an intrapulmonary infusion, including a 0.6 mg/kg 2-minute infusion of rt-PA and a 1 mg/kg 10-minute infusion of rt-PA. Preliminary studies suggest that a single bolus infusion of a fibrinolytic agent locally can provide effective clot lysis without producing the major bleeding complications associated with continuous higher dose infusion therapy. However, larger confirmatory studies are needed before this nonstandard approach can be recommended for general use.

Selection of Thrombolytic Agent

Choice of a fibrinolytic agent depends on patient characteristics, drug availability, physician familiarity with the different agents, and differences in rates of complications and adverse effects. The Global Utilization of Streptokinase and Tissue Plasminogen Activator for Occluded Coronary Arteries (GUSTO) investigators studied 41,000 patients, providing important data regarding relative safety profiles of streptokinase and rt-PA. The incidence of hemorrhagic strokes was found to be slightly higher in the rt-PA group. Risk of major bleeding outside the cranium was comparable for both agents. The risk of hypotension and anaphylactic reactions, however, was much higher with streptokinase. Urokinase and rt-PA are preferred treatments when readministration of thrombolytic therapy is necessary. Major and minor contraindications to administration of thrombolytic therapy for major pulmonary embolism are presented in Table 76–2.

Pearls and Pitfalls of Thrombolytic Therapy

Streptokinase is most frequently associated with hypotension and anaphylactic reactions. If such a reaction is encountered, the drug should be stopped immediately. Antihistamines and corticosteroids should be administered as needed and pressors used to reverse hypotension. However, one must be careful to avoid *hypertension* to prevent potential bleeding complications. Although urokinase is also associated with febrile-type reactions, it has a lesser rate of true allergic reactions.

Table 76–2. Contraindications to Thrombolytic Therapy

Major Contraindications

Active internal bleeding
Recent cerebrovascular accident (within 2 mo)
Intracranial processes, including neoplasm, aneurysm, or arteriovenous malformation

Minor Contraindications

Recent major surgery, obstetric delivery, organ biopsy, puncture of noncompressible blood vessel
Recent serious gastric bleeding
Recent serious trauma
Severe arterial hypertension
Recent minor trauma, including cardiopulmonary resuscitation
Presence of left heart thrombus
Bacterial endocarditis
Hemostatic defects
Pregnancy
Age >75 yr
Diabetic hemorrhagic retinopathy

Once a decision has been made to initiate thrombolytic therapy, large-bore intravenous (IV) access should be obtained. If continuous arterial access is required, it is prudent to establish it before starting the infusion. Attempts to insert IV catheters bigger than 18 gauge should be avoided during the infusion, and all phlebotomy procedures should be reduced to a minimum. If a patient is a potential candidate for lytic therapy, any IV access sheath placed during angiography should be left in place. It can provide large-bore IV access as well as tamponade the vein to decrease the risk of bleeding at the angiography site.

Interventional Radiologic Therapy for Major Pulmonary Embolism

Rapid restoration of blood flow to the affected pulmonary segments is important in patients with major pulmonary emboli. Recently developed techniques of mechanical clot disruption with various catheter devices can be effective in dispersing the clot to more distal locations within the pulmonary arterial tree, thus reducing the obstruction of the pulmonary vasculature. This technique, when combined with the thrombolytic therapy, potentially facilitates faster clot resolution. Techniques of clot extraction, including transvenous catheter embolectomy, have also been developed and successfully employed, although large series are lacking.

Surgical Therapy for Major Pulmonary Embolism

A surgical approach to major pulmonary embolism was first proposed by Trendelenburg in 1908, with the first successful embolectomy performed by Kirschner in 1924. Cardiopulmonary bypass was first used as an adjunct to open chest embolectomy by Sharp in 1961 and immediately improved the previously dismal survival rates.

Despite the availability of cardiopulmonary bypass, open chest pulmonary embolectomy continues to have high mortality. In the most extensive review of this procedure, del Campo reported a mortality rate of 40% with the use of cardiopulmonary bypass in 537 patients. Gray and associates reported a mortality rate of 30% in the 71 patients who underwent pulmonary embolectomies. Soyer and colleagues reported a 30% mortality rate in 17 patients who underwent open chest embolectomy for major pulmonary embolism on long-term follow-up. More recently, Schmid and colleagues reported a mortality rate of 44% in 27 patients. Thus, pulmonary embolectomy should serve as an alternative to thrombolytic therapy mainly in patients who have contraindications to medical therapy or who seem too hemodynamically unstable to await the outcome of a trial of thrombolytic therapy.

Inferior Vena Cava Interruption

A meta-analysis of 24 case series of inferior vena cava (IVC) filter insertion has shown that recurrent pulmonary embolism is rare after filter placement, with only eight deaths reported among 2557 filter recipients. In a review of the PIOPED data by Carson and associates, of the 375 patients who received standard treatment (anticoagulation alone) for pulmonary embolism, only 10 of the patients died of pulmonary embolism. Nine of these patients were suspected of having recurrent pulmonary embolism, which could have been prevented by filter placement. This emphasizes the importance of assessing residual peripheral deep venous thrombosis in the management of patients with pulmonary emboli of all sizes (see Chapter 47). There are no situations in which IVC plication or ligation should be routinely employed considering the high mortality rates associated with both procedures (6 to 27% and 7 to 21%, respectively). Instead, angiographic insertion of an IVC filter is the procedure of choice to interrupt the IVC because of the low associated morbidity and mortality of this procedure. A listing of indications for IVC filter placement is given in Table 76–3. Placement of an IVC filter is not a contraindication to subsequent thrombolytic therapy. The introducer sheath should be left in place to both tamponade the vein and serve as a large-caliber intravenous access site. Leaving the sheath in situ also provides convenient access for repeat angiography to assess the results of thrombolytic therapy.

Table 76–3. Indications for Inferior Vena Cava Filter Placement

Pulmonary embolism or proximal deep venous thrombosis, or both, with contraindications to anticoagulation

Complications of anticoagulation leading to premature discontinuation

Recurrent thromboembolism while on appropriate therapy (embolization of pre-existing thrombus does not represent anticoagulation failure)

Prophylaxis in high-risk patients with contraindications to anticoagulation

Caval and iliofemoral vein thrombosis, especially if proximal end of clot is free-floating or if thrombolytic therapy is anticipated

Medical Versus Surgical Therapy of Major Pulmonary Embolism

Only two studies comparing medical and surgical treatment of major pulmonary embolism are available. In 1987, Lund and collegues compared 20 patients who underwent open chest embolectomy with 22 patients who received streptokinase and 32 patients who received only heparin. Patients with major central emboli and irreversible hemodynamic compromise as well as those who were hemodynamically stable but had contraindications to thrombolytic use were included in the embolectomy group. Streptokinase was given to patients who were hemodynamically stable with central or lobar emboli. Finally, patients with peripheral emboli received heparin. The mortality rate at 30 days was 21% in the streptokinase group, 6% in the heparin group, and 20% in the embolectomy group. Of the 30-day survivors, the 5-year survival rate was 100% in the embolectomy group as compared with 75% survival rate in the medical groups. The treatment groups were not significantly different at follow-up when compared according to right-sided heart catheterization data, degree of pulmonary artery obstruction, right ventricular diameter and wall thickness, ventilatory functions, and electrocardiographic changes. This study has severe limitations, not only because the patients were not randomly assigned to therapies but also because the therapies were not even compared in the same classes of patients.

Gulba and associates compared the efficacy of embolectomy and thrombolysis in 37 patients who presented in shock because of major pulmonary embolism. A 77% survival rate was documented in the surgical arm of the study, which included routine clipping of the inferior vena cava. This was not statistically different from the 67% survival rate for the patients treated with rt-PA followed by heparin. However, there was a 28% incidence of major hemorrhage in the rt-PA group, and 20% of the medically treated patients had a subsequent embolism. Results of this trial suggest that open chest surgical embolectomy or other invasive approach, for example, angiographic clot disruption or embolectomy, should be considered in unstable patients with major pulmonary embolism, especially if such techniques are readily available and performed by experienced interventional radiologists or surgeons.

BIBLIOGRAPHY

Arcasoy SM, Kreit JW: Thrombolytic therapy of pulmonary embolism. A comprehensive review of current evidence. Chest 115:1695–1707, 1999.
This is a recent, comprehensive review that provides evidence-based guidelines for use of thrombolytic therapy and discusses practical aspects of thrombolysis for pulmonary embolism.
Carson JL, Kelley MA, Duff A, et al: The clinical course of pulmonary embolism. N Engl J Med 326:1240–1245, 1992.
This is a prospective follow-up of the 399 patients with confirmed pulmonary embolism in the PIOPED study. During follow-up, the majority of deaths were due to the patients' underlying diseases. Only 2.5% died of pulmonary embolism almost all of which were from recurrent embolic events.

del Campo C: Pulmonary embolectomy: A review. Can J Surg 28:111–113, 1985.
This review of the literature shows that surgical embolectomy can be successful in patients who

had contraindications to, or who were unlikely to survive, medical therapy. Recommendations for indications for embolectomy and patient management are offered.

Goldhaber SZ. Pulmonary embolism. N Engl J Med 339:93–104, 1998.
This is a comprehensive review article about pulmonary emboli in general by one of the authorities in the field.

Goldhaber SZ, Agnelli G, Levine MN: Reduced dose bolus alteplase vs. conventional alteplase infusion for pulmonary embolism thrombolysis. An international multicenter randomized trial. Chest 106:718–724, 1994.
This describes a randomized trial of bolus injection of rt-PA (0.6 mg/kg/15 min) vs. the standard 100 mg of rt-PA administered by continuous intravenous infusion over 2 hours. No significant differences were detected with respect to bleeding complications, adverse clinical events, or imaging studies but those in the bolus treatment group had less depression of fibrinogen.

Gray HH, Miller GA, Paneth M: Pulmonary embolectomy: Its place in the management of pulmonary embolism. Lancet 1:1441–1445, 1988.
This reports a large series of hemodynamically unstable patients who underwent pulmonary embolectomy. Of the patients who had sustained significant periods of cardiac arrest before surgery, two thirds died. However, if patients survived hospitalization, most (70%) had no long-term morbidity.

Gulba DC, Schmid C, Borst HG, et al: Medical compared with surgical treatment for major pulmonary embolism. Lancet 343:576–577, 1994.
This is a retrospective review of patients in shock with massive pulmonary embolism who were treated either surgically (13 patients) or with rt-PA followed by heparin (24 patients). Seventy-seven percent of surgical patients survived as compared to 67% of the medically treated patients. Major bleeding occurred in 28% of the medically treated patients.

Lund O, Nielsen TT, Ronne K, et al: Pulmonary embolism: Long-term follow-up after treatment with full-dose heparin, streptokinase or embolectomy. Acta Med Scand 221:61–71, 1987.
This reports on long-term follow-up of 74 patients alive 30 days after treatment for pulmonary embolism with embolectomy (20), streptokinase (22), or heparin (32). The 5-year survival was 100% in the embolectomy group vs. 75% (±7%) in the medically treated groups.

Schmid C, Zietlow S, Wagner TOF, et al: Fulminant pulmonary embolism: Symptoms, diagnostics, operative technique, and results. Ann Thorac Surg 52:1102–1107, 1991.
This is an analysis of 27 patients who underwent pulmonary embolectomy for massive pulmonary embolism. Overall mortality was 44%, with two thirds of deaths due to intractable right heart failure; other deaths were due to anoxic encephalopathy and sepsis.

Soyer R, Brunet AP, Redonnet M, et al: Follow-up of surgically treated patients with major pulmonary embolism with reference to 12 operated patients. Thorac Cardiovasc Surg 30:103–108, 1982.
Twelve of 17 (71%) patients who underwent embolectomy for massive pulmonary embolism survived to hospital discharge. Two of these had limitations due to pulmonary hypertension, while the others had minimal or no residual vascular occlusion.

The GUSTO Investigators: An international randomized trial comparing four thrombolytic strategies for acute myocardial infarction. N Engl J Med 329:673–692, 1993.
Evaluation of the results of a study of 41,021 patients with myocardial infarction allows for a comparison of the risks and differences between streptokinase and rt-PA (alteplase). Alteplase had more rapid thrombolysis (and had significantly fewer deaths due to myocardial infarction). However, it had a higher rate of hemorrhagic stroke than streptokinase (0.72% vs. 0.54%).

The UKEP Study: Multicenter clinical trial of two local regimens of urokinase in major pulmonary embolism. Eur Heart J 8:2–10, 1987.
Intrapulmonary infusion of urokinase by two different protocols (2000 IU/kg/h with heparin for 24 h vs. 4400 IU/kg/h for 12 h followed by heparin) were compared for efficacy and complications. An average of 66% of the pulmonary vascular bed was occluded in each group. There were similar and significant degrees of resolution of the emboli. Likewise, the two groups had a similar frequency of bleeding complications (approximately 25%) with severe bleeding rates of 4.5% and 3.0%, respectively.

77

Obesity Hypoventilation Syndrome

Frank Trudo
Richard J. Schwab

Sleep-disordered breathing is a common clinical problem that may affect intensive care unit (ICU) patients. For example, obesity hypoventilation syndrome (OHS) may precipitate a patient's admission to the ICU. In addition, OHS or obstructive sleep apnea (OSA) may exacerbate a pre-existing cardiopulmonary disorder. Since identification of ICU patients with sleep-disordered breathing is critical to initiating appropriate treatment, this chapter presents the pathophysiologic features of OSA and OHS, the differential diagnosis of chronic alveolar hypoventilation, and a diagnostic and management strategy for these conditions in the ICU.

SPECTRUM OF SLEEP-DISORDERED BREATHING

Although sleep-disordered breathing has only recently been recognized as a specific syndrome affecting many individuals, features of these disorders were first described in ancient Greek literature and later by Charles Dickens. His novel, *The Posthumous Papers of the Pickwick Club,* is recognized as the classic literary depiction of the *pickwickian syndrome* in the character of Joe. Joe manifested the typical features of OHS: obesity, daytime sleepiness, and signs of right-sided congestive heart failure. The term *pickwickian syndrome* is synonymous with OHS. As such, it should be reserved for patients who demonstrate daytime hypersomnolence, hypercapnia, and hypoxemia in addition to nocturnal hypoventilation. Sleep-disordered breathing should be considered a continuous spectrum of conditions ranging from snoring to life-threatening disorders of hypoventilation and right-sided heart failure (Table 77–1). It is not fully understood why some patients move along this continuum and develop the more severe forms of sleep-disordered breathing. However, significant weight gain, an important risk factor for both OSA and OHS, is likely to be a key factor.

OBSTRUCTIVE AND CENTRAL SLEEP APNEAS

Obstructive sleep apena (OSA) is characterized by loud snoring, excessive daytime sleepiness, and episodic arterial desaturation during sleep. Other features include witnessed apneas by bed partners, intellectual impairment, irritability, morning headaches, and an increased risk of automobile accidents as a result of chronic sleep deprivation and associated daytime hypersomnolence. In contrast to OHS, patients with OSA do *not* have daytime hypercapnia. OSA is defined as recurrent episodes of apnea during sleep caused by occlusion of the upper airway. Anatomic narrowing of the upper airway is a major factor in its pathogenesis. In addition to this anatomic abnormality, a neural component with reduction in the activity of

Table 77–1. Spectrum of Sleep-Disordered Breathing

DEGREE OF SEVERITY	FORM	COMMENT
Mild	Snoring	Worsens with alcohol.
Mild	Upper airway resistance syndrome	Snoring with arousals* and associated sleep fragmentation† and daytime hypersomnolence.
Moderate	Hypopneas	Episodes in which airflow decreased by $\geq$50% associated either with $\geq$4% fall in arterial oxygen saturation or with arousals ($\geq$10 sec in duration). It may be due to partial occlusion of upper airway or decreased central neuronal respiratory drive. More than five such episodes/h is abnormal.
Moderate	Obstructive sleep apnea (OSA)	Breathing stops for 10 seconds or more with >5 episodes/h but $\leq$20/h.
Severe	OSA	Breathing stops for >10 sec or more >20 times/h.
Severe	Obesity hypoventilation syndrome (OHS)	Usually combines features of severe OSA plus chronic daytime $Paco_2$ elevation.

*Arousals, an electroencephalographic defined change in state from a deeper stage of sleep to a lighter stage of sleep or to wakefulness, often manifested by the presence of alpha activity.
†Sleep fragmentation, disruption of normal sleep stages and their sequence and cycles.

the upper airway dilator muscles during sleep is likely involved. This predisposes the upper airway to collapse during sleep. Repeated apneic events result in arousals (change in sleep state from a deeper stage of sleep to a higher stage of sleep or wakefulness, often manifested by the presence of an alpha pattern on the electroencephalogram), sleep fragmentation (disruption of normal sequence of sleep stages and cycling), and sleep deprivation (decreased total time asleep per 24 hours), especially decreased rapid eye movement (REM) sleep.

Central sleep apnea is defined as repeated episodes of apnea during sleep in the absence of any respiratory muscle effort. The pathogenesis of central sleep apnea is related to transient loss of central nervous system drive to the respiratory muscles. In contrast, in obstructive apneas, respiratory effort is preserved but airflow is prevented by upper airway occlusion.

An overnight polysomnogram (which monitors the electroencephalogram, extraocular muscles, airflow at mouth and nose, and movements of the chest wall, abdomen, and extremities) can differentiate central from obstructive apnea. It may also demonstrate hypopneas (defined as 50% or greater decrement in airflow associated with a fall of 4% or more in oxygen saturation or an arousal). Mixed apneas are common and occur when a patient demonstrates both central and obstructive events during polysomnography.

OBESITY HYPOVENTILATION SYNDROME

Obesity hypoventilation syndrome (OHS) is defined by the presence of obesity and chronic hypoventilation, that is, hypercapnia with a $Paco_2$ greater than 45 mm Hg, when awake. Other features of OHS include hypersomnolence, resting hypoxemia, and pulmonary hypertension with chronic right-sided heart failure (Table 77–2). Approximately 10% of patients with OSA also have OHS. Conversely, OSA occurs frequently among patients diagnosed with OHS. OHS is often identified in those patients who are morbidly obese (see Table 77–2). OHS should be considered in any patient who is obese and hypersomnolent and demonstrates hypercapnia while awake. Hypoxemia while awake is another feature of this syndrome and results from hypercapnia, with the additional effects of basilar atelectasis resulting from obesity and shallow breathing. Despite the hypercapnia and hypoxemia, patients with OHS characteristically are not dyspneic or tachypneic at rest, indicating a loss of normal ventilatory response to hypercapnia and a blunting or a complete loss of response to hypoxemia.

Patients with OHS have a characteristic pattern on nocturnal oximetry that distinguishes this disorder from OSA (Fig. 77–1). The clinical diagnosis of OHS can be confirmed by demonstrating a greater than 10 mm Hg increase in $Paco_2$ when a patient falls asleep. The exact cause of OHS is likely multifactorial. It includes impaired central respiratory drive, adverse effects of obesity on pulmonary function, ventilation-perfusion mismatch, and compromised respiratory muscular capacity. It is important to recognize OHS in the ICU in order to differentiate this syndrome from other causes of alveolar hypoventilation and chronic hypercapnia.

Diagnosis

In order to appropriately evaluate the obese hypercapnic patient, it is important to understand the physiologic determinants of alveolar ventilation and $Paco_2$ (see Chapter 1, Table 1–1) as well as to rule out other causes of chronic alveolar hypoventilation, especially those cases due to chronic airway obstruction.

Distinguishing chronic obstructive pulmonary disease (COPD) from OHS is particularly important because the treatment for these conditions is different. For example, in both conditions, patients can present with hypercapnia and right-sided congestive heart failure. Likewise, laboratory data in both disorders may demonstrate compensated respiratory acidosis, polycythemia, and hypoxemia. Al-

Table 77–2. Clinical Signs and Symptoms of Obesity Hypoventilation Syndrome

Obesity (often morbid obesity*)
Daytime symptoms of hypercapnia
Chronic fatigue
Morning headache
Daytime hypersomnolence
Lower extremity edema often unresponsive to diuretics due to right-sided congestive heart failure (cor pulmonale)

*Morbid obesity = $\geq 200\%$ ideal body weight or body mass index ≥ 40.

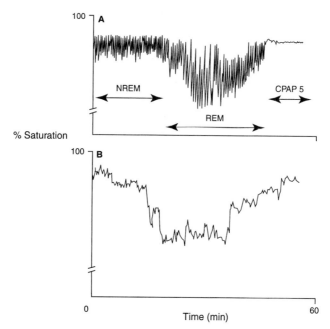

% Saturation

Figure 77–1. *A,* Nocturnal oximetry in a patient with severe obstructive sleep apnea demonstrating recurrent desaturations in non–rapid eye movement (NREM) and rapid eye movement (REM) sleep. Each apneic event results in an oxyhemoglobin desaturation that improves as the apnea is terminated. The degree of desaturation is greater in REM sleep and resolves when continuous positive airway pressure (CPAP) of 5 cm H_2O is applied. *B,* In contrast to *A,* this nocturnal oximetry demonstrates prolonged desaturation in a patient with obesity hypoventilation syndrome (OHS). The desaturation corresponds to periods of prolonged hypoventilation. Although not diagnostic, this pattern is highly suggestive of OHS.

though OHS and COPD may coexist, OHS should be considered in the obese patient who has daytime hypersomnolence, loud snoring, witnessed apneas, and evidence of pulmonary hypertension or right ventricular failure on examination. Absence of significant tobacco use and lack of hyperinflation on chest radiographs makes COPD less likely. Although the presence of normal airflow on pulmonary function tests can reliably exclude COPD, such studies may be difficult to perform in ICU patients, especially if patients are intubated. The diagnosis of OHS can be

Table 77–3. Laboratory Findings in Obesity Hypoventilation Syndrome

Hypercapnia while awake ($Paco_2$ >45 mm Hg)
Resting arterial desaturation while awake (Sao_2 <90%)
>10 mm Hg increase in $Paco_2$ when going from awake to sleep
Respiratory acidosis during sleep (pH < 7.3)
Nocturnal oximetry demonstrating persistent oxyhemoglobin desaturations (Sao_2 <90%)
Polysomnography demonstrating concomitant obstructive sleep apnea or evidence of central hypoventilation

confirmed by demonstrating progressive hypercapnia (>10 mm Hg $Paco_2$ increase from baseline during sleep) (Table 77–3). In order to diagnose OHS and to assess the severity of nocturnal hypercapnia, it is recommended that arterial blood gas determinations be obtained about every 2 hours during sleep via an arterial catheter. If an arterial catheter is not used, at a minimum, arterial blood gas measurements must be obtained before and after sleep.

Therapy

The management of OHS requires assisted ventilation while treating coexisting medical problems. Giving only supplemental oxygen may prolong apneas and worsen respiratory acidosis in patients with OHS. Although diuretics may help improve leg edema resulting from right-sided congestive heart failure, the treatment of choice for patients with OHS is nocturnal noninvasive ventilation administered via a nasal or oral face mask. If patients are unable to tolerate noninvasive ventilation, conventional mechanical ventilation via an uncuffed (or rarely a cuffed) tracheostomy should be considered.

If successful, nocturnal noninvasive ventilation in patients with OHS should correct daytime hypercapnia and hypoxemia, reduce pulmonary artery pressure, and improve right ventricular function. It can be applied with conventional volume- or pressure-cycled ventilators (Table 77–4). Volume-cycled nasal ventilation is usually more effective than pressure-cycled ventilation because the latter may not provide sufficient inspiratory pressure to generate adequate tidal volumes in mor-

Table 77–4. Protocol for Nocturnal Noninvasive Ventilation

Set-up phase: admission to ICU/step-down unit

Arterial catheter insertion to guide adjustment of ventilator settings
Obtain appropriately fitting CPAP mask, nasal pillows, or oronasal mask
Chin strap may be necessary to keep the mouth closed

Volume-cycled ventilator parameters

Tidal volume: for obese patients (>100 kg), use 5–7 mL/kg
Respiratory rate
   Start with 6 breaths per minute
   Adjust rate to obtain appropriate $Paco_2$ (not >10 mm Hg drop during first night)
   Aim for an ultimate $Paco_2$ of 40–50 mm Hg, but may need to accept 50–60 mm Hg
Supplemental oxygen
   In patients with a normal (A-a) gradient, ambient air is usually sufficient
   Aim to keep O_2 saturations ≥ 92% with supplemental oxygen if needed
Mode: Assist control mode or intermittent mandatory ventilation

Pressure-cycled ventilator or bilevel systems

Pressure settings
   Initial inspiratory positive airway pressure (IPAP) of 6 cm H_2O and expiratory positive
     airway pressure (EPAP) of 2 cm H_2O
   Inspiratory pressure may need to be raised to 25–30 cm H_2O to decrease $Paco_2$ effectively
Respiratory rate: same as for volume ventilators but to decrease $Paco_2$, increase IPAP or the
   respiratory rate, or both
Supplemental oxygen: same as for volume ventilators

Table 77–5. Monitoring Noninvasive Ventilation

Exhaled volume
  Although exhaled volume should theoretically equal the tidal volume (V_T) delivered by the
    ventilator, it is usually less because of leaks in the system
  Increase the V_T delivered until exhaled volume (measure on the ventilator or with a hand-
    held spirometer with bilevel systems) equals the desired V_T
Sao_2
  Pulse oximetry is used to adjust supplemental oxygen to keep $Sao_2 \geq 92\%$
$Paco_2$
  An in-dwelling arterial catheter should be used
  Arterial blood gases ($Paco_2$) should be checked every 2 h during sleep to guide ventilator
    adjustments

bidly obese patients. In either mode, supplemental oxygen can be added (Table 77–5). Air leaks can be managed by increasing the delivered tidal volume, using a chin strap, or utilizing a full face mask. It is important not to correct the $Paco_2$ too rapidly (no more than 10 mm Hg from baseline) during the first night of ventilation. Otherwise, a posthypercapnic metabolic alkalosis will result.

After starting noninvasive ventilation, most patients experience symptomatic improvement. This includes a reduction in daytime hypersomnolence, increased energy levels, relief of morning headaches, and improvement in pulmonary hypertension and right-sided heart failure.

Significant weight reduction also improves the signs and symptoms of both OSA and OHS, and it should be encouraged in all obese patients.

Pharmacologic interventions with respiratory stimulants such as medroxyprogesterone or acetazolamide have had minimal success in limited clinical trials. Frequent side effects and a lack of demonstrated long-term benefits of these medications limit their usefulness.

CONCLUSION

The life-threatening consequences of OHS are reversible with correction of nocturnal hypoventilation. OHS should be suspected in obese patients who have hypercapnia while awake and a history of witnessed apneas, daytime hypersomnolence, or morning headaches, or a combination of these factors. Demonstrating a greater than 10 mm Hg increase in $Paco_2$ during sleep compared with wakefulness is diagnostic of this syndrome. A polysomnogram should be performed to identify concomitant central or obstructive apnea. Therapy should start with a trial of noninvasive nocturnal ventilation. If not successful, nocturnal ventilation should be performed through an uncuffed tracheostomy tube. If treated appropriately, patients with OHS will have improved symptoms and fewer life-threatening complications, such as pulmonary hypertension and right-sided heart failure.

BIBLIOGRAPHY

Hillberg RE, Johnson DC: Noninvasive ventilation. N Engl J Med 337:1746–1752, 1997.
  Review of positive and negative pressure ventilatory techniques, indications, and limitations in acute and chronic respiratory failure.

Krachman S, Criner GJ: Hypoventilation syndromes. Clin Chest Med 19:139–155, 1998.
Review of multiple disorders associated with hypoventilation. The pathophysiology, assessment, and treatment of these disorders are discussed.

Kryger MH: Fat, sleep, and Charles Dickens: Literary and medical contributions to the understanding of sleep apnea. Clin Chest Med 6:555–562, 1985.
This article describes the literary accounts of OSA and the pickwickian syndrome, emphasizing Charles Dickens' work. In addition, this article reviews the historical clinical descriptions and the development of diagnostic and therapeutic approaches to these disorders.

Martin TJ, Sanders MH: Chronic alveolar hypoventilation: A review for the clinician. Sleep 18:617–634, 1995.
This is an extensive review of the pathophysiology, differential diagnosis, and therapeutic options for chronic alveolar hypoventilation. Techniques of diaphragmatic pacing, noninvasive ventilation, pharmacologic therapy, and ventilatory assistance via tracheostomy are discussed.

Rapoport DM, Garay SM, Epstein H, et al: Hypercapnia in the obstructive sleep apnea syndrome. Chest 89:627–635, 1986.
A study of eight patients with OSA and chronic awake hypercapnia who were evaluated before and after therapy with either tracheostomy or nocturnal continuous positive airway pressure. Chronic hypercapnia was corrected in half of the subjects with treatment. There was no difference in pulmonary function, residual apnea, or ventilatory chemoresponsiveness between the two groups. The fact that sustained hypoventilation can persist despite correction of apneas indicates that these patients had OHS as well as OSA.

Schwab RJ, Getsy JE, Pack AI: Central respiratory failure, including sleep disorders. In: Carlson RW, Geheb MA (eds): Principles and Practice of Medical Intensive Care. Philadelphia: WB Saunders, 1993, pp 773–786.
This is a comprehensive review of sleep-disordered breathing that includes diagnostic strategies and therapeutic interventions for OSA and OHS. The role of primary sleep disorders in respiratory failure in the ICU and the detrimental effects of sleep on respiratory disorders (including asthma and COPD) are detailed.

78

Acute Renal Failure and Rhabdomyolysis

Linda Fried
Paul M. Palevsky

Acute renal failure (ARF) is defined as an abrupt decline in renal function and is manifested by increases in the plasma creatinine and blood urea nitrogen (BUN) concentrations. Usually, an increase in the serum creatinine concentration of more than 0.5 to 1.0 mg/dL (45 to 90 μmol/L) over one to several days is deemed clinically significant. The frequency of ARF ranges from 2 to 5% in hospitalized general medical-surgical patients to 10 to 15% in patients in the intensive care unit (ICU). Although ARF frequently develops as a direct complication of the patient's underlying disease process, the majority of episodes are partly iatrogenic.

ARF increases morbidity and the length and cost of hospitalization. Patients with ARF have an overall mortality rate of 40 to 60%. However, for those who require dialysis for ARF, mortality rates increase to 60 to 90%. Death in patients with ARF is attributable not to ARF itself but rather to infections and cardiovascular or respiratory complications. Mortality increases when ARF occurs with sepsis, respiratory failure, oliguria (urine volume <400 mL/day), and hypotension requiring inotropic support (but not age per se).

DIFFERENTIAL DIAGNOSIS

ARF can be divided into three broad pathophysiologic categories: decreased renal perfusion (prerenal ARF), obstruction to urine flow (postrenal ARF), or a renal parenchymal insult (intrinsic ARF). This last category can be further divided into vascular, glomerular, interstitial, and tubular disease.

Prerenal Acute Renal Failure

Any decrease in renal perfusion activates physiologic processes designed to maintain glomerular filtration and solute excretion. Moderate decreases in perfusion activate both neural and hormonal factors (primarily angiotensin II, prostaglandins, catecholamines, aldosterone, and vasopressin), producing selective postglomerular (efferent) arteriolar vasoconstriction. This efferent vasoconstriction results in maintenance of glomerular filtration and enhances renal sodium reabsorption. However, with more severe and prolonged renal hypoperfusion, these regulatory processes are unable to maintain a normal glomerular filtration rate (GFR), culminating in prerenal ARF (Table 78–1). As GFR falls to less than normal, nitrogenous wastes accumulate in the blood.

True intravascular volume depletion or states producing depletion of effective arteriolar volume, for example, congestive heart failure, cirrhosis, and the nephrotic syndrome, can lead to prerenal ARF. In these latter states, renal perfusion may be

877

Table 78–1. Causes of Prerenal Acute Renal Failure

Volume depletion	Renal vasoconstriction
Decreased effective blood volume	Cyclosporin A
Congestive heart failure	Hepatorenal syndrome
Cirrhosis	Hypercalcemia
Nephrotic syndrome	Nonsteroidal anti-inflammatory drugs (NSAIDs)
	Tacrolimus

further compromised by diuretic therapy, which superimposes a component of true volume depletion. Drugs that block homeostatic responses to renal hypoperfusion (angiotensin-converting enzyme [ACE] inhibitors, angiotensin-receptor antagonists, and nonsteroidal anti-inflammatory drugs [NSAIDs]) may worsen renal function. Vasoconstrictors, such as catecholamines, cyclosporine, or tacrolimus, potentially decrease renal perfusion and exacerbate prerenal ARF. The hepatorenal syndrome results from severe renal vasoconstriction associated with end-stage liver disease (see Chapter 19) and does not improve with volume loading. In the critically ill patient, multiple factors usually contribute to prerenal ARF.

The hallmarks of prerenal ARF are the excretion of a concentrated urine (urine osmolality >700 mOsm/kg [700 mmol/kg], urine specific gravity >1.020) with a relatively low sodium concentration (urine sodium <20 mEq/L [20 mmol/L]), fractional excretion of sodium less than 1% (see Chapter 37), and its rapid reversibility with correction of the underlying cause. Although prerenal ARF is typically oliguric, in patients with underlying renal insufficiency or renal concentrating defects, urine volumes may exceed 500 mL/day. In addition, diuretic therapy or a solute diuresis from hyperglycemia or protein loading may increase renal sodium excretion, impair renal concentration, and result in nonoliguric ARF.

Postrenal Acute Renal Failure

Obstruction to urine flow at any level of the urinary collecting system may produce ARF (Table 78–2). Obstruction of the lower urinary tract may occur at the level of the bladder, bladder outlet, or urethra, and upper urinary tract obstruction may occur at the level of the ureter or the renal pelvis. Upper tract obstruction must be bilateral to cause ARF unless there is only a single functioning kidney or baseline renal insufficiency. Complete obstruction produces anuria; with partial obstruction, urine output is variable, with polyuria or fluctuation between polyuria and anuria characteristic. Postrenal causes should be ruled out in all patients with ARF, as obstructive renal failure is potentially reversible if promptly diagnosed and decompressed.

Intrinsic Acute Renal Failure

Intrinsic renal parenchymal injury producing ARF may be characterized into five broad categories on the basis of the underlying pathogenesis: acute tubular necrosis

Table 78–2. Causes of Postrenal Acute Renal Failure

Lower tract obstruction
  Benign prostatic hypertrophy
  Bladder cancer
  Bladder stones
  Blood clot
  Neurogenic bladder
  Prostate cancer
  Urethral stricture
Upper tract obstruction (must be bilateral unless there is only one functioning kidney)
  Aortic aneurysm
  Blood clot
  Kidney stone
  Pelvic malignancy
  Renal papillary necrosis
  Retroperitoneal fibrosis
  Retroperitoneal tumor
  Transitional cell carcinoma

(ATN), acute interstitial nephritis (AIN), acute glomerulonephritis (AGN), intratubular obstruction, and acute vascular syndromes (Table 78–3). Of these categories, ATN is the most common cause of intrinsic ARF.

Acute Tubular Necrosis

ATN is characterized pathologically by injury and death of renal tubular epithelial cells. Intratubular obstruction by exfoliated necrotic cells, back leakage of glomerular filtrate through the damaged tubular epithelium, and decreased glomerular filtration from reactive vasoconstriction all contribute to renal excretory failure.

ATN can be divided into ischemic and nephrotoxic injuries. Renal ischemia accounts for approximately half of all ATN cases. Substantial variability exists in the renal response to ischemia: in some patients a few minutes of ischemia may produce ATN, whereas in others, prolonged renal hypoperfusion produces only transient prerenal azotemia. Any cause of prerenal ARF, if prolonged and severe enough, may produce ATN. However, most cases of ischemic ATN are associated with a period of frank hypotension. Factors that increase the risk of ischemic ATN developing include sepsis, major surgery (especially after cardiopulmonary bypass, abdominal aortic aneurysm repair, and biliary tract surgery), and treatment with ACE inhibitors, angiotensin-receptor antagonists, and NSAIDs. Among the agents that can produce nephrotoxic ATN are the aminoglycoside antibiotics, amphotericin B, acetaminophen, cisplatin, radiocontrast material, free hemoglobin, and myoglobin. In many patients in the ICU, ATN is multifactorial, resulting from a combination of nephrotoxic and ischemic insults.

Patients with pre-existing renal insufficiency and older patients are at increased risk for the development of ATN and are less likely to experience the ultimate recovery of renal function after onset of ATN. Similarly, volume depletion and vasoconstricting agents increase the risk of ATN from other causes.

Table 78–3. Causes of Intrinsic Acute Renal Failure

....

Acute Tubular Necrosis

Ischemic
  Cardiopulmonary arrest
  Hypotension
  Hypovolemic shock
  Sepsis
Nephrotoxic
Drug-induced (acetaminophen, aminoglycosides, amphotericin B, cisplatin, radiocontrast agents)
Pigment nephropathy (hemoglobin, myoglobin)

Acute Interstitial Nephritis

Drug-induced
  Cephalosporins
  Furosemide
  Nonsteroidal anti-inflammatory drugs (NSAIDs)
  Penicillins
  Phenytoin
  Sulfonamides
Infection-related
  Bacterial infection
  Mycobacterial infection
  Rickettsial infection
  Viral infection

Acute Glomerulonephritis

Endocarditis-associated glomerulonephritis
Hemolytic uremic syndrome, thrombotic thrombocytopenic purpura
Postinfectious glomerulonephritis
Rapidly progressive glomerulonephritis (including Goodpasture's syndrome, poststreptococcal
  glomerulonephritis)
Systemic vasculitis (acute lupus nephritis, polyarteritis nodosa, Henoch-Schönlein purpura, Wegener's
  granulomatosis, cryoglobulinemia)

Intratubular Obstruction

Ethylene glycol
Multiple myeloma
Tumor lysis syndrome

Acute Vascular Syndromes

Cholesterol emboli
Malignant hypertension
Renal artery thromboembolism
Renal vein thrombosis
Scleroderma renal crisis

....

Depending on the severity of parenchymal injury, ATN may be either oliguric or nonoliguric. Because of the loss of tubular integrity, both urinary concentrating and diluting ability are lost. Thus, urine osmolality is approximately 300 mOsm/kg (300 mmol/kg) (isosthenuria) and urine specific gravity is approximately 1.010. Similarly, tubular sodium reabsorption is impaired, resulting in a urine sodium concentration that is generally greater than 40 mEq/L (40 mmol/L) and a FEN (fractional excretion of sodium) greater than 2%.

Acute Interstitial Nephritis

AIN is characterized by inflammation of the renal interstitium and tubules, with a lymphocytic and eosinophilic infiltrate typically seen on biopsy. The clinical triad of fever, rash, and eosinophilia is classically associated with AIN, but one or more components are frequently absent. Most cases of AIN result from drug hypersensitivity. The most commonly associated agents include penicillins, cephalosporin and sulfa antibiotics, diuretics, and anticonvulsants, although almost any medication can be implicated. Less commonly, AIN develops as the result of an immune reaction to an infection. Patients with AIN usually are not oliguric and generally have a much less abrupt increase in serum creatinine concentrations than do patients with ATN. The urine sediment usually demonstrates pyuria, hematuria, and white blood cell casts. Eosinophiluria may be present and is best demonstrated using a Hansel stain.

AIN associated with NSAIDs commonly presents without an associated fever, rash, or eosinophilia. In addition, nephrotic-range proteinuria, which is not associated with other causes of AIN, may be present.

Acute Glomerulonephritis

A variety of glomerular syndromes may present with acute (progressing over hours to days) or subacute (progressing over days to weeks) renal failure (see Table 78–3). Goodpasture's syndrome is a specific syndrome of anti–glomerular basement membrane antibody (anti-GBM)–associated, rapidly progressive (crescentic) glomerulonephritis associated with pulmonary hemorrhage. The characteristic feature of the glomerulonephritides is the presence of a nephritic urine sediment with hematuria and red blood cell casts. Measurement of serum complement and serologic studies (e.g., antinuclear antibody, antineutrophil cytoplasmic antibody, cryoglobulins, and anti–glomerular basement membrane) may suggest a diagnosis. However, renal biopsy is usually necessary for definitive diagnosis.

Intratubular Obstruction

Intratubular obstruction by crystal deposition or paraproteins may also produce ARF. Acute uric acid nephropathy most commonly occurs in the *tumor lysis syndrome* after chemotherapy of sensitive tumors. The tumor lysis syndrome is usually associated with hyperkalemia, hyperphosphatemia, and severe hyperuricemia (serum uric acid concentrations >20 mg/dL [1200 μmol/L]). Characteristically, the urine uric acid:creatinine ratio, measured in milligrams per deciliter, is greater than 1 (>0.7 when measured in μmoles per liter), and microscopic examination of the urine invariably demonstrates many uric acid crystals. Ethylene glycol ingestion or, less commonly, the anesthetic methoxyflurane, may produce acute oxalate nephropathy, which is characterized by heavy oxalate crystalluria. Intratubular precipitation of methotrexate and acyclovir may also produce ARF.

Patients with *multiple myeloma* are at risk for ARF from a number of causes, including hypercalcemia, hyperuricemia, and direct nephrotoxicity from immunoglobulin light chains. They may also have an increased risk of radiocontrast nephropathy, especially in association with hypercalcemia or volume depletion. The classic pathology in acute myeloma of the kidney is the presence of widespread intratubular precipitation of light chains and tubular atrophy. The diagnosis is usually suggested by demonstration of a serum paraprotein or light chains in the urine.

Acute Vascular Syndromes

Partial or complete renovascular occlusion from renal artery thromboembolism, arteriolar spasm in malignant hypertension, and scleroderma renal crisis as well as atheroembolic (cholesterol embolic) disease may cause ARF. In atheroembolic disease, renal failure is frequently associated with fever, livedo reticularis, lower extremity petechiae, eosinophilia, and hypocomplementemia. Although atheroembolic ARF occurs most commonly after angiography and aortic surgery, spontaneous atheroemboli may develop in patients with severe atherosclerotic disease. Acute renal vein thrombosis is also a rare cause of ARF.

DIAGNOSTIC EVALUATION

The evaluation and management of the patient with falling urine output or rising serum creatinine is presented in detail in Chapter 37 and is only briefly summarized here. The first step is to categorize the renal failure as prerenal, postrenal, or intrinsic. Prerenal ARF is suggested by clinical evidence of renal hypoperfusion (e.g., relative hypotension, orthostatic hypotension, decreased central venous and pulmonary artery wedge pressures, or decreased cardiac output), a sodium avid state (urine sodium concentration <20 mEq/L [20 mmol/L], fractional excretion of sodium <1%), and a bland urine sediment. The diagnosis of prerenal ARF may be confirmed by the clinical response to volume resuscitation or improved cardiac function.

Postrenal (obstructive) ARF should be ruled out in all patients who are unresponsive to volume resuscitation or augmentation of cardiac output. Demonstrating residual bladder volume after voiding of greater than 100 mL by bladder catheterization is diagnostic of bladder outflow obstruction or a neurogenic bladder. Renal ultrasonography should be performed to rule out upper tract obstruction.

The differential diagnosis of intrinsic ARF should be guided by the clinical history and physical examination. Careful attention must be paid to medications administered preceding the onset of renal failure, episodes of sepsis or hypotension, and the administration of intravenous radiocontrast material. Examination of the urine sediment is useful to narrow the differential diagnosis. The urine in ATN usually contains many tubular epithelial cells and granular casts, frequently described as "muddy brown" in appearance. A positive dipstick test for blood in the absence of red blood cells on microscopy is suggestive of rhabdomyolysis or intravascular hemolysis. Red blood cell casts indicate glomerulonephritis. In AIN, the urine usually contains red cells, white cells, and white cell casts. Although bacteria may not be seen, a urine culture should be performed to exclude pyelonephritis or lower urinary tract infection. The presence of eosinophiluria, although suggestive of interstitial nephritis, is not diagnostic. The presence of heavy crystalluria may also guide the diagnosis: bipyramidal (envelope-shaped) calcium oxalate crystals suggest ethylene glycol poisoning; rhomboidal uric acid crystals suggest tumor lysis syndrome. A positive sulfosalicylic acid test result for protein in the setting of a negative dipstick test result for protein suggests the diagnosis of myeloma kidney. Renal biopsy is rarely necessary in the diagnosis of ARF. It should be limited to patients in whom a diagnosis of glomerulonephritis is considered and to patients with persistent unexplained ARF.

MANAGEMENT

Prerenal Acute Renal Failure

The treatment of prerenal ARF is the restoration of normal renal perfusion. Hypovolemic patients should receive fluid resuscitation with blood products, colloid, or isotonic crystalloid as appropriate. When poor cardiac function produces ARF, inotropic support and afterload reduction may be required. In patients with severe cirrhosis, effective volume depletion may occur despite total body volume overload. Volume replacement in cirrhotic patients must be monitored carefully. On clinical presentation, it may not be possible to differentiate between simple prerenal azotemia and the hepatorenal syndrome. The use of central venous or pulmonary artery pressure monitoring may help guide fluid therapy and prevent excessive replacement and iatrogenic pulmonary edema. In all patients with prerenal azotemia, diuretics and NSAIDs should be discontinued, and ACE inhibitors and angiotensin-receptor antagonists used only with extreme caution.

Postrenal Acute Renal Failure

The treatment of postrenal ARF consists of relief of the obstruction. In patients with bladder outlet obstruction or neurogenic bladder, this can be accomplished with bladder catheterization. When upper tract obstruction is present, ureteral stents or percutaneous nephrostomies are necessary.

After relief of the obstruction, a postobstructive diuresis may occur. To the extent that volume overload developed during the course of the ARF, the polyuria is physiologic and results in correction of the volume overload. In some patients, however, residual tubular injury results in urinary concentrating defects or renal salt wasting, or both. Urine output and volume status must therefore be monitored closely after relief of obstruction. In volume overload, urine output should be only partially replaced to permit negative fluid balance. In euvolemic patients, urine output should be more completely replaced while ensuring that excessive fluid administration does not drive the polyuria. The electrolyte composition of the replacement fluid should be guided by the urine electrolyte composition. In the absence of such measurements, 0.45% saline is an appropriate initial replacement solution. After relief of obstruction, patients may have potassium secretory deficits or renal potassium wasting, leading to hyperkalemia or hypokalemia, respectively. Such patients may also have an acquired renal tubular acidosis or renal phosphate wasting. Potassium, bicarbonate, and phosphate replacement must therefore be guided by serum and urine electrolyte measurements.

Intrinsic Acute Renal Failure

Supportive Measures

Supportive measures are the mainstay of therapy for all forms of intrinsic ARF. Fluids may be necessary to correct hypovolemia and then replace obligate losses. Diuretic administration may facilitate the treatment of volume overload in nonoliguric ARF. Serum electrolytes must be monitored closely and bicarbonate replaced to treat metabolic acidosis. Routine potassium supplements should be discontinued and hyperkalemia treated (see Chapter 36). Phosphate intake should be restricted and oral binders (e.g., calcium carbonate or aluminum hydroxide) given to reduce elevated phosphate levels.

Nephrotoxins such as aminoglycoside antibiotics and intravenous radiocontrast dyes should be discontinued or avoided, if possible. Medications that reduce renal perfusion, such as ACE inhibitors, angiotensin-receptor antagonists, and NSAIDs, should also be avoided. All medication dosages should be adjusted for renal failure, and blood levels should be monitored (see Chapter 12).

ARF is a hypercatabolic state. Protein loading does not, however, result in positive or even neutral nitrogen balance. It may exacerbate azotemia and accelerate the need for dialysis. The optimal nutritional protein prescription is therefore controversial, with protein recommendations generally ranging between 1.2 and 1.5 g/kg/day. When parenteral nutrition is used, careful attention must be paid to the selection of electrolyte formulations. Most standard electrolyte formulations contain excessive potassium, phosphate, and magnesium for a patient with renal failure.

Many patients require renal replacement therapy during the course of their ARF. Intermittent hemodialysis, peritoneal dialysis, and the continuous renal replacement therapies (continuous arteriovenous or venovenous hemofiltration, hemodialysis, or hemodiafiltration) are all efficacious for the treatment of ARF (see Chapter 16). Indications for initiation of dialysis include diuretic-resistant volume overload, metabolic acidosis or hyperkalemia unresponsive to medical therapy, uremic symptoms (e.g., mental status changes, pericarditis), and severe azotemia. Although no level of BUN serves as an absolute requirement for the initiation of dialysis, a BUN of greater than 100 mg/dL is generally accepted as an indication for dialysis. Neither early initiation of dialysis nor "intensive" dialysis has been demonstrated to improve survival or recovery from ARF. The dialysis procedure may, in fact, prolong the course of renal failure, both as the result of transient mild hypotension occurring during the dialysis procedure and as the result of complement and cytokine activation by contact of blood with the dialysis membrane.

Acute Tubular Necrosis

No therapy has been proved effective for ATN, and management is primarily supportive. Although oliguric ATN carries a higher mortality rate than does nonoliguric ATN, it is controversial whether inducing diuresis in an oliguric patient with diuretics or dopamine improves outcome or merely selects for patients with less severe tubular injury. Conversion to a nonoliguric state does, however, simplify fluid management and may help delay the need for dialysis. Since loop-acting diuretics (e.g., furosemide, bumetanide) act from the luminal side of the tubule, high doses (e.g., 160 to 200 mg of intravenous furosemide as a bolus or 20 to 40 mg/hour as a continuous infusion) may be required to achieve diuresis in patients with reduced glomerular filtration. There is no evidence that any of the newer loop-acting diuretics are more efficacious than furosemide at equipotent doses, and all are substantially more expensive. The combination of a loop-acting diuretic with oral metolazone or an intravenous thiazide diuretic (e.g., chlorothiazide) may be synergistic. If dopamine is used, it should be tried early during the course of ATN and at low doses (<2.5 μg/kg/min). Higher doses are vasoconstrictive, may increase the risk of bowel ischemia, and should only be used when a pressor response is desired. The combination of dopamine and a loop-acting diuretic may also be synergistic.

In many circumstances, the best treatment for ATN is prevention. Nephrotoxic agents should be avoided whenever possible. Aminoglycoside dosing should be monitored closely to ensure that toxic drug levels do not occur. Many agents, including aminoglycosides, amphotericin B, and radiocontrast media, are more likely to cause ATN in the setting of volume depletion. Saline loading may therefore decrease the risk of aminoglycoside- and amphotericin B–induced ATN. This was demonstrated in a prospective trial to be more effective than either furosemide or mannitol in preventing contrast nephropathy in high-risk patients undergoing coronary angiography. Saline loading combined with urinary alkalinization should be instituted to prevent ATN in patients with rhabdomyolysis. NSAIDs should be avoided in all patients at risk for the development of ATN.

Acute Interstitial Nephritis

The treatment of AIN consists of the discontinuation of any offending medication or therapy for an underlying infection. If treated before the development of interstitial fibrosis, the renal failure is usually reversible. Steroid therapy has been proposed to hasten and lead to a more complete recovery of renal function. However, this recommendation is based only on anecdotal case series rather than on controlled trials. The steroid doses used have varied from pulse intravenous methylprednisolone (500 to 1000 mg daily for 3 to 4 days) to short courses of oral prednisone (60 mg/day for 2 weeks with a rapid taper).

Acute Glomerulonephritis

The treatment of acute glomerulonephritis depends on the underlying cause and should be guided by renal biopsy results. ARF associated with poststreptococcal, postinfectious, and endocarditis-associated glomerulonephritis usually is self-limited and requires no specific therapy other than treatment of the underlying infection. Acute glomerulonephritis associated with lupus or systemic vasculitis and rapidly progressive (crescentic) glomerulonephritis is usually treated with steroids and cytotoxic agents. Plasmapheresis is of benefit in patients with anti-GBM disease, hemolytic uremic syndrome, and thrombotic thrombocytopenic purpura (see Chapter 63).

Intratubular Obstruction

Ethylene glycol poisoning should be treated with intravenous sodium bicarbonate to correct the metabolic acidosis, ethanol administration (intravenous or by gavage) to inhibit its metabolism, and emergent hemodialysis. 4-Methylpyrazole may be used as an alternative to ethanol, but it is much more expensive. Prompt initiation of therapy may prevent or attenuate ARF. In the tumor lysis syndromes, ARF may be prevented by pretreatment with allopurinol and induction of a forced alkaline diuresis. Intensive hemodialysis to lower serum uric acid levels should be initiated in patients in whom acute urate nephropathy develops.

Acute myeloma kidney should be treated by induction of an alkaline diuresis and initiation of chemotherapy. The associated hypercalcemia and hyperuricemia should also be treated. Acute lowering of circulating paraproteins by plasmapheresis may also be beneficial in reversing the ARF.

Acute Vascular Syndromes

There is no effective therapy for atheroembolic (cholesterol embolic) ARF. Anticoagulation is of no benefit and may exacerbate the condition. Thrombolytic therapy of acute renal artery thrombosis and thromboembolism may permit revascularization but is frequently associated with persistent renal dysfunction. ARF associated with malignant hypertension should be treated with prompt antihypertensive therapy. Scleroderma renal crisis should be treated with ACE inhibitors.

RHABDOMYOLYSIS

Rhabdomyolysis is the clinical syndrome that results from skeletal muscle injury and the release of muscle cell contents. Most cases are subclinical, and the diagnosis is generally made on the basis of elevations in the serum concentrations of released cellular contents, particularly creatine phosphokinase (CPK), lactic dehydrogenase, or serum aspartate aminotransferase (AST). In severe cases, overt myoglobinuria (manifested as red or brown urine testing positive for blood on dipstick but without red blood cells on microscopic examination) may be seen. Acute tubular necrosis is the most serious potential complication of rhabdomyolysis but fortunately develops in only a minority of patients as the result of intratubular obstruction from myoglobin casts, arteriolar vasoconstriction, and direct tubular cell toxicity.

Etiology and Clinical and Laboratory Features

The causes of rhabdomyolysis can be broadly divided into traumatic and nontraumatic categories (Table 78–4). Although the classic description of myoglobinuric ARF by Bywaters and Beal during the London blitz was associated with severe trauma and crush injuries, the majority of cases of rhabdomyolysis are nontraumatic, developing as complications of alcohol abuse, passive muscle compression from immobilization (e.g., drug-induced coma), and seizures. Presenting symptoms usually reflect the primary disease process, with superimposed weakness, myalgia, and muscle tenderness. Physical findings consist of tender, "doughy" feeling muscles, edema, and muscle weakness. In severe cases, compartmental compression syndromes may develop with signs and symptoms of neurovascular compromise. A sustained intracompartmental pressure of greater than 40 mm Hg indicates the need for fasciotomy (see Chapter 95).

Severe hyperkalemia, hyperphosphatemia, and hyperuricemia are commonly seen in patients in whom ARF develops from rhabdomyolysis. Profound hypocalcemia develops as the result of deposition of calcium salts in injured muscle and as the result of changes in vitamin D and parathyroid hormone metabolism induced by severe hyperphosphatemia. However, the hypocalcemia does not require specific therapy unless it is symptomatic.

Elevations in the CPK level to greater than 5000 IU/L (80 μkat/L) are associated with an increased risk of renal failure developing, although there is no clear relationship between the absolute level of CPK and the risk of renal failure. Volume depletion and acidemia appear to be important contributory factors in the development of renal failure. Although myoglobin is believed to be the most

Table 78–4. Causes of Rhabdomyolysis

Traumatic	Immobilization, passive compression
Burns	Infections
Crush injuries	Gangrene, myonecrosis
	Viral myositis
Nontraumatic	Medications, drugs
Electrolyte disorders	Alcohol
Hyperglycemia	Cocaine
Hypokalemia	Gemfibrozil
Hypophosphatemia	HMG CoA reductase inhibitors
Excessive muscular activity	Muscle ischemia
Heat stroke	Carbon monoxide poisoning
Malignant hyperthermia	Vascular occlusion
Neuroleptic malignant syndrome	Metabolic disorders
Seizures	McArdle's disease
Vigorous exercise	Carnitine palmitoyl transferase

Table 78–5. Causes of a Low Fractional Excretion of Sodium in Acute Renal Failure

Acute glomerulonephritis	Prerenal azotemia
Contrast nephropathy	Rhabdomyolysis
Early obstructive uropathy	

important tubular toxin in rhabdomyolysis, purified myoglobin is relatively non-toxic in the absence of volume depletion.

Therapy

Initial therapy of patients with rhabdomyolysis should be directed at preventing the development of ARF. The most important therapeutic intervention is aggressive volume expansion, with many liters of crystalloid required to compensate for third spacing of fluid in the injured muscle. Urinary alkalinization is also believed to be of benefit by inhibiting precipitation of myoglobin in the renal tubules, although metabolic alkalosis may exacerbate symptoms of hypocalcemia. Mannitol and loop-acting diuretics are not proved to be of benefit in preventing the development of ARF. In patients in whom significant renal failure develops, early dialysis is frequently necessary to control hyperkalemia and other metabolic disturbances.

CLINICAL PEARLS AND PITFALLS

1. The fractional excretion of sodium is useful in differentiating prerenal azotemia from other causes of ARF. However, in patients taking diuretics or in those with underlying renal insufficiency, the fractional excretion of sodium can be elevated despite volume depletion. In addition, other forms of ARF may be associated with a low fractional excretion of sodium (Table 78–5).
2. Not all azotemia is renal failure. The BUN can be elevated in a number of conditions in the absence of significant reduction in GFR (Table 78–6).
3. Patients with renovascular disease and baseline hypertension may require a higher blood pressure in order to maintain renal perfusion. This is also true for patients with accelerated or malignant hypertension. In these situations, the blood pressure should not be decreased too rapidly or to normal.

Table 78–6. Causes of Azotemia (Increased Blood Urea Nitrogen)

Corticosteroid therapy	Protein overfeeding
Gastrointestinal hemorrhage	Renal failure
Hypercatabolic state	Tetracycline antibiotics

4. The addition of $NaHCO_3$ to 0.9% saline results in a hypertonic solution and should not be used for urinary alkalinization. A better choice is to add 50 to 75 mEq (50 to 75 mmol) of $NaHCO_3$ to a liter of 0.45% saline, yielding slightly hypotonic to isotonic alkaline fluid.

BIBLIOGRAPHY

Bennett WM, Aronoff GR, Golper TA, et al: Drug Prescribing in Renal Failure, 2nd ed. Philadelphia: American College of Physicians, 1991.
This is an excellent guide for adjusting drug dosing in patients with renal failure.

Better OS, Stein JH: Early management of shock and prophylaxis of acute renal failure in traumatic rhabdomyolysis. N Engl J Med 322:825–829, 1990.
This is a good review of the pathophysiology and treatment of rhabdomyolysis.

Conger JD: Interventions in acute renal failure: What are the data? Am J Kidney Dis 26:565–576, 1995.
This article is a critical review of treatments for ARF (e.g., diuretics, dopamine, dialysis, nutrition), concentrating on controlled trials.

Gabow PA, Kaehny WD, Kelleher SP: The spectrum of rhabdomyolysis. Am J Med 61:141–152, 1982.
This is a classic paper on the causes, presentation, and course of rhabdomyolysis.

Galpin JE, Shinaberger JH, Stanley TM, et al: Acute interstitial nephritis due to methicillin. Am J Med 65:756–765, 1978.
This is a classic paper on the presentation and course of AIN.

Linton AL, Clark WF, Driedger AA, et al: Acute interstitial nephritis due to drugs. Ann Intern Med 93:735–741, 1980.
This article provides a classic review of AIN.

Menasche PI, Ross SA, Gottlieg JE: Acquired renal insufficiency in critically ill patients. Crit Care Med 16:1106–1109, 1988.
This article describes a study of 315 patients admitted to a medical-surgical ICU to determine the frequency and prognosis of ARF.

Myers BD, Moran SM: Hemodynamically mediated acute renal failure. N Engl J Med 314:97–105, 1986.
This is an excellent review of the pathophysiology of ischemic ATN.

Solomon R, Werner C, Mann D, et al: Effects of saline, mannitol, and furosemide on acute decreases in renal function induced by radiocontrast agents. N Engl J Med 331:1416–1420, 1994.
This article describes a prospective, randomized trial comparing three modalities to prevent ARF in patients receiving contrast. The study found that 0.45% saline was the most efficacious regimen.

Thadhani R, Pascual M, Bonvente JV: Acute renal failure. N Engl J Med 334:1448–1459, 1996.
An excellent recent review of the causes, pathophysiology, and treatment of acute renal failure.

79

Diabetic Ketoacidosis, Nonketotic Hypertonic Hyperglycemia, and Alcoholic Ketoacidosis

Harold M. Szerlip

Diabetic ketoacidosis (DKA), nonketotic hypertonic hyperglycemia (NKHH), and alcoholic ketoacidosis (AKA) are three common fluid and electrolyte disorders that often precipitate admission to the intensive care unit (ICU). All typically have an abrupt onset with symptoms that bring patients rapidly to medical attention. An understanding of the pathophysiology of these distinct but related conditions should enable the ICU clinician to make a rapid diagnosis, initiate proper therapy, and avoid major pitfalls.

DIABETIC KETOACIDOSIS

Definition

The diagnosis of diabetic ketoacidosis is made if an individual presents with a defining set of laboratory parameters (Table 79–1): hyperglycemia (usually >250 mg/dL), metabolic acidosis (arterial blood pH <7.35 with bicarbonate <16 mEq/L), and ketonemia (serum ketones present in at least a 1:2 dilution). Although DKA is considered pathognomonic of type 1 (insulin-dependent) diabetes, 5 to 30% of type 2 diabetics also present with parameters meeting this definition. In addition, alcoholic ketoacidosis may on occasion have a presentation similar to that of DKA.

Pathogenesis

DKA arises because of decreased insulin (either absolute or relative) in combination with an abundance of counterregulatory hormones—in particular, glucagon and catecholamines (Fig. 79–1). The hyperglycemia results in an osmotic diuresis and volume depletion. As renal perfusion and the glomerular filtration rate (GFR) fall, the kidney excretes less glucose, which exacerbates the hyperglycemia. An increase in ketoacid production secondary to fatty acid oxidation produces the acidosis. Approximately 90% of patients with DKA have been previously diagnosed with diabetes, and 10% are new-onset diabetics. Common precipitating factors are noncompliance with insulin regimen, stressors such as infection and myocardial ischemia, drugs and alcohol, and renal failure.

Table 79–1. Comparison of Diabetic Ketoacidosis, Nonketotic Hypertonic Hyperglycemia, and Alcoholic Ketoacidosis

VARIABLE	DIABETIC KETOACIDOSIS	NONKETOTIC HYPERTONIC HYPERGLYCEMIA	ALCOHOLIC KETOACIDOSIS
Serum glucose	250–600 mg/dL	>600 mg/dL	Low or normal (but 10% with glucose >250 mg/dL)
Serum ketones	+ in 1:2 or greater dilution	Minimal	May be absent when testing only for acetoacetate
Acidosis	Present (pH <7.35 with serum $[HCO_3{}^-]$ <16 mEq/L)	Absent or mild	Present (but pH may be normal or elevated)
Type of acidosis	Anion gap alone (or mixed anion gap, hyperchloremic)	Anion gap due to ketoacidosis or lactate acidosis (due to poor perfusion)	Anion gap often with respiratory and metabolic alkaloses (see text for details)
History	90% with diabetes (most often type I)	50% with diabetes (most often type II)	Nondiabetic chronic alcohol users who binge and then fast 1–2 days

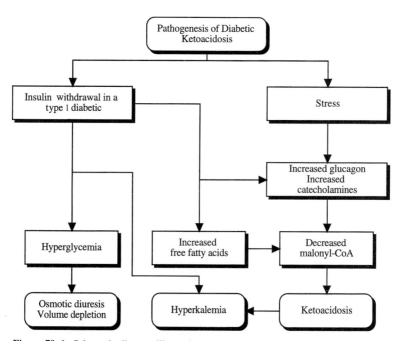

Figure 79–1. Schematic diagram illustrating the pathogenesis of diabetic ketoacidosis.

Evaluation

Symptoms of DKA are related to hyperglycemia and acidosis. Patients with DKA usually present complaining of polyuria and polydipsia (from the hyperglycemia), nausea, vomiting and abdominal pain (emetic effects of acidosis), and shortness of breath (secondary to the acidosis-induced increase in respiratory drive—called *Kussmaul respirations).*

The physical examination is remarkable for signs of volume depletion (e.g., orthostatic hypotension and dry mucous membranes), Kussmaul respirations, and mild abdominal tenderness. Temperature is normal or mildly hypothermic. Fever is not characteristically present unless there is a concurrent infection. Finally, the patient's breath has the fruity odor of acetone. The presence of acetone, however, is not unique to DKA. Other disorders in which acetone is present include *alcoholic ketoacidosis* and *isopropyl alcohol* ingestion. (The latter is metabolized to acetone without the formation of ketoacids and, therefore, acidosis is not present.) Because patients with DKA rarely present with decreased sensorium, other complicating conditions should be actively sought if a patient with DKA is comatose or unresponsive.

Laboratory analysis demonstrates hyperglycemia. The serum glucose level is typically between 250 and 600 mg/dL (14 to 33 mmol/L). Higher levels are uncommon in DKA because the acidosis causes these patients to present early in the course of their illness, that is, before more significant volume depletion and hyperglycemia occur. A pure metabolic acidosis with respiratory compensation is typically present. Although the acidosis is most commonly an anion gap acidosis, a mixed anion gap and hyperchloremic acidosis, or rarely a pure hyperchloremic acidosis may be found (see Chapter 80). The *type of acidosis* depends on the *intravascular volume* of the patient. If fluid intake is adequate, the kidney excretes ketones, thus reducing unmeasured anions without affecting the acidosis.

By definition, serum ketones must be present in at least a 1:2 dilution, but unlike in AKA, the ratio of the reduced form of nicotinamide-adenine dinucleotide (NADH) to nicotinamide-adenine dinucleotide (NAD) is rarely at such a high level that ketoacid metabolism is driven almost exclusively toward production of beta-hydroxybutyrate (which is not measured by the standard laboratory assay).

Because of the lack of insulin, hyperkalemia is usually present. It is important to remember that despite initial elevation in serum potassium levels, the ongoing osmotic diuresis results in substantial *total body potassium depletion.* When insulin therapy is begun, hypokalemia may develop as insulin increases the transport of potassium into cells. Similar to potassium, phosphate levels are initially elevated but fall dramatically with treatment. Although leukocytosis is common in ketoacidosis, *white blood cell counts greater than 25,000/µL* should raise suspicion of an *underlying infection.*

Treatment

The evaluation and management of DKA are outlined in Figure 79–2. It is important to look for precipitating factors and to rule out other causes of acidosis. The initial management of DKA should be directed toward intravascular volume

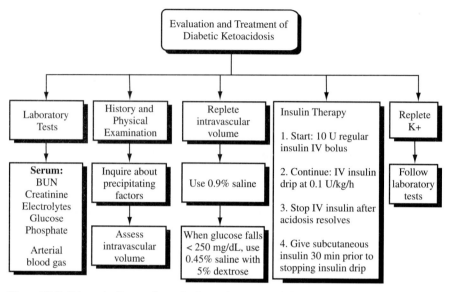

Figure 79–2. Schematic diagram for evaluation and treatment of diabetic ketoacidosis.

repletion. Depending on the degree of volume contraction, 1 to 2 L of 0.9% saline should be infused rapidly. If there is no evidence of renal failure and the patient has good urine output (>60 mL/hour), potassium repletion by mouth or intravenously should be initiated.

Insulin therapy should begin only after initial volume replacement. Because the osmotic effects of the hyperglycemia hold water in the intravascular space, premature administration of insulin before adequate volume repletion causes this intravascular water to move intracellularly and may produce significant hypotension. Although this is more likely to occur in patients with nonketotic hypertonic hyperglycemia (NKHH), it can also occur in patients with DKA. Since there is no convincing evidence that withholding insulin for the first 15 to 30 minutes of volume resuscitation has any adverse effects on outcome, premature administration of insulin during this period should be avoided. After adequate repletion of the intravascular volume (as judged clinically), intravenous fluid therapy can be changed to 0.45% saline.

After initial volume repletion, between 10 and 15 units of regular insulin should be given intravenously and a maintenance infusion begun at 0.1 units/kg/hour. Despite significant acidosis, *bicarbonate therapy is rarely, if ever, necessary.* Even with severe acidemia (pH <7.0), there is no proven advantage to using alkali therapy. Such therapy may even be detrimental because it can cause hypertonicity, elevate mixed venous carbon dioxide and intracellular acidosis. The latter may occur when the increased blood pH (due to alkali therapy) decreases respiratory drive, which, in turn, allows $Paco_2$ to rise. Elevated $Paco_2$ equilibrates within cells rapidly, whereas the anionic base does not, resulting in an intracellular acidosis.

Capillary blood glucose should be monitored every hour (and verified by frequent measurements of serum glucose). When *serum glucose falls to 250 mg/*

dL (14 mmol/L) or less, one should *change intravenous fluids* to *include 5% dextrose*. Because the serum glucose normalizes before ketoacid production stops, however, it is important to *continue the insulin drip* to avoid worsening acidosis. Insulin may need to be decreased to 2 to 4 units/hour to avoid hypoglycemia.

The acidosis should be monitored by following the anion gap and total carbon dioxide. Initially, *ketones may appear to increase* as the beta-hydroxybutyrate (which is not measured by the standard assay) is converted to acetoacetate (which is). This apparent increase in serum ketones should not alarm the well-informed clinician. It is more important to follow the anion gap than the ketonemia. As insulin shuts off production of ketoacids and the kidney excretes those already present, the anion gap normalizes and a hyperchloremic metabolic acidosis becomes evident. As bicarbonate is regenerated by the kidney over 12 to 24 hours, the acidosis resolves. When it is evident that ketoacid production has been suppressed and the bicarbonate is normalizing, the insulin infusion can be discontinued. At least 0.5 hour before stopping the infusion, however, the patient should be given subcutaneous insulin to prevent the recurrence of the acidosis.

Whether or not phosphate should be replaced is controversial. No controlled studies have demonstrated any advantage to phosphate repletion. Theoretical concerns, for example, decreased 2,3-diphosphoglycerate or rhabdomyolysis, suggest that if the deficiency is severe (<1 mg/dL (0.32 mmol/L)), phosphate should be administered. This should be accomplished by giving one third of the potassium replacement as potassium phosphate (see also Chapter 35).

Since the advent of insulin therapy, mortality from DKA has been low (less than 5% of patients with DKA die). Mortality increases in the geriatric population and is usually secondary to comorbid events, such as sepsis or myocardial infarction. Although cerebral edema has been reported occasionally as a complication of DKA in children, it is rare in adults.

NONKETOTIC HYPERTONIC HYPERGLYCEMIA

The entity of NKHH has a pathogenesis similar to that of DKA (Fig. 79–3). Hyperglycemia and volume contraction predominate, however, with absent or relatively mild acidosis. NKHH occurs most frequently in type 2 diabetics. Why there is minimal ketosis is unclear. It has been traditional teaching that circulating insulin levels are adequate for the prevention of ketosis but not high enough to prevent hyperglycemia. Measurements of plasma insulin, however, do not support this theory. In all likelihood, the lack of ketosis is related more to the levels of counterregulatory hormones, which are lower in NKHH than in DKA.

This disorder has been called *hypertonic hyperglycemic nonketotic coma*. Coma due to hyperosmolality usually occurs when serum tonicity (or effective osmolality $= \{2[Na^+] + [glucose]/18\}$) is greater than 340 mOsm/kg. Since coma is actually uncommon, this term should be abandoned. Effective osmolality includes osmotically active solutes that are confined to the extracellular space (i.e., sodium and glucose in the absence of insulin). Urea nitrogen freely crosses cell membranes and therefore does not contribute to serum tonicity.

The hallmark of NKHH is hyperglycemia and volume contraction. The elevated blood glucose causes an osmotic diuresis with the loss of hypotonic fluid. If the patient can maintain adequate volume intake, the GFR remains normal and glucose

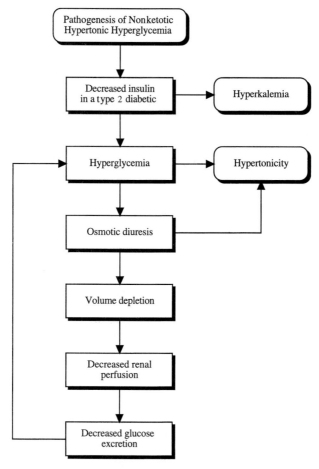

Figure 79–3. Schematic diagram illustrating the pathogenesis of nonketotic hypertonic hyperglycemia (NKHH).

is excreted. In this case, serum glucose levels rarely rise to greater than 400 mg/ dL and, except for polyuria and polydipsia, there are no significant sequelae. When volume intake is inadequate, however, GFR and glucose excretion decrease, resulting in a greater degree of hyperglycemia (increasing osmotic diuresis) and more significant volume contraction (see Fig. 79–3). The loss of hypotonic fluid combines with the hyperglycemia to produce severe hypertonicity.

Evaluation

Patients with NKHH present with signs and symptoms of volume contraction and hypertonicity. Orthostatic hypotension is universal as are dry mucous membranes and skin tenting. There is often a change in mental status and central nervous system symptoms secondary to hypertonicity. These symptoms may range from mild confusion and agitation to seizures and coma. As mentioned earlier, coma is unusual unless serum tonicity is greater than 340 mOsm/kg.

Laboratory analysis (see Table 79–1) usually reveals a glucose concentration greater than 600 mg/dL. The serum sodium may be low, normal, or elevated, depending on water intake, but a normal or elevated serum sodium indicates profound hypertonicity and a worse prognosis. Hyperglycemia osmotically "pulls" water out of the intracellular compartment and dilutes the serum sodium. As in DKA, total body potassium depletion is common in NKHH. The serum potassium, however, is often elevated secondary to the relative lack of insulin and the hypertonicity. An anion gap metabolic acidosis may be present secondary either to ketoacidosis or to increased lactate production as a consequence of poor organ perfusion. Because of the volume contraction and decreased renal perfusion, blood urea nitrogen and creatinine are elevated in a prerenal pattern with the blood urea nitrogen:creatinine ratio frequently greater than 20. If volume contraction is severe enough, acute renal failure may occur.

A thorough history and physical examination are necessary to define precipitating events, although as many as 50% of patients presenting with NKHH will not have been previously diagnosed with diabetes. Infections, especially pulmonary and urinary, are common, but even subtle infections may be enough to precipitate NKHH. As with DKA, cardiac ischemia should be ruled out. Drugs such as corticosteroids are frequent causative agents. Other drugs which have been implicated in NKHH are cimetidine, beta-adrenergic blockers, and phenytoin.

Treatment

Volume Resuscitation

The therapy of NKHH is outlined in Figure 79–4. Because the major morbidity associated with NKHH is secondary to intravascular volume depletion, volume resuscitation is the mainstay of therapy. If the patient is hypotensive, 1 to 2 L of 0.9% saline should be rapidly infused intravenously until the blood pressure is stabilized. Intravenous 0.9% saline should be continued at a rate of 250 to 500 mL/h until intravascular volume is repleted as confirmed by blood pressure and urine output. Most patients with NKHH require between 4 and 6 L of saline. In the elderly and in patients with underlying heart disease, one should closely monitor for the presence of physical examination findings of congestive heart failure (basilar crackles, gallop rhythm, jugular venous distention and hepatojugular reflex) during fluid resuscitation to avoid iatrogenic volume overload.

Hyperglycemia

Volume repletion by itself frequently lowers the serum glucose by as much as 50% as renal perfusion and GFR improve enabling the excretion of glucose. Insulin therapy should wait until volume resuscitation is complete because the osmolality provided by glucose helps support the vascular space in the face of volume depletion. *Premature use of insulin can result in vascular collapse* as glucose and water move out of the extracellular compartment into the intracellular

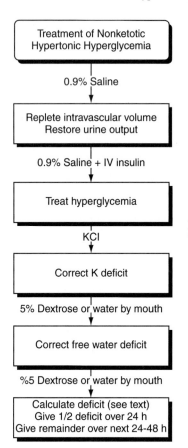

Figure 79–4. Schematic diagram for therapy of NKHH (see text for details). IV, intravenous.

space. After volume repletion is confirmed, regular insulin should be given as an intravenous bolus of 10 units. Although a maintenance insulin infusion at 0.1 units/kg/hour is most convenient, it is not mandatory. This therapy should lower the glucose by 100 to 200 mg/dL/hour, during which time glucose concentration should be monitored frequently.

Hypertonicity

Once the volume contraction is corrected, therapeutic attention should be turned to the hypertonicity. Significant quantities of free water can be lost during the osmotic diuresis. If the patient has not been able to replete these losses orally, hypernatremia occurs. By pulling water out of the intracellular space, hyperglycemia, by itself, causes hyponatremia, often masking the underlying hypernatremia. Every 100 mg/dL of glucose greater than 100 mg/dL decreases the serum sodium by approximately 1.6 mEq/L. Therefore, a normal or elevated serum sodium concentration implies significant hypernatremia. To estimate the amount of free water necessary to treat this, serum sodium should be corrected for the hyperglycemia. For example, if the serum sodium is 140 mEq/L and the serum glucose is 1000 mg/dL, the corrected sodium will be 154 mEq/L ($= 1.6 \times 9 + 140$). Once this is calculated, the free water deficit can be estimated by the following:

Current total body water $\times$ current [Na$^+$]
$$= \text{normal total body water} \times \text{normal [Na}^+] \qquad (1)$$

where [Na$^+$] is the serum sodium concentration, normal total body water equals 60% of body weight and normal [Na$^+$] = 140 mEq/L.

For example, if a man who weighs 70 kg has a serum sodium of 160 mEq/L, his normal total body water would equal 42 L (0.6×70 kg) and his current total body water would equal 36.75 L ($42 \times 140/160$). His water deficit is, therefore, 5.25 L ($42 - 36.75$).

Despite being based on several inaccurate assumptions, this formula provides a fairly good approximation of the underlying water deficit. One half of the calculated free water deficit plus any ongoing losses should be replaced over the first 24 hours and the remainder over the next 48 hours. More rapid correction of the hypernatremia is dangerous and might result in cerebral edema. During periods of hypertonicity, brain cells increase intracellular solute ("idiogenic osmoles") to prevent shrinkage. Correcting the extracellular hypertonicity too rapidly may cause water to flow into brain cells and produce swelling.

Potassium Deficit

Finally, attention should be paid to correcting the potassium deficit. As soon as urine output is established, potassium repletion can be initiated. Potassium deficits may be as high as 500 mEq. Potassium supplementation can be given orally or intravenously over several days.

Complications

Complications of NKHH are usually related to treatment. As discussed earlier, premature administration of insulin may cause vascular collapse. Overzealous correction of the hypertonicity can result in cerebral edema and central pontine myelinolysis (see Chapter 81). In addition, an increased risk of thrombotic events has been noted. This hypercoagulability is most likely secondary to volume contraction and sludging of blood. Routine prophylaxis against deep venous thrombosis (not full anticoagulation) is recommended. Because of improved understanding of the pathophysiology of NKHH, the mortality of this disorder, which had been as high as 50%, has decreased to less than 10%. Present-day mortality relates more to the presence of underlying conditions than to the hypertonicity itself.

ALCOHOLIC KETOACIDOSIS

Alcohol ketoacidosis, which was first described in 1940, is an increasingly recognized cause of ketoacidosis. Although initially considered a rare disorder occurring predominantly in female alcoholics, it is apparent that it is more common than previously believed and can be seen in chronic alcoholics of both genders.

Several reasons for the previous lack of recognition of this acid-base disorder include the camouflaging of the acidosis by *concurrent respiratory and metabolic alkalosis,* which are common in alcoholics, and the fact that beta-hydroxybutyrate is the predominant ketone (and hence not measurable by the standard ketone assay, as noted earlier). Today's physicians are less easily fooled by these physiologic occurrences and more readily recognize AKA.

Diagnosis

Alcoholic ketoacidosis is diagnosed in nondiabetic chronic alcohol abusers who present with an anion gap acidosis and ketonemia, but without significant hyperglycemia. Typically patients have had an alcohol binge and stopped eating because of the development of abdominal pain or nausea and vomiting. They usually present 24 to 48 hours into their fast with a chief complaint of nausea, vomiting, abdominal pain, and shortness of breath. Alcohol is usually unmeasurable or present at nonintoxicating levels.

The pathophysiology of AKA has not been clearly defined. The key components are alcohol intake and starvation (Fig. 79–5). Starvation leads to decreased glycogen stores, decreased levels of insulin, and increased levels of glucagon. The

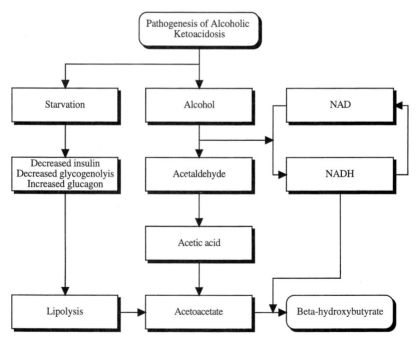

Figure 79–5. Schematic diagram illustrating the pathogenesis of alcoholic ketoacidosis (AKA). NAD, nicotinamide-adenine dinucleotide; NADH, nicotinamide-adenine dinucleotide (reduced form).

metabolism of alcohol to acetaldehyde via alcohol dehydrogenase converts NAD to NADH. Similar to DKA, there is an increase in fatty acid oxidation. Because the NADH:NAD ratio is high and much greater than in DKA, the predominant ketone is beta-hydroxybutyrate.

Evaluation

Evaluation of the patient with suspected AKA should include a thorough history and physical examination. In an *alcoholic with a metabolic acidosis,* one must rule out other causes for the acidosis, such as *hemorrhagic pancreatitis, sepsis, or ingestion of ethylene glycol or methanol.* Fever is uncommon in AKA unless there is an underlying infection or evidence of alcohol withdrawal. Abdominal pain is commonly present, but the abdominal examination is typically benign.

Although laboratory analysis (see Table 79–1) usually reveals an anion gap metabolic acidosis, the pH may be normal or even alkalemic (secondary to a respiratory alkalosis from chronic liver disease or a metabolic alkalosis from vomiting). Initially, ketones may not be detected in the serum or urine because the high NADH:NAD ratio causes a shift of acetoacetate to beta-hydroxybutyrate. If ketone levels are normal, serum lactate should be measured to rule out lactic acidosis, and a toxicology screen performed for ethylene glycol and methanol.

Potassium levels may be normal on presentation, but total body potassium depletion often is present. Hypophosphatemia and hypomagnesemia are also common, whereas the glucose concentration is normal or low. Approximately 10% of patients with AKA have a glucose level greater than 250 mg/dL (14 mmol/L), making it difficult to distinguish these individuals from those with true DKA. Alcohol bingeing and lack of a prior history of diabetes should lead the clinician to suspect AKA. Not until the episode has resolved and glucose tolerance is found to be normal can diabetes be definitively discounted.

Treatment

The treatment of AKA begins with volume repletion using 0.9% saline. Because starvation and lack of glycogen stores are contributing factors to AKA, 5% dextrose should be included for all patients who are not frankly hyperglycemic. Insulin is not indicated except if the blood glucose is greater than 250 mg/dL (14 mmol/L). To avoid precipitation of Wernicke encephalopathy, *thiamine must be given before the infusion of dextrose.*

Attention should also be directed at correcting underlying electrolyte abnormalities. Potassium replacement is often necessary and can be given intravenously or orally if tolerated. Hypophosphatemia less than 1 mg/dL (0.32 mmol/L) should be treated with potassium phosphate. Hypomagnesemia is also routinely treated, although no convincing data exist demonstrating benefit of this therapy. If the magnesium is less than 1 mg/dL (0.41 mmol/L), 2 to 4 g magnesium sulfate (8 to 16 mmol) can be infused every 6 hours. Half that dose may be repeated over the next 24 hours.

Finally, because these patients are at high risk for the development of alcohol withdrawal syndrome, empirical use of benzodiazepines for prophylaxis is warranted. The mortality of AKA is not well documented but appears to be low. When it occurs, death is usually secondary to underlying disease or from alcohol withdrawal syndrome.

BIBLIOGRAPHY

Adrogue HJ, Madias NE: Management of life-threatening acid-base disorders. N Engl J Med 338:26–34, 1998.
    This is a recent, concise review of all major types of metabolic acidoses, including diabetic ketoacidosis and alcoholic ketoacidosis.

Feig PU, McCurdy DK: The hypertonic state. N Engl J Med 297:1444–1454, 1977.
    This is a classic article on hypertonicity—must reading for all students and house officers. Discusses normal osmoregulation and describes the classic approach to understanding hypertonicity.

Fleckman AM: Diabetic ketoacidosis. Endocrinol Metab Clin North Am 22:181–207, 1993.
    This is a well-written, entertaining, easy-to-read review. It covers all aspects of DKA, from pathophysiology to treatment and complications. It is highly recommended.

Fulop M: Alcoholic ketoacidosis. Endocrinol Metab Clin North Am 22:209–219, 1993.
    This article reviews all major publications on AKA and puts it all together.

Halperin ML, Hammeke M, Josse RG, Jungas RL: Metabolic acidosis in the alcoholic: A pathophysiologic approach. Metabolism 32:308–315, 1983.
    This is a complicated review of the pathogenesis of AKA. It is an important paper for those clinicians wishing to "know it all."

Lorber D: Nonketotic hypertonicity in diabetes mellitus. Med Clin North Am 79:39–52, 1995.
    This is a good, easy-to-read review of NKHH.

Piniés JA, Cairo G, Gaztambide S, Vazquez JA: Course and prognosis of 132 patients with diabetic nonketotic hyperosmolar state. Diabetes Metab 20:43–48, 1994.
    This is a prospective study of NKHH. It reviews the causes of mortality in hypertonic hyperglycemia and points out that mortality is related more to the presenting hemodynamics than to the degree of hypertonicity.

Wachtel TJ, Tetu-Mouradjian LM, Goldman DL, et al: Hyperosmolarity and acidosis in diabetes mellitus: A three-year experience in Rhode Island. J Gen Intern Med 6:495–502, 1991.
    This is an epidemiologic study of diabetes that demonstrates the frequency of overlap between DKA and NKHH and the difficulty the clinician often has in distinguishing these syndromes.

Wrenn KD, Slovis CM, Minion GE, Rutkowski R: The syndrome of alcoholic ketoacidosis. Am J Med 91:119–128, 1991.
    This is the largest case series published examining AKA. It discusses presenting signs and symptoms as well as common laboratory findings.

80

Metabolic Acidoses and Alkaloses

George M. Feldman

Acidosis and *alkalosis* are terms that refer to the pathophysiologic processes that cause the body to accumulate or lose H^+ ions, whereas the terms *acidemia* and *alkalemia* refer to the actual changes in arterial blood pH. *Metabolic* acid-base disorders are those disturbances that primarily affect serum HCO_3^- concentration, whereas *respiratory* acid-base disorders primarily affect Pa_{CO_2}.

Acid-base disorders in the patient in the intensive care unit (ICU) often cause widespread physiologic changes of clinical importance. For example, acute acidemia increases pulmonary vascular resistance, decreases the affinity of hemoglobin for oxygen ("shift to the left") (Fig. 1, Appendix A), and increases the free concentration (and potential for toxicity) of many drugs by decreasing their protein binding (see Chapter 12). Acutely, acidemia can also induce hyperkalemia, promote cardiac arrhythmias, and depress mental status, whereas chronically it can cause protein catabolism.

In contrast, acute alkalemia reduces cerebral blood flow and tissue delivery of oxygen by increasing hemoglobin's affinity for oxygen ("shift to the right"; Fig. 1, Appendix A). Alkalemia also increases calcium binding to proteins, which may precipitate tetany, seizures, and arrhythmias.

PATHOPHYSIOLOGY

Acid-Base Physiology

Metabolism of food ultimately produces acid (H^+) and base (HCO_3^-). Basic organic anions, for example, citrate and acetate, are equivalent to HCO_3^- because they produce HCO_3^- when oxidized. Complete oxidation of carbon-containing compounds yields a volatile acid, carbonic acid (H_2CO_3), as shown by Equation 1.

$$H^+ + HCO_3^- = H_2CO_3 = CO_2 + H_2O \qquad \text{(Equation 1)}$$

Incomplete oxidation produces nonvolatile organic acids (e.g., lactic, beta-hydroxybutyric, and acetoacetic acids). Oxidation of sulfur-containing amino acids yields sulfuric acid (H_2SO_4). The effect of these metabolic events on acid-base homeostasis is influenced by respiration and the exhalation of CO_2. The H^+ from nonvolatile acids (e.g., sulfuric and lactic acids) are excreted by the kidneys. A typical American diet produces slightly more acid than base, equal to approximately 1 mmol H^+/kg body weight per day; in contrast, a strict vegetarian diet produces a net base.

Buffers minimize pH changes that result from the addition or removal of H^+. Equation 1 can be rewritten in the Henderson-Hasselbalch format:

$$pH = pK + \log [HCO_3^-] / [CO_2] \qquad \text{(Equation 2)}$$

903

where pK = 6.1 (equilibrium constant for carbonic acid) and $[CO_2]$ is the concentration (mmol/L) of CO_2 dissolved in blood.

$[CO_2]$ is determined by measuring $Paco_2$ and multiplying it by the solubility coefficient (0.03 mm Hg/mmol/L). Thus, a normal $Paco_2$ of 40 mm Hg equals 1.2 mmol/L of CO_2. With this value and a normal $[HCO_3^-]$ of 24 mmol/L, the ratio of $[HCO_3^-]/[CO_2]$ normally equals 20:1 (and log 20 = 1.3). Thus, this ratio corresponds to a pH of 7.40.

The $[HCO_3^-]/[CO_2]$ buffer pair is the most important because of the abundance of their components and how the relationship between them can be influenced independently by the kidneys and lungs. For example, by Equation 1, in metabolic acidosis the addition of H^+ increases $[H^+]$ (which, at equilibrium, proportionately decreases $[HCO_3^-]$). By the Law of Mass Action, the increased $[H^+]$ drives the reaction to the right, increasing the production of CO_2. Under normal conditions, this increased CO_2 production does not result in a rise in $[CO_2]$ or $Paco_2$ because of a compensatory increase in ventilation. If there were no such increase, the resulting hypercapnia would have aggravated the drop in pH caused by the metabolic acidosis. In addition to buffering by $[HCO_3^-]/[CO_2]$, inorganic phosphates, plasma and intracellular proteins, and hemoglobin help to buffer changes in pH.

Renal Acid-Base Handling

Normally functioning kidneys regulate the serum HCO_3^- concentration in two ways. First, they reabsorb the filtered load of HCO_3^- (= GFR × serum $[HCO_3^-]$), 1 mmol of which, if lost in the urine, would be equivalent to gaining 1 mmol of H^+. Second, they excrete H^+ at a rate equal to the metabolic production of H^+. HCO_3^- reabsorption occurs in the proximal portion of the nephron by a mechanism that depends on carbonic anhydrase. This enzyme accelerates the hydration reaction of CO_2 (Equation 1) and is stimulated by angiotensin II.

H^+ is excreted by the distal nephron and its excretion is stimulated by distal Na^+ delivery and aldosterone. Effective excretion of H^+ utilizes urinary buffers, phosphate, and ammonium. Urinary phosphate excretion depends on dietary intake, whereas urinary ammonium is produced by renal metabolism. Ammonium production is stimulated by metabolic acidosis, hypokalemia, and glucocorticoids and, conversely, is suppressed by metabolic alkalosis, hyperkalemia, and glucocorticoid deficiency.

Compensatory Mechanisms

After the onset of a primary acid-base disturbance, homeostatic events, that is, compensation, occur that tend to return blood pH toward normal values. Ventilation changes in response to primary metabolic abnormalities, whereas renal acid-base handling changes in response to primary respiratory abnormalities. Although the effects of compensation tend to normalize blood pH, in general, it should never correct blood pH fully, that is, to a pH of exactly 7.4.

Respiratory Compensation for Metabolic Disorders

The respiratory response to metabolic acid-base disturbances begins immediately but takes up to 24 hours to achieve full effect. Hyperventilation compensates for metabolic acidosis. This pattern of ventilation, called Kussmaul respirations, is characterized by increased tidal volume and to a lesser extent increased respiratory rate. The magnitude of the compensation varies with the degree of acidosis but can be accurately predicted by "Winters's formula" for acute metabolic acidosis:

$$Pa_{CO_2} \text{ (predicted) (mm Hg)} = 1.5 \text{ (mm Hg/mmol/L)} \times [HCO_3^-]$$
$$\text{(measured) (mmol /L)} + 8 \ (\pm \ 2) \text{ (mmol/L)} \qquad \text{(Equation 3)}$$

where Pa_{CO_2} (predicted) is the Pa_{CO_2} expected if its level results only from respiratory compensation, and $[HCO_3^-]$ (measured) is the value measured in an arterial blood sample. (This is shown graphically in Fig. 1, Appendix D.)

Hypoventilation compensates for metabolic alkalosis and the elevation of P_{CO_2} increases with the severity of the alkalosis. However, the hypoventilatory response is more variable than the hyperventilatory response and may be limited by hypoxemia due to hypercapnia (Equation 12, Table 1–1). Consequently, the compensatory Pa_{CO_2} is often difficult to predict accurately (see also Fig. 1, Appendix D).

Renal Compensation for Respiratory Disorders

Respiratory acid-base disorders elicit metabolic (renal) compensation. In compensation for respiratory alkalosis, the serum $[HCO_3^-]$ decreases 2 to 4 mEq/L for each 10 mm Hg decrease in the Pa_{CO_2} and takes 12 to 24 hours to complete. The serum $[HCO_3^-]$ rises in compensation for respiratory acidosis; it takes 3 to 5 days to achieve a 1 to 3 mEq/L increase for every 10 mm Hg rise in Pa_{CO_2}. These relationships are shown graphically in Figure 1, Appendix D.

METABOLIC ACIDOSES

Metabolic acidoses occur when the rate of nonvolatile acid intake (or production), or HCO_3^- loss, exceeds the rate of renal H^+ excretion. They are classified into anion gap acidoses and hyperchloremic (non–anion gap) metabolic acidoses.

Anion Gap Acidoses

The anion gap (expressed in mEq/L) is the difference between measured serum cations and anions, as in Equation 4:

$$\text{Anion gap} = [Na^+] - \{[Cl^-] + [tCO_2]\} \qquad \text{(Equation 4)}$$

where $[tCO_2]$ is the total serum bicarbonate as measured on a venous blood sample as part of the same chemistry panel giving values (mEq/L) for serum $[Na^+]$ and $[Cl^-]$. The anion gap consists of negatively charged proteins, for example, albumin, and small anions, for example, urate and phosphate. Its normal range is 8 to 14

Table 80–1 Metabolic Acidoses: Anion Gap Acidoses

TYPE OF ANION	ETIOLOGY
Ketones	Diabetic ketoacidosis
	Alcoholic ketoacidosis
Toxins, poisons	Salicylates
	Methanol
	Ethylene glycol
Lactate	Lactic acidosis
Phosphates and sulfate	Chronic renal failure

and increases when nonvolatile acids accumulate because of increased net production (e.g., lactate, acetoacetate, or beta-hydroxybutyrate) or decreased renal excretion (e.g., phosphate and sulfate in chronic renal failure).

Lactic acidosis and diabetic ketoacidosis (DKA) are common causes of an anion gap acidosis (Table 80–1). In DKA, metabolism of fatty acids produces H^+ and the anion acetoacetate (which is detected by the nitroprusside reaction). Starvation produces ketosis but only minimal acidosis. In contrast, alcoholic ketoacidosis (AKA), which includes aspects of starvation, can produce a severe anion gap acidosis. After binge drinking, it is often characterized by vomiting episodes, and it generates the anion beta-hydroxybutyrate (which is not detected by the nitroprusside reaction for ketones). (See Chapter 79 for a detailed discussion of DKA and AKA.)

Several toxins induce anion gap acidoses (see also Chapter 57). For example, salicylates induce lactic acid production while also affecting central nervous system respiratory centers to produce a second primary disorder, a respiratory alkalosis. Methanol and ethylene glycol are metabolized by hepatic alcohol dehydrogenase. Methanol yields formaldehyde and formic acid, whereas ethylene glycol yields glycolic, oxalic, and formic acids. Formic acid damages the optic nerve, leading to scotomas and blindness, whereas oxalate crystals can damage kidneys, brain, heart, and lungs.

Hyperchloremic (Non-Anion Gap) Metabolic Acidoses

In hyperchloremic metabolic acidosis (HCMA), the anion gap is not widened because the decrement in serum HCO_3^- is "matched" by an increment in serum $[Cl^-]$. For example, ingestion or administration of HCl yields a hyperchloremic acidosis. Intake of the chloride salts of ammonium, arginine, and lysine also causes HCMA because their metabolism yields HCl. Impaired renal H^+ excretion as occurs in renal failure or other renal disorders can also result in HCMA (Table 80–2).

The most common cause of loss of HCO_3^- via the gastrointestinal tract is diarrhea of almost any cause, including infections and laxative abuse. Ingestion of anion exchange resins, for example, cholestryamine, causes HCO_3^- loss, as does

Table 80–2 Metabolic Acidoses: Hyperchloremic (Non-Anion Gap) Acidoses

MECHANISM OF DISORDER	ETIOLOGY
Addition of equimolar H^+ and Cl^-	Ingestion or administration of HCl, NH_4Cl, lysine or arginine HCl
Loss of HCO_3^- with equimolar gain of Cl^-	Secretory diarrhea (cholera-like) due to infections or laxatives; other GI loss of base (pancreatic fistula)
Inability to excrete daily load of H^+	Renal tubular acidosis (see Table 80–3) Chronic renal failure
Inability to maintain serum $[HCO_3^-]$ due to renal losses of HCO_3^-	Renal tubular acidosis (see Table 80–3) Acetazolamide use
Dilution of serum $[HCO_3^-]$	Volume expansion with fluid loading with NaCl

GI, gastrointestinal.

the ingestion of $CaCl_2$ or $MgCl_2$. Ureteral diversion, that is, ureterosigmoidostomy and ileal conduit, results in HCO_3^- loss in the diverted urine. External loss of biliary and pancreatic secretions, for example, pancreas transplants draining into the bladder, also result in net loss of HCO_3^-.

Loss of HCO_3^- leading to HCMA can occur via the kidneys in some renal diseases, with the use of carbonic anhydrase inhibitors (e.g., acetazolamide and methazolamide), and in hyperparathyroidism. Renal tubular acidosis refers to one of several renal tubular defects that impair reclamation of filtered HCO_3^- or H^+ excretion (Table 80–3).

Table 80–3 Categories of Renal Tubular Acidosis

CATEGORY	DESCRIPTION
Proximal RTA	Defective reabsorption of filtered HCO_3^- by the proximal tubule is frequently associated with glycosuria and amino aciduria (Fanconi's syndrome). It can be inherited or acquired (amphotericin B, renal transplants). Since HCO_3^- is continually excreted, urine pH is often > 5.5, but it can be lower. HCO_3^- administration exaggerates HCO_3^- potassium losses.
Distal RTA	Limitations in H^+ secretion in the distal nephron results in accumulation of H^+ and severe HCMA. Distal RTA can be inherited or acquired (autoimmune diseases or many drugs). It is associated with hypercalciuria, nephrocalcinosis, and nephrolithiasis. The urine pH is always > 5.5.
Decreased synthesis of ammonia	Decreased synthesis of ammonia reduces urinary buffer content, decreasing net H^+ excretion. Tubular mechanisms of H^+ secretion, however, are intact and urine pH is frequently < 5.5. Ammonia synthesis is inhibited by hyperkalemia and glucocorticoid deficiency. Some hyperkalemic patients also have low renin hypoaldosteronism (also called type IV RTA). Hyperkalemia in these patients fails to stimulate aldosterone secretion; they also tend to be unresponsive to exogenous aldosterone. Decreased ammonia synthesis due to reduced renal mass also contributes to the acidosis of chronic renal insufficiency.

RTA, renal tubular acidosis; HCMA, hyperchloremic metabolic acidosis.

Finally, dilution of serum HCO_3^- can occur subsequent to large volumes of NaCl, and this may result in a HCMA ("expansion acidosis"). Its severity, however, is limited by nonbicarbonate buffers.

METABOLIC ALKALOSES

Excess addition of alkali (e.g., HCO_3^-, lactate, or citrate) or excess excretion or loss of H^+ (via either the gastrointestinal tract or the kidneys) can generate metabolic alkaloses.

In either case, however, the elevated $[HCO_3^-]$ is maintained because the kidneys fail to excrete it. Several mechanisms can reduce renal HCO_3^- excretion. First, renal failure decreases HCO_3^- excretion because of a decreased glomerular filtration rate. Second, volume depletion also reduces HCO_3^- excretion (and its equivalent, increasing H^+ excretion) by the following: (1) angiotensin II stimulates the proximal tubule to increase HCO_3^- reabsorption; (2) aldosterone acts to increase H^+ secretion in the distal nephron; (3) aldosterone-induced hypokalemia stimulates ammoniagenesis and increases H^+ secretion.

Patients with volume depletion and alkalosis are depleted of Cl^- and have low urinary $[Cl^-]$ (<20 mEq/L). They are considered to have "chloride-sensitive metabolic alkalosis" because NaCl and KCl repletion correct their abnormality. In certain types of metabolic alkaloses, however, the volume status plays no role in pathogenesis and the urine $[Cl^-]$ is normal (>30 mEq/L). As expected, these patients with a "chloride-resistant metabolic alkalosis" do not improve with NaCl or KCl administration (Table 80–4).

Chloride-Sensitive Metabolic Alkaloses

Vomiting-Nasogastric Suction. Loss of H^+-rich gastric secretions generates an alkalosis. The associated volume depletion maintains the alkalosis. Between vomiting episodes, however, urinary HCO_3^- excretion is virtually nonexistent and urinary pH is low.

Chloridorrhea. Chloride-rich diarrhea can cause alkalosis because the diarrheal fluid is also rich in ammonium and potassium and has virtually no HCO_3^-. This occurs in a rare congenital condition, infrequently in some viral infections, and in villous adenomas. Volume depletion maintains the alkalosis.

Diuretics. Thiazides and loop diuretics cause alkalosis by depleting potassium and volume.

Posthypercapnic Alkalosis. Alkalosis may occur in patients after correction of hypercapnia if they become volume depleted or hypokalemic, or both, due to diuretic therapy.

Antibiotic-Related Alkalosis. Antibiotics such as carbenicillin are anions that are not reabsorbed by the kidneys, so that their excretion obligates cation loss, for example, Na^+, K^+, H^+, and NH_4^+. Such antibiotics cause alkalosis when simultaneous NaCl administration is limited for other reasons.

Table 80–4 Metabolic Alkaloses

CATEGORY	CHLORIDE-SENSITIVE ALKALOSIS		CHLORIDE-RESISTANT ALKALOSIS	
Urinary [Cl⁻]	<20 mEq/L		>30 mEq/L	
Extracellular fluid volume	Decreased	Increased	Euvolemic or decreased	
Site of problem	Renal	Renal	Renal	
Causes	Gastrointestinal	Excess mineralocorticoid states	Bartter's syndrome	
	Vomiting		K^+ depletion (severe)	
	Nasogastric suction		Exogenous HCO_3^- load in presence of renal failure	
	Chloride-rich diarrhea		Nonreabsorbable anion	
	Villous adenoma			
	After chronic hypercapnia			
	Diuretics			
	K^+ depletion (mild-moderate)			
	After organic acidosis			
	Refeeding alkalosis			

Chloride-Resistant Metabolic Alkaloses

Mineralocorticoid Excess. Mineralocorticoid excess (whether primary or secondary) increases net H^+ excretion directly and via hypokalemia. These patients are volume-expanded rather than volume-contracted.

Bartter's Syndrome. This uncommon alkalosis occurs in normotensive, euvolemic patients who have potassium depletion, hypomagnesemia, hyperreninemia, hyperaldosteronism, and juxtaglomerular apparatus hyperplasia on kidney biopsy. The disorder usually presents in childhood, but an acquired form associated with gentamicin has been reported in adults.

Recovery from Organic Acidosis. Alkalosis can occur after resolution of an organic acidosis (e.g., ketoacidosis or lactic acidosis) if HCO_3^- was administered during the acidosis. During recovery, metabolism of lactate and ketoacids regenerates HCO_3^- and, if hypovolemia or hypokalemia coexist, the administered HCO_3^- plus the regenerated HCO_3^- can result in severe, prolonged metabolic alkalosis. Administration of large quantities of organic anions such as citrate (in transfusions) can have similar effects. Transient "refeeding" alkalosis can follow prolonged starvation because ketoacid anions accumulate during starvation.

Renal Failure. In renal failure, because HCO_3^- is not excreted, excessive alkali ingestion or administration can lead to severe metabolic alkalosis. In addition, ingestion of large amounts of calcium carbonate can lead to renal failure, metabolic alkalosis, and hypercalcemia, a triad known as *milk-alkali syndrome.*

DIAGNOSTIC EVALUATION

Since patients can have two or more acid-base disorders at the same time, a systematic approach for diagnosing complex or mixed acid-base disturbances is recommended (Fig. 80–1). This approach relies on the use of all available data rather than the *isolated* use of arterial blood gas measurements with or without an acid-base nomogram (Fig. 1, Appendix D).

The patient's *history* and *physical examination* are the foundation of the diagnostic approach. First, one should consider how symptoms (vomiting, diarrhea, and polyuria), history (diabetes mellitus, congestive heart failure, and emphysema), medications (diuretics, laxatives, and sedatives), treatments (mechanical ventilation, nasogastric suction, intravenous fluid), and physical observations (signs of extracellular volume contraction or expansion, hypotension, tetany, jaundice, hyperpnea, and cyanosis) might have affected acid-base balance. One should then review not only the patient's serum and urinary electrolytes and the arterial blood gas measurements but also common tests such as complete blood count, liver and renal function tests, urinalysis, and chest film for the presence of lung or renal disease. The laboratory evidence can be used to support or refute one's initial impression of the likely acid-base abnormalities to be encountered (Table 80–5). After the data-gathering phase, one can formulate a *differential diagnosis* of the particular acid-base disorders (see Tables 80–1 to 80–4). Finally, one needs *to rule in or out* each diagnosis in the differential diagnosis.

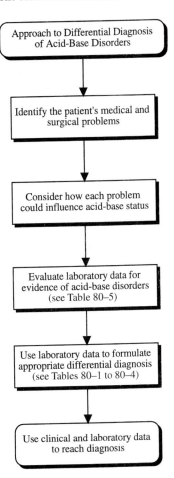

Figure 80–1. Schematic representation of the recommended process to evaluate and diagnose acid-base disturbances (see text for details).

Both serum and urine laboratory data can help in the diagnosis of acid-base disorders. For example, in anion gap acidoses due to toxins such as ethanol, methanol, and ethylene glycol, the toxins (and their metabolites) accumulate in the serum and contribute to the measured osmolality (see Chapter 57). However, the estimated osmolality, derived from the serum electrolytes, blood urea nitrogen, and glucose, "misses" the new osmols, and an "osmolar gap" can be detected. It is also valuable to compare changes in the anion gap with changes in the tCO_2 or to calculate the delta (Δ) gap. For example, in acute lactic acidosis due to seizures, the anion gap increases as much as the tCO_2 falls because the lactic acid contributes equimolar quantities of the unmeasured anion that widens the anion gap and the H^+ that titrates HCO_3^- down. In contrast, in alcoholic ketoacidosis, the anion gap is often wider than the tCO_2 is depressed because vomiting, a common occurrence in alcoholic ketoacidosis, induces a concomitant metabolic alkalosis. Thus, the lack of stoichiometry between the changes in the anion gap and the tCO_2, that is, a large Δ gap, can provide evidence for an otherwise overlooked metabolic

Table 80–5 Interpretation of Laboratory Data in Acid-Base Disorders

LABORATORY TEST	NORMAL RESULT	ABNORMAL RESULTS
Serum total CO_2 (tCO_2)	There may be two or more offsetting acid-base disturbances	There is at least one acid-base disturbance
Serum AG*	Consistent with HCMA or respiratory alkalosis Hypoalbuminemia may obscure a wide AG	Wide AG suggests metabolic acidosis Small AG suggests presence of paraprotein
Serum OG†		Large OG alone with wide AG suggests toxin-induced acidosis (see Chapter 57)
Delta gap (Δ gap)‡		Positive Δ gap (>6) suggests presence of metabolic alkalosis Negative Δ gap (<−6) suggests presence of HCMA
Serum K^+		1. In acute acid-base disorders, changes in $[K^+]$ may predict pH: ↓ $[K^+]$ in alkalemia, ↑ $[K^+]$ in acidemia. 2. Chronic ↓ $[K^+]$ → ↑ NH_4^+ synthesis. 3. Chronic ↑ $[K^+]$ → ↓ NH_4^+ synthesis.
Urine AG§		Urine AG in HCMA is typically negative Positive urine AG in HCMA suggests reduced urinary NH_4^+ excretion Positive urine AG in setting of an AG acidosis is consistent with excess unmeasured urinary anion (the same anion as in serum)

*[AG = Na − (Cl + tCO_2)]; normal AG = 8 to 14 mEq/L.
†OG = measured osmolality − estimated osmolality, where estimated osmolality = 2 × (Na + K) + BUN/2.8 + glucose/18; normal OG = <10 mOsm/kg.
‡Delta gap = ΔAG − ΔtCO_2, where ΔAG = [observed anion gap − normal AG (= 12)] and ΔtCO_2 = [normal tCO_2 (= 28) − observed tCO_2]; normal Δgap = 0 ± 6 mEq/L.
§Urine anion gap (UAG) = Na + K − Cl.
AG, anion gap; HCMA, hyperchloremic metabolic acidosis; OG, osmolar gap; BUN, blood urea nitrogen; ↓, decreased; ↑, increased.

alkalosis. Combined acid-base disorders are often called double or triple disturbances.

The urine anion gap can provide an estimate of urinary ammonia excretion (see Table 80–5). In metabolic acidosis, unmeasured NH_4^+ usually generates a negative urine anion gap. In patients with decreased ammonia excretion, however, the urine anion gap is positive. In ketoacidosis or ethylene glycol ingestion, the unmeasured anions appear in the urine, generating a positive urine anion gap.

MANAGEMENT

Metabolic Acidosis

In general, the treatment for all acid-base disorders is to determine and correct the primary cause. Thereafter, therapy for severe acute acidosis is aimed at increasing the pH to greater than 7.2 and the serum [HCO$_3^-$] to greater than 10 mEq/L. Since the volume of distribution of HCO$_3^-$ varies inversely with the plasma [HCO$_3^-$], the dose of HCO$_3^-$ to be administered can be calculated:

$$\text{Dose (mEq) of HCO}_3^- = \{0.4 + 2.4/[\text{HCO}_3^-] \text{ (current)}\} \times \text{ weight (kg)}$$
$$\times \{10 - [\text{HCO}_3^-] \text{ (current)}\} \qquad \text{(Equation 5)}$$

The equation makes its calculation for a desired plasma HCO$_3^-$ of 10 mEq/L. This formula does not account for continued production of acid, and thus the effects of therapy should be monitored closely. The large sodium load associated with NaHCO$_3$ administration may be limiting, especially in states of volume overload, and hemodialysis should be considered (see Chapter 16). Other limitations of HCO$_3^-$ therapy are discussed further on.

Although the treatment of methanol and ethylene glycol intoxication follows the preceding paradigm, it is also important to decrease the metabolism of these toxins (see Chapter 57). Because ethanol is also a substrate for hepatic alcohol dehydrogenase, intravenous ethanol slows the breakdown of methanol and ethylene glycol. Alkalemia should be avoided because it accelerates metabolism of methanol and ethylene glycol. Hemodialysis removes the toxins effectively.

Correcting chronic hyperkalemia that has resulted in reduced renal ammoniagenesis increases net H$^+$ excretion. Strategies include increasing NaCl intake with or without a diuretic, providing a K$^+$-removing resin, for example, sodium polystyrene sulfonate (Kayexalate), or administering the synthetic mineralocorticoid fludrocortisone acetate. Diuretic use alone can be counterproductive when Na intake is limited because the consequent reduction in extracellular fluid volume reduces urine flow in the distal nephron, limiting net H$^+$ and potassium excretion.

Metabolic Alkalosis

In most cases of alkalosis, the cause (e.g., vomiting or diuretics) is obvious. When extracellular volume depletion exists, treatment is centered on repleting volume as NaCl and, if necessary, as KCl. If the cause is less obvious, urine chloride measurements can help in deciding whether repleting volume will be beneficial (see Table 80–5 and Fig. 1). In cases of mineralocorticoid excess, treatment with K$^+$-sparing diuretics such as spironolactone (an aldosterone receptor blocker) or amiloride or triamterene (blockers of aldosterone-stimulated Na$^+$ reabsorption) is useful. In cases of suspected diuretic and laxative abuse, urine chloride values can be misleading and drug screens are helpful.

When the alkalemic patient is acutely symptomatic (having seizures or tetany), rapid correction of the alkalosis can be achieved with the administration of HCl, arginine hydrochloride, and NH$_4$Cl. The latter two should be avoided in patients with liver disease. HCl may be administered in a 0.1 to 0.2 M solution into a central vein, and arterial blood gases should be monitored frequently. Oral administration of CaCl$_2$ or MgCl$_2$ has been successful in patients with cirrhosis.

In patients on ventilators, correcting metabolic alkalosis by repleting potassium and volume deficits can assist weaning (see Chapter 3). Treatment with HCO$_3^-$-losing diuretics, that is, carbonic anhydrase inhibitors, may also help, although K$^+$ losses may increase, and the inhibitor's ability to induce bicarbonaturia is blunted by volume depletion. Correction of potassium deficits in patients with liver disease reduces renal ammoniagenesis and may ameliorate hepatic encephalopathy.

CLINICAL PEARLS AND PITFALLS (see Table 80–5)

1. **The anion gap**

   Plasma proteins affect the anion gap. Hypoalbuminemia decreases it; hyperalbuminemia increases it. Paraproteinemias can affect the gap depending on the charge of the paraprotein, and a negative gap suggests multiple myeloma. By increasing the net negative charge of albumin, alkalemia widens the gap; acidemia has the opposite effect. Marked elevations of $[Ca^{2+}]$, $[Mg^{2+}]$, and lithium reduce the gap, as does bromide. High levels of anionic antibiotics, for example, carbenicillin, increase the gap.

   Renal disease causes an anion gap acidosis and an HCMA. Initially, the acidemia results from the reduction in net H^+ excretion causing the HCMA. However, the anion gap acidosis occurs in later stages of renal failure and results from the retention of poorly cleared anions. In earlier stages of renal insufficiency, clearance of the unmeasured anions is adequate.

2. **tCO_2 and HCO_3^-**

   The tCO_2 is the total CO_2 in serum (ionic HCO_3^- + dissolved CO_2) and is usually measured in venous samples, whereas the HCO_3^- is usually measured in arterial samples. In normal individuals, the venous tCO_2 should be 2 to 5 mEq/L higher than the arterial HCO_3^-; the difference increases in patients with CO_2 retention. The tCO_2 is used to calculate the anion gap, whereas the arterial HCO_3^- is used in Winter's formula. Newer instrumentation has affected the reliability of tCO_2 and HCO_3^- determinations, improving that of HCO_3^- and worsening that of tCO_2.

3. **Dilution and contraction**

   Because non-HCO_3^- buffers are effective, saline administration has a minimal effect on serum tCO_2 levels. Indeed, "dilutional acidosis" does not explain the appearance of HCMA during recovery from diabetic and alcoholic acidoses. Rather, ketoacid anions (anions that can be converted to HCO_3^-) are excreted during the development of the acidoses and their loss is exacerbated by improved renal perfusion due to the saline. Non-HCO_3^- buffers also mitigate the effect of extracellular fluid volume contraction on the tCO_2 levels.

4. **Potassium and pH**

   In acute HCMA, intracellular potassium can shift into the extracellular fluid. However, serum K^+ is unaltered in some acute anion gap acidoses, for example, seizure-induced lactic acidosis. In other anion gap acidoses, such as diabetic ketoacidosis and lactic acidosis due to shock or sepsis, the serum K^+ is influenced by factors including volume status, insulin deficiency, poor tissue oxygenation, impaired aldosterone secretion, and reduced renal potassium excretion.

5. **Compensation for respiratory alkalosis**

   Some patients with chronic respiratory alkalosis break the usual rule and compensate completely and have normal arterial pH.

6. NaHCO₃ therapy

$NaHCO_3$ treatment can be harmful. Besides its ability to expand extracellular fluid volume, it is hypertonic. The Na^+ concentration is 1 mEq/mL or 1000 mEq/L and the osmolality is 2000 mOsm/kg. It can cause hypokalemia and hypocalcemia. Rebound alkalosis can occur if excessive HCO_3^- is given to patients with ketoacidoses and lactic acidosis. Alkalemia increases the production rate of many organic acids, including lactic acid, ketoacids, formic acid, and oxalic acid. Alkalemia also increases hemoglobin's affinity for O_2, reducing oxygen delivery to tissues. As HCO_3^- is administered, it is titrated by non-HCO_3^- buffers, increasing $Paco_2$ and the demand for ventilation. Also, the rise in $Paco_2$ may depress central nervous system function, because CO_2 (but not HCO_3^-) enters the cerebrospinal fluid rapidly and decreases cerebrospinal fluid pH.

In studies of patients with acute mild to moderate metabolic acidosis, HCO_3^- therapy has *not* been shown to improve patient outcome. HCO_3^- therapy is not beneficial during cardiac resuscitation and may be harmful (see Appendix E). Thus, the role of HCO_3^- therapy in acutely ill patients is controversial and deserves further study.

BIBLIOGRAPHY

Adrogue HJ, Madias NE: Management of life-threatening acid-base disorders. Part 1. N Engl J Med 338:26–34, 1998.
Adrogue HJ, Madias NE: Management of life-threatening acid-base disorders. Part 2. N Engl J Med 338:107–111, 1998.
  This two-part series reviews recent literature and recommendations to manage severe acid-base disorders.
Alpern RJ, Rector FC Jr: Renal acidification mechanisms. In: Brenner BM (ed): The Kidney, 5th ed. Philadelphia: WB Saunders, 1996, pp 408–471.
  This chapter is a modern detailed review of renal and cell acid-base physiology.
Davenport HW: The ABC's of Acid-Base Chemistry, 6th ed. Chicago: University of Chicago Press, 1974.
  This is a solid review of clinically relevant acid-base chemistry.
DuBose TD Jr, Cogan MG, Rector FC Jr: Acid-base disorders. In: Brenner, BM (ed): The Kidney, 5th ed. Philadelphia: WB Saunders, 1996, pp 929–998.
  This chapter is a modern detailed review of human acid-base pathophysiology.
Emmett M, Narins RG: Clinical use of the anion gap. Medicine 56:38–54, 1977.
  This is a classic review of the anion gap.
Fernandez PC, Cohen RM, Feldman GM: The concept of bicarbonate distribution space: The crucial role of body buffers. Kidney Int 36:747–752, 1989.
  This is a description of how buffers interact and affect HCO₃⁻ administration.
Harrington JT, Cohen JJ: Measurement of urinary electrolytes—indications and limitations. N Engl J Med 293:1241–1243, 1975.
  This is a classic review of the clinical utility of urinary electrolytes.
Hills AG: Acid-base balance: Chemistry, physiology, pathophysiology. Baltimore: Williams & Wilkins, 1973.
  This is an outstanding reference on acid-base physiology and chemistry with an extensive pre-Medline bibliography.
Kaehny WD, Anderson RJ: Bicarbonate therapy of metabolic acidosis. Crit Care Med 22:1525–1527, 1994.
  This is a thoughtful commentary on the use of HCO₃⁻ therapy.
McCurdy DK: Mixed metabolic and respiratory acid-base disturbances: Diagnosis and treatment. Chest 62:35S–44S, 1972.
  The classic description of how to diagnose acid-base disorders.

81

Disorders of the Serum Sodium Concentration

Malcolm Cox

Disorders of the serum sodium concentration are manifestations of abnormal water (tonicity) homeostasis. They frequently accompany serious illness and can cause significant morbidity. *Hyponatremia* (serum sodium concentration <135 mEq/L) is usually associated with hypotonicity (hypotonic hyponatremia) but can also coexist with normal (isotonic hyponatremia) or elevated (hypertonic hyponatremia) body fluid tonicity. *Hypernatremia* (serum sodium concentration >145 mEq/L) is always associated with hypertonicity.

Hypotonic hyponatremia almost always reflects impaired renal diluting ability. Hypotonic hyponatremia is the defining feature of the syndrome of inappropriate antidiuretic hormone (SIADH) and is also commonly seen in patients with edematous disorders (cardiac failure, hepatic failure), sodium depletion (due to gastrointestinal fluid losses or diuretic use), and renal failure. This chapter, unless otherwise qualified, uses the term hyponatremia as synonymous with hypotonic hyponatremia.

Isotonic hyponatremia (also known as factitious or pseudohyponatremia) is a laboratory artifact seen with analytic methods that measure the amount of sodium per unit volume of serum sampled. In the presence of marked hypertriglyceridemia or paraproteinemia (producing an increased nonaqueous volume of the serum sample), the amount of sodium in the sample volume is reduced. This is reflected as a low serum sodium concentration, even though the concentration of sodium in serum water (and therefore plasma osmolality) is normal. Direct potentiometry (which uses an ion selective electrode in undiluted serum) avoids this problem and is becoming the most common method for measuring the serum sodium concentration clinically.

Hypertonic hyponatremia results from the presence in extracellular fluid of large amounts of osmotically effective solutes other than sodium—for example, glucose and mannitol. The osmotic pressure exerted by the nonsodium solutes leads to redistribution of water from the intracellular to the extracellular fluid compartment and thereby to hyponatremia. Hyperglycemia in association with poorly controlled diabetes mellitus is the most common cause of hypertonic hypernatremia (see Chapter 79).

Hypernatremia occurs most commonly in patients without free access to water (intubated, obtunded, or comatose) in whom excessive insensible and gastrointestinal water losses and defects in renal concentrating ability (due to solute diuresis, diuretic use, diabetes insipidus, or renal failure) frequently complicate the picture.

RESPONSE OF BRAIN CELLS TO TONICITY CHANGES

The clinical manifestations of hyponatremia and hypernatremia are largely attributable to changes in cell volume. Hypotonic hyponatremia is associated with hypotonicity and intracellular volume expansion, whereas hypernatremia results in intracellular volume contraction. Changes in cell water content are of greatest consequence in the brain, where the associated changes in metabolism are perhaps most critically expressed. In addition, because of the rigid calvarium, hyponatremia can increase intracranial pressure, leading to cerebral herniation. Conversely, the reduction in brain volume in patients with hypernatremia may predispose to intracerebral, subarachnoid, or subdural hemorrhage.

Well-developed regulatory mechanisms mitigate tonicity-related changes in brain volume. Volume changes are generally maximal 1 to 2 hours after the onset of acute hyponatremia or hypernatremia. Thereafter, cell volume returns toward normal over many hours. Thus, brain cells do not act as true osmometers, since changes in volume are less than those predicted by the change in the serum sodium concentration. This occurs because brain cells adapt to changes in tonicity by changing their intracellular solute content.

In adapting to *hyponatremia*, cells give up electrolytes to the extracellular fluid during the first 6 to 12 hours of adaptation. Over the next 24 to 72 hours, organic solutes (largely amino acids) are lost more slowly or are osmotically inactivated. Thus, full adaptation may take several days.

In the early phases of adaptation to *hypernatremia*, extracellular sodium chloride moves into cells. Over time, the brain also gains organic osmolytes, such as inositol from the extracellular fluid, as well as generates new organic solutes (so-called idiogenic osmoles), such as glutamine, glutamate, and taurine. Rates of new solute accumulation vary considerably among individuals and in different clinical situations, with full equilibration taking up to a week.

HYPONATREMIA

Presentation

The morbidity and mortality associated with hyponatremia are influenced by the magnitude and rate of development of the hyponatremia, the age and gender of the patient, and the nature and severity of any underlying diseases. At particular risk are the very young and very old, premenopausal women, and chronic alcoholics.

Neurologic symptoms usually do not occur until the serum sodium concentration falls to less than 125 mEq/L, at which point patients typically complain of anorexia, nausea, or generalized malaise. Between concentrations of 120 and 110 mEq/L, headache, lethargy, confusion, agitation, and obtundation are seen. More severe symptoms (seizures, coma, respiratory arrest) occur with levels less than 110 mEq/L. Focal neurologic findings are unusual.

Although symptoms generally resolve with correction of the hyponatremia, hyponatremia developing in less than 24 hours can be associated with residual neurologic deficits and may have a mortality rate as high as 50%. In contrast, when hyponatremia develops more gradually, symptoms are less frequent and less severe, so much so that some patients with chronic hyponatremia may be completely asymptomatic.

Pathophysiology and Differential Diagnosis

The primary abnormality in patients with (hypotonic) hyponatremia is the inability of the kidney to excrete sufficient electrolyte-free water to match water intake. This may be due to (1) excessive water ingestion in a setting of normal renal diluting ability or (2) impaired renal diluting ability with or without excessive water ingestion. Diluting defects may result from decreased delivery of fluid to the renal diluting segment (ascending limb of the loop of Henle and early distal convoluted tubule), abnormalities in the generation of electrolyte-free water in the diluting segment, or persistently elevated plasma vasopressin levels despite hyponatremia (Table 81–1).

The normal response to water ingestion producing even slight hyponatremia is the excretion of maximally dilute urine (urine osmolality < 100 mOsm/kg). Hence, a urine osmolality less than 100 mOsm/kg points to excessive water intake as the cause of the hyponatremia (Fig. 81–1). In contrast, a urine osmolality greater than 100 mOsm/kg in the face of hyponatremia signifies impaired renal diluting ability (with or without excessive water ingestion).

Hyponatremia may be associated with normal, decreased, or increased extracellular volume. Because the bedside determination of extracellular fluid volume is not always reliable, urinary indices of renal sodium handling (urinary sodium concentration, fractional excretion of sodium) are commonly used to supplement the clinical impression (see Fig. 81–1). Distinguishing between euvolemic and hypovolemic patients is a particular problem. In the absence of disorders that impair renal tubular sodium reabsorption, natriuresis provides strong evidence for euvolemic hyponatremia.

Syndrome of Inappropriate Antidiuretic Hormone

SIADH is the most common cause of hyponatremia in hospitalized patients and has many causes (Table 81–2). It is characterized by elevated circulating vasopressin levels in the absence of osmotic or hemodynamic stimuli to vasopressin release. Persistent secretion of vasopressin from the hypothalamic-pituitary axis, unregulated release of vasopressin or related peptides from extrahypothalamic sites

Table 81–1. Renal Diluting Defects

Decreased Delivery to Diluting Segment

Sodium depletion
Effective arterial hypovolemia

Diluting Segment Dysfunction

Loop diuretics
Thiazide diuretics

Elevated Plasma Vasopressin

Sodium depletion
Effective arterial hypovolemia
Syndrome of inappropriate antidiuretic hormone (SIADH)

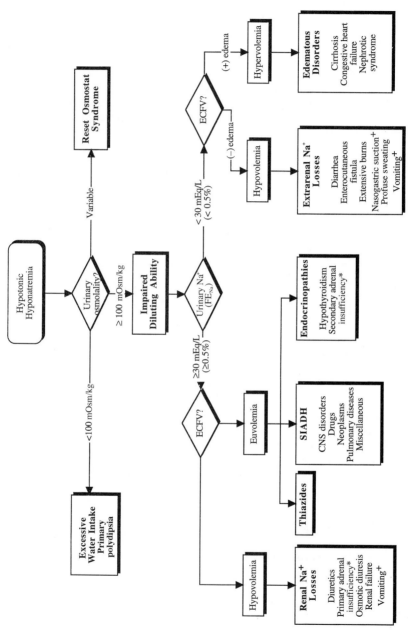

Figure 81–1. *See legend on opposite page*

Table 81–2. Causes of Syndrome of Inappropriate Diuretic Hormone (SIADH)
....

Central Nervous System Disorders

Head trauma, stroke, subdural hematoma, subarachnoid hemorrhage, brain tumors, encephalitis, meningitis, multiple sclerosis

Pulmonary Diseases

Pneumonia, tuberculosis, bronchiectasis, lung abscess, aspergillosis, asthma, cystic fibrosis

Neoplasms

Bronchogenic carcinoma, pancreatic carcinoma, duodenal carcinoma, prostatic carcinoma, lymphoma, thymoma

Drugs

Vasopressin analogs (e.g., desmopressin), oxytocin, opioids, apomorphine, barbiturates, general anesthetics, phenothiazines, tricyclic antidepressants, chlorpropamide, carbamazepine, clofibrate, vincristine, cyclophosphamide, thiazide diuretics, nonsteroidal anti-inflammatory agents

Miscellaneous

Pain, nausea, stress, positive-pressure ventilation, acquired immunodeficiency syndrome, hypokalemia
....

(ectopic SIADH), and renal hypersensitivity to vasopressin together with persistent vasopressin secretion all produce clinically identical pictures.

The diagnosis of SIADH is made on the basis of hypotonic hyponatremia (plasma osmolality < 280 mOsm/kg, serum sodium concentration < 135 mEq/L), and an inappropriately concentrated urine (urine osmolality > 100 mOsm/kg) after excluding other medical conditions (see Fig. 81–1). Water loading is unnecessary (and dangerous if the patient is severely hyponatremic) and plasma vasopressin levels are not useful in differentiating SIADH from other causes of hyponatremia. With the exception of primary polydipsia and the "reset osmostat syndrome," all sustained hyponatremia is associated with elevated vasopressin levels.

Reset Osmostat Syndrome

The reset osmostat syndrome may account for as many as one third of cases that at first sight appear to be classic SIADH. A formal water load can distinguish the

---

Figure 81–1. Schematic flow diagram to evaluate (hypotonic) hyponatremia. Because the normal kidney has an enormous capacity to excrete water, impaired renal diluting ability is the underlying cause of most hyponatremia. ECFV, extracellular fluid volume; FE_{Na}, fractional excretion of sodium = $100 \times (U_{Na} \times S_{Cr})/(S_{Na} \times U_{Cr})$, where S_{Na} is the serum sodium concentration, U_{Na} is the urine sodium concentration, and S_{Cr} and U_{Cr} are the serum and urine creatinine concentrations, respectively. The cutoff value for urine sodium concentration (30 mEq/L) is derived from hyponatremic patients proved to be either hypovolemic or euvolemic by their response to intravenous isotonic saline.

*Cortisol deficiency is associated with elevated plasma vasopressin levels, accounting for the euvolemic hyponatremia characteristic of secondary adrenal insufficiency; in patients with primary adrenal insufficiency (with glucocorticoid *and* mineralocorticoid deficiency), however, lack of aldosterone leads to renal sodium wasting and extracellular volume contraction.

†Vomiting and nasogastric suction are associated with sodium chloride depletion and metabolic alkalosis. In steady state metabolic alkalosis, U_{Na} is low, reflecting hypovolemia; during episodes of vomiting (or intermittent nasogastric suction), however, acute elevations in the serum bicarbonate concentration lead to bicarbonaturia and obligate urinary cation (sodium and potassium) loss.

two conditions but, again, this is dangerous to perform in severely hyponatremic patients. Unlike SIADH, patients with a reset osmostat defend body fluid tonicity around a depressed set point and usually have only mild to modest hyponatremia. Because their hyponatremia does not worsen on an "as wanted" fluid intake, water restriction is not required.

Thiazide-Induced Hyponatremia

Thiazide diuretics can produce severe, symptomatic hyponatremia in the absence of overt signs of volume depletion. Thiazide-induced hyponatremia is some four-fold more common in women than in men and usually develops within a few days of starting the diuretic. Although its cause is uncertain, subclinical volume contraction, inhibition of diluting segment function, primary polydipsia in the face of impaired renal diluting ability, SIADH, and potassium depletion have all been implicated. Aside from discontinuing the diuretic and any other drugs that may affect renal diluting ability (see Tables 81–1 and 81–2), treatment may also need to be directed at restoring extracellular fluid volume and body potassium stores.

Treatment of Asymptomatic Hyponatremia

The vast majority of patients with mild to moderate hyponatremia (serum sodium concentration between 120 and 135 mEq/L) are asymptomatic, and treatment should be directed at the underlying cause.

Euvolemic hyponatremia represents pure water excess, so treatment depends on restricting water intake to less than daily insensible stool and urinary water losses. In SIADH, potentially offending drugs should be discontinued and treatable causes identified (see Table 81–2). If water restriction alone is insufficient to maintain the serum sodium concentration at greater than 130 mEq/L, adjunctive therapy with demeclocycline may be of benefit. This agent blocks vasopressin-mediated water reabsorption in the collecting duct.

Hypovolemic hyponatremia arises when renal or extrarenal solute and water losses are replaced with electrolyte-free water. Treatment should be directed at repleting body sodium and potassium stores while identifying and correcting the cause of the excessive solute loss. If intravenous therapy is indicated, isotonic (0.9%) saline should be employed to restore intravascular volume and stabilize the blood pressure. Volume repletion readily elicits a water diuresis by increasing the delivery of fluid to the renal diluting segment and suppressing vasopressin release.

Resolution of the hyponatremia associated with any of the edematous disorders *(hypervolemic hyponatremia)* ultimately depends on correction of the process responsible for the intense sodium retention in these disorders. Unfortunately, this is rarely possible, so the mainstay of therapy for the hyponatremic edematous patient remains salt and water restriction. Diuretics are often a double-edged sword. They may be needed to treat pulmonary vascular congestion, peripheral edema, and ascites, but if used to excess can worsen effective arterial hypovolemia and exacerbate water retention. Strategies directed at increasing effective arterial blood volume (e.g., afterload reduction with angiotensin-converting enzyme inhibitors), however, have had some success in ameliorating hyponatremia in patients with congestive heart failure.

Treatment of Symptomatic Hyponatremia

Severe hyponatremia (serum sodium concentration < 120 mEq/L) can be life-threatening, and immediate therapy is usually required. Irrespective of cause, therapy is aimed at the same objective: to raise body fluid tonicity and shift water out of the intracellular space, thereby ameliorating cerebral edema. The rate of correction must be carefully regulated. Overly rapid correction has been associated with *central pontine myelinolysis*. Rapid correction is particularly risky in patients with chronic hyponatremia in whom cell volume adaptations are complete.

Osmotic demyelination typically occurs 2 to 6 days after treatment is initiated and is characterized by dysarthria, dysphagia, incoordination, quadriplegia and, in severe cases, coma. The cause of this devastating syndrome is controversial, but three factors have been implicated: (1) the duration of the hyponatremia, (2) the rate of correction of the hyponatremia, and (3) the magnitude of the change in the serum sodium concentration. Osmotic demyelination occurs most commonly during the treatment of chronic hyponatremia, following the rapid correction of hyponatremia, and especially if hyponatremia is *over*corrected.

In most circumstances, especially in patients with chronic hyponatremia or hyponatremia of unknown duration, *the serum sodium concentration should be raised by no more than 10 mEq/L in the first 24 hours, and by no more than 18 mEq/L in the first 48 hours (i.e., at a rate of approximately 0.5 mEq/L per hour).* In grave situations (serum sodium concentration < 105 mEq/L), initial therapy can be more aggressive—targeting a change in the serum sodium concentration of 1 to 2 mEq/L per hour for the first few hours, but the recommended daily target should not be exceeded. Full correction should take place over several days, and hypernatremia should be assiduously avoided.

Treatment is best accomplished with hypertonic (3%) saline. The amount of solute to be administered can be estimated as follows: A 70-kg man with a serum sodium concentration of 105 mEq/L has a total body water of 42 L (assumed to be equal to 60% of body weight). The amount of sodium needed to raise his serum sodium concentration by 10 mEq/L is 420 mEq (10 mEq/L × 42 L). Three percent saline has a sodium concentration of 513 mEq/L; therefore, about 820 mL of 3% saline (420/513 × 1000 mL) would be required in the first 24 hours.

Because it takes no account of ongoing solute and water losses, this calculation provides at best a rough estimate. Consequently, frequent measurements of the serum sodium concentration (initially every 2 to 4 hours) are mandatory, and these should be used to adjust the rate of correction. One should also be aware that rapid extracellular volume expansion with hypertonic saline can easily precipitate pulmonary edema, especially in patients with underlying heart disease. If this is a consideration, a loop diuretic (furosemide) can be administered simultaneously with the 3% saline.

Isotonic saline alone should never be used to treat hyponatremia in patients with SIADH. Water is retained and salt excreted so that the hyponatremia may actually worsen. The use of isotonic saline and furosemide in SIADH is also not recommended. Although effective, the rise in the serum sodium concentration is less predictable than with 3% saline, and large urinary potassium and magnesium losses often complicate the clinical picture.

HYPERNATREMIA

Presentation

The manifestations of hypernatremia depend on both the magnitude and the rate of rise of the serum sodium concentration. In general, the higher the serum sodium concentration, the greater the depression of the sensorium, and acute changes are generally less well tolerated than chronic changes. Central nervous system symptoms range from agitation, restlessness, confusion, and lethargy to stupor and coma, whereas other signs and symptoms also include nausea, vomiting, muscle weakness or fasciculations, and seizures.

Symptoms are unusual until the serum sodium concentration rises to greater than 150 to 155 mEq/L. The very young and the very old are at particular risk. Comorbidity must be taken into account when considering published mortality rates, which are as high as 40 to 60% in this often seriously ill group of patients. Symptoms generally resolve with correction of the hypernatremia, but permanent neurologic deficits may occur, particularly in acute, severe hypernatremia, when the brain's volume regulatory defenses are overwhelmed. When hypernatremia develops more gradually, symptoms are both less frequent and less severe and, as in chronic hyponatremia, some patients with chronic hypernatremia may be completely asymptomatic.

Changes in extracellular fluid volume and the presence of comorbid conditions commonly modify the presentation of hypernatremia, and may even dominate the clinical picture. For example, hypernatremia secondary to excess salt frequently is associated with symptoms of volume overload, whereas hypernatremia that results from the loss of hypotonic fluids is associated with signs of extracellular volume depletion. Changes in extracellular fluid volume may be of such significance that their treatment must take priority over the treatment of the hypernatremia itself.

Pathophysiology and Differential Diagnosis

Although renal water conservation serves as a first line of defense, the ultimate defense against dehydration is progressive thirst leading to water intake. Thus, the primary abnormality in most patients with hypernatremia is inadequate electrolyte-free water intake relative to the prevailing rate of cutaneous, gastrointestinal and renal losses (Fig. 81–2). Insufficient free water intake may be due to impaired thirst (hypodipsia) or an inability to obtain adequate amounts of water (obtunded or bedridden adults). Rarely, hypernatremia is due to a gain of sodium in excess of water.

Renal concentrating ability is rarely normal in the seriously ill, promoting hypernatremia in hospitalized patients. Concentrating ability may be impaired because of defects in the generation or maintenance of the corticopapillary osmotic gradient (protein malnutrition, diuretics, osmotic diuresis, renal failure), the synthesis or release of vasopressin (hypothalamic diabetes insipidus), or the action of vasopressin (nephrogenic diabetes insipidus).

Sodium Excess

Although uncommon in the general hospital population, sodium excess is an important iatrogenic cause of hypernatremia in the intensive care unit (ICU), particularly after treatment of hyponatremia or metabolic acidosis. The 3% saline solution commonly employed in the treatment of severe hyponatremia contains 513 mEq of sodium per liter. Even more hypertonic is the 7.5% sodium bicarbonate solution (890 mEq/L) sometimes used during cardiopulmonary resuscitation; this contains 44.5 mEq of sodium per ampule.

Hypodipsia

Isolated hypodipsia is rare; more commonly, hypodipsia coexists with abnormalities in vasopressin secretion. Some patients have partial hypothalamic diabetes insipidus, a combination that may produce severe, life-threatening hypernatremia. Others (with so-called essential hypernatremia) have selective osmoreceptor dysfunction, with vasopressin release being governed primarily by changes in extracellular fluid volume rather than by body fluid tonicity. These patients have more modest, nonprogressive hypernatremia and normal renal concentrating ability.

Many elderly individuals have impaired thirst. Furthermore, when dehydrated, even otherwise healthy elderly individuals sense less thirst and drink less than younger individuals, putting them at increased risk for hypernatremia should intercurrent illness stress the osmoregulatory system. The cause of this so-called geriatric hypodipsia has yet to be elucidated.

Diabetes Insipidus

Any pathologic process involving the hypothalamus above the sella turcica or near the base of the third ventricle may lead to vasopressin deficiency (Table 81–3); however, 80 to 85% of the vasopressin-secreting neurons must be destroyed for symptoms to be clinically significant.

Diabetes insipidus after head trauma or surgery may be transient, permanent, or even follow a triphasic course. The transient form is most common, with an abrupt onset within the first 24 hours and then resolution within several days or weeks. The permanent form also has an abrupt onset within the first 24 hours but does not resolve. In the triphasic pattern, there is an initial period of vasopressin deficiency, lasting 2 to 4 days (resulting from axonal injury), a 5- to 7-day period of inappropriate vasopressin release (due to leakage from the degenerating neurons) and, finally, permanent diabetes insipidus.

The diagnosis of diabetes insipidus is usually obvious if the patient presents with hypernatremia and dilute urine (osmolality less than 250 to 300 mOsm/kg). Although more subtle forms of diabetes insipidus occur (with polyuria as the only complaint in the patient's history), these would likely be difficult to diagnose in a

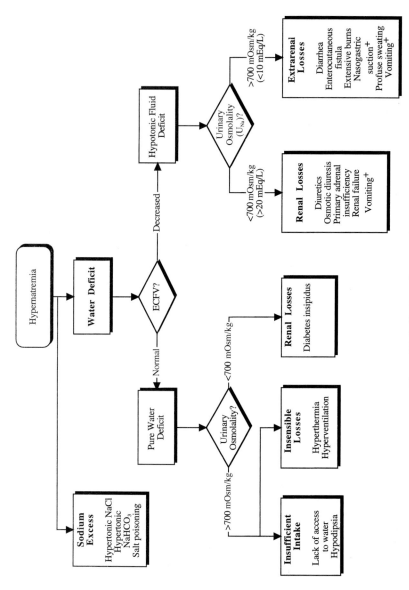

Figure 81-2. *See legend on opposite page*

Table 81–3. Causes of Hypothalamic Diabetes Insipidus

Head trauma
Pituitary surgery
Neoplasia
    Pituitary adenoma, craniopharyngioma, dysgerminoma, pinealoma, glioma, metastatic carcinoma
       (breast, lung), leukemia, lymphoma
Vascular lesions
    Ruptured aneurysm, cavernous sinus thrombosis, hypertensive encephalopathy, Sheehan's syndrome
       (postpartum pituitary infarction)
Infections
    Encephalitis, meningitis, tuberculosis, syphilis
Granulomatous diseases
    Sarcoidosis, histiocytosis X
Miscellaneous
    Hypoxic encephalopathy, idiopathic, hereditary forms

critically ill patient in the ICU setting. The diagnosis would require provocative tests that stress the osmoregulatory system—usually a simple overnight dehydration test, which would be difficult to perform or interpret in the typical ICU patient.

Nephrogenic diabetes insipidus also has many causes (Table 81–4). It can usually be readily differentiated from hypothalamic diabetes insipidus by the patient's failure to respond to exogenous vasopressin.

Treatment of Hypernatremia

The effective management of hypernatremia requires consideration of intravascular volume status and an appreciation of the cerebral adaptation to hypertonicity. Unless large, pure water losses are usually not associated with intravascular volume depletion. In contrast, tachycardia and hypotension are common when hypernatremia arises from hypotonic fluid losses, and the prompt restoration of adequate tissue perfusion is paramount. Optimal therapy is isotonic (0.9%) sodium chloride solution administered intravenously at a rate sufficient to stabilize the blood pressure.

Once intravascular volume status has been addressed, attention can be turned to the treatment of the hypernatremia itself. Although the rate of new intracellular

---

Figure 81–2. Schematic flow diagram to evaluate hypernatremia. Because hypernatremia is a potent stimulus to thirst, sustained hypernatremia always implies inadequate water intake. The cutoff value for renal concentrating ability (700 mmol/kg) is derived from hospitalized patients with no evidence of neurohypophyseal or renal disease. Precise cutoff values for the urine sodium concentration in hypernatremic patients with renal or extrarenal hypotonic fluid losses are not available; those provided should be considered approximations. ECFV, extracellular fluid volume; U_{Na}, urine sodium concentration.

†Vomiting and nasogastric suction are associated with sodium chloride depletion and metabolic alkalosis. In steady state metabolic alkalosis, U_{Na} is low, reflecting hypovolemia; during episodes of vomiting (or intermittent nasogastric suction), however, acute elevations in the serum bicarbonate concentration lead to bicarbonaturia and obligate urinary cation (sodium and potassium) loss.

Table 81–4. Causes of Nephrogenic Diabetes Insipidus

....

Drugs

Lithium, demeclocycline, amphotericin B, methoxyflurane

Electrolyte Disorders

Hypercalcemia, hypokalemia

Renal Disorders

Obstructive nephropathy, postobstructive diuresis, diuretic phase of acute tubular necrosis, renal transplant

Miscellaneous

Sjögren's syndrome, amyloidosis, multiple myeloma, sickle cell anemia, hereditary forms

....

solute generation in the brain has not been precisely defined, full adaptation to hypertonicity may take several days. Consequently, acute hypernatremia is poorly tolerated and should be treated more aggressively than chronic hypernatremia.

Before attempting rapid correction, it is important to establish firmly that the hypernatremia is *acute* in origin. Identifying acute hypernatremia is usually straightforward in patients with hypernatremia secondary to salt poisoning or iatrogenic hypertonic fluid administration but may be more difficult in other situations. Because the rapid correction of chronic hypernatremia is dangerous, aggressive therapy should *never* be employed when the duration of the hypernatremia cannot be established with reasonable certainty.

The rate at which new brain solute is removed (or inactivated) during therapy is even less well understood than its rate of generation. Cells that contain this new solute have a greater volume at any given body fluid tonicity than would be the case with a normal intracellular solute content. Consequently, rapidly returning tonicity to normal may produce cerebral edema and precipitate seizures, coma, permanent neurologic sequelae, or death. Therefore, the correction of chronic hypernatremia (or hypernatremia of *unknown duration*) should always proceed over a period of several days.

In general, no more than half the estimated deficit should be replaced during the first 24 hours, with careful monitoring of the patient's neurologic status and the serum sodium concentration. The remainder of the deficit can then be replaced over the ensuing 24 to 48 hours. The oral route is always preferable provided that the patient is alert and there is no risk of pulmonary aspiration. In other cases, 5% dextrose in water should be administered intravenously.

Calculation of the magnitude of an isolated water deficit (Equation 1) is based on total body sodium not changing so that the resultant hypernatremia is directly proportional to the deficit in total body water.

$$\text{Current TBW} \times \text{current } [\text{Na}^+] = \text{normal TBW} \times \text{normal } [\text{Na}^+] \quad \text{(Equation 1)}$$

where TBW = total body water, normal TBW = 60% of body weight, and normal $[\text{Na}^+]$ = 140 mEq/L.

For example, by Equation 1, in a patient weighing 60 kg with a serum sodium concentration of 160 mEq/L, current TBW = $(0.6 \times 60) \times (140/160) = 31.5$ L. Thus, the free water deficit is 4.5 L (36 L − 31.5 L).

Despite inherent inaccuracies in estimating normal total body water (using current rather than predehydration weight because the latter is rarely known and assuming total body water is 60% of body weight), this calculation provides an approximate value that can be used in planning therapy. The same calculation is often used to estimate the water deficit in hypernatremic patients with hypotonic fluid losses but, because of the associated electrolyte losses, it may underestimate the true water deficit. An accurate reflection of the residual water deficit, however, can be obtained once sodium and potassium deficits have been corrected.

In patients in whom hypernatremia is caused by excess salt (salt poisoning), the amount of water needed to correct the hypernatremia can be estimated in an analogous fashion. Of course, in this situation, there is no water deficit, and the water administered to correct body fluid tonicity will increase total body water to greater than normal. If it is clear that the hypernatremia is acute (<12 hours in duration), correction can be rapid; otherwise, the more conservative recommendations provided for the treatment of chronic hypernatremia should be followed. The rapid administration of electrolyte-free water should continue only until neurologic symptoms improve. Because many of these patients are also receiving potent diuretics, hemodialysis, or hemofiltration (treatment modalities that have their own unique effects on solute and water balance), close monitoring of neurologic status and the serum sodium concentration is mandatory. Frequent adjustments in the rate of water administration may be needed.

Once water repletion is under way, consideration should be given to estimating and replacing ongoing water losses. Both insensible (cutaneous and pulmonary) and renal water losses need to be considered. In addition, therapy for hypodipsia (prescription of an adequate water intake) and specific therapy for hyperthermia, hyperventilation, and diabetes insipidus should be initiated.

Treatment of Diabetes Insipidus

Water ingestion in sufficient quantity to maintain water balance and prevent hypernatremia is the mainstay of therapy for diabetes insipidus. Hormone replacement in hypothalamic diabetes insipidus has the goal of decreasing the polyuria and permitting maintenance of water balance with a more tolerable level of water intake. Because of the short duration of action and undesired pressor and coronary vasospastic effects of vasopressin itself, replacement therapy is best accomplished with the synthetic analog 1-deamino-8-D-arginine vasopressin (desmopressin or DDAVP). Desmopressin is usually administered intranasally at a dose of 5 to 20 µg, has an onset of action within 30 minutes, and a duration of action of 12 to 24 hours. Intravenous or subcutaneous administration is useful in patients in the ICU when intranasal insufflation may be difficult; when used in this manner, the usual dose is 5 to 20% of the intranasal nose.

Nephrogenic diabetes insipidus does not respond to hormone replacement therapy. Offending drugs should be discontinued, electrolyte disorders corrected, and any other underlying disorders addressed, if possible (see Table 81–4). Thiazide diuretics, in combination with salt and protein restriction, are important adjuncts to the therapy of nephrogenic diabetes insipidus. Volume depletion increases proximal tubular fluid reabsorption and decreases delivery of fluid to the distal nephron. Protein restriction reduces daily obligate solute excretion, thereby attenuating polyuria. Nonsteroidal anti-inflammatory agents, which block renal prostaglandin synthesis and enhance vasopressin-independent water reabsorption, have been used in selected patients with nephrogenic diabetes insipidus. Likewise, amiloride, which blocks the uptake of lithium by the renal collecting duct, has been used with some success in lithium-induced nephrogenic diabetes insipidus.

BIBLIOGRAPHY

Anderson RJ, Chung HM, Kluge R, Schrier RW: Hyponatremia: A prospective analysis of its epidemiology and the pathogenetic role of vasopressin. Ann Intern Med 102:164–168, 1985.
A prospective analysis of the incidence, etiology, clinical characteristics, and outcomes of hospitalized patients with hyponatremia.

Buonocore CM, Robinson AG: The diagnosis and management of diabetes insipidus during medical emergencies. Endocrinol Metab Clin North Am 22:411–423, 1993.
A practical review of the diagnosis and treatment of diabetes insipidus.

Chung HM, Kluge R, Schrier RW, Anderson RJ: Clinical assessment of extracellular fluid volume in hyponatremia. Am J Med 83:905–908, 1987.
The classic article describing the utility of the urine sodium concentration in the differential diagnosis of hyponatremia.

Kovacs L, Robertson GL: Syndrome of inappropriate antidiuresis. Endocrinol Metab Clin North Am 21:859–875, 1992.
A practical review of the diagnosis and treatment of the syndrome of inappropriate antidiuretic hormone.

Lauriat SM, Berl T: The hyponatremic patient: Practical focus on therapy. J Am Soc Nephrol 8:1599–1607, 1997.
A practical description of the evaluation and management of the different categories of hyponatremia.

McManus ML, Churchwell KB, Strange K: Regulation of cell volume in health and disease. New Engl J Med 333:1260–1266, 1995.
A review of the cellular and molecular events underlying cell volume homeostasis and their relevance to clinical practice.

Palevsky PM, Bhagrath R, Greenberg A: Hypernatremia in hospitalized patients. Ann Intern Med 124:197–203, 1996.
A prospective analysis of the incidence, etiology, clinical characteristics, and outcomes of hospitalized patients with hypernatremia.

Rose BD: New approach to disturbances in the plasma sodium concentration. Am J Med 83:905–908, 1986.
A classic review of the pathogenesis of hyponatremia and hypernatremia.

Szerlip H, Palevsky PM, Cox M: Sodium and water. In: Rock RC, Noe DA (eds): Laboratory Medicine: The Selection and Interpretation of Clinical Laboratory Studies. Baltimore, Williams and Wilkins, 1994, pp 692–731.
An exhaustive review of disorders of sodiuim and water homeostasis.

Zerbe RL, Robertson GL: A comparison of plasma vasopressin measurements with a standard indirect test in the differential diagnosis of polyuria. New Engl J Med 305:1539–1546, 1981.
The classic article describing the physiologic basis for the differential diagnosis and classification of polyuria.

82

Thyroid and Adrenal Disorders

Kelly D. Davis

Adaptive endocrine and metabolic responses are important components of any medical illness. However, failure to treat hormonal diseases appropriately in critically ill patients usually results from failure to recognize the disorder. This chapter discusses the clinical presentation, diagnosis, and management of hypothyroidism, thyrotoxicosis, and adrenal insufficiency in the intensive care unit (ICU).

THYROID FUNCTION IN NONTHYROIDAL ILLNESS

Nonthyroidal illness (NTI), also called the *euthyroid sick syndrome,* is the most common hormonal abnormality in the ICU, affecting more than 50% of critically ill patients. During illness, thyroid function and the concentration of biologically active thyroid hormones are reduced in proportion to the severity of the illness. Despite extensive descriptions of NTI, the physiologic significance and cause remain unknown. Teleologically, NTI is adaptive, slowing metabolism and conserving energy in the setting of physiologic stress or starvation.

Under normal conditions, thyroxine (T_4) is 5'-monodeiodinated to triiodothyronine (T_3), the most active thyroid hormone. In NTI, however, deiodination is shifted to an alternative pathway, resulting instead in biologically inactive reverse T_3 (rT_3) production. Therefore, the earliest and most universal abnormality in sick patients is a low serum T_3 concentration. The mechanism for inhibition of the 5'-monodeiodinase enzyme is poorly understood. In some patients in the ICU, drugs known to inhibit the enzyme may also contribute to this inhibition (glucocorticoids, propranolol in high doses and amiodarone).

In the critically ill patient, the serum total T_4 is often low (<1 to 2 mg/dL). Poor nutrition augments T_4 diminution by producing reductions in serum levels of thyroid-binding globulin (TBG) and other thyroid hormone–binding proteins (prealbumin and albumin). The commonly high-normal or increased T_3 resin uptake can be explained by the low serum levels of TBG and possibly by a circulating inhibitor of T_4 binding to TBG. T_4 production by the thyroid gland remains low because the hypothalamic-pituitary axis fails to respond by increasing thryrotropin-releasing hormone and thyroid-stimulating hormone (TSH). Administration of drugs, such as glucocorticoids and dopamine, can also suppress TSH secretion. Therefore, the TSH level is typically normal or even subnormal, indicating an inappropriate pituitary response to the low T_3–low T_4 state. A minority of patients have TSH levels elevated to the 5 to 20 µIU/mL range, especially during recovery from illness. A TSH level greater than 20 µIU/mL strongly suggests the diagnosis of primary hypothyroidism. Euthyroid hypothyroxinemia in the setting of severe illness has a dismal prognosis. It is often a challenge to exclude or confirm concurrent hypothyroidism in severely ill patients (especially secondary or central hypothyroidism, in which the TSH would be expected to be low). Therefore, it is important to limit evaluation of thyroid function to patients in

931

whom there is reasonable suspicion on clinical grounds. As shown in Figure 82–1, the best way to distinguish hypothyroidism and NTI is to measure free T_4 levels, which are usually normal or even slightly high in NTI and low in hypothyroidism. The rT_3 levels can also be helpful and are generally increased in NTI and low in hypothyroidism. Treating NTI in critically ill patients with thyroid hormone not only is ineffective in improving the outcome but also may be harmful.

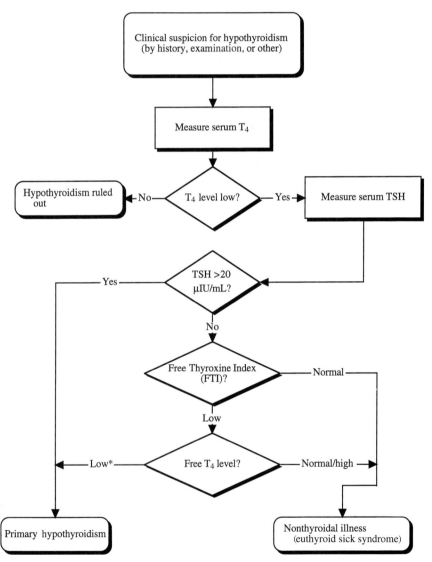

Figure 82–1. Laboratory evaluation in nonthyroidal illness of the critically ill. *Also consider secondary hypothyroidism with these results. T_4, thyroxine; TSH, thyroid-stimulating hormone.

MYXEDEMA COMA

Myxedema coma is a medical emergency that represents the end-stage of severe decompensated hypothyroidism. Fortunately, it is now a rare presentation of hypothyroidism because improved and widely available laboratory tests for measurement of T_4 and TSH allow diagnosis earlier in the course of disease. Most patients with myxedema coma are elderly and have alterations in mental status as well as hypothermia and hypotension. These are usually precipitated by an acute illness or event. Early recognition and therapy are essential because the untreated disorder is associated with a high mortality rate.

Pathophysiology

Virtually every organ system and many metabolic pathways are altered in severe hypothyroidism. To compensate for diminished thermogenesis, peripheral blood vessels constrict. Blood is therefore shunted centrally to maintain a normal core body temperature. Hypothyroidism also decreases beta-adrenergic responsiveness. In long-standing untreated hypothyroidism, these adaptive responses lead to diastolic hypertension and a reduction in blood volume. Eventually these hypothyroid-induced changes become so severe that the patient cannot compensate for the decreased cardiac output, which results in decreased cerebral blood flow. Myxedema coma may be the culmination of severe, long-standing hypothyroidism but is usually hastened by an acute event such as infection, myocardial infarction, cold exposure, or sedative administration.

Epidemiology and Etiology

Since older women have the highest incidence of hypothyroidism, they also have the highest incidence of myxedema coma. The latter may result from any of the usual causes of hypothyroidism, usually chronic autoimmune thyroiditis or postsurgical or postablative hypothyroidism (Table 82–1). Observing a thyroidec-

Table 82–1. Causes of Hypothyroidism Relevant to Patients in the Intensive Care Unit

....

Primary (thyroidal)
  Chronic autoimmune thyroiditis
  Drugs (antithyroid thionamides, amiodarone,
    lithium, interferon-alfa, interleukin-2,
    perchlorate)
  Infiltrative diseases of the thyroid gland
  Iodine (deficiency or excess)
  After radioiodine therapy or external irradiation
  After thyroidectomy
  Recovery from thyroiditis
Hypothalamic or pituitary disease
Generalized thyroid hormone resistance

....

tomy scar on the neck or discovering a history of iodine-131 therapy or previous hypothyroidism provide clues to the diagnosis. When a history can be obtained from family members, there have often been antecedent symptoms of thyroid dysfunction followed by progressive lethargy, stupor, and coma.

Clinical Picture

The hallmarks of myxedema coma are decreased mental status and hypothermia, but hypotension, bradycardia, hyponatremia, hypoglycemia, and hypoventilation are frequently present. One should also always search for a precipitating infection or acute illness. Decreased thermogenesis observed in the hypothyroid state results in hypothermia. Severe hypothermia may not be recognized because many thermometers do not register frankly hypothermic body temperatures. Approximately half of myxedema coma patients have hyponatremia that may be severe and contribute to the abnormal mental status. Most patients have impairment in renal free water excretion due to inappropriately high serum levels of vasopressin, which reverses after thyroid hormone replacement. Thus, myxedema is one cause of the syndrome of inappropriate antidiuretic hormone secretion.

Hypoventilation with respiratory acidosis results primarily from central depression of ventilatory drive, but mechanical obstruction by a large tongue or respiratory muscle weakness, or both, may also contribute. Hypoglycemia may be caused by hypothyroidism alone or it may coexist with adrenal insufficiency. Although a decrease in functional beta-adrenergic receptors seen in chronic hypothyroidism leads to bradycardia and decreased myocardial contractility, frank congestive heart failure is rare. Pericardial effusions may contribute to diminished auscultated heart sounds, low voltage seen on the electrocardiogram, and a large cardiac silhouette on chest radiography. All the cardiac abnormalities are reversible with appropriate thyroid hormone replacement, administered cautiously because of the risk of precipitating arrhythmias or myocardial infarction.

Treatment

Myxedema coma is an endocrine emergency that needs aggressive treatment. The diagnosis is based on the history, physical examination, and exclusion of other causes of coma. Emergent treatment should be instituted in any patient suspected of having the condition, even before confirmatory laboratory results are available. Before treatment, serum should be drawn for measurement of T_4, TSH, and cortisol (because of the possibility of associated adrenal insufficiency or hypopituitarism causing both thyroid and adrenal dysfunction). The T_4 level is usually extremely low and an elevated TSH concentration confirms the diagnosis of primary hypothyroidism. However, in myxedema coma from secondary hypothyroidism (hypothalamic or pituitary dysfunction), the TSH concentration is usually normal or low.

The exact mode of thyroid hormone replacement in myxedema coma is controversial, largely because the condition is so rare that there are no controlled clinical trials comparing the efficacy of different regimens. Immediate restoration of serum thyroid hormone levels is essential but carries a risk of precipitating myocardial infarction or cardiac arrhythmias. Many experts prefer treatment with intravenous

T_4 (levothyroxine sodium), allowing the patient's deiodinase to produce T_3. An initial dose of 0.3 to 0.6 mg should be followed by daily doses of 0.05 to 0.1 mg. After clinical improvement, the daily replacement can be converted to an equivalent oral dose. The serum T_4 and TSH concentrations should be monitored to avoid overtreatment. Although levothyroxine sodium administration produces a smooth clinical response, other authors advocate administration of T_3 (liothyronine sodium) because of its greater biologic activity. Also, patients with myxedema coma and superimposed NTI theoretically have low serum levels of the 5'-deiodinase required to convert T_4 to T_3. Recommended dosing of liothyronine sodium is 25 mg intravenously every 8 hours for the first 24 to 48 hours. Therapy with levothyroxine sodium (0.05 to 0.1 mg/day) may be initiated once the patient tolerates oral medication.

General supportive measures are tremendously important in the management of patients with myxedema coma. Hypotension may take hours to days to be corrected by thyroid hormone. Therefore, severe hypotension that does not respond to fluids should be managed with vasopressors until the levothyroxine sodium has time to act. Passive rewarming is preferred over active external rewarming because of the risk of vasodilatation and worsening hypotension. Until coexisting adrenal insufficiency is excluded, patients with life-threatening hypothyroidism should receive glucocorticoids in stress doses (hydrocortisone given intravenously, 100 mg every 8 hours).

Chronically hypothyroid patients hospitalized in the ICU setting may have their oral levothyroxine sodium discontinued for several days without significant adverse effects. If it is necessary for the patient to be fasting for a more lengthy period, levothyroxine sodium can be administered intravenously. However, the dosage should be adjusted to approximately 75% of the oral dose to compensate for differences in absorption of the parenteral and oral preparations.

HYPERTHYROIDISM

The clinical syndrome of thyrotoxicosis results from the body's response to excessive serum concentrations of T_4 or T_3. Most commonly, autonomous overproduction of T_4 and T_3 by the thyroid gland (primary hyperthyroidism) produces thyrotoxicosis with an increased radioactive iodine uptake. In others, however, the thyroid gland is inactive, with excessive T_3 and T_4 either released from a damaged gland or ingested. In these individuals, the radioactive iodine uptake is low. Excessive pituitary secretion of TSH (secondary or central hyperthyroidism) is a rare cause of thyrotoxicosis. Most hyperthyroid patients are young and able to tolerate the hypermetabolic state such that evaluation and treatment as a rule occur in the outpatient setting. Rarely, however, a patient presents with life-threatening, decompensated hyperthyroidism ("thyroid storm") in which the usual manifestations of thyrotoxicosis are accompanied by fever, tachycardia, and altered mental status (agitation, delirium, psychosis, stupor, or coma).

Clinical Manifestations

Because thyroid hormone accelerates metabolic processes in every tissue, thyrotoxicosis affects multiple organ systems (Table 82–2). Many thyroid hormone effects

Table 82–2. Signs, Symptoms, and Laboratory Abnormalities in Hyperthyroidism

Signs	Hyperreflexia; hypertension; lid retraction; muscle weakness; restlessness; smooth, warm, moist skin; stare; tachycardia; tremor
Symptoms	Dyspnea, heat intolerance, hyperdefecation, increased appetite, insomnia, mood changes, nervousness, palpitations, sweating tremulousness, weakness and fatigue, weight loss
Hemodynamics	Decreased systemic vascular resistance, increased stroke volume, tachycardia
Laboratory Findings	Increased T_4 levels, low TSH (in primary hyperthyroidism), hypercalcemia, increased transaminase levels, low cholesterol

TSH, thyroid-stimulating hormone.

suggest activation of the adrenergic nervous system, mediated by increased sensitivity to catecholamines rather than elevated catecholamine concentrations. Elderly thyrotoxic patients may present with isolated weight loss, atrial fibrillation, congestive heart failure, or muscle weakness without prominent signs of increased metabolism. This syndrome of *apathetic hyperthyroidism* should be considered in the differential diagnosis of any patient who presents with one of these conditions.

Causes

One should always identify the underlying cause of hyperthyroidism (Table 82–3). The clinical evaluation can provide important diagnostic clues (duration of symptoms, recent exposure to radioiodine contrast agents, thyroid size or tenderness, or extrathyroidal manifestations of Graves' disease) that can help formulate the best form of therapy. Most patients requiring intensive care have severe thyrotoxicosis due to Graves' disease, toxic multinodular goiter, or overdosage with exogenous liothyronine sodium or levothyroxine sodium.

Table 82–3. Causes of Hyperthyroidism and Associated Findings

CAUSE	CLUES	RADIOACTIVE IODINE UPTAKE
Graves' disease	Ophthalmopathy, thyroid bruit	High
Toxic adenoma	Palpable thyroid nodule	High
Toxic multinodular goiter	Goiter, usually elderly patients	High
Ingestion of T_4	No goiter, low thyroid-binding globulin	Low
Subacute thyroiditis	Thyroid usually tender, erythrocyte sedimentation rate high	Low

T_4, thyroxine.

Treatment

Treatment of severe thyrotoxicosis requires the use of several drugs to decrease thyroid hormone production, inhibit release of stored thyroid hormone from the gland, block conversion of T_4 to T_3, and antagonize catecholaminergic effects (Table 82–4). Antithyroid drugs, which inhibit thyroid hormone synthesis by blocking organification and coupling reactions, are not available in parenteral forms and must therefore be given by nasogastric tube in emergency situations. Propylthiouracil is preferred over methimazole because it also inhibits T_4 to T_3 conversion. Iodides acutely block both release and synthesis of thyroid hormones from the gland. Antithyroid drugs *must* be administered 1 to 2 hours before giving iodides in order to prevent acute hyperthyroidism if thyroid synthetic function was not adequately inhibited. Therefore, beta-blockers should be given initially, followed by propylthiouracil, glucocorticoids and, finally, iodide.

ADRENAL INSUFFICIENCY

De novo adrenal insufficiency is an uncommon clinical problem, occurring in less than 5% of patients admitted to an ICU setting. However, many critically ill patients (>30% in one study) are either receiving glucocorticoid therapy for another condition or have known adrenal insufficiency. Therefore, familiarity with the management of this condition is essential.

Table 82–4. Treatment of Severe Hyperthyroidism

DRUG	DOSE	MECHANISM
Beta-Blockers		
Propranolol	40–80 mg orally every 6 h or 2–4 mg IV every 4 h (adjust to maintain control of heart rate)	Antagonizes adrenergic effects Inhibits $T_4 \rightarrow T_3$ conversion
Antithyroid Agents		
Propylthiouracil	200–300 mg orally every 4–6 h	Blocks T_4-T_3 synthesis Inhibits $T_4 \rightarrow T_3$ conversion
Methimazole	30 mg orally every 6 h	Blocks T_4-T_3 synthesis
Glucocorticoids		
Dexamethasone	2 mg IV every 6 h	Inhibits $T_4 \rightarrow T_3$ conversion
Iodide	Lugol's solution (SSKI) 5–8 drops orally every 6 h	Interferes with release of T_4-T_3 Inhibits $T_4 \rightarrow T_3$ conversion
Plasmapheresis		Reduces circulating T_3 and T_4
Exchange Transfusion		Reduces circulating T_3 and T_4

IV, intravenously; SSKI, saturated solution of potassium iodide; T_4, thyroxine; T_3, triiodothyronine.

Etiology

The adrenal gland is composed of two functionally and anatomically distinct parts, the cortex and medulla. The cortex produces mineralocorticoids (e.g., aldosterone), glucocorticoids (e.g., cortisol), and adrenal androgens. The adrenal medulla is derived from neuroendocrine tissue and secretes catecholamines in concert with the sympathetic nervous system. Approximately 90% of adrenal cortical function must be lost before the deficiency becomes clinically apparent.

Although tuberculosis was the most common cause of adrenal insufficiency in the first half of the 20th century, *autoimmune adrenalitis* now causes the majority of cases. This may occur as an isolated deficiency or as part of a familial autoimmune polyglandular syndrome. Other causes seen in patients in the ICU (Table 82–5) include hemorrhage and infarction (associated with septic shock, anticoagulation, or the antiphospholipid antibody syndrome) and infection (systemic fungal infections or, in patients with acquired immunodeficiency disease, opportunistic infections). Secondary adrenal insufficiency (deficiency of corticotropin-releasing hormone or adrenocorticotropic hormone [ACTH], or both) occurs with underlying hypothalamic or pituitary disease or adrenal axis suppression from chronic glucocorticoid therapy.

Clinical Manifestations

The symptoms of adrenal insufficiency (weakness, fatigue, orthostatic dizziness and hypotension, anorexia, weight loss, nausea, vomiting, abdominal cramps, diarrhea, and fever) are nonspecific and often attributed to other causes. Hyperpigmentation of the skin and mucous membranes may provide important clues to primary and chronic hypoadrenalism but are absent in patients with secondary adrenal insufficiency or acute primary adrenal insufficiency, for example, adrenal

Table 82–5. Selected Causes of Adrenal Insufficiency

Primary Adrenal Insufficiency

AIDS (opportunistic infections or Kaposi's sarcoma)
Autoimmune adrenalitis (isolated or associated with autoimmune polyglandular syndrome)
Bilateral adrenal hemorrhage or infarction (anticoagulation, septic shock)
Fungal infections (blastomycosis, histoplasmosis, cryptococcosis)
Metastatic carcinoma or lymphoma
Tuberculosis

Secondary Adrenal Insufficiency

Head trauma
Histiocytosis X
Hypothalamic, pituitary mass lesions
Pituitary apoplexy
Pituitary surgery or irradiation
Sarcoidosis
Sheehan's syndrome

AIDS, acquired immunodeficiency syndrome.

hemorrhage. ACTH does not primarily regulate mineralocorticoid secretion, and therefore hyperkalemia (indicating aldosterone deficiency) suggests primary rather than secondary adrenal insufficiency. Hypoadrenalism should be considered in any critically ill patient with unexplained hypotension resistant to pressors, fever, hyponatremia, or hyperkalemia. In addition, the diagnosis of bilateral adrenal hemorrhage or infarction may be an underling factor in any patient with upper abdominal pain and hypotension, especially in the setting of anticoagulation, sepsis, or the antiphospholipid antibody syndrome.

Diagnosis

The simplest screening test for adrenal insufficiency is the rapid ACTH stimulation test, which tests the adrenal glands' output of cortisol in response to a pharmacologic bolus of synthetic ACTH. Plasma cortisol is measured before and 30 to 60 minutes after the intravenous or intramuscular injection of 0.25 mg of cosyntropin. The peak response should exceed 20 mg/dL. Patients with high basal cortisol levels may have little further increase because of pre-existing maximal adrenal stimulation. Although a subnormal response indicates adrenal insufficiency in most cases, patients with secondary adrenal insufficiency may normally respond to the rapid ACTH stimulation test because the amount of cosyntropin used in the test is at least 100 times normal physiologic concentrations.

Development of an accurate assay for ACTH has been important in the evaluation of patients with suspected adrenal insufficiency. The ACTH concentration can now be used to distinguish primary from secondary adrenal insufficiency in the same way as TSH is used in the evaluation of hypothyroidism. If there is a high index of suspicion for adrenal insufficiency on clinical grounds and the patient will be treated with glucocorticoids while awaiting the results of the cosyntropin test, the ACTH level should be determined before institution of exogenous glucocorticoids (which suppress ACTH production).

Therapy

Adrenal crisis consists of severe hypotensive shock that is poorly responsive to fluids and pressors and may be accompanied by nausea, vomiting, and hyponatremia. Fluid resuscitation should be initiated with normal saline containing 5% dextrose as the first step, followed by a rapid cosyntropin test with basal and 30-minute measurements of cortisol and an ACTH level. Therapy with glucocorticoids (hydrocortisone, 100 mg intravenously every 8 hours) should be continued until the cortisol results are available. If normal, glucocorticoid therapy may be discontinued abruptly. If abnormal, stress steroids should be continued until the patient begins to improve, and then the dose may be tapered over several days to a maintenance dose, usually 30 mg of oral hydrocortisone daily (20 mg in the morning and 10 mg with lunch).

BIBLIOGRAPHY

Annane D, Sébille V, Troché G, et al: A 3-level prognostic classification in septic shock based on cortisol levels and cortisol response to corticotropin. JAMA 283:1038–1045, 2000.
This observational study of 189 consecutive ICU admissions with septic shock showed that three categories based on baseline cortisol levels and responses to corticotropin correlated with different risks of death at 28 days. The highest risk of death was in patients with a baseline cortisol >34 μg/dL and a rise not greater than 9 μg/dL after corticotropin.

Chopra IJ: Euthyroid sick syndrome: Is it a misnomer? J Clin Endocrinol Metab 82:329–334, 1997.
This review describes how to evaluate abnormalities in thyroid function tests in critically ill patients and argues to avoid use of "euthyroid sick syndrome" (with 98 references).

Drucker D, Shandling M: Variable adrenocortical function in acute medical illness. Crit Care Med 13:477–479, 1985.
This report described measured plasma ACTH and cortisol levels and response to ACTH administration in 40 severely ill patients. It found plasma cortisol levels were commonly elevated but with considerable variability and no evidence of occult adrenocortical insufficiency.

Franklyn JA: The management of hyperthyroidism. N Engl J Med 330:1731–1738, 1994.
This is a comprehensive review of the topic by an authority in the field (with 89 references).

Hylander B, Rosenquist U: Treatment of myxedema coma—Factors associated with a fatal outcome. Acta Endocrinol 180:65–71, 1985.
This analysis of the causes of death of 11 myxedema coma patients emphasized the importance of using a cautious replacement regimen.

McIver B, Gorman CA: Euthyroid sick syndrome: an overview. Thyroid 7:125–132, 1997.
This is a review of euthyroid sick syndrome (with 120 references).

Monig H, Arendt T, Meyer M, et al: Activation of the hypothalamo-pituitary axis in response to septic or non-septic diseases—implications for the euthyroid sick syndrome. Intensive Care Medicine 25:1402–1406, 1999.
This study found that the changes in thyroid function tests indicating NTS were present in patients with sepsis upon ICU admission.

Nicoloff JT, LoPresti JS: Myxedema coma: A form of decompensated hypothyroidism. Endocrinol Metabol Clin North Am 22:279–290, 1993.
This is a review of myxedema coma describing its major pathophysiological alterations and the use and limitations of thyroid hormone therapy for its treatment (with 27 references).

Oelkers W: Adrenal insufficiency. N Engl J Med 335:1206–1212, 1996.
This is a comprehensive review of the topic, including testing with corticotropin and emergency therapy (with 34 references).

Utiger RD: Altered thyroid function in nonthyroidal illness and surgery—To treat or not to treat? N Engl J Med 333:1562–1563, 1995.
This is an editoral on nonthyroidal illness and its treatment with triiodothyronine.

How to Read and Understand the Anesthesia Record

83

Stuart J. Weiss
David Fish

The introduction of the anesthesia record into medical practice is attributed to Harvey Cushing. In 1895, he devised a graphic chart of the pulse and blood pressure during ether anesthesia at the Massachusetts General Hospital. Today, the anesthesia record continues to provide a graphic picture of hemodynamic measurements as well as accounts of significant intraoperative events and interventions. All too often, the "brief" surgical note includes scanty information and usually concludes that "the patient tolerated the procedure and was transferred to the PACU (postanesthesia care unit) or intensive care unit (ICU) in stable condition." Under these circumstances, the anesthesia record can be a key source for information about the patient during the surgical procedure. The anesthesia record, with its timeline of events and data, should be used to supplement the even more important direct communication between anesthetist and intensivist ("doctor-to-doctor report") about clinically significant intraoperative events.

ORGANIZATION OF THE TRADITIONAL ANESTHESIA RECORD

The appearance and organization of the anesthesia record varies among institutions but retains the same basic format and elements (Fig. 83–1 and Table 83–1). Common elements include a brief review of preoperative data, patient demographics, diagnosis, surgical procedure, names of health care professionals, charting, and annotative description of the intraoperative course. The record documents events, hemodynamics, and pharmacotherapy from the period before induction of anesthesia until arrival in the postanesthesia care unit or ICU. Under most circumstances, vital signs are recorded every 5 minutes.

The *event narrative section* is frequently the most useful but also one of the most difficult areas of the record to interpret. In this section, the anesthetist records intraoperative events, often in a manner that may be difficult to read and understand because of space limitations, legibility, or both. Nevertheless, crucial data that are not recorded elsewhere, such as interpretation of hemodynamic changes and intraoperative complications, can be found in this section. Many postoperative problems result from, or relate to, intraoperative events or management strategies.

REVIEWING THE ANESTHESIA RECORD ON THE PATIENT'S ADMISSION TO THE INTENSIVE CARE UNIT

On the patient's arrival in the ICU, the intensivist should review the preoperative data section and confirm the diagnosis and surgical procedure. It is important to

941

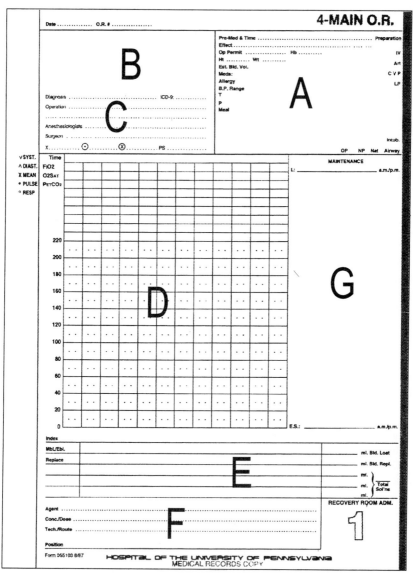

Figure 83–1. Common elements of a typical traditional anesthesia record include preoperative patient demographic data *(A)*; name, hospital identification number *(B)*; surgical procedure, times, personnel, and diagnosis *(C)*; a graphic record of monitored parameters (heart rate, systolic and diastolic blood pressure, oxygen saturation by pulse oximetry, and body temperature) *(D)*; fluid balance (blood loss, urine output, and volume and type of fluids administered) *(E)*; totals of drugs administered *(F)*; and annotation of operative events *(G)*.

Table 83–1. Common Elements of the Anesthesia Record

Patient demographics	Name
	Hospital identification number
	Date of birth
Preoperative data	Synopsis of past medical history
	Height, weight
	Medications
	Drug allergies
	Baseline blood pressure
	Physical status classification (I-V, E)*
Surgical procedure	Date of surgery
	Times (start, completion)
	Diagnoses
	Names of surgeon and anesthesiologist
	Operation or operations performed
Graphic record section	
Hemodynamic monitors	Systolic and diastolic BP, CVP, PA pressure, PAWP, cardiac output
Respiratory monitors	End-tidal P_{CO_2} by capnography
	Sa_{O_2} by pulse oximetry
	F_{IO_2}
	Peak inspiratory pressure
	Minute ventilation, respiratory rate, tidal volume
Miscellaneous data	Body temperature
	Urine output
	Blood loss
Drugs administered	Anesthetic agents (inhaled anesthetic, opioids, sedatives, epidural infusions)
	Vasoactive agents
	Neuromuscular blocking agents
Totals	Estimated blood loss
	Fluids (crystalloid, colloid, blood products)
	Urine output
	Summation of drug quantities
Annotations	Location and type of intravenous access
	Airway (ease of mask ventilation, intubation)
	Type of laryngoscope used for intubation
	Size of endotracheal tube and distance from tip and location where it was secured
Events	Induction
	Intubation (degree of difficulty)
	Placement of nerve block
	Start surgery
	Acute critical events, e.g., aortic cross-clamp applied
	Drug administration (antibiotics, neuromuscular blocking agent and reversal agent)
	Laboratory data (arterial blood gas, Na^+, K^+, CBC)

BP, blood pressure; CVP, central venous pressure; PA, pulmonary artery; PAWP, pulmonary artery wedge pressure; CBC, complete blood count.

*American Society of Anesthesiologists (ASA): New classification of physical status. Anesthesiology 24:111, 1963 (ASA I, healthy patient; ASA II, mild systemic disease; ASA III, severe systemic disease; ASA IV, severe systemic disease that is a constant threat to life; ASA V, moribund patients unlikely to survive 24 h with or without surgery; the suffix "E" is added if surgery is an emergency, e.g., ASA IVE).

read the event narrative section, noting any critical events such as the response to anesthesia and any difficulties with airway management. The hemodynamic response to the induction of anesthesia, intubation of the trachea, and surgical stresses provide clues as to the inadequacy of the patient's intravascular volume or the presence of myocardial dysfunction or reduced cardiac reserve. Occurrence of cardiac dysrhythmias or myocardial ischemia will also be noted in the event narrative section. Although a rhythm strip is unlikely to be part of the anesthesia record, specific ST-segment and electrocardiographic lead information may be described. The relationship of dysrhythmias to intraoperative events, for example, bradycardia during traction on the viscera, and the rhythm's response to therapeutic intervention can help guide postoperative management.

If new clinical problems occur in the immediate postoperative period after the patient's admission to the ICU, the anesthetic record can provide important information to consider as part of the differential diagnosis (Tables 83–2 to 83–5).

Choices of Intraoperative Monitoring

The choice and aggressiveness of intraoperative monitors reflects the anesthesiologist's expectations regarding the invasiveness of the surgical procedure, intraopera-

Table 83–2. Respiratory Distress Occurring in the Immediate Postoperative Period

POSSIBLE CAUSES	DIFFERENTIAL DIAGNOSIS AND COMMENTS
Aspiration	Review documentation of induction and emergence for critical events, placement of nasal gastric tube
Central respiratory depression	Residual anesthetic agents, central effects of systemic or epidural opioids
Congestive heart failure	History of cardiac dysfunction preoperatively, review net fluid balance and totals
Diaphragmatic dysfunction	Phrenic nerve dysfunction during cold cardioplegia or mobilization of internal mammary artery, site of surgery (upper abdominal or thoracic surgery)
Endobronchial intubation	Check presence of bilateral breath sounds and where tube was secured during intubation and obtain chest radiograph
Exacerbation of pre-existing pulmonary disease	Check past medical history, preinduction arterial blood gas results, check for use of beta-blockers in patient with prior obstructive airway disease
Inspiratory stridor	Laryngeal (supraglottic) edema (due to local trauma), localized hematoma
Pneumothorax	Site of surgery, placement of central venous catheter
Pulmonary embolism (air, fat, thrombus)	Type of surgical procedure, review notation of critical events
Respiratory muscle weakness	Inadequate reversal of neuromuscular blockage (as determined by "train of four" nerve stimulation test), "high" spinal anesthetic effects
Vocal cord dysfunction	Injury to cord during intubation or to recurrent laryngeal nerve during surgery (neck dissection or aortic arch procedure)

Table 83–3. Hypotension Occurring in the Immediate Postoperative Period

POSSIBLE CAUSE	DIFFERENTIAL DIAGNOSIS AND COMMENTS
Arrhythmia	New-onset atrial fibrillation due to endogenous or exogenous catecholamines
Hypovolemia	Sympathectomy related to epidural, spinal anesthesia
	Bleeding
	"Third spacing" after certain surgical procedures
	Vasodilatation during rewarming
Myocardial ischemia	Check preoperative medical history
	Check events section for ST-segment changes or administration of nitroglycerin (see Chapter 34)
Pulmonary embolism	Type of surgery
	Were pneumatic compression devices used?
Sepsis	Bowel surgery
	Abscess drainage
Tension pneumothorax	Site of surgery
	Insertion of central venous catheter

Table 83–4. New Onset of Tachycardia in Immediate Postoperative Period

POSSIBLE CAUSE	DIFFERENTIAL DIAGNOSIS AND COMMENTS
Arrhythmia	New-onset atrial fibrillation
Hypovolemia	See Table 83–3
Iatrogenic	Drug reactions
	Pain
	Anticholinesterase medication
	Inotropic infusion

Table 83–5. Confusion Occurring in the Immediate Postoperative Period

POSSIBLE CAUSE	DIFFERENTIAL DIAGNOSIS AND COMMENTS
Drug-induced	Residual anesthetics
	Scopolamine
Operative factors	Emergence delirium
	Pain
	Paradoxical embolism
Preoperative factors	Advanced age
	History of carotid artery disease
	Preoperative cognitive impairment

tive hemodynamic changes, and severity of fluid shifts during the postoperative period. Although most hemodynamic measurements recorded intraoperatively reflect the conditions of the patient while anesthetized, they can guide initial ICU fluid management, for example, to optimize left ventricular preload and cardiac function.

Fluid and Drug Therapies

The anesthesia record has a section for reporting total blood loss, intravenous and other fluid administration, urine output, and drug administration. The fluid administered typically reflects the estimated preoperative fluid deficit, maintenance requirements, insensible losses due to evaporation and edema, urine output, and blood loss. As volume replacement for blood loss, blood products and colloid (albumin, Hetastarch) are generally given at a ratio of 1:1, whereas crystalloid is given at a ratio of 3:1 (crystalloid:blood loss).

Intraoperative Airway Management

Details of intraoperative airway management may be critical when formulating plans for terminating mechanical ventilation and extubation. The anesthesia record should be reviewed for details of airway management (the size and type of endotracheal tube, the depth of insertion, and the type of laryngoscope blade used for intubation) and whether difficulties were encountered in placing the artificial airway. Any intraoperative problems in airway management are often exacerbated during the initial postoperative period.

Repeated instrumentation of the airway may cause sufficient laryngeal and tracheal edema that may delay safe extubation by 1 day or more. In order to decrease this edema, the anesthetist may administer steroids (although the efficacy of this therapy is unproved) and raise the head of the bed (to facilitate venous drainage). If a difficult reintubation in the ICU is judged likely based on knowledge of events occurring in the operating room, it should be performed with appropriate additional equipment readily available (fiberoptic bronchoscope, a tube changer through which oxygen can be delivered, and endotracheal tubes with small diameters, for example, 6 mm) by personnel with expertise and experience in management of difficult airways (see Chapter 28).

Postoperative Respiratory Failure

Postoperative respiratory insufficiency may relate to intraoperative events or therapeutic interventions (see Table 83–2). Respiratory function is monitored intraoperatively by pulse oximetry, end-tidal capnography, peak inspiratory pressure (PIP), and associated tidal volumes. Increases in PIP for the same tidal volume reflect decreases in the patient's airway resistance or decreases in lung and chest wall compliance, or both. Acute falls in oxygen saturation may reflect intraoperative events such as embolization (air, fat, thrombus), congestive heart failure, endobronchial intubation with contralateral lobar atelectasis, pulmonary edema, or aspiration.

In order to differentiate among these diagnoses, the physician should review the anesthesia record, examining the time course of changes in pulse oximetry, capnography, and PIP. For example, intraoperative development of increased inflation pressures associated with a decrease in oxygen saturation and blood pressure may reflect an acute tension pneumothorax. Conversely, increased inflation pressures associated with decreased oxygen saturation without blood pressure changes may indicate bronchial intubation, acute bronchospasm, airway secretions, or onset of pulmonary edema. If the oxygenation problems persist into the postoperative period, the operative record, physical examination, chest radiograph, and fiberoptic bronchoscopy are often useful diagnostic tools.

THE "AUTOMATED" ANESTHESIA RECORD

A number of difficulties and inconsistencies may exist with the traditional anesthesia record. As noted previously, the records are institution-specific, and their usefulness is limited by the availability of space, legibility, and variable priorities of the record. Because hemodynamic data are recorded every 5 minutes in most situations, anesthetists may often "smooth" a record and ignore (for record-keeping purposes) transient periods of hypertension or hypotension, since such an "event" does not represent the general trend of the case. In addition, the anesthetist is often burdened with performing multiple simultaneous tasks. Because of lack of time during particularly eventful periods, documentation may be incomplete when reconstructing and recording the information from memory.

Automated anesthesia record keeping can circumvent many of these dilemmas. Microprocessor-based recording devices, linked directly to all available data as output from the anesthesia machine, can monitor and capture the information electronically. Problems due to smoothing should disappear. A narrative is easily written with the use of preformatted statements or direct keyboard entry of free text. As a result, a more complete and legible record will be available for review postoperatively.

Until such records are common, the ICU clinician will need to interpret the handwritten anesthesia record for data pertinent to the care of the critically ill patient. Once understood, the record can serve not only as a source of intraoperative historical data but also as a guide to postoperative management in the ICU.

BIBLIOGRAPHY

Vacanti CJ, VanHouten RJ, Hill RC: A statistical analysis of the relationship of physical status to postoperative mortality in 68,388 cases. Anesth Analg 49:564–566, 1970.
  This large cohort study validated the relationship of the American Society of Anesthesiologists classification of physical status (see Table 83–1) to postoperative mortality.

84

Perioperative Approach to the High-Risk Surgical Patient

Michael W. Russell
Clifford S. Deutschmann

The changes in organ system, cellular, and biochemical functions that accompany and follow major surgery differ from most others encountered in medical practice in that they follow a predictable pattern, a so-called response trajectory. These changes become even more important clinically when the patient undergoing surgery is "high risk." High-risk patients are those with pre-existing conditions, such as disease or advanced age, that markedly limit their physiologic reserves.

STRESS RESPONSE TO ACUTE INJURY

Acute injury results in a characteristic biphasic set of physiologic and metabolic changes, collectively described as the stress (or inflammatory) response (Fig. 84–1). The initial period, which Cuthbertson termed the *ebb phase,* is associated with the reduction in blood flow to the periphery, hypothermia, and an overall decrease in the resting energy expenditure (REE). The subsequent period, or *flow phase,* is accompanied by fever, an increase in blood flow to most tissues, and an increased REE. Virtually all variables associated with acute inflammation peak on about postinjury day 3 and then decline to baseline by postinjury day 7 (Table 84–1). Deviations from this expected pattern indicate the influence of pre-existing medical conditions or postoperative complications.

Hypermetabolic Phase

The increase in energy expenditure (hypermetabolism) reflects repair processes of damaged tissue primarily driven by the metabolic activities of inflammatory cells, especially white blood cells. Skeletal and visceral (smooth) muscles are catabolized to provide amino acids to be used as substrate for white blood cells, for hepatic gluconeogenesis, and for the synthesis of structural proteins and enzymes. Energy needs of other organs are met by oxidation of fatty acids. This global increase in metabolism is reflected in a rise in REE, oxygen consumption, and carbon dioxide production. In the flow phase, cardiac output and minute ventilation normally increase proportionately to the increase in carbon dioxide production, which keeps $Paco_2$ in the normal range.

In addition, the regional vasculature dilates and capillaries are recruited to support the delivery of substrate to damaged tissue. Injured tissue, however, is essentially avascular at first and substrate delivery is primarily a function of diffusion across the interstitium. To increase substrate delivery to a wound, nearby

949

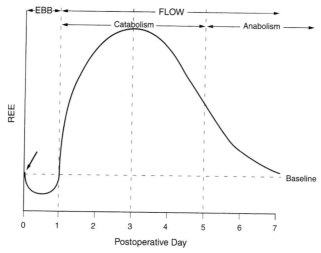

Figure 84–1. Changes in resting energy expenditure (REE) over time following injury. Other "stress" indicators follow a similar time course (see text and Table 84–1). The arrow indicates onset of injury or surgical procedure.

capillaries become "leaky" and fluid is lost to the extracellular compartment. This results in intravascular fluid loss, accompanied by increased salt and water retention, and fluid translocation from the intracellular compartment (Fig. 84–2).

Unchecked, the hypermetabolic process would eventually result in death. By the fourth to fifth postoperative day, however, neovascularization permits the

Table 84–1. Increases in Organ System Parameters After Major Surgery

ORGAN SYSTEM	PARAMETER
Cardiovascular	Cardiac output-index
	Heart rate
	Systemic vascular resistance
Pulmonary	Minute ventilation
	CO_2 production ($\dot{V}O_2$)
	Work of breathing
Nutritional-metabolic	Resting energy expenditure (REE)
	Inflammatory mediators
	Cytokines
	Interleukins
	Tissue necrosis factor
	Oxygen consumption ($\dot{V}O_2$)
	Lipolysis (respiratory quotient)
	Gluconeogenesis
Neuroendocrine	Catecholamines
	Corticosteroids
	Renin-angiotensin-aldosterone

The time course of these changes parallels the response trajectory described in Figure 84–1.

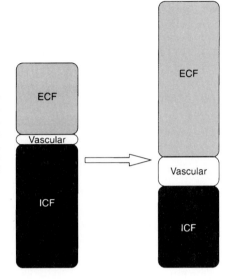

Figure 84–2. Schematic changes in fluid compartments following major surgery with postoperative exogenous fluid therapy. Note that an obligatory expansion of the extracellular fluid (ECF) compartment occurs and this must be supported by exogenous fluid administration to limit depletion of intravascular or intracellular fluid (ICF) volumes.

restoration of blood flow into the wound and the enhanced delivery of substrate reverses the hypermetabolic process. This subdivision of the hypermetabolic phase was first recognized by Francis Moore. He called the preneovascularization period *the catabolic phase* (reflecting the catabolism of endogenous protein and loss of cellular water, described earlier), and the postneovascularization period the *anabolic phase*.

The anabolic phase is characterized by restitution of body cell mass; movement of water, potassium, magnesium, and phosphate back into cells; vasoconstriction; and mobilization of extracellular fluid. Clinically, there is a brisk diuresis, resolution of anasarca as the capillary leak resolves, and a decrease in serum levels of K^+, Mg^{2+}, and PO_4^{-3} (resulting in the need for replacement therapy). The time required to reverse the catabolic changes is proportional to the degree of injury; this typically takes weeks to months after a major surgery or trauma.

The hypermetabolic *flow phase* is driven by the energy required for tissue repair. Attempts to prevent this phase completely are ineffective. For example, the use of epidural anesthesia to block the sympathetic nervous system delays its onset, but once the anesthetic is removed, hypermetabolism begins. Similarly, drugs such as beta-adrenergic blockers (which limit a patient's ability to achieve the metabolic and physiologic changes of the hyperdynamic phase) can reduce the peak hypermetabolic response, but they also prolong its duration.

Postoperative Issues

Concurrent diseases may have their greatest impact by limiting responses during the hyperdynamic phase. The magnitude of these changes depends on the extent of the initial injury as well as on pre-existing diseases (Table 84–2). Three important factors have an impact on the patient's ultimate outcome. The *first factor* is the ability of the patient to mount a hypermetabolic response. In some cases,

Table 84–2. Disease States Compromising the Extent of the Hyperdynamic Response

ORGAN SYSTEM	DISEASE
Cardiovascular	Coronary artery disease
	Myocardial pump dysfunction
	Valvular heart disease
	Peripheral vascular disease
	Rhythm disturbance with reduced cardiac output
Pulmonary	Emphysema
	Restrictive lung disease
	Reactive airway disease
Neuromuscular	Altered mental status, confusion
	Stroke
	Myopathies
	Myasthenia gravis
	Muscular deconditioning
Gastrointestinal: metabolic	Nutritional deficiencies
	Malabsorption syndromes
	Renal insufficiency
	Hepatic synthetic disorder, cirrhosis
Endocrine	Addison's disease (or inadequate adrenal cortical function due to chronic corticosteroid use)
	Hypothyroidism

this requires high levels of hemodynamic support. In others, however, the intensive care unit (ICU) physician's role in management is simply to support the hypermetabolic response, particularly by replacing ongoing fluid losses (especially those lost into the "third space"). This allows the cardiovascular system to become hyperdynamic, which, in turn, supports blood flow and oxygen delivery to the wound and major organ systems, such as the liver and kidneys.

The *second factor* is the ability of the ICU clinician to recognize when the patient's response deviates from the expected pattern. The patient who remains hypermetabolic—that is, neither manifesting a brisk diuresis nor requiring replacement of potassium, magnesium, or phosphate—by postoperative day 6, is not following the expected response trajectory. He or she likely has a complication, such as sepsis. The *third factor* is the extent of pre-existing disease and therapy for those problems, which often alter the ability of the patient to tolerate hypermetabolism or to resolve the hypermetabolic state. For example, beta-blockade may alter the patient's ability to become hypermetabolic, thus limiting or prolonging the expected response.

Preoperative Issues: Preparing the High-Risk Patient for Surgery

Response to surgical trauma should be viewed within the context of the stress response. In this paradigm, the intraoperative and immediate postoperative period is the ebb (hypometabolic) phase and the ensuing postoperative period is the flow (hypermetabolic) phase. Preparing the high-risk patient for surgery requires anticipating this pattern and how the patient's physiologic limitations will interfere with the hypermetabolic phase.

The hallmark of this perioperative approach to the high-risk surgical patient is to ensure the optimal functioning of physiologic systems when they are activated in response to surgical stress. Many surgical interventions can be anticipated well in advance, allowing time to plan a course of action. When dealing with a critically ill patient, however, only hours rather than days may be available for this preparation.

Fortunately, even with limited time, a great deal can be done to support the cardiopulmonary and metabolic reserves of the patient preoperatively. Key interventions are (1) restoration of fluid volume stores, (2) correction of important electrolyte abnormalities, (3) limitation of exogenous catecholamine administration, (4) correction of reversible impairment of pulmonary mechanics, particularly bronchospasm, and (5) initiation of other exogenous therapy, such as mechanical ventilation and metabolic support, when indicated.

SPECIFIC PERIOPERATIVE INTERVENTIONS

Correcting Volume Deficits

The preoperative management of the critically ill or high-risk surgical patient begins with ensuring adequate *intravascular, interstitial,* and *intracellular* fluid volumes. Since the delivery of substrate for repair of damaged tissue is accomplished in part by the development of capillary leak, fluid shifts from the intravascular and intracellular compartments into the interstitial compartment occur even in undamaged tissue. As a result, any pre-existing deficit in intravascular or intracellular fluid volume will be exaggerated postoperatively without appropriate interventions. Further, adequate intravascular volume is essential for the development of the hyperdynamic cardiovascular response. Repleting intravascular volumes permits supranormal hemodynamics to be achieved without excessive tachycardia and associated myocardial oxygen demand.

Assessing and achieving proper fluid balance in critically ill patients can be difficult. This difficulty is amplified in patients with major pre-existing medical disorders (see Table 84–2). Further, some patients appear to be in fluid balance or even overloaded when, in fact, a relative intravascular volume deficit exists. For example, the use of diuretics in patients with congestive heart failure or hypertension can lead to total body deficits of water, sodium, and potassium. These may result in an inability to mount an adequate postoperative hyperdynamic response.

A number of surgical factors can be expected to exaggerate the tendency toward relative preoperative hypovolemia. Critically ill patients taken to the operating room from the ICU or the emergency department may have unrecognized intravascular volume deficits due to infection, fever, or bleeding. The acute vasodilatory and anti-inotropic effects of anesthetics can compound the hemodynamic consequences of preoperative hypovolemia, placing the patient at even greater risk. Pulmonary artery monitoring is useful to diagnose hypovolemia and to assess how well it is corrected (Fig. 84–3).

In short, the safe conduct of surgical intervention and the requirements of postoperative physiology demand that hypovolemia be avoided or rapidly corrected

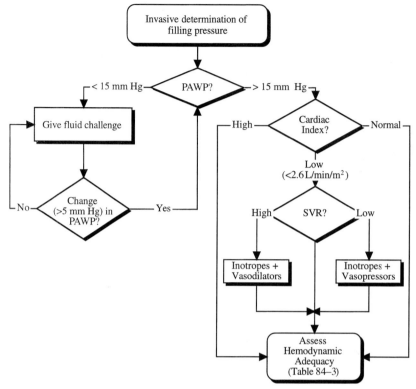

Figure 84–3. Schematic flow diagram illustrating steps in invasive assessment of effective intravascular volume (as represented by pulmonary artery wedge pressure) and adequacy of hemodynamics. PAWP, pulmonary artery wedge pressure; SVR, systemic vascular resistance.

in the preoperative and intraoperative periods. Sympathomimetic agents should be instituted only as a temporizing measure.

Optimizing Cardiac Performance

The normal physiologic response after injury requires the development of a hyperdynamic cardiovascular state proportional to the degree of injury. Pre-existing myocardial dysfunction may limit the patient's ability to increase cardiac output. Cardiomyopathy of any type eventually results in a dilatation of the left ventricular cavity and a corresponding increase in myocardial wall tension. Impaired contractility leads to a reduction in ejection fraction and stroke volume. In the chronically stressed myocardium, increased catecholamine stimulation results in changes in adrenergic receptor populations that are further altered by surgical intervention per se. This may decrease the response to endogenous or exogenous catecholamines. At this point, increases in cardiac output are primarily accomplished by increases in heart rate.

Patients with coronary artery disease frequently require surgery and may experience postoperative myocardial ischemia, leading to myocardial infarction and death. Based on the timing of the stress response, one can predict how and when this ischemia occurs. Assuming appropriate fluid resuscitation to ensure that the hyperdynamic response can develop, the demanded increase in cardiac output may well outstrip the ability of diseased coronary arteries to supply the myocardium by postoperative day 2. Not surprisingly, the peak incidence of postoperative myocardial infarction is on postoperative day 2 or 3.

Several approaches for limiting the occurrence of ischemia should be used: (1) adequately controlling pain (see Chapter 85) to limit increases in metabolic and heart rates due to pain; (2) avoiding hypotension, especially diastolic hypotension, by liberal fluid administration to prevent underperfusing coronary vessels; and (3) preventing increases in heart rate by beta-adrenergic blockade. The last alters the metabolic response essential to the inflammatory response, thus prolonging the catabolic phase. This tradeoff is worth it, however, because perioperative myocardial infarction and ischemia are such serious complications. Indeed, several randomized controlled clinical trials have studied patients with, or at high risk for, coronary heart disease who undergo noncardiac major surgery. Those treated with beta-blockers (started 2 days before surgery and continuing for at least 5 days postoperatively) have significantly better outcomes. Improved outcomes included decreased mortality rates, myocardial ischemias, and infarctions not only in the *perioperative period* but also in the *2-year postoperative period.*

Preoperative tachycardia should prompt a search for contributory factors amenable to correction (pain, hypovolemia, hypoxia, and so on). Primary treatment with beta-blockers requires careful assessment of hemodynamic status to avoid unmasking hypovolemia or impaired ventricular ejection. Any mechanical factor that reduces cardiac compliance or efficiency also limits maximal cardiac performance. Pericardial effusion, tamponade, or trauma-induced decreases in ventricular compliance ("stiff heart") reduce diastolic filling and stroke volume. Arrhythmias may result in uncoordinated atrioventricular activity or an inadequate diastolic interval for ventricular filling. Efforts should be made to stabilize acute (or chronic) arrhythmias to attempt to increase cardiac performance.

If high filling pressures have been reached and the patient remains unstable or has evidence of hypoperfusion, ventricular performance must be addressed (see Fig. 84–3). Improved myocardial performance from inotropic support may result in a reduction of abnormally high systemic vascular resistance. As cardiac output changes, preload can also decrease, which, in turn, may necessitate administration of additional fluid. Optimal hemodynamics are those necessary to perfuse key organ systems and to match oxygen delivery to oxygen consumption (Tables 84–3 and 84–4). As a rule, using a pulmonary artery catheter to assess the hemodynamic status and mixed venous oxygen saturation ($S\bar{v}O_2$) should be part of preoperative and postoperative management of the high-risk patient.

Pulmonary Dysfunction

Postinjury responses require a level of pulmonary function that a patient with intrinsic lung disease may not be able to achieve—for example, being able to clear the increased production of carbon dioxide. It is, therefore, important to identify individuals with baseline hypercapnia or those with severe obstructive airway

Table 84–3. Methods to Assess Hemodynamic Inadequacy

Clinical Parameter	Consistent with Inadequate Hemodynamic Status
Systolic blood pressure	<90 mm Hg or >40 mm Hg drop from baseline hypertension
Mean blood pressure	<60 mm Hg
Slow capillary filling on digits	>2 sec (>3 sec in elderly)
Skin appearance	Mottling of skin of lower extremity, livedo reticularis
Urine output	<30 mL/h
Invasive Parameter	
Cardiac index	<2.6 L/min/m^2
Use of mixed venous oxygen saturation or $\dot{D}O_2/\dot{V}O_2$	See Table 84–4

disease or neuromuscular weakness who may experience hypercapnic respiratory failure postoperatively despite normal baseline arterial blood gases.

Preoperative pulmonary care should concentrate on improving reversible conditions. *Bronchospasm* should be treated aggressively with a combination of beta-agonist and ipratropium bromide via metered-dose inhalers or nebulizers (see Chapter 74). If bronchospasm persists despite these agents, systemic steroid therapy is indicated. *Inhaled* steroids are not useful in the acute setting because 2 to 4 weeks of use is needed for their effects. Aggressive pulmonary toilet including mucolytics, postural drainage, and nasotracheal or endotracheal suctioning should

Table 84–4. Use of $\dot{D}O_2/\dot{V}O_2$ and Mixed Venous Oxygen Saturation to Assess Hemodynamic Adequacy

$\dot{D}O_2/\dot{V}O_2$	MIXED VENOUS OXYGEN SATURATION*	OXYGEN EXTRACTION	LIKELY CARDIAC INDEX	COMMENTS
4–5:1	>75%	Low	Normal/high	If serum lactate level–anion gap is elevated or patient needs inotropes or vasopressors, consider sepsis, liver failure, arteriovenous fistula, adrenal failure, or anaphylaxis. If not, hemodynamics are adequate-to-optimal for $\dot{V}O_2$.
2–3:1	<70%	Moderate	Low/normal/high	Inconclusive data; consider both extremes while observing trend.
<2:1	<50%	High	Low/normal	Inadequate cardiac index for $\dot{V}O_2$ (see Chapter 6); increase in $\dot{V}O_2$ may be due to shivering, fever, or major wound healing.

*Assumes $SaO_2 = 100\%$.

be included as appropriate. Simple methods of pulmonary preparation should not be overlooked. Deep breathing and splinted cough instruction are inexpensive ways to avoid expensive postoperative pulmonary complications. Finally, high-risk patients undergoing elective surgery should be strongly urged to stop smoking 1 month or more in advance.

Patients should be given as much information as possible when a period of postoperative mechanical ventilation is a likely possibility. This should include the rationale for its use and reassurance that it is intended as a temporary supportive measure only. Many misunderstandings regarding patient preferences against long-term mechanical ventilation can be avoided by having such discussions with the patient and family prior to surgery.

Malnutrition

It may not be possible to correct metabolic and nutritional deficits acutely in critically ill patients prior to surgery. Postoperatively, hypermetabolism will place additional demands on a nutritionally depleted patient. Postoperative caloric and protein requirements may exceed basal requirements considerably, but empirically increasing calories by some arbitrary factor may result in overfeeding. This, in turn, can increase respiratory loads by increasing the respiratory quotient (RQ) ($RQ = \dot{V}_{CO_2}/\dot{V}_{O_2}$), which, in some cases, can result in a RQ greater than 1.0. Accurate bedside measurements of REE to define nonprotein caloric requirements should be used to guide therapy (see Chapter 13).

Renal Dysfunction

Patients with elevated BUN and creatinine levels should be evaluated for renal, prerenal or postrenal azotemia, and correctable causes of pre- and postrenal azotemia should be treated (see Chapters 37 and 78). If the azotemia is found to be based on decreased renal function, the need for preoperative dialysis should be considered. Finally, the likely need for postoperative dialysis in the setting of preoperative azotemia should be discussed with the patient and family prior to surgery.

Several caveats apply to the assessment of renal function in the critically ill patient. Surgical trauma results in activation of the renin-angiotensin-aldosterone system. As a result, sodium uptake and water reabsorption increase in the immediate postoperative period. Urinary output then becomes an unreliable indicator of adequate intravascular volume or tissue perfusion. Intraoperative urine output also correlates poorly with postoperative renal function. Conversely, increased solute loads occurring after tissue disruption, absorption of hematoma, perioperative hyperglycemia, or administration of exogenous solutes may result in an artificial elevation in urine output as obligate water loss accompanies excretion of solutes. Finally, the effects of vasoactive agents on afferent and efferent glomerular blood flow and dilution of medullary concentration gradients may change urine flow independent of effective intravascular volume.

Perioperatively, the indiscriminate use of diuretics should be avoided. Once a loop diuretic is administered, urine output becomes unreliable for assessing the renal response to physiologic changes. Low or "renal" dose dopamine may be warranted, but its effectiveness in preventing postoperative renal failure remains to be determined. The relevant variable is not urine output per se, but the ability of the kidney to handle the increased solute load presented to it in the postoperative period. Therefore, measures of concentrating ability, such as the fractional excretion of sodium or, more simply, the urine sodium, give a more reliable indicator of normal renal function (see Chapters 37 and 78). The first response to a falling urine output (<0.5 mL/kg per hour) should always be clinical assessment of intravascular volume and whether it improves after a fluid challenge in the absence of unequivocal signs of volume overload. Even in the setting of high filling pressures, cardiac output and afterload should be optimized before diuretics are given (see Fig. 84–3).

Electrolyte Abnormalities

Hypomagnesemia and *hypocalcemia* may play a role in depressed cardiac performance in some critically ill patients. Hypomagnesemia can contribute to ventricular and supraventricular tachyarrhythmias, which may be resistant to traditional antiarrhythmic therapy. Magnesium is also required as a cofactor in the enzymatic reactions of the coagulation cascade. Severe *hypophosphatemia* can impair intracellular generation of high-energy phosphates. Cardiac and respiratory arrest have been reported in association with severe phosphate depletion. Since the risk of normalizing serum phosphate levels is small (if carried out enterally), treatment of documented deficiencies is warranted.

Hypokalemia is often seen preoperatively as a result of diuretic therapy or inadequate replacement of renal or gastrointestinal losses. Although preoperative hypokalemia was associated with cardiac arrhythmias in the past, more recent observations suggest that the risk of a serious rhythm disturbance in patients with *chronic* hypokalemia is only slight. Because potassium is lost intracellularly as well as extracellularly, the transmembrane gradient may be near normal in states of chronic K^+ losses. The rapid correction of chronic mild or moderate hypokalemia may *increase* the risk of arrhythmias. Delaying urgently needed surgery for hypokalemia in the absence of life-threatening arrhythmias is unwarranted. Most anesthesiologists currently recommend replacing potassium losses gradually (0.2 mEq/kg/h). If hypokalemia is severe (<2.5 mEq/L) or associated with significant arrhythmias, it may be repleted at 0.4 mEq/kg/h with continuous electrocardiographic monitoring.

Hematologic and Coagulation Function

Preoperative abnormalities of coagulation may be mild, moderate, or severe. Although severe elevations of prothrombin time (PT) and partial thromplastin time (PTT) should obviously be corrected, the correction of mild elevations is controversial, with little evidence for excessive bleeding for an international normalization ratio (INR) less than or equal to 1.8. More important are the number of circulating platelets. Although not a risk factor for spontaneous bleeding, platelet counts of 50,000 to 75,000/μL are associated with increased surgical bleeding.

Accordingly, preoperative platelet transfusions to achieve counts of 80,000 to 100,000/μL are indicated. Qualitative abnormalities of platelet function alone caused by drugs (aspirin, nonsteroidal anti-inflammatory drugs) or disease (uremia) do not correlate well with excessive surgical bleeding.

PERIOPERATIVE INVASIVE MONITORING—WHEN AND FOR HOW LONG?

No invasive monitoring method is without risks, which generally fall into two categories. The first is technical and relatively time-independent. Examples are arrhythmias, bleeding, or pneumothorax at the time of insertion of pulmonary artery catheters. The second includes inherent complications of foreign bodies, which are time-dependent. The most common of these is catheter-related infection. Some complications such as pulmonary artery rupture associated with balloon inflation fall between these groups. It is axiomatic that before attempting a procedure in critical care, as in all medicine, that the benefit of the procedure needs to exceed its risk.

Although controversial, some studies suggest that aggressive monitoring, including pulmonary artery catheters, improves patient outcome in certain high-risk surgical populations. Even more controversial is whether augmenting the hyperdynamic stress response (so-called supercharging) improves outcomes. Studies can be cited that support either position. Without controversy, however, is the observation that failure to mount a hyperdynamic hemodynamic response *spontaneously* in the postoperative period indicates a poor prognosis.

Because postoperative morbidity, especially cardiac morbidity, peaks on the second or third day after operation, it seems prudent to monitor the high-risk patient's cardiovascular response at least through this period. As a practical rule, once invasive monitoring is established in high-risk patients, it should be continued until the hyperdynamic phase is clearly resolving (in the absence of specific indications to stop it earlier).

BIBLIOGRAPHY

Berlauk JF, Abrams JH, Gilmour IJ, et al: Preoperative optimization of cardiovascular hemodynamics improves outcome in peripheral vascular surgery: A prospective randomized clinical trial. Ann Surg 214:289–299, 1991.
This article supports the use of pulmonary artery catheterization to "optimize" hemodynamics in a high-risk group of patients, demonstrating improved mortality with normalization of hemodynamics in this population.

Boyd O, Grounds M, Bennett ED: A randomized clinical trial of the effect of deliberate perioperative increase of oxygen delivery on mortality in high-risk surgery patients. JAMA 270:2699–2707, 1993.
This article describes a prospective randomized study showing improved morbidity and mortality with deliberate increases in preoperative oxygen delivery.

Cuthbertson D, Tustone W: Metabolism in the post-injury period. Adv Clin Chem 12:1–55, 1977.
This is a summary of Cuthbertson's classic description of the metabolic response to injury.

Garrison RN, Wilson MA, Matheson PJ, Spain DA: Preoperative saline loading improves outcome after elective, noncardiac surgical procedures. Am Surg 62:223–231, 1996.

This article demonstrates the ability of simple crystalloid volume expansion to reduce intraoperative instability and postoperative complications.

Gattinoni L, Brazzi L, Pelosi P, et al: A trial of goal-oriented hemodynamic therapy in critically ill patients. N Engl J Med 330:1025–1032, 1995.
This article describes a prospective controlled clinical trial of "supercharging" that found no significant benefit in survival.

Goldman L: Cardiac risk in noncardiac surgery: An update. Anesth Analg 80:810–820, 1995.
This is an update on the original Goldman and Caldera criteria, including subsequent modifications and newer diagnostic (thallium scintigraphy) and therapeutic (percutaneous transluminal coronary angioplasty [PTCA]) options.

Goldman L, Caldera DL, Southwick FS, et al: Cardiac risk factors and complications in non-cardiac surgery. Medicine 57:357–370, 1978.
This is a classic description of risk factors for cardiac morbidity in noncardiac procedures.

Mangano DT, Layug EL, Wallace A, et al: Effect of atenolol on mortality and cardiovascular morbidity after noncardiac surgery. N Engl J Med 335:1713–1720, 1996.
This randomized controlled clinical trial showed improved survival and reduced cardiovascular morbidity for up to 2 years in patients treated with atenolol starting 2 days before and continuing for at least 5 days after noncardiac surgery.

Palda VA, Detsky AS: Clinical Guideline, Part II. Perioperative assessment and management of risk from coronary artery disease. Ann Intern Med 127:313–328, 1997.
This article is an evidence-based review of the literature and represents the official practice guidelines endorsed by the American College of Physicians.

Poldermans D, Boersma E, Bax JJ, et al: The effect of bisoprolol on perioperative mortality and myocardial infarction in high-risk patients undergoing vascular surgery. N Engl J Med 341:1789–1794, 1999.
In this study high-risk patients (defined as those who had positive results on dobutamine echocardiography) were treated with a beta-adrenergic blocker (5 or 10 mm Hg) for 1 week prior to, and for 1 month after, surgery. The drug was titrated in the ICU to keep the heart rate below 80. (The drug was held for heart rates below 50 or systolic blood pressure below 100 mm Hg). Death from cardiac causes or myocardial infarction within 30 days of surgery significantly decreased from 34% in the untreated group to 3.4% in the treated group

Shoemaker WC, Kram HB, Appel PL, Fleming AW: The efficacy of central venous and pulmonary artery catheters and therapy based upon them in reducing mortality and morbidity. Arch Surg 125:1332–1338, 1990.
This study is frequently quoted to support hemodynamic "supercharging" as defined by supranormal values of cardiac index and oxygen delivery-consumption.

Wallace A, Layug B, Tateo I, et al: Prophylactic atenolol reduces postoperative myocardial ischemia. Anesthesiology 88:2–5, 1998.
This randomized, placebo-controlled, double-blind clinical trial showed a significant reduction in postoperative myocardial ischemia in patients with, or at risk for, coronary heart disease when atenolol was administered for 1 week following noncardiac surgery.

Wolfe BM, Moore PG: Preparation of the intensive care patient for major surgery. World J Surg 17:184–191, 1993.
This is a short, practical review of the basic steps in the perioperative care of the high-risk patient.

85

Management of Postoperative Pain

Mitchell D. Tobias
F. Michael Ferrante

Since postoperative pain can be anticipated, it is a unique form of acute pain. It thereby lends itself to the use of pre-emptive analgesia and offers the potential for complete control. This chapter focuses on current understanding of the mechanisms of pain and practical methods of pain ablation and acute pain management in the intensive care unit (ICU) setting.

UNDERMEDICATING POSTOPERATIVE PAIN

Historically, *pro re nata* (prn, as needed) opioids have been administered parenterally for acute postoperative pain. Time has proved this to be a safe method that requires no special equipment or hospital support, and with which health care providers are comfortable. Unfortunately, a majority of patients treated in this manner are not relieved of pain, and they recall moderate to severe distress postoperatively. Undermedication to treat this pain continues to be a problem.

The causes of postoperative undermedication are multiple. The most common reason is lack of knowledge of the pharmacology of commonly employed medications. In one survey of ICU-based physicians and nurses, a large majority of physicians held the misconception that benzodiazepines provided analgesia. Shockingly, many doctors and nurses endorsed pancuronium as an anxiolytic and some even believed it provided analgesia. Another problem relates to lack of clinical experience, for example, management of postoperative pain is often relegated to the least trained members of the surgical house staff.

These barriers to effective pain management are compounded by excessive fears of both patients and staff regarding addiction and side effects of opioids. There is abundant evidence that the extremely subjective nature of pain and bilateral miscommunication also contribute to undermedication. Fears of side effects (particularly respiratory depression) and failure to appreciate the severity of pain have classically led to administration of only 25% of an already overconservative prn prescription.

Finally, there is a lag time in the delivery of prn opioids between when the patient requests pain relief and when they actually receive that relief. First, a nurse responds to a patient's call bell and locates, prepares, and administers the opioid, after which the patient must await the therapeutic effect of the opioid. This lag time becomes even more problematic when, as is typical, the patient does not request relief until the pain is overwhelming. *Pro re nata* administration is more effective if frequent small doses of intravenous (IV) analgesic are immediately available; this is the basis of patient-controlled analgesia (PCA).

ASSESSMENT OF PAIN

Pain involves a subjective perception of a sensory stimulus and an emotional reaction to it. The subjective nature of pain renders it difficult to quantify in terms of severity. In conscious patients, this assessment may be made by analysis of a patient's verbal and behavioral expressions. Interpreting these expressions can be challenging in patients with extremely stoic or emotive personalities. In unconscious, sedated, or paralyzed patients, vital signs and provocative tests must be relied on. Assessment of pain in the unresponsive patient may be undertaken by (1) noting changes in continuously monitored arterial pressure and pulse rate in response to palpation or percussion of injury or incision sites and (2) measuring tidal volume and respiratory rate in an intubated patient. Bedside spirometry before and after analgesic administration can provide valuable insights in pain management for patients who are able to perform these maneuvers.

In alert, conscious patients, pain can be assessed using a visual analog pain scale (VAPS) (Fig. 85–1). This easy-to-understand system avoids much misinterpretation. Patients generally do not choose either extreme and a VAPS score of 3.0 (or less) generally represents acceptable pain control in an ICU setting because there is usually always some discomfort, even if unrelated to the surgery (intravenous catheters, nasogastric tube, bed-bound status, tape, and so on). The choice of one extreme or the other generally implies a stoic or emotive personality.

RATIONALE FOR USING PRE-EMPTIVE ANALGESIA

Effective preoperative analgesia may decrease postoperative pain in a manner that exceeds expectations. Studies support a concept of postinjury *peripheral* and *spinal* nerve hypersensitization and spinally mediated *neuroplasticity* following pain perception (nociception). Neuroplasticity implies that the central nervous system and the dorsal horn cells adapt in response to noxious stimulation. For example, repetitive stimulation of small pain fibers produces a progressive increase in action potential discharge (wind-up) and a prolonged increase in the excitability of spinal neurons with which they synapse. Central sensitization predisposes dorsal horn nociceptive neurons to respond to the input of normally innocuous A_b afferent fibers. Spinal sensitization seems dependent upon N-methyl- D-aspartic acid receptor stimulation and may be prevented by N-methyl- D-aspartic acid receptor antagonists administered before or after the peripheral injury. These antagonists may be key to the alleviation of pain and the prevention of pain syndromes in the future.

The prevention of central sensitization can be achieved through the pre-emptive use of local anesthetics, opioids, and to a degree, nonsteroidal anti-inflammatory

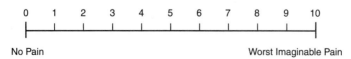

Figure 85–1. Typical visual analog pain scale (VAPS) in which patients are asked to indicate by voice or by pointing where their pain is located on the scale. A score of 3 is usually acceptable in ICU patients.

drugs. Interventions following injury are much less effective and volatile anesthetics neither provide pre-emptive analgesia nor prevent central sensitization.

METHODS OF CONTROLLING POSTOPERATIVE PAIN

Intercostal Nerve Blocks

Percutaneous intercostal nerve blocks with local anesthetics can be performed for patients with unilateral chest or abdominal wall somatic pain. This simple technique has been found to give superior analgesia compared with systemic opioids. Multiple intercostal nerve injections are usually given. A shortcoming of the technique, especially in the ICU setting, is the relatively brief duration of action of the block, despite the use of a long-acting local anesthetic with epinephrine. This necessitates repeated injections, increasing the risks of pneumothorax and intravascular injection. When local anesthetics are effective, continuous intercostal catheterization can be performed, obviating the need for repetitive injections.

Patient-Controlled Analgesia

Patient-controlled analgesia (PCA) is a modality designed to accommodate an approximate fourfold variation in analgesic requirements among patients for the same noxious stimulus. PCA permits patients to treat their pain by direct activation of a microprocessor-controlled programmable infusion device that administers intermittent predetermined aliquots (demand doses) of analgesic. Often there is concurrent continuous infusion of the same drug (basal rate) delivered by the same device.

The demand dose is immediately responsive to the patient's perceived pain and permits titration of analgesics to the minimal effective analgesic concentration, thus reducing periods of excessive pain or sedation. Patients act as their own "nocistat" with frequent small prn (demand) boluses. Analgesic administration is reduced to a simple feedback loop: The patient's request for analgesia is rapidly honored by the PCA pump, which minimizes the "lag time." In effect, PCA optimizes the traditional prn opioid cycle. The frequency of administration of the demand dose is determined by a preset interval (lockout time), which is predicated on the pharmacokinetics of the medication being used (Table 85–1).

In theory, the basal continuous infusion prevents significant decreases in the serum level of opioid while patients sleep, so they can avoid awakening with

Table 85–1. Intravenous Opioid Patient-Controlled Analgesia (PCA) Guidelines

OPIOID	BOLUS	LOCKOUT	BASAL INFUSION
Fentanyl	20–50 μg	5–10 min	20–100 μg/h
Hydromorphone	0.1–0.5 mg	5–15 min	0.2–0.4 mg/h
Morphine	0.5–3.0 mg	10–20 min	1.0–10 mg/h

severe pain. The use of a basal infusion, however, has been demonstrated to increase opioid use without improving overall patient satisfaction or VAPS score. Still, respiratory depression has only rarely been reported with reasonable doses of PCA, and ICU patients on positive-pressure ventilators are generally safe with continuous basal infusions. Respiratory depression has been reported following postoperative hemorrhage because of a reduction in the volume of distribution that resulted in relatively high opioid concentrations. One report of meperidine overdose was attributable to a "runaway" malfunction of the PCA pump. Even when given by a functioning IV PCA pump, meperidine is not recommended for PCA because of the potential for accumulation of normeperidine, a central nervous system (CNS) excitatory metabolite with a long half-life. Normeperidine toxicity is more likely in patients with renal dysfunction. If a basal infusion is used, it must be appreciated that sleep and coadministered sedatives (see Chapter 4) are synergistic in their respiratory depressant effects.

Compared with patients receiving traditional prn opioids, patients using IV PCA achieve earlier ambulation, better cooperation with physiotherapy, and shorter ICU and hospital lengths of stay.

Neuraxial Analgesia

Perispinal (subarachnoid or epidural) deposition of local anesthetics and opioids in combination or separately can provide high-quality analgesia. These two classes of analgesics act at differing sites along the nociceptive pathway, and they have differing profiles of side effects (Table 85–2). Local anesthetics and opioids are often combined to permit synergism with less untoward effects. It is a good rule to place the catheter within the desired dermatomal area to be treated in an effort to minimize the volume of infusion required for analgesia (see Appendix F for dermatomal distributions).

As an example of the effectiveness of this approach, Yeager and colleagues compared outcomes of high-risk surgical patients randomly assigned to two groups.

Table 85–2. Comparative Profile of Local Anesthetics and Perispinal Opioids

CHARACTERISTICS	LOCAL ANESTHETICS	OPIOIDS
Site of action	Nerve roots	Dorsal horn
Inhibition	Global-axonal conduction	C and Aδ fibers*
Side Effects		
Cardiovascular	Hypotension, bradycardia	None
Central nervous system	None (unless overdosed)	Sedation, somnolence
Respiratory	None (unless overdosed)	Depressed respiration
Gastrointestinal	Nausea with hypotension	Central nervous system–mediated nausea
Genitourinary	Urinary retention	Urinary retention
Peripheral nervous system	Motor or sensory block, or both	Pruritus

*Spares motor, autonomic, and proprioceptive fibers.

One group received general anesthesia and conventional prn systemic opioids. The other group received epidural anesthesia and postoperative epidural analgesia. The epidural group not only had significantly lower mortality and morbidity rates but also had significantly shorter ICU stays and reduced hospital costs.

Local Anesthetics in Neuraxial Analgesia

The earliest description of the placement of an epidural (caudal) catheter for postoperative pain management dates to 1949. The technique involved intermittent boluses of local anesthetic, which can cause unwanted effects like motor weakness and sensory and autonomic blockade. ICU patients with hypotension or hypovolemia are not good candidates for what, in effect, is a widely distributed sympathectomy. Continuous slow infusions (3 to 8 mL/h) of low concentration of local anesthetic (0.05 to 0.15% bupivacaine) without any bolus administration prevents profound sympathetic blockade and permits time to counteract undesirable reductions in sympathetic tone. Potent analgesia can be achieved in many patients with a neuraxial local anesthetic alone. This is a time-tested regimen that can be especially recommended for ICU patients who are hypertensive or could otherwise benefit from a reduction in blood pressure.

Perispinal Opioids

The first clinical use of epidural and subarachnoid opioids in humans occurred in 1979. Neuraxially administered opioids act by selective suppression of the activity of substantia gelatinosa nociceptors. Compared with local anesthetics, the use of opioids in this manner minimizes sensory motor and autonomic blockade and causes fewer physiologic cardiovascular changes (no changes in cardiac preload, output, or peripheral vascular resistance). In addition, a nontoxic reversal agent (naloxone) is available. Compared with systemic opioids, perispinal opioids show a reduction in side effects, such as somnolence, sedation, and ileus, and no evidence of spasm of the sphincter of Oddi or CNS or cardiovascular system excitability or toxicity. Perispinal administration of opioids markedly increases their potency and the duration of their analgesic effect.

Patient-Controlled Epidural Analgesia

Patient-controlled epidural analgesia (PCEA) combines the superior analgesic qualities of spinal local anesthetics or opioids and the increased patient satisfaction of PCA (Table 85–3). Studies have shown superior analgesia with significantly less sedation and anxiety with morphine administered by PCEA compared with IV PCA morphine. The rapid onset (3 to 5 minutes) of lipophilic opioids like fentanyl makes them the logical agent of choice for PCEA, using small doses with short lockout intervals. This lipophilic property, however, can also result in substantial systemic uptake. Because, intravenous, subcutaneous, or epidural fentanyl provides similar analgesia with comparable serum levels at 18 and 24 hours, the specificity of neuraxial administration of lipophilic opioids, like fentanyl, has been questioned.

Table 85–3. Patient-Controlled Epidural Analgesia (PCEA) Dosing Guidelines

DRUG CONCENTRATION	BOLUS (mL)	LOCKOUT (min)	BASAL INFUSION (mL/h)
Morphine 0.01% with 0.05% bupivacaine	Abdominal: 5–7 Thoracic: 2–5	20–30	Abdominal: 4–10 Thoracic: 2–7
Fentanyl 0.0002% with 0.05% bupivacaine	Thoracic: 2–5	10–20	Thoracic: 2–5
Fentanyl 0.0005%	Thoracic: 2–7	10	Thoracic: 2–5

Side Effects of Patient-Controlled Epidural Analgesia

The following sections discuss a variety of side effects of PCEA. Their management is summarized in Figure 85–2.

Nausea and Vomiting. Although opioids may stimulate the chemoreceptor trigger zone of the medulla, causing nausea and vomiting, these are common postoperative events even in the absence of opioid administration. Visceral traction, ileus, anticholinergic therapy, vagal innervation, increased intracranial pressure, and nasogastric (NG) tube displacement also contribute to postoperative nausea and emesis. Treatment may be prophylactic (NG tube suction and administration of ondansetron, metoclopramide, or droperidol) or responsive (naloxone, NG tube repositioning, prochlorperazine).

Pruritus. The mechanism of pruritus is unclear but may be related to opioid modulation of normal cutaneous afferent sensory integration at the spinal level. It is not seen for a period of 2 to 6 hours after administration. Diphenhydramine has been used as initial treatment even though the mechanism of pruritus does not involve histamine release. Naloxone may be administered intermittently (40 μg bolus intravenously) or by continuous low-dose infusion (40 to 100 μg/h) for refractory symptoms.

Urinary Retention. The true frequency of urinary retention following postoperative spinal opioid administration is masked by the common presence of a Foley catheter for the first 1 to 2 postoperative days. Similar to nausea and vomiting, urinary retention is a common postoperative occurrence, whether or not spinal opioids have been used. Activation of spinal opioid receptors, however, is known to cause detrusor muscle relaxation, which, in turn, increases bladder capacity. These changes are reversed by naloxone, and bethanechol has also been reported to induce contractile responses. In addition to the use of neuraxial opioids and local anesthetics, intraoperative use of anticholinergic drugs may potentiate urinary retention.

Many patients do not have detrusor dysfunction with epidural analgesia, depending on the level of the catheter, the composition and rate of the infusate, and patient sensitivity.

Somnolence. The use of potent anesthetic agents and adjunctive drugs are a common cause of somnolence in the postoperative period. Spinal opioid–induced somnolence is related to central effects on the reticular activation system by rostral spread in the cerebrospinal fluid. Somnolence is a serious side effect of spinal opioids and must be treated to prevent respiratory depression. The possibility of

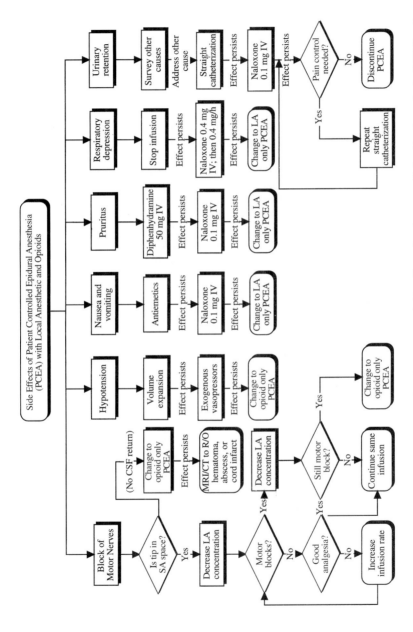

Figure 85–2. Schematic flow diagram illustrating the spectrum of side effects of patient-controlled epidural anesthesia (PCEA) and their management. SA, subarachnoid space; LA, local anesthetic; CSF, cerebrospinal fluid; MRI/CT, magnetic resonance imaging/computed tomography; R/O, rule out; IV, intravenously.

hypercapnia from respiratory depression should be entertained in any somnolent patient.

A four-point observer sedation score should be used to evaluate ICU patients receiving spinal opioids (Table 85–4). An observer sedation score of 2 warrants close observation, whereas a score of 3 warrants intervention. A score of 4 obviously should never be reached. Somnolence is treated with oxygen therapy, continuous pulse oximetry, cessation of continuously infused sedatives or opioids, and specific reversal agents (flumazenil, physostigmine, or naloxone) as appropriate.

Respiratory Depression. Intraspinal morphine administration has been associated with delayed onset of respiratory depression. This problem is related to the hydrophilic nature of the morphine sulfate molecule, which predisposes it to remain in the cerebrospinal fluid and be slowly transported to supraspinal centers. The more lipid-soluble drugs (fentanyl and sufentanil) may be associated with a lower incidence of hypoventilation, but they are limited in their duration of analgesia and spread within the neuraxis. Occurrence of respiratory depression following spinal morphine is rare: 1 in 1000 for mild cases (respiratory rate <12/min) and 1 in 10,000 for severe cases (respiratory rate <8/min). Risk factors for the development of this complication are related to patient, drug, and technique. First, patients older than 60 years of age and patients with respiratory disease or severe debilitation are at higher risk. Second, the use of hydrophilic opioids in large doses or in large volumes increases the risk of respiratory depression. Finally, the concomitant use of parenteral opioids and the use of thoracic (versus lumbar) epidural or subarachnoid administration also increases the risk of respiratory depression.

The potential for respiratory depression necessitates the immediate availability of oxygen and reversal agents (naloxone) at any site where patients are being so treated. Severe respiratory depression should be treated with an IV loading dose of 0.4 mg of naloxone followed by a continuous IV infusion at 0.4 mg/h.

CONCLUSIONS

Many patients now see adequate analgesia as a right rather than a privilege, and major improvements in pain management make that possible. With knowledge of the expected hemodynamic and CNS side effects of the many different analgesic regimens, one can design a stable and effective regimen, even in the most critically ill patient. The psychologic trauma of unrelenting pain in a paralyzed and ventilated

Table 85–4. Sedation Score to Evaluate Patients Receiving Spinal Opioids

SCORE	CLINICAL MANIFESTATIONS
1	Alert, oriented, initiates conversation
2	Drowsy, oriented, conversant
3	Very drowsy, disoriented, but respondent
4	Stuporous to unarousable, disoriented, nonrespondent

patient is unique to the operating room and the ICU. Failure to treat pain for fear of eliminating adrenergic stimulation is an archaic and inappropriate response. In this circumstance, one should be give exogenous catecholamines and relieve the pain rather than rely on pain to maintain hemodynamics. Moreover, the physiologic effects of untreated pain can harm the cardiovascular and renal systems through tachycardia and decreased regional blood flow.

There is now no reason for ICU patients to suffer severe pain postoperatively. The increasing and appropriate expectations of patients and family compel adoption of effective analgesic regimens.

BIBLIOGRAPHY

Choiniere M, Melzack R, Girard N, et al: Comparison between patients' and nurses' assessments of pain and medication efficacy in severe burns and injuries. Pain 40:143–152, 1990.
  This article exemplifies miscommunication between patients and staff; a reason for continuing undermedication.

Gottschalk A, Smith DS, Jobes DR, et al: Preemptive epidural analgesia and recovery from radical prostatectomy: A randomized controlled trial. JAMA 279:1076–1082, 1998.
  This is a classic landmark study on this important subject.

Loper KA, Butler S, Nessly M, Wild L: Paralyzed with pain, the need for education. Pain 37:315–317, 1989.
  This presents a frightening study of the lack of knowledge of pharmacology in the ICU.

Marks RM, Sacher EJ: Undertreatment of medical patients with narcotic analgesics. Ann Intern Med 78:173–181, 1973.
  Another important landmark study documenting undermedication.

Owen H, McMillan V, Rogowski D: Postoperative pain therapy: A survey of patients' expectations and their experiences. Pain 41:303–307, 1990.
  This article is a follow-up reference to the article by Choiniere and colleagues.

Owen H, Szekely SM, Plummer JL, et al: Variables of patient-controlled analgesia. 2. Concurrent infusion. Anesthesia 44:11–13, 1989.
  This article shows that the risks of side effects increase with continuous-infusion PCA intravenous morphine.

Rawal N, Mollefors K, Axelsson K, et al: An experimental study of urodynamic effects of epidural morphine and of naloxone reversal. Anesth Analg 62:641, 1983.
  This article discusses dose-dependent naloxone reversible detrusor relaxation from epidural morphine.

Walmsley PNH: Patient-controlled epidural analgesia. In: Sinatra RS, Hord AH, Ginsberg JS, et al (eds): Acute Pain, Mechanisms and Management. St. Louis: CV Mosby, 1992.
  This is a good basic overview of subject in a useful textbook.

Warfield CA, Kahn CH: Acute pain management. Programs in U.S. hospitals and experiences and attitudes among U.S. adults. Anesthesiology 83:1090–1094, 1995.
  This article documents the continued problems in acute pain management and a newly awakened patient recognition of this problem.

Woolf CJ: Evidence for a central component of post injury pain hypersensitivity. Nature 306:686–688, 1983.
  This is a seminal article on an important concept regarding central pain generation with intense peripheral nociception.

Woolf CJ, Thompson SW: The induction and maintenance of central sensitization is dependent on

N-methyl-D-aspartic acid receptor activation; implications for the treatment of post-injury pain hypersensitivity states. Pain 44:293–299, 1991.
This article provides further important elucidation of the mechanisms of neuroplasticity and sensitization, the subject of intensive clinically related research in pain.

Yeager MP, Glass DD, Neff RK, et al: Epidural anesthesia and analgesia in high risk surgical patients. Anesthesiology 66:729–736, 1987.
This important article documents decreased morbidity and costs with epidural analgesics.

86

Cardiac Surgery

Michael Acker
Alberto Pochettino

Over the last two decades, cardiac surgery has experienced dramatic growth fueled by the high prevalence of atherosclerotic disease involving the coronary arteries plus improved outcomes of complex cardiac surgical procedures. The latter can be attributed to multiple improvements in surgical technique, cardiopulmonary bypass (CPB) technology, cardiac anesthesia, and postoperative care.

Before the 1950s, cardiac surgery was limited to closed-chamber procedures, such as closed mitral commissurotomy, or short procedures, such as closure of an atrial septal defect. Development of CPB and the use of hypothermia allowed more complex procedures so that today most cardiac operations are performed on CPB, during moderate hypothermia (28 to 32° C), with the heart quiet and bloodless. These conditions allow complex surgical procedures to be performed with relatively low morbidity and mortality.

EFFECTS OF CARDIOPULMONARY BYPASS

Most "open" operations on the heart require that CPB substitute for physiologic cardiac function. The CPB machine has been designed to receive all venous return of the body, pass it through a membrane oxygenator where oxygen is added and carbon dioxide is removed and return this blood to the arterial system at a physiologic pressure to perfuse all organs adequately.

Since much of the morbidity and mortality encountered after heart surgery results from the use of CPB, it is important to be familiar with the functioning of CPB, its limitations, and especially the reactions resulting from a patient's blood interacting with its artificial surfaces.

The basic CPB circuit is composed of a venous catheter, a reservoir, a centrifugal or roller pump, an oxygenator, a heat exchanger, a debubbler, and an arterial catheter. Blood is "returned" from one or two venous catheters to the reservoir by gravity. Blood shed in the operative field is collected by pump suckers and also returned to the reservoir. Reservoir blood is then pumped through the oxygenator and heat exchanger. In turn, the warmed and oxygenated blood is infused into the arterial system via a cannula positioned in a large artery, usually the distal ascending aorta or aortic arch.

In order to commence CPB, the blood needs to be anticoagulated well beyond what might be sufficient to conduct a vascular surgical procedure without "pump assist" (CPB). Heparin dosage is titrated by following activated clotting times (ACTs). Traditionally heparin is given before cannulation, and the ACT is verified to be greater than 400 seconds before initiation of CPB. More recently, heparin titration protocols have been developed based on the ACT response of an aliquot of the patient's blood to a fixed dose of heparin.

Exposure of blood to the CPB circuit can have profound effects on blood components and other organs; these effects often become manifested in the early postoperative period in the intensive care unit (ICU). *Complement activation* induced by exposure of plasma to CPB causes a generalized inflammatory reaction characterized by the release of a cascade of multiple cytokines, lymphokines, and proteases. *Platelet disruption* occurs as a result of direct contact with the circuit's inner surface, especially at the level of the oxygenator. Platelet dysfunction also occurs as a consequence of complement-induced opsonization and the generalized inflammatory state. The *fibrinolytic pathway* is activated by CPB, which contributes to a bleeding diathesis sometimes seen postoperatively. *Red blood cell disruption* leading to hemoglobinuria correlates with the intensity of pump sucker use as well as with the total duration of CPB. *White blood cell sequestration* can occur in the lungs during full CPB. When combined with complement activation and high levels of circulating cytokines, this can lead to pulmonary injury and, in some instances, postoperative acute respiratory distress syndrome (so-called postpump lung injury).

Hypothermia is used during CPB to minimize tissue oxygen demand. A 10° C decrease from normal core temperature decreases tissue oxygen consumption by approximately 50%. At the extreme, temperatures less than 20° C can be used when a period of circulatory arrest is required, for example, during reconstruction of the aortic arch. When electroencephalographic monitoring is available, cooling should be continued until electroencephalographic silence has been documented. When electroencephalographic monitoring is not available, data suggest that almost all patients achieve electroencephalographic silence at a nasopharyngeal temperature of approximately 15° C.

EVALUATION OF CARDIAC FUNCTION IN THE INTENSIVE CARE UNIT

As a rule, patients are routinely admitted to the ICU after heart surgery and they commonly arrive with invasive hemodynamic monitoring in place (see Chapters 5 and 9). Systemic arterial and pulmonary arterial catheters provide important information to guide postoperative fluid and cardiac management in the ICU setting. Some cardiac surgeons employ the following precaution: to specifically order the ICU nursing staff not to perform routine inflation, for example, every 4 hours, of the balloon of the pulmonary arterial catheter in order to measure the pulmonary artery wedge pressure (PAWP). These patients usually have several factors that put them at higher risk for balloon-induced rupture of the pulmonary artery, including pulmonary hypertension and a bleeding diathesis induced by heparin, antiplatelet agents, and CPB-induced platelet dysfunction. In addition to invasive hemodynamic monitoring, a number of noninvasive methods to monitor cardiac function postoperatively serve as important sources of information.

Chest Radiographs

Chest radiographs are essential in any postoperative cardiac surgery patient. They provide information on the degree of lung expansion and the presence of undrained pleural fluid, pneumothorax, fluid overload, or pulmonary edema. A dramatic enlargement in cardiac silhouette should also raise the possibility of cardiac tamponade (see Chapter 53). The location of all invasive catheters, tubes, and the tip of the endotracheal tube should be documented by chest radiograph.

Electrocardiograms

The 12-lead electrocardiogram can provide valuable information on postoperative ischemia, partial or complete atrioventricular blocks, interventricular conduction abnormalities, or significant ventricular hypertrophy, or can suggest a myocardial infarction in evolution. Any of these signs may indicate the need for therapeutic maneuvers, including pacing via temporary wires, administering a coronary vasodilator, performing an emergency echocardiogram or cardiac catheterization, or returning the patient to the operating room. For these reasons, it is imperative that a postoperative electrocardiogram be obtained promptly in the ICU and followed up as clinically indicated.

Echocardiograms

Echocardiograms are important evaluative tools used in the intraoperative and the early postoperative period. An echocardiographic examination can be performed via the transthoracic or transesophageal route. Transthoracic echocardiography (TTE) has the advantage of being noninvasive, but its use is limited postoperatively because of the lack of "acoustic windows." In the perioperative period, transesophageal echocardiography (TEE) allows excellent imaging in almost all patients in whom the esophagus can be safely intubated. Furthermore, imaging with TEE can proceed without interruption of surgery. Similarly, a rapid and accurate cardiac evaluation can be obtained by TEE in the ICU setting. This includes anatomic information about chamber sizes, valvular structures, presence of intracardiac air or thrombus, pericardial effusion, aortic size, and disease. It also provides physiologic information about valvular stenosis or regurgitation, regional or global wall motion abnormalities, degree of cardiac filling and diastolic function, estimates of chamber pressures, and presence of intracardiac shunts. The TEE results can then be correlated with invasive hemodynamic measurements.

POSTOPERATIVE COMPLICATIONS

Myocardial Stunning and Cardiogenic Shock

As noted earlier, most cardiac surgical procedures result in a period of cardiac ischemia when the heart is kept cold and mechanically quiescent by the use of cardioplegia and topical cooling. Despite the low temperature and diastolic arrest, cardiac metabolic demand continues, albeit at a low rate, so that cardiac demand for metabolic substrates exceeds their supply. As a result, the heart may demonstrate postoperative stunning that is manifested by poor cardiac performance and requires inotropic support.

Inotropic Support

If inotropic support is required, the patient is commonly given a combination of catecholamines and afterload reducing agents whose dosage is guided by invasive hemodynamic data. The goal is to maximize cardiac index by improving preload, afterload, and myocardial contractility. High-dose inotropic agents can cause significant arrhythmias, especially in a patient with a residual ischemic focus. Supraventricular arrhythmias are common in all patients after CPB with cardioplegic arrest. In the hemodynamically unstable patient, cardioversion and intravenous procainamide or amiodarone should be used (see Chapter 31). If the patient is stable, digoxin and beta-blockade can often treat these arrhythmias effectively.

Mechanical Assist Devices

If left ventricular failure persists despite maximal medical therapy, an intra-aortic balloon pump (IABP) is often used to increase diastolic coronary perfusion and further decrease afterload. The IABP will not, however, ameliorate right ventricular failure (except when due to left ventricular failure). If pulmonary vasodilators are not sufficient to reverse right ventricular failure, a right ventricular assist device (RVAD) is often used. Cannulas are placed in the right atrium and the pulmonary artery and an external pump acts in parallel to the right ventricle. If the left ventricle is still failing despite IABP, a similar left ventricular assist device (LVAD) can be placed. A cannula is placed in the left atrium or the left ventricle and blood is returned by a second cannula to the aorta. When significant pulmonary dysfunction is also present, extracorporeal membrane oxygenation can be used to maintain the patient on continuous CPB until adequate recovery occurs. In this circumstance, blood is drained from the right atrium or vena cava and passed through a membrane oxygenator before being returned to the systemic arterial system.

When recovery fails to occur in a patient who is otherwise a cardiac transplant candidate, a permanent assist device can be placed. Currently, permanent LVADs approved by the U.S. Food and Drug Administration (FDA) include the TCI Heartmate® (Thermo Cardiosystems, Inc.) and the Novocor® (Baxter Healthcare Corporation). A third device (from Thoratec Laboratories Corporation) is FDA approved as an interim therapy and can be used as either a RVAD or a LVAD. The TCI Heartmate® has a textured surface on all parts in contact with blood, which allows the formation of a thrombus-resistant pseudointima to minimize risk of neurologic complications. At present, all these devices are primarily used as a "bridge" to cardiac transplantation, with device infection being the most common complication.

Respiratory Problems

Cardiopulmonary bypass causes significant fluid accumulation, which may contribute to pulmonary edema in the early postoperative period. This may be compounded in a patient with preoperative congestive heart failure. As noted earlier, the lungs are also one of the major targets of the inflammatory activation caused by CPB. These adverse effects, which are dependent on the length of CPB and are aggravated by intraoperative hypothermia, may cause postoperative acute respiratory distress syndrome.

Many patients who have cardiovascular disease are also at risk for pulmonary disease because of advanced age and a heavy exposure to cigarette smoking. Chronic obstructive pulmonary disease places patients at risk for complications after cardiac surgery, including prolonged dependence on mechanical ventilation and postoperative pneumonia. In order to minimize the need for postoperative mechanical ventilation and its complications, an anesthetic regimen that minimizes opioid administration is typically used. This allows the patient to be awake and spontaneously breathing early after surgery and leads to early extubation, often using respiratory therapist–driven weaning protocols. If the disease process does not allow an early extubation and the patient remains ventilator-dependent, early tracheostomy should be considered to provide an easy and secure access for pulmonary toilet, to simplify the weaning process, and to enhance patient comfort compared with the continued use of an endotracheal tube.

Preoperative chronic right ventricular overload can result in postoperative right ventricular failure. Although most of the pulmonary hypertension reverses after surgical closure of a shunt, improvement in left ventricular function, or mitral valve replacement, the pulmonary vasculature usually remains highly reactive in the early postoperative period. During this period, *pulmonary hypertensive crises* can be catastrophic and may be triggered by carbon dioxide retention, tracheal suctioning, or hypoxia. Patients with pulmonary hypertension should be kept well sedated and ventilated for longer than usual. The use of pharmacologic pulmonary vasodilators such as prostacyclin or inhaled nitric oxide can be helpful in treating these crises.

Bleeding Problems

In the early postoperative period, the cardiac surgery patient is particularly susceptible to significant bleeding, and close monitoring is mandatory. Patients undergoing cardiac surgery are typically treated preoperatively with antiplatelet agents, such as aspirin, and undergo anticoagulation for prolonged periods. Furthermore, during CPB, clotting factors are diluted and platelets are damaged. Not surprisingly, bleeding remains one of the most common early complications after cardiac surgery. Preoperative liver dysfunction due to liver congestion, alcohol use, viral hepatitis, or other causes also increases the risk of bleeding.

Postoperative chest tube drainage must be monitored closely, and output greater than 500 mL in 1 hour or greater than 200 mL/h in 3 hours mandates surgical reexploration. Conversely, an abrupt decrease in chest tube drainage with deterioration of cardiac function suggests the development of cardiac tamponade. Repeat sternotomies for reoperations carry a higher postoperative bleeding risk because of the need to dissect the scarred mediastinum. Pharmacologic agents such as aminocaproic acid and aprotinin can be used to decrease bleeding. Although aprotinin appears to be effective, on occasion it may cause thrombotic complications. Although its mechanism of action is not completely understood, it may work by activating platelets as well as inhibiting the fibrinolytic pathway. Arginine vasopressin can also be used to decrease bleeding, but its usefulness appears highest in patients with renal failure (see Chapter 20).

Factor and platelet deficiencies should be corrected in the early postoperative period if clinically indicated. The patient who continues to bleed significantly after correction of coagulation parameters requires re-exploration.

Neurologic Problems

Cardiopulmonary bypass is associated with global neurologic impairment in a small but significant number of patients. Focal deficits can also occur and are usually due to embolic events. Many patients with coronary artery disease also have significant artherosclerotic disease involving the extracranial and intracranial cerebral circulation. Nonpulsatile flow at lower mean arterial pressure during CPB may cause ischemia to a brain region distal to a vessel with critical stenosis. When significant carotid artery disease is suspected, full carotid evaluation should be carried out when feasible. If the patient has clinical symptoms due to the carotid disease and has compensated cardiac disease, carotid endarterectomy should be performed first, followed by cardiac surgery. If the cardiac disease is poorly compensated, simultaneous carotid and cardiac surgery should be performed.

Although the factors that contribute to global neurologic dysfunction are not fully understood, embolization of particulate matter and microbubbles likely occur during CPB (despite the use of in-line filters) and play an important role in its pathogenesis. Furthermore, aortic disease is often underestimated, and intraoperative embolization from aortic plaques can result from cannulation, aortic cross-clamping, or resumption of pulsatile flow after an open chamber procedure. In the postoperative period, embolic strokes are most commonly due to atrial fibrillation, the presence of new significant ventricular dyskinesia (leading to a left ventricular thromboembolus), or a residual intracardiac shunt (allowing a paradoxical embolus). Patients with atrial fibrillation or a left ventricular aneurysm should undergo systemic anticoagulation to decrease the frequency of embolism.

Renal Problems

Renal function can be affected by the complement activation and generalized inflammatory response to CPB. Nonpulsatile flow during CPB may be particularly deleterious in the patient with poor preoperative renal function or severe renal vascular disease. Free hemoglobin caused by red cell damage in CPB can also contribute to acute renal injury, especially when combined with severe acidemia. Hematuria alone is not necessarily a marker of renal dysfunction but is most often related to a prolonged period on CPB. Postoperatively, prolonged periods of low cardiac output combined with catecholamine administration can also contribute to acute renal failure.

Hepatic Dysfunction

Because of its role in producing coagulation factors, liver dysfunction can profoundly affect the outcome of any cardiac operation. Conversely, cardiac dysfunction can contribute to liver dysfunction and hepatic failure. Venous hypertension due to severe right ventricular failure and low cardiac output act synergistically to cause hepatic dysfunction resulting from congestion and arterial ischemia. The institution of mechanical circulatory support (ventricular assist device [VAD], IABP) is appropriate when inotropic support has failed. Cirrhosis predating a cardiac procedure confers significantly increased morbidity and mortality to the cardiac procedure. Cirrhotic patients typically have increased cardiac outputs due to shunting, and if high cardiac outputs cannot be maintained during the perioperative period, liver function can deteriorate further, leading to hepatic encephalopathy, the hepatorenal syndrome, variceal bleeding, and death.

Gastrointestinal Problems

Pancreatitis and splanchnic ischemia have been described after prolonged CPB, typically when vasopressors are used to maintain arterial pressure during bypass. Pressors shunt blood flow away from the pancreas and the gut, leading to variable degrees of pancreatitis and, on occasion, to patchy necrosis of the bowel.

Patients requiring prolonged postoperative ventilatory support are at risk for stress ulcers and gastritis, and all should receive appropriate stress ulcer prophylaxis (see Chapter 10). Furthermore, early institution of nutritional therapy is appropriate in many patients because of postoperative catabolism. Recent studies suggest that enteral feedings are preferable to the parenteral route (see Chapter 13). If prolonged ventilator dependency is expected and aspiration risk is significant, a jejunostomy tube should be placed when the tracheostomy is performed.

Infectious Complications

Endocarditis and mediastinitis are the most important infectious issues in the postoperative period. Endocarditis is broadly defined as the infection of cardiac endocardial lining. The cardiac valves are most commonly affected, with an anatomically abnormal valve being the predisposing factor. The endocardium near a ventricular septal defect or a patent ductus arteriosus may also become infected. Most commonly, organisms enter the blood stream from dental manipulation, skin or mucosal injuries, or low-grade infections elsewhere, for example, cholecystitis. Contaminated intravenous lines can also be a source of bacteremia in the ICU setting.

Wound inflammation or drainage and sternal pain and instability are suggestive of mediastinitis, especially when accompanied by systemic signs of infection. Echocardiography, computed tomography, and magnetic resonance imaging are often suggestive, but rarely conclusive, in diagnosing mediastinitis. Historically, mediastinitis was managed by opening the wound and débriding the mediastinum. This resulted in excessive bleeding and substantial mortality. A preferable approach is to re-explore the mediastinum as soon as a deep infection is suspected. On exploration, multiple Gram stains and cultures are obtained and, if infection is confirmed, débridement of devitalized tissue is performed, followed by closure with muscle flaps or omentum. This approach allows early mobilization; protects vital structures with healthy, infection-resistant tissue; and results in decreased mortality.

BIBLIOGRAPHY

Baumgartner WA, Owens SG, Cameron DE, Reitz BA: The Johns Hopkins Manual of Cardiac Surgical Care. St Louis: CV Mosby, 1994.
This is a practical manual for care of the cardiac surgery patient.
Edmunds LH Jr (ed): Cardiac Surgery in the Adult. New York: McGraw Hill, 1997.
This is a well-illustrated text showing the major adult cardiac procedures and covering postoperative decision making and management.
Kirklin JW, Barratt-Boyes BG (eds): Cardiac Surgery. 2nd ed. New York: Churchill Livingston, 1993.
This is a classic text covering the scope of the discipline from a surgical perspective.
Salgo IS, Savino JS: Cardiothoracic intensive care. Seminars in Anesthesia, Perioperative Medicine and Pain 18:135–148, 1999.
This review of postoperative ICU care of patients undergoing cardiac surgery gives practical examples of ICU admission and discharge criteria as well as descriptions and examples of fast-track weaning protocols for uncomplicated open-heart surgery patients.
Waldhausen JA, Orringer MB (eds): Complications in Cardiothoracic Surgery. St. Louis: Mosby-Year Book, 1991.
This text describes perioperative complications of cardiac surgery, many of which become apparent during the postoperative period in the ICU.

87 Craniotomy

Kevin D. Judy

Injuries of the brain have been described since medical antiquity. Trephined skulls have been found that date back to 7000 to 3000 BC. One of the earliest recordings of craniotomies was in the Hippocratic writings *De Capitis Vulneribus* (ca. 460 to 370 BC), which discussed evaluation and treatment of head injuries. Today craniotomy is a routine procedure, and many patients requiring craniotomy are admitted to the intensive care unit (ICU) for diagnosis, initial management, and postoperative care.

COMMON INDICATIONS FOR CRANIOTOMY

Tumors

Patients with brain tumors present with headache, neurologic deficits, and seizures. New-onset seizures should be investigated by brain computed tomography (CT) or magnetic resonance imaging. Supratentorial tumors typically cause cranial nerve dysfunction or motor or sensory changes. Patients with optic chiasm and temporal, parietal, and occipital tumors should have a neuro-ophthalmologic examination to evaluate visual fields. Hydrocephalus is a major complication of supratentorial tumors, which, if left untreated, can cause rapid decompensation, herniation, and death. If the tumor is proximate to the sella or suprasellar region, the patient's hormonal status should be investigated, including prolactin, follicle-stimulating hormone, luteinizing hormone, thyroid, cortisol, and growth hormone levels.

Tumors in the posterior fossa should be evaluated for evidence of cranial nerve dysfunction or brain stem compression. An altered level of consciousness, hypertension, or bradycardia or an altered respiratory pattern can indicate brain stem compression. Acoustic neuromas arising from the eighth cranial nerve can cause loss of hearing, and these patients should be evaluated with an audiogram.

Hematomas

Subdural and epidural hematomas are often associated with significant head trauma necessitating direct admission to the ICU. Bleeding, however, may result from minor head trauma or spontaneous hemorrhage in the elderly because of shrinkage of the brain and traction on bridging veins from the surface of the brain to the dura. Hematomas are extra-axial collections that cause compression of the brain. In general, subdural hematomas arise from a venous injury, whereas epidural hematomas are arterial in nature. For this reason, epidural hematomas can progress more rapidly than subdural hematomas.

Epidural hematomas have been described as having a classic presentation of an interval of unconsciousness followed by a lucid interval followed by unconsciousness. In clinical practice, however, a patient rarely presents in this fashion.

979

The overwhelming majority of subdural and epidural hematomas arise in the supratentorial space, although they can occur in the posterior fossa. Subdural hematomas often cause headaches, confusion, aphasia, hemiparesis, or seizures. Epidural hematomas more commonly present with a decrease in level of consciousness. Chronic subdural hematomas occur most often in the elderly and present with a decrease in the level of consciousness, focal hemiparesis, severe headaches, or new-onset seizures.

Aneurysms and Arteriovenous Malformations

Aneurysms and arteriovenous malformations typically present with subarachnoid hemorrhage and headache that is often described as the "worst headache of my life." Seizure, focal neurologic deficit, and coma are other presenting symptoms. Hemorrhage may occur during physical activity, bowel movement, or sexual intercourse.

Patients with *subarachnoid hemorrhage* present with varying levels of consciousness, ranging from fully alert to comatose. The Hunt and Hess classification is used to estimate severity and prognosis (Table 87–1). Hunt and Hess grades 1 to 3 are considered to be surgical candidates; grades 4 and 5 are treated medically unless they improve to a higher grade because the frequency of meaningful survival for these grades is less than 10%. Management is dictated by the initial neurologic deficit and is described further on.

INTENSIVE CARE EVALUATION AND MANAGEMENT

Subdural and Epidural Hematomas

Small subdural hematomas with no mass effect may be treated conservatively with observation and a repeat CT of the head in 24 hours (Table 87–2). If the patient experiences progressive neurologic deficit or the size of the clot increases with time, surgical intervention is indicated.

Epidural hematomas usually expand more rapidly because of the arterial bleeding and need to be evacuated quickly. A clot that causes mass effect and shift of the midline or a significant neurologic deficit should be evacuated immediately.

Table 87–1. Hunt-Hess Classification of Subarachnoid Hemorrhage

GRADE	DESCRIPTION
0	Unruptured
1	Asymptomatic, mild headache
2	Moderate severe headache, cranial nerve findings
3	Focal neurologic deficit, lethargy, confusion
4	Stupor, hemiparesis
5	Coma, extensor posturing

Table 87–2. Evaluation of Various Types of Intracranial Pathology

SUSPECTED PATHOLOGY	RADIOGRAPHIC STUDY
Hematoma (subdural and epidural)	Noncontrast computed tomography
Intracranial tumor	Magnetic resonance imaging with and without contrast
Aneurysm and arteriovenous malformation	Computed tomography to confirm subarachnoid hemorrhage and rule out hydrocephalus
	Cerebral angiogram to diagnose aneurysm, arteriovenous malformation
Vasospasm	Transcranial Doppler or cerebral angiogram

Patients with chronic subdural hematomas can be treated in an expectant fashion. If the only symptom is headache, the patient can be observed, permitting the hematoma to resolve spontaneously. Occasionally, burr hole drainage is required.

Subarachnoid Hemorrhage

Patients presenting with *aneurysm* or *arteriovenous malformation* and *subarachnoid hemorrhage* are admitted to the ICU for close neurologic monitoring. Hydrocephalus is treated by placement of a ventriculostomy, which may effect dramatic improvement in patients who are Hunt and Hess grade 3 or worse. Patients with sizable hematomas require urgent operative decompression. Rapid preoperative performance of a cerebral angiogram is preferable to define vascular anatomy and determine the presence and location of intracerebral aneurysms. Subarachnoid hemorrhage can cause electrocardiographic abnormalities such as T-wave abnormalities, QT prolongation, ST segment changes, permanent U waves and rhythm abnormalities. These electrocardiographic changes are reflective of subendocardial ischemia, hemorrhage, or focal areas of myocardial necrosis.

Vasospasm

Clinical Manifestations

Vasospasm is a poorly understood complication of subarachnoid hemorrhage that can lead to cerebral infarction or death. Blood in the subarachnoid space, that is, on the external surface of the cerebral arteries, may cause vasospasm and ischemia of the tissue supplied by the artery. Vasospasm usually does not occur until 4 to 5 days after the subarachnoid hemorrhage and is usually resolved by 2 weeks after the hemorrhage. The development of a delayed focal neurologic deficit or decreased level of consciousness not attributable to hydrocephalus suggests vasospasm. A cerebral angiogram shows narrowing or complete cutoff of involved arterial vessels. A noncontrast head computed tomographic scan should also be obtained to diagnose infarction, hydrocephalus, or hemorrhage.

Transcranial Doppler offers a noninvasive method to record blood flow velocity

Table 87–3. Treatment of Vasospasm after Subarachnoid Hemorrhage

> Increase systolic blood pressure to 160–180 mm Hg
>   Intravenous volume loading
>   Intravenous vasopressors
> Relax arterial smooth muscle
>   Nimodipine (60 mg q4h orally or by nasogastric tube)
> If vasospasm persists:
>   Papaverine (administered directly into the offending vessel via angiographic catheter)
>   Angioplasty (via interventional radiology)

in vessels at risk for vasospasm. High-velocity blood flow (>120 cm/sec) is diagnostic of vasospasm. Daily or alternate-day evaluation may reveal trends toward improvement or deterioration.

Treatment

Vasospasm is treated by volume loading, vasopressor-induced hypertension, and nimodipine therapy (Table 87–3). Colloids and crystalloids are infused to increase central venous pressure. Young, otherwise healthy patients often eliminate infused fluids through normal renal function. They may require volumes in excess of 10 L/day or administration of drugs such as desmopressin acetate and fludrocortisone acetate that result in renal fluid retention.

If infusion of fluids fails to correct the neurologic deficit, vasopressors are infused to increase systolic blood pressure to 160 to 180 mm Hg. Blood pressure is increased to a level that results in resolution of the neurologic deficit, but the systolic blood pressure should not exceed 200 mm Hg. Many patients have a blood pressure threshold below which they develop a profound neurologic deficit that resolves when the blood pressure increases.

Nimodipine is a calcium channel blocker that has been shown to improve outcomes in patients with subarachnoid hemorrhage and vasospasm. These therapies for vasospasm may cause congestive heart failure, and placement of a pulmonary artery catheter is indicated in older patients.

When hypervolemic and hypertensive therapy and calcium channel blocking drugs fail to improve the neurologic deficit, angiography is indicated to identify the offending vessel or vessels. Papaverine can then be injected directly into the vessel to decrease the vasospasm. The beneficial effects of papaverine, however, are transient and typically last only hours. Balloon angioplasty of the offending vessel is a more durable alternative. It obviously cannot be applied within the region of an aneurysm clip because it may dislodge the clip.

Surgery for Aneurysm

The ideal timing of surgery for intracranial aneurysms has evolved over the past several decades. The current consensus is that operative therapy should not be delayed. The risk of rebleeding is 4% within the first 24 hours and then 1.5%/day for the following 2 weeks.

Hypothermia is often intentionally induced during surgery for intracranial aneurysm and patients should be rewarmed before postoperative neurologic evaluation. The discovery of a new focal neurologic deficit mandates performance of head CT. If the computed tomographic scan is normal, the patient should undergo angiography to determine if there is a problem with the placement of the aneurysm clip. Hydrocephalus, causing a decreased level of consciousness, can occur up to 2 weeks after the subarachnoid hemorrhage.

Postoperative Care in the Intensive Care Unit

The neurologic examination is the ideal way to evaluate brain *function*. Headaches may be the presenting symptom of a postoperative hematoma. Agitation and hypertension are consistent with posterior fossa herniation syndrome after posterior fossa surgery but may be incorrectly attributed to postoperative pain and treated with opioids. Patients with these symptoms should be promptly evaluated with CT.

In contrast, supratentorial herniation syndromes typically progress more slowly, with lethargy, contralateral hemiparesis, a dilated pupil, and respiratory compromise. Nevertheless, patients with these symptoms after supratentorial craniotomy should also be investigated with CT before treatment with opioids. The brain has no sensation, and the only sources of pain from a craniotomy are the dura, scalp, and underlying facial muscles, which are adequately treated with acetaminophen.

Patients who have had posterior fossa surgery are at risk for injury to cranial nerves IX, X, and XII, which innervate the pharynx and tongue and are consequently at risk for airway obstruction. They should be observed closely at the time of extubation after surgery. If there is concern regarding the function of these lower cranial nerves, the patient should remain intubated until pharyngeal function is evaluated. When pharyngeal dysfunction persists, tracheostomy should be performed for airway protection.

Coagulation profiles and platelet counts are followed closely after intracranial hemorrhage (subarachnoid, subdural, epidural) and corrected when necessary to prevent any further bleeding. Postoperative head CT is performed within 24 hours to look for any other evidence of bleeding within the brain. It is common that once an acute subdural or epidural hematoma is evacuated, a contusion of the underlying brain can swell, creating significant mass effect. Contusions that develop after evacuation of an epidural or subdural hematoma may require re-exploration and evacuation in some patients.

Steroids are of no value in treating edema after traumatic brain injury. Serum osmolality is therapeutically increased to 290 to 310 mOsm/kg to reduce the frequency of brain edema after brain injury. The head of the patient should be elevated to 30 degrees to reduce venous engorgement of the brain. Routine postoperative medications include corticosteroids (which are then rapidly tapered over the next week) to prevent meningismus from subarachnoid blood or brain swelling after surgery for tumor. Anticonvulsants are used to prevent seizures, H_2 histamine receptor blocker to prevent gastrointestinal bleeding, and antiemetics for postoperative nausea. Antifibrinolytic agents, such as aminocaproic acid (once used to reduce the incidence of rebleeding), have been shown to cause persistence of blood clot within the subarachnoid space. Because they may increase the incidence of vasospasm, their use has fallen out of favor.

The patient undergoing an uncomplicated craniotomy for tumor may resume oral intake later on the evening of surgery or by the next day. Patients are encouraged to get out of bed the morning after surgery. In most cases, the patient can be safely transferred out of the ICU the day after surgery. Early ambulation is essential to prevent deep venous thrombosis and subsequent pulmonary emboli.

BIBLIOGRAPHY

Allen GS, Ahn HS, Preziosi TJ, et al: Cerebral arterial spasm—a controlled trial of nimodipine in patients with SAH. N Engl J Med 308:619–624, 1983.
This article describes a well-controlled clinical trial that proved the efficacy of nimodipine in improving the outcome of patients who suffer a subarachnoid hemmorhage.

Bedford R: Supratentorial masses. In: Coltrell J, Smith DS (eds): Anesthetic Considerations in Anesthesia and Neurosurgery, 3rd ed. St. Louis: CV Mosby, 1994, pp 312–314.
This textbook chapter contains a thorough discussion of the neuroanesthetic techniques used for most craniotomies.

Bergstorm NI, Ericson K, Levander B, et al: Computed tomography of cranial subdural and epidural hematomas: Variation of attenuation related to time and clinical events such as rebleeding. J Comput Assist Tomogr 1:449–455, 1977.
This classic article was the first to delineate the time course of resolving blood in subdural and epidural hematomas. This provided the ability to determine the age of hematomas, which has a significant impact on clinical management.

Dearden NNI, Gibson JS, McDowall DG, et al: Effect of high-dose dexamethasone on outcome from severe head injury. J Neurosurg 64:81–88, 1986.
This article put to rest the ongoing controversy of using steroids to treat head trauma. It proved that the use of steroids did not improve outcome and contributed to poor blood glucose control and perhaps impaired wound healing.

Fischer CNI, Kistler JP, Davis JM: Relation of cerebral vasospasm to SAH visualized by CT scanning. Neurosurgery 6:1–9, 1980.
This classic article proposed an association between the amount of subarachnoid blood and the incidence and severity of vasospasm. This has provided the basis for the development of therapies designed to remove blood from the subarachnoid space such as basal cistern irrigation and infusion of alteplase into the cisterns.

Galicich JH, French LA: Use of dexamethasone in the treatment of cerebral edema resulting from brain tumors and brain surgery. Am Pract Dig Treat 12:164–174, 1961.
This was an early definitive article on the use of dexamethasone to treat brain edema from tumors.

Hunt WE, Hess RM: Surgical risk as related to time of intervention in the repair of intracranial aneurysms. J Neurosurg 28:14–20, 1968.
This classic article established a grading scale for patients who suffered a subarachnoid hemorrhage. The Hunt and Hess classification is still the gold standard for determining the severity of subarachnoid hemorrhage and is used to determine whether a patient is a surgical candidate for clipping of the aneurysm.

Inagawa T, Kamiya K, Ogasawara H, et al: Rebleeding of ruptured intracranial aneurysms in the acute stage. Surg Neurol 28:93–99, 1987.
This widely quoted paper defined the incidence of rebleeding from aneurysms over the life span of the individual.

Kassell NF, Peerless SI, Durward QJ, et al: Treatment of ischemic deficits from vasospasm with intravascular volume expansion and induced arterial hypertension. Neurosurgery 11:337–343, 1982.
This article provides a succinct discussion regarding the use of hypervolemic and hypertensive therapy for the treatment of vasospasm.

Marion DW, Segal R, Thompson ME: Subarachnoid hemorrhage and the heart. Neurosurgery 18:101–106, 1986.
This article explored all the electrocardiographic abnormalities seen in patients with subarachnoid hemorrhage. There are many such abnormalities seen, and until this article the electrocardiographic

changes were not felt to be indicative of real cardiac injury. This article showed that the heart does suffer injury associated with subarachnoid hemorrhage.

Nehls DC, Flom RA, Carter LP, et al: Multiple intracranial aneurysms: Determining the site of rupture. J Neurosurgery 63:342–348, 1985.

When presented with a patient with subarachnoid hemorrhage and multiple aneurysms on the angiogram, how does one determine which aneurysm bled? Nehls and colleagues present a logical evaluation process using vasospasm, location, and size to decide which aneurysm is probably the offending one.

Nishioka H, Torner JC, Graf CJ, et al: Cooperative study of intracranial aneurysms and SAH: III. SAH of undetermined etiology. Arch Neurol 41:1147–1151, 1984.

This article discusses the possible causes and predicted incidence of recurrence in patients with subarachnoid hemorrhage and normal angiograms.

88

Major Abdominal Surgery: Postoperative Considerations

Michael D. Grossman
Patrick M. Reilly

Intensivists frequently care for patients undergoing major abdominal surgery, the majority of whom have surgery for intra-abdominal malignancies or infection. Many are elderly with multiple comorbid conditions, including atherosclerotic cardiovascular disease, chronic obstructive airway disease (COPD), and diabetes mellitus. Exacerbation of these chronic conditions resulting from the stress of critical illness and surgery is the rule and should be expected in postoperative care.

If patients undergo surgery electively, one has the opportunity to treat comorbid conditions, which has been shown to improve outcomes. Although operations performed under emergency circumstances do not allow for a complete preoperative evaluation and treatment of comorbidities, all high-risk patients should be evaluated and *physiologically optimized* prior to surgery (see Chapter 84). This may include preoperative intravascular fluid loading for optimal preload, correction of anemia, coagulopathy and electrolyte disorders, placement of invasive monitoring catheters and, in some cases, intubation to treat respiratory failure. Failure to intervene preoperatively in this manner may lead to intraoperative hemodynamic instability and a stormy postoperative course.

When being transferred to the intensive care unit (ICU) after major abdominal surgery, the patient should be accompanied by the anesthesiologist and one or more members of the surgical team. An immediate dialog should be established between the intensivist and operating team (a so-called doctor-to-doctor report), which serves as the foundation for all subsequent care delivered in the ICU. This dialog should first include details of the patient's history and preoperative evaluation. Next, the intensivist should carefully review the anesthetic record with the anesthesiologist before he or she leaves the ICU (see Chapter 83). Third, the intensivist should discuss with the surgeon details of the operation that might influence postoperative management, including placement of drains, tubes, or stomas; the potential for third space fluid shifts; and the degree to which a septic focus was manipulated, removed, or retained.

OPERATIVE PROCEDURES (Table 88–1)

Pancreaticoduodenectomy (Whipple Procedure)

Whipple procedures are performed most often for carcinoma of the pancreas. Patients whose tumors are resectable are not usually jaundiced or malnourished. The operation lasts from 4 to 10 hours, depending on the experience of the

987

Table 88–1. Major Abdominal Surgery and Its Common Complications

PROCEDURE	COMPLICATIONS
Whipple procedure	Third space losses into retroperitoneum; if total pancreatectomy is performed, diabetes and hyperglycemia; anastomotic breakdowns occur on postoperative days 5–10.
Hepatic lobectomy (>50% of liver resected)	Jaundice is common, peaks on postoperative days 3–4 and needs investigation if it persists beyond postoperative day 10. Hypoglycemia is also common; patients need 10% dextrose postoperatively; hepatic failure may occur in cirrhotic patients.
Esophagogastrectomy	Complications occur commonly in 10–25% of cases. Pulmonary complications are frequent, often due to gastric aspiration. Anastomotic leaks in chest cause mediastinitis or empyema, or both.
Intestinal and reoperative surgery	Preoperative severe dehydration, contraction alkalosis, hypokalemia, and marked third space losses into obstructed bowel. Continued third space losses occur postoperatively as well as intra-abdominal infection or fistula formation due to inadvertent enterotomies or anastomotic leaks.

surgeon. The pancreatic head and entire duodenum are resected en bloc, and two or three anastomoses are required to re-establish gastrointestinal (GI) tract continuity. When performed without undue technical difficulty, the degree of physiologic perturbation is moderate, involving mostly third space losses into the retroperitoneum. If total pancreatectomy is carried out, the patient will immediately become diabetic and glucose may be difficult to control. Major complications are related to the anastomoses and these usually occur between 5 and 10 days postoperatively. There are drains and possibly a T-tube stenting the biliary anastomosis. The specific location of each drain or tube should be illustrated in the patient's record. Mortality rates in centers performing more than 50 cases per year are less than 5%.

Hepatic Lobectomy

Resection of 50% or more of hepatic parenchyma may result in hyperbilirubinemia, jaundice, hypoglycemia, hypoalbuminemia, hypophosphatemia, and hypokalemia. Jaundice and hypoglycemia are the most common sequelae. Jaundice usually peaks between 3 and 4 days postoperatively and should be investigated if it persists beyond 10 days. Hypoglycemia is often severe enough to warrant infusion of 10% dextrose, and its resolution is frequently followed by hyperglycemia. Aside from early bleeding, the most feared complication of major liver resection is liver failure. This may occur in patients with cirrhosis who cannot tolerate resection of a significant volume of liver tissue.

Esophagogastrectomy

There are three principal approaches to esophageal resection, and the postoperative course and complications differ depending on which is employed. Common to all is an upper midline laparotomy incision. Some patients will also have a thoracotomy, whereas others have a left cervical incision. In general, complications following esophageal resection are more common than in other abdominal or thoracic operations, occurring in 10 to 25% of cases. Pulmonary complications may be related to the thoracotomy or to loss of the lower esophageal sphincter, which predisposes the patient to aspiration of gastric contents. Many patients with esophageal carcinoma have malnutrition and chronic obstructive airway disease as comorbid conditions. Infection is also a significant cause of postoperative morbidity and mortality and is often due to an anastomotic leak. When the leak occurs at an anastomosis that is placed in the chest, mediastinitis and empyema may develop. Although less common than leakage from a cervical anastomosis, leaks in the chest are less well tolerated.

Intestinal and Reoperative Abdominal Surgery

Because reoperative abdominal surgery is frequently performed to treat intestinal obstruction, these topics are presented together. Physiologic derangements frequently accompany intestinal obstruction. Severe dehydration, contraction alkalosis, hypokalemia, and marked third space losses into the obstructed intestine may be encountered prior to surgery. Reasonable attempts to correct these abnormalities are warranted in order to avoid substantial postoperative problems. Reoperative surgery that is often required to treat bowel obstruction may be prolonged and may itself involve massive losses of third space fluids due to extensive lysis of adhesions. It is common for an extensive lysis of adhesions to take between 4 and 8 hours. Postoperative intra-abdominal infection or fistula formation, or both, may occur because of inadvertent enterotomies or anastomotic leaks. In general, morbidity rates following surgery for intestinal obstruction are 25 to 30%. Advanced age, delay in operative intervention, and comorbid conditions increase complication rates. Malignant obstruction and obstruction due to radiation enteritis also result in higher morbidity and mortality rates. If infarcted intestine is encountered, massive small bowel resection may be required and short-gut syndrome may result.

POSTOPERATIVE MANAGEMENT

Fluid Management

Fluid losses during abdominal surgery are a function of the extent of surgical dissection, length of operation, blood or extravascular fluid lost during surgery, and presence or absence of infection and fever. Formulas exist that attempt to define "ideal" maintenance fluids for patients undergoing major abdominal surgery. These are based on estimation of the degree of evaporative or insensible losses associated with laparotomy. These are only approximations, however, and are not a substitute for fluid management guided by urine output, measured or estimated blood loss (usually a "low" estimate), acid-base status, hemodynamic data, and clinical assessment of perfusion (see Chapter 84).

Like other patients undergoing major surgery, patients undergoing major abdominal surgery experience a stress or inflammatory response that favors fluid sequestration into the extravascular fluid compartment (see Chapter 84). The presence of peritonitis may add dramatically to fluid loss into the peritoneum both intraoperatively and postoperatively.

"Third-spacing" of fluid decreases intravascular volume, which, in turn, decreases glomerular filtration rate. This effect plus elevated levels of circulating catecholamines, aldosterone, and antidiuretic hormone enhance tubular resorption of Na^+ and water with the end result of increased fluid retention. The degree to which this fluid remains in the intravascular space depends on the presence of an inflammatory component that produces a capillary leak and loss of fluid into the "third space." This type of inflammation occurs with all major surgery, but its severity is proportional to the magnitude of the operation, degree of blood loss, and presence and degree of other sites of inflammation, such as peritonitis.

Postoperative fluid management can be simplified by separating maintenance fluids from all other fluid requirements. Early in the postoperative course, patients require a maintenance IV rate that is generally 100 mL/h in a 70-kg patient. Fluids are usually isotonic crystalloids and contain 5% dextrose unless salt restriction is indicated such as in cirrhotic patients. Supplemental fluids, including those required to replace measured and insensible losses, should *not* contain glucose and may be in the form of colloid or crystalloid.

It is practical to devote a separate IV line for these nonmaintenance fluids and to deliver "bolus" fluids as required to replace measured and unmeasured losses. Using concentrated albumin solutions is not indicated for routine fluid replacement. Measured losses include blood from drains and GI contents from nasogastric (NG), intestinal, or biliary tubes and ileostomies. Unmeasured losses include ongoing third space losses and evaporative losses due to fever and open wounds. Since the determination of the degree of insensible loss may be difficult, monitoring of end-organ perfusion via urine output and acid-base status plus hemodynamic monitoring are recommended to guide fluid replacement therapy accurately (see Fig. 84–3 and Tables 84–3 and 84–4).

Pain Control

Pain management plays an important role especially in the prevention of postoperative pulmonary complications and in decreasing demands on the cardiovascular system. Historically, parenteral opioids have been the mainstay in providing postoperative pain control (see Chapter 85). Patient-controlled analgesia delivered parenterally has been shown to be more effective than intermittent opioid dosing by care providers. Caution must be exercised when continuous or basal rate patient-controlled opioids are used, however, as the incidence of respiratory depression is somewhat higher than with intermittent dosing alone.

Epidural analgesia has emerged as the preferred method of pain control for patients undergoing major abdominal operations (see Chapter 85). This method allows delivery of opioid and local anesthetic directly to receptors in the spinal cord. Because it achieves pain control at much lower serum concentrations of opioid, less respiratory and central nervous system depression is observed. Active participation by patients in their own respiratory care, for example, performing deep breathing exercises and coughing, is crucial in the postoperative period and with epidural analgesia, they can better participate in these postoperative respiratory maneuvers as well as be mobilized in general earlier. Complications of epidural analgesia are rare and include infection, bleeding into the epidural space, postspinal headaches, and vasodilation and accompanying hypotension when local anesthetics are used (see Fig. 85–2).

Nonsteroidal anti-inflammatory drugs are also useful in postoperative pain management because they, like epidural opioids, have little or no respiratory or central nervous system depression. They may be administered parenterally (ketorolac) or by suppository (indomethacin) in patients who are receiving nothing by mouth.

Management of Tubes, Drains, and Stomas

Drainage Considerations

The performance of abdominal surgery is often associated with the placement of drains or tubes in various positions within the digestive tract, biliary ducts, or peritoneal cavity. Stomas, which are openings of the digestive tract onto the abdominal wall, may also be required. It is less important for the intensivist to understand the precise indications and technical features of these drainage and diverting methods than to have an appreciation of their practical management.

Two basic modalities of drainage are employed: passive and active. A passive drain relies on a wick effect to remove fluid, whereas an active drain usually employs suction. When suction is employed, a "sump" is often present alongside the drain tube to prevent the suction port from clogging. Drains may be open or closed and, depending what it is draining, a closed system is *theoretically* sterile because there is no ongoing communication with the environment. Today, most surgeons employ active closed drainage systems to drain blood, bile, pancreatic juice, or infected material from an abscess cavity.

As a rule, one should assume that the operating surgeon has a clear purpose for any drainage tube, and it is therefore axiomatic that no such device should be removed or manipulated without the express permission of the surgeon. Accordingly, drain tubes should be carefully secured, usually by sutures, to the patient's skin. When the patient returns from the operating room, one should note whether this has been carried out and, if not, one should notify the surgeon.

Nasogastric Tubes

NG tubes deserve special mention because they are used so commonly. A number of studies demonstrate that the routine use of an NG tube following abdominal surgery is not indicated. Nonetheless, advocates of their use believe that vomiting and aspiration, as well as suture line or abdominal wound disruption, occur more frequently when they are not routinely placed. When an NG tube is in place, care must be taken to prevent it becoming retroflexed over the patient's forehead because this position can exert pressure against the nasal ala and lead to ulceration and, in some cases, necrosis of the nasal ala. The prolonged presence of a NG tube is also a risk factor for ipsilateral sinusitis and nosocomial pneumonia.

Removal of NG tubes usually follows evidence of return of bowel function, normally 3 to 5 days after surgery. Occasionally, high NG outputs in excess of 1 L/day persist beyond 3 to 5 days. It may be useful to remove the tube from suction for several hours followed by a check of residual gastric contents ("clamping trial"). If "residuals" (fluid that remains in the stomach after a certain time) are less than 150 to 200 mL/4 h, one can assume antegrade passage of gastric contents and consider removing the NG tube.

Intestinal Stomas

Intestinal stomas are created to divert the intestinal stream. They may be permanent or temporary and consist of a side hole in a loop of intestine or a free end. The principal acute complications associated with intestinal stomas are bleeding, necrosis, and separation from the abdominal wall. Bleeding can usually be controlled locally with a suture. Ischemia and necrosis are diagnosed by appearance of the stoma. A useful technique to assess the stoma is to insert a test tube into the opening and, with a penlight, examine the mucosa for viability (it should appear pink or red). Ileostomies or proximal small bowel stomas can cause skin excoriation because their effluent is caustic. Colostomies are less likely to cause excoriation, but both small bowel and large bowel stomas should be adequately protected with a base plate and collecting bag.

Nutrition

A comprehensive discussion of surgical nutrition is well beyond the scope of this chapter (see Chapter 13), but a few select points are particularly germane to the intensivist caring for postoperative abdominal surgery patients. Many patients undergoing abdominal surgery are elderly and have malignancies. These patients often have depletion of baseline visceral protein stores and associated impaired immunologic competence. They are at high risk for multiple complications and have increased mortality rates when compared with patients whose nutritional status is adequate. Early, aggressive nutritional support is therefore important.

Enteral nutrition is preferred over parenteral nutrition. It is believed that even low levels of enteral feeding (which do not meet protein and caloric needs) may be helpful in preserving the gut–mucosal barrier function and maintaining immunologic function. Daily nitrogen and carbohydrate requirements can be met by administration of parenteral nutrition in such patients. Enteral nutrition can be provided by nasoenteric tubes placed beyond the pylorus or via an NG tube in the stomach. An NG tube is preferable to smaller diameter feeding tubes for gastric feeds because residuals can be checked more easily. Surgically placed feeding tubes that are distal to the ligament of Treitz have a lower incidence of aspiration in populations at high risk for this problem, but they may have other complications. Postoperative patients generally have caloric requirements in the range of 25 to 40 Kcal/kg/day and protein requirements between 1.5 and 2.5 g/kg/day.

The timing of nutritional support is somewhat controversial. In trauma patients, several studies have demonstrated the safety and efficacy of low-volume enteral feeds begun in the operating room. Experimental work suggests that intestinal anastomoses can heal well under these circumstances. However, many surgeons operating on an older, more chronically debilitated group of patients are less willing to feed patients until there is evidence of bowel function. Total parenteral nutrition can theoretically be started at any time following surgery, but in the immediate postoperative period (when patients are in the midst of an acute stress response), repletion of carbohydrate and protein stores is not possible. The value of early enteral feeding during this early postoperative time period is hypothesized to be due to its beneficial effects on the immune and "barrier" function of the gut.

POSTOPERATIVE COMPLICATIONS

Pulmonary Complications

The most common complications of upper abdominal surgery are pulmonary, occurring in 5 to 50% of cases. Patients at high risk for such complications are smokers or those with dyspnea on exertion, cough, and sputum production. The precise role of preoperative pulmonary function studies prior to abdominal surgery is unclear, but patients with a maximal voluntary ventilation less than 50% of predicted have significantly more pulmonary complications than those with a normal maximal voluntary ventilation.

Lung volumes are reduced after all types of abdominal surgery. For example, functional residual capacity and vital capacity may fall to less than 50% of preoperative values on the first postoperative day, with a gradual recovery over the next week. Lack of sighs (due to opioids and splinting) and shallow tidal breathing prevent re-activation of surfactant, which, in turn, decreases functional residual capacity (FRC). As a result, segmental, lobar, or even multilobar atelectasis often occurs. Pain also compromises the patient's ability to cough and clear respiratory secretions

Respiratory compliance is reduced because of a reduction in FRC and splinting resulting from incisional pain. The work of breathing increases because of this reduced compliance, low tidal volumes, and higher rates, which are also associated with increased $\dot{V}{CO_2}$ during the postoperative response to stress (see Chapter 84). The extent of these abnormalities is related to preoperative status, type of incision, duration of the anesthesia, and quality of postoperative pain control.

The incision used by the operating surgeon is an extremely important factor in postoperative care. *Thoracoabdominal* and *combined thoracic and midline incisions*, as encountered in some patients undergoing esophagectomy or reoperative surgery of the gastroesophageal junction, produce the greatest reductions in lung volumes (splinting) postoperatively. Upper midline incisions and subcostal or bilateral subcostal incisions are commonly used in the treatment of a variety of upper gastrointestinal and hepatobiliary procedures. Because *subcostal incisions* actually divide muscle in the upper abdomen, they are more likely to result in postoperative discomfort than are upper abdominal midline incisions.

Incisions centered around or below the umbilicus are typically used in elective lower GI and pelvic surgery. They have much less of an impact on postoperative pulmonary function than do subcostal or upper midline incisions. *Laparoscopic* procedures produce the least postoperative pain and the lowest occurrence of pulmonary complications in the postoperative period. They may, however, produce a marked decrease in FRC (which predisposes to basilar atelectasis) during the intraoperative period if high gas insufflation pressures are used.

Patient participation in postoperative respiratory care is essential. Regular performance of deep breathing exercises (with or without an incentive spirometer) decreases the frequency of pulmonary complications following laparotomy from 30 to 10%. *Routine* administration of oxygen is not prophylactic against pulmonary complications, but it may suppress the drive to breath and impair V/Q matching by releasing hypoxic pulmonary vasoconstriction. Stimulation or induction of coughing is effective by itself only in patients with secretions to be cleared. Since it produces low lung volumes at the end of expiration, coughing tends to aggravate atelectasis unless combined with deep breathing exercises.

Fever

Fever is common in the postoperative period. It is stimulated by release of inflammatory cytokines, predominantly interleukin-1, from macrophages at sites of tissue injury and infection (see Chapter 84). Figure 88–1 lists common sources of postoperative fever and their temporal relationship to surgery. The mnemonic "wind, water, wound, walking" applies to this set of relationships where walking refers to deep venous thrombosis of the lower extremities (encountered most commonly between days 5 and 7 postoperatively). For the intensivist managing postoperative patients, one fundamental problem is to know when to pursue an expensive work-up of a postoperative fever aggressively. In general, blood cultures are of little value in the first 48 hours following surgery, even more so if the patient is on antibiotics.

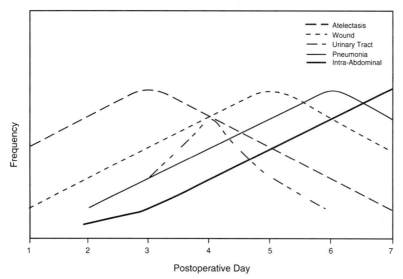

Figure 88–1. Schematic illustration of the time course and frequency of common causes of fever following major abdominal surgery.

Urinary Tract Infection

Urinary tract infection is the most common postoperative nosocomial infection, with gram-negative bacteria the predominant pathogens. Most of these occur following bladder catheterization. Ten to 25% of patients with long-term catheterization (>3 days) become infected and 1 to 5% of patients having short-term catheterization (immediate operative period) become infected. Urinary catheterization and urinary tract infection are the predisposing factors most often associated with gram-negative bacteremia, which is twice as likely to originate from the urinary tract as from any other site. Diagnosis is based on greater than 10^5 bacteria/mL of catheterized urine or greater than 100 bacteria/mL of urine aspirated from a suprapubic tap.

Pneumonia

Pneumonia is the second most common nosocomial infection encountered in the postoperative period. Multiple associated risk factors have been identified, including age greater than 70 years, upper abdominal surgery, depressed level of consciousness, use of H_2 histamine receptor blockers, and exposure to improperly sterilized respiratory care devices. Occult aspiration of neutralized gastric contents and colonization of the oropharynx by hospital-acquired bacteria have been proposed as theories to account for the overwhelming proportion of gram-negative pneumonias encountered postoperatively. Diagnosis requires the presence of fever, leukocytosis, infiltrate on the chest radiograph, and isolation of a predominant, pathogenic organism in the sputum (or specimen from the lower respiratory tract) (see Chapter 11).

Wound Infections

Wound infections occur in 2 to 40% of abdominal operations. Operations may be classified as clean, clean-contaminated, contaminated, and dirty, with increasing infection rates correlating with their order. Obesity, old age, other sites of infection, and duration of surgery also correlate with increased rates of wound infection. Redness, pain, swelling, fever, and drainage from the wound site indicate the presence of an infection, usually between the third and seventh postoperative days. *Staphylococcus aureus* remains the most common isolate, although gram-negative and mixed infections are seen frequently after abdominal surgery. Opening the wound to facilitate drainage is the mainstay of therapy. Antibiotics are indicated only if significant cellulitis is observed or a major soft tissue infection is suspected.

Aggressive, necrotizing *abdominal wall infections* caused by hemolytic streptococci and clostridial species may produce high fevers in the early postoperative period (see Fig. 88–1). These may be devastating if not diagnosed promptly. The infected wound may weep a thin tan fluid, bullae may appear in the surrounding skin, or the skin may become dusky and crepitant. Such infections are rare, but when present require parenteral antibiotics and, more importantly, prompt surgical intervention (see Chapter 66).

Ileus

An ileus is defined as a delay in the return of prograde intestinal peristalsis. It is an operational definition because the time course to return of function varies. The small bowel is usually first to recover motility after major abdominal surgery, followed by the stomach and finally the colon. Preoperative peritonitis, extensive retroperitoneal dissection, reoperative surgery, and pancreatitis are associated with increased delay in return of peristalsis. High-dose opioids, phenothiazines, and anticholinergic medications are also associated with ileus (see Chapter 41). The patient may have a distended abdomen, usually with diminished to absent bowel sounds, but rarely with substantial associated pain. Treatment is largely supportive. Prokinetic agents such as metoclopramide, cisapride, and erythromycin may be helpful as may cessation of agents predisposing to ileus (see Chapter 41).

Thromboembolic Disorders

Deep vein thrombosis may complicate abdominal surgery in as many as 30% of patients. All patients undergoing abdominal surgery should receive appropriate prophylaxis against deep vein thrombosis, ideally beginning *before* the patient is anesthetized. The presence of malignancy, preoperative bed rest, multiple trauma, pelvic surgery, and prior history of thromboembolic disease are additional risk factors. Prophylaxis with subcutaneous heparin (or enoxaparin) or use of a pneumatic compression device on the lower extremities is indicated. Prophylaxis should be continued until the patient is ambulating. In high-risk patients, routine surveillance in the postoperative period using duplex ultrasound may be warranted and, in very high-risk trauma patients, prophylactic vena cava interruption may be warranted.

Hemorrhage and Hypotension

Bleeding following abdominal surgery is usually not subtle. It may manifest as a GI bleed (bloody NG drainage, hematemesis, or hematochezia). Bleeding from an intestinal suture line may be observed for a time postoperatively and is not unusual in most anastomoses. Intra-abdominal bleeding is harder to diagnose and may necessitate a return to the operating room if hemodynamic instability or a steadily falling hemoglobin is evident. Any coagulopathy must be corrected if postoperative bleeding is noted because even minor bleeding points may not stop in the presence of a coagulopathy. A systemic approach to postoperative hypotension is recommended (see Fig. 91–1).

Intra-Abdominal Sepsis

Patients undergoing major abdominal surgery occasionally experience postoperative *intra-abdominal sepsis*. Those at greatest risk are the immunosuppressed, malnourished, or elderly. The intra-abdominal infection may also be related to the initial operation, that is, abscess, or disrupted anastomosis. An infection following a primary procedure performed for peritonitis is referred to as "secondary" peritonitis. Some patients acquire "tertiary" peritonitis, a diffuse peritoneal infection with no radiographic correlate and very high associated mortality, following repeated operations for peritonitis. The intra-abdominal process may also be acquired but unrelated (except temporally) to the primary abdominal operation, for example, acute acalculous cholecystitis or postoperative pancreatitis.

Clinical manifestations include high fever beyond 5 days postoperatively, persistent leukocytosis, a failure to mobilize third space fluid, unexplained obtundation and "remote" organ system dysfunction, such as acute respiratory distress syndrome. Some patients may localize a new abdominal complaint (even in the presence of a fresh incision), which helps to direct diagnostic studies.

Diagnostic studies directed by clinical findings or laboratory abnormalities yield a higher success rate than those performed in response to nonspecific elevations of fever, white blood cell count, and organ system failure. The presence of two gram-negative enteric organisms in blood cultures suggests an intra-abdominal process if suspicion for pneumonia is low.

If acalculous cholecystitis is suspected, portable right upper quadrant ultrasonography should be performed first, which, if suspicious, should be followed by an abdominal computed tomographic scan or ultrasound-guided drainage, depending on the clinical urgency.

Nondirected computed tomographic scans performed within the first 7 to 10 days after surgery are unlikely to provide useful information. Occasionally, diagnostic laparotomy is advocated as "diagnostic and therapeutic." In the absence of specific information on an imaging study or a focal finding on physical examination, however, the yield of nondirected surgical explorations is low.

When an intra-abdominal focus is discovered, attempts to perform computed tomographically guided catheter drainage are warranted. Percutaneous drainage of the gallbladder in suspected cases of acalculous cholecystitis has become well established and may be the preferred therapy in critically ill ICU patients.

Clinical Pearls

1. The metabolic response to major abdominal surgery is predictable (see Chapter 84). Patients should begin mobilizing fluid and have decreasing fever curves within a week. If not, one should be suspect complications and begin to search for a source of infection.
2. Immediate attention to postoperative pain control including liberal use of epidural analgesia is likely to result in fewer major pulmonary complications.
3. Patients who undergo extensive lysis of adhesions should be *expected* to have a prolonged ileus, which may extend well into the second postoperative week. Conservative management with attention to fluid balance, electrolyte abnormalities, and nutrition is usually effective.
4. In the patient at high-risk for the development of postoperative intra-abdominal infection, repeated physical examination by the same clinician represents a useful diagnostic modality by itself with the potential to provide as much information as a nondirected abdominal computed tomographic scan in the early postoperative period.

BIBLIOGRAPHY

Bessey PQ: Metabolic response to critical illness. In: Wilmore WD, Cheung LY, Harken AH, et al (eds): Scientific American Surgery, vol 1: Critical Care. New York, Scientific American, 1994, II-11:1–27.
This is a superb review of neuroendocrine, humoral, and cytokine response to critical surgical illness. This review emphasizes the time course of events. It contains excellent graphic illustrations.

Cheatham ML, Chapman WC, Key SP, et al: A meta-analysis of selective versus routine nasogastric decompression after elective laparotomy. Ann Surg 221:469–476, 1995.
This article reviews all randomized trials of selective versus mandatory NG tube decompression.

Dougherty SH, Simmons RL: The biology and practice of surgical drains. Part I. Current Problems in Surgery 29:559–623, 1992.

Dougherty SH, Simmons RL: The biology and practice of surgical drains. Part II. Current Problems in Surgery 29:633–730, 1992.
These are definitive reviews of a topic that is extremely controversial among surgeons.

Jayr C, Thomas H, Rey A, et al: Postoperative pulmonary complications: Epidural analgesia using bupivacaine and opioids versus parenteral opioids. Anesthesiology 78:666–676, 1993.
This article documents the beneficial effect of reduced postoperative pain on pulmonary complications.

Moore FA, Moore EE: Clinical benefits of early post-injury enteral feeding [review]. Clin Intensive Care 6:21, 1995.
This is a concise review of trials measuring clinical outcomes in patients receiving early enteral feeding.

Practice guidelines for acute pain management in the perioperative setting: A report by the American Society of Anesthesiologists Task Force on Pain Management, Acute Pain Section. Anesthesiology 82:1071–1081, 1995.
This article describes the current recommendations regarding available modalities for treatment of postoperative pain. Very well referenced with special emphasis on safety of different regimens.

Sinnanan M, Maier RV, Carrico CJ: Laparotomy for intra-abdominal sepsis in the ICU. Arch Surg 119:652–658, 1984.
This describes one of several studies from the early and middle 1980s examining the role of various diagnostic tests in the detection of intra-abdominal infection in the ICU. Somewhat dated, it reports a limited role for computed tomographic scanning in this setting.

89

Major Orthopedic Procedures

Edward J. Vresilovic, Jr.
R. John Naranja

The vast majority of elective orthopedic procedures require intensivist management only for perioperative complications involving organ systems other than the musculoskeletal system. When patients are treated in the intensive care unit (ICU) for primary orthopedic problems, they usually have multiple trauma. These patients frequently sustain injuries to both the axial and appendicular musculoskeletal systems (Table 89–1). Although an isolated extremity injury is not life-threatening in general and would not warrant ICU admission by itself, if extremity injuries occur in combination, they can cause hypotension and injury to distant organ systems. Conversely, axial injuries are frequently life-threatening in isolation or combination and require intensive management.

Axial injuries to the spine are covered as a separate topic in Chapter 98. This chapter addresses musculoskeletal injuries to the appendicular skeleton and pelvis and the associated orthopedic procedures.

MUSCULOSKELETAL INJURIES IN EXTREMITY TRAUMA

Occult Blood Loss

The patient with extremity trauma requires resuscitation for evident and occult blood loss. Table 89–2 summarizes the estimated occult blood loss for different long bone fractures and for fracture of the pelvis. Fluid resuscitation can be guided by these estimates. Furthermore, certain fractures are associated with major vascular injuries that can cause additional blood loss (see Chapter 95).

Musculoskeletal Survey

Following initial resuscitation, a secondary survey of all organ systems is necessary. A systematic review of extremity osseous and ligamentous structures should

Table 89–1. Major Musculoskeletal Injuries and Complications with Multiple Trauma

Extremity trauma
  Compartment syndrome
  Dislocations
  Gunshot wounds
  Long bone fractures
  Open fractures
  Traumatic amputation
Pelvic trauma

Table 89–2. Occult Blood Loss of Various Fractures

FRACTURED BONE	BLOOD LOSS (UNITS)
Ankle	0.5–1.5
Elbow	0.5–1.5
Femur	1.0–2.0
Forearm	0.5–1.0
Hip	1.5–2.5
Humerus	1.0–2.0
Knee	1.0–1.5
Pelvis	1.5–4.5
Tibia	0.5–1.5

be performed. Failure to diagnose fractures results in delayed management and exacerbation of the initial injury. Early stabilization and repair of musculoskeletal injuries has a beneficial effect on long-term outcome in patients who initially survive multiple trauma.

The musculoskeletal survey begins with observation. All long bones should be palpated and joint range of motion examined. Clues to injury include swelling, ecchymosis, crepitus, malalignment and, of course, pain. Any region that demonstrates any of these signs or symptoms requires further radiographic imaging (taken in at least two planes and including the joint proximal and, if applicable, distal to the area of suspected injury).

Open Fractures

After a systematic examination of major osseous and ligamentous structures, open injuries are assessed. Fractures and dislocations adjacent to soft tissue wounds and lacerations are considered open injuries until proved otherwise. Open injuries are orthopedic emergencies requiring surgical irrigation and débridement within 6 hours of injury. Immediate priorities include the acquisition of cultures, betadine dressing for the wound, and intravenous antibiotics (culture, betadine, and antibiotics represent the so-called CBA mnemonic).

Prophylactic antibiotic treatment is guided by a grading system for open fractures (Table 89–3). Critical factors include the degree of soft tissue injury, the mechanism, and the degree of contamination. Open fractures can occur through an "inside-out" mechanism in which fracture fragments cause a skin laceration from within the skin envelope, or an "outside-in" mechanism, which is typically more severely contaminated. Segmental fractures, farm yard injuries occurring in a highly contaminated environment, shotgun wounds, or high-velocity gunshot wounds are automatically classified as grade III injuries. Grade III injuries require both Gram-positive and Gram-negative coverage with a cephalosporin and an aminoglycoside. Penicillin may be added in agricultural injuries where clostridial infection is a greater risk, and tetanus prevention should be considered in all patients with open fractures (Table 89–4).

The neurovascular status should also be evaluated as part of the examination

Table 89–3. Antibiotics for Grades of Open Fractures

GRADE	SKIN LACERATION	DESCRIPTION	ANTIBIOTICS
I	< 1 cm	Relatively "clean" "inside-out" mechanism	First-generation cephalosporin
II	1–10 cm	"Outside-in" mechanism	First-generation cephalosporin
IIIa	>10 cm	Contaminated with potential for soft tissue coverage of the bone	First-generation cephalosporin with an aminoglycoside
IIIb	>10 cm	Contaminated; no potential for soft tissue coverage of the bone	First-generation cephalosporin with an aminoglycoside
IIIc	>10 cm	Same as IIIb plus vascular injury	First-generation cephalosporin with an aminoglycoside

Note: See Chapter 14 for examples of first-generation cephalosporins and Chapter 12 for examples of aminoglycosides.

and, when compromised, reduction of the fracture or dislocation may make assessment more reliable and result in clinical improvement.

Long Bone Fractures

The fracture pattern, the degree of soft tissue injury, and associated injuries determine the treatment of long bone fractures. The fracture *location* is generally described as diaphyseal, metaphyseal, or intra-articular, whereas the fracture *pattern* is described as transverse, oblique or spiral, and simple or comminuted. Long bone fractures occur when energy imparted to the extremities cannot be dissipated in the soft tissues. Comminuted fractures are more likely with open fractures. The type and rate of stress loading determine the fracture pattern. Slow torque causes

Table 89–4. Indications for Tetanus Prophylaxis

TETANUS IMMUNIZATION (PRIOR DOSES OF TETANUS TOXOID)	CLEAN, MINOR WOUNDS		CONTAMINATED WOUNDS	
	Tetanus Toxoid	Tetanus Immune Globulin	Tetanus Toxoid	Tetanus Immune Globulin
Uncertain or <2	Yes	No	Yes	Yes
2	Yes	No	Yes	No*
≥3	No†	No	No‡	No

*Yes, if wound greater than 24 h old.
†Yes, if more than 10 yr since last dose.
‡Yes, if greater than 5 yr since last dose.
From Behrens F: A primer of fixator devices and configurations. Clin Orthop 241:5–14, 1989.

a spiral fracture, whereas a high-energy, direct blow causes a comminuted transverse fracture.

Splints are used for initial immobilization because of their ease of application and ability to readily reassess the injury. Immobilization, traction, external fixation, and a variety of techniques of internal fixation are used for definitive stabilization. Casts are applied to immobilize the joint above and below a fracture. Complications from casting include cast burns and compartment syndromes. Both complications are more likely to occur in the unconscious or insensate patient who cannot complain of pain.

Skeletal traction involves the application of longitudinal stabilization forces using a pin or wire through bone distal to the fracture site. Currently, the trend is to use skeletal traction only in the preliminary treatment of some adult fractures until definitive stabilization may be completed. One reason for this is that prolonged skeletal traction is not conducive to early mobilization. In contrast, *external fixation* of fractures is a definitive, percutaneous stabilization technique that allows rapid stabilization of a fracture without further soft tissue injury resulting from open surgery. This technique also avoids the implantation of hardware at a site that is at risk for bacterial colonization and infection. Finally, external fixation facilitates wound care and patient mobilization.

Internal fixation has been advocated in the multiply injured patient because it permits direct reduction of the fracture, early motion of joints, and patient mobilization. The latter improves pulmonary toilet, decreasing the risk of infection, and reduces the risk of deep venous thrombosis. When long bone fractures are stabilized within 48 hours, there is improved mortality, shorter ICU and hospital stays, and lower costs. A disadvantage of internal fixation is the requirement for surgery, with additional tissue trauma and blood loss. Internal fixation with intramedullary rodding may increase the risk for fat embolism syndrome and post-traumatic acute respiratory distress syndrome.

Although fracture mechanisms are the same for open and closed fractures, open fractures are at much greater risk for infection and nonunion because of injury to the soft tissue envelope surrounding the bone. Surgical treatment of open fractures should be performed within 6 hours of injury to minimize the risk of osteomyelitis, gangrene, and sepsis. These injuries require surgical débridement of foreign material and necrotic tissues as well as irrigation to decontaminate viable tissues. Open fractures should be treated by either delayed primary closure or a split-thickness skin graft in 3 to 5 days. Immediate postoperative management involves surveillance of the wound for evidence of infection and gangrene.

Dislocations

Joint dislocations require early reduction to minimize complications of neurovascular injury, avascular necrosis, and post-traumatic arthritis. Careful documentation of pre- and postreduction neurovascular status is essential. In some cases, an angiogram may be required to determine the status of blood vessels, for example, in all knee dislocations (see Chapter 95). Joint reduction is usually performed outside the operating room except when open dislocations necessitate débridement and irrigation or when closed reduction is unsuccessful, necessitating general anesthesia to facilitate treatment. Neurovascular status must be monitored after reduction.

Neurovascular Injuries

The most important factors determining extremity viability are injuries to vessels, nerves, and surrounding soft tissues (see Chapter 95). Advances in microvascular surgery, soft tissue reconstruction, and nerve grafting have significantly expanded the potential for limb salvage in severely traumatized extremities.

Traumatic Amputation

Patients with traumatic amputation require immediate evaluation for limb salvage surgery. Lower extremity injuries with irreparable sciatic or posterior tibial nerve deficits, massive necrotic soft tissue, significant bone loss, losses of plantar skin, or a combination of these are indications against limb salvage. Traumatic amputations of the upper extremity and hand are preferred for reimplantation because of the greater disability from these injuries. Limb reperfusion may lead to myoglobinuria and renal failure after reimplantation.

Compartment Syndrome

Compartment syndrome is a serious complication that may result from an extremity injury and compression from dressings or plaster casts and is discussed in Chapter 95.

PELVIC FRACTURES

Pelvic fractures may be defined as stable, rotationally unstable, or rotationally and vertically unstable. All unstable injuries involve disruption of the posterior portion of the pelvic ring. Unstable pelvic fractures result from high-energy injuries in the setting of multiple trauma and are associated with 50% mortality in the multiple trauma patient. They require rapid assessment for stabilization and triage. The pelvis is the supporting structure for the peritoneal contents and retroperitoneal structures. Because the pelvis lies in close proximity to vessels, the colon, and genitourinary structures, pelvic injuries are associated with retroperitoneal bleeding and neurologic, bowel, and bladder injuries.

Posterior pelvic disruption can result in 3 to 4 L of blood loss and hemodynamic instability (see Table 89–2). Pneumatic antishock garments have been used in cases of shock with pelvic fractures, but their use remains controversial because of complications and the difficulties they present in examination and treatment of the patient. Complications include lactic acidosis, cardiac collapse after deflation, diaphragmatic herniation, and lower extremity compartment syndrome. Another option for the extremity management of bleeding associated with pelvic fractures is percutaneous external fixation. External fixation is a temporary measure before definitive open reduction and internal fixation, which have superior stabilization properties. When pelvic stabilization is not possible or bleeding continues despite application of external fixation, angiography and embolization are therapeutic alternatives.

The anterior and posterior pelvis should be inspected for open wounds. In males, the scrotal contents are palpated for testicular displacement and the penile meatus is examined for blood, which would suggest urethral injury. Rectal examination is completed for assessment of possible laceration and prostate displacement. Female patients should undergo both bimanual and speculum examinations to rule out vaginal, urethral, and bladder injury. Vaginal or rectal laceration requires specific treatment. Radiographic assessment includes an anteroposterior view of the pelvis, a lateral view of the sacrum, and inlet and outlet views. Further evaluation of identified fractures is obtained with pelvic computed tomography, and a cystogram and retrograde urethrogram may also be indicated.

The patient with an unstable pelvic fracture is often admitted to the ICU after application of a pelvic external fixator. This fixation, although often adequate to reduce the fracture and control bleeding, does not provide extraordinary mechanical stability. Caution must be used in mobilizing the patient with this as the sole stabilization given the potential for resumption of bleeding with disruption of clot. Vigilance in assessment of associated injuries should be maintained until the patient has stabilized.

Postoperative Management

Once patients are stabilized hemodynamically, they should return to the operating room for definitive care of pelvic fractures. Stabilization of these fractures leads to earlier patient mobilization, minimizing the risk of pulmonary complications.

After stabilization of fractures, one should aggressively mobilize the patient as much as possible given the stability of the pelvic reconstruction. Large forces occur across the pelvis because it serves as a platform for transmitting the lower extremity forces to the torso. Often patients with pelvic fracture are unable to ambulate immediately. This is not only because of the severe nature of these injuries but also because of the associated injuries. Mobilization starts with range of motion exercise to the extremities as soon as possible after injury. This is followed with upright sitting and transfer to a chair. Ambulation is advanced depending on the pelvic stability and other injuries.

After pelvic stabilization, the patient is subject to normal orthopedic postoperative complications directly related to treatment, such as infection, loss of fixation, malunion, and nonunion. In addition, there are more severe complications particularly related to these injuries and include neurologic impairment, pulmonary embolism, and sepsis.

Neurologic injury occurs in 1 to 5% of pelvic fractures. It is most frequently due to nerve root traction or avulsion. Therapeutically, the patients are initially treated with observation. Electrodiagnostic studies (electromyography and nerve conduction testing) are typically considered at approximately 3 weeks after injury to help determine the long-term treatment plan.

Pelvic trauma predisposes the patient to deep venous thrombosis, and prophylaxis for pulmonary embolism must be administered. However, because anticoagulants must be used with caution in the setting of severe retroperitoneal bleeding, a vena cava filter is often placed angiographically to prevent pulmonary embolism.

Open Pelvic Fractures

Open pelvic injuries are associated with high-energy trauma and have higher morality rates than do closed injuries. Initially, these open injuries are life-threatening because of bleeding, but later they become potential sources of deep-seated infection. Greater risk for infection is associated with disruption of the bladder and urethra as well as rectal and vaginal lacerations. Urologic injuries are generally treated with urinary diversion and rectal lacerations with a diverting colostomy, whereas vaginal injuries are treated in an open procedure. These measures, along with antibiotic therapy and surgical débridement, can decrease the risk of deep abscess, osteomyelitis, and sepsis.

BIBLIOGRAPHY

Bone L, Johnson K: Early versus delayed stabilization of femoral fractures: A prospective randomized study. J Bone Joint Surg 71A:336–340, 1989.
This study prospectively evaluated the results of early versus delayed stabilization of femoral fractures in 178 patients. When fracture stabilization was delayed in patients with multiple injuries, the incidence of pulmonary complications was higher.

Bone L, McNamara K, Shine B, et al: Mortality in multiple trauma patients with fractures. J Trauma 37:262–264, 1994.
This multicenter study demonstrated that mortality was significantly reduced in patients with multiple injuries if they underwent early fracture stabilization.

Cayten C, Berendt B, Bryne D, et al: A study of pneumatic antishock garments in severely hypotensive trauma patients. J Trauma 34:728–733, 1993.
An analysis of the effectiveness of the pneumatic antishock garment in severely hypotensive (systolic blood pressure < 50 mm Hg) patients found improved mortality rates when used in this setting. Those patients, however, whose systolic blood pressure was greater than 50 mm Hg did not have improved mortality rates when compared with patients in whom pneumatic antishock garments were not used.

Green N, Allen B: Vascular injuries associated with dislocation of the knee. J Bone Joint Surg 59A:236–239, 1977.
This article describes a study in which 245 knee dislocations were reviewed. Those dislocations associated with vascular injury required early repair (within 6 to 8 hours) to obtain optimal results.

Gustilo R, Anderson J: Prevention of infection in the treatment of one thousand and twenty-five open fractures of long bones. J Bone Joint Surg 58A:453, 1976.
This combined retrospective and prospective analysis of open long bone fractures found a 70.3% incidence of positive cultures. Sensitivity studies demonstrated that a first-generation cephalosporin is the best single antibiotic for open fractures.

Gustilo R, Mendoza R, Williams D: Problems in the management of type III (severe) open fractures: A new classification of type III open fractures. J Trauma 24:742–746, 1984.
This study demonstrated the importance of a first-generation cephalosporin and an aminoglycoside in the treatment of type III open fractures.

Heppenstall R, Sapega A, Scott R, et al: The compartment syndrome: An experimental and clinical study of muscular energy metabolism using phosphorus nuclear magnetic resonance spectroscopy. Clin Orthop 226:138–155, 1988.
This study introduces the concept of delta P as a guide for fasciotomy based on muscular energy metabolism.

Rorabeck C, Castle G, Hardie R, Logan J: Compartmental pressure measurements: An experimental investigation using the slit catheter. J Trauma 21:446, 1981.
A comparison of the accuracy of the slit catheter, wick catheter, and needle manometer in measuring pressures demonstrated that the slit and wick catheters are the most accurate in an experimental canine model.

Robertson P: Prediction of amputation after severe lower limb trauma. J Bone Joint Surg 73B:816–818, 1991.
This study demonstrated the high specificity of a mangled extremity severity score (MESS) greater than 7 for predicting ultimate amputation, but additionally noted that some patients with a MESS less than 7 eventually underwent amputation, indicating a limited sensitivity with this scoring system.

Wozasek G, Thurnher M, Redl H: Pulmonary reaction during intramedullary fracture management in traumatic shock: An experimental study. J Trauma 37:249–254, 1994.
Using a sheep model, the authors demonstrated that intramedullary nailing resulted in moderate increases in pulmonary pressure but not in lung permeability. If, however, an additional insult such as hemorrhagic shock overlies the injury, even after adequate resuscitation, lung disturbances may be expected postoperatively.

90 Major Tissue Flaps

David W. Low

Patients undergoing a wide variety of major flap reconstructions warrant postoperative monitoring in an intensive care unit (ICU) setting to monitor flap viability, provide adequate hemodynamic support, and rapidly recognize compromised flaps. Because early recognition can result in the salvage of ischemic flaps in most patients, the ICU clinician must be able to diagnose when a flap is "in trouble," necessitating a return to the operating room.

FLAP TYPES

A flap refers to a surgically created tongue or lip of tissue attached at one end but otherwise cut away from its surroundings. It is a commonly used technique to repair defects in plastic surgery. Tissue types for flaps include skin and subcutaneous tissue, fascia, muscle, bowel, omentum, or bone, or combinations of several tissues, such as a myocutaneous flap. The anatomic vascular supply to these flaps influences the method of flap transfer and dictates which parameters must be monitored postoperatively to ensure flap viability.

Skin (and its subcutaneous tissue) that is transposed to an adjacent area without being detached is a *skin flap*. Generally, the width of a skin flap should equal its length to provide adequate perfusion. If there is no known vessel running within the flap, it is a *random flap*. If there is a vascular pedicle running through the flap, either in the subcutaneous layer or just above the fascial plane, it is an *axial pattern flap*, and its length can be significantly longer than its width. If the skin receives its blood supply from the underlying muscle via perforating vessels, it is a *myocutaneous flap*, and the skin can survive as an island. *Skin grafts* are not considered to be flaps because they survive initially by diffusion rather than by direct perfusion.

Muscle or myocutaneous flaps, when mobilized with preservation of the vascular supply and transposed to the desired site without disrupting their vessels, are *pedicled flaps*. Alternatively, when muscle or myocutaneous flaps are moved to distant sites, but their vessels are divided and reanastomosed to recipient vessels, they are referred to as *microvascular free flaps*. Other tissues can also be transferred as pedicled flaps or as free flaps, including omentum, fasciocutaneous flaps (radial forearm), bone (fibula), and bowel (jejunum). The success of the operation depends on establishing a reliable arterial inflow and venous outflow.

Replantation usually involves the reattachment of a finger or thumb; scalp, ears, lips, hands, feet, and penises have also been salvaged. If the amputation is incomplete, but the vessels are transected, the repair is a *revascularization*. As with a microvascular free flap, success depends on restoring adequate arterial and venous flow.

COMPLICATIONS OF FLAP SURGERY

Both the recipient and donor sites of flaps are subject to the problems of any operative wound, such as bleeding, hematoma formation, suture line dehiscence, infection, and localized edema (Table 90–1). Since many patients receive perioperative anticoagulation, *hematoma formation* is a distinct risk because flap "harvests" result in large raw surfaces at the donor site. The use of surgical drains will not prevent hematoma formation if significant bleeding occurs or if clots occlude the drains. In the ICU, drains should be "stripped" hourly, that is, compressing the drain manually along its length from a proximal to distal direction to remove clots and enhance drainage. The aim of "stripping" is to decrease the risk of hematoma and seroma formation and to promote obliteration of the donor site dead space. An unexplained drop in hemoglobin may be secondary to unrecognized donor site bleeding. Hematoma formation at the recipient site can occlude venous outflow, leading to venous congestion and flap loss.

Postoperative edema can severely compromise flap perfusion and stress suture lines. The operated site should be elevated above the level of the heart, if possible. The use of corticosteroids during flap harvest and early postoperatively to decrease flap edema remains controversial.

Flap ischemia is the most significant complication that can occur in flap surgery and can be due to arterial or venous obstruction, or both. In the case of pedicled flaps, ischemia may result from torsion of the vascular pedicle, increased tension on the pedicle as the tissues swell, or improper postoperative positioning that stretches the pedicle. The surgeon should clearly specify any restrictions in activity or positioning in the ICU postoperative orders. With microvascular free flaps and replantations, flap ischemia in the first 48 hours may be due to a technical problem that is correctable, and a prompt return to the operating room for re-exploration is usually the best course of action.

FLAP MONITORING

There are many subjective and objective approaches to monitoring flaps, each with its own advantages and problems. Some require expensive technology that may

Table 90–1. Risk Factors for Flap Ischemia in the Immediate Postoperative Period

Hematoma, bleeding	Malpositioning of patient
Donor site or sites	Increased tension on vascular pedicle
Recipient site	Compression of vascular pedicle
Anticoagulation-related	Increased dependent edema
Ischemia due to arterial obstruction	Potential pressure necrosis
Vasoconstriction, vasospasm	Other generic factors
Twisted or kinked pedicle	Anemia
Excessive traction	Edema
Thrombosed anastomosis	Infection
Ischemia due to venous obstruction	Hypothermia
Twisted or kinked pedicle	Hypovolemia with hypotension
Excessive traction	
Compression by hematoma or flap edema	
Thrombosed anastomosis	

not be readily available; others may be too sensitive and falsely indicate flap compromise because of patient movement, probe dislodgment, or corrosion of the sensing fiber. Although a combination of clinical judgment and objective monitoring usually results in a diagnosis of flap ischemia, if made too late, flap salvage may be unsuccessful. For example, free flaps that are ischemic for more than 6 to 8 hours usually cannot be saved.

Subjective Methods

Color

A skin flap or a skin island of a myocutaneous flap (Fig. 90–1) should be the same color (or slightly more pink) as the adjacent skin from which it was harvested. If it is hyperemic and purple, however, the venous outflow may be occluded. If it is mottled or extremely pale, the arterial inflow may be compromised. In contrast, color is not a reliable indicator for skin-grafted muscle flaps.

Capillary Refill

It should normally take about 1 to 2 seconds for the color to return after blanching the skin with a finger or the circular handle of a hemostat or scissors. (The circular

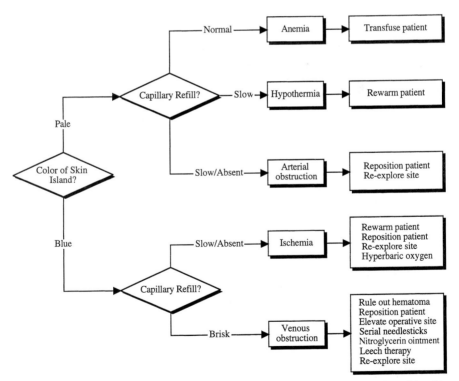

Figure 90–1. Schematic flow diagram for evaluation and management of a threatened flap with a skin island visible.

pattern is easier to discern with pale skin.) Flaps with venous congestion show instantaneous (brisk) refill, whereas flaps that are slow to fill may have compromised arterial inflow. Capillary refill may be difficult to assess in patients with darkly pigmented skin. A skin graft has no capillary refill initially, as it takes 4 to 5 days for vessels to reperfuse the graft.

Temperature

Flaps are often cooler than the surrounding native skin, making absolute temperature an unreliable indicator. A change in temperature, however, may indicate vascular compromise, and a temperature probe is more reliable than palpation alone.

Tissue Turgor and Flap Contour

Most flaps become edematous in the immediate postoperative period, with edema reaching a maximum at 24 to 48 hours. Flaps that appear extremely tense and protruding may have venous congestion or an underlying expanding hematoma that requires evacuation. Previously swollen flaps that appear soft or desiccated may have an arterial occlusion.

Pulse

A palpable pulse is not usually present in most flap reconstructions because the vessels are usually too deep or too small to be detected. Occasionally, when a large-diameter vein graft, for example, the saphenous vein, is used to connect a flap with a distant blood supply, the vein graft may have a palpable pulse.

Objective Methods

Needle Stick

Bright red oozing from a punctured skin island or muscle flap suggests continued normal perfusion. Cyanotic blood that then becomes more red suggests venous engorgement. Absence of pinprick bleeding and a persistent hole after withdrawal of the needle signals a lack of arterial flow and reduced tissue turgor.

Flow Monitor

Intermittent or continuous ultrasonic Doppler flow monitoring (Fig. 90–2) is a frequently used method for assessing arterial patency in flap surgery. Doppler probes are widely available in the ICU for monitoring patients undergoing peripheral vascular surgery, and the same instrument can be used to follow flap patients. The surgeon should identify and clearly mark a reliable site so that ICU personnel can easily assess the pulse, at least hourly for the first 48 hours operatively. A loss of Doppler signal mandates immediate notification of the surgical team. Use of the Doppler may be less reliable in areas such as the head and neck where other

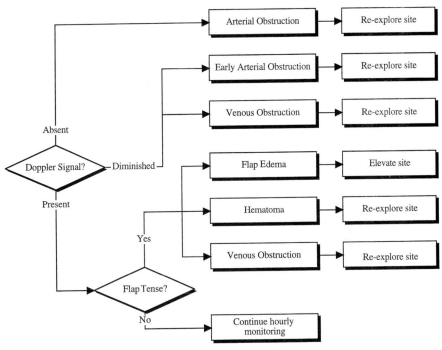

Figure 90–2. Schematic flow diagram for evaluation and management of a threatened microvascular free flap that is buried or skin grafted.

regional arteries may give a false signal that may be mistaken for the flap pedicle. In some cases, a venous Doppler signal can also be monitored (venous "hum"); this varies with respiration and can be augmented by compressing the flap. Implantable ultrasonic Doppler probes give a continuous waveform that can record both arterial and venous flow, but probe dislodgment or mechanical failure can give rise to false alarms.

Some institutions have laser Doppler instruments, which use light instead of sound waves to detect red blood cell motion. They are placed on the surface of, or implanted next to, the vascular pedicles to provide continuous monitoring. However, their sensitive fibers may give false alarms if they become encrusted with blood and secretions or if the patient moves. Implantable Doppler probes may have their greatest utility for monitoring buried flaps because such flaps cannot be reliably followed with surface probes.

Pulse Oximeter

Pulse rate and oxygen saturation can be continuously monitored in digital replants with a fingertip pulse oximeter. A loss of pulsations indicates arterial occlusion, and a drop in saturation ($<85\%$) suggests venous obstruction.

Monitoring Partial Pressure of Oxygen

Transcutaneous Po_2 monitoring with a surface electrode is available in some institutions (e.g., for neonatal monitoring) and has applicability in monitoring skin flaps or myocutaneous flaps. It is not useful for skin-grafted muscle flaps or for buried flaps. Additionally, the electrode heats up the skin and must be moved periodically to prevent possible burn injuries.

Surface Temperature Probe

Temperature-sensing electrodes, or even adhesive temperature strips, can be used to document temperature changes. A fall of 1 to 2° C may indicate vascular compromise. Surface temperature monitoring is more accurate with replanted digits when compared with flaps, which can be warmed by heat transfer from the underlying bed. Accuracy is also improved if the adjacent skin is monitored for temperature changes as well, since environmental factors and local hemodynamic changes can greatly affect cutaneous temperature readings at both sites. Thermocouple probes can also be implanted adjacent to vascular pedicles to monitor buried flaps. In most centers, however, temperature monitoring has been abandoned in favor of alternative monitoring devices.

Fluorescein

Intravenous administration of fluorescein (10 to 20 mg/kg) and use of a Wood lamp to assess fluorescence may have utility in intraoperative flap assessment, particularly in determining peripheral flap viability. Routine ICU use for flap monitoring (1.5 mg/kg intravenously, assessed every 2 hours with a dermal fluorometer), however, is unusual and can only be performed with skin flaps or myocutaneous flaps. Side effects of fluorescein include nausea, vomiting, hypotension, and, rarely, anaphylaxis.

GENERIC POSTOPERATIVE MANAGEMENT

Fluid Management and Blood Transfusions

Patients must remain well hydrated to maintain adequate perfusion pressure and fluid volume in the microvasculature of the flap. They must also be kept warm to decrease peripheral vascular resistance and vasoconstriction. The use of pressors to maintain blood pressure is deleterious to flaps because they cause peripheral vasoconstriction. Use of colloids, such as hydroxyethyl starch, may help maintain intravascular volume longer than do crystalloids and may help decrease perioperative flap edema.

With microvascular surgery, a certain degree of hemodilution is desirable to decrease blood viscosity. Isovolemic hemodilution is the goal. Previously, one tried to maintain, but not exceed, a hemoglobin of 10 g/dL. More recently, concerns have surfaced regarding infectious risks with multiple transfusions, and hemoglobin levels as low as 7 or 8 g/dL are tolerated as long as patients remain asymptomatic.

Anticoagulation and Thrombolysis

Anticoagulation is not routinely used for pedicled flaps, aside from prophylaxis against deep venous thrombosis, nor do many microsurgeons routinely use anticoagulation for free flap surgery, unless there is a problem intraoperatively, the patient is at high risk (traumatized or irradiated tissues), or the patient requires re-exploration for vascular occlusion. Others always use some form of postoperative anticoagulation with various regimens and doses. The risk of bleeding complications must be considered and weighed against the risk of vascular thrombosis.

Heparin

Heparin binds with antithrombin III and inhibits thrombosis by inactivating activated Factor X; this inhibits the conversion of prothrombin to thrombin. Once thrombosis has occurred, heparin hampers the conversion of fibrinogen to fibrin and prevents the formation of stable clots by inhibiting activation of fibrin-stabilizing factor. It also decreases platelet adhesiveness. Patients are usually given a bolus intraoperatively at the time of vascular anastomosis and a continuous drip postoperatively at therapeutic or subtherapeutic doses. The partial thromboplastin time should be followed if heparin is given in therapeutic doses (see Chapter 12).

Aspirin

Aspirin inhibits the release of cyclooxygenase from platelets, blocking the subsequent formation of thromboxane A_2. As an antiplatelet agent, low-dose aspirin (3 to 5 mg/kg/day) may be given for up to a month beginning on the day of surgery. The desirable effect of aspirin is offset by its inhibition of prostacyclin generation by endothelial cells at higher doses.

Low Molecular Weight Dextran (10% Dextran 40)

As a polysaccharide available with a mean molecular weight of 40,000 d, low molecular weight dextran was initially used as a colloid for intravascular volume expansion. In addition to decreasing blood viscosity, it has an antiplatelet effect and also depresses Factor VIII activity. It is started intraoperatively with a loading dose of 40 mL then given as a continuous drip at 20 to 30 mL/h. Duration and tapering schedule vary according to surgeon, for example, 20 mL/h for 3 days, 10 mL/h for 2 days and then discontinue, or 20 to 25 mL/h for 5 days and then discontinue with no taper.

Pentoxifylline

Pentoxifylline is a vasoactive drug derived from xanthine. It increases red blood cell flexibility, may cause smooth muscle relaxation, and also has an antiplatelet effect. It is usually started several weeks preoperatively (orally) to achieve its effects on red blood cells and continued postoperatively until the operative site is healed. It may be useful in the difficult diabetic patient undergoing flap surgery.

Urokinase

Urokinase is a thrombolytic agent produced by human kidney cells that converts plasminogen to plasmin, a fibrinolytic enzyme. It is usually reserved for localized infusion during intraoperative free flap re-exploration. Although it is commonly used as a continuous drip in the ICU for patients with occluded peripheral vascular grafts, it is rarely, if ever, administered in this manner for flaps. After successful thrombolysis with urokinase, heparin is usually given as a continuous systemic infusion.

MANAGING THE COMPROMISED FLAP

Positioning

Pedicled flaps are rarely subject to arterial occlusion, but they may suffer arterial vasospasm, venous congestion, or distal ischemia. Malpositioning that places tension on the flap and hypothermia should be corrected to decrease vasospasm. If the flap remains purple or blue but with brisk capillary refill, elevation of the flap may improve venous return and decrease flap edema.

Vasodilators

Persistent engorgement may respond to nitroglycerin, a vascular smooth muscle relaxant with a greater effect on the venous than the arterial vasculature. Topical application, rather than intravenous infusion, is the usual mode of delivery, for example, nitroglycerin ointment 1/4 inch applied every 8 hours. Intermittent pricking of the skin island usually demonstrates oozing of dark venous blood, and a transient improvement in color.

Other Interventions

Additional maneuvers include the application of small felt pads soaked in heparin to promote continued venous oozing between needle pricks and application of *medicinal leeches.* Leeches (*Hirudo medicinalis*) are usually available through the hospital pharmacy. They avidly attach to the site of a needle stick and begin to suck. After the leech detaches, the site bleeds because of a natural anticoagulant (hirudin) that inactivates thrombin. New leeches are applied when the oozing subsides if the flap remains engorged. Hemoglobin should be monitored during the course of leech therapy (which may last more than 5 days), as blood loss can be significant. Patients receiving leech therapy require antibiotic coverage against *Aeromonas hydrophila,* a symbiotic bacterium in the leech gut.

Surgical Maneuvers

Distal ischemia is usually allowed to demarcate, requiring later flap débridement. Other maneuvers to maximize flap viability include the use of hyperbaric oxygen, if available. To date, calcium channel blockers have been disappointing in their effectiveness to relieve vasospasm and decrease flap ischemia. In the future, administration of free oxygen radical scavengers may diminish the effects of toxic oxidant species.

Venous occlusion in the patient with a microvascular free flap usually requires intraoperative re-exploration and revision of the anastomosis, sometimes with vein grafts. While waiting for the operating room to receive the patient, however, the surgeon may elect to remove sutures to decompress a possible hematoma that may be occluding the vessels. This maneuver alone may restore flow if the vessels are not thrombosed.

If there is an obvious clot in the vein, transecting the vein and administering a bolus (5000 units) of intravenous heparin may flush out the clot and restore normal circulation. The venous anastomosis can then be revised in the operating room. If no suitable vein repair can be performed, as may be the case with digital replants, leech therapy is usually instituted. Alternatively, removing the nail bed and applying heparin-soaked felt pledgets may permit venous drainage if no leeches are immediately available.

If the arterial Doppler signal becomes fainter but is still present, adequate systemic pressure and fluid status should be confirmed, and the flap should be kept warm to diminish vasospasm and constriction of the peripheral vasculature. If capillary refill is sluggish or absent and the pulse does not improve, patients should be readied for immediate re-exploration. If there is suspicion of an expanding hematoma compressing the vascular pedicle, however, removal of a few key sutures at the bedside by the surgeon may result in restoration of a pulse.

BIBLIOGRAPHY

Buncke HJ: Microsurgery: Transplantation-Replantation: An Atlas-Text. Philadelphia, Lea & Febiger, 1991.
Chapter 37 has a detailed table listing many methods of flap monitoring, the mechanism of action, technique of application, clinical applications, and complications.

Daniel RK, Kerrigan CL: Principles and physiology of skin flap surgery. In: McCarthy JG (ed): Plastic Surgery. Philadelphia, WB Saunders, 1990, pp 275–328.
A truly comprehensive chapter describing skin and muscle flaps, physiologic manipulation, and monitoring strategies.

Furnas H, Rosen JM: Monitoring in microvascular surgery. Ann Plast Surg 26:265–272, 1991.
This is an excellent discussion of monitoring systems, detailing the advantages and disadvantages of each method with 75 references.

Jones NF: Intraoperative and postoperative monitoring of microsurgical free tissue transfers. Clin Plast Surg 19:783–797, 1992.
This is an encyclopedic discussion of monitoring techniques, with the author's preferred approaches explained along with 102 references.

Sigurdsson GH: Perioperative fluid management in microvascular surgery. J Reconstr Microsurg 11:57–65, 1995.
This is a good discussion of intravenous fluid therapy in the perioperative period, including a detailed description of dextran and hydroxyethyl starch administration, with 115 references.

91 Major Vascular Procedures

Marc E. Mitchell
Jeffrey P. Carpenter

The care of patients with vascular disease in the intensive care unit (ICU) is challenging and requires an in-depth understanding of cardiovascular physiology and critical care. Aortic reconstruction, lower extremity revascularization, and carotid endarterectomy are the most frequently performed major vascular procedures, and the majority of these patients are admitted to the ICU postoperatively. This chapter focuses on the preoperative, intraoperative, and postoperative care of the vascular surgery patient in general, as well as on aspects specific for these three major procedures.

GENERAL APPROACH TO THE VASCULAR PATIENT

Preoperative Evaluation

Peripheral vascular disease (PVD) occurs most commonly in elderly patients with significant coexisting diseases. Since atherosclerosis is a systemic disease, it must be assumed that patients with PVD also suffer from coronary artery disease (CAD). Furthermore, patients with vascular disease frequently have a history of tobacco abuse, which results in significant underlying respiratory disease. Hypertension and diabetes mellitus are additional conditions commonly associated with PVD, often accompanied by some degree of renal insufficiency. Because these comorbid conditions frequently cause morbidity and mortality after major vascular reconstruction, the preoperative evaluation and preparation of the vascular surgery patient should address both the underlying vascular disease and these associated conditions.

As part of the preoperative evaluation, all patients require an imaging study to assess the extent of the vascular disease. Although duplex ultrasound scans, computed tomograpy (CT) scans, and contrast arteriography are most commonly used, magnetic resonance angiography (MRA) has recently gained favor for the evaluation of all types of vascular disease. It provides excellent anatomic detail noninvasively while avoiding the risks of iodinated contrast agents.

Coronary Artery Disease

Complications of CAD account for 25 to 70% of the early and late morbidity and mortality after vascular reconstructive surgery and occur in up to 25% of patients undergoing major vascular reconstructions. Atherosclerosis is a disease affecting all arteries, and it is unusual for a patient to have normal coronary arteries in the face of significant PVD. The frequency of triple-vessel CAD in patients undergoing surgery for PVD ranges from 15% in asymptomatic patients to 44% in those with symptoms. In addition to a thorough history and physical examination, all patients

1017

with vascular disease should undergo electrocardiography as part of the preoperative evaluation.

Because of the high prevalence of asymptomatic CAD, most vascular surgeons also require a formal evaluation of cardiac function before proceeding with elective major vascular reconstruction. The most commonly used noninvasive tests to evaluate cardiac function include exercise testing, radionuclide ventriculography, echocardiography, dobutamine stress echocardiography, and dipyridamole thallium scintigraphy. Coronary angiography is performed if noninvasive testing shows evidence of myocardial dysfunction or ischemia. If angiography demonstrates significant CAD, coronary angioplasty or bypass grafting may be performed before proceeding with elective vascular reconstruction. Recently, the benefits of preoperative coronary revascularization have been questioned. The combined morbidity and mortality of coronary artery bypass grafting followed by major vascular surgery may be higher than elective vascular reconstruction in the patient with uncorrected CAD. At this time, however, complete cardiac evaluation followed by coronary revascularization, if indicated, remains the standard approach.

Respiratory Dysfunction

Because vascular reconstructive procedures are frequently long, require a general anesthetic, and use abdominal or thoracic incisions, postoperative respiratory complications are common. Patients with vascular disease often have pre-existing chronic obstructive pulmonary disease (COPD) from tobacco abuse, which can worsen in the postoperative period. A careful preoperative history and physical examination must be performed in all patients to screen for COPD and other pulmonary diseases. All patients undergoing major vascular reconstruction should undergo chest radiography. If there is clinical or radiographic evidence of underlying pulmonary disease, arterial blood gas determinations and bedside spirometry or formal pulmonary function testing should be performed. Preoperative treatment with bronchodilators or inhaled or systemic corticosteroids is used to optimize the functional status of patients with COPD before elective surgery. Finally, smokers should be strongly encouraged to abstain from tobacco use before elective surgery.

In patients with significant pulmonary dysfunction, it may be preferable to avoid general anesthesia, if possible. Spinal or epidural anesthesia is a frequently used alternative, particularly for lower extremity revascularization. A retroperitoneal approach can be used instead of the standard transabdominal approach for some aortic procedures. The retroperitoneal incision results in less postoperative pain and pulmonary dysfunction compared with an abdominal incision. Effective postoperative pain control is essential in order to prevent postoperative pulmonary complications. Pulmonary toilet, including coughing and incentive spirometry, is critically important in the postoperative period, but is not possible without effective relief of postoperative incisional pain. Epidural analgesia has become the method of choice for pain control postoperatively in patients undergoing thoracic or abdominal vascular procedures (see Chapter 85).

Renal Insufficiency

Hypertension and renal insufficiency are frequently present in patients with PVD. This may be the result of atherosclerotic renal artery occlusive disease, diabetic nephropathy, or essential hypertension. Renal artery stenosis has a reported prevalence of up to 40% in patients with PVD. Since iodinated contrast agents used in arteriography or CT scans can result in an acute deterioration of renal function, patients must be hydrated before and after undergoing these diagnostic procedures. If possible, the use of iodinated contrast agents should be avoided in patients with known renal insufficiency. If there is a deterioration in renal function after a diagnostic procedure, elective surgery should be delayed in order to allow renal function to return to baseline.

Laboratory Studies

All patients undergoing vascular reconstruction should have a focused laboratory evaluation preoperatively. Many patients are taking medications, such as diuretics, which can result in electrolyte disturbances. Electrolytes, glucose, blood urea nitrogen, and creatinine should be evaluated in all patients. Many patients with PVD take aspirin, other antiplatelet drugs, or warfarin. A complete blood count and coagulation studies should be performed in all patients. Patients with a history of arterial or venous thrombosis should be screened for a hypercoagulable condition. A blood sample should be sent for type and screen or crossmatch, depending on the procedure to be performed. Patients may donate autologous blood for use in the perioperative period before elective aortic reconstruction.

Intraoperative Care

All patients should receive an antibiotic that is effective against normal skin flora within 1 hour prior to the incision being made. If a prosthetic graft is placed, the antibiotic should be continued for 24 hours postoperatively. Massive blood loss can occur during vascular reconstruction, and it is mandatory that adequate venous access be available for resuscitation. It is important to maintain body temperature close to normal during the procedure because hypothermia is associated with coagulation abnormalities and cardiac dysfunction. Warming blankets, humidification of the anesthesia circuit, and warming of intravenous fluids are techniques used to maintain normothermia during the procedure. An autotransfusion system should be used to scavenge shed blood during aortic reconstruction. Patients undergo systemic anticoagulation with heparin before arterial clamping. If bleeding is a problem after completion of the vascular reconstruction, the effects of heparin can be reversed with protamine sulfate. If a coagulopathy develops during the procedure, it must be treated aggressively with blood products and clotting factors.

Because of the potential for hemodynamic instability, patients undergoing aortic or carotid surgery should have continuous blood pressure monitoring with an indwelling arterial catheter. The decision for pulmonary artery pressure monitoring is based on the patient's cardiac status and the magnitude of the operative procedure to be performed. Transesophageal echocardiography is sometimes used to monitor cardiac function intraoperatively. Patients with CAD often require a continuous infusion of nitroglycerin during the procedure to optimize coronary blood flow. Inotropic agents such as dobutamine or dopamine are frequently used to augment cardiac output.

Postoperative Care

Most patients require monitoring in an ICU during the postoperative period after major vascular reconstruction. Many patients also require mechanical ventilation, invasive hemodynamic monitoring, and support with inotropic agents or vasoactive drugs. Because CAD is so prevalent among vascular patients, cardiac performance is of primary concern in the postoperative period. A postoperative electrocardiogram should be obtained in all patients to look for ischemic changes that may have occurred during the procedure. Many patients require a chest radiograph to verify endotracheal tube, central venous catheter, pulmonary artery catheter, or thoracostomy drainage tube placement. Hemoglobin, hematocrit, platelet count, and coagulation studies must also be monitored closely during the postoperative period. Blood pressure must be tightly controlled to avoid the complications of hypertension or hypotension (Fig. 91–1).

PROCEDURE-SPECIFIC CARE: AORTIC RECONSTRUCTION

Preoperative Care

Aortoiliac reconstruction is commonly undertaken for aneurysmal disease or atherosclerotic occlusive disease. Even with improvements in imaging using MRA, the contrast-enhanced CT scan remains the gold standard for evaluation of abdominal aortic aneurysms (AAAs). It provides accurate information regarding aneurysm size, wall integrity, proximal and distal extent of the aneurysm, relationship of the aneurysm to renal and visceral arteries, venous anomalies, and renal anomalies, and also detects inflammatory aneurysms. In addition to the CT scan, many surgeons routinely use preoperative angiography in the evaluation of AAA. Angiography provides detailed anatomic information about the proximal and distal extent of the aneurysm, associated visceral and iliac artery occlusive disease, and associated arterial anomalies such as accessory renal arteries. Aortoiliac occlusive disease is also routinely evaluated by angiography.

Intraoperative Care

The aorta can be approached through a midline or left retroperitoneal incision. The retroperitoneal approach is frequently used for exposure of the suprarenal aorta, but access to the right iliac system and the right renal artery is limited. The retroperitoneal approach is often used for patients with significant underlying respiratory disease. This approach is also preferred with inflammatory aneurysms, in the presence of a horseshoe kidney, and in obese patients and patients with a "hostile" abdomen that would make a transabdominal approach difficult.

Aortic cross-clamping and unclamping produce marked changes in cardiac afterload and can cause significant hemodynamic instability. Since the aneurysm is limited to the infrarenal aorta and iliac arteries in 95% of patients with AAA, the aorta can usually be clamped below the renal arteries. When suprarenal aortic clamping and unclamping are required, the hemodynamic changes are more

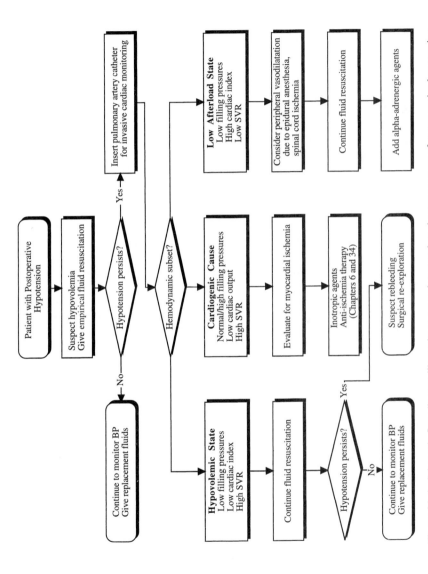

Figure 91–1. Schematic flow diagram illustrating a general approach to the management of postoperative hypotension. BP, blood pressure; SVR, systemic vascular resistance.

pronounced and present an even greater challenge for the anesthesiologist to maintain the blood pressure in an acceptable range. Fluids and vasoactive drugs are used to optimize preload and afterload at the time of aortic clamping and unclamping.

It is important to maintain adequate urine output during the time that the aorta is clamped. Osmotic diuretics (mannitol) or loop diuretics (furosemide) can be given before clamping to maintain adequate urine output. Renal dose dopamine is also frequently used to optimize renal blood flow during aortic cross-clamping.

Postoperative Care

All patients require monitoring in the ICU after aortic reconstruction, with many patients requiring mechanical ventilation overnight. Cardiac complications are a major cause of postoperative morbidity and mortality, as previously described. Invasive hemodynamic monitoring with a pulmonary artery catheter is required to direct fluid resuscitation and optimize cardiac function. Significant intraoperative blood loss and fluid shifts can result in hypotension in the postoperative period. Postoperative fluid requirements after aortic reconstruction frequently are large because of fluid sequestration and third spacing from extensive retroperitoneal dissection. Volume resuscitation is the initial treatment for *postoperative hypotension* (see Fig. 91–1). Once the patient's volume status has been optimized, cardiac function can be augmented with inotropic drugs if hypotension persists.

Postoperative hypertension may result in suture line bleeding and may increase myocardial oxygen consumption. Hypertension should be treated with vasodilators such as nitroglycerin or sodium nitroprusside. Occasionally, hypertension can be the result of postoperative pain, which can be treated with intravenous opioids or other modalities (see Chapter 85).

Postoperative hemorrhage is a relatively uncommon complication of aortic reconstruction, occurring in less than 2% of patients. Hemorrhage is usually the result of either a technical problem or an abnormality of the coagulation mechanism. Many factors contribute to postoperative coagulopathy after aortic surgery. Hypothermia can result from a long operation with a large abdominal or thoracic incision. Platelet dysfunction from preoperative antiplatelet therapy can cause significant postoperative bleeding. Thrombocytopenia from large intraoperative blood losses without replacement of platelets can occur. Inadequate reversal of the effects of heparin with protamine sulfate can result in a coagulopathy. Coagulation abnormalities from hepatic ischemia can occur if the aorta is cross-clamped above the celiac axis.

Dilutional coagulopathy from large intraoperative blood losses and replacement with banked blood is the most common cause of *postoperative coagulopathy.* Replacement of clotting factors and platelets and normalization of body temperature are the first steps in the treatment of postoperative bleeding. If the patient has excessive blood losses or if the bleeding continues in the face of a normal coagulation system, reoperation to look for a technical cause of the bleeding is indicated.

Limb ischemia due to embolization or thrombosis is an occasional complication of aortic reconstruction, occurring in 1 to 3% of patients. Limb ischemia is usually secondary to distal thromboembolization during the procedure or thrombosis of the graft resulting from a technical problem with the graft. The status of lower extremity pulses should be documented preoperatively and serve as a baseline. In the postoperative period, they should be checked frequently. The loss of peripheral pulses demands urgent exploration and restoration of blood flow to the ischemic limb.

Clinically significant *intestinal ischemia,* most commonly affecting the rectosigmoid colon, occurs in up to 2% of patients after aortic reconstruction. The frequency of ischemic changes is higher in studies in which routine colonoscopy was performed. Ischemia occurs most frequently in patients with occlusive disease of the mesenteric vessels, resulting from interruption of collateral blood flow to the intestine. The rectosigmoid colon is affected most commonly because of the frequency of disease in the inferior mesenteric and hypogastric arteries. The diagnosis can be difficult because patients are often sedated and the incisional pain can mask the abdominal pain. The most common clinical findings include bloody diarrhea, abdominal distention, peritonitis, metabolic acidosis, and sepsis. Since the sigmoid colon and rectum are almost always involved, the diagnosis can usually be made by sigmoidoscopy. A high index of suspicion is the key to early diagnosis. Cases of ischemia limited to the mucosa can be treated with supportive care, antibiotics, and close observation. Abdominal exploration with resection of ischemic bowel and colostomy formation is required for transmural ischemia. The overall mortality for aortic surgery complicated by clinically significant intestinal ischemia exceeds 50% and may approach 90% in cases of transmural ischemia.

Acute renal failure after aortic reconstruction is also a relatively uncommon occurrence, even though many patients have some degree of underlying renal insufficiency preoperatively. Iodinated contrast used during preoperative arteriography often contributes to postoperative renal insufficiency. Myoglobin from reperfusion of ischemic lower extremities and intraoperative hypotension are risk factors for the development of postoperative renal failure. Thromboembolization from manipulation and clamping of the aorta as well as suprarenal aortic clamping are technical factors that also increase the risk of renal failure. Normally perfused kidneys should tolerate up to 45 minutes of warm ischemia. Chronically ischemic kidneys, however, usually tolerate longer periods of ischemia because of the presence of collateral blood flow. Maintaining renal blood flow by optimizing fluid status and cardiac output is the most effective way to both prevent and treat postoperative renal failure.

Spinal cord ischemia resulting in paraplegia is an uncommon but devastating complication after infrarenal aortic reconstruction. The frequency of spinal cord ischemia is 1 in 400 after AAA repair and 1 in 5000 after aortoiliac reconstruction for occlusive disease. The complication rate is higher for repair of ruptured AAA and thoracoabdominal aneurysms. Infarction of the spinal cord can result from disruption of blood supply to the spinal cord or systemic hypotension during the procedure. The artery of Adamkiewicz is the major blood supply to the lower spinal cord, usually arising as a branch of an intercostal artery between T8 and Ll. Occasionally, it may originate from the infrarenal aorta, accounting for the rare occurrence of spinal cord ischemia after infrarenal aortic reconstruction. If a patient develops paraplegia after aortic reconstruction, magnetic resonance imaging of the spinal cord should be performed to confirm cord ischemia and to rule out a compressive lesion such as a hematoma.

PROCEDURE-SPECIFIC CARE: CAROTID ARTERY SURGERY

Intraoperative Care

Carotid endarterectomy is indicated to prevent stroke in patients with symptomatic carotid artery stenoses or with high-grade asymptomatic stenoses. Surgery on the carotid artery is often complicated by significant hemodynamic instability. Manipulation of the baroreceptors in the carotid body can result in bradycardia with associated hypotension. This can be blocked by injecting the carotid body with lidocaine during the dissection. It is not uncommon for patients to have large variations in blood pressure during the procedure, which can result in myocardial or cerebral ischemia. Vasopressors or vasodilators are frequently required to maintain blood pressure in the normal range during the procedure.

Controversy exists about the best method for maintaining cerebral perfusion during carotid surgery. Since anesthesia reduces the metabolic requirements of the brain and increases cerebral tolerance of ischemia, many patients can tolerate clamping of the carotid artery with no adverse effects. Other patients experience cerebral ischemia during carotid clamping, which may result in a permanent neurologic deficit. The use of a temporary shunt to maintain antegrade flow through the internal carotid artery is the most reliable method of cerebral protection during carotid clamping. Some surgeons always use a shunt, whereas others do so on a selective basis. The latter use several methods to determine the adequacy of collateral cerebral blood flow during carotid artery clamping. If flow is determined to be suboptimal or if ischemic changes occur, a shunt is placed.

Postoperative Care

Blood pressure control is extremely important in the postoperative period after carotid endarterectomy. *Hypertension* (systolic blood pressure >200 mm Hg or mean blood pressure >35 mm Hg greater than baseline) occurs in up to 50% of patients. Intracerebral hemorrhage is a devastating complication that can result from postoperative hypertension. Bleeding with neck hematoma formation and possible airway compromise can also result from uncontrolled hypertension. Preoperative hypertension and carotid stenosis greater than 90% are risk factors for the development of postoperative hypertension. Vasodilating agents such as nitroglycerin or sodium nitroprusside are the drugs of choice because they allow for rapid control and easy titration of blood pressure. Intravenous beta-blockers, such as esmolol or labetalol, are also effective in controlling postoperative hypertension. As soon as the patient is awake and neurologic function has been evaluated and found to be normal, patients who chronically take oral antihypertensives may resume their medications.

Hypotension can also occur after carotid endarterectomy, although less commonly than hypertension. Hypotension is usually the result of hypovolemia (see Fig. 91–1). It is important to treat hypotension aggressively because internal carotid thrombosis, neurologic changes, or myocardial ischemia can result. Volume resuscitation is usually the initial treatment for postoperative hypotension. If the hypotension does not respond to fluids, cardiac function must be evaluated to rule out myocardial ischemia or other cardiac dysfunction. If cardiac ischemia is determined to be the cause of the hypotension, it should be aggressively treated.

It is surprising that *bleeding* is an uncommon complication after carotid endarterectomy, considering that all patients undergo systemic anticoagulation with heparin and many receive antiplatelet drugs preoperatively. Less than 2% of patients require reoperation for bleeding after carotid endarterectomy. Most surgeons do not reverse the effects of heparin with protamine sulfate after carotid surgery, as it has been demonstrated to increase the rate of perioperative stroke. A closed suction drain may be placed at the time of surgery to evacuate any blood that accumulates in the neck. If a significant hematoma develops, airway obstruction or neurologic insult may result. Because hematoma is uncomfortable for the patient and may act as a nidus for infection, if one develops, it should be surgically evacuated.

Postoperative stroke is perhaps the most devastating complication after carotid endarterectomy. The purpose of carotid endarterectomy is to prevent stroke, but the procedure itself has a 2% risk of stroke. Postoperative neurologic deficits can be the result of cerebral ischemia during carotid clamping, atheromatous or platelet emboli during the procedure, or thrombosis of the internal carotid artery. The patient should not leave the operating room until he or she has emerged from anesthesia and has moved all extremities. If the patient awakens with a neurologic deficit, the neck should be explored immediately to verify the patency of the internal carotid artery. Neurologic function must be monitored closely in the postoperative period. A patient who experiences a neurologic deficit in the early postoperative period that is appropriate to the operated side should have the patency of the internal carotid artery evaluated immediately. This can be carried out by carotid duplex scanning, arteriography, or neck exploration. If noninvasive testing or arteriography cannot be obtained quickly, a neck exploration should be performed. Rapid restoration of cerebral blood flow is the only way to reverse a neurologic deficit if the internal carotid artery is thrombosed. Neck exploration should not be delayed in order to obtain diagnostic testing.

Patients who experience *transient ischemic attacks* (TIAs) postoperatively should have the patency of the internal carotid artery evaluated with carotid duplex scan. If this shows a patent artery, an arteriogram should be obtained to look for an anatomic or technical cause of the TIA. If a correctable lesion is demonstrated, exploration of the internal carotid artery is performed. If none is found, a CT scan of the head should be obtained to look for intracerebral hemorrhage. Anticoagulation with heparin is begun if there is no evidence of hemorrhage. If the duplex scan or arteriogram demonstrates thrombosis of the internal carotid artery, the best treatment is unclear. If the TIA resolves completely, the patient may be treated with anticoagulation. If symptoms persist, exploration of the artery is indicated.

Cranial nerve injury is another potential complication after carotid endarterectomy. Injury to the vagus or recurrent laryngeal nerve has been reported in up to 8% of patients undergoing carotid endarterectomy. The result is hoarseness, with the majority of cases resolving within a few months. The hypoglossal nerve crosses the internal carotid artery above the bifurcation and has been reported to be injured in up to 8% of patients undergoing carotid endarterectomies. Injury to this nerve results in ipsilateral deviation of the tongue, inarticulate speech, and difficulty with mastication. The superior laryngeal nerve and marginal mandibular branch of the facial nerve are also at risk for injury.

All patients should be given aspirin as *antiplatelet therapy* before surgery; the aspirin is then continued after surgery to prevent platelet emboli. Patients not receiving aspirin preoperatively should receive low molecular weight dextran during surgery and postoperatively until aspirin therapy can be started. Most patients are observed in the postanesthesia care unit or ICU for at least 6 hours postoperatively after carotid endarterectomy. If the postoperative course is uncomplicated, the patient can be transferred to a step-down unit the evening of surgery and discharged from the hospital the evening of the day after surgery.

PROCEDURE-SPECIFIC CARE: INFRAINGUINAL RECONSTRUCTION

Intraoperative Care

Revascularization of the lower extremities is indicated for severe lifestyle-limiting claudication and limb-threatening ischemia. Although intraoperative hemodynamic instability is not as frequent in these patients as in patients undergoing aortic or carotid surgery, the frequency of perioperative cardiac complications is similar. In order to avoid the potential complications of general anesthesia, these procedures are frequently performed using regional anesthesia. Revascularization is usually performed with a saphenous vein graft or with a prosthetic material such as polytetrafluoroethylene. If the limb is severely ischemic, reperfusion can result in acidosis and electrolyte abnormalities, which can affect cardiac function. Myoglobinuria can also occur and cause renal injury. This is best treated with hydration.

Postoperative swelling can be severe, and the patient is at risk for the development of a compartment syndrome. When extremities that have been severely ischemic for an extended period are revascularized, fasciotomies should be performed.

Postoperative Care

The postoperative care of these patients is similar to that of other vascular patients, with particular attention to the optimization of cardiac function. The leg operated on should be elevated and the neurovascular status evaluated frequently. The character and quality of the pulses should be documented immediately postoperatively, with any deterioration requiring exploration. The development of a neurologic change, severe pain in the extremity, or a change in the perfusion are signs of compartment syndrome. Compartment pressures can be measured, but if there is any question of a compartment syndrome, fasciotomies should be performed. Most patients receive aspirin, and some patients with distal bypasses are anticoagulated with warfarin. The exact indications for anticoagulation are not well established.

BIBLIOGRAPHY

Hertzer NR, Bevan EG, Young JR, et al: Coronary artery disease in peripheral vascular patients. A classification of 1000 coronary angiograms and results of surgical management. Ann Surg 199:223–323, 1984.
This is a classic study documenting the high prevalence of CAD in vascular patients.

Huber TS, Harward TRS, Flynn TC, et al: Operative mortality rates after elective infrarenal aortic reconstructions. J Vasc Surg 22:287–294, 1995.
This article describes a study identifying the frequency of major complications after aortic surgery and the mortality rate of aortic surgery.

Knipslci WC, Layug EL, Reilly LM, et al: Comparison of cardiac morbidity between aortic and infrainguinal operations. J Vasc Surg 15:354–365, 1992.
This study documented a similar risk of cardiac morbidity and mortality in patients undergoing aortic and infrainguinal reconstruction.

North American Symptomatic Carotid Endarterectomy Trial Collaborators: Beneficial effect of carotid endarterectomy in symptomatic patients with high-grade carotid stenosis. N Engl J Med 325:445–453, 1991.
A large study documenting the benefits, complications, and mortality of carotid surgery.

Olsen PS, Schroeder T, Perko M, et al: Renal failure after operation for abdominal aortic aneurysms. Ann Vasc Surg 4:580–583, 1990.
This large study reported the frequency of postoperative renal failure after aortic surgery and the mortality.

Owen RS, Carpenter JP, Baum RA, et al: Magnetic resonance imaging of angiographically occult runoff vessels in peripheral arterial disease. N Engl J Med 326:1577–1581, 1992.
This study showed that MRA was equivalent to contrast angiography as a diagnostic imaging modality.

Taylor LM, Yeager RA, Moneta GL, et al: The incidence of perioperative myocardial infarction in general vascular surgery. J Vasc Surg 15:52–6l, 1991.
This article reports a study demonstrating the incidence of myocardial infarction in vascular surgery patients.

Wong T, Detsky AS: Preoperative cardiac risk assessment for patients having peripheral vascular surgery. Ann Intern Med 116:743–753, 1992.
This is an overview of the preoperative cardiac evaluation of patients undergoing vascular surgery.

Zelenock GB, Strodel WE, Knol JA, et al: A prospective study of clinically and endoscopically documented colonic ischemia in 100 patients undergoing aortic reconstructive surgery with aggressive colonic and pelvic revascularization, compared with historic controls. Surgery 106:771–780, 1989.
This large study documented the frequency and mortality of intestinal ischemia after aortic reconstruction.

92 Thoracic Surgical Patient

John R. Roberts
Bruce R. Rosengard

Important elements of the perioperative care of thoracic surgical patients include careful patient selection, preoperative patient evaluation and management, pain control, and postoperative fluid management.

PATIENT SELECTION

Pulmonary function tests are commonly obtained during preoperative evaluation of patients undergoing a pulmonary resection. Complete pulmonary function tests should include spirometry with expiratory flows and volumes, and measurement of lung volumes, arterial blood gas, and diffusing capacity. Although a generally accepted rule holds that patients should be left with a minimal forced expiratory volume in 1 second (FEV_1) of approximately 800 mL after resection, improved postoperative management with limited and muscle-sparing incisions, epidural catheters, and patient-controlled analgesia (PCA) has permitted pulmonary resections in patients with increasingly severe lung disease. For example, some patients with limited ventilation or perfusion to the operative lung can tolerate a pneumonectomy despite the fact that their predicted postoperative FEV_1 may be less than 800 mL. Quantitative ventilation/perfusion scans that separately measure perfusion and ventilation to right lung and left lung can help estimate the lung function that would remain if pneumonectomy becomes necessary. Thoracoscopic resection of small peripheral cancers or nodules and lung volume reduction for treatment of emphysema can be safely performed in patients with severe chronic obstructive pulmonary disease.

Improved postoperative outcomes have led to increasingly aggressive thoracic surgical procedures in more compromised patients. Consequently, those patients who require postoperative intensive care and mechanical ventilation are often critically ill with poor physiologic cardiopulmonary reserves.

Patients who retain carbon dioxide have historically been considered poor candidates for pulmonary resection. Although the combination of carbon dioxide (CO_2) retention and impaired pulmonary function still increases the risk of surgery, many patients with preoperative arterial carbon dioxide tension ($Paco_2$) of 50 to 60 mm Hg can safely undergo limited resections.

Diffusing capacity is a useful measure of the overall available pulmonary vascular bed. Destruction of the vascular bed, which occurs in emphysema or interstitial fibrosis, reduces diffusing capacity and is manifested as a decrease in oxygen saturation (Sao_2) with exercise. Patients with diffusing capacities of less than 50% are at substantially increased risk for surgical procedures. Finally, excellent cardiac capacity can compensate to some extent for diminished ventilatory capacity or diffusing capacity. Despite diminished capacity in one of these three measures, some patients may have good exercise tolerance (as demonstrated by the capacity to climb stairs) and should still be considered as candidates for pulmonary resection.

After the decision is made for a surgical resection, preparing the patient appropriately is important. Smokers benefit from abstinence from cigarettes (preferably for more than 3 to 4 weeks), bronchodilator therapy, inhaled and systemic corticosteroids, and empirical antibiotics. Patients with severely compromised pulmonary function may benefit from a course of pulmonary rehabilitation or conditioning before elective surgery.

PERIOPERATIVE MANAGEMENT

The thoracic surgical patient is at particular risk from perioperative volume overload, pulmonary secretions, incisional pain, cardiac dysrhythmias, and malnutrition.

Volume Overload

Lung resection increases the risk of perioperative pulmonary edema by three mechanisms: (1) intraoperative lung manipulation can injure the lung; (2) mediastinal lymphadenectomy disrupts lymphatic drainage; and (3) extensive lung resection decreases the pulmonary vascular bed so that the remaining lung receives increased blood flow, typically at higher pressure. This increased blood flow results in increased pulmonary capillary pressures and increased transcapillary fluid flux. Limitation of intraoperative volume administration, the use of volume-sparing inotropes or vasopressors (such as dopamine), and postoperative diuresis are appropriate management strategies. The goals of postoperative diuretic management should be to achieve serum sodium levels of about 145 mEq/L, or a blood urea nitrogen:creatinine ratio of about 30 to 40:1, with a urine output of about 0.5 mL/kg per hour. Overdiuresis increases the risk of electrolyte abnormalities, renal insufficiency, and inspissation of pulmonary secretions.

Pulmonary Secretions

Pulmonary secretions predispose the patient to the development of mucous plugging, atelectasis, and pneumonia. Conservative measures include early postoperative mobilization, incentive spirometry, chest physiotherapy, and nasotracheal suctioning (if the patient has a poor cough). An alternative to nasotracheal suctioning is to place a small-bore catheter through the cricothyroid membrane at the end of the procedure in the operating room. This can be used to stimulate coughing by injections of small boluses of sterile saline and for suctioning secretions directly. Bronchoscopy permits directed pulmonary toilet and is indicated for patients with mucous plugs and lobar collapse. Finally, expeditious performance of a tracheostomy is appropriate in some patients who are unable to clear secretions by nasotracheal suctioning or coughing. Antibiotics should be administered to patients with infected secretions.

Table 92–1. Methods to Decrease Postoperative Thoracic Surgery Pain

....

Limited incisions using video assisted thoracoscopic surgery (VATS)
Muscle-sparing incisions (e.g., not cutting the latissimus dorsi)
Intraoperative and postoperative rib blocks with local anesthetics
Intravenous patient-controlled analgesia (see Chapter 85)
Patient-controlled epidural analgesia with opioid and local anesthetic (see Chapter 85)

....

Perioperative Pain Management

Splinting due to incisional pain decreases the effectiveness of coughing and predisposes to the development of atelectasis. The use of modified incisions (e.g., thoracoscopic, muscle sparing) and advances in pain control (e.g., epidural catheters, patient-controlled analgesia) (see Chapter 85) have demonstrably lowered perioperative mortality in thoracic surgical patients (Table 92–1).

Malnutrition

Patients with poor pulmonary function are often malnourished either from increased work of breathing or chronic deconditioning. Parenteral or preferably enteral feeds should be instituted early (see Chapter 13). Enteral feeds should be administered *postpylorically* to decrease the risk of aspiration, since this is a particularly catastrophic complication in patients with marginal pulmonary function.

Cardiac Arrhythmias

Supraventricular dysrhythmias are common in postoperative thoracic surgical patients, resulting from diuresis, secondary electrolyte abnormalities (hypokalemia, hypomagnesemia), and atrial irritation. Beta-blockers are contraindicated in patients with severe obstructive lung disease because of the potential for exacerbation of bronchospasm. Digoxin and calcium channel blocking agents are preferable for rate control.

POSTOPERATIVE COMPLICATIONS

Pneumonia

Pneumonia is the most common cause of serious infection and sepsis in these postoperative patients. Several variables have been independently associated with nosocomial pneumonia (Table 92–2). The diagnosis is suggested by leukocytosis, fever, and a characteristic appearance on chest radiography. Gram-negative bacilli are the most common pathogens. The mechanism of most nosocomial pneumonias is subclinical aspiration of oropharyngeal or gastric contents, which can occur

Table 92–2. Risk Factors for Postoperative Nosocomial Pneumonia

Age >70 yr
Depressed level of consciousness
Chronic obstructive pulmonary disease
Tracheal intubation (endotracheal or tracheostomy tube)
Duration of mechanical ventilation
Documented gastric aspiration
Mechanical factors that promote gastric reflux, e.g., horizontal position
Medications that allow gastric colonization, e.g., H_2 histamine receptor blockers

even if the patient has a cuffed endotracheal tube in place. Aspiration pneumonia may be complicated by hypoxemia, bacterial pneumonia, lung abscess, or empyema.

Gastric aspiration can be mild, with minimal clinical changes, or severe, resulting in acute respiratory distress syndrome requiring intubation and mechanical ventilation. The risk of nosocomial pneumonia after aspiration is greater in patients who receive acid-suppressing medication, whether antacids, H_2-blockers, or proton pump inhibitors. Acid suppression results in bacterial colonization of the stomach and oropharynx.

Lung Abscess

Aspiration pneumonia does not typically develop into lung abscess, although aspirated anaerobic bacteria can facilitate abscess formation by other bacteria. A lung abscess is an intraparenchymal collection of pus that results from liquefactive necrosis of the lung, usually due to a subacute pulmonary infection. The chest radiograph shows a cavity within the lung parenchyma. Lung abscesses are rare in postoperative patients but may develop in resected patients who have pre-existing chronic aspiration or who aspirate secondary to gastric distention from ileus. Intensivists commonly care for patients with lung abscesses secondary to pneumonia or chronic aspiration—typically patients with alcoholism or seizure disorder or those who have undergone gastric or esophageal surgery. Most lung abscesses can be treated with antibiotics and chest physiotherapy. Large, complicated, poorly drained abscesses or lung abscesses in immunocompromised patients may require radiologic, bronchoscopic, or surgical drainage. Patients may be stabilized with a course of intravenous antibiotics and then undergo elective rather than emergent surgery.

Empyemas

Empyemas are infected pleural collections that typically develop as an extension of pneumonia. Nonpurulent collections are considered infected if they demonstrate low pH, low glucose, or high lactate dehydrogenase (LDH) in the pleural fluid (Table 92–3). Positive Gram stains and cultures of the pleural fluid should be

Table 92–3. Guidelines for Chest Tube Insertion in Patients with Nonpurulent Parapneumonic Effusions

PLEURAL FLUID FINDINGS	MANAGEMENT
pH <7.0 or glucose <40 mg/dL	Insert chest tube
pH 7.0–7.2 or LDH >1000 IU/L	Insert chest tube for large or loculated effusions
pH >7.2 and glucose >40 mg/dL and LDH <1000 IU/L	Start antibiotics and repeat thoracentesis if effusion increases or clinical situation worsens (any clinical deterioration is an indication for chest tube placement)

Note: Grossly purulent effusions should always be treated initially with placement of chest tube.
LDH, lactate dehydrogenase.

considered diagnostic of an infected pleural effusion and warrant consideration of prompt surgical management.

Appropriate treatment of an empyema requires both drainage and antibiotics. An early infected parapneumonic effusion, with thin serous fluid and relatively high pH and glucose levels, may respond to antibiotic treatment alone (see Table 92–3). Thin, free-flowing collections may be adequately drained with multiple thoracenteses or tube thoracostomy. Empyemas with loculations, lower pH and glucose levels, and higher LDH levels are less likely to respond to intravenous antibiotics or to multiple thoracenteses, and most of these patients require tube thoracostomy. For some of these patients, this will be adequate treatment, whereas others will require further surgical intervention. Limited empyemas may be evacuated thoracoscopically. Larger empyemas typically require a full thoracotomy with decortication or parietal pleurectomy, or both, to effect complete drainage.

Computed tomography (CT) of the chest is useful to clarify anatomy but not necessary prior to initial chest tube placement. When the empyema fluid is thin and without significant loculations, tube thoracostomy may result in complete drainage. Evaluation of a chest CT scan after initial thoracostomy may reveal a single remaining loculation that can be drained by a second chest tube or extensive disease necessitating surgical intervention.

Patients with chest tubes in place and inadequate drainage may benefit from direct instillation of streptokinase into the chest tube to break down loculations and improve drainage. The technique requires daily instillation of 250,000 units of streptokinase with 100 mL of saline into the chest tube, which is then clamped for 4 hours. The treatment is repeated daily until the drainage falls to less than 150 mL/day or until the chest radiograph no longer improves. Contraindications include suspected allergy to streptokinase, bronchopleural fistula, trapped lung, and multiple large loculations that are unlikely to respond. This technique should be considered for patients in poor medical condition who would not tolerate surgery well, but not if it just delays necessary surgery.

Postpneumonectomy Empyema and Bronchopleural Fistula

Postpneumonectomy empyemas generally present in a chronic fashion. These patients return to clinic as long as 12 months after surgery with weight loss, fatigue, and general malaise, suggesting a diagnosis of recurrent cancer. Thoracentesis is critical to make the diagnosis. Fluid should be sent for culture and cell count; LDH and albumin levels; pH; and glucose levels. With this information, the diagnosis is generally straightforward.

The empyema may be associated with a bronchopleural fistula. Patients with a bronchopleural fistula have an air-fluid level either at the level of the carina or below, whereas all patients without a fistula should have an air-fluid level that is either higher than the carina or there should be none whatsoever.

Treatment of a postpneumonectomy empyema requires drainage of the loculated collection with a thoracostomy (so-called Clagett window) and intravenous antibiotics. Infections in postpneumonectomy empyemas involve multiple organisms, including anaerobes, and patients should be covered with antibiotics appropriate for anaerobes (even if the culture for anaerobes is negative). The patients are treated with antibiotics and open packing until the infectious process resolves. At that point, the chest can be closed primarily if the fistula has healed. Patent fistulas must be covered with vascularized tissue, either a muscle flap (latissimus muscle, serratus muscle, or pectoralis muscle) or an omental flap.

Esophageal Perforation

Esophageal perforation typically presents in patients with a history of esophageal cancer, vomiting or retching, or recent endoscopy. Substernal or back pain, fever and leukocytosis, and a chest radiograph with subdiaphragmatic air, pneumomediastinum, or pleural effusion are the hallmarks of diagnosis. Such a diagnosis should be confirmed by esophagogram (using water-soluble contrast) to detect the site of perforation. If the perforation is limited and is well drained into the gastrointestinal tract, it can be followed with serial examinations and intravenous antibiotics and may not require surgery.

Endoscopic perforations most commonly occur at a site of iatrogenic dilatation or at the three areas where the esophagus naturally narrows: (1) the gastroesophageal junction, (2) the aortic arch, or (3) the cricopharyngeus. Many injuries can be managed conservatively (with intravenous antibiotics and observation) if the tear is small and there is no contamination. Most iatrogenic perforations, however, require surgical repair.

Patients with esophageal perforation from a nonendoscopic cause ultimately require surgical management. Although drainage of the perforation is urgent, the repair can occasionally be delayed. For example, patients with a remote perforation (>48 hours) can be drained and resuscitated initially. If drainage is thorough and sepsis does not develop, immediate surgery is not necessary and should be delayed, particularly in patients who will require esophagectomy to treat underlying disease.

SUMMARY

Preoperative preparation, advances in surgical techniques and pain management, and improved postoperative care now permit thoracic surgery in patients with severe lung disease. The inevitable consequence of doing this increasingly aggressive surgery is that some of these patients require prolonged postoperative mechanical ventilation, eventually becoming "challenge to wean" patients (see Chapter 23).

BIBLIOGRAPHY

Heffner JE: Pneumonia and empyema. In: Niederman MS, Sarosi GA, Glassroth J (eds): Respiratory Infections: A Scientific Basis for Management. Philadelphia: WB Saunders, 1994.
This is a comprehensive review article focusing on the diagnosis and management of infected pleural effusions.

Light RW: Pleural Diseases, 2nd ed. Philadelphia: Lea & Febiger, 1990.
This is the definitive monograph that comprehensively covers the pleura and its disorders and diseases.

Light RW: Management of parapneumonic effusions. Chest 100:892–893, 1991.
This is a review article on the management of pleural effusions by the author of much of the definitive literature on this topic.

Mark JBD, Rizk NW: Pneumonia, bronchiectasis, and lung abscess. In: Baue AE, Geha AS, Hammond GL, Laks H, Naunheim KS (eds): Glenn's Thoracic and Cardiovascular Surgery. Norwalk CT: Appleton & Lange, 1996.
This chapter covers diagnosis and treatment of pneumonia complicated by empyema.

Strange C, Sahn S: Management of parapneumonic pleural effusions and empyema. Infect Dis Clin North Am 5:539–559, 1991.
This chapter, written by a thoracic surgeon and a pulmonologist, reviews the medical and surgical management of pulmonary infections.

93

Approach to the Trauma Patient

C. William Hanson, III
Paul S. Brown, Jr.

Trauma is the leading cause of death in the first three decades of life, accounting for more deaths in the United States than all other diseases combined. Despite decreasing mortality rates over the past 100 years, the number of deaths due to trauma still remains high, approximately 140,000/year. In addition, 50 million injuries occur each year, and 20% of these are disabling. To illustrate the dimensions of effects on the U.S. health system, trauma patients occupy 12% of hospital beds and account for 75 billion to 100 billion dollars of health care expenditures.

PATTERNS OF MORTALITY FROM TRAUMA

Death from trauma has a trimodal distribution. The first peak occurs within seconds to minutes of the injury. These deaths are usually due to lacerations of the brain, brainstem, spinal cord, heart, aorta, or other large vessels. The second peak occurs in the immediate minutes to hours after injury. These deaths represent the greatest opportunity for lifesaving intervention and are usually due to subdural and epidural hematomas, hemopneumothorax, ruptured spleen, lacerated liver, pelvic fractures, or multiple injuries associated with major blood loss. The third peak of death occurs in the days to weeks after trauma. These deaths result from infection, acute respiratory distress syndrome, and multiple organ system failure.

One factor in the reduction of morbidity and mortality from trauma has been the development of rapid transport networks that deliver injured patients to regional trauma centers. Emergency medical personnel are trained to perform triage on patients and transport them to hospitals that are equipped to handle their injuries. This means that more trauma patients with potentially fatal injuries arrive in the emergency department during what is called the "golden hour" and can be saved with rapid assessment and treatment.

STRUCTURED MANAGEMENT OF THE TRAUMA PATIENT

The initial management of the injured patient involves a structured, prioritized approach using two surveys to evaluate and manage injuries. The *primary survey* is shown in Table 93–1. Life-threatening conditions are treated as soon as they are identified during the primary survey. Resuscitation is initiated immediately with crystalloid or blood, or both, depending on the estimated blood loss. The *secondary survey* follows the primary survey, during which the body is examined by regions for injuries. After the primary and secondary surveys and resuscitation are undertaken, injuries are managed definitively.

Definitive care of the severely injured patient may or may not involve immediate

1037

Table 93–1. Primary Survey of Trauma Patient in Emergency Department

THE "ABC'S" PLUS "D AND E"	SPECIFIC AREA SURVEYED
A	Airway maintenance with cervical spine control
B	Breathing and ventilation
C	Circulation with hemorrhage control
D	Disability: check neurologic status
E	Exposure: completely undress the patient

surgery. Patients who have sustained blunt injuries, for example, may have closed head injuries, pulmonary contusions, visceral lacerations, or pelvic fractures requiring intracranial pressure monitoring and treatment, mechanical ventilation, and hemodynamic resuscitation, and yet these patients have no need for surgery. Some patients who do require immediate intra-abdominal surgery are best managed with staged procedures. The term *damage control* has been used to describe a surgical approach wherein major exsanguinating injuries are treated immediately. The abdomen is left open and packed to tamponade bleeding, and the patient is transferred to the intensive care unit (ICU) for rewarming and resuscitation. The patient then returns to the operating room in 24 to 48 hours for definitive management of any remaining injuries and abdominal closure.

The principles and practices guiding ICU management of patients with specific injuries are described in the following five chapters. No matter the type of injury, successful treatment of any severely injured trauma patient, who is often young with the great potential for functional recovery, is one of the most satisfying experiences in clinical medicine.

When The Trauma Patient Arrives In The Intensive Care Unit

Initial Evaluation

A complete reassessment of all trauma patients coming to the ICU should be performed on their arrival, regardless of whether the patient had an operation or not (Table 93–2). There may be a tendency for all concerned to rest easy when the patient gets to the ICU. Trauma patients, however, typically continue to reveal new injuries over the next several days and have injuries that are still in the process of being evaluated. The ICU physician should obtain a history of the patient's accident and hospital course, perform a complete physical examination, and survey the patient's current status. There should be one team of physicians responsible for the overall care of the patient in order to coordinate the sometimes conflicting desires of the multiple consulting surgical subspecialties.

Obtaining a past medical history from family members or friends is important in all trauma patients, but especially so for older ones. It is useful to tell families that it is common for other injuries to present themselves over the next few days. All laboratory tests ordered up to this point should be reviewed. All radiographs and especially computed tomographic scans should be carefully re-examined to

Table 93–2. Trauma Patient Evaluation on Arrival at the Intensive Care Unit

History

Obtain a history of the patient's accident
Review prior hospital course and anesthesia record
Obtain past medical history from family members and friends

Physical Examination

Perform a physical examination

Laboratory and Radiographic Tests

Review all laboratory tests and make an inventory of outstanding results
Review and inventory all radiographs and computed tomographic scans
List all radiographs that are outstanding or need to be repeated
List all radiographs without official interpretation and review them with radiologist

Ongoing Therapies

Survey the patient's current status, medications, and treatments

List of All Known and Potential Injuries

List all *known and evaluated* injuries with a treatment plan
List all *known and partially evaluated or unevaluated* injuries with a time line for evaluation
List all *potential* injuries with a surveillance plan to diagnose them

Coordination and Consultation

Designate a single coordinating physician
Obtain appropriate consultations

look for missed injuries, and a list should be made of all films that are outstanding or still need official interpretation by a radiologist.

An inventory of injuries should be made. First, all known injuries should be listed along with the treatment given and the expected plan for outcome and further treatment. Second, all injuries in the process of being evaluated should be documented (such as an uncleared cervical spine) and re-evaluated and a time frame for definitive evaluation outlined. Appropriate precautions should be set in place for the patient until full evaluations have been peformed because some ICU personnel may falsely assume that the cervical spine has been cleared. Third, one should always have an open mind about the possibility of new injuries that were missed or not yet evident, such as a fractured pancreas, broken hand and facial bones, delayed subdural hematomas, bowel injuries, or complications of treatments of known injuries, such as fat emboli from a broken femur.

Immediate Priorities

In the immediate postoperative period, the priorities for management of the trauma patient are similar to those of any postoperative or critically ill patient (Table 93–3). Most importantly, one needs to make sure that cardiac function is adequate, that there is appropriate treatment of ongoing bleeding or coagulopathy, and that all organs are adequately perfused. Once the patient is reasonably stable, one should continue the process of diagnosing and treating other injuries. A plan for weaning from ventilatory support should be developed and implemented.

The use of inotropic drugs in trauma patients *without* myocardial injury usually

Table 93–3. Intensive Care Unit Management Pearls for Trauma Patients

Airway and Breathing

Formulate a plan for weaning patients from ventilatory support

Circulation

Ensure adequate cardiac function
Correct acidosis
Ensure that all organs are adequately perfused
Wean from inotropic support
Minimize the amount of fluids administered
Maximally concentrate medications

Diagnosis and Treatment

Control ongoing bleeding or coagulopathy
Diagnose and treat other injuries
Early operative fixation of fractures
Avoid prophylactic antibiotic administration
Monitor for infections

Nutrition

Start nutrition early

Disposition

Consult discharge planner early

means that there has not been adequate volume resuscitation or correction of acidosis. Every attempt should be made to wean the patient from inotropic support. One should consider early initiation of nutritional support and always be looking for infection. Early operative treatment of all fractures is desirable because it allows earlier mobilization of the patient.

The care of the trauma patient does not end when the patient leaves the ICU. Consideration must be given to how the trauma could have been prevented in the first place and reviewed with the patient and family. Finally, if appropriate, discussions should be held to try to persuade the patient to make lifestyle changes to avoid further preventable trauma.

BIBLIOGRAPHY

Advanced Trauma Life Support Program Instructor Manual. Chicago: American College of Surgeons, 1990.

94   Abdominal Trauma

Michael L. Nance
Michael F. Rotondo

Trauma is the leading cause of death in Americans less than 44 years of age. It is also responsible for the greatest total number of years of life lost and the highest lifetime cost per death. Blunt trauma such as that due to a motor vehicle accident is the predominant mechanism in most regions of the country. In urban centers, however, penetrating trauma such as that due to a gunshot wound may represent about half of all admissions due to trauma.

Classically, death due to trauma occurs in three distinct periods. The first peak occurs immediately or in the first few minutes following injury as a result of severe head or spinal cord injuries or major vascular disruptions. These patients usually die at the scene or shortly thereafter. The second peak occurs minutes to hours following injury, during the so-called golden hour. Advanced trauma life support (ATLS) programs were designed to affect this subset of trauma patients by designing ATLS protocols in which these patients undergo rapid assessment, resuscitation, and treatment. The third peak occurs days to weeks following the injury and is typically the result of organ failure or sepsis. In the intensive care unit (ICU), the clinician can have an impact on the outcome of patients in the second period through aggressive resuscitation and treatment, and in the third period through recognition and prevention of sepsis and multiple organ failure.

INITIAL ASSESSMENT

The initial assessment of a trauma patient begins at the scene of an injury with information provided by paramedics, family, or the patient. Knowledge of the extent of damage to vehicles, ejection from the vehicle, and the use of safety devices are important in the evaluation of the patient with blunt trauma, as are descriptions of weapons or the number of shots fired in the case of penetrating trauma. This information, when considered in the context of the physical examination, may provide additional clues to potential injury and direct the course of treatment in abdominal trauma. Past medical and surgical histories as well as known allergies are also important and should be sought. Previous intra-abdominal surgery has particular importance because it may alter diagnosis and therapy.

After evaluation and stabilization of the airway, breathing, and circulation as directed by ATLS protocol, a directed neurologic examination is performed. Resuscitation begins concomitantly and continues as the secondary survey (completion of physical examination) is performed to determine other potential life-threatening injuries. Warmed saline is used for initial volume resuscitation. Hemodynamic instability despite the administration of 2 L of crystalloid in the adult patient is an indication for blood transfusion and suggests that operative intervention may be necessary. Type O, Rh(-)blood should be administered if type-specific blood is not yet available. In the patient with abdominal trauma, persistent hemodynamic instability despite volume therapy requires emergent laparotomy.

1041

Physical examination of the abdomen should include inspection, making careful note of findings such as ecchymosis from seat belts, tire marks, bullet entry and exit sites, or stab wound depth and direction. Abdominal distention may suggest intra-abdominal hemorrhage, whereas a scaphoid abdomen suggests a ruptured diaphragm. Palpation should be directed to detect areas of tenderness or masses, whereas auscultation should assess bowel sounds and the presence of bruits.

Initial laboratory work should include a complete blood count, serum electrolyte determination, coagulation studies, blood typing, and antibody screen (or cross-match), serum pregnancy test (as indicated), and a urinalysis. Other studies of possible benefit in the initial evaluation and management may include liver function tests, amylase and lipase determinations, and toxicology screens.

Radiologic studies obtained on most patients with major blunt trauma include lateral cervical spine films, supine chest radiographs, and pelvic views. Conventional abdominal radiographs are rarely helpful in the assessment of blunt abdominal trauma. In the case of penetrating trauma, all foreign bodies must be accounted for by examination or radiologic study, or both. Entrance and exit sites are identified with radiopaque markers on the patient prior to exposure of the film to help determine trajectory and therefore potential injured organs. Included in the initial assessment is a determination of the need for operation. Many patients have absolute indications for surgery that are apparent early in the evaluation (Table 94–1).

Most instances of hypotension in the immediate peritrauma period should be treated aggressively with volume, typically warmed saline, or, if needed, blood products. Severely injured patients with possible cardiac injury or comorbid disease may benefit from the placement of a pulmonary artery catheter.

Because of the life-threatening nature of the injuries in many trauma patients or an altered level of consciousness, a thorough secondary survey is not always possible. On arrival in the ICU and after the patient is stabilized, it is imperative to review the injuries identified and the completeness of the diagnostic work-up. A tertiary survey (follow-up complete physical examination) should be performed in the ICU to identify any missed injuries. Despite primary and secondary surveys,

Table 94–1. Indications for Immediate Operative Intervention

Blunt Abdominal Trauma

Hemodynamic instability despite volume resuscitation
Signs of peritonitis
Positive peritoneal lavage
Evidence of diaphragmatic rupture

Penetrating Abdominal Trauma

All gunshot wounds (nontangential)
Stab wounds with
    Evisceration
    Blood per rectum or nasogastric tube
    Positive peritoneal lavage
    Hemodynamic instability despite volume resuscitation
    Signs of peritonitis
    Mental status changes precluding reliable serial abdominal examination

Table 94–2. Comparison of Utility of Diagnostic Modalities

SITE TO BE ASSESSED	PERITONEAL LAVAGE	ABDOMINAL-RETROPERITONEAL COMPUTED TOMOGRAPHY	ULTRASONOGRAPHY
Free fluid	+ + +	+ +	+ +
Hollow viscus	+	+	+
Retroperitoneum	0	+ + +	+
Solid viscus	+ +	+ + +	+ +

0, no utility; +, fair utility; + +, good utility; + + +, excellent utility.

a missed injury rate of 9% or more can be expected. Although these injuries are usually non–life threatening, they may be clinically debilitating and compromise the patient's long-term outcome.

All patients with either blunt or penetrating abdominal trauma should be given tetanus prophylaxis. If laparotomy is planned, a preoperative dose of broad spectrum antibiotics, typically a second-generation cephalosporin is given prior to the incision. If no enteric contamination has occurred, no further antibiotics are required. In the event of enteric spillage, however, a short, 24-hour postoperative course of antibiotics should be continued.

As a routine, all lines placed in the trauma admitting area should be removed within 24 hours of arrival in the ICU and new sites accessed as necessary.

DIAGNOSTIC EVALUATION OF THE PATIENT WITH BLUNT ABDOMINAL TRAUMA

In the stable patient with blunt abdominal trauma, additional diagnostic studies are often indicated to assess the need for operative intervention. The choice of study depends on the availability of equipment, information sought, stability of patient, and preference of the clinician responsible for the patient (Table 94–2). Diagnostic evaluation should never cause delay in any patient with a clear indication for abdominal exploration.

Diagnostic Peritoneal Lavage

Many trauma surgeons favor diagnostic peritoneal lavage (DPL) as the primary diagnostic tool in evaluation of the abdomen following blunt trauma. A closed, guide wire technique is preferred because of shorter procedure time, lower complication rate, and results comparable to an open technique. Prepackaged, sterile DPL kits are available commercially. Controversy exists regarding the threshold values (red and white blood cell counts and presence of particulate matter) in the effluent that constitute a positive study. In general, however, a red blood cell (RBC) count greater than 100,000/μL is considered an indication for laparotomy. There may be a high negative laparotomy rate in blunt abdominal injuries (up to 28%) if intervention is based on DPL RBC counts alone, since the presence of blood in the lavage fluid is a nonspecific indication of injury. White blood cell counts are unreliable indicators of injury, particularly if obtained soon after the injury (before white blood cells have had time to enter the peritoneal cavity). Additionally, DPL does not allow evaluation of the retroperitoneal structures, plus it is usually contraindicated in the patient who has undergone prior abdominal surgery.

DPL is indicated in the unstable patient in whom an abdominal-retroperitoneal computed tomographic scan cannot be obtained without delay or in the setting of a patient who requires emergent operative intervention for associated trauma. Moreover, DPL may be performed in the operating room or ICU to evaluate the abdomen of a patient in whom examination is unreliable (e.g., because the patient is anesthetized, intoxicated, or has received a head injury) in the setting of clinical deterioration.

Computed Tomography

The advent of computed tomography (CT) has virtually revolutionized the care of patients with abdominal trauma. It allows the clinician to grade the severity of solid organ injury, identify intra-abdominal fluid or air, thereby helping to determine the necessity of laparotomy. CT is also useful in the patient with concomitant head or thoracic injury; it readily visualizes the retroperitoneum, including genitourinary and major vascular structures. CT of the abdomen also provides information about injuries to adjacent extra-abdominal sites such as the bony pelvis or lower mediastinum. Improvements in technology have increased the resolution and reduced scan acquisition time, increasing the attractiveness and applicability of this modality. Ultrafast and spiral scanners have been shown to be as accurate as conventional machines and require as little as one fifth the scan time.

Ultrasonography

Ultrasonography is increasing in popularity in the initial assessment of trauma patients because of the immediate availability of information, ease of use, and absence of radiation exposure. Ultrasonography is most useful in detecting specific abnormalities, such as the presence of intraperitoneal fluid or significant injury to a solid organ. It is ideal in the assessment of the pregnant trauma patient, providing information on fetal viability, placental integrity, and maternal injuries. Increasingly, trauma surgeons have acquired sufficient proficiency with ultrasonography to rely solely on the information it provides to guide therapy.

DIAGNOSTIC EVALUATION OF THE PATIENT WITH PENETRATING ABDOMINAL TRAUMA

Over the past several decades, the handgun has replaced the knife as the weapon of choice in violent crime. The evaluation of the penetrating abdominal trauma patient differs based on the mechanism of injury (stab wound versus gunshot wound). In the patient with a stab wound to the abdomen, it is important to consider the location of the wound, the length of the weapon, and the depth of the wound in determining the diagnostic approach. The major diagnostic hurdle in evaluation of the stab wound patient is determining if the peritoneum has been violated because that implies potential intra-abdominal injury.

In contrast, for the patient with a gunshot wound, it is routinely assumed that the peritoneum has been violated and that intra-abdominal injury has occurred. In gunshot wound cases, it is imperative to determine the path of the projectile prior to laparotomy because trajectory determination is a fundamental part of injury identification. The type of weapon (e.g., handgun or rifle), distance from the weapon, or special ammunition are important factors in arriving at a management plan.

Diagnostic Peritoneal Lavage

DPL has been advocated by some authors as a method to determine if intra-abdominal injury has occurred in the patient with an abdominal stab wound or in the rare gunshot wound patient with stable hemodynamics. In this setting, the values accepted as a positive study are much lower than those for the patient with blunt trauma but, again, the best threshold has not been conclusively established. DPL is limited because of the inability to assess rupture of the diaphragm or injury to the retroperitoneal structures, which can be a large reservoir for blood loss.

Laparoscopy

The use of laparoscopy has been recommended in the stable patient with penetrating abdominal trauma (due to a stab wound or gunshot wound) to determine if peritoneal penetration has occurred. This method provides a reliable look at the peritoneal surface but is less effective at assessing for other injuries such as bowel perforation or retroperitoneal injury. The laparoscope may be particularly useful in patients with low thoracic wounds to assess for diaphragmatic injury, which, if present, would necessitate operative repair.

Computed Tomography

CT is uncommonly used in the setting of penetrating abdominal trauma but may be of some value in isolated circumstances. Its major drawback is the poor recognition of small bowel injuries, the second most frequent organ injured in abdominal gunshot wounds. In the hemodynamically stable patient with a gunshot wound in the right upper quadrant in whom an isolated hepatic injury is suspected, CT may provide an adequate assessment of the bullet's trajectory to prevent a nontherapeutic laparotomy. CT, with the addition of rectal contrast, also provides a good look at the rectum and may be useful in the evaluation of a patient with a transpelvic gunshot wound. Useful information about injury to retroperitoneal structures can be obtained using CT, but it is not recommended for routine use.

MANAGEMENT

Patient with Blunt Abdominal Trauma

Like its impact on the diagnostic evaluation, CT has drastically altered how blunt abdominal trauma patients are managed. With rapid, high-resolution images of the abdomen available, the surgeon can reliably determine the extent of solid viscus injuries and formulate a management strategy. For example, a nonoperative management protocol (based on CT, hemodynamic status, and associated injury) is now the standard of practice for splenic injuries in the pediatric population. This strategy, developed by the pediatric surgical group at the Hospital for Sick Children in Toronto, demonstrated that more than 85% of splenic injuries could be managed nonoperatively in the hemodynamically stable child. These principles were then successfully extended to adult patients with a splenic injury. More recently, similar strategies have been adopted for the management of stable patients with blunt abdominal trauma and liver injuries as well.

This trend is likely to continue as trauma surgeons become more comfortable with the technique and as imaging modalities improve. The patient managed nonoperatively with a solid viscus injury proven by CT is typically admitted to the ICU for observation. The patient is kept on strict bed rest and given nothing by mouth. Serial abdominal examinations by an experienced surgeon, as well as serial hemoglobin checks, are necessary. Abnormalities in clotting factors should be corrected with blood products. A preset limit on the number of transfused packed RBCs that will be tolerated before laparotomy is performed should be decided on admission to the ICU. Deterioration in the clinical status, such as hemodynamic instability or change in abdominal examination, warrants investigation with either follow-up CT or laparotomy.

Patient with Penetrating Abdominal Trauma

All patients with a penetrating abdominal injury and hemodynamic instability or peritoneal signs require urgent exploratory laparotomy. However, in the absence of peritoneal signs in the hemodynamically stable, cooperative patient with an abdominal *stab* wound, many surgeons elect to observe these injuries. This practice requires serial abdominal examinations by an experienced surgeon, with laparotomy indicated if clinical deterioration occurs. Except in the rare case, most surgeons explore the abdomen of the patient with an abdominal *gunshot* wound.

Damage Control

"Damage control" is a new, evolving technique used in the management of critically ill patients with blunt or penetrating trauma. Patients with severe multisystem trauma are particularly susceptible to the development of a coagulopathic state secondary to hypothermia, acidosis, hemodilution, and ongoing blood loss. Without interruption, this state will continue in a downward spiral and have a fatal outcome. Damage control is designed to break the spiral and salvage these most critically injured patients.

Damage control has three phases. Initially, patients undergo an expeditious exploratory laparotomy to stop obvious hemorrhage and limit the contamination from bowel perforation. Laparotomy packs may be left in the abdomen for tamponade and hemostasis.

In the second phase, patients are aggressively resuscitated in the ICU by volume repletion, support of hemodynamics, correction of clotting abnormalities, and rewarming. Large-bore central catheters for volume repletion are used and all fluid and blood products should be warmed to restore normal core temperature as rapidly as can be safely achieved. Additional measures to rewarm the patient include warm sterile saline bladder irrigation, warm fluid lavage through tube thoracostomy, and warming of ventilation circuits. Rapid correction of the coagulopathic state with specific blood products as determined by measured hematologic deficiencies is essential. These patients frequently are managed with the aid of a pulmonary artery catheter to determine the appropriate balance of volume and vasoactive medications. Only after achieving normothermia, a normal coagulation profile, and resolution of metabolic acidemia should the patient return to the operating room, unless obvious surgical bleeding or intra-abdominal hypertension threatens the immediate survival of the patient. Resuscitation and rewarming in the ICU usually requires 24 to 48 hours.

The third phase of damage control involves re-exploration; removal of packing; repair; resection or reconstruction of injured organs, or both; placement of tubes for enteral access for feeding (if indicated); and definitive wound closure. More than one packing change may be necessary to achieve hemostasis and allow dissipation of bowel edema. Preliminary reports from centers using the damage control techniques reveal improved survival rates that approach 50% in this severely injured subset of patients.

POSTOPERATIVE AND POST-TRAUMATIC COMPLICATIONS

Complications in the postoperative period may prolong the ICU stay and add to the complexity of the management. Prompt recognition and aggressive treatment of these complications is the foundation of good ICU care.

Missed Injuries

All surgeons worry about the possibility of a missed injury in the trauma patient. Nowhere is this more challenging than in the management of abdominal trauma. In patients managed nonoperatively, hollow viscus and pancreatic injuries are notoriously difficult to diagnose and must always be considered in the patient who fails to improve, has unexplained sepsis, or acquires the acute respiratory distress syndrome. Patients who undergo abdominal exploration for a life-threatening injury frequently have abnormal anatomy because of destruction of tissues or the distortion of normal planes by surrounding hematoma or edema. Such distortion makes thorough assessment difficult and increases the potential for missed injury. For example, it may be difficult to determine whether an organ is injured beyond salvage or simply blood-stained from adjacent injury. It is not surprising that the more complex the injury or the more unstable the patient, the more likely the possibility of a missed injury.

Hemorrhage

Continued bleeding in the postoperative period is an all too frequent phenomenon, often manifested by saturation of wound dressings or copious bloody output from abdominal drains. A distinction must be made rapidly between true "surgical" bleeding that requires additional operative intervention and coagulopathic bleeding that will abate with correction of clotting factor deficiencies. The postoperative patient should be warmed and resuscitated, and deficiencies of coagulation factors corrected when possible, *prior* to the decision to re-explore the abdomen for bleeding. Premature return to the operating room in a coagulopathic patient may have devastating results.

Infection

Infection is another common complication of the postoperative ICU trauma patient. In the setting of abdominal trauma, often there is free perforation of unprepared bowel with gross contamination of the peritoneal cavity. Despite perioperative antibiotics and lavage of the abdomen at the time of injury, abscesses may develop, typically 5 to 7 days following the injury. They may present insidiously as low-grade recurrent fevers or more dramatically as profound sepsis and organ failure. Diagnosis is commonly made with the assistance of CT. Drainage of intra-abdominal collections is required by an open operative approach or by a radiologically guided catheter approach. These patients are also susceptible to infections that complicate invasive monitoring and intensive care therapy.

Abdominal Hypertension

Although the concept of abdominal hypertension or abdominal compartment syndrome is not new, the clinical significance has only recently been appreciated. Severe abdominal trauma with associated visceral edema; intra-abdominal or retroperitoneal hemorrhage, or both; and intra-abdominal packs (such as following damage control) are risk factors for the development of increased intra-abdominal pressure and an abdominal compartment syndrome. The possible consequences of this complication include decreased renal perfusion with resultant oliguria, elevated peak airway pressures due to decreased abdominal compliance, and low cardiac output due to a decrease in venous return from vena cava obstruction. Intra-abdominal pressures are usually determined indirectly as a reflection of the intravesicular pressure. Bladder pressures can be measured easily at the bedside using sterile water and an indwelling Foley catheter. The normal intra-abdominal pressure is zero or less. Clinically significant effects of intra-abdominal hypertension may be seen with pressures as low as 10 to 15 mm Hg, but pressures greater than 20 mm Hg should be cause for concern. Management of an abdominal compartment syndrome requires decompression by laparotomy. If the cause was hemorrhage, evacuation of hematoma and closure of the abdomen may resolve the problem. Severe bowel swelling may require delayed abdominal closure following diuresis and resolution of the edema.

Acalculous Cholecystitis

In recent years, increasing attention has been given to the clinical entity of *acalculous cholecystitis*. This condition, characterized ultrasonographically by increased gallbladder wall thickness, biliary sludge, and hydrops of the gallbladder, has been demonstrated prospectively in up to 18% of patients with multiple trauma. Acalculous cholecystitis may present insidiously with a gradual increase in the white blood cell count or fever curve. In the alert patient, right upper quadrant pain can typically be elicited. In this setting, ultrasonographic evaluation of the hepatobiliary tree is indicated. Clinical signs of cholecystitis plus ultrasonographic evidence suggestive of cholecystitis are indications for a percutaneous cholecystostomy or operative cholecystectomy (see also Chapter 38).

BIBLIOGRAPHY

Advanced Trauma Life Support Student Manual. Chicago: American College of Surgeons, 1993.
This is the basic manual outlining standard management algorithms used in caring for the trauma patient.

Morris JA Jr, Eddy VA, Blinman TA, et al: The staged celiotomy for trauma. Ann Surg 217:576–586, 1993.
This article reviews the rationale behind and experience with damage control in the trauma population.

Nance ML, Nance FC: Blunt abdominal trauma. In: Cameron JC (ed): Current Surgical Therapy, 5th ed. Philadelphia: BC Decker, 1995.
This is a summary of the initial evaluation and management of the blunt abdominal trauma patient.

Schein M, Wittmann DH, Aprahamian CC, Condon RE: The abdominal compartment syndrome: The physiologic and clinical consequences of elevated intra-abdominal pressure. J Am Coll Surg 180:745–753, 1995.
This article provides a description of the pathophysiology of abdominal hypertension.

Thal ER, Meyer DM: The evaluation of blunt abdominal trauma: Computed tomography scan, lavage, or sonography? Adv Surg 24:201–228, 1991.
This is a thorough review of diagnostic modalities used in the evaluation of the patient with blunt abdominal trauma. It includes strengths, weaknesses, and application of the various techniques.

95

Extremity and Major Vascular Trauma

William S. Hoff
James F. Reilly

EXTREMITY TRAUMA

Both penetrating and blunt injury to the extremities can result in a spectrum of injuries involving three important tissues: vessels, nerves, and soft tissue within fascial compartments. When the patient with extremity trauma arrives in the intensive care unit (ICU), these three areas demand the continued focused attention of the ICU team.

Peripheral Vascular Injuries

Penetrating trauma of extremities produces injuries of vessels ranging from partial disruption to complete transection. The trajectory of penetrating injuries determines which vascular structures are in jeopardy. In addition, the "blast effect" of gunshot wounds may result in injuries to vessels both proximal and distal to the obvious points of injury. In blunt trauma of extremities, compression, traction, and deceleration forces can produce thrombosis, intimal disruption, and avulsion of vessels. After blunt injury, fractures and dislocations can also injure and lacerate vessels.

Diagnosis

Regardless of the mechanism of injury, the affected extremity should be examined for active hemorrhage, hematoma, or a palpable thrill. Perfusion is evaluated by palpation of distal pulses, assessment of venous refilling, and time for capillary refilling; skin color; and determination of neurologic function. Areas of paresthesia, hypesthesia, or paralysis usually correlate with arterial injuries. Table 95–1 lists "hard" and "soft" signs of vascular injury.

The ankle-brachial index (ABI) is determined by dividing the systolic pressure in the traumatized extremity by the systolic pressure at the brachial artery. An ABI of less than 0.9 is indicative of major vascular injury but should be considered a "soft" sign because it does not mandate surgical exploration by itself.

Patients who present with "hard" signs require no additional diagnostic testing. In patients with "soft" signs, especially those with an ABI of less than 0.9, the diagnostic modality of choice is arteriography. An arteriogram confirming vascular injury can be anticipated in up to 35% of patients with "soft" signs. In the absence of other findings, proximity of the injury to a major vessel is not an absolute indication for arteriography. Regardless of the vascular examination, however, arteriography is recommended after knee dislocation to rule out blunt injury to the popliteal artery, as well as after shotgun wounds because of the multiple small projectiles.

1051

Table 95–1. Signs of Peripheral Vascular Injury

....

"Hard" Signs

Distal pulse deficit
Expanding or pulsatile hematoma
Palpable thrill or audible bruit
Visible arterial hemorrhage

"Soft" Signs

Adjacent nerve injury
Diminished pulse (or ankle-brachial index <0.9)
Injury in proximity to major artery
Moderate visible hemorrhage
Small to moderate size, nonexpanding hematoma

....

Noninvasive studies are used with increased frequency for the evaluation of vascular trauma, primarily for patients with seemingly minimal injuries. Duplex ultrasonography is appropriate in those with "soft" signs and an ABI greater than 0.9. Many noninvasive modalities are not universally available, may be difficult to perform and interpret, and depend on operator skill and experience.

Operative Interventions

Patients with "hard" signs should be transported directly to the operating room for surgical exploration and repair. An intraoperative arteriogram may be performed if necessary. Other patients may require surgery, depending on the results of further diagnostic studies. Arterial injuries are initially controlled with vascular clamps, the injured segment of artery is resected, and an interposition graft is placed to restore flow. Occasionally, a small injury may be amenable to simple repair, resection, and primary anastomosis or use of a vein patch. An intraluminal shunt may be used to perfuse the extremity temporarily while other injuries are addressed (e.g., unstable fracture). Arterial reconstructions should be evaluated after completion with an intraoperative arteriogram.

When possible, major venous injuries should be repaired but, aside from the popliteal vein, all other veins may be ligated if necessary. The decision to ligate is based on the overall patient condition and complexity of the injury.

Fasciotomy should also be performed when there has been a significant delay in restoration of perfusion, preoperative hypotension, significant swelling or crush injury of the extremity, combined arterial and venous repairs, or ligation of a major vein.

Postoperative Care

The goals of postoperative care are resuscitation of intravascular volume, rewarming, and correction of acidosis. Acidosis, hyperkalemia, and edema result from reperfusion of the ischemic extremity. Antihypertensive therapy (sodium nitroprusside, labetalol) (see Chapter 52) is indicated when necessary to avoid disruption of vascular repairs. Serial assessments of distal perfusion are important to detect early thrombotic complications. Because pulses may not be easily palpable as a result of vasoconstriction and hypothermia, capillary refill is used to assess adequacy of perfusion in the early postoperative period. Elevation of the extremity is useful to limit edema formation, and elastic wrapping of the extremity helps reduce edema after venous ligation or repair. The extremity must be evaluated frequently for signs and symptoms of compartment syndrome if a fasciotomy was not performed.

Thrombosis of an arterial reconstruction should be suspected when a discrepancy exists between pulses or when the ABI falls to less than 0.9 in the normothermic patient. These patients may require immediate return to the operating room. Although edema is a universal complication, especially after venous ligation, edema may also indicate thrombosis at the site of a venous repair.

Bleeding in the postoperative period may be due to coagulopathy, incomplete ligation of small vessels, or dehiscence of an arterial suture line. Coagulopathy should be reversed with appropriate blood component therapy as guided by coagulation parameters (see Chapter 15). Routine anticoagulation is unnecessary in the presence of a technically adequate reconstruction. Careful inspection of the wound and estimation of the degree of hemorrhage help to differentiate simple wound bleeding from suture line dehiscence.

Graft infection rarely complicates the early postoperative period. Wound infection, however, must be considered in the febrile patient because groin incisions are frequently used for lower-extremity vascular trauma. Proximity to the perineum and interruption of the lymphatics are factors predisposing to infection.

Peripheral Nerve Injuries

Categories of Nerve Injuries

Injuries to peripheral nerves often accompany vascular trauma, and they are classified by their histologic changes and associated neurologic insults.

Neurapraxia occurs most frequently after blunt trauma and is characterized by local physiologic loss of axonal conduction. Patients typically present with motor paralysis, but sensory and autonomic function are spared. Because the distal axon remains intact and there is preservation of electrical conductivity, full recovery with conservative management is the rule.

Axonotmesis results from disruption of the axon with preservation of its endoneurium (connective tissue elements) after blunt trauma or traction. Wallerian degeneration produces motor, sensory, and autonomic dysfunction with subsequent distal muscle atrophy. Nerve regeneration occurs at a rate of 1 mm/day. Recovery is influenced by age, associated injuries, and the peripheral level of injury (proximal versus distal). Surgery may be indicated for patients who fail to recover function.

Complete or partial transection of the nerve is defined as *neurotmesis* and is characterized by complete loss of motor, sensory, and autonomic function and distal muscle atrophy. Lack of connective tissue support results in misrouting of regenerating nerves and formation of painful neuromas. Surgical intervention is required for patients who are expected to have a meaningful overall functional recovery from their other traumatic injuries, particularly head injuries.

Diagnosis

The diagnosis of peripheral nerve injury is based on a careful history and physical examination. Determination of sensory deficits helps to delineate the level of the injury (see Appendix F for sensory dermatomes). Electromyographic testing defines the injury type and has prognostic value, but the electromyogram should be delayed until 3 to 4 weeks after injury. Treatment may involve surgery in severe injuries. Since injured extremities are at risk for muscle atrophy, joint stiffness, fibrosis, and trophic skin changes, early physical therapy is essential for an optimal outcome (see Chapter 25).

Compartment Syndrome

Since the muscles of the extremities are enveloped in fascial compartments (Fig. 95–1), edema may prevent effective venous return from the compartment after injury (Table 95–2). When pressure within a fascial compartment exceeds capillary perfusion pressure, tissues in that compartment are subject to ischemia and ultimately to cell death. Although compartment syndrome occurs most often in the lower leg, other compartments—for example, those in the arm or buttocks—are also at risk.

Diagnosis

In conscious patients, early clinical features include weakness, hypesthesia, palpable fullness, and pain out of proportion to that expected by the clinical setting or with passive stretch (dorsiflexion). Assessment of distal pulses alone is *insufficient* as a monitoring modality because pulse deficits develop well *after* irreversible

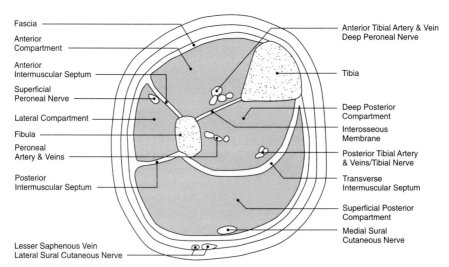

Figure 95–1. Cross-section of the lower leg showing the four major fascial compartments and their associated nerves and vessels.

Table 95–2. Risk Factors for Compartment Syndrome

Arterial injury or combined arteriovenous injury
Burns (circumferential or electrical) (see Chapter 56)
Crush injury (extensive soft tissue trauma)
External compression (casts, splints, and so on)
Fracture (open or closed)
Prolonged ischemia of the extremity (vascular occlusion, hypotension)
Severe venous occlusive disease

muscle damage has occurred. The same applies to paralysis and sensory deficits, which are *late findings* and suggest muscle necrosis.

If compartment syndrome is suspected in an unconscious patient, compartment pressures should be measured. Pressures are measured in a standardized manner by inserting a fluid-filled catheter connected to a pressure transducer into each of the compartments in question.

Management

Fasciotomy is indicated for compartment pressures greater than 40 mm Hg, for pressures between 30 and 40 mm Hg for 4 hours or more, or for pressures less than 30 mm Hg with concomitant clinical findings. The extremity should be placed at the level of the heart, and external devices (compression boots) that may compromise perfusion should be removed. Limb salvage requires prompt fasciotomy.

VASCULAR INJURIES OF THE NECK

Diagnosis

Blunt injuries to the carotid artery may be difficult to diagnose for a number of reasons. First, overt signs of neck trauma may be absent; second, clinical signs of carotid artery injury may be insidious (Table 95–3); and third, neurologic assessments are limited in these patients because of associated head trauma. Under these circumstances, one must rely on physical examination and a high index of suspicion based on the mechanism of injury. Suspicion of blunt carotid injury should prompt an arteriographic evaluation.

In contrast, penetrating neck trauma is usually clinically apparent. Focal neuro-

Table 95–3. Neurologic Signs of Blunt Injury to Carotid Artery

Ipsilateral Horner's syndrome
Limb paresis in an otherwise neurologically intact patient
Lucid postinjury period before onset of neurologic signs
Transient attacks of cerebral ischemia

logic deficits must be sought and documented, and injuries to the trachea or esophagus must be excluded. A large or expanding hematoma requires early definitive airway control. Hemodynamically unstable patients require prompt operative evaluation.

Treatment

The anatomic zones of the neck determine the diagnostic and therapeutic approach. Zone I of the neck includes those tissues that lie above the transverse plane at the level of the angle of the mandible. Zone III lies below the same plane at the level of the cricoid cartilage, whereas zone II is everything between zones I and III.

In stable patients with neck injuries, the diagnostic modality of choice is selective arteriography. For all patients with surgically inaccessible injuries, that is, injuries in zones I and III, arteriography also affords the possibility of embolization. Collateral perfusion is assessed by visualization of the contralateral carotid and both vertebral arteries. This becomes important if ligation or embolization is a therapeutic consideration. Traditionally, mandatory exploration of zone II injuries has been recommended. A selective approach, consisting of arteriography, bronchoscopy, and esophagoscopy, has recently been advocated for zone II injuries without absolute surgical indications, such as an expanding hematoma.

Hemorrhage control mandates surgical repair for many penetrating carotid injuries. The natural history of nonhemorrhagic carotid lesions, for example, intimal disruptions, is not fully known. Except in the presence of evidence of a profound brain injury (severe stroke, dense coma), all carotid injuries should be repaired. Repair may involve débridement and simple repair or excision of an injured segment with graft interposition; when reconstruction is performed, an autogenous vein graft is preferred. Because surgical exposure of the vertebral arteries is difficult, if adequate collateral flow is documented, embolization or ligation is the preferred approach.

Postoperative Care

In the absence of significant hematoma, patients should be extubated and sedation minimized in order to permit accurate neurologic evaluations. The surgical site requires careful surveillance for the development of swelling or a hematoma, which may precede respiratory compromise. In order to facilitate venous drainage, the head of the bed should be elevated. Pharmacologic therapy is indicated to avoid extremes in blood pressure.

Postoperative stroke may result from occlusion or thrombosis. Early occlusion is often due to a technical error. The surgeon should evaluate changes in neurologic examination, and prompt return to the operating room should be considered. Wound infection is uncommon in the absence of associated injuries to the aerodigestive tract. Duration of antibiotic coverage is based on the presence of associated injuries.

INJURIES TO THE ABDOMINAL AORTA AND VISCERAL BRANCHES

Hemodynamic instability after penetrating or blunt abdominal trauma suggests major vascular injury. Penetrating wounds are detected on physical examination.

Blunt injuries may exhibit abdominal wall contusion or a "seat belt sign." Distal pulse deficits may be present in injuries to the pelvic vessels. In the awake patient, the organs injured influence the symptoms present.

Diagnosis and Treatment

Exploratory laparotomy remains the primary diagnostic modality in unstable patients with penetrating injury (see Chapter 94). In stable patients with gunshot wounds, preoperative radiographs facilitate trajectory determination. Laparoscopy, diagnostic peritoneal lavage, local wound exploration, and simple observation may be elected for stable patients with stab wounds and tangential gunshot wounds. Diagnostic peritoneal lavage and ultrasonography are used to exclude hemoperitoneum in the unstable patient with blunt trauma. In the hemodynamically stable patient with blunt trauma, computed tomography offers a noninvasive diagnostic modality (see Chapter 94).

Arteriography is indicated for nonvisualization of a kidney on computed tomography. Arteriography may be both diagnostic and therapeutic when an area of high density (suggestive of active hemorrhage) is seen in the liver or spleen. Lower-extremity pulse deficits unexplained by extremity injuries require arteriographic evaluation.

The primary concern at laparotomy is hemorrhage control. In the presence of massive exsanguination, control is achieved by clamping the aorta at the level of the diaphragm. Once the specific injury is identified, all attempts should be made to reposition the clamps in order to limit ischemia of the kidneys, liver, splanchnic bed, and lower extremities.

Small, simple injuries to the abdominal aorta can be repaired primarily. Extensive injuries may require a prosthetic graft, which is less desirable because of the associated enteric injuries. Survival rates are greater in infrarenal than suprarenal aortic injuries (50% versus 35% survival rate). Celiac vessels should be repaired when possible, although collateral flow permits ligation in the unstable patient. Definitive repair of the superior mesenteric artery is required to prevent lethal bowel necrosis. Extensive collateral flow permits safe ligation of the inferior mesenteric artery. Simple repair is usually successful for the inferior vena cava. Ligation of the infrarenal vena cava is reserved for unstable patients with multiple injuries. Injuries to the retrohepatic vena cava are frequently lethal because exposure, control, and repair are extremely difficult.

Simple penetrating wounds of the renal vessels are often amenable to repair. In the unstable patient with renovascular injuries, nephrectomy offers the best surgical option, but the structure and function of the contralateral kidney should be assessed before nephrectomy. Intimal disruption and thrombosis secondary to blunt injury requires complex reconstruction and, depending on the ischemic time from injury, nephrectomy may be considered.

Distal control of iliac vessels may require a groin incision and exposure of the femoral vessels. Primary repair or interposition grafting should be considered, particularly for injuries to the common iliac artery and external iliac artery. Ligation of either of these arteries is associated with a high amputation rate (40 to 50%). Ligation of the internal iliac artery is safe and preferable to complex reconstruction in an unstable patient. Simple repairs for injuries to the major pelvic veins are indicated in stable patients, but ligation should be considered for extensive venous injuries in the presence of hemodynamic instability.

Postoperative Care

After surgery for major vascular injuries, large fluid shifts (i.e., third spacing) are expected. In this population, active resuscitation continues after admission to the ICU. Monitoring cardiac filling pressures by use of a central venous or pulmonary arterial catheter facilitates fluid management. Normothermia, correction of acidosis, and replacement of coagulation factors are the goals of resuscitation, and these are best achieved by judicious administration of warm crystalloids and blood components, careful electrolyte management, and intravascular volume loading to support increases in oxygen delivery (Chapters 7 and 84). Complications due to inadequate resuscitation include renal failure, hepatic failure, acute respiratory distress syndrome, and multiorgan system failure.

Since dehiscence of a vascular repair may result in rapid hemorrhage, suspicion of dehiscence requires surgical re-evaluation. The lower extremities of the patient with injured common or external iliac vessels must be carefully monitored for edema, compartment syndrome, and perfusion deficits indicative of thrombosis. If ligation of the common iliac or external iliac vein has been performed, the involved extremity should be wrapped with an elastic wrap and elevated to reduce edema.

Intestinal infarction may result after superior mesenteric artery repair secondary to graft thrombosis. Shock, increased fluid requirement, leukocytosis, and metabolic acidosis suggest the diagnosis. If this diagnosis is suspected, an arteriogram should be performed to evaluate the patency of the repair.

Oliguria may indicate stenosis of a renal artery repair. Although other causes for oliguria (hypovolemia, acute tubular necrosis, radiographic contrast, or aminoglycoside-induced nephropathy) are often possibilities in this clinical setting, the presence of hypertension supports the diagnosis of graft stenosis. To avoid nephrotoxic contrast material, digital subtraction angiography or other noncontrast methods (magnetic resonance angiography) should be considered to evaluate vascular patency.

Graft infection may occur, especially with associated enteric injuries. Although autologous graft material should be used when possible, for extensive injuries to larger structures prosthetic graft may be the only option.

BIBLIOGRAPHY

Blaisdell FW, Trunkey DD: Trauma to extremities: General principles. In: Wilmore DW, Cheung LY, Harken AH, et al (eds): Care of the Surgical Patient. New York, Scientific American, 1988–1995, pp 1–13.
This is a self-descriptive chapter in a definitive text.

Bongard F: Thoracic and abdominal vascular trauma. In: Rutherford RB (ed): Vascular Surgery, 4th ed. Philadelphia, WB Saunders, 1995.
This chapter describes the evaluation and management of aortic injuries.

Clarke D, Richardson P: Peripheral nerve injury. Curr Opin Neurol 7:415–421, 1994.
This review article addresses the pathophysiology of nerve injury and current surgical and nonsurgical management alternatives.

Hurst JM, Fowl RJ: Vascular surgery and trauma. In: Civetta JM, Taylor RW, Kirby RR (eds): Critical Care, 2nd ed. Philadelphia, JB Lippincott, 1992, pp 707–723.
This is a review chapter that addresses extremity trauma, specific vascular repairs, and postoperative management issues.

Mabee JR: Compartment syndrome: A complication of acute extremity trauma. J Emerg Med 12:651–656, 1994.
This is a review of the setting, clinical findings, diagnosis, and treatment of compartment syndrome.

Perry MO: Injuries of the brachiocephalic vessels. In: Rutherford RB (ed): Vascular Surgery, 4th ed. Philadelphia, WB Saunders, 1995.
This chapter describes the evaluation and management of injuries to the brachiocephalic vessels.

Shackford SR, Rich NH: Peripheral vascular injury. In: Feliciano DV, Moore EE, Mattox KL (eds): Trauma, 3rd ed. Stamford, CT: Appleton & Lange, 1996.
This chapter describes the evaluation and management of injuries to the peripheral vessels.

96 Head Trauma

Matthew F. Philips
Mark J. Kotapka

Each year in the United States approximately 600,000 individuals (about one a minute) are hospitalized for head trauma. It accounts for close to 60% of all trauma-related deaths, with gunshot wounds to the head carrying the highest death rate (75 to 80%) of all mechanisms of head trauma. Motor vehicle accidents contribute about two thirds of all head injuries (66%), followed by falls and gunshot wounds. In contrast, falls are the most likely mechanism of head injuries in the pediatric and elderly populations.

CLASSIFICATION OF HEAD TRAUMA

Scalp Injury

The head is a multilayered structure composed of the scalp, skull, dura, and brain. The strains that each layer can tolerate depend on its tissue composition. The first layer of brain protection is the scalp. Because the scalp is a highly vascular structure, scalp lacerations can result in dramatic blood loss and even hypotension. Violation of the scalp with concomitant violation of the skull and dura can lead to intracranial infection. Irrigation, local débridement, and primary closure are the usual steps of treatment for lacerations. In cases of scalp avulsion with moderate to severe scalp loss, rotational flaps, skin grafting, microsurgical reimplantation, or free tissue transfers may be required. More recently, the process of tissue expansion has greatly enhanced scalp reconstruction. Implantation of a subcutaneous silicon reservoir, followed by serial injections of sterile saline into the reservoir over several weeks, can sufficiently stretch the scalp skin for flapping purposes. Up to 50% of the scalp can be replaced with this method.

Skull Injury

When the force sustained by the skull is greater than the strength of the skull, the skull fractures. Cranial vault fractures can be classified as open or closed, depending on the integrity of the overlying scalp and underlying dura. Among the various types of fractures, the *linear fracture* is the most common. A simple linear fracture with no scalp violation may only require brief observation to rule out intracranial injury. If the fracture violates perinasal air cavities, however, the risk of cerebrospinal fluid (CSF) rhinorrhea or otorrhea increases; meningitis can also develop when the fracture exposes the epidural space to sinus contents. These fractures may require surgical intervention. Finally, injury to vascular structures, such as the middle meningeal artery or venous sinuses, can complicate skull fractures and result in potentially lethal epidural hematomas or sinus thromboses.

  Depressed fractures result from impact with small surface area objects (<2 in^2)

1061

at high velocities. They may be open or closed and involve vascular structures. At the time of injury, both dura and cortex may be violated, with resulting hematoma formation or intracranial contamination from bone fragments or foreign bodies, or both. The management of depressed skull fractures is controversial. From a series of 284 patients with depressed fractures, only 2.8% of those treated nonoperatively developed infectious complications. From those data, van den Heever and van der Merwe concluded that the majority of these fractures are best treated conservatively. In this study, surgical management was indicated for those fractures with gross contamination, established infection, presence of CSF or brain tissue in the wound, an intracranial lesion requiring surgery, undue bleeding from the wound, frontal sinus involvement, cosmetically unacceptable depressions, as well as for severely comminuted fractures.

Skull base fractures can be so small that they are radiographically inapparent, and their diagnosis must be made on clinical grounds. The presence of "raccoon's eyes" (periorbital ecchymoses) or Battle's sign (retromastoid hematoma) reliably signifies a skull base fracture. CSF otorrhea or rhinorrhea, hemotympanum, or blood in the external auditory meatus without evidence of direct ear trauma is also a hallmark of these fractures. Skull base fractures can involve the carotid canal and result in carotid rupture, dissection, or thrombosis. When this is suspected, cerebral angiography is indicated to evaluate vessel integrity.

Fractures through any of the skull base foramina can cause specific cranial nerve injuries. The delicate neurons of the olfactory nerves that pass through the cribriform plate are especially prone to disruption. As with the linear fractures, operative repair is usually not indicated for skull base fractures unless there is persistence of CSF leak or compromise of vascular or neural tissue. Pulsatile exophthalmos, ophthalmoplegia, chemosis, or a bruit with visual loss should alert the examiner to a possible carotid-cavernous sinus fistula, which may require immediate operative or endovascular treatment.

Meningeal Injury

Injury or violation of the meninges rarely occurs without violation of the skull. Bridging veins from the pial surface of the brain to the dura and its venous structures are easily torn, resulting in subdural hematoma formation. As discussed earlier, violation of the dura, particularly at the cranial base, may include vascular structures or lead to CSF rhinorrhea or otorrhea.

Brain Injury

Focal Brain Injuries

How focal injuries present neurologically relates directly to the specific brain areas involved. Global neurologic deficits or coma with focal injuries are a result from brainstem compression and require urgent diagnosis and treatment.

In 1448 patients with mild head injury (Glasgow Coma Scale [GCS] score of 13 to 15, Table 96–1), the most common lesion was a *contusion*. Contusions often involve the surface of the brain beneath vault fractures, at points at which the

Table 96–1. Scoring for Glasgow Coma Scale*

EYE OPENING		VERBAL		MOTOR	
Best Function	Score	Best Function	Score	Best Function	Score
Spontaneous	4	Oriented	5	Follows commands	6
To voice	3	Disoriented	4	Localizes	5
To pain	2	Inappropriate	3	Withdraws	4
No response	1	Incomprehensible	2	Flexes	3
		No response	1	Extends	2
				No response	1

*Glasgow Coma Scale is calculated as the sum of the highest scores from each of the three categories listed. Maximal score is 15 and minimal score is 3.

brain surface collides with bony surfaces of the middle and frontal fossae, or at areas of the cortex where high surface strains are produced by the inner table of the skull. Of patients with focal injuries, those with contusions tend to fare best. *Intracerebral hematomas* result from torn blood vessels in deeper brain structures. They are not contiguous with the cortical surface and typically occur in the deep white matter of the frontal and temporal lobes. Injuries in which the pial surface is violated with parenchymal disruption are termed *cerebral lacerations.*

Epidural hematomas are focal injuries that result from direct contact forces occurring at the time of impact. These cause disruption of dural vessels, sinuses, or diploic channels, which allows blood to dissect into the epidural space. The middle meningeal artery is frequently injured with temporal bone trauma, resulting in an epidural hematoma.

Epidural hematomas can occur in the setting of a relatively minor head injury, with few presenting neurologic signs or symptoms. Although they occur in less than 3% of head-injured patients, rapid diagnosis and evacuation are crucial in preventing life-threatening complications from brain compression. Prognosis with epidural hematomas is intermediate and is related to age, GCS score at presentation, and timing of evacuation. Concomitant intracranial injury, such as subdural hematoma, adversely affects outcome.

About 5% of epidural hematomas occur in the posterior fossa. Because of the small volume of that space and its proximity to the brainstem, treatment of any expanding lesion in the posterior fossa must be urgent. Bounded posteriorly and laterally by bone and superiorly by the tentorium cerebelli, posterior fossa hematomas can cause tonsillar herniation and brainstem compression with rapid deterioration to coma and death.

Subdural hematomas are focal lesions that result from contact or acceleration and inertial forces. When vascular structures of the pial surface are disrupted, bleeding occurs into the subdural space. When the head undergoes rapid deceleration, as in a motor vehicle accident, cortical bridging veins can tear and bleed into the subdural space. In general, subdural hematomas have a poor prognosis because, in contrast to epidural hematomas, they are usually accompanied by a significant parenchymal injury. The morbidity and mortality associated with subdural hematomas is related to the GCS on presentation, age, intracranial pressure (ICP), and mechanism of injury. Decreased level of consciousness results from impending herniation and compressive effects on the brainstem, making rapid recognition and treatment essential. This was confirmed in the landmark study by Seelig and colleagures, who reported that patients who underwent craniotomy and evacuation of subdural hematomas within 4 hours of injury had a significantly lower mortality rate than did those who received treatment after the 4-hour window (30% versus 90% mortality).

Diffuse Brain Injury

Concussion and diffuse axonal injury are the two opposite ends of the spectrum of diffuse brain injury. In this category of brain injury there are no grossly evident intracranial lesions. As a result, alterations in level of consciousness result from global or diffuse disruption of the anatomic and physiologic neural substrates rather than brainstem compression. The perturbation lies at the level of the neuronal cell membranes and axolemmas and can be widespread in both the cerebrum and brainstem.

Concussion is a mild form of global neurologic dysfunction. The exact mechanism and pathophysiology of concussion remains an enigma. Both temporary and permanent neurologic disturbances seen in concussive syndromes may relate to the magnitude and site of head injury. Although concussion may or may not be associated with loss of consciousness, amnestic periods and long-term higher cognitive deficits have been reported. In classic concussion, associated with a "reversible" neurologic deficit and temporary loss of consciousness, it is theorized that the reticular activating system may experience a temporary neurophysiologic perturbation. Although there are no grossly evident radiographic or neuropathologic lesions, neurochemical and ultrastructural changes have been observed.

Diffuse axonal injury (DAI) is the most severe form of diffuse brain injury. When the tensile strain from angular acceleration and deceleration forces act on the brain parenchyma, axons and small vessels tear. For example, DAI was reported in more than 48% of closed head injuries in one study. Characteristically, the head-injured patient presents with a low GCS score (3 to 8) but there are no gross neuroradiographic abnormalities evident. Placement of an ICP monitor may reveal intracranial hypertension that may require intensive medical therapy over the following days (see Chapter 42).

Unlike concussive syndromes, DAI is evident histologically throughout the callosal, periventricular, internal capsular, basal ganglia, and brainstem white matter. Tissue tear hemorrhages can occasionally be appreciated on the presenting computed tomographic scan. In fact, a grading system based on initial computed tomography (CT) results has demonstrated a correlation between computed tomographic severity of DAI and clinical outcome. When no intraparenchymal hemorrhage has occurred, T2-weighted magnetic resonance imaging demonstrates multifocal and hyperintense foci in the deep white matter structures. In postmortem studies, histologic evaluation reveals evidence of axonal injury and white matter tract disruption. Ultrastructural and immunohistochemical investigations have revealed several different mechanisms of axonal injury resulting in irreversible disruption of the structural integrity of the axons. Patients with DAI who remain comatose for greater than 24 hours after the initial injury tend to have a worse prognosis and, in comparison to other types of head injury, survivors of DAI have the highest frequency of permanent neurologic disability.

EVALUATION OF THE HEAD-INJURED PATIENT

History

The first key to the delivery of appropriate care for the head-injured patient is recognition and triage of the central nervous system injury. At the time of initial resuscitation and primary survey, a brief, pertinent history is obtained. Knowledge of the mechanism of injury may provide insight into the degree of intracranial injury. Reports by the paramedics or other prehospital personnel of initial neurologic status often prove useful. For example, a history of a transient improvement in mental status, that is, the so-called lucid interval, in transit between the field and the trauma bay can be vital in estimating the degree and time of onset of secondary brain injury. In patients with multiple trauma, information about hypoxic or hypotensive episodes should be sought because they may have a significant bearing on clinical outcome. When sedation or paralytic agents are used to establish the patient's airway or for safety during transportation to the hospital, information about the prehospital neurologic examination can be crucial. Recent drug or alcohol use complicates the diagnosis of severe brain injury, and a brief history of these should also be sought.

Physical Examination

During the general examination, evaluation of the head and face for obvious external injury is important. Physical findings provide the examiner with an idea of how much energy was transferred to the head. Because the face and its sinuses are capable of absorbing a moderate amount of energy, however, the amount of facial deformation may not be a reliable indicator of underlying brain injury. Facial fractures should alert the examiner to the possibility of an associated skull base fracture. Scalp lacerations or puncture sites may point to focal skull or brain injuries. A depressed skull fracture itself suggests the mechanism of injury because high-velocity, small-surface-area objects are required for penetration. In contrast, contact with larger objects such as the ground or a windshield cause global vault fractures, often with skull base fractures. Periorbital or retromastoid hematomas or frank blood, CSF, or brain tissue observed in ears or nose signal a cranial base pathologic condition.

The GCS (see Table 96–1) provides a universal and reproducible method of characterizing brain injury. It provides a numerical score derived from the patient's eye opening, verbal response, and motor abilities. In general, the GCS score correlates with the severity and relative prognosis of the head injury. A patient who is awake and neurologically intact on presentation receives the highest score of 15. A neurologically devastated individual in flaccid coma receives the lowest score of 3. Mild traumatic brain injury is usually considered to be GCS 13 to 15. Moderate injury falls in the 9 to 12 range, whereas a score less than 8 indicates coma. Confounding variables such as time between injury and assessment, interexaminer differences, body temperature, the presence of central nervous system depressants, such as alcohol, or hypotension at the time of presentation may result in an inaccurate assessment of the severity and prognosis of the head injury.

Of equal importance to the GCS score in establishing the severity of the injury is the recognition of both focal and global signs of neural injury. For example, a dilatated, nonreactive pupil ("blown pupil"), the hallmark of the life-threatening transtentorial herniation of the medial temporal lobe structures, indicates pressure on the ipsilateral third cranial nerve by an expanding intracranial lesion. In addition, compression of the cerebral peduncle directly by the temporal lobe results in contralateral hemiparesis. A Kernohan notch syndrome occurs when the contralateral third cranial nerve and peduncle are forced against the tentorial edge, causing a contralateral dilatated pupil and ipsilateral hemiparesis. Because acute uncal herniation is accompanied by changes in mental status, the awake and otherwise neurologically intact patient with pupillary irregularities is likely to have a direct ocular injury. In contrast, in the stuporous or obtunded patient with these ocular findings, primary ocular injuries should be considered only after intracranial pathology has been ruled out.

Signs and symptoms of *posterior fossa lesions* include headache, vomiting, hypotonia, dysmetria, and nystagmus. The patient may rapidly deteriorate to cardiorespiratory instability, coma, and death as an expanding lesion exerts pressure on the lower brainstem. Bilateral abnormal pupils—for example, midposition and fixed—can indicate severe brainstem injury, especially in the presence of obtundation or long tract signs. Any history of paralytics, depressants, or toxin use or ingestion is important. Finally, bilateral limb weakness, a defined sensory level, and bowel or bladder dysfunction characterize a spinal cord injury (see Chapter 98). In any head-injured patient, concomitant cervical spine injury should be suspected. A cross-table lateral cervical spine radiograph, including C7–T1, should be obtained at initial presentation. In general, focal signs are indicative of focal, potentially reversible injuries, and urgent diagnosis and intervention are essential.

Computed Tomography

With the availability and the rapid speed of spiral CT scanners, plain skull radiographs rarely provide any additional, relevant information in an acutely head-injured patient and are unwarranted. Most clinicians would agree that computed tomographic evaluation of the head is the most essential tool in the rapid diagnosis and delivery of care to the head-injured patient. This imaging technique accurately represents both soft tissue and bone trauma, and it specifically displays acute intracranial hemorrhage better than other radiographic modalities. For example, CT has demonstrated an 8 to 21% prevalence of intracranial pathology in pedestrians and bicyclists with a GCS score of 13 to 15 who were hit by automobiles. The high sensitivity of CT to detect acute intracranial pathology in mildly head-injured patients has convinced most clinicians to have a low threshold for computed tomographic scanning in this population.

CT can identify skull fractures, including skull base and facial fractures. Foreign objects and their relationship to vital neural or vascular structures are readily appreciated. With regard to high-velocity missile injuries, CT often displays the bullet's intracranial trajectory and relative involvement of hemispheres, multiple lobes, or the ventricular system, or a combination. Also readily visualized are traumatic communications between cranial sinuses, the middle and inner ear compartments, and orbital or globe injuries. Pneumocephalus on the presenting computed tomographic scan is obvious and pathognomonic of a skull fracture.

Initial Management

Initial management, triage, and rapid treatment of the head-injured patient begins in the field or emergency department. Patients with a GCS score less than 9 and those with localizing signs should be intubated and have intravenous mannitol (1 g/kg) administered to reduce the ICP. In the hypotensive patient, fluid resuscitation is imperative to maintain adequate cerebral perfusion. Recent studies suggest that resuscitation with hypertonic solution (hypertonic lactate solution rather than normotonic crystalloids, such as lactated Ringer solution) may be advantageous in the setting of head injury because raising serum osmolarity can lower ICP. Immediate radiographic evaluation by CT should follow to ascertain whether the lesion is focal or diffuse. Focal lesions, such as intracranial hematomas, often require emergent operative decompression, whereas patients with nonoperative lesions, such as DAI, are admitted for intensive ICP management (see Chapter 42). ICP monitoring is mandatory with a GCS score of 8 or less or when prolonged extracranial procedures under anesthesia are planned.

In many patients, the majority of brain damage does not occur at the time of injury, but rather is the result of a pathophysiologic cascade that occurs after trauma and culminates in cerebral ischemia. Treatment therefore should be directed at reduction of ICP, ensuring adequate oxygen delivery, and maintaining adequate tissue perfusion pressure to meet the metabolic needs of the injured brain.

In the less severely injured patient, a full examination should be performed, with particular regard to a history of loss of consciousness, skull fractures, CSF rhinorrhea or otorrhea, and intoxication. Because of the potential for delayed deterioration due to slowly expanding intracranial lesions and possible complications from open wounds or an intracranial-extracranial communication, the threshold for hospital admission and observation should be low.

OUTCOMES

Outcomes correlate with a variety of factors, including mechanism of injury, examination on presentation, age, hypotension, anoxia, head CT results, level of ICP, timing of delivery of care, and the neurotrauma experience of the hospital. These studies, however, only grossly predict an individual's specific outcome, and no gold standard for brain injury prognosis exists.

A standard instrument, the Glasgow Outcome Scale (GOS) (Table 96–2), was initially developed to describe the outcome of patients with head injury. In the GOS, patients are scored based on their level of disability, and, in general, the GOS correlates with the GCS.

Head injury has an overall mortality of approximately 14%, with many more patients having post-traumatic disability as measured by functional independent measures. The morbidity and mortality due to head trauma continue to tax the medical, financial, and social structure of society. Early recognition, triage, rapid delivery of care, and a systematic, multidisciplinary approach to the trauma patient

Table 96–2. Scoring for the Glasgow Outcome Scale

OUTCOME	FUNCTION	SCORE
Good recovery	Normal life	5
Moderate disability	Disabled but independent for daily activities	4
Severe disability	Dependent for daily activities	3
Persistent vegetative state	Unresponsive and bedridden	2
Death		1

at designated trauma centers have been major advances in treating patients with acute head injuries. Furthermore, as the pathophysiology and molecular mechanisms of secondary brain injury are better understood, hypothesis-driven treatments can be tested. However, improved understanding of the myriad variables that affect outcome should not diminish educational efforts to modify behaviors to prevent head trauma in the first place.

BIBLIOGRAPHY

Gennarelli TA: Mechanisms of cerebral concussion, contusion, and other effects of head injury. In: Youmans JR (ed): Neurological Surgery, 3rd ed. Philadelphia: WB Saunders, 1990, p 1953.
Chapter by one of the pioneers in head injury research reviewing the pathophysiology of various types of head injury.

Gentry LR, Godersky JC, Thompson B, Dunn VD: Prospective comparative study of intermediate-field MR and CT in the evaluation of closed head trauma. AJR 150:673–682, 1988.
A prospective study evaluating the relative strengths and weaknesses of CT and MRI in the evaluation of acute head injury.

Luerssen TG, Klauber MR, Marshall LF: Outcome from head injury related to patient's age. J Neurosurg 68:409–416, 1988.
A large study evaluating the relative outcomes of patients younger than 15 compared with older patients after head injury, which showed that pediatric patients had a significantly better outcome.

Marshall LF, Gautille T, Klauber MR, et al: The outcome of severe closed head injury. J Neurosurg 75:S28–S36, 1991.
Review of outcome after closed head injury

Rivas JJ, Lobato RD, Sarabia R, et al: Extradural hematoma: Analysis of factors influencing the courses of 161 patients. Neurosurgery 23:44–51, 1988.
Older study evaluating the CT and clinical findings in a series of patients operated on for extradural hematoma. Compares comatose and noncomatose subgroups.

Seelig JM, Becker DP, Miller JD, et al: Traumatic acute subdural hematoma: Major mortality reduction in comatose patients treated within four hours. N Engl J Med 304:1511–1518, 1981.
Classic study suggesting that acute surgical intervention (within 4 hours of injury) for traumatic subdural hematoma improves outcome.

Sosin DM, Sniezek JE, Waxweiler RJ: Trends in death associated with traumatic brain injury, 1979 through 1992. Success and failure. JAMA 273:1778–1780, 1995.
Retrospective analysis of national trends in traumatic brain injury indicating that there has been a 25% decline in death rates associated with motor vehicle accidents while there has been a concurrent 13% increase in firearm deaths.

Teasdale G, Jennett B: Assessment of coma and impaired consciousness. Lancet 2:81–84, 1974.
Classic article first describing the Glasgow Coma Scale.

Wilberger JE, Harris M, Diamond DL: Acute subdural hematoma: Morbidity, mortality, and operative timing. J Neurosurg 74:212–218, 1991.
Recent study suggesting that ICP management is more critical to outcome after traumatic subdural hematoma than the timing of subdural blood removal.

97 Thoracic Trauma

Paul S. Brown, Jr.

As with all trauma care, the initial evaluation and management of the thoracic trauma patient includes assessment of the airway, breathing, and circulation. This is followed by a secondary assessment of all injuries. Based on the initial survey, airway management and volume resuscitation are undertaken. Radiographic evaluation precedes the secondary survey for additional injuries. The chest radiograph should be evaluated for pneumothorax, subcutaneous or mediastinal emphysema, rupture of the diaphragm, widened mediastinum, and intrathoracic foreign bodies. This information determines whether chest tube placement or immediate surgical intervention is indicated. Hypotension in the absence of an obvious source of bleeding—that is, open wounds, fractures, intra-abdominal hemorrhage, or a massive hemothorax—should immediately alert one to the possibility of other causes of "traumatic hypotension" that need diagnosis and treatment (Table 97–1).

SPECTRUM OF INJURIES AND THEIR MANAGEMENT

Chest Wall Injuries

Chest wall injuries include fractures of ribs, clavicles, sternum, and flail chest. Each may be accompanied by hemopneumothorax from lacerations of chest wall muscles, intercostal vessels, or pulmonary parenchyma. Children have flexible chest walls and a reduced frequency of chest wall injuries when compared with adults; the force of impact is, however, more likely to injure intrathoracic organs. Conversely, elderly patients have fragile chest walls that fracture easily, but intrathoracic organs are less likely to be injured.

A flail chest wall segment results when multiple ribs are broken in two or more places, as occurs in severe blunt chest trauma. Although the flail segment may give rise to paradoxical chest wall motion, this rarely causes a problem with respiratory mechanics by itself; instead, its presence should be viewed as an indicator of underlying pulmonary contusion.

Clavicular fractures are common in blunt injuries but of little consequence. Scapular fractures are rare and suggest severe force to the chest wall, as do fractures of the first and second ribs, the thoracic spine, and sternum. Fractures of

Table 97–1. Causes of Shock After Trauma

Blood loss (intrathoracic, intra-abdominal, soft tissue, external)	Ruptured diaphragm
	Spinal shock
Cardiac tamponade	Tension pneumothorax
Embolus (air or pulmonary)	Traumatic septal defect or valvular
Myocardial contusion or infarction	incompetence
Profound acidosis	

the sternum generally occur as a result of steering wheel injuries and are usually missed on initial radiographic and physical examination. Treatment is generally conservative. Reduction and internal fixation, however, are indicated if they contribute to respiratory insufficiency. Myocardial contusion may also accompany sternal fracture.

Lung and Myocardial Contusion

Treatment of uncomplicated *myocardial contusion* is supportive. Patients with low cardiac output, arrhythmias, or electrocardiographic changes require directed therapy for these problems. Although it is common practice to monitor for arrhythmias, treatment is rarely required and overnight evaluation probably also is not required. Echocardiographic evaluation is useful to assess murmurs or low cardiac output and can diagnose traumatic (e.g., tricuspid) valvular insufficiency. Unless required by a clinical emergency, the surgical repair should be performed electively after the patient has recovered substantially from the trauma.

Pulmonary contusion is the result of severe blunt chest wall trauma causing intraparenchymal hemorrhage and localized edema. The contusion is usually evident on the initial chest radiograph, although it may not become apparent until 24 to 48 hours later. Mechanical ventilation is occasionally required to treat associated hypoxemia. Fluids should be limited as much as possible to prevent worsening lung dysfunction caused by capillary leakage. *Hematomas* of the lung are usually caused by penetrating injury. They are more localized than contusions and usually develop into isolated masses that resolve spontaneously.

Aortic Disruption

Blunt chest trauma may cause traumatic disruption of the thoracic aorta; however, 90% of patients with this type of deceleration injury die at the scene of the accident. The rest acquire a contained hematoma that will likely rupture if left untreated. A disrupted aorta is diagnosed by having a high degree of suspicion in conjunction with a chest radiograph showing a widened mediastinum or one of the many other signs suggestive of disrupted thoracic aorta (Table 97–2). When this injury is suspected, definitive diagnostic evaluation should be performed quickly to avoid the risk of rupture during preoperative evaluation for other injuries. The "gold standard" for the diagnosis of traumatic aortic disruption has been an aortogram. Computed tomography with contrast dye may also be used to

Table 97–2. Conditions Suggestive of Traumatic Aortic Disruption

Apical pleural cap	Obliteration of aortic knob
Depression of left mainstem bronchus	Obliteration of aortopulmonary window
First and second rib fracture	Widened mediastinum (width >8 cm on supine
Fractured sternum or thoracic spine	chest radiograph just above aortic knob)
Massive hemothorax	

diagnose the injury, but there are false-negative results associated with computed tomographic scanning. Another modality is transesophageal echocardiography, which is reliable and can give a diagnosis immediately.

If the patient has other primary indications for left thoracotomy, no further diagnostic studies are needed because the diagnosis of a disrupted aorta, if present, will be immediately apparent on direct intraoperative inspection of the aorta. Repair of this injury is usually performed with aortic cross-clamping and left atrial–descending thoracic aortic bypass. The diagnosis and treatment of traumatic injury to the thoracic aorta is described in Chapter 50.

Pneumothorax and Air Leaks

Although pneumothorax is common after chest injuries, mediastinal and subcutaneous emphysema are not. They may indicate more severe injuries to the tracheobronchial tree or esophagus. Massive air leaks through the chest tubes should also alert one to the possibility of bronchial or esophageal injury, which should be evaluated with bronchoscopy and esophagoscopy. Air leaks generally seal in less than 72 hours. A prolonged air leak suggests the formation of a bronchopleural fistula or missed bronchial injury.

The best evidence of tracheal injury is massive air leakage with an inability to expand the lung. Patients with suspected bronchial injuries should undergo immediate bronchoscopy to evaluate the injury. Most major bronchial injuries are located within 2 cm of the carina; although of these, only about 50% have an associated pneumothorax. Treatment is early diagnosis and repair. Small tracheobronchial injuries involving less than one third of the circumference are managed nonoperatively if the lung can be expanded without pneumothorax; otherwise, surgical repair is required. Small bronchial tears may go unnoticed at initial injury but may be evident later as a bronchial stenosis requiring resection.

Pain Management

Much of the morbidity from chest wall trauma comes from pain, which results in poor respiratory effort. This, in turn, leads to retained secretions, pneumonia, and the need for mechanical ventilation. Severe pain is also a major cause of hypoventilation in the patient with flail chest. Adequate analgesia alone usually improves ventilation and eliminates the need for mechanical ventilation. However, this usually requires close attention to "walking" the fine line between adequate pain relief (thereby allowing the patient to breath deeply) and hypoventilation (from oversedation). Multiple rib fractures are a serious problem in the elderly and carry up to a 20% mortality. The older, more fragile thoracic trauma patient may require more than systemic opioids for pain control, for example, epidural analgesia or an intercostal nerve block, to permit comfortable breathing and coughing. Chest splinting or wrapping is not recommended. Approaches to pain management that are applicable to these injuries are described in Chapter 85.

Hemothorax

Large-bore (at least 36 Fr) chest tubes are inserted to drain hemopneumothoraces and are then used to monitor subsequent hourly drainage. Complete lung re-expansion with thorough fluid drainage is the goal of treatment. Thresholds for blood loss suggesting the need for immediate surgical exploration are listed in Table 97–3. Although some injuries with lesser bleeding eventually require thoracotomy, significant bleeding usually indicates injury to a major or minor structure with bleeding that will not clot on its own. The bleeding source is usually a torn intercostal artery or lacerated lung tissue that can be repaired with simple sutures. It is not unusual, however, to enter the chest and find no major active bleeding. Nonetheless, evacuation of blood clots allows the lung to fully expand, which tamponades any continued oozing. Pulmonary parenchymal injuries usually stop bleeding spontaneously, seldom require sutures or lobectomy, and rarely require pneumonectomy. Pneumonectomy for trauma has an almost universally fatal outcome and should be avoided if at all possible. An algorithm for the management of hemothorax can be found in Figure 97–1.

Delayed hemothorax or persistent hemothorax in the otherwise stable patient can usually be evacuated by video-assisted thoracoscopic surgery, but it may require a thoracotomy. Penetrating trauma lateral to the mediastinum does not necessarily require a thoracotomy unless the bleeding requirement is met or there are massive air leaks suggestive of bronchial injury.

Emergency Thoracotomy

The pulseless patient who has sustained *penetrating trauma* and has had documented signs of life after injury should undergo immediate left anterior thoracotomy through the fourth intercostal space in the trauma bay. This incision is readily extended across the midline sternum to give access to both chest cavities and the mediastinum. Although the chance for survival in this setting is slim, it is possible. In these cases, cardiac tamponade from injury to the heart or mediastinum can be temporally controlled by finger pressure pending definitive repair. In contrast, emergency department thoracotomy in the *blunt trauma* patient is usually a futile endeavor.

Penetrating wounds of the heart most commonly involve the right atrium and ventricle, as they are the most anterior structures. Cardiopulmonary bypass may occasionally be required to effect repair. These major injuries, however, are seen rarely because they are usually fatal in the field.

Table 97–3. Indications for Thoracotomy in Treatment of Hemothorax

Immediate drainage >1500 mL
Drainage >250 mL/h over 3–4 h
Large hemothorax remains despite well-placed chest tube

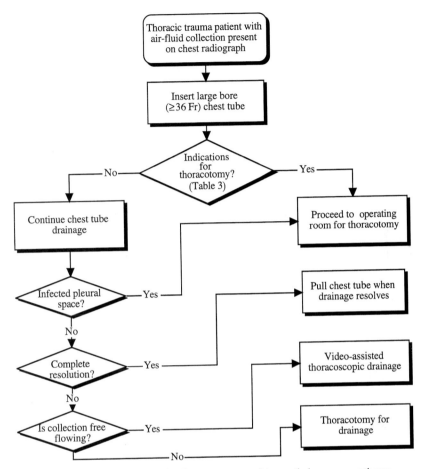

Figure 97–1. Schematic algorithm for the management of traumatic hemopneumothorax.

Complications in the Intensive Care Unit

Air embolism can occur in patients with injuries to a bronchus or lung parenchyma after initiation of positive-pressure ventilation. Air enters the left atrium through the pulmonary venous system and is ejected into the aorta. The patient may experience a stroke or myocardial infarction. Treatment is the same as that indicated for other types of severe air embolism, that is, compression in a hyperbaric chamber.

The most significant complications after thoracic injury are acute respiratory distress syndrome and infection. Evaluation and management of acute respiratory distress syndrome are described in Chapter 73.

Small, undrained pleural fluid collections are well tolerated and usually reabsorb on their own. However, because blood and serous fluid collections often stimulate an exudative process, moderate to large collections often enlarge and, if complicated by infection, may lead to empyema or fibrothorax with trapped lung. Large or enlarging pleural collections should be treated by placement of a chest tube, drainage, and complete expansion of the lung. Giving antibiotics prophylactically is controversial because of the risk of selecting out resistant organisms. Many intensivists believe that antibiotics should be reserved for treatment of infected pleural effusions rather than given prophylactically.

Undrained collections become loculated and turn to a gelatinous consistency. If this occurs, video-asisted thoracoscopic drainage is indicated. If untreated, however, the collection may subsequently organize and form a fibrous peel entrapping the lung. This later stage requires a thoracotomy and decortication with the risk of persistent air leaks. The chest cavity can become infected (empyema) at any time, requiring either long-term chest tube drainage or open drainage.

A bronchopleural fistula results from parenchymal injury near a bronchus or bronchial stump dehiscence and presents as a persistent air leak, pneumothorax, or empyema. This complication is treated with antibiotics, placement of chest tubes, and re-expansion of the lung. Bronchoscopy is performed to assess large airway disruption, and computed tomographic scanning is indicated to assess for undrained pleural fluid collections. If the lung is completely expanded with fluid collections drained, a small fistula can usually heal without surgery. Otherwise thoracotomy, resection, and closure with a muscle flap or Eloesser open drainage is required. As a rule, the bronchus never heals in the presence of positive-pressure ventilation and repair should not be attempted until the patient is extubated or on minimal ventilatory settings. The only exception should be in the patient who cannot be ventilated secondary to large air losses. Fortunately the latter is rarely the case. In these circumstances, a lobectomy or completion pneumonectomy with open drainage may be required.

BIBLIOGRAPHY

Battistella F, Benfield JR: Blunt and penetrating injuries of the chest wall, pleura and lungs. In: Shields TW (ed): General Thoracic Surgery, 4th ed. Philadelphia: Lea & Febiger, 1995.
This is a review chapter on chest injuries and their surgical and perioperative management

Haenel JB, Moore FA, Moore EE: Pulmonary consequences of severe chest trauma. Respir Clin North Am 2:401–424, 1996.
The epidemiology, pathophysiology, and management of flail chest and pulmonary contusion are discussed.

LoCicero J, Mattox KL: Epidemiology of chest trauma. Surg Clin North Am 69:15–19, 1989.
This article discusses the epidemiology and etiology of thoracic injuries as well as postoperative management and indications for surgery.

Mandal AK, Thadepalli H, Chettpalli U, et al: Posttraumatic empyema thoracis: A 24-year experience at a major trauma center. J Trauma 43:764–771, 1997.
This is a review of the experience with 5500 patients admitted for chest injury, microbiology, antibiotic management; 1.6% experienced empyema.

Nakayama DK, Ramenofsky ML, Rowe MI: Chest injuries in childhood. Ann Surg 210:770, 1989.
This is a review of 105 pediatric admissions for chest trauma and their causes and outcomes.

Shackford SR: Blunt chest trauma: The intensivist's perspective. J Intensive Care Med 1:125, 1986.
This is a self-descriptive review of intensive care management of blunt injuries.

Wisner DH: A stepwise logistic regression analysis of factors affecting morbidity and mortality after thoracic trauma: Effect of epidural analgesia. J Trauma 30:799, 1990.
This is a statistical analysis of risk factors affecting outcome after trauma.

Wisner DH, Reed WH, Riddick RS: Suspected myocardial contusion. Ann Surg 212:82, 1990.
This is a report of a series of admissions for "rule-out" myocardial contusion, demonstrating that significant contusions will be apparent on initial evaluation and that observation is unnecessary.

Woodring JH, Dillon ML: Radiographic manifestations of mediastinal hemorrhage from blunt chest trauma. Ann Thorac Surg 37:171–178, 1984.
This article discusses radiologic findings of intrathoracic hemorrhage.

Yee ES, Verrier ED, Thomas AN: Management of air embolism in blunt and penetrating thoracic trauma. J Thorac Cardiovasc Surg 85:661–668, 1983.
This article discusses air embolism in trauma and management approaches.

98 Spinal Injury

Paul Marcotte
Andrew Freese

The intensivist managing the patient with major trauma in the intensive care unit (ICU) setting must be vigilant for the presence of a coexistent injury to neural or osteoligamentous components of the spine. The history and neurologic examination determine the functional status and level of the neurologic injury, whereas imaging studies determine the integrity and stability of the osteoligamentous complex. Despite the advances of imaging investigations, plain films remain of value for defining instability, especially in the cervical spine. Computer-assisted imaging (computed tomography and magnetic resonance imaging) are complementary studies, each of which contributes valuable information to the assessment and management of the patient with a spinal injury (Table 98–1).

Three goals guide the ICU management of patients with spinal injuries: (1) preventing neurologic injury or progression of an existing neurologic deficit, (2) enhancing the physiologic environment in which neurologic recovery takes place, and (3) stabilizing the spinal column. This chapter presents the management principles and the pharmacologic, nonsurgical, and surgical interventions used to achieve these goals.

PATHOPHYSIOLOGY AND BIOMECHANICS OF SPINAL INJURY

Spinal cord injury can be subdivided into primary and secondary injures. In the setting of trauma, the *primary injury* results from the application of force to the spinal cord, causing vascular injury or direct injury to the neuronal and non-neuronal cell populations. The severity of the primary spinal cord injury remains the strongest predictor of neurologic outcome.

Table 98–1. Imaging Studies for Spinal Injury

STUDY	ADVANTAGES	DISADVANTAGES
Plain radiograph	Performed rapidly as a portable study; can be used to determine stability in flexion and extension	Poor resolution
Computed tomography	Shows bony structure well, can be used to reconstruct cervicothoracic junction	Worse than magnetic resonance imaging for tissue densities; not portable
Magnetic resonance imaging	Excellent tissue definition (cord, ligament, hematomas)	Poor bone definition, not portable, more time required for study compared with computed tomography

Secondary spinal cord injury results from a cascade of physiologic and bio-chemical events that follow the primary injury. The cascade involves the formation of oxygen free radicals, cell membrane disruption, and cell death. Factors, such as ischemia and hypoxia, can accelerate local metabolic injury, emphasizing the need for rigid control of systemic blood pressure and oxygenation in the management of a patient with a spinal cord injury.

The cervical spine (C-spine) consists of the atlantoaxial complex and the subaxial C-spine. The major articulation at the atlantoaxial complex involves the odontoid process and the anterior arch of C1, which is stabilized by the transverse ligament. Direct ligamentous injury and bony injuries that cause incompetence of the transverse ligament complex produce atlantoaxial instability. These include some C1 fractures, most odontoid fractures, transverse ligament injuries, and complex atlantoaxial fractures. Unstable subaxial cervical spine injuries are diagnosed on lateral cervical spine films obtained in a neutral position and during flexion and extension.

Unstable injuries of the thoracic spine are more likely to occur at the thoracolumbar junction or in the lumbar spine because of the stabilizing capabilities of the rib cage and sternum.

ASSESSMENT OF SPINAL CORD INJURY

The first priority with respect to managing any critically injured patient remains assessment and stabilization of the airway, breathing, and circulation. Unnecessary manipulation of the patient's spine, however, should be avoided before radiographic confirmation of stability.

Inspection of the body for superficial abrasions and contusions can assist in the differential diagnosis of the neurologic injury, localizing it either centrally or to the periphery. Palpation of the entire spine may provoke pain, which can assist in localization of the level of a significant spinal injury. Pain, however, does not determine the extent and stability of the spinal injury. Any pain identified by manual examination requires imaging of that segment of the spine to assess for an osteoligamentous injury. On occasion with extreme spinal trauma, widening of the interspinous space or step-offs between adjacent vertebrae can be appreciated by palpating posteriorly. Such findings occur rarely in isolation and patients with them often have severe neurologic deficit or localized pain, or both.

The emphasis of the neurologic examination is on peripheral neural function. A limited assessment of cognitive and cranial nerve function should be performed to determine the presence of intoxication, hypothermia, or brain injury since these processes can interfere with the interpretation of the examination of the peripheral nervous system. The presence of a *unilateral* neurologic deficit, except in the instance of penetrating spinal injury, is more typical of an intracranial abnormality or involvement of a peripheral nerve, or nerve root or plexus. Acceleration and deceleration injuries of the spinal cord generally produce symmetric deficits.

A complete assessment of spinal cord function necessitates a thorough examination of sensory, motor, and reflex function. In particular, a segment-by-segment assessment of each dermatome and myotome must be made in order to determine the level and completeness of the spinal cord injury.

Sensory Examination

The sensory examination should include both pain perception and proprioception because these two modalities travel through distinct anatomic tracts in the spinal cord (spinothalamic tracts and posterior columns, respectively). Appreciation of noxious stimulus requires a dermatome-by-dermatome assessment from the highest cervical to the lower sacral levels (see Appendix F, Fig. 1).

The lower cervical and upper thoracic dermatomes (C5–T2) are not represented on the anterior torso. The upper cervical dermatomes (C3–4) extend to the supramammary region, immediately superior to the T3–4 dermatome. Examination of the torso alone results in a sensory assessment that makes the transition from the C4 to the T4 levels, not directly testing the intervening dermatomes. Because of this, a detailed examination must be carried out in the arms and hands to assess these areas. Otherwise, a patient with a low cervical injury can be misdiagnosed as having an upper thoracic injury by a sensory assessment limited to the torso.

The upper extremity sensory assessment must include all six dermatomes represented on the arm for adequate localization of a deficit (see Appendix F). Individual leg dermatomes should also be assessed, although disparity in sensory function in a dermatomal pattern after a spinal cord injury is less common in the legs.

The sacral dermatomes, located within the perineal region, should also be tested (see Appendix F). The presence of perineal sensation alone ("sacral sparing") in a patient who otherwise has no demonstrable neurologic function represents an incomplete spinal cord injury, which may have a better prognosis for recovery of spinal cord function than a patient with a complete injury.

The assessment of posterior column function involves position or vibration sense testing, or both. Since pain and proprioceptive fibers travel within the same peripheral sensory nerves, posterior column testing can involve the distal aspects of the upper and lower extremities alone, after the detailed noxious stimulus assessment. A disparity in the results of sensory assessments between proprioceptive and pain appreciation occurs only in a patient with a partial cord injury affecting either the posterior or anterior aspects of the cord alone. Transverse injury, or an injury involving the peripheral nerve, should affect spinothalamic and posterior tracts with equal severity.

Motor Examination

Like the sensory examination, the motor examination must be meticulously performed, assessing individual myotomes of the upper and lower extremities. Proximal arm and forearm motion observed by a cursory examination can obscure the presence of a lower cervical injury involving the triceps and intrinsic hand functions. In the lower extremities, thoracic spinal cord compression can manifest itself as proximal motor weakness in the legs with sparing of distal muscle groups.

Reflex Examination

The reflex examination includes deep and superficial reflex assessments. The deep tendon reflexes are tested in the arms and legs. The significance of abnormal reflexes depends on the location and time course of the injury.

In the presence of an acute complete spinal cord injury, the deep tendon reflexes below the level of the lesion are hypoactive. In some instances, normal reflex activity may be seen in the hyperacute state. Hyperactive reflexes develop in the subacute phase (4 to 6 weeks) after an injury because of the loss of inhibition from descending corticospinal pathways. The Babinski reflexes follow the time course of the deep tendon reflexes. In the acute phase of an injury to the spinal cord, they remain unreactive, or a flexor response is occasionally identified. Extensor plantar response develop from chronic compression of the spinal cord or in the subacute phase of an injury.

In acute trauma, the differential diagnosis of hypoactive reflexes includes nerve root injury, plexus injury, and spinal shock. The underlying cause of hyporeflexia is determined by the pattern of the patient's neurologic symptoms and associated motor and sensory deficits. In addition, hypoactive reflexes may be due to a preexisting condition such as peripheral neuropathy or chemotherapy use, or they may be a normal variant.

Focal hypoactive reflexes in the *upper extremities* are often the result of a nerve root or brachial plexus abnormality. If the motor and sensory deficits correspond to multiple, adjacent motor or sensory root levels, a plexus injury is likely the underlying cause. Contusions or abrasions of the skin, or underlying fractures involving the shoulder girdle structures, pelvis, or transverse processes, can be associated with these deficits and their presence should be sought to confirm the diagnosis.

Spinal shock is a phenomenon that is present after a complete spinal cord injury. The patient has absence of all volitional and reflex neurologic activity below the level of the lesion. In contrast, *neurogenic shock* is a hemodynamic phenomenon. After spinal cord injury at or above the T5 vertebral level, patients may become hypotensive. Characteristically, patients have a relative bradycardia in the presence of low blood pressure. The shock results from the loss of sympathetic outflow. This causes peripheral vasodilation and pooling of blood, which, in turn, impairs venous return to the heart. Loss of sympathetic outflow also has negative inotropic and chronotropic effects on the heart.

Superficial reflexes are diminished in the presence of a spinal cord injury. Nerves from T6–9 and T10–12 subserve the upper and lower superficial abdominal reflexes, respectively. The absence of both upper and lower superficial abdominal reflexes indicates that the lesion is above T6. The absence of lower and preservation of upper superficial abdominal reflexes indicates that the lesion is below T9. Likewise, the L1–2 segmental nerves mediate the cremasteric reflex, and loss of this reflex is pathologic.

The tone of the anal sphincter should also be assessed as part of a full neurologic work-up. It is usually diminished or absent in the presence of a complete acute spinal cord injury.

Radiographic Examination

Indications for spinal imaging (see Table 98–1) include (1) history of trauma, (2) neurologic deficit, (3) local spinal tenderness, and (4) a nonresponsive or unconscious patient. Imaging is performed to determine the integrity of the osteoligamentous complex, assess the presence and cause of ongoing neural compression, and determine the optimal surgical approach to a spinal lesion.

Despite advances in computer-assisted imaging, plain radiographs remain an integral part of the imaging assessment of the spine. They are particularly useful in the ICU setting because portable radiographs are readily available, requiring little manipulation or transportation of the patient. Plain radiographs give an initial indication of the potential for osteoligamentous injury. In particular, lateral radiographs are essential because the criteria for determining stability of a spinal segment are based on these projections, particularly in the C-spine.

A complete C-spine study includes a view incorporating the occiput to the C7–T1 junction. The shoulders can obscure the cervicothoracic junction. Techniques available in the surgical intensive care unit to augment visualization of this region include manual downward traction on the arms and a swimmer's view. If the junction cannot be seen adequately despite these supplementary techniques, computer-assisted imaging is required. Plain cervical radiographs in flexion and extension enable dynamic imaging for the assessment of stability. These views can be obtained in the ICU with plain films for a conscious, cooperative patient, or with fluoroscopy in an unconscious patient. Because there is a 5% frequency of noncontiguous spinal fractures in trauma patients, visualization of the entire spine must be obtained in the presence of trauma, even if an unstable injury is found at one segment of the spine.

MANAGEMENT

Stabilization of the Injured Spine

When the mechanism of injury to a patient is consistent with a possible spinal injury, the spine is stabilized while cardiorespiratory resuscitation is undertaken.

Immobilization of the spine in a neutral position generally protects the neural elements from further injury in the presence of an unstable injury. Protection of the cervical spine often begins in the field during transportation of an injured patient. Techniques include application of a rigid cervical collar or immobilization of the head and torso on a rigid spinal board with lateral props, such as sandbags or rigid foam inserts. If the head is fixed to the backboard, the rest of the patient's body should be rigidly secured to the board. This approach to stabilization should be viewed as temporary because an unconscious or spine-injured patient who has lost sensation can quickly acquire pressure ulcers if left immobilized on a rigid backboard even for only a few hours.

Although a cervical collar is adequate for a cooperative, calm patient, it is insufficient in an uncooperative, active patient with a potentially unstable cervical spine. An effective alternative in the ICU is cervical traction. Traction is useful for realigning the spine, and it protects against movement that could compromise the spinal canal. Patients in traction should be carefully followed by serial cervical spine films and neurologic examinations. Cervical traction is inappropriate, however, for patients with unstable atlantoaxial injuries. Instead, they should be placed in a cervical collar or a halo ring and vest. The latter is less effective at the cervicothoracic junction.

In some circumstances, the halo ring and vest can be an impediment to the care of the ICU patient. They restrict access for central line placement, chest tube placement, airway management, and cardiac compression. The instrument required for removal of the halo should be readily accessible and accompany the patient at all times. If appropriate and necessary, traction can be a temporary alternative.

There are fewer good techniques for immobilization of the thoracolumbar spine. Backboard positioning is first initiated empirically in the field. Subsequently, if the patient is relatively immobile on a standard mattress, he or she is unlikely to incur further neurologic injury. Firm mattresses are preferable to soft ones. A thoracolumbosacral orthosis or cast enhances immobilization and prevents flexion in an uncooperative patient.

Thoracolumbar traction is more cumbersome and is less effective for reducing deformity, and halo-pelvic traction is rarely used.

Nonoperative Treatment

In the presence of an existing neurologic deficit, there are limited means of augmenting neurologic recovery. General care of the patient, including maintaining blood pressure, oxygenation, and nutrition, provides an environment in which neurologic recovery can potentially take place and may contribute to the prevention of progressive secondary spinal cord injury. Also, it is important to identify and treat related medical complications associated with a spinal cord injury, which can be life-threatening and increase morbidity and the duration of in-hospital recovery.

Pharmacologic means of augmenting spinal cord recovery are under active investigation. The use of high-dose steroids has demonstrated some efficacy for acute spinal cord injury. The National Acute Spinal Cord Injury Study II assessed the benefits of steroid administration after spinal cord injury. It had two treatment arms and a placebo group. One treatment group received high-dose methylprednisolone (30 mg/kg intravenous bolus over the first hour, followed by 5.4 mg/kg/h of a continuous infusion over the subsequent 23 hours), and the other treatment group received naloxone. When the steroids were given at these doses within 8 hours after the injury, a statistically significant improvement in neurologic outcome without increased morbidity was found. The neurologic outcome with naloxone was found to be the same as with placebo.

In view of these results, most agree that a patient presenting with a partial spinal cord injury within 8 hours of the injury should receive high-dose methylprednisolone. The merits of high-dose steroids in a setting of a complete spinal cord injury are less certain, although some also advocate their use in this situation.

In the ICU, nonoperative techniques are usually sufficient to stabilize an injured spinal segment. Postural reduction or segmental immobilization with collars and braces is usually sufficient in a noncombative patient to prevent induction or progression of a spinal cord injury. The priority in the ICU setting should be to stabilize the patient's cardiorespiratory function and treat other acute medical conditions. Since nonoperative techniques can be used to stabilize osteoligamentous injuries, definitive treatment should be undertaken on an elective basis.

Operative Treatment

In contrast to the limitations in enhancing neurologic recovery after spinal cord injury, techniques for spinal stabilization have greatly improved. As a result, except for some atlantoaxial injuries, most unstable spinal injuries are treated operatively.

The principles of spinal surgery, regardless of cause, include decompression, reduction, and stabilization. These principles are most clearly illustrated in the setting of acute trauma.

Decompression

Spinal cord compression results from retropulsion of bone or soft tissue (disk, hematoma) into the spinal canal. The effectiveness of acute or subacute spinal cord decompression after the initial spinal injury is controversial. Most would agree that the effect of compression on the neural elements is maximal at the time of impact. During this interval, the compressive fragment or spinal translation occurs with the encroaching element being accelerated into the spinal cord, thereby imparting force on the neural elements. It is uncertain if the ongoing compression after the initial impact continues to promote injury via a primary or secondary mechanism. Theoretically, the presence of ongoing compression could increase local tissue pressure and thereby alter regional perfusion, promoting secondary injury. Those authors who advocate early decompression cite this theoretical concern.

Others recommend elective, delayed decompression based on the concern of incurring a secondary injury at the time of surgery, for example, operating on a patient who is unstable from a cardiac or respiratory point of view. With refined operative techniques, including anterior approaches, and advances in neuroanesthesia, early intervention for decompression has become safer and its efficacy is being re-evaluated.

One clear indication for emergent spinal cord decompression is a patient who has progressive neurologic deficit and ongoing neural element compression. Decompression of a patient with a complete deficit is considered elective and some would deem it unnecessary. The patient with a stable, partial cord deficit could be considered for a neural decompressive procedure at the time of definitive stabilization. As discussed earlier, the timing of this intervention remains controversial. Reports of clinical improvement in groups of patients who have chronic deficits after delayed spinal cord decompressions indicate the potential merits of neural element decompression.

Reduction and Stabilization

Depending on the nature of the injury and the segment of the spine involved, reduction can be performed by external or internal techniques. Although cervical traction is effective for realigning translational deformity in the cervical spine, thoracolumbar traction is relatively ineffective. Open, internal reduction is feasible along all segments of the spine. In order to achieve reduction, a force must be applied to the spine to counteract the deforming force and to prevent subsequent deformity after the initial reduction.

Stabilization of the spine must be considered in terms of immediate and long-term stability. In the setting of acute trauma, immediate stabilization is provided by application of a rigid immobilizing device, either internally or externally. Long-term stabilization is achieved by bony healing or fusion.

Significant innovations have been made in the development of internal fixation devices. The purpose of such spinal instrumentation is to achieve short-term fixation of the spine and, in some cases, deformity correction. In addition to stabilizing the involved segment of the spine, some devices have dynamic properties that enable the application of force to the spine for deformity correction. A major advantage of this type of instrumentation is that it achieves immediate stabilization of the spine. The patient is able to commence physical and rehabilitation therapy without risking neurologic injury. Early rehabilitation reduces the likelihood of complications that can result from prolonged recumbency. The disadvantages of a fixation device include added operative time and risk, immobilization of segments with normal motion in order to achieve adequate fixation, and imaging artifact obscuring anatomic detail on postoperative studies

BIBLIOGRAPHY

Bracken MB, Shepard MJ, Collins WF, et al: A randomized controlled trial of methylprednisolone or naloxone in the treatment of acute spinal cord injury. Results of the second National Acute Spinal Cord Injury Study. N Engl J Med 322:1405–1411, 1990.
This article describes the first major randomized controlled study demonstrating the efficacy of steroids in spinal cord injury.

Chestnut RM, Marshal LF: Early assessment, transport and management of patients with post-traumatic spinal instability. In: Cooper PR (ed): Management of Post-Traumatic Spinal Instability. Park Ridge, IL: American Association of Neurologic Surgeons, 1990, pp 1–17.
This is an expert-devised review of early management of patients with spinal trauma.

Davidoff J, Hoyt D, Rosen P: Distal cervical spine evaluation using swimmer's flexion/extension radiograph. J Emerg Med 11:55–59, 1993.
This article describes radiographic C-spine clearance.

Donovan WH, Dwyer AP: An update on the early management of traumatic paraplegia (nonoperative and operative management). Clin Orthop 189:12–21, 1984.
This is a review of the management considerations in traumatic paraplegia.

Lewis LM, Dougherty M, Ruoff BE, et al: Flexion/extension views in the evaluation of cervical spine injuries. Ann Emerg Med 20:117–121, 1991.
This article describes radiographic C-spine clearance.

Tator CH, Fehlings MG: Review of the secondary injury theory of acute spinal cord trauma with emphasis on vascular mechanisms. J Neurosurg 75:15–26, 1991.
This article describes the mechanism of secondary injury to the spinal cord.

Appendix

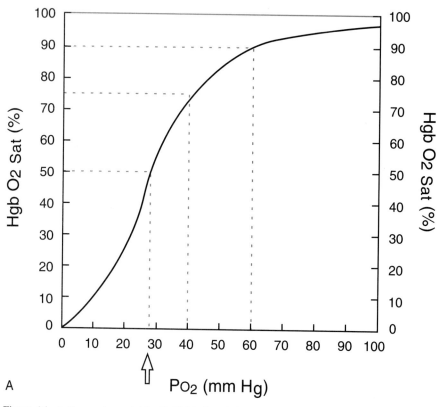

Figure A1. *A*, Oxygen-hemoglobin (O$_2$-Hgb) dissociation curve under normal conditions (pH, Pco$_2$, and temperature). The oxygen (O$_2$) saturation of hemoglobin is 50% at a Po$_2$ of 26 mm Hg *(open arrow and dashed lines above the arrow)*. Mixed venous blood (and systemic capillary blood) typically has a Po$_2$ of 40 mm Hg with a corresponding O$_2$ saturation of 75% *(second set of dashed lines)*. The transition from the flat part to the steep part of the O$_2$-Hgb curve, below which decreases in Po$_2$ results in clinically relevant falls in O$_2$ saturation, occurs at Po$_2$ of about 60 mm Hg with a corresponding O$_2$ saturation of 90% *(third set of dashed lines)*.

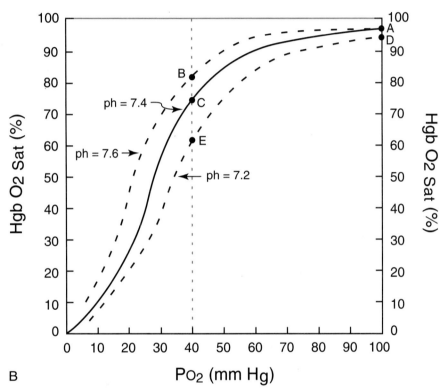

B

Figure A1 *Continued. B,* The solid curve is the same O₂-Hgb curve under normal conditions ("normal") as in A. The dashed curve to the left of the normal curve represents a "shift to the left" of the O₂-Hgb curve due to alkalosis. The dashed curve to the right of the normal curve represents a "shift to the right" of the O₂-Hgb curve due to acidosis (the same shift to the right would occur with elevated temperature or PCO₂). At PO₂ of 40 mm Hg the O₂ saturations of the three curves are markedly different. Note that the curve shifted to the left can "unload" *less* oxygen at 40 mm Hg than the normal curve (note the change in O₂ saturation in going from Points A to B vs. Points A to C). In contrast, the curve shifted to the right can "unload" more oxygen at 40 mm Hg (note the change in O₂ saturation going from Points A to C vs. Points D to E).

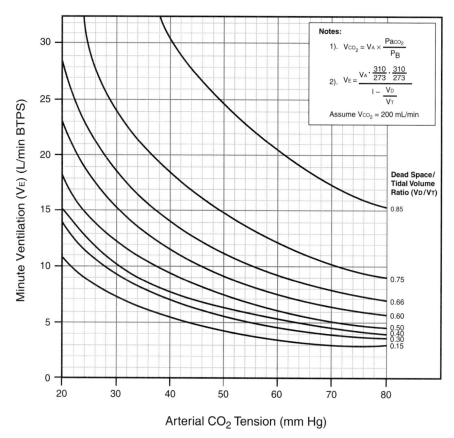

Figure B1. Each curved line is an isopleth with a certain dead space-to-tidal volume ratio [VD/VT] (right ordinate). The curves illustrate the relationship between $Paco_2$ (abscissa) and minute ventilation (left ordinate) for different values of VD/VT but at the same $\dot{V}co_2$ (200 mL/min). (The curves can be derived from Equation 11, Table 1–1, Chapter 1). One can use this graph to adjust the level of mechanical ventilation for a patient without "overshooting" ($Paco_2$ too low) or "undershooting" ($Paco_2$ too high). To use this, first measure the $Paco_2$ and the corresponding $\dot{V}E$ of a ventilated patient. These values will identify which isopleth the patient is "on," that is, the patient's $\dot{V}D/\dot{V}T$. Then follow that curve to the desired $Paco_2$ and note the $\dot{V}E$ corresponding to that $Paco_2$. Then change the ventilator's respiratory rate (assuming that the patient is not breathing faster than the ventilator's rate) to achieve the new $\dot{V}E$.

For example, consider a patient with chronic obstructive pulmonary disease (COPD) and chronic CO_2 retention who has recently been started on invasive mechanical ventilation for acute respiratory failure. With a $\dot{V}E$ of 10 L/min, the patient's $Paco_2$ equals 70 mm Hg. This corresponds to the isopleth with VD/VT of 0.75. You want to decrease his $Paco_2$ to 50 mm Hg (his baseline) so follow the 0.75 isopleth to where it intersects 50 mm Hg and find that the corresponding $\dot{V}E$ is 15 L/min. Thus, you increase the ventilator's rate to achieve a $\dot{V}E$ of 15 L/min, which should result in a $Paco_2$ of about 50 mm Hg. Do not increase the *tidal volume* to increase $\dot{V}E$ since that would change VD/VT (and invalidate the assumption of keeping the VD/VT the same). Note: you can use Equation 3, Chapter 3 to arrive at the same result. (From Selecky PA, Wasserman K, Klein M Ziment I: A graphic approach to assessing interrelationships among minute ventilation, arterial carbon dioxide tension and the ratio of physiologic dead space to tidal volume in patients on respirators. Am Rev Respir Dis 177:181–184, 1978.)

Palliative Drug Therapy for Terminal Withdrawal of Mechanical Ventilation

Paul N. Lanken
Eric T. Wittbrodt

Table 1. Stepwise Approach to Palliative Drug Therapy for Terminal Withdrawal of Mechanical Ventilation

Step 1. Select agents to be used and route of administration. In general, one should use a **combination** of opioid and benzodiazepine because of their complementary pharmacological effects: **opioid** to control air hunger and pain and the **benzodiazepine** to sedate and to control anxiety. In order to rapidly titrate their doses to the desired effect, the agents, in general, should be given as intravenous (IV) **bolus** injections followed by **continuous** IV infusions.

Step 2. If the patient is receiving a neuromuscular blocking agent, stop its administration. Allow its effects to wear off or reverse the effects if possible (see Chapter 4) prior to extubation or start of terminal weaning.

Step 3. Anticipate that additional opioid or sedative will be needed for palliation after withdrawal of mechanical ventilation. In this case, at least 30 min *before* extubation or start of terminal weaning, give an IV bolus of the agent followed by continuous IV infusion. The IV infusion rate should be a certain fraction of the last bolus dosage given, depending on the agent chosen (see Tables 2 to 5).

If no additional opioid or sedative is judged to be needed before withdrawal from assisted ventilation, continue current level of palliative drug therapy and proceed to Step 7.

Step 4. Titrate the dose of agent (Steps 5 and 6) to desired effect. Judge adequacy of palliation by lack of patient responsiveness and lack of signs or symptoms of pain, anxiety, fear, dyspnea, tachypnea (e.g., respiratory rate <20/min), or other discomfort. Whenever additional doses are given, document in the medical record that the dose was given in order to control specific signs and symptoms of distress, that is, it was being titrated to effect.

Step 5. If desired effect is not achieved by 20–30 min (depending on the agent used), repeat IV bolus of drug at *double* the dosage of the prior bolus and also *double* the rate of the continuous infusion. See Step 10 if this results in a respiratory rate <10/min.

Step 6. If desired effect is still *not* achieved, repeat Step 5. If using a combination of an opioid and benzodiazepine, alternate between them when doubling the agent when repeating Step 5.

Step 7. When desired effect *is* achieved, continue the IV infusion at the same rate and extubate the patient or begin the terminal wean.

Step 8. Reassess level of palliation, using signs listed in Step 4, every 15 min (or at shorter or longer intervals as the clinical condition of the patient dictates).

Step 9. If the patient exhibits discomfort, repeat bolus at double the dosage of the most recent bolus and also double the IV infusion rate. If discomfort persists, repeat this Step until desired effect is again achieved.

Step 10. If the respiratory rate falls below 10/min, continue at the same IV infusion rate but do not give more boluses or increase the IV infusion rate unless the patient is clearly in pain or distress. Anticipate that the family may misinterpret agonal respirations as representing patient discomfort and prepare them accordingly. If the patient's blood pressure or pulse falls, do not decrease dose or rate but continue as indicated in Steps 4 through 9.

Table 2. Morphine Sulfate Dosing for Terminal Withdrawal from Mechanical Ventilation

EXPOSURE TO AGENT OVER PRIOR 24 h*	BOLUS DOSING	CONTINUOUS INTRAVENOUS (IV) INFUSION
0–10 mg/h	1. If patient is not at desired level of palliation (see Step 3, Table 1), give 5–10 mg IV "push" at least 30 min before extubation or start of terminal wean. 2. Bolus may be repeated at double the prior dosage. 3. Repeat Step 2 as needed until desired end point of symptom control is reached (see Steps 4–6, Table 1). 4. If Step 3 is reached, consider using combination therapy with benzodiazepine as described in Table 1.	Immediately after bolus, start a continuous IV infusion at a rate of 2–10 mg/h, using 150 mg in 150 mL normal saline or 5% dextrose solution, yielding a concentration of 1 mg/mL.
>10 mg/h	1. If patient is not at desired level of palliation, double the dose of morphine administered in the prior 2 h and give it as an IV bolus. 2. After 20–30 min, if desired effect is still not achieved, double the dose again and give it as IV bolus. 3. Repeat Step 2 until goal of palliation is reached. 4. If Step 3 is reached, use combination therapy with benzodiazepine as described in Table 1.	After the bolus, start a continuous IV infusion at rate of one half of the dosage of IV bolus given per hour. Appropriate solutions can be made up by dissolving 250 mg of morphine in 250 mL normal saline or 5% dextrose, yielding a concentration of 1 mg/mL.

*Mean hourly dose over prior 24 hours.

Table 3. Fentanyl Dosing for Terminal Withdrawal from Mechanical Ventilation

EXPOSURE TO AGENT OVER PRIOR 24 h*	BOLUS DOSING	CONTINUOUS INTRAVENOUS (IV) INFUSION
0–100 μg/h	1. If patient is not at desired level of palliation, give 200–300 μg as IV push (as described in Table 2).	After bolus, start at a rate of 100–400 μg/h using 4 mg of fentanyl in 250 mL normal saline or 5% dextrose, yielding a concentration of 16 μg/mL.
>100 μg/h	1. If patient is not at desired level of palliation, take the maximal hourly dosage during the past 24 h, multiply it times 4 and give as IV push (as described in Table 2). 2. If, after 20 min, one still has not achieved desired palliative effect, double the dosage again and give as a bolus. 3. Repeat Step 2. 4. If Step 3 is reached, use combination therapy with benzodiazepine as described in Table 1.	After bolus, start IV infusion at a rate of one half of the bolus given per hour. Appropriate solutions can be made up by dissoving 4 mg of fentanyl in 250 mL normal saline or 5% dextrose solution, yielding a standard fentanyl concentration of 16 μg/mL. If desired, for example, to concentrate fluids, fentanyl can be given in higher concentrations: 20 μg/mL (5 mg in 250 mL); 50 μg/mL (12.5 mg in 250 mL); 100 μg/mL (25 mg in 250 mL).

*Mean hourly dose over prior 24 hours.

Table 4. Lorazepam Dosing for Terminal Withdrawal from Mechanical Ventilation

EXPOSURE TO AGENT OVER PRIOR 24 h*	BOLUS DOSING	CONTINUOUS INTRAVENOUS (IV) INFUSION
0–2 mg/h	1. If patient is not at desired level of sedation, take the maximal hourly dosage in the past 24 h, double it and give as an IV bolus. 2. After 20–30 min, if desired level of sedation is still not achieved, then double the prior dosage and give as a repeat bolus. 3. Repeat Step 2 until desired endpoint is reached. 4. If Step 3 is reached, use combination therapy with opioid as described in Table 1.	After bolus, start at a rate of 2–4 mg/h using 100 mg of lorazepam in 250 mL normal saline or 5% dextrose solution, yielding a concentration of 0.4 mg/mL, or 200 mg in 500 mL normal saline or 5% dextrose solution, also yielding a concentration of 0.4 mg/mL.
>2 mg/h	1. If patient is not at desired level of sedation, take the maximal hourly dosage in the past 24 h, double it and give as an IV bolus. 2. After 20–30 min, if desired level of sedation is still not achieved, then double the prior dosage and give as a repeat bolus. 3. Repeat Step 2 until desired end is reached. 4. If Step 3 is reached, use combination therapy with opioid as described in Table 1.	After bolus, start at a rate of one half of the bolus dosage per hour. Appropriate concentrations can be made by dissolving 100 mg in 250 mL normal saline or 5% dextrose solution (0.4 mg/mL) or 200 mg in 500 mL normal saline or 5% dextrose solution (0.4 mg/mL).

*Mean hourly dose over prior 24 hours.

Table 5. Diazepam Dosing for Terminal Withdrawal from Mechanical Ventilation

EXPOSURE TO AGENT OVER PRIOR 24 h*	BOLUS DOSING	CONTINUOUS INTRAVENOUS (IV) INFUSION
0–60 mg/h	1. If patient is not at desired level of sedation, give a 20 mg IV bolus. 2. After 30 min, if desired level of sedation is still not achieved, then give 40 mg as an IV bolus. 3. If desired effect is seen at 30 min post-bolus, repeat boluses of same dose q2h. Repeat this step until desired endpoint is reached. 4. If patient "breaks through" with signs of discomfort prior to 2 h, repeat Steps 1 and 2 and give routine boluses every hour.	Diazepam is not recommended for use as a continuous infusion due to the long half-lives of the parent compound and its active metabolite (see Chapter 4).
>60 mg	1. If patient is not at desired level of sedation, give as an IV bolus the maximal bolus given over the past 8 h. 2. After 30 min, if desired level of sedation is still not achieved, then double the prior dosage and give as a repeat bolus. 3. If desired effect is reached after 30 min, repeat bolus at same dosage at 2 h intervals. 4. If patient "breaks through" with signs of discomfort prior to 2 h, repeat Steps 1 and 2 and repeat routine boluses every hour.	Diazepam is not recommended for use as a continuous infusion due to the long half-lives of the parent compound and its active metabolite (see Chapter 4).

*Mean hourly dose over prior 24 hours.

Acid-Base Map

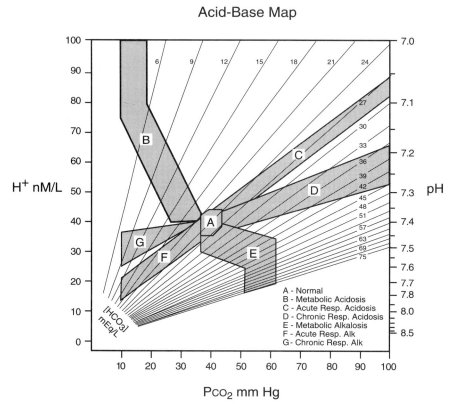

Figure D1. This acid-base map identifies the normal range of values for arterial pH, $Paco_2$ and arterial bicarbonate (HCO_3^-) and six domains representing 95% confidence limits of these values for the six simple acid-base disorders listed as A–G (defined in body of the figure). Numbered lines represent isopleths for arterial bicarbonate. If the patient has a *simple* acid-base disorder, you should be able to plot the results of the patient's arterial blood gas (ABG) analysis into one of the six domains A–G. If the results plot to a region in-between two domains, you should then suspect that the patient has a *mixed* (double or triple) acid-base disturbance. If values for pH, $Paco_2$, and HCO_3^- from the patient's ABG analysis do not fall on the same point, then there is an error in one or more numbers since they are not internally consistent, that is, noncompatible with the Henderson-Hasselbalch equation (see Chapter 80). Because this acid-base map has important limitations (e.g., it does not distinguish between anion gap and non-anion gap metabolic acidosis), it should never take the place of a thoughtful, systematic analysis of acid-base disorders, such as described in Chapter 80. (From Goldberg M, Green SB, Moss ML, et al: Computer-based instuction and diagnosis of acid-base disorders. A systematic approach. JAMA 223:269–275, 1973.)

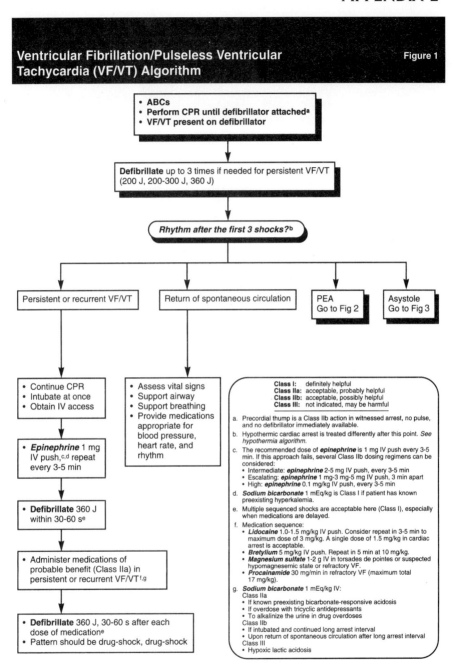

Figure E1. Advanced cardiac life support (ACLS) algorithm for ventricular fibrillation (VF) or pulseless ventricular tachycardia (VT). ABCs, airway, breathing and circulation; CPR, cardiopulmonary resuscitation; IV, intravenous; J, joules.

Pulseless Electrical Activity (PEA) Algorithm   Figure 2
(Electromechanical Dissociation [EMD])

Includes
- Electromechanical dissociation (EMD)
- Pseudo-EMD
- Idioventricular rhythms
- Ventricular escape rhythms
- Bradyasystolic rhythms
- Postdefibrillation idioventricular rhythms

- Continue CPR
- Intubate at once
- Obtain IV access

- Assess blood flow using Doppler ultrasound, end-tidal CO_2, echocardiography, or arterial line

---

Consider possible causes
(Parentheses = possible therapies and treatments)

- Hypovolemia (volume infusion)
- Hypoxia (ventilation)
- Cardiac tamponade (pericardiocentesis)
- Tension pneumothorax (needle decompression)
- Hypothermia (see hypothermia algorithm)
- Massive pulmonary embolism (surgery, ***thrombolytics***)

- Drug overdoses such as tricyclics, digitalis, β-blockers, calcium channel blockers
- Hyperkalemia[a]
- Acidosis[b]
- Massive acute myocardial infarction (see Chapter 49)

- ***Epinephrine*** 1 mg IV push,[a,c] repeat every 3-5 min

- If absolute bradycardia (<60 BPM) or relative bradycardia, give ***atropine*** 1 mg IV
- Repeat every 3-5 min to a total of 0.03-0.04 mg/kg[d]

Class I: definitely helpful
Class IIa: acceptable, probably helpful
Class IIb: acceptable, possibly helpful
Class III: not indicated, may be harmful

a. ***Sodium bicarbonate*** 1 mEq/kg is Class I if patient has known preexisting hyperkalemia.
b. ***Sodium bicarbonate*** 1 mEq/kg:
   Class IIa
   - If known preexisting bicarbonate-responsive acidosis
   - If overdose with tricyclic antidepressants
   - To alkalinize the urine in drug overdoses
   Class IIb
   - If intubated and continued long arrest interval
   - Upon return of spontaneous circulation after long arrest interval
   Class III
   - Hypoxic lactic acidosis
c. The recommended dose of ***epinephrine*** is 1 mg IV push every 3-5 min. If this approach fails, several Class IIb dosing regimens can be considered:
   - Intermediate: ***epinephrine*** 2-5 mg IV push, every 3-5 min
   - Escalating: ***epinephrine*** 1 mg-3 mg-5 mg IV push, 3 min apart
   - High: ***epinephrine*** 0.1 mg/kg IV push, every 3-5 min
d. The shorter ***atropine*** dosing interval (3 min) is possibly helpful in cardiac arrest (Class IIb).

Figure E2. ACLS algorithm for treatment of pulseless electrical activity (PEA) (previously called electromechanical dissociation [EMD]). CPR, cardiopulmonary resuscitation; IV, intravenous.

Asystole Treatment Algorithm

Figure 3

- **Continue CPR**
- **Intubate at once**
- **Obtain IV access**
- **Confirm asystole in more than one lead**

↓

Consider possible causes
- Hypoxia
- Hyperkalemia
- Hypokalemia
- Preexisting acidosis
- Drug overdose
- Hypothermia

↓

Consider immediate transcutaneous pacing (TCP)[a]

↓

- ***Epinephrine*** 1 mg IV push,[b,c] repeat every 3-5 min

↓

- ***Atropine*** 1 mg IV, repeat every 3-5 min up to a total of 0.03-0.04 mg/kg[d,e]

↓

Consider termination of efforts[f]

Class I: definitely helpful
Class IIa: acceptable, probably helpful
Class IIb: acceptable, possibly helpful
Class III: not indicated, may be harmful

a. TCP is a Class IIb intervention. Lack of success may be due to delays in pacing. To be effective TCP must be performed early, simultaneously with drugs. Evidence does not support routine use of TCP for asystole.

b. The recommended dose of ***epinephrine*** is 1 mg IV push every 3-5 min. If this approach fails, several Class IIb dosing regimens can be considered:
   - Intermediate: ***epinephrine*** 2-5 mg IV push, every 3-5 min
   - Escalating: ***epinephrine*** 1 mg-3 mg-5 mg IV push, 3 min apart
   - High: ***epinephrine*** 0.1 mg/kg IV push, every 3-5 min

c. ***Sodium bicarbonate*** 1 mEq/kg is Class I if patient has known preexisting hyperkalemia.

d. The shorter ***atropine*** dosing interval (3 min) is Class IIb in asystolic arrest.

e. ***Sodium bicarbonate*** 1 mEq/kg:
   Class IIa
   - If known preexisting bicarbonate-responsive acidosis
   - If overdose with tricyclic antidepressants
   - To alkalinize the urine in drug overdoses
   Class IIb
   - If intubated and continued long arrest interval
   - Upon return of spontaneous circulation after long arrest interval
   Class III
   - Hypoxic lactic acidosis

f. If patient remains in asystole or other agonal rhythm after successful intubation and initial medications and no reversible causes are identified, consider termination of resuscitative efforts by a physician. Consider interval since arrest.

Figure E3. ACLS algorithm for treatment of asystole. CPR, cardiopulmonary resuscitation; IV, intravenous.

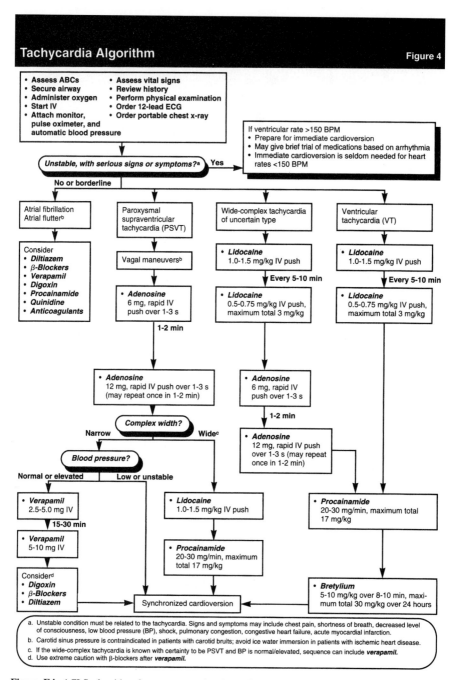

Tachycardia Algorithm Figure 4

- **Assess ABCs**
- **Secure airway**
- **Administer oxygen**
- **Start IV**
- **Attach monitor, pulse oximeter, and automatic blood pressure**

- **Assess vital signs**
- **Review history**
- **Perform physical examination**
- **Order 12-lead ECG**
- **Order portable chest x-ray**

If ventricular rate >150 BPM
- Prepare for immediate cardioversion
- May give brief trial of medications based on arrhythmia
- Immediate cardioversion is seldom needed for heart rates <150 BPM

Unstable, with serious signs or symptoms?[a] — Yes

No or borderline

| Atrial fibrillation Atrial flutter[b] | Paroxysmal supraventricular tachycardia (PSVT) | Wide-complex tachycardia of uncertain type | Ventricular tachycardia (VT) |

Consider
- *Diltiazem*
- *β-Blockers*
- *Verapamil*
- *Digoxin*
- *Procainamide*
- *Quinidine*
- *Anticoagulants*

Vagal maneuvers[b]

- *Lidocaine* 1.0-1.5 mg/kg IV push

Every 5-10 min

- *Lidocaine* 1.0-1.5 mg/kg IV push

Every 5-10 min

- *Adenosine* 6 mg, rapid IV push over 1-3 s

1-2 min

- *Lidocaine* 0.5-0.75 mg/kg IV push, maximum total 3 mg/kg

- *Lidocaine* 0.5-0.75 mg/kg IV push, maximum total 3 mg/kg

- *Adenosine* 12 mg, rapid IV push over 1-3 s (may repeat once in 1-2 min)

- *Adenosine* 6 mg, rapid IV push over 1-3 s

1-2 min

Complex width?

Narrow — Wide[c]

Blood pressure?

- *Adenosine* 12 mg, rapid IV push over 1-3 s (may repeat once in 1-2 min)

Normal or elevated — Low or unstable

- *Verapamil* 2.5-5.0 mg IV

15-30 min

- *Verapamil* 5-10 mg IV

- *Lidocaine* 1.0-1.5 mg/kg IV push

- *Procainamide* 20-30 mg/min, maximum total 17 mg/kg

Consider[d]
- *Digoxin*
- *β-Blockers*
- *Diltiazem*

- *Procainamide* 20-30 mg/min, maximum total 17 mg/kg

Synchronized cardioversion

- *Bretylium* 5-10 mg/kg over 8-10 min, maximum total 30 mg/kg over 24 hours

a. Unstable condition must be related to the tachycardia. Signs and symptoms may include chest pain, shortness of breath, decreased level of consciousness, low blood pressure (BP), shock, pulmonary congestion, congestive heart failure, acute myocardial infarction.
b. Carotid sinus pressure is contraindicated in patients with carotid bruits; avoid ice water immersion in patients with ischemic heart disease.
c. If the wide-complex tachycardia is known with certainty to be PSVT and BP is normal/elevated, sequence can include *verapamil*.
d. Use extreme caution with β-blockers after *verapamil*.

Figure E4. ACLS algorithm for treatment of tachycardia. ABCs, airway, breathing and circulation; BPM, beats per minute; CPR, cardiopulmonary resuscitation; ECG, electrocardiogram; IV, intravenous.

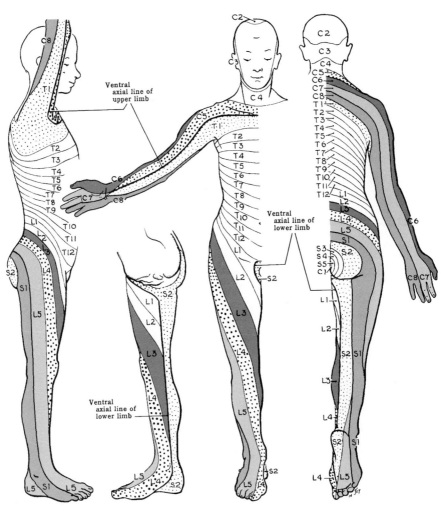

Figure F1. Typical location of dermatomes. When transmission via a dorsal nerve root is interrupted, the result is a diminution of sensation (pin prick, light touch, or temperature) in the associated dermatone. (From Grant JCB: Grant's Atlas of Anatomy, 5th ed. Baltimore: Williams & Wilkins, 1962.)

INDEX